Surgery of the Thyroid and Parathyroid Glands

Surgery of the Thyroid and Parathyroid Glands

THIRD EDITION

Editor

Gregory W. Randolph, MD, FACS, FACE, FEBS (Endocrine)

Professor of Otolaryngology Head and Neck Surgery,
The Claire and John Bertucci Endowed Chair in Thyroid Surgical Oncology,
 Harvard Medical School
Director of the Comprehensive Otolaryngology Division and the
 Thyroid & Parathyroid Endocrine Surgical Division,
Department of Otolaryngology Head and Neck Surgery,
 Massachusetts Eye and Ear Infirmary,
Member Division of Surgical Oncology, Department of Surgery,
 Massachusetts General Hospital,
Boston, Massachusetts

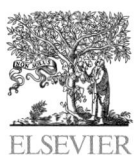

ELSEVIER

1600 John F. Kennedy Blvd.
Ste 1600
Philadelphia, PA 19103-2899

SURGERY OF THE THYROID AND PARATHYROID GLANDS, THIRD EDITION   ISBN: 978-0-323-66127-0
Copyright © 2021 by Elsevier, Inc. All rights reserved.

Original illustrations reused from the second edition © Gregory W. Randolph.

No part of this publication may be reproduced or transmitted in any form or by any means, electronic or mechanical, including photocopying, recording, or any information storage and retrieval system, without permission in writing from the publisher. Details on how to seek permission, further information about the Publisher's permissions policies and our arrangements with organizations such as the Copyright Clearance Center and the Copyright Licensing Agency, can be found at our website: www.elsevier.com/permissions.

This book and the individual contributions contained in it are protected under copyright by the Publisher (other than as may be noted herein).

Notice

Practitioners and researchers must always rely on their own experience and knowledge in evaluating and using any information, methods, compounds or experiments described herein. Because of rapid advances in the medical sciences, in particular, independent verification of diagnoses and drug dosages should be made. To the fullest extent of the law, no responsibility is assumed by Elsevier, authors, editors or contributors for any injury and/or damage to persons or property as a matter of products liability, negligence or otherwise, or from any use or operation of any methods, products, instructions, or ideas contained in the material herein.

Library of Congress Control Number: 2019957955

Content Strategist: Jessica McCool
Content Development Manager: Kathryn DeFrancesco
Senior Content Development Specialist: Rae Robertson
Publishing Services Manager: Deepthi Unni
Project Manager: Haritha Dharmarajan
Design: Ryan Cook

Printed in Canada

Last digit is the print number: 9 8 7 6 5 4 3 2 1

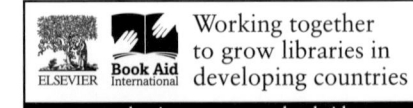

My wife, **Lorraine**
whose living faith and love have given me strength. Your faith, hard work, and selfless devotion
to others have always been my guiding light on this our path.
Without you, Lorraine,
none of this would have been worthwhile.
I will love you forever.

Gregory, Benjamin, and **Madeline**
Gregory, your sensitivity, artistic expertise, and hard work have gotten the job done.
Benjamin, I am so proud of the man you are, your strength, and your abiding concern for others.
Madeline, your intelligence, accomplishments, and grace through all inspire me.
My beautiful children, I could not love you more.

My mother, **Frances**
who fostered a hopeful strength and a desire to learn, I love you.

CONTRIBUTORS

Devaprabu Abraham, MD, MRCP(UK), ECNU, FACE
Professor of Medicine
Department of Medicine
University of Utah
Salt Lake City, Utah

Nikita R. Abraham, BS
Instructor
Center for Math and Science
University of Utah
Salt Lake City, Utah

Amit Agarwal, MS, FICS, FACS, FAMS
Professor of Endocrine Surgery
Sanjay Gandhi Postgraduate Institute
 of Medical Sciences
Lucknow, Uttar Pradesh, India

Mahsa S. Ahadi, MD
Department of Anatomical Pathology
Royal North Shore Hospital
Sydney, Australia

Ehab Alameer, MD
Endocrine Surgery Fellow
Department of Surgery
Tulane University
New Orleans, Louisiana

Wilson Alobuia, MD
General Surgery Resident
Department of Surgery
Stanford University
Palo Alto, California

Eran E. Alon, MD, MBA
Chairman
Department of Otolaryngology Head
 and Neck Surgery
Chaim Sheba Medical Center
Tel Hashomer, Israel

Anuwong Angkoon, MD, FRCST, FACS
Department of Surgery
Minimally Invasive and Endocrine Surgery
 Division
Police General Hospital
Bangkok, Thailand

Zaid Al-Qurayshi, MBChB, MPH
Resident Physician
Department of Otolaryngology - Head
 and Neck Surgery
University of Iowa Hospitals and Clinics
Iowa City, Iowa

Trevor E. Angell, MD
Assistant Professor of Clinical Medicine
Department of Endocrinology, Diabetes, and Metabolism
Keck School of Medicine
University of Southern California
Associate Director of the Thyroid Center
Keck Hospital of University of Southern California
Los Angeles, California

Peter Angelos, MD, PhD, FACS
Linda Kohler Anderson Professor of Surgery and Surgical Ethics
Chief
Endocrine Surgery
Associate Director
MacLean Center for Clinical Medical Ethics
The University of Chicago
Chicago, Illinois

Jung Hwan Baek, MD, PhD
Professor
Department of Radiology
Asan Medical Center
Seoul, South Korea

Zubair W. Baloch, MD, PhD
Professor
Department of Pathology & Laboratory Medicine
University of Pennsylvania Medical Center
Philadelphia, Pennsylvania

Marcin Barczyński, MD, PhD, FEBS-ES
Professor
Department of Endocrine Surgery
Third Chair of General Surgery
Jagiellonian University Medical College
Krakow, Poland

Andrew J. Bauer, MD
Director
The Thyroid Center
Department of Endocrinology and Diabetes
The Children's Hospital of Philadelphia
Associate Professor of Pediatrics
Perelman School of Medicine
University of Pennsylvania
Philadelphia, Pennsylvania

Rocco Bellantone, MD
Professor of Surgery
Endocrine and Metabolic Surgery
Agostino Gemelli University Polyclinic
Institute of Surgical Semeiotics
Catholic University of the Sacred Heart
Rome, Italy

CONTRIBUTORS

Amandine Berdelou, MD
Department of Adult Medicine
Institut Gustave Roussy
Villejuif, France

Anders Bergenfeltz, MD, FEBS
Professor and Consultant Surgeon in Endocrine
 and Sarcoma Surgery
Skåne University Hospital
Lund, Sweden

Victor J. Bernet, MD
Chair
Division of Endocrinology
Mayo Clinic
Associate Professor of Medicine
Mayo Clinic School of Medicine
Jacksonville, Florida

Keith C. Bible, MD, PhD
Professor
Department of Oncology
Mayo Clinic
Rochester, Minnesota

John Paul Bilezikian, MD
Professor of Medicine and Professor
 of Pharmacology
Department of Medicine
Columbia University
New York, New York

Juliana Bonilla-Velez, MD
Assistant Professor
Department of Otolaryngology Head
 and Neck Surgery
University of Washington
Seattle Children's Hospital
Seattle, Washington

Laura Boucai, MD, MSc
Associate Professor
Department of Medicine
Memorial Sloan Kettering Cancer Center
Weill Cornell Medical College
New York, New York

Gregory A. Brent, MD
Professor of Medicine and Physiology
Chief
Division of Endocrinology
David Geffen School of Medicine at UCLA
Chair
Department of Medicine
VA Greater Los Angeles Healthcare System
Los Angeles, California

Ingrid Breuskin, MD, PhD
Département de Cancérologie Cervico-Faciale
Institut Gustave Roussy
Villejuif, France

James Duncan Brierley, MBBS, MRCP, FRCR, FRCP (C)
Radiation Oncologist
Princess Margaret Cancer Centre
Professor
Department of Radiation Oncology
University of Toronto
Toronto, Ontario, Canada

Simon Brisebois, MD, MSc
Associate Professor
Department of Surgery
Université de Sherbrooke
Sherbrooke, Quebec, Canada

Jennifer Brooks, MD
Attending Physician
Department of Pediatric Otolaryngology
Boston Children's Hospital
Boston, Massachusetts

Kevin T. Brumund, MD
Associate Professor
Division of Otolaryngology-Head
 and Neck Surgery
Department of Surgery
Moores Cancer Center
UC San Diego Health System
San Diego, California

Mijenko Bura, MD, PhD
Ear, Nose, Throat, and Head
 and Neck Department
University Hospital Center ZAGREB
Zagreb, Croatia

Jean Gabriel Bustamante Alvarez, MD, MS
Fellow
Department of Medical Oncology
The Ohio State University Wexner Medical Center
Columbus, Ohio

Denise Carneiro-Pla, MD, FACS
Professor of Surgery
Department of Surgery
Medical University of South Carolina
Charleston, South Carolina

Claudio R. Cernea, MD, PhD
Professor of Surgery
Head and Neck Service
University of São Paulo School of Medicine
São Paulo, Brazil

Rita Yuk-kwan Chang, FRCS (Edin), FCSHK, FHKAM
Department of Surgery
Queen Mary Hospital
Hong Kong

Amy Chen, MD, FACS
Professor and Vice Chair
Department of Otolaryngology Head
 and Neck Surgery
Emory University
Atlanta, Georgia

CONTRIBUTORS

Feng-Yu Chiang, MD
Department of Otolaryngology–Head and Neck Surgery
Kaohsiung Medical University Hospital
Kaohsiung Medical University
Kaohsiung, Taiwan

Ashish V. Chintakuntlawar, MD, PhD
Assistant Professor
Department of Medical Oncology
Mayo Clinic
Rochester, Minnesota

Nancy L. Cho, MD
Associate Surgeon
Department of Surgery
Brigham & Women's Hospital
Boston, Massachusetts

Woong Youn Chung, MD
Department of Surgery
Open NBI Convergence Technology Research Laboratory
Severance Hospital
Yonsei Cancer Center
Yonsei University College of Medicine
Seoul, Korea

Edmund S. Cibas, MD
Director of Cytopathology
Department of Pathology
Brigham and Women's Hospital
Professor of Pathology
Harvard Medical School
Boston, Massachusetts

Carolyn Dacey, MD, MAS
Clinical Instructor
Department of Surgery
University of California, San Francisco
San Francisco, California

Louise Davies, MD, MS, FACS
Associate Professor of Otolaryngology - Head & Neck
Geisel School of Medicine at Dartmouth
Associate Professor
The Dartmouth Institute for Health Policy & Clinical Practice
Dartmouth College
Hanover, New Hampshire
Physician
VA Outcomes Group
White River Junction VA Medical Center
White River Junction, Vermont

Carmela De Crea, MD, PhD
Professor
U.O. Chirurgia Endocrina e Metabolica
Fondazione Policlinico Universitario A. Gemelli IRCCS,
Roma – Università Cattolica del Sacro Cuore
Rome, Italy

Leigh Delbridge, MD
Emeritus Professor of Surgery
Department of Surgery
University of Sydney
Sydney, Australia

Gillian Diercks, MD, MPH
Instructor
Department of Otolaryngology-Head & Neck Surgery
Harvard Medical School
Boston, Massachusetts

Gerard M. Doherty, MD
Moseley Professor and Chair of Surgery
Department of Surgery
Harvard Medical School
Surgeon-in-Chief and Crowley Family Chair
Department of Surgery
Brigham and Women's Hospital
Boston, Massachusetts

Henning Dralle, MD, PhD
Professor
Department of General, Visceral and Transplantation Surgery
University Hospital Essen
Essen, Nordrhein-Westfalen, Germany

Quan-Yang Duh, MD
Professor
Chief Section of Endocrine Surgery
University of California San Francisco
Attending Surgeon
Department of Surgery
VA Medical Center
San Francisco, California

Quinn Alexander Dunlap, MD
Resident Physician
Department of Otolaryngology-Head and Neck Surgery
University of Arkansas for Medical Sciences
Little Rock, Arkansas

Cosmio Durante, MD, PhD
Department of Internal Medicine and Medical Specialties
Sapienza University of Rome
Rome, Italy

Ahmad Mohamed Eltelety, MBBCh, MSc, MD-PhD, MRCS(ENT)
Clinical Fellow Endocrine Head and Neck Surgery
Otolaryngology
Medical College of Georgia, Augusta University
Augusta, Georgia
Lecturer in Otolaryngology
Faculty of Medicine, Cairo University
Cairo, Egypt

Douglas B. Evans, MD
Professor and Chair
Department of Surgery
Medical College of Wisconsin
Milwaukee, Wisconsin

Guido Fadda, MD, MIAC
Division of Anatomic Pathology
 and Histology
Catholic University
Foundation "Agostino Gemelli" University
 Hospital
Rome, Italy

William C. Faquin, MD, PhD
Professor of Pathology
Harvard Medical School
Director, Head and Neck Pathology
Department of Otolaryngology
Massachusetts Eye and Ear
Pathologist
Department of Pathology
Massachusetts General Hospital
Boston, Massachusetts

Erin Felger, MD
Department of Surgery
Medstar Washington Hospital Center
Washington, DC

Robert L. Ferris, MD, PhD
Director
UPMC Hillman Cancer Center
Hillman Professor of Oncology
Associate Vice-Chancellor for Cancer Research
Co-Director
Tumor Microenvironment Center
Professor of Otolaryngology, Immunology,
 and Radiation Oncology
University of Pittsburgh Medical Center
Pittsburgh, Pennsylvania

Sebastiano Filetti, MD
Professor of Internal Medicine
Department of Internal Medicine and Medical
 Specialties
Sapienza University of Rome
Rome, Italy

Jeremy L. Freeman, MD, FRCSC, FACS
Professor
Department of Otolaryngology-Head and Neck Surgery
University of Toronto
Toronto, Ontario, Canada

Christopher Fundakowski, MD
Associate Professor
Department of Otolaryngology Head & Neck Surgery
Thomas Jefferson University
Philadelphia, Pennsylvania

Ian Ganly, BSc, MD, PhD, MS, FRCS, FRCS-ORL
Professor
Department of Head and Neck Service
Memorial Sloan Kettering Cancer Center
Department of Otolaryngology Head and Neck Surgery
Weill Cornell Medical College
New York, New York

Benjamin Joseph Gigliotti, MD
Assistant Professor of Medicine
University of Rochester School of Medicine & Dentistry
Rochester, New York

Anthony J. Gill, MD, FRCPA
Professor
Sydney Medical School
University of Sydney
Sydney, Australia
Staff Specialist
Department Anatomical Pathology, Royal North Shore Hospital
NSW Health Pathology
St. Leonards, Australia

Thomas J. Giordano, MD, PhD
Henry Clay Bryant Professor of Pathology
Department of Pathology
University of Michigan
Ann Arbor, Michigan

Meredith E. Giuliani, MBBS, MEd, FRCP (C)
Radiation Oncologist
Princess Margaret Cancer Centre
Assistant Professor
Department of Radiation Oncology
University of Toronto
Toronto, Ontario, Canada

Zhen Gooi, MBBS
Section of Otolaryngology-Head and Neck Surgery
University of Chicago Medicine
Chicago, Illinois

Raj K. Gopal, MD, PhD
Assistant in Medicine
Departments of Hematology & Oncology
Massachusetts General Hospital
Boston, Massachusetts

Joanne Guerlain, MD
Département de Carcinologie Cervico-Faciale
Institut Gustave Roussy
Villejuif, France

Julien Hadoux, MD, PhD
Department of Endocrine Oncology
Institut Gustave Roussy
Villejuif, France

Nathan Hales, MD
Private Practice, Otolaryngology, Head and Neck Surgery
San Antonio Head and Neck
San Antonio, Texas

Dana Hartl, MD, PhD
Department of Head and Neck Oncology
Institut Gustave Roussy
Villejuif, France

Bryan R. Haugen, MD
Professor of Medicine and Pathology
Head, Division of Endocrinology, Metabolism and Diabetes
University of Colorado School of Medicine
University of Colorado Cancer Center
Aurora, Colorado

CONTRIBUTORS

Megan R. Haymart, MD
Nancy Wigginton Endocrinology Research Professor
  of Thyroid Cancer
Associate Professor of Internal Medicine
University of Michigan Medical School
Ann Arbor, Michigan

William B. Inabnet, III, MD, MHA
Johnston-Wright Endowed Professor and Chair
Dept of Surgery
University of Kentucky College of Medicine

Jonathan Irish, MD, MSc, FRCSC, FACS
Professor and Head
Division of Head and Neck Oncology
  and Reconstructive Surgery
Department of Otolaryngology-Head and Neck Surgery
University of Toronto
Toronto, Ontario, Canada

Ayaka Iwata, MS, MD
Thyroid and Parathyroid Fellow
Massachusetts Eye and Ear Infirmary
Boston, Massachusetts

Dipti Kamani, MD
Research Director
Division of Thyroid and Parathyroid Endocrine Surgery
Massachusetts Eye and Ear
Boston, Massachusetts

Emad Kandil, MD, MBA
Professor of Surgery
Department of Surgery
Tulane University School of Medicine
New Orleans, Louisiana

Edwin L. Kaplan, MD
Professor
Department of Surgery
University of Chicago Pritzker School of Medicine
Chicago, Illinois

Ken Kazahaya, MD, MBA
Associate Director
Department of Pediatric Otolaryngology
Children's Hospital of Philadelphia
Associate Professor of Clinical Otorhinolaryngology Head
  and Neck Surgery
Department of Otorhinolaryngology Head and Neck Surgery
University of Pennsylvania
Philadelphia, Pennsylvania

Electron Kebebew, MD
Professor and Chief
Department of Surgery
Stanford University
Stanford, California

Matthew I. Kim, MD
Associate Physician
Division of Endocrinology, Diabetes
  and Hypertension
Brigham and Women's Hospital
Boston, Massachusetts

Kevin J. Kovatch, MD
Resident Physician
Department of Otolaryngology-Head and Neck Surgery
University of Michigan
Ann Arbor, Michigan

Brian H.H. Lang, MS, FRACS
Clinical Professor
Department of Surgery
University of Hong Kong
Hong Kong

Sophie Leboulleux, MD, PhD
Department of Nuclear Medicine and Endocrine Oncology
Institut Gustave Roussy
Villejuif, France

Angela M. Leung, MD, MSc
Associate Professor of Medicine
Division of Endocrinology, Diabetes, and Metabolism
David Geffen School of Medicine at UCLA
VA Greater Los Angeles Healthcare System
Los Angeles, California

Robert A. Levine, MD
Adjunct Assistant Professor of Medicine
Department of Endocrinology
Geisel School of Medicine at Dartmouth College
Hanover, New Hampshire

Whitney Liddy, MD
Assistant Professor
Department of Otolaryngology - Head and Neck Surgery
Northwestern University
Chicago, Illinois

Virginia A. LiVolsi, MD
Professor of Pathology
Department of Pathology & Laboratory Medicine
Perelman School of Medicine
University of Pennsylvania
Philadelphia, Pennsylvania

Celestino Pio Lombardi, MD
Professor of Surgery
Endocrine and Metabolic Surgery
Agostino Gemelli University Polyclinic
Institute of Surgical Semeiotics
Catholic University of the Sacred Heart
Rome, Italy

Carrie C. Lubitz, MD, MPH
Associate Professor of Surgery
Massachusetts General Hospital
Boston, Massachusetts

Andreas Machens, MD
Associate Professor
Department of Visceral, Vascular and Endocrine Surgery
Martin Luther University Halle-Wittenberg
Halle (Saale), Germany

Ellie Maghami, MD, FACS
Clinical Professor and Chief, Division of Head and Neck Surgery
Department of Surgery
City of Hope
Duarte, California

Susan J. Mandel, MD, MPH
Professor of Medicine and Associate Chief
Division of Endocrinology, Diabetes, and Metabolism
Perelman School of Medicine
University of Pennsylvania
Philadelphia, Pennsylvania

Anastasios Maniakas, MD, MSc
Fellow, Head & Neck Surgery
The University of Texas MD Anderson Cancer Center
Houston, Texas

Douglas J. Mathisen, MD
Chief of Thoracic Surgery
Department of Surgery
Massachusetts General Hospital
Boston, Massachusetts

Aarti Mathur, MD
Endocrine Surgery Fellow
Department of Surgery, Division of Endocrine Surgery
The Johns Hopkins Hospital
Baltimore, Maryland

Albert Merati, MD
Professor & Chief
Department of Otolaryngology - Head & Neck Surgery
University of Washington
Seattle, Washington

Mira Milas, MD
Professor of Surgery and Chief of Endocrine Surgery
Division of Endocrine Surgery
University of Arizona College of Medicine
Banner University Medical Center Phoenix
Phoenix, Arizona

Akira Miyauchi, MD, PhD
Department of Surgery
Kuma Hospital
Kobe, Japan

Eric Monteiro, MD, MSc, FRCSC
Assistant Professor
Department of Otolaryngology-Head & Neck Surgery
University of Toronto (Mount Sinai Hospital)
Toronto, Ontario, Canada

James L. Netterville, MD
Mark C. Smith Professor
Head & Neck Surgical Oncology
Executive Vice Chair, Bill Wilkerson Center
Vanderbilt Medical Center
Nashville, Tennessee

Yuri E. Nikiforov, MD, PhD
Professor of Pathology
Director, Division of Molecular & Genomic Pathology
Department of Pathology
University of Pittsburgh Medical Center
Pittsburgh, Pennsylvania

Lisa A. Orloff, MD
Professor of Otolaryngology-Head and Neck Surgery
Stanford University
Director, Thyroid Tumor Program
Stanford Cancer Center
Stanford, California

T.K. Pandian, MD, MPH
Endocrine Surgery Fellow
BWH/MGH Harvard Combined Endocrine Surgery Program
Boston, Massachusetts
Chief Resident of Surgery
Mayo Clinic
Rochester, Minnesota

Sareh Parangi, MD
Professor of Surgery
Department of Surgery
Massachusetts General Hospital
Harvard Medical School
Boston, Massachusetts

Sanjay Parikh, MD, FACS
Associate Professor of Otolaryngology-Head and Neck Surgery
University of Washington
Medical Director
Surgical Services
Bellevue Clinic and Surgery Center
Department of Surgery
Seattle Children's Hospital
Seattle, Washington

Auh Whan Park, MD
Associate Professor
Department of Radiology
University of Virginia
Charlottesville, Virginia

Elizabeth N. Pearce, MD, MSc
Professor of Medicine
Section of Endocrinology, Diabetes, and Nutrition
Boston University School of Medicine
Boston, Massachusetts

Phillip K. Pellitteri, DO, FACS
Chair, Otolaryngology/Head & Neck Surgery
Guthrie Health System
Sayre, Pennsylvania
Clinical Professor of Otolaryngology/Head & Neck Surgery
Temple University School of Medicine
Philadelphia, Pennsylvania
Clinical Professor
Department of Surgery
Geisinger Commonwealth School of Medicine
Scranton, Pennsylvania

Francesco Pennestrì, MD
Endocrine and Metabolic Surgery
Agostino Gemelli University Polyclinic
Institute of Surgical Semeiotics
Catholic University of the Sacred Heart
Rome, Italy

Roma Pradhan, MS, MCh
Department of Endocrine Surgery
Dr. Ram Manohar Lohia Institute of
 Medical Sciences
Lucknow, Uttar Pradesh, India

Ruth Prichard, MB, BAO, BCh, MCh, FRCSI
Department of Endocrine Surgery
St. Vincent's University Hospital
Dublin, Ireland

Marco Raffaelli, MD
Professor
U.O. Chirurgia Endocrina e Metabolica
Fondazione Policlinico Universitario A. Gemelli
Istituto di Semeiotica chirurgica
Università Cattolica del Sacro Cuore
Rome, Italy

Gregory W. Randolph, MD, FACS, FACE, FEBS (Endocrine)
Professor of Otolaryngology Head and Neck Surgery
The Claire and John Bertucci Endowed Chair in Thyroid Surgical
 Oncology, Harvard Medical School
Director of the Comprehensive Otolaryngology Division and the
 Thyroid & Parathyroid Endocrine Surgical Division
Department of Otolaryngology Head and Neck Surgery,
 Massachusetts Eye and Ear Infirmary
Member Division of Surgical Oncology, Department of Surgery,
 Massachusetts General Hospital
Boston, Massachusetts

Jeff Rastatter, MD, FAAP, FACS
Associate Professor
Department of Otolaryngology - Head and Neck Surgery
Northwestern University Feinberg School of Medicine
Division of Pediatric Otolaryngology - Head
 and Neck Surgery
Ann & Robert H. Lurie Children's Hospital
 of Chicago
Chicago, Illinois

Lisa M. Reid, MD
Associate Professor of Clinical Surgery
Department of Surgery
Cooper University Hospital
Camden, New Jersey

Sara L. Richer, MD, FACS
Otolaryngologist - Head and Neck Surgeon
Department of Surgery
Bridgeport Hospital - Yale New Haven Health
Bridgeport, Connecticut

Jeremy D. Richmon, MD, FACS
Associate Professor
Department of Otolaryngology
Massachusetts Eye and Ear Infirmary
Harvard Medical School
Boston, Massachusetts

Matthew D. Ringel, MD
Professor of Internal Medicine
The Ohio State University
Columbus, Ohio

Benjamin R. Roman, MD, MSHP
Assistant Attending Surgeon
Department of Surgery, Head & Neck Division
Memorial Sloan Kettering Cancer Center
New York, New York

Anatoly F. Romanchishen, MD
Chief of Hospital Surgery
St. Petersburg State Pediatric Medical University
St. Petersburg, Russia

Douglas S. Ross, MD
Professor of Medicine
Harvard Medical School
Co-Director
Thyroid Associates
Massachusetts General Hospital
Boston, Massachusetts

Jonathon O. Russell, MD
Assistant Professor
Director of Endoscopic and Robotic Thyroid and Parathyroid Surgery
Department of Otolaryngology-Head and Neck Surgery
Johns Hopkins University
Baltimore, Maryland

Marika D. Russell, MD, FACS
Associate Professor of Otolaryngology - Head and Neck Surgery
University of California, San Francisco
San Francisco, California

Mabel Ryder, MD, MS
Assistant Professor of Medicine
Division of Endocrinology, Diabetes, Metabolism, Nutrition and
 Division of Medical Oncology
Mayo Clinic
Rochester, Minnesota

Mona M. Sabra, MD
Professor of Clinical Medicine
Memorial Sloan Kettering Cancer Center
Professor of Clinical Medicine
Weill Cornell School of Medicine
New York, New York

Uma M. Sachdeva, MD, PhD
Fellow in Cardiothoracic Surgery
Division of Thoracic Surgery, Department of Surgery
Massachusetts General Hospital
Boston, Massachusetts

Peter M. Sadow, MD, PhD
Director, Head and Neck Pathology
Massachusetts General Hospital
Massachusetts Eye and Ear
Associate Professor
Department of Pathology
Harvard Medical School
Boston, Massachusetts

Joseph Scharpf, MD
Associate Professor of Surgery
Head and Neck Institute
Cleveland Clinic
Cleveland, Ohio

Martin Schlumberger, MD
Chair
Department of Nuclear Medicine and Endocrine Oncology
Institut Gustave Roussy
Villejuif, France
Professor of Oncology
University Paris-Sud
Orsay, France

Rick Schneider, MD
Department of General, Visceral, and Vascular Surgery
Martin Luther University Halle-Wittenberg
Halle (Saale), Germany

David Scott-Coombes, MS, FRCS, FEBS
Consultant Endocrine Surgeon
Department of Endocrine Surgery
University Hospital of Wales
Cardiff, United Kingdom

Andrew B. Sewell, MD
Surgical Oncology Fellow
Department of Otolaryngology – Head and Neck Surgery
University of Toronto
Toronto, Ontario, Canada

Jatin Shah, MD, PhD, DSc, FACS, FRCS(Hon), FDSRCS(Hon), FRCSI(Hon), FRACS(Hon), FRCSDS(Hon)
Professor of Surgery
E.W. Strong Chair in Head and Neck Oncology
Memorial Sloan Kettering Cancer Center
New York, New York

Manisha H. Shah, MD
Professor of Internal Medicine
The Ohio State University Comprehensive Cancer Center
Columbus, Ohio

Maisie Shindo, MD
Professor
Department of Otolaryngology-Head and Neck Surgery
Oregon Health & Science University
Portland, Oregon

David Shonka, MD
Associate Professor
Department of Otolaryngology-Head and Neck Surgery
University of Virginia
Charlottesville, Virginia

Shonni Joy Silverberg, MD
Professor
Department of Medicine
Columbia University College of Physicians & Surgeons
New York, New York

John Randall Sims, MD
Fellow
Department of Head and Neck Surgery
Mount Sinai Beth Israel
New York, New York

Catherine F. Sinclair, MBBS (Hons), BSc (Biomed), FRACS, FACS
Associate Professor
Icahn School of Medicine at Mount Sinai
Director, Division of Head and Neck Surgery
Mount Sinai West
New York, New York

Michael C. Singer, MD, FACS, FACE
Director, Division of Thyroid & Parathyroid Surgery
Department of Otolaryngology – Head and Neck Surgery
Henry Ford Health System
Detroit, Michigan

Allan E. Siperstein, MD
Professor and Chair
Department of Endocrine Surgery
Cleveland Clinic
Cleveland, Ohio

Jennifer A. Sipos, MD
Professor of Medicine
Division of Endocrinology and Metabolism
Wexner Medical Center, The Ohio State University
Columbus, Ohio

Cristian Martin Slough, MD
Attending Physician
Department of Otolaryngology
Willamette Valley Medical Center
McMinnville, Oregon

Julie A. Sosa, MD, MA
Leon Goldman, MD Distinguished Professor and Chair
Department of Surgery
University of California San Francisco-UCSF
San Francisco, California

Brendan C. Stack, Jr., MD, FACS, FACE
Professor and Chairman
Dept of Otolaryngology Head and Neck Surgery
Southern Illinois University School of Medicine
Springfield, Illinois

Nikolaos Stathatos, MD
Instructor in Medicine
Massachusetts General Hospital
Harvard Medical School
Boston, Massachusetts

Michael James Stechman, MD, FRCS
Department of Endocrine Surgery
University Hospital of Wales
Cardiff, United Kingdom

Antonia E. Stephen, MD
Assistant Professor of Surgery, Dept of Surgery
Massachusetts General Hospital
Boston, Massachusetts

David L. Steward, MD
Professor of Otolaryngology and Neck Surgery
Division of Endocrinology, Departrment of Medicine
University of Cincinnati College of Medicine
Cincinnati, Ohio

Hyun Suh, MD, FACS
Attending Physician
Department of Surgery
Assistant Professor of Surgery
Icahn School of Medicine at Mount Sinai
New York, New York

Mark Sywak, MBBS, MMed Sci (Clin Epi), FRACS
Associate Professor of Surgery
Department of Endocrine Surgery
Royal North Shore Hospital
University of Sydney
Sydney, Australia

Alice Tang, MD
Assistant Professor
Department of Otolaryngology- Head and Neck Surgery
University of Cincinnati College of Medicine
Cincinnati, Ohio

David J. Terris, MD
Regents' Professor
Department of Otolaryngology - Head & Neck Surgery
Augusta University
Augusta, Georgia

Geoffrey Bruce Thompson, MD
Professor of Surgery
Department of Surgery
Mayo Clinic
Rochester, Minnesota

Neil Tolley, MD, FRCS, DLO
Professor
Department of Otolaryngology-Head & Neck Surgery
Imperial College Healthcare NHS Trust
London, United Kingdom

Yoshihiro Tominaga, MD, PhD
Thyroid, Parathyroid, and Bone Division
Noa Imaike Clinic
Director, Division of Endocrine Surgery
Nagoya Second Red Cross Hospital
Nagoya, Japan

Frédéric Triponez, MD
Professor
Department of Thoracic and Endocrine Surgery
University Hospitals of Geneva
Geneva, Switzerland

Richard W. Tsang, MD, FRCP(C)
Radiation Oncologist
Princess Margaret Cancer Centre
Professor
Department of Radiation Oncology
University of Toronto
Toronto, Ontario, Canada

R. Michael Tuttle, MD
Clinical Director
Endocrinology Service
Memorial Sloan Kettering Cancer Center
New York, New York

Mark L. Urken, MD, FACS
Professor
Department of Otolaryngology-Head and Neck Surgery
Albert Einstein College of Medicine
Chief of Head and Neck Surgical Oncology
Beth Israel Medical Center
New York, New York

Kristina V. Vabalayte, PhD
Associate Professor
Hospital Surgical Department
St. Petersburg State Pediatric Medical Department
St. Petersburg, Russia

Andrew M. Vahabzadeh-Hagh, MD
Assistant Professor
Department of Surgery
Division of Otolaryngology
University of California, San Diego
La Jolla, California

Erivelto Martinho Volpi, MD, PhD
Head and Neck Surgeon
Oncology Center at Oswaldo Cruz German Hospital
Professor of Surgery
Medical School of Nove de Julho University
Sao Paulo, Brazil

Tracy S. Wang, MD, MPH, FACS
Professor of Surgery and Chief
Section of Endocrine Surgery
Department of Surgery
Medical College of Wisconsin
Milwaukee, Wisconsin

Che-Wei Wu, MD, PhD
Associated Professor of Otorhinolarygology
Kaohsiung Medical University
Director of Otorhinolarygology
Kaohsiung Municipal Hsiao-Kang Hospital
Kaohsiung Medical University Hospital
Kaohsiung, Taiwan

Lori J. Wirth, MD
Assistant Professor
Department of Medicine
Harvard Medical School
Massachusetts General Hospital
Boston, Massachusetts

Ian Witterick, MD, MSc, FRCSC
Professor and Chair
Department of Otolaryngology-Head & Neck Surgery
University of Toronto
Otolaryngologist-in-Chief
Sinai Health System
Toronto, Ontario, Canada

Richard J. Wong, MD
Head and Neck Service
Department of Surgery
Memorial Sloan Kettering Cancer Center
New York, New York

Gayle E. Woodson, MD
Adjunct Professor
Department of Otolaryngology
Drexel University
Philadelphia, Pennsylvania
Professor
Department of Communication Sciences and Disorders
University of Central Florida
Orlando, Florida

Cameron D. Wright, MD
Professor of Surgery
Massachusetts General Hospital
Harvard Medical School
Boston, Massachusetts

Mark E. Zafereo, MD
Associate Professor
Department of Head and Neck Surgery
MD Anderson Cancer Center
Houston, Texas

Fermin M. Zubiaur, MD
Director, Voice and Swallowing Clinic
Surgical Otolaryngology Group
Professor
Panamerican University School of Medicine
President, Mexico Chapter of the Voice Foundation
Mexico City, Mexico

FOREWORD TO THE SECOND EDITION

I had the pleasure of reading Gregory Randolph's first edition of *Surgery of the Thyroid and Parathyroid Glands* from cover to cover in 2004. I was very impressed with the comprehensive coverage by an array of truly outstanding authors from multidisciplinary fields of expertise. Not only was the written content excellent and as up-to-date as a textbook will allow, but the illustrations by Robert Galla also were superb and enhanced each of the procedures or the description of the anatomy especially well. Obviously a great deal of thought and exceptional editing went into the creation of this text. Having had the opportunity to review most of the other surgical texts in this field for the past three decades, I considered this one the most outstanding that had been published about the thyroid and parathyroid glands.

Now that the second edition has been produced, one might wonder whether any significant improvements or additions would be made. Dr. Randolph has not disappointed us. He has both revised and added to the text in content with many new authors and produced several videos that are included on a website that accompanies the book. Because of his activities as a clinical surgeon, researcher, educator, and frequent guest speaker both in the U.S. and overseas, Dr. Randolph has been able to evaluate and select the very best individuals to contribute chapters to this edition. He has chosen well. Where there were 46 chapters in the first edition, there are 70 in this one. No areas in which new developments have occurred have been neglected. Two of the new chapters that are noteworthy are those by Angelos and Heller on "Ethics and Malpractice in Thyroid and Parathyroid Surgery" and by Scott-Coombes and Bergenfelz on "Endocrine Quality Registers: Surgical Outcome Measurement." These topical subjects should be of interest to all readers regardless of discipline.

Once again, Dr. Randolph has achieved his goal of producing a comprehensive review of state-of-the-art knowledge in endocrine pathophysiology, surgical anatomy, techniques, preoperative and postoperative care, and the very latest technological advances provided by the very best in their areas of expertise. Although this is a second edition, considering updates, new authors, new chapters, and editing, it can almost be considered a new text on its own merits. It is a book that most endocrinologists, pathologists, radiologists, and *all* surgeons interested in the thyroid and parathyroid glands will want to have readily available as an authoritative reference. Dr. Randolph has shown that there is always room for improvement, even when the original was very good.

Norman W. Thompson, MD
*Professor of Surgery Emeritus, University of Michigan,
Ann Arbor, Michigan*

In this new second edition of the classic textbook *Surgery of the Thyroid and Parathyroid Glands*, Dr. Gregory W. Randolph has put forth an impressive effort to build on and improve his first edition. He has expanded the content and added new chapters and authors appropriate for such a comprehensive review of diseases of and surgery for the thyroid and parathyroid glands. All previous chapters have been updated with overall improvement in the figures and tables and, of course, updated references. As quality and outcomes now define patient care, a specific chapter focusing on this topic has been added. Another excellent addition has been the discussion of medical ethics related to thyroid and parathyroid disease.

I believe the exhaustive coverage of these topics, provided by authors who cross multiple specialties, including otolaryngology, general surgery, and thoracic surgery, provides the most comprehensive text ever to address surgery of the thyroid and parathyroid glands. The book is a tribute to Dr. Randolph and his coauthors and will be a valuable addition to the library of anyone who practices endocrine surgery.

Keith D. Lillemoe, MD
*W. Gerald Austen Professor of Surgery,
Harvard Medical School,
Surgeon-in-Chief and Chief of Surgery,
Massachusetts General Hospital, Boston, Massachusetts*

The first edition of this text, written by experts in a variety of specialties, including otolaryngology, general surgery, endocrinology, and pathology, was published in 2003 and has quickly become a classic. The second edition not only is an update and revision, but also contains 24 new chapters. Dr. Randolph is to be congratulated in attracting more than 140 internationally respected authors. In addition, 17 video clips illustrating surgical anatomy and technique are included with the text.

Surgery of the Thyroid and Parathyroid Glands provides a thorough treatment of benign and neoplastic disease of thyroid and parathyroid glands, surgical management, its complications, and postoperative medical considerations. The text and outstanding illustrations provide a comprehensive treatise on best practice and surgical techniques.

This text, as was the first edition, is clearly destined to be the authoritative source for disorders of the thyroid and parathyroid glands.

Joseph B. Nadol, MD, Jr
*Walter Augustus LeCompte Professor and Chairman,
Department of Otology and Laryngology, Harvard Medical School,
Chief of Otolaryngology, Massachusetts Eye and Ear Infirmary, Boston,
Massachusetts*

FOREWORD

> Please go to expertconsult.com to view related video:
> **Video F.1** Prelude to Surgery of the Thyroid and Parathyroid Glands, Third Edition.

The third edition of *Surgery of the Thyroid and Parathyroid Glands*, edited by Dr. Gregory Randolph, is a timely sequel to the previous editions. The editor has done a splendid job in assembling the world leaders in thyroid and parathyroid diseases to contribute to this up-to-date opus on the subject of surgery of the thyroid and parathyroid glands. The landscape of head and neck endocrinology is constantly changing with the evolution of new insights into the etiopathogenesis of thyroid diseases; newer methods of diagnosis, molecular/genetic testing, imaging, surgical approaches; and completely new concepts in nonsurgical management of low-risk lesions. To conform to these shifts of knowledge and paradigms, the content of this text is maintained in lockstep with this evolution. Chapters from previous editions have been added and deleted, and there are extensive additions by the original authors regarding the epidemiology and genetics of thyroid cancer; the preoperative workup for both thyroid and parathyroid diseases; the addition of the new AJCC 8th Edition staging; and chapters on the new Bethesda 2017 system and on NIFTP. Also new to this edition is an extensive chapter on nonsurgical management of thyroid nodules with radio frequency, lasers, and alcohol ablation. The chapter on nerve monitoring has been expanded with newer techniques, and complete coverage of newer minimally invasive surgical techniques and robotic and transoral approaches is also included in the chapter on surgical approaches.

To his credit the editor has diplomatically disposed of territorial differences and creatively produced a multidisciplinary array of highly scientific and state-of-the-art chapters, leaving no subject in the specialty unattended. The well-edited and highly scrutinized chapters are written in a clear fashion and bring to light evidence-based science, techniques, controversies, and management algorithms. Dr. Greg Randolph, a recognized global leader in thyroid and parathyroid surgery, and an energetic and indefatigable ambassador and colleague, has accomplished an outstanding task in putting together this third edition of *Surgery of the Thyroid and Parathyroid Glands*, with contributions from world experts covering all aspects of the specialty. This book will be a "must" in the libraries of medical schools and academic departments of surgery and otolaryngology, and an essential *read* for surgical trainees and practicing surgeons and endocrinologists. It is an honor and a privilege for us to write this foreword for this opus magnum of thyroid and parathyroid surgery.

Jeremy L. Freeman, MD, FRCSC, FACS
Professor of Otolaryngology—Head and Neck Surgery
Professor of Surgery
Temmy Latner/Dynacare Chair in Head and Neck Oncology
Mount Sinai Hospital
University of Toronto
Toronto, Ontario, Canada

Jatin Shah, MD, MS (Surg), PhD (Hon), DSc(Hon), FACS, FRCS (Hon), FRCSI(Hon), FRACS(Hon), FDSRCS(Hon), FRCSDS(Hon)
Professor of Surgery, E W Strong Chair in Head and Neck Oncology
Memorial Sloan Kettering Cancer Center
New York, New York

PREFACE

 Please go to expertconsult.com to view related video:
Video P.1 Introduction to Surgery of the Thyroid and Parathyroid Glands, Third Edition.

Surgery of the Thyroid and Parathyroid Glands is a comprehensive review of state-of-the-art knowledge of endocrine pathophysiology, surgical anatomy and techniques, preoperative and postoperative evaluation, and the latest technological advances relating to the thyroid and parathyroid glands, representing a substantial update and expansion of our second edition.

Thyroid and parathyroid surgery is seen in the context of a broad head and neck surgical perspective, and therefore chapters on associated neurolaryngology, anatomy of the lateral neck, and airway considerations are included. Throughout, emphasis is given to thorough preoperative workup and informed intraoperative decision making. Recent advances within the field, including preoperative localization, recurrent laryngeal nerve monitoring, intraoperative parathyroid hormone analysis, parathyroid autofluorescence, preoperative and prognostic mutational testing, and minimally invasive approaches, are all thoroughly reviewed. An attempt has been made throughout the text to present controversies, such as extent of nodal surgery for thyroid cancer or conservative shave procedures for invasive thyroid cancer, and also to provide clear-cut summary recommendations.

The strength of the whole relates to the quality of each part. Each contributor, drawn from the very best in the world in the fields of endocrine, head and neck, and thoracic surgery, as well as endocrinology, oncology, radiology, and pathology was selected because of his or her clinical activity and research contributions in the medical literature within the chapter topic area. These contributors provide an overarching unique orientation to their respective topics that goes beyond the individual disparate facts. It has been gratifying to work with such a group. In numerous chapters collaborators were paired from different areas of the world and in some circumstances different specialties to provide a blending of various heterogeneous elements.

Chapter length in the text involved necessary page limitations. However, many chapters contain additional material available online. When the reader sees the online icon in the margin 📶, additional material can be found in the online version of *Surgery of the Thyroid and Parathyroid Glands*.

This book represents a comprehensive surgical text blended with a surgical atlas. Many chapters that focus on surgical anatomy and maneuvers are heavily illustrated by Robert Galla, medical illustrator. The operative realism of Mr. Galla's handsome images is impressive and represents one of the real strengths of this text. Our third edition is also decorated with wonderful new images from new talented artists Zach Zuffante and Sophia D'Abate.

In addition, the book now is associated with a video library, which highlights numerous complex surgical maneuvers and procedures by leaders in the field. Where the reader sees the video icon ▶, online video material is available. Also this edition contains introductory videos for numerous key chapters wherein the main author orients and familiarizes the reader to the chapter's content and key pivotal issues. The introductory videos of this work were produced, edited, and organized by Gregory William Randolph, Jr., our surgical text video Editor in Chief.

The book is intended for surgeons and endocrinologists, as well as oncologists, radiologists, and pathologists with an interest in thyroid and parathyroid disease. It is my intention that the book be a resource to both the surgeon in training and the experienced surgeon.

Enjoy the read!

Gregory W. Randolph, MD

ACKNOWLEDGMENTS

I would like to thank the many people without whom this project would not have been possible. Substantial thought and effort went into the development of each image in this text. Virtually every image is the result of a collaborative effort. Robert Galla and I reviewed initial sketches and ideas from contributors and then revised each drawing multiple times. It has been a pleasure to work with Mr. Galla. His drawings truly represent the backbone of this text. They are as informative as they are beautiful. We are also very pleased to include and showcase the artwork of Zach Zuffante and Sophia D'Abate. Art is so important in surgery.

In addition, I would like to thank the tireless research assistance of my friend and colleague, Dr. Dipti Kamani. I would also like to thank John and Claire Bertucci and Mike and Eliz Ruane for their ongoing support through the years and for their friendship.

Finally, I would like to thank some of the physicians who have been important in the development of this book, including Dr. Brad Welling, my chairman, friend, and mentor, who supported the initial development and continuing evolution of my thyroid surgical practice in Boston. I would like to thank Drs. Keith Lillemoe and Ken Tanabe for their belief in a true collaborative environment and commitment to modern endocrine surgery, and Dr. Lori Wirth for her oncologic perspective and friendship. I am indebted to Dr. Gil Daniels, whose instruction over the years has provided framework and grounding for my thyroid and parathyroid surgical practice. For your teaching and friendship, Gil, I am grateful.

I am most grateful to my family, Lorraine, Greg Jr., Benjamin, and Madeline who have borne the burden of the days of work in this and many other work endeavors. Thank you for your patience with me.

Gregory W. Randolph, MD

To Bob Sofferman, friend, artist and champion.

Then I heard the voice of the Lord saying "Whom shall I send and who will go for us?" And I said, "here I am; send me"

Isaiah Chapter 6 Verse 6.

To Michael Brauckhoff, his life and work.

The early lilacs became part of this child and grass and white and red morning glories and white and red clover and the song of the Phoebe bird.... All became part of him.

Leaves of Grass, *Walt Whitman.*

CONTENTS

SECTION 1 Introduction

1. **History of Thyroid and Parathyroid Surgery**, 2
   Cristian M. Slough, Whitney Liddy, Jennifer Brooks, Edwin L. Kaplan, Mijenko Bura, Anatoly F. Romanchishen, Kristina Vabalayte, and Gregory W. Randolph
2. **Applied Embryology of the Thyroid and Parathyroid Glands**, 15
   Roma Pradhan, Amit Agarwal, Celestino P. Lombardi, and Marco Raffaelli
3. **Thyroid Physiology and Thyroid Function Testing**, 26
   Angela M. Leung and Gregory A. Brent

SECTION 2 Benign Thyroid Disease

4. **Thyroiditis**, 40
   Trevor E. Angell, Matthew I. Kim, and Victor J. Bernet
5. **Thyroglossal Duct Cysts and Ectopic Thyroid Tissue**, 50
   Christopher Fundakowski, Erin Felger, and Ellie Maghami
6. **Surgery of Cervical and Substernal Goiter**, 53
   Whitney Liddy, James L. Netterville, and Gregory W. Randolph
7. **Approach to the Mediastinum: Transcervical, Transsternal, and Video-Assisted**, 70
   Uma M. Sachdeva, Cameron D. Wright, and Douglas J. Mathisen
8. **Surgical Management of Hyperthyroidism**, 79
   Lisa A. Orloff and Maisie L. Shindo
9. **Reoperation for Benign Thyroid Disease**, 89
   Mark Sywak, Ruth Prichard, and Leigh Delbridge

SECTION 3 Preoperative Evaluation

10. **The Evaluation and Management of Thyroid Nodules**, 100
    Kevin J. Kovatch, Elizabeth N. Pearce, and Megan R. Haymart
11. **Fine-Needle Aspiration of the Thyroid Gland: The 2017 Bethesda System**, 108
    William C. Faquin, Guido Fadda, and Edmund S. Cibas
12. **Fine-Needle Aspiration and Molecular Analysis**, 118
    Benjamin J. Gigliotti, Marika D. Russell, David Shonka, and Nikolaos Stathatos
13. **Ultrasound of the Thyroid and Parathyroid Glands**, 132
    Kevin T. Brumund and Susan J. Mandel
14. **Preoperative Radiographic Mapping of Nodal Disease for Papillary Thyroid Carcinoma**, 149
    Sara L. Richer, Dipti Kamani, Robert Levine, Zaid Al-Qurayshi, and Gregory W. Randolph
15. **Laryngeal Examination in Thyroid and Parathyroid Surgery**, 156
    Neil Tolley, Ian Witterick, and Gregory W. Randolph
16. **Radiofrequency and Laser Ablation of Thyroid Nodules and Parathyroid Adenoma**, 163
    Jung Hwan Baek and Auh Whan Park

SECTION 4 Thyroid Neoplasia

17. **Differentiated Thyroid Cancer Incidence**, 174
    Quinn Dunlap and Louise Davies
18. **Molecular Pathogenesis of Thyroid Neoplasia**, 181
    Matthew D. Ringel and Thomas J. Giordano
19. **Papillary Thyroid Cancer**, 186
    Jennifer A. Sipos and Bryan R. Haugen
20. **Papillary Thyroid Microcarcinoma**, 194
    Douglas S. Ross
21. **Papillary Carcinoma Observation**, 199
    Akira Miyauchi and R. Michael Tuttle
22. **Follicular Thyroid Cancer**, 204
    Cosimo Durante and Sebastiano Filetti
23. **Noninvasive Follicular Thyroid Neoplasm With Papillary-Like Nuclear Features (NIFTP)**, 213
    Yuri E. Nikiforov and Robert L. Ferris
24. **Dynamic Risk Group Analysis and Staging for Differentiated Thyroid Cancer**, 218
    Laura Boucai and R. Michael Tuttle
25. **Hürthle Cell Tumors of the Thyroid**, 225
    Raj K. Gopal, Peter M. Sadow, and Ian Ganly
26. **Sporadic Medullary Thyroid Carcinoma**, 229
    Benjamin R. Roman and Richard J. Wong
27. **Syndromic Medullary Thyroid Cancer: MEN 2A and MEN 2B**, 235
    Henning Dralle and Andreas Machens
28. **Anaplastic Thyroid Cancer and Primary Thyroid Lymphoma**, 246
    Ashish V. Chintakuntlawar, Mabel Ryder, and Keith C. Bible
29. **Pediatric Thyroid Cancer**, 255
    Gillian Diercks, Andrew J. Bauer, Jeff Rastatter, Ken Kazahaya, and Sanjay Parikh
30. **Familial Nonmedullary Thyroid Cancer**, 264
    Wilson Alobuia, Aarti Mathur, and Electron Kebebew

SECTION 5 Thyroid and Neck Surgery

31. **Principles in Thyroid Surgery**, 272
    Whitney Liddy, Juliana Bonilla-Velez, Frédéric Triponez, Dipti Kamani, and Gregory Randolph
32. **Robotic and Extracervical Approaches to the Thyroid and Parathyroid Glands**, 294
    Emad Kandil, Ehab Alameer, Woong Youn Chung, Hyun Suh, and David J. Terris
33. **Transoral Thyroidectomy**, 301
    Jeremy D. Richmon, Angkoon Anuwong, Zhen Gooi, and Jonathon O. Russell
34. **Minimally Invasive Video-Assisted Thyroidectomy**, 311
    Rocco Bellantone, Francesco Pennestrì, and Celestino Pio Lombardi
35. **Surgical Anatomy and Monitoring of the Superior Laryngeal Nerve**, 316
    Marcin Barczyński, Claudio R. Cernea, and Catherine F. Sinclair

36 **Surgical Anatomy and Monitoring of the Recurrent Laryngeal Nerve,** 326
Gregory W. Randolph, Dipti Kamani, Che-Wei Wu, and Rick Schneider

37 **Surgery for Locally Advanced Thyroid Cancer: Larynx, Tracheal Invasion, and Esophageal,** 360
Mark L. Urken, John R. Sims, Eran E. Alon, and Joseph Scharpf

38 **Central Neck Dissection: Indications and Technique,** 372
Alice L. Tang, Lisa M. Reid, Gregory W. Randolph, and David L. Steward

39 **Lateral Neck Dissection: Indications and Technique,** 379
Anastasios Maniakas, Amy Chen, Feng-Yu Chiang, and Mark E. Zafereo

40 **Incisions in Thyroid and Parathyroid Surgery,** 386
David J. Terris and Ahmad M. Eltelety

41 **Surgical Pathology of the Thyroid Gland,** 391
Zubair W. Baloch and Virginia A. LiVolsi

SECTION 6 Postoperative Considerations

42 **Pathophysiology of Recurrent Laryngeal Nerve Injury,** 404
Gayle Woodson

43 **Management of Recurrent Laryngeal Nerve Paralysis,** 410
Simon Brisebois, Andrew M. Vahabzadeh-Hagh, Fermin Zubiaur, and Albert Merati

44 **Nonneural Complications of Thyroid and Parathyroid Surgery,** 419
William B. Inabnet, III, David Scott-Coombes, and Erivelto Volpi

45 **Quality Assessment in Thyroid and Parathyroid Surgery,** 426
Eric Monteiro, Carolyn Seib, Julie A. Sosa, and Jonathan Irish

46 **Ethics and Malpractice in Thyroid and Parathyroid Surgery,** 433
Peter Angelos

SECTION 7 Postoperative Management

47 **Postoperative Management of Differentiated Thyroid Cancer,** 440
Dana Hartl, Sophie Leboulleux, Julien Hadoux, Amandine Berdelou, Ingrid Breuskin, Joanne Guerlain, and Martin Schlumberger

48 **Postoperative Radioactive Iodine Ablation and Treatment of Differentiated Thyroid Cancer,** 447
Mona M. Sabra

49 **External Beam Radiotherapy for Thyroid Malignancy,** 452
Meredith E. Giuliani, Richard W. Tsang, and James D. Brierley

50 **Reoperative Thyroid Surgery,** 461
Jeremy L. Freeman, Andrew B. Sewell, Nathan W. Hales, and Gregory W. Randolph

51 **Nonsurgical Treatment of Thyroid Cysts, Nodules, Thyroid Cancer Nodal Metastases, and Hyperparathyroidism: The Role of Percutaneous Ethanol Injection,** 472
Devaprabu Abraham and Nikita R. Abraham

52 **Medical Treatment Horizons for Metastatic Differentiated and Medullary Thyroid Cancer,** 479
Jean G. Bustamante Alvarez, Lori J. Wirth, and Manisha H. Shah

SECTION 8 Parathyroid Surgery

53 **Primary Hyperparathyroidism: Pathophysiology, Surgical Indications, and Preoperative Workup,** 486
Shonni J. Silverberg and John P. Bilezikian

54 **Guide to Preoperative Parathyroid Localization Testing,** 494
Carrie C. Lubitz and Quan-Yang Duh

55 **Principles in Surgical Management of Primary Hyperparathyroidism,** 502
Nancy L. Cho and Gerard M. Doherty

56 **Standard Bilateral Parathyroid Exploration,** 517
Allan E. Siperstein, Antonia E. Stephen, and Mira Milas

57 **Minimally Invasive Single Gland Parathyroid Exploration,** 529
Sareh Parangi, T.K. Pandian, and Geoffrey Thompson

58 **Minimally Invasive Video-Assisted Parathyroidectomy,** 537
Rocco Bellantone, Marco Raffaelli, Celestino Lombardi, and Carmela De Crea

59 **Intraoperative PTH Monitoring During Parathyroid Surgery,** 546
Denise Carneiro-Pla and Phillip K. Pellitteri

60 **Surgical Management of Multiglandular Parathyroid Disease,** 553
Michael Stechman, Anders Bergenfeltz, and David Scott-Coombes

61 **Surgical Management of Secondary and Tertiary Hyperparathyroidism,** 564
Yoshihiro Tominaga

62 **Parathyroid Management in the MEN Syndromes,** 576
Tracy S. Wang and Douglas B. Evans

63 **Revision Parathyroid Surgery,** 585
Michael C. Singer, Ayaka Iwata, and Brendan C. Stack

64 **Parathyroid Carcinoma,** 591
Rita Y.K. Chang and Brian H.H. Lang

65 **Surgical Pathology of the Parathyroid Glands,** 597
Mahsa S. Ahadi and Anthony J. Gill

Index, 605

VIDEO CONTENTS

Foreword
Video F-1 Prelude to *Surgery of the Thyroid and Parathyroid Glands,* Third Edition – Jatin P. Shah

Preface
Video P-1 Introduction to *Surgery of the Thyroid and Parathyroid Glands,* Third Edition – Gregory W. Randolph

SECTION 2 Benign Thyroid Disease

Chapter 6 Surgery of Cervical and Substernal Goiter
Video 6-1 Surgery for Cervical and Substernal Goiter – Gregory W. Randolph

SECTION 3 Preoperative Evaluation

Chapter 10 The Evaluation and Management of Thyroid Nodules
Video 10-1 Introduction to Chapter 10, the Evaluation and Management of Thyroid Nodules – Megan R. Haymart

Chapter 11 Fine-Needle Aspiration of the Thyroid Gland: The 2017 Bethesda System
Video 11-1 Thyroid Nodule Fine-Needle Aspiration – Erik K. Alexander
Video 11-2 Fine-Needle Aspiration Slide Preparation – William C. Faquin

Chapter 12 Fine-Needle Aspiration and Molecular Analysis
Video 12-1 Introduction to Chapter 12, Fine-Needle Aspiration and Molecular Analysis – Bryan McIver

Chapter 13 Ultrasound of the Thyroid and Parathyroid Glands
Video 13-1 Ultrasound of the Thyroid and Parathyroid Glands: Equipment and Techniques – Robert A. Sofferman

Chapter 15 Laryngeal Examination in Thyroid and Parathyroid Surgery
Video 15-1 Fiberoptic Laryngeal Exam: Laryngeal Anatomy and Function – Gregory W. Randolph

Chapter 16 Laser and Radiofrequency Treatment of Thyroid Nodules and Parathyroid Adenoma
Video 16-1 Laser and Radiofrequency Treatment of Thyroid Nodules and Parathyroid Adenoma – Roberto Valcavi, Giorgio Stecconi Bortolani
Video 16-2 RFA of a Thyroid Nodule Using the Trans-isthmic Approach and the Moving Shot Technique – Jung Hwan Baek, Auh Whan Park
Video 16-3 RFA of a Recurrent Tumor in the Subcutaneous Location with Hydrodissection and the Moving Shot Technique – Jung Hwan Baek, Auh Whan Park

SECTION 4 Thyroid Neoplasia

Chapter 17 Differentiated Thyroid Cancer Incidence
Video 17-1 Introduction to Chapter 17, Differentiated Thyroid Cancer Incidence – Louise Davies

Chapter 20 Papillary Thyroid Microcarcinoma
Video 20-1 Introduction to Chapter 20, Papillary Thyroid Microcarcinoma – Douglas S. Ross

Chapter 21 Papillary Carcinoma Observation
Video 21-1 Introduction to Chapter 21, Papillary Carcinoma Observation – R. Michael Tuttle

Chapter 23 Noninvasive Follicular Thyroid Neoplasm with Papillary-Like Nuclear Features (NIFTP)
Video 23-1 Introduction to Chapter 23, Noninvasive Follicular Thyroid Neoplasm with Papillary-Like Nuclear Features – Yuri E. Nikiforov

Chapter 25 Hürthle Cell Tumors of the Thyroid
Video 25-1 Introduction to Chapter 25, Hürthle Cell Tumors of the Thyroid – Peter M. Sadow

Chapter 26 Sporadic Medullary Thyroid Carcinoma
Video 26-1 Introduction to Chapter 26, Sporadic Medullary Thyroid Carcinoma – Richard J. Wong

Chapter 29 Pediatric Thyroid Cancer
Video 29-1 Introduction to Chapter 29, Pediatric Thyroid Cancer – Gillian Diercks

SECTION 5 Thyroid and Neck Surgery

Chapter 31 Principles in Thyroid Surgery
Video 31-1 Basic Thyroid Surgical Maneuvers – Gregory W. Randolph
Video 31-2 Advanced Thyroid Cancer Surgery – Gregory W. Randolph
Video 31-3 Total Thyroidectomy: Autofluorescence and Parathyroid Angiography – Whitney Liddy, Juliana Bonilla-Velez, Gregory W. Randolph, Frédéric Triponez

Chapter 32 Robotic and Extracervical Approaches to the Thyroid and Parathyroid Glands
- Video 32-1 Transaxillary Robotic Thyroidectomy – Ronald B. Kuppersmith
- Video 32-2 Postauricular Robotic Thyroidectomy – David J. Terris

Chapter 33 Transoral Thyroidectomy
- Video 33-1 Introduction to Chapter 33, Transoral Thyroidectomy – Jeremy D. Richmon
- Video 33-2 Transoral Endoscopic Thyroidectomy: Vestibular Approach – Jeremy D. Richmon

Chapter 34 Minimally Invasive Video-Assisted Thyroidectomy
- Video 34-1 Minimally Invasive Video-Assisted Thyroidectomy – Paolo Miccoli, Carlo Enrico Ambrosini, Gabriele Materazzi

Chapter 35 Surgical Anatomy and Monitoring of the Superior Laryngeal Nerve
- Video 35-1 Introduction to Chapter 35, Surgical Anatomy and Monitoring of the Superior Laryngeal Nerve – Marcin Barczyński
- Video 35-2 Superior Laryngeal Nerve Anatomy and Monitoring – Gregory W. Randolph
- Video 35-3 Stimulation of the Right-Sided External Branch of the Superior Laryngeal Nerve During Thyroidectomy – Marcin Barczyński, Claudio R. Cernea, Catherine F. Sinclair

Chapter 36 Surgical Anatomy and Monitoring of the Recurrent Laryngeal Nerve
- Video 36-1 Introduction to Chapter 36, Surgical Anatomy and Monitoring of the Recurrent Laryngeal Nerve – Gregory W. Randolph
- Video 36-2 Recurrent Laryngeal Nerve Monitoring – Gregory W. Randolph
- Video 36-3 Continuous Vagal Nerve Monitoring – Gregory W. Randolph

Chapter 37 Surgery for Locally Advanced Thyroid Cancer: Larynx, Tracheal Invasion, and Esophageal
- Video 37-1 Tracheal Resection for Locally Advanced Carcinoma of the Thyroid Gland – Jatin P. Shah

Chapter 38 Central Neck Dissection: Indications and Technique
- Video 38-1 Introduction to Chapter 38, Central Neck Dissection: Indications and Technique – Alice L. Tang, David L. Steward
- Video 38-2 Central Compartment Dissection – James I. Cohen

Chapter 39 Lateral Neck Dissection: Indications and Technique
- Video 39-1 Lateral Neck Dissection for Differentiated Thyroid Cancer – Randal S. Weber

Chapter 40 Incisions in Thyroid and Parathyroid Surgery
- Video 40-1 Introduction to Chapter 40, Incisions in Thyroid and Parathyroid Surgery – David J. Terris

SECTION 6 Postoperative Considerations

Chapter 43 Management of Recurrent Laryngeal Nerve Paralysis
- Video 43-1 Vocal Fold Augmentation Using Transcricothyroid Membrane Submucosal Approach – Simon Brisebois, Andrew M. Vahabzadeh-Hagh, Fermin Zubiaur, Albert Merati

Chapter 45 Quality Assessment in Thyroid and Parathyroid Surgery
- Video 45-1 Introduction to Chapter 45, Quality Assessment in Thyroid and Parathyroid Surgery – Julie A. Sosa

Chapter 46 Ethics and Malpractice in Thyroid and Parathyroid Surgery
- Video 46-1 Introduction to Chapter 46, Ethics and Malpractice in Thyroid and Parathyroid Surgery – Peter Angelos

SECTION 7 Postoperative Management

Chapter 48 Postoperative Radioactive Iodine Ablation and Treatment of Differentiated Thyroid Cancer
- Video 48-1 Introduction to Chapter 48, Postoperative Radioactive Iodine Ablation and Treatment of Differentiated Thyroid Cancer – Mona M. Sabra

Chapter 50 Reoperative Thyroid Surgery
- Video 50-1 Introduction to Chapter 50, Reoperative Thyroid Surgery – Jeremy L. Freeman

Chapter 51 Nonsurgical Treatment of Thyroid Cysts, Nodules, Thyroid Cancer Nodal Metastases, and Hyperparathyroidism: The Role of Percutaneous Ethanol Injection
    Video 51-1 Floating Debris – Devaprabu Abraham, Nikita R. Abraham
    Video 51-2 Percutaneous Ethanol Injection: Cyst Injection – Devaprabu Abraham, Nikita R. Abraham
    Video 51-3 Percutaneous Ethanol Injection: Toxic Adenoma – Devaprabu Abraham, Nikita R. Abraham
    Video 51-4 Percutaneous Ethanol Injection: Metastasis – Devaprabu Abraham, Nikita R. Abraham
    Video 51-5 Ultrasound Cord Check – Devaprabu Abraham, Nikita R. Abraham

Chapter 52 Medical Treatment Horizons for Metastatic Differentiated and Medullary Thyroid Cancer
    Video 52-1 Introduction to Chapter 52, Medical Treatment Horizons for Metastatic Differentiated and Medullary Thyroid Cancer – Lori J. Wirth

SECTION 8 Parathyroid Surgery

Chapter 54 Guide to Preoperative Parathyroid Localization Testing
    Video 54-1 Introduction to Chapter 54, Guide to Preoperative Parathyroid Localization Testing – Carrie C. Lubitz

Chapter 56 Standard Bilateral Parathyroid Exploration
    Video 56-1 Introduction to Chapter 56, Standard Bilateral Parathyroid Exploration – Antonia E. Stephen

Chapter 57 Minimally Invasive Single Gland Parathyroid Exploration
    Video 57-1 Minimally Invasive Parathyroidectomy – T.K. Pandian, Sareh Parangi, Geoffrey Thompson

Chapter 61 Surgical Management of Secondary and Tertiary Hyperparathyroidism
    Video 61-1 Total Parathyroidectomy with Forearm Autograft for Patients with Advanced Secondary Hyperparathyroidism – Yoshihiro Tominaga
    Video 61-2 Total Parathyroidectomy with Forearm Autograft for Patients with Advanced Secondary Hyperparathyroidism: Usefulness of IONM – Yoshihiro Tominaga

Chapter 64 Parathyroid Carcinoma
    Video 64-1 Parathyroid Carcinoma: Management Principles with an Illustrative Case – Rita Y.K. Chang, Brian H.H. Lang

Surgery of the Thyroid and Parathyroid Glands

SECTION 1

Introduction

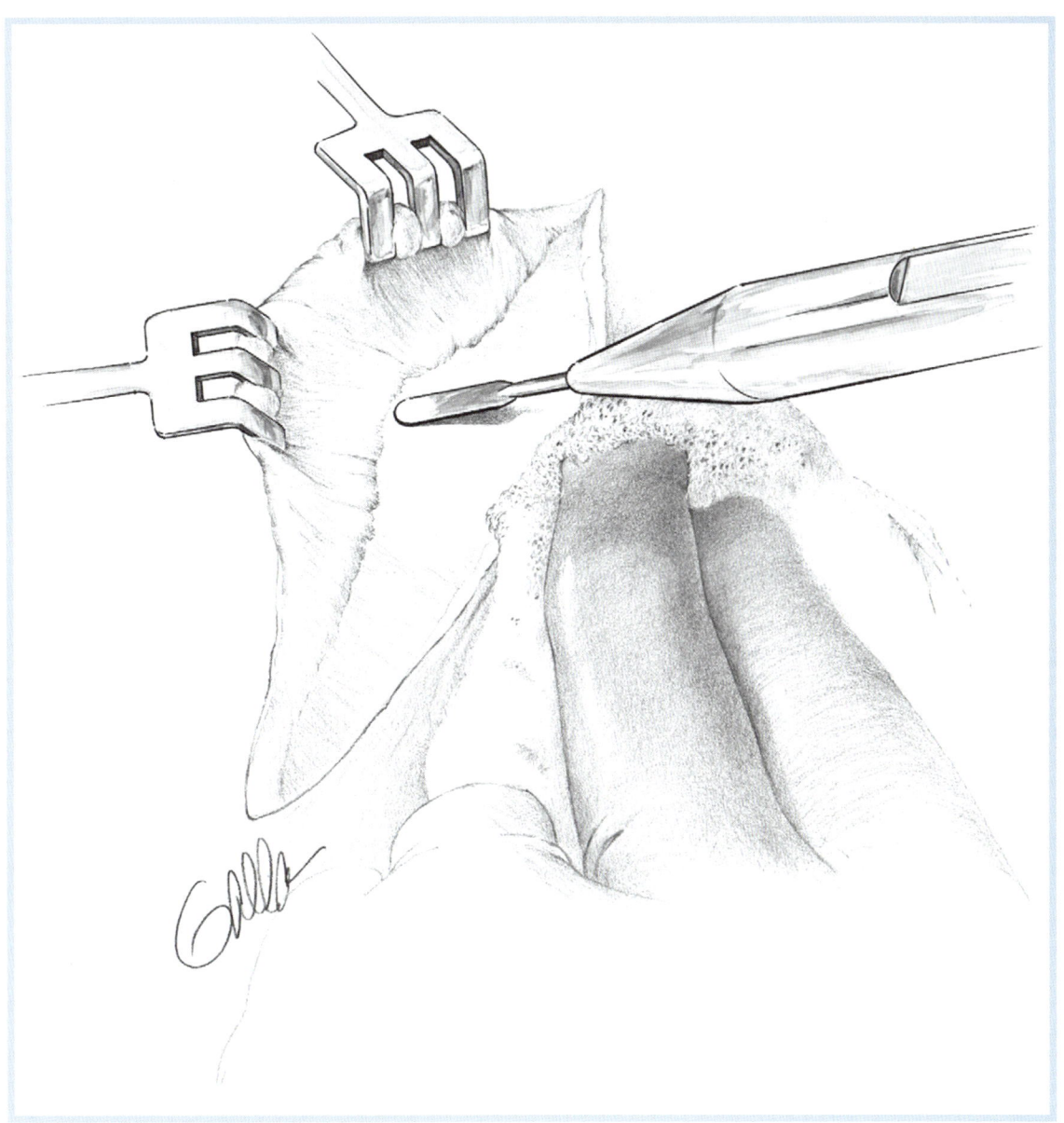

History of Thyroid and Parathyroid Surgery

Cristian M. Slough, Whitney Liddy, Jennifer Brooks, Edwin L. Kaplan, Mijenko Bura, Anatoly F. Romanchishen, Kristina Vabalayte, Gregory W. Randolph

"Only the man who is familiar with the art and science of the past is competent to aid in its progress in the future."

—T. Billroth, 1862[1]

The history of thyroid surgery closely parallels the evolution of modern surgical techniques and the synthesis of our understanding of anatomy, physiology, endocrinology, and pathology. The evolution of thyroid surgical techniques has been convoluted. Even when thyroid and parathyroid disorders were first recognized as discrete entities, they were misunderstood. Initially, Graves' disease was considered to represent a cardiac illness; hypothyroidism, a neurologic and dermatologic disorder; and hyperparathyroidism, a primary bone disorder. One of the first thyroid procedures in the 1600s resulted in the imprisonment of the surgeon.[2] Fortunately, the anatomist and physiologist embraced the initial morbid surgical misadventures, ultimately rendering the applied art of thyroid surgery a safe and even triumphant treatment form. As Halsted has written, "The extirpation of the thyroid gland for goiter typifies perhaps better than any other operation the supreme triumph of the surgeon's art."[3] The surgical story begins with the treatment of iodine deficiency.

THE EARLY YEARS

Goiter has been recognized as a discrete disease entity since the earliest recorded history. The first mention of goiters in China occurs as early as 2700 B.C. Although goiter has been endemic in several parts of the world throughout history, it was not until 500 A.D. that Abdul Kasan Kelebis Abis, in Baghdad, performed the first recorded goiter excision. The patient survived despite massive postoperative bleeding. Other early remedies included the application of toad's blood to the neck and stroking of the thyroid gland with a cadaverous hand.

In Europe, Abu al-Qasim is credited with performing and describing the technique of goiter excision where the patient just avoids exsanguination, as recorded in his surgical tome, *Al-Tasrif*, in 952 A.D. Early developments in thyroid surgery came from the school of Salerno, Italy, in the 12th and 13th centuries (Figure 1.1). The typical operation involved insertion of two heated iron setons at right angles into the offending mass. These were then manipulated at the skin surface twice a day until they pierced the flesh. In cases in which arterial supply of the goiter was thought not to be excessive, the surface of the goiter was cut, the tumorous tissue was grasped with a hook, and the skin was dissected away from it. Once exposed, the section of encapsulated goiter would be removed with a finger. Pedunculated goiters would be ligated en masse with a bootlace and removed.[4] During such procedures, patients were tied down to a table and held firmly. Although these procedures sometimes reduced goiter size, patients often died from sepsis or hemorrhage.[4]

The anatomy of the normal thyroid gland was not generally understood until the Renaissance, with the work of Leonardo da Vinci (Figure 1.2). He drew the thyroid as two globular glands, which he speculated filled up empty spaces in the neck (Figure 1.3).[5] Others pondered the function of the thyroid gland, speculating that its role was to lubricate the neck or make it more aesthetically pleasing. Caleb Hillier Parry of Bath, England, recognizing the thyroid gland's vascularity, considered the gland a blood buffer to protect the brain from sudden increases in blood flow from the heart.[6] In Roman times, increased neck girth was believed to herald the onset of puberty.[7] Bartholomaeus Eustachius of Rome in the 16th century characterized the gland as "glandulam thyroideam" with two lobes connected via an isthmus.[4] The term *thyroid gland* (glandulae thyreoidea) is attributed to Thomas Wharton (described in his work *Adenographia*, 1646), who gave it this name either because of the gland's own shield-like shape (*thyreos*: Greek "shield") or because of the shape of the thyroid cartilage, with which it is closely associated.[8]

In 1646 Wilhelm Fabricius reported the first thyroidectomy performed using scalpels. However, the patient, a 10-year-old girl, died and the surgeon was imprisoned.[2] In 1791 Pierre Joseph Desault performed a successful partial thyroidectomy in Paris.[2] Guillaume Dupuytren followed in Desault's footsteps and in 1808 performed the first "total" thyroidectomy. Unfortunately, despite little intraoperative blood loss, the patient died of "shock."[2] The most successful thyroid surgeon of that time was Johann Hedenus, a German surgeon from Dresden. By 1821 he had reported on the successful removal of six large obstructing goiters. His remarkable series of successes would not be equaled for nearly 40 years.[5] In the 1850s a variety of incisions—longitudinal, oblique, and occasionally Y-shaped—were performed for thyroidectomy. Collar incisions had been introduced by Jules Boeckel of Strasbourg in 1880.[2] After skin incisions, most surgeons at this time performed blunt dissection. Bleeding was generally inadequately controlled. Bloodletting was performed for postoperative complications, despite perioperative blood loss. Typically, wounds were left open and dead spaces were either packed or left to fill with blood.[4]

The progress of early thyroid surgery is intertwined with initial advances in our understanding of thyroid endocrinology. It had been known empirically for some time that seaweed kelp and marsh seawater reduced goiter size. In 1811 Bernard Courtois discovered iodine in burned seaweed.[5] By 1820 Johann Straub and Francois Coindet, both Swiss, systematically studied the use of iodine to treat goiter. Coindet went on to recommend the use of iodine preoperatively to reduce the size and vascularity of goiters and consequently to lessen operative risks.[4] The use of iodine preparations became widespread. Considered miracle drugs, iodine medications were abused, and toxicity often resulted.[9] In the 1830s Robert Graves and Karl von Basedow initially described toxic diffuse goiter through recognition of the "Merseburg

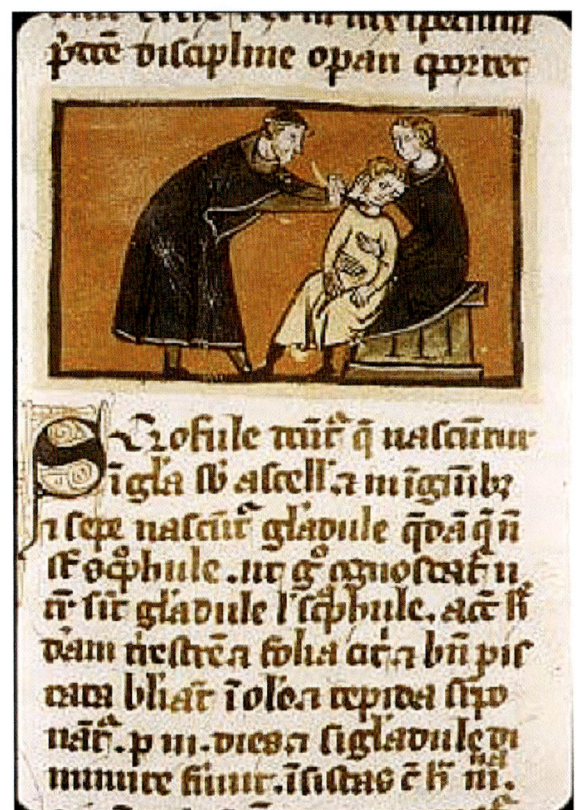

Fig. 1.1 The assistant holds the patient as the surgeon cuts scrofula (goiter) from the patient's neck. Rogerius Salernitanus (Ruggero Frugardo): Chirurgia (1180). (From Ignjatović M: The thyroid gland in works of famous old anatomists and great artists. *Langenbecks Arch Surg.* 2010;395[7]:973–985.)

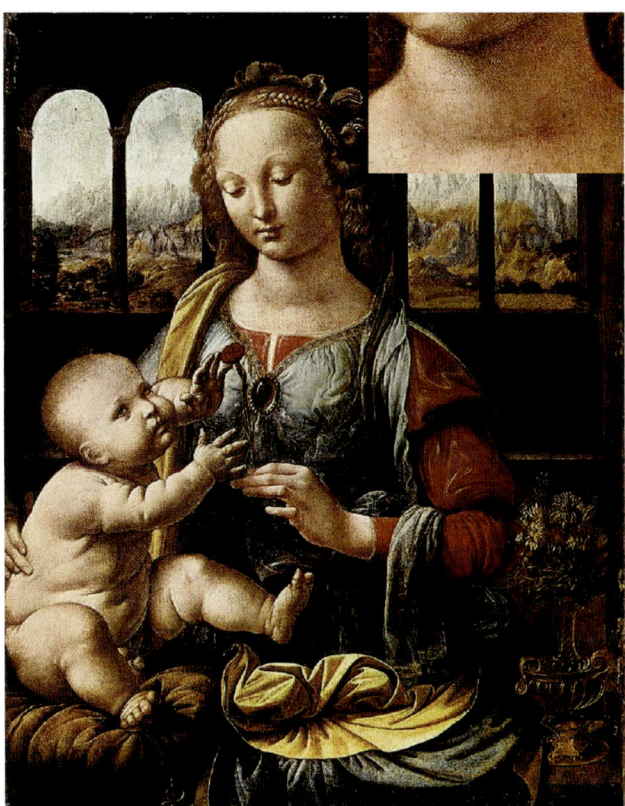

Fig. 1.2 Leonardo da Vinci: "The Madonna of the Carnation" or "Madonna with a Rose" ca. 1478. Madonna with the goiter. (From Ignjatović M: The thyroid gland in works of famous old anatomists and great artists. *Langenbecks Arch Surg.* 2010;395[7]:973–985.)

triad" of goiter, exophthalmos, and palpitations.[10,11] Interestingly, despite being attributed to Graves and Basedow, the association of goiter and orbital disease was initially described in the 11th century by two Persian physicians, Avicenna and Aj-Jurjani.[12]

By the 1850s the mortality rate after thyroid surgery was still high, at approximately 40%. The French Academy of Medicine at this time condemned any operative intervention on the thyroid gland. At about this time Samuel David Gross, a prominent American surgeon, wrote in 1866:

> *Can the thyroid gland, when in a state of enlargement, be removed with a reasonable hope of saving the patient? Experience emphatically answers NO.... If a surgeon should be so foolhardy as to undertake it ... every step of the way will be environed with difficulty, every stroke of his knife will be followed by a torrent of blood, and lucky will it be for him if his victim lives long enough to enable him to finish his horrid butchery. No honest and sensible surgeon would ever engage in it!*[13]

THE SURGICAL REVOLUTION

Landmark developments in surgery and medicine that occurred in the mid-1800s onward helped convert surgery of the thyroid gland from a bloody and condemned procedure to a modern, safe surgical intervention. Foremost among these developments were anesthesia, antisepsis, and surgical hemostatic instrumentation.

The surgical revolution began with the pivotal discovery of anesthesia, as it was subsequently termed by Oliver Wendell Holmes.[14] In 1842 Crawford W. Long, from Georgia, was the first to use sulfuric ether as an anesthetic during surgery.[9] The era of modern surgical anesthesia truly began with William Morton's demonstration of ether's efficacy at Massachusetts General Hospital (MGH) in Boston in 1846.[9]

Thyroid surgery was simultaneously blossoming in other parts of the world. Nikolaiy Ivanovich Pirogov, a Russian surgeon, presented his understanding of the structure, function, and morphology of the thyroid while defending his doctorate at the age of 20 in 1831. Pirogov wrote: "Prior to extirpation, ligation of the superior thyroid artery should be performed and preferably on both sides. Regarding the inferior thyroid artery, due to its deep location under the gland, it has to be ligated after the lower end of the thyroid is lifted..."[1A]

Pirogov, after his experiments with ether anesthesia, performed one of the first thyroid resections under general anesthesia less than a year after the beginning of clinical use of ether by John Warren.[15] The patient was a 17-year-old girl with a goiter causing compression of the trachea. The surgery was complicated by the goiter size, the need of more than 30 ligatures, and postoperative infection. The outcome of the surgery was nevertheless a success. Pirogov continued to perform thyroid surgeries in St. Petersburg and developed the habit of never placing sutures at the wound edges for fear of erysipelas and "purulent pockets."[16]

The introduction of antisepsis by Joseph Lister in 1867 was the second step in the surgical revolution. Lister's concept was quickly adopted in continental Europe but was met with some resistance in Great Britain and the United States.[5] Theodor Kocher and Albert Theodor Billroth, fathers of modern thyroid surgery, adopted Lister's antisepsis concepts in the 1870s. Gustav Neuber introduced the concept of

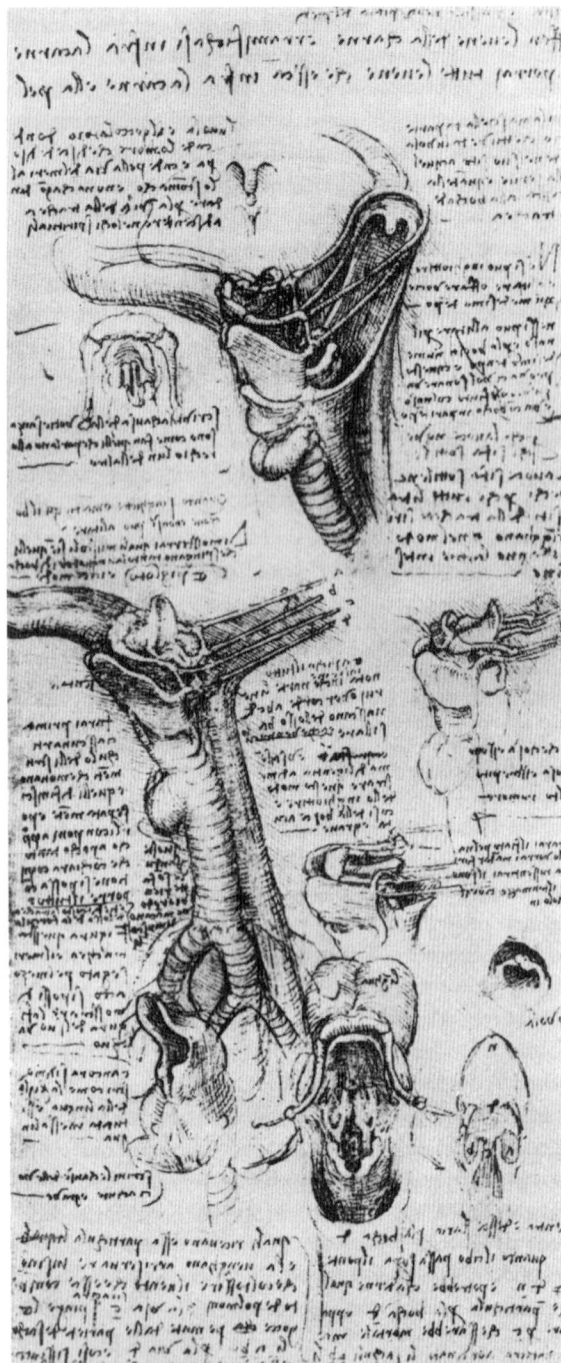

Fig. 1.3 The first illustration of a thyroid is attributed to Leonardo da Vinci in 1503. (From O'Malley CD, de CM Saunders JB: *Leonardo on the Human Body*. New York: Dover Publications; 1983:169.)

intraoperative asepsis in 1883 when he wore a cap and gown into the operating theater. In 1886 Ernst von Bergmann of Berlin introduced steam sterilization of surgical instruments.[17]

The final step in the development of modern surgery was improved hemostasis, made possible because of new surgical instrumentation introduced by Spencer Wells. He devised a simple, self-retaining arterial forceps with a catch in 1872 and reported on its use in 1874.[18] Additional improvements of the forceps, such as reduction in its weight and inclusion of more ratcheted catches, transformed surgical technique by reducing operative bleeding and, ultimately, mortality.

With patient factors controlled by anesthesia and hemostasis improved by enhanced hemostatic forceps, surgeons had more time to attend to the underlying anatomy, allowing for more successful thyroidectomies with safe, nonseptic postoperative courses. Consequently, from 1850 to 1875, mortality from thyroid surgery was reduced by half.[2]

DEVELOPMENT OF MODERN THYROID SURGERY

Albert Theodor Billroth (1829-1894)

Albert Theodor Billroth is generally regarded as the most distinguished surgeon of the 19th century. He was born the son of a German clergyman in 1829 (Figure 1.4). Appointed at the age of 31 to be the Chair of Clinical Surgery at the University of Zurich, he cautiously undertook the surgical treatment of obstructive goiters endemic to this area. During his first 6 years in Zurich, he performed 20 thyroidectomies. He courageously published the results, noting a mortality rate of approximately 40%. Mortality was primarily due to postoperative sepsis and intraoperative hemorrhage. Billroth considered this mortality rate disastrous, and he virtually abandoned the procedure for almost a decade.[13] He regained confidence in performing thyroid surgery in 1877 after the advent of antisepsis (which he was initially slow to embrace) and improved instrumentation. At that time, the mortality rate of his procedure fell to 8%. Billroth's procedure typically involved division of the sternocleidomastoid muscle and incision and drainage of any thyroid cysts. Hemostasis was achieved through arterial ligation

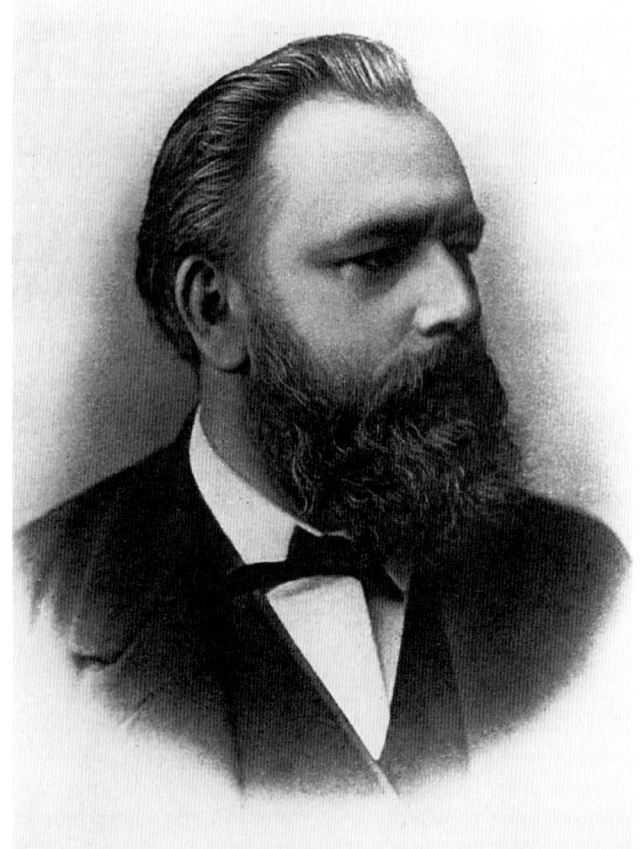

Fig. 1.4 Albert Theodor Billroth, 1867. (Reproduced with permission from Institut für Medizingeschichte, Universität Bern, Buehlstrasse 26, CH 3012 Bern.)

and the use of aneurysmal needles and an Indian vegetable styptic, punghawar djambi.

Billroth's accomplishments were impressive. By the time he accepted the chair at Vienna in 1867, he had already published his textbook, *General Surgical Pathology and Therapeutics*, and had founded the Archives of Clinical Surgery. He became the most experienced thyroid surgeon in the world at that time. He was also a renowned teacher and was influential in establishing a school of surgery. Many notable surgeons studied under him, including Jan Mikulicz, Anton von Eiselsberg, and Anton Wölfler. Coincidentally, in 1880 Billroth was asked to examine Nikolai I. Pirogov, a forefather of Russian thyroid surgery. Billroth diagnosed an inoperable maxillary cancer in the 70-year-old Pirogov. Billroth's other notable contributions to head and neck surgery included performing the first successful laryngectomy in 1873 and the first esophagectomy in 1881.

Theodor Kocher (1841-1917)

It is, however, Theodor Kocher who stands alone in the annals of thyroid surgery. The work of Kocher (Figure 1.5) was instrumental in the development of modern thyroidectomy. After graduation in 1865 from the University of Bern, Kocher spent a year visiting and studying at foreign clinics. He visited Glasgow, where he witnessed Lister's revolutionary antisepsis work; Paris, where he met Louis Pasteur and Auguste Verneuil; and Zurich, where he met with Billroth. He became well versed in current developments in surgery, and in 1872 at the age of 31, he was appointed surgical chair at the University of Bern. Halsted observed that "a greater advance was made in the operative treatment of goiter in the decade from 1873 to 1883 than any in the forgone years, and I may say in all the years that have followed ... during which period the art of operating for goiter by Billroth and Kocher and men of their school had been almost perfected, relatively minor problems remain to be solved."[2]

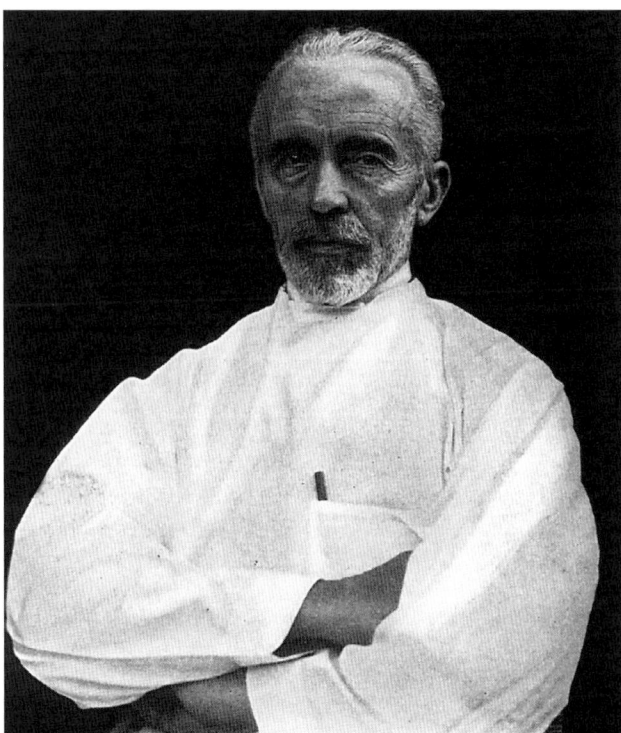

Fig. 1.5 Theodor Kocher, 1912. (Reproduced with permission from Institut für Medizingeschichte, Universität Bern, Buehlstrasse 26, CH 3012 Bern.)

At the time of Kocher's appointment to Bern, goiters were endemic in Switzerland. Kocher noted that up to 90% of schoolchildren in Bern were afflicted with goiter.[19] He quickly acquired remarkable experience in thyroid surgery and eventually performed more than 5000 thyroidectomies over the course of his career. He was a meticulous surgeon who paid careful attention to hemostasis. He introduced initial ligation of the inferior thyroid arteries, which substantially reduced the risk of hemorrhage. His advocacy of the use of antisepsis and hemostasis, evident in his textbook of surgery, was manifest in his mortality rates. He reported a reduction in mortality from 12.6% in the 1870s to 0.2% in 1898.[20] During Kocher's tenure, Bern became the world capital of goiter surgery (Figure 1.6). Kocher's surgical technique differed from Billroth's in that Kocher preserved the strap muscles and usually used a collar incision, whereas Billroth typically used an oblique and more restrictive incision.[13] Kocher also paid close attention to the available anesthesia methods. One of Kocher's few mortalities was secondary to chloroform anesthesia. From that point onward, he used only local anesthesia with cocaine.[8]

In 1867 Kocher learned that one of his early patients, 10-year-old Marie Bischel, had developed slowness of affect, stunted growth, mental retardation, thickened fingers, and other manifestations of cretinism after bilateral thyroidectomy. He called this unknown condition *cachexia strumipriva*.

In 1882 when Kocher became familiar with the work of Jacques-Louis Reverdin of Geneva, who described similar symptoms of myxedema after total thyroidectomy, he began a concerted effort to recall all his goiter patients.[21] Of the 18 thyroidectomy patients Kocher was able to review, 16 displayed varying degrees of myxedema. Kocher was so appalled at the outcome epitomized by Marie Bischel (Figure 1.7) that he resolved to never again perform a total thyroidectomy for benign disease. This observation served as the first evidence of the thyroid's physiologic role in growth and development.

In 1883 Kocher presented to the Fifth German Surgical Congress his historic paper in which he described the adverse effects of total thyroidectomy (termed *cachexia strumipriva*) and evidence that the thyroid gland in fact had a function.[22] About this time, Felix Semon, a Prussian otolaryngologist, in a meeting of the Clinical Society of London, also suggested similarities between English myxedematous patients and patients who had undergone total thyroidectomy.[23,24]

An interesting comparative observation between Billroth's and Kocher's surgical technique was made by William Halsted (Figure 1.8; see also Figure 1.6) who, as a student, visited the clinics of both surgeons.[2] Halsted noted that most of Kocher's thyroidectomy patients developed myxedema postoperatively but rarely tetany. The reverse was true of Billroth's patients. Halsted proposed that the origin of this phenomenon lay in Kocher's and Billroth's different surgical techniques. Whereas Kocher was known for his bloodless operative field, attention to detail, and removal of most of the thyroid with the preservation of surrounding structures, Billroth was known for a more rapid approach, resulting in parathyroid injury and larger retained segments of thyroid. Kocher was a versatile and astute surgeon whose accomplishments extended beyond that of endocrine surgery. Kocher's achievements included the development of a method of shoulder dislocation reduction, use of the right subcostal incision in cholecystectomy, work with gunshot wounds and osteomyelitis, localization of spinal cord lesions, and development of the surgical mobilization maneuver of the duodenum that bears his name.[13] In 1908 Kocher was awarded the Nobel Prize for his work on the physiology, pathology, and surgery of the thyroid gland, and he has been called "the father of modern thyroid surgery."[3]

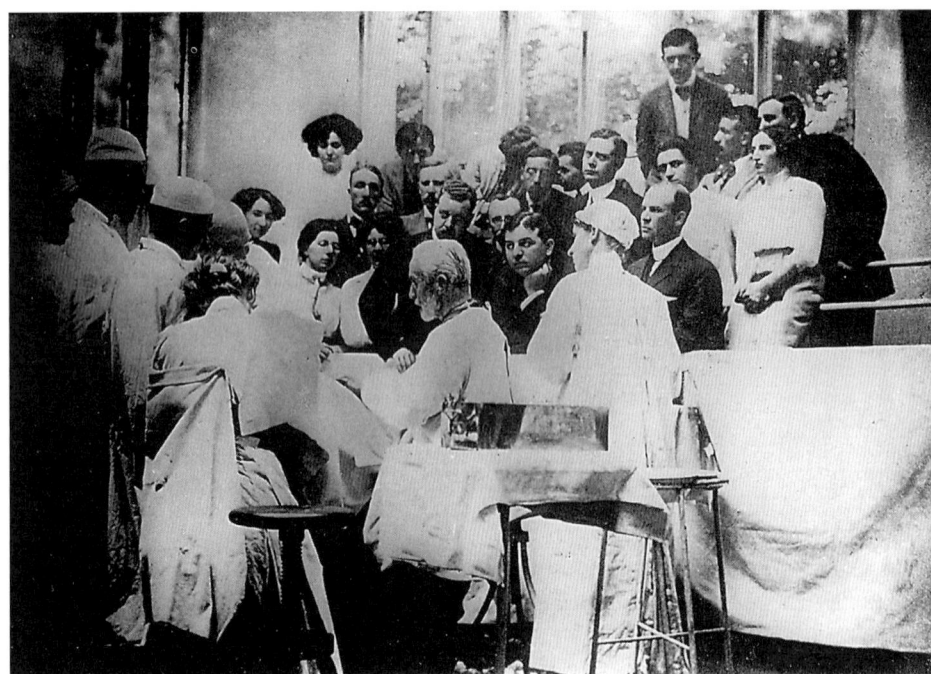

Fig. 1.6 Kocher in the operative theater. This unique photograph of Kocher also shows his student, William Halsted, present in the audience (fourth from the left at the head of the table facing Kocher). (Reproduced with permission from Institut für Medizingeschichte, Universität Bern, Buehlstrasse 26, CH 3012 Bern.)

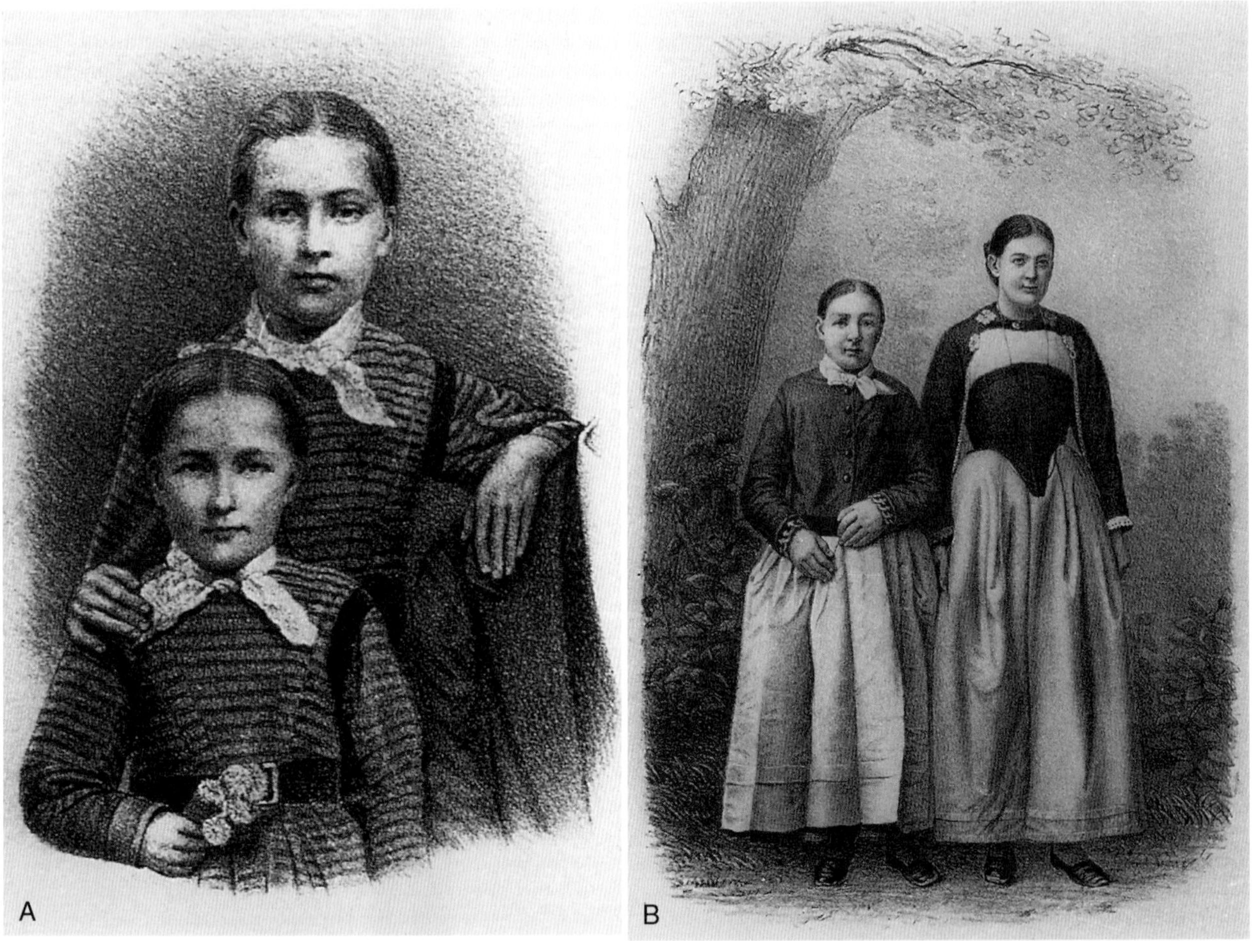

Fig. 1.7 A, Marie Bichsel *(right)* as an 11-year-old in 1873 with her younger sister. **B,** Marie Bichsel *(left)* as a 20-year-old with her younger sister. (Reproduced with permission from Institut für Medizingeschichte, Universität Bern, Buehlstrasse 26, CH 3012 Bern.)

CHAPTER 1 History of Thyroid and Parathyroid Surgery

Beyond Kocher and Billroth

William Halsted (1852-1922; see Figure 1.8), a student and close acquaintance of Kocher, brought Kocher's surgical philosophy to the American surgical arena. After his graduation from Yale in 1879, Halsted studied for 2 years in well-known German and Austrian clinics, where he was influenced by the work of both Billroth and Kocher. On returning from Europe, Halsted was shocked at the state of thyroid surgery in the United States. In fact, little thyroid surgery was done at all in the United States at that time. In 1881 in New York, Halsted assisted Henry Sands at Roosevelt Hospital with the resection of a right thyroid mass. The patient sat awake in a dental chair with a rubber bag tied around his neck to catch the blood. The two hemostats available at the hospital at that time were both used.[3] Halsted was quick to use the knowledge of antisepsis and modern hemostatic forceps in the United States.[4] In 1881 he wrote that the confidence "acquired from masterfulness in controlling hemorrhage gives to the surgeon the calm which is so needed for clear thinking and orderly procedure at the operative table."[2] His early work, however, was not without peril. While experimenting with local infiltration anesthetic agents, Halsted became addicted to cocaine.[25] His work "The Operative Story of Goiter," published in 1920, describes advances made in thyroid surgery from the earliest days to the revolutionary work of Billroth and Kocher, whose techniques he held in great esteem.

Halsted helped found the auspicious Johns Hopkins Hospital, where he was named the first Johns Hopkins professor of surgery. There he introduced residency training and trained many surgeons, including Harvey Cushing, Walter Dandy, Walter Reed, and a number of respected thyroid surgeons, including Charles Horace, Frank Lahey, and George Crile.[25] Crile's contributions extended to early studies of shock and the surgical treatment of hyperthyroidism. Roswell Park used a pneumatic antishock suit, devised by Crile, to help prevent shock in hyperthyroid patients undergoing thyroid operations (Figure 1.9).

Charles Mayo adopted Kocher's technique of partial thyroidectomy for patients with Graves' disease. In 1913 his medical counterpart, Henry Plummer, established the value of iodine use preoperatively in Graves' disease. Adoption of these practices at Mayo Clinic resulted

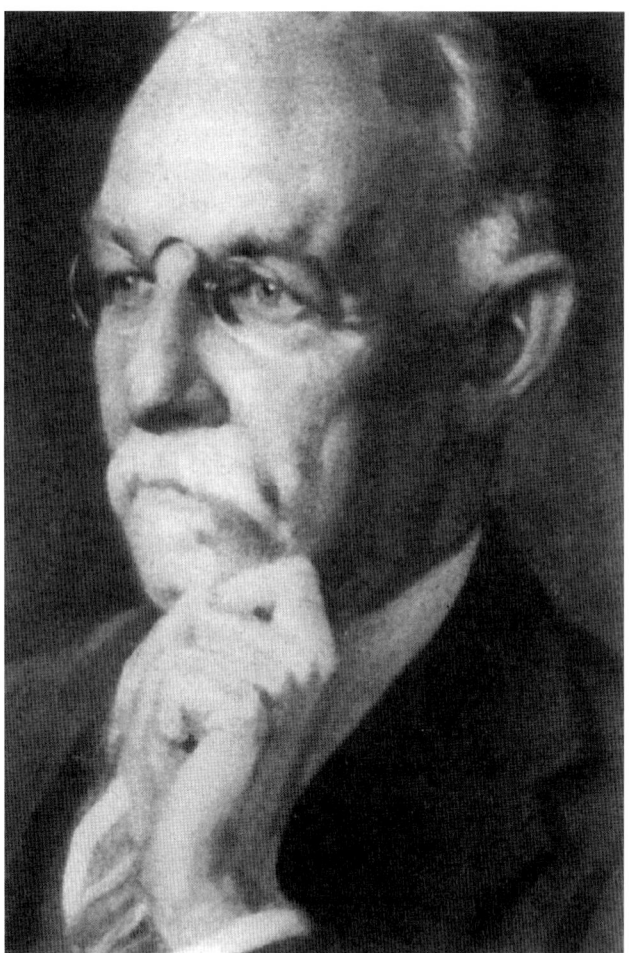

Fig. 1.8 William S. Halsted. (From Organ CH Jr. The history of parathyroid surgery, 1850-1996: the Excelsior Surgical Society 1998 Edward D Churchill Lecture. *J Am Coll Surg.* 2000;191[3]:284–299, Fig. 11. Used with permission.)

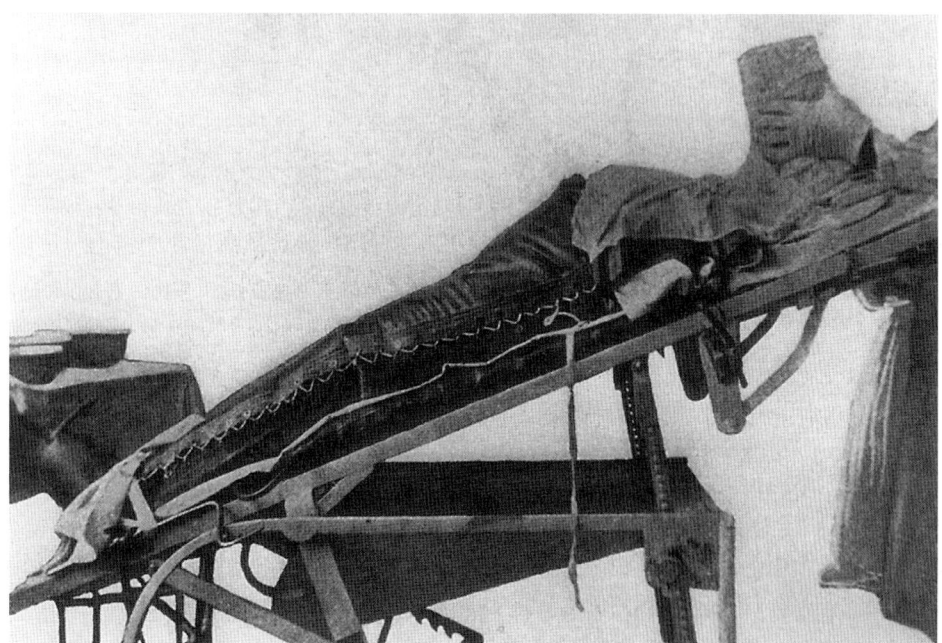

Fig. 1.9 Crile's pneumatic suit used to prevent shock in thyroid operations. (From Park R. *Principles and Practice of Modern Surgery,* Philadelphia: Lea and Brothers; 1907. Used with permission.)

in a drop in the mortality rate in surgery for Graves' disease from 3% to 4% to under 1%.[3]

Thomas Peel Dunhill adopted the technique of total lobectomy on one side and subtotal resection on the other for toxic patients. He practiced total lobectomy by a pericapsular dissection technique. Dunhill also described the operative method of retrosternal goiter resection through a sternotomy.[8]

Jan Mikulicz was one of the first to demonstrate the feasibility and value of partial thyroid resection; he also showed that thyroid parenchyma can be crushed, divided, and ligated without fear of uncontrollable hemorrhage or impairment of wound healing, thereby forming the basis of modern unilateral and bilateral subtotal lobectomy.[3]

Once the major obstacles of hemorrhage and infection had been addressed, thyroid surgeons recognized and investigated the peculiar entity of postthyroidectomy tetany. Billroth's pupils Anton Wölfler and Jan Mikulicz Radecki were the first to seek a solution to this problem. Wölfler, while employed as Billroth's first assistant, first described postoperative tetany in 1879.[26] Eiselsberg later succeeded Wölfler as first assistant and continued the work on postoperative tetany in Billroth's clinic. In 1886 Wölfler, who was then the chair of surgery of Graz, described tetany in further detail. However, it was Radecki a few years earlier in 1882 who devised a new approach to thyroidectomy to prevent tetany by preserving the posterior aspects of both the lobes.[2A]

The etiology of postoperative tetany, however, was unknown until 1891 when Eugéne Gley reported that the cause could be attributed to removal of the parathyroid glands or to interference with their blood supply.[3] It was not until the 1920s that low calcium was recognized as the clear physiologic cause of tetany.

It is also noteworthy to mention Harold Foss, who adopted the use of motion pictures to teach surgical techniques. A film he produced of a thyroid operation in 1935, in color, was shown at a national meeting.[27]

Our understanding of the surgical treatment of thyroid cancer has evolved over time as well. Ironically, both ends of the treatment spectrum have been the "standard of care" at one time or another, characterized by either insufficient treatment or excessive treatment. For instance, metastatic papillary carcinoma of the thyroid initially was regarded as an embryologic migration error and termed *lateral aberrant thyroid*. It was believed that such patients did not require thyroid surgery. However, when the high rate of cervical lymph node metastasis in papillary carcinoma was ultimately appreciated, the response was to perform a radical neck dissection.[28] With time, enthusiasm for more appropriately conservative neck treatment prevailed.

Further Advances in Endocrine Surgery

Further advances in miniaturization and endoscopy have allowed thyroid surgeons to push the envelope of what is possible. Minimally invasive surgical techniques have been introduced into the field of thyroid surgery, including video-assisted techniques, endoscopic techniques, and robotic techniques.

One of the first surgeons to attempt an endoscopic approach for endocrine surgery in the neck was Michel Gagner from the Cleveland Clinic Foundation, who in 1995 performed a three-and-a-half-gland parathyroidectomy for primary hyperparathyroidism. Using four 5-mm trocars through 1-cm incisions above the clavicle and sternal notch, carbon dioxide was insufflated to 15 mm Hg to create a space above the strap muscles. Employing a 5-mm endoscopic scissor and dissector and a 5-mm 30-degree endoscope, the anterior and lateral borders of the trachea and thyroid were dissected. Three and one-half parathyroid glands were removed, and their blood supply was ligated with 5-mm titanium clips. The procedure took 5 hours, and the patient had tachycardia and hypercarbia necessitating hyperventilation. Subcutaneous emphysema was present from the eyelids to the scrotum, resolving on day 3 after surgery. He ultimately did well after the operation, discharging from the hospital on post of day 4 with a serum calcium level decreasing to normal.[3A,4A] Gagner and his group were able to show that this approach was feasible, cosmetically appealing, and provided another surgical approach for patients with primary hyperparathyroidism.

Several other surgeons around the world expanded on these techniques, with some continuing to use carbon dioxide insufflation, others developing endoscopic gasless techniques, and still others developing open, lateral, radio-guided, and video-assisted minimally invasive approaches.[5A-10A] These approaches were primarily directed at the management of hyperparathyroidism. These techniques were additionally aided by the development of rapid intraoperative parathyroid assays, which allowed confirmation of the success of targeted parathyroidectomy.

Soon thereafter the focus shifted from using these techniques solely for parathyroidectomy to exploring the feasibility of these endoscopic techniques in thyroid surgery. Hüscher et al. were the first to describe the endoscopic approach to thyroid lobectomy and used a lateral approach with carbon dioxide insufflation for a benign 4-mm adenoma.[11A] Hüscher's work demonstrated the feasibility of endoscopic thyroid lobectomy. This work was quickly followed by several others employing various techniques to remove the thyroid endoscopically or via video-assistance.[12A-15A] The endoscopic technique and minimally invasive technique also led the way for endocrine surgery via the anterior chest, axilla, breast, and most recently, the oral cavity.[16A-19A]

These various approaches were initially limited to smaller, benign lesions of the thyroid. Miccoli and colleagues expanded their technique to include thyroid lobectomy for carcinomas.[20A] Subsequent work by the same group and others demonstrated the use of a minimally invasive, video-assisted approach to perform a total thyroidectomy that was equivalent to a conventional approach.[20A, 21A] This technique, although initially confined to low-risk carcinomas, was successfully used in patients with intermediate-risk lesions as well.[22A] Rocco Bellantone soon thereafter established the feasibility and safety of a central neck dissection via a minimally invasive approach.[23A]

LARYNGEAL NERVES

The history of the recurrent laryngeal nerve (RLN) and its relationship to the voice is a fascinating story, beginning in in antiquity. The earliest reference to the voice and structures in the neck that we have discovered is found in the *Sushruta Samhita* written in India in the sixth century B.C. An injury in the neck near the angle of the jaw was considered critical and caused hoarseness and a change in taste. This was thought to be due to damage to the vessels of the neck.[29] By the first century A.D., Rufus the Ephesian wrote that it was nerves and not vessels that were responsible for the faculty of voice.[30] About the same time, Leonides recognized the importance of avoiding injury to the "vocal" nerves during operations of the head and neck. He warned that if the nerves were cut, the voice would be lost.[4]

However, it was Galen who first described the RLNs in detail during the second century. Although Greek philosophy and medicine held the heart to be most important—the seat of intellect and learning—Galen recognized the importance of the brain. He was delighted when he found a nerve from the brain on each side of the neck that went down toward the heart and then reversed course and ascended to the larynx. Nerves were thought to contract similarly to tendons and muscles. To contract the laryngeal muscles, the pull had to be from below, he thought, and here was just such a nerve that came from the brain. He called these two nerves the *recurrent nerves* (or reversivi).[31]

He took great pride in this wonderful finding and said that he was the first to discover these nerves. He felt that the recurrent nerves gained great mechanical advantage by a pulley action, similar to a glossocomion, which was a popular device of that day for reducing fractures. He dissected these nerves in many animals—even swans, cranes, and ostriches because of their long necks—and marveled at the mechanical advantage of the pulley system that was able to open and close the muscles of the larynx.

Galen recognized in studies on the living pig that "if one compresses the nerve with the fingers or a ligature" or if one cuts the nerve, the pig stopped squealing and the muscles of the larynx on that side ceased to work.[32]

He gathered the elders of Rome and, to impress them with his greatness and knowledge, operated on the neck of a live, squealing pig. When he cut the RLN, the pig stopped squealing. This was thought to be wondrous. His dissection on the living pig is depicted in a beautiful medieval illustration (Figure 1.10).

Galen described two children who were operated on by surgeons ignorant of anatomy. One surgeon tore out swollen lymph nodes from the neck with his nails and apparently removed the surrounding nerves at the same time. The slave was rendered mute.

Similarly, another surgeon, while performing an operation on another child rendered him "half mute," evidently having damaged only one of the nerves. "Everybody found it strange that the voice was damaged, although the larynx and trachea remained intact. But when I demonstrated to them the phonetic nerve [i.e., the recurrent nerve], their astonishment abated."[33]

Because of Galen's fame over the ages and the spread of his teachings, the RLN was discussed by many surgeons and anatomists thereafter. Aetius, in the sixth century, wrote that "In the case of the throat glands, the vocal nerves must be carefully avoided ... (otherwise) the patient is bereft of his voice."[34] Paulus Aeginetus, in the seventh century, again stressed that when operating in the neck, "avoiding in particular the carotid arteries and recurrent nerves" must be exercised.[35]

Arabic medical literature of the ninth to 12th centuries also contains references to the RLN. Abul Kasim (Albucassis, 1000 A.D.) is credited by some with the first recorded description of a thyroidectomy. He echoed the same warnings as Aeginetus with regard to the RLN: "Be most careful not to cut a blood-vessel or nerve."[36] He also describes a slave girl who stabbed herself in the neck. The artery and vein had not been cut, but she developed hoarseness.

In the Middle Ages, the same experiments on the RLNs in pigs that were done by Galen were repeated in the Salernitan demonstrations. During the Renaissance, in 1503, Leonardo da Vinci drew what may be the first anatomic representation of the RLN, possibly in an ape. The first drawing of the thyroid gland is attributed to da Vinci as well (see Figure 1.3).

Vesalius, in 1543, was particularly interested in the RLN because, as he wrote, "nothing is more delightful to contemplate than this great miracle of nature." His drawing of Cupid operating on the neck of the pig is reminiscent of Galen's former operations. He also produced excellent anatomic drawings of the RLNs.

Other anatomists in the 16th and 17th centuries produced excellent dissections of the RLNs and the muscles of the larynx (Figure 1.11). Hence, by the 17th or 18th century, a great deal was known not only about the anatomy of the RLNs, but also about the complications when one or both of them were cut or damaged and ways to avoid these problems. Thus in 1724, Fulvio Gherli could write:

Although there are other complications more terrible and frightening, the cutting of the recurrent nerves is dangerous in the highest degree (for when) this unfortunately occurs, either the patient

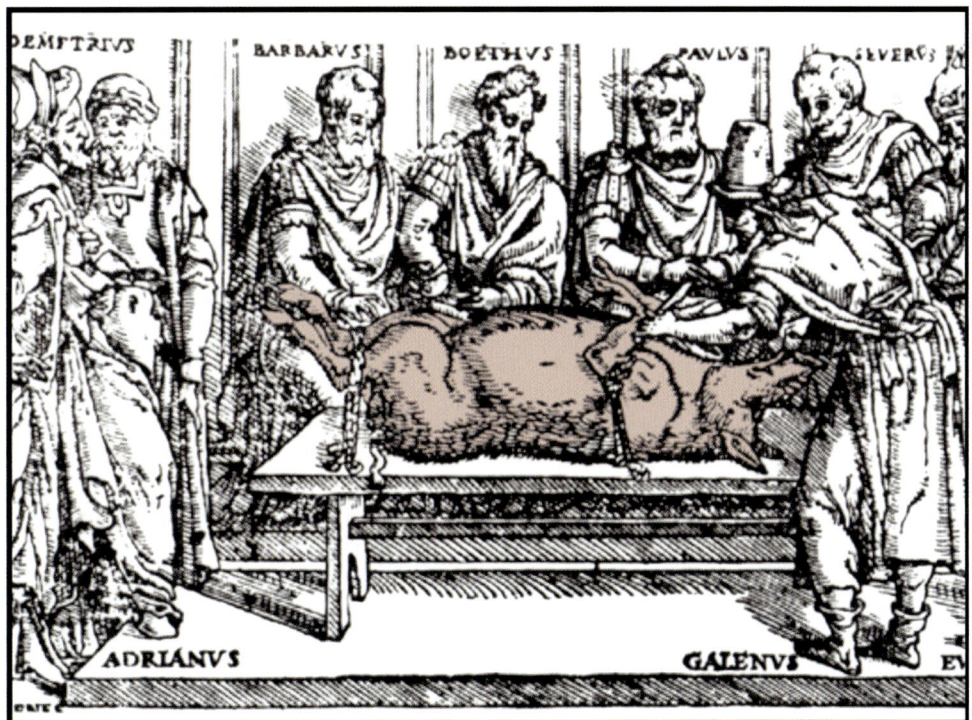

Fig. 1.10 Galen demonstrating the recurrent laryngeal nerve in the living pig to the elders of Rome. When the nerve was divided, the pig's squealing ceased and it became mute. (From Galeni Librorum Quinta Classis EAM Medicinae Partem, edited by Fabius Paulinus. Published by Guinta Family of Venice, 1625. IM Rutkow. *Surgery: An Illustrated History*. St. Louis: Mosby; 1993:40.)

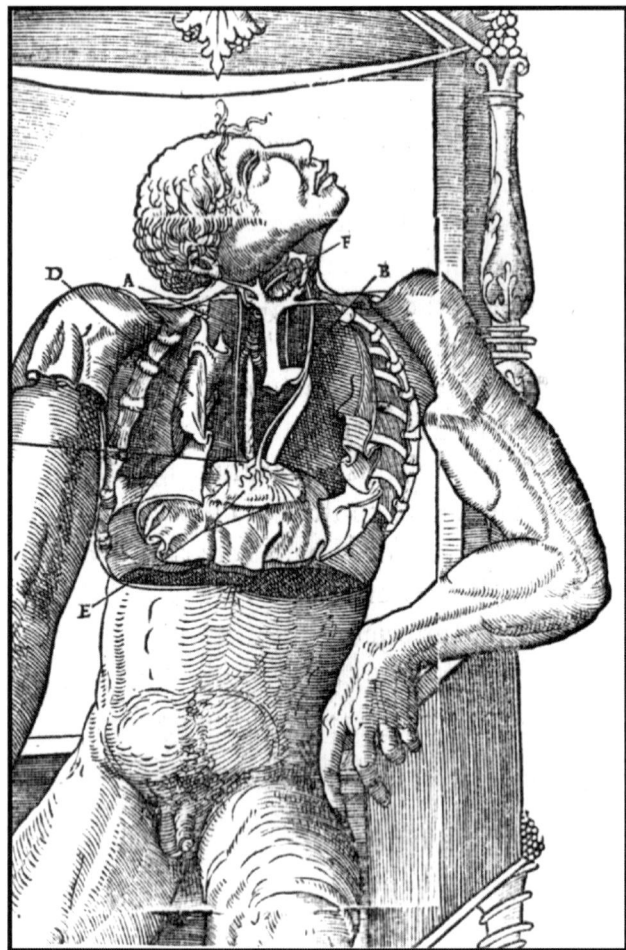

Fig. 1.11 Taken from the beautiful anatomic dissection of Charles Estienne, 1546. The recurrent laryngeal nerves are shown. (From Estienne C: *La dissection des parties du corps humain divisee en trios livres*. Paris: Simon Colinaeus; 1545. From the Special Collections Research Center, University of Chicago Library.)

dies of it miserably or at least loses for the rest of his life the most beautiful prerogative given to man by God, which is (la favella) speech; but this danger can easily be avoided by that Surgeon who, with the provision of Anatomy, knows the site of these nerves.[37]

Although the 19th century brought great advances in surgery in general and in operations on the thyroid, eminent surgeons continued to have problems not only with bleeding, infection, and tetany (which some thought was due to hysteria), but also with recurrent nerve injuries. Karl von Klein of Stuttgart, for example, reported the loss of voice during removal of a goiter in 1820.[38]

Billroth's group, reported by Wölfler, his chief assistant in 1882, had a 40% mortality rate for thyroidectomy for goiter while he was in Zurich before 1867 and an 8.3% mortality rate for goiter during the antiseptic period, from 1877 to 1881.[39] Five out of 48 patients (10.5%) required a tracheostomy. Unilateral nerve injuries were reported in 25% (11/44) and bilateral nerve injuries in 4.5% (2/44) of the latter group.

Jankowsky reported a 14% incidence (87/620 patients) of recurrent nerve injuries for goiter operations before 1885.[40] Undoubtedly, the number was far greater because laryngeal examinations were not routine.

It was Theodor Kocher of Bern who brought his operative mortality of thyroidectomy from 14.8% in 1882 to an eventual level of less than 0.18% in 1898.[41] His meticulous technique resulted in an incidence of recurrent nerve injury similar to that of surgeons today.

Billroth, Kocher, and others appreciated the need to avoid injury to the RLN during thyroid surgery. At that time, the common practice for preserving the nerve was to identify the inferior thyroid artery, isolate it, and ligate it laterally away from the nerve in a bloodless field. In 1882 Mikulicz recommended leaving a posterior portion of the thyroid capsule to cover the distal course of the nerve and therefore preserve it.[21] Kocher also preferred to leave a small posterior remnant of the thyroid to avoid damage. Once he perfected this technique, hoarseness became the exception after his operations.[38]

Credit for the advent of the ability to visualize and properly diagnose an RLN injury goes to the Spanish singer Manuel Garcia who introduced the mirror examination of the larynx in 1854. In September of that year during a visit to Paris, he visited a famous instrument-maker in search of a thin mirror with a long shaft that could be used to inspect the throat. After the instrument-maker gave him a small dental mirror, to place in the back of his mouth, he used an additional small pocket mirror to cast in light and saw his larynx wide open before him.[24A]

In the early 1900s a debate over the proper operative approach for thyroidectomy ensued. Professor Vasiliy I. Razumovsky from Saratov published a monograph in 1903 that advocated leaving residual thyroid tissue intact to prevent damage to the recurrent nerves and a bilateral palsy of the vocal cords. He also recommended visualization of the larynx in all patients before the surgery to determine the possibility of damage to the RLN preoperatively. In his text, Razumovsky also described "a puncture and removal of goiter fragments for diagnostic purposes," representing some of the earliest techniques to biopsy the thyroid, now a standard practice.[25A] In 1904 a fellow Russian, Alexandr A. Bobrov, described the technique of recurrent nerve visualization during thyroidectomy in 106 operations.[42] August Bier of Berlin (1911) preferred to expose the RLNs routinely, but most surgeons opposed this method.[43] George Crile, the founder of the Cleveland Clinic, wrote in 1932 that "The greatest tragedies that follow thyroidectomies pertain to these nerves, not because of their anatomy but because of their specific vulnerability to trauma.[44]

As compared with peripheral nerves, the recurrent nerves are exceedingly soft ... and the slightest direct or even indirect pressure on the recurrent nerve interferes with nerve conduction. ... And it is this extreme vulnerability that is the first and the most important factor in the production of abductor paralysis. ... if the nerve trunk is directly exposed in the course of the operation, the exposed nerve will be covered with scar formation. Scar tissue is capable of producing a block in the action current, hence, causing a physiologic severance of the nerve.[44]

Crile recommended leaving the posterior capsule of the thyroid in each thyroid resection. He called the area near the nerve *no man's land*. "It is not to be palpated; it is subjected to the least possible traction and no division of tissue is made. By these precautions temporary and permanent injury of the recurrent laryngeal nerve may be completely eliminated."

Prioleau wrote in 1933, "a nerve if seen is injured."[45] This philosophy of purposely not seeing the recurrent nerves, which influenced an entire generation of surgeons, still exists today in the minds of some inexperienced surgeons.

In 1938 Lahey reported on more than 3000 thyroidectomies performed by his fellows and staff during a 3-year period.[46] The RLN was dissected in virtually every case. Careful dissection would "not increase but definitely decrease the number of injuries to the recurrent laryngeal nerves," he wrote. Lahey's work with its emphasis on anatomy set the course and direction for modern thyroid surgery.

Later, in 1970, Riddell wrote that when the nerve is identified and carefully followed throughout its course, a nerve injury may occur, but the paralysis is nearly always transient. When the nerve is not identified, however, permanent paralysis of the vocal cord occurs in at least a third of cases.[46]

Finally, to paraphrase Professor William Halsted, thyroidectomy may be the supreme triumph of the surgeons' art.[2] However, to perform it safely, the greatest care must be exercised to preserve the integrity of the RLN. It is clear that our knowledge of the anatomy and physiology of this nerve began close to 2000 years ago.

Despite work on the avoidance of RLN injury, little attention was paid to the surgical importance of the external branch of the superior laryngeal nerve (SLN). Kocher did not even mention the external branch of the SLN in his book, which for many years was considered the cornerstone of thyroid surgery. It was not until 1935, after world-famous operatic soprano Amelita Galli-Curci underwent goiter surgery, with resultant loss of her upper vocal registry, that the SLN came into the limelight. The media at the time wrote, "the surprising voice is gone forever. The sad specter of a ghost replaces the velvety softness."[47]

The objective to protect the RLN continued to evolve as technology evolved. Knut Flisberg and T. Lindholm were the first to describe the use of electrical stimulation of the RLN during thyroid surgery.[26A] Several other authors expanded on this work and proposed several varying methods of stimulating the nerve and intraoperatively observing the resulting action potential of this stimulation to help protect the nerve during thyroidectomy. These methods included direct palpation, direct and indirect needle electrode placement, direct visualization and via endolaryngeal/endotracheal electrodes.[27A-30A] Work by Torkil Hvidegaard first described the use of endotracheally attached electrodes in 1984.[31A] In 1998 Alberto Echeverri and Phillip Flexon published one of the first large series describing their experience with 70 patients undergoing thyroidectomy and the pair's use of electrophysiologic nerve stimulation for identification of the RLN during that procedure.[32A] However, it was work by Brennan et al. that brought intraoperative nerve monitoring to the forefront of thyroid surgery through a prospective analysis of the efficacy of continuous intraoperative nerve monitoring during thyroid and parathyroid surgery.[33A] Intraoperative nerve monitoring has continued to evolve with new systems for continuous nerve monitoring of not only the RLN but also the vagus nerve during thyroid surgery.[34A-36A] Extensive work by Randolph et al. revealed that intraoperative nerve monitoring of the RLN during thyroid and other neck surgeries can aid in nerve mapping, nerve identification, and prognostication of postoperative vocal cord function, as well as influence the surgeon's decision to proceed with bilateral surgery.[37A] Consolidation of this work has led to several consensus statements and guidelines concerning the use of intraoperative nerve monitoring during neck endocrine surgery, which is now widely adopted.[38A,39A]

PARATHYROID GLANDS

Parathyroid Anatomy and Physiology

The parathyroid glands were first identified in 1850 in an Indian rhinoceros in a London zoo by Richard Owen, then professor of anatomy at the Hunterian Museum of the Royal College of England.[26] His work, published in 1862, went unnoticed for several years.

Credit for recognition and identification of the parathyroid glands in humans went to Ivar Sandström (Figure 1.12), a medical student at Uppsala University in Sweden. In 1887 Sandström came across the parathyroid glands while dissecting the neck of a dog; he subsequently identified these glands in cats, rabbits, oxen, and horses. Later, Sandström dissected 50 human cadavers, illustrating the anatomic

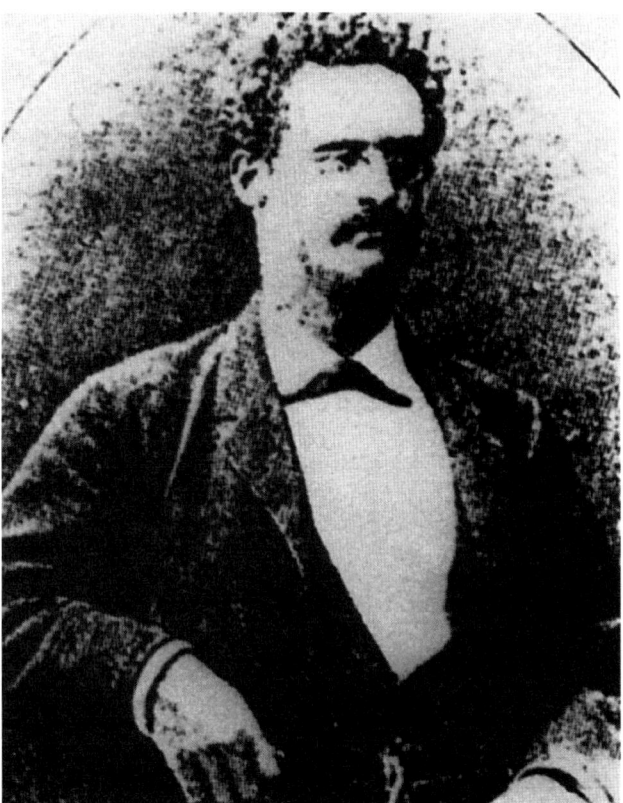

Fig. 1.12 Ivar V. Sandström, Upsaala, Sweden. (From Organ CH Jr. The history of parathyroid surgery, 1850-1996: the Excelsior Surgical Society 1998 Edward D Churchill Lecture. *J Am Coll Surg.* 2000;191[3]: 284–299, Fig. 4. Used with permission.)

position, blood supply, and variability of the location of the parathyroid glands. This work led to his monograph, *On a New Gland in Man and Fellow Animals*.[26] Sandström was also the first to suggest that these glands be named "glandulae parathyreoidae." His manuscripts, initially rejected by a German journal as too long, were finally published in a Swedish medical journal.[26] In 1890, Gley, a French pathologist, came across Sandström's work in two abstracts published in a German yearbook. Unfortunately, Sandström committed suicide before his fundamental work had been rediscovered by Gley. Although the parathyroid glands were observed independently by Cresswell Baber in 1881 in England, it was not until Gley's work in the 1890s that the parathyroid glands and their function became widely appreciated.[4] Wölfler observed tetany in Billroth's patients after total thyroidectomy but attributed this development to hyperemia of the brain.[26] Gley observed that animals whose parathyroid glands were removed subsequently developed tetany.[48] Two Italians, Giulio Vassale and Francesco Generali, later duplicated this work, confirming that tetany followed parathyroidectomy.[4] As a result of these observations, surgeons understood that it was vital to treat the parathyroid glands with great care during thyroidectomy.

In 1905 William George McCallum found that he could relieve tetany that followed parathyroidectomy by injecting animals with parathyroid extract.[49] Subsequently, McCallum and Carl Voegtlin of Baltimore, in 1909, helped elucidate the connection between the parathyroid gland and calcium regulation. They found that tetany after parathyroidectomy was accompanied by calcium deficiency in tissues and that this condition could be relieved by injections of crude parathyroid extract or of calcium. They further were able to identify the cause of tetany as hypocalcemia resulting from insufficient parathyroid secretion.[50] In 1907 Halsted also reported the use of parathyroid extracts to treat tetany after thyroidectomy.[26] Halsted and a Johns Hopkins medical student, Herbert Evans, together detailed human parathyroid blood supply.[51]

Frederick von Recklinghausen, then professor of pathology at Strasbourg, presented seven patients with bone disease in a book written in honor of Rudolf Virchow in 1891. However, only in 1906 was the connection between parathyroid glands and bone disease established by the work of Jakob Erdheim in Vienna. When he cauterized the parathyroid gland in rats, he noted that not only did tetany become manifest but also defective calcification in their teeth occurred.[4] He went on to examine the parathyroid glands of patients who had died of skeletal disease and in 1907 reported enlargement of the glands after bone diseases such as osteomalacia and osteitis fibrosa cystica.[26] Erdheim himself regarded this gland enlargement to be compensatory, secondary to the bone disease. This view persisted for several years. Friedrich Schlagenhaufer of Vienna was the first physician to suggest that parathyroid glandular enlargement was primary, with bone disease a secondary effect. He suggested that surgery be performed to remove the enlarged glands and therefore cure the bone condition.[4]

Henry Dixon and colleagues in St. Louis, Missouri, coined the term *hyperparathyroidism*, describing its features, including bone disease, muscular weakness, hypercalciuria, renal stones, and a high serum calcium level.[4] However, it was only in 1963, with the development of the immunoassay measurement of parathyroid hormone (PTH) by Solomon Berson and Rosalyn Yalow, that a clear understanding of PTH and calcium metabolism emerged.[52] In 1977 Yalow received the Nobel Prize in Physiology or Medicine for her and Berson's work. Because Nobel Prizes are only given to the living, Yalow received the award without Berson, who died in 1972.

Parathyroid Surgery

Many physicians in the early 1900s thought that parathyroid glandular enlargement was associated with parathyroid hypofunction, analogous to goiter and myxedema. As a result, patients with hyperparathyroidism were treated with parathyroid gland extracts in the hope of correcting a presumed parathyroid deficiency. As previously noted, it was Schlagenhaufer in 1915 who first suggested removal of enlarged parathyroid glands as an appropriate treatment for von Recklinghausen's disease. It was not until 1925 that Felix Mandl (Figure 1.13) of Vienna actually performed the first parathyroidectomy on Albert Gahne, a tram car conductor.[4] The patient had been previously treated with parathyroid extract and implantation of parathyroid glands, consistent with contemporary thinking. In desperation, Mandl extracted a 2.1 × 1.5 × 1.2 cm parathyroid gland, believed in retrospect to represent parathyroid carcinoma. The procedure was initially successful and changed the current thinking and practice of the day. Unfortunately, Gahne developed recurrent hypercalcemia and died soon after a second surgical exploration.[26]

Less than 6 months after the operation performed by Mandl, E.J. Lewis performed the first parathyroidectomy in the United States at Cook Hospital in Chicago.[53] Four months later, additional lessons in the surgical management of hyperparathyroidism were learned through the experiences of sea captain Charles Martell at MGH in Boston. In 1931 James Walton of London advocated that during parathyroid surgery "wide exposure is essential, for not only is it necessary to explore all the parathyroid glands, but also sometimes to search behind the trachea and in the mediastinum."[54]

Further Parathyroid Advances and Autotransplantation

Eiselsberg, one of Billroth's pupils, first attempted to transplant a parathyroid gland in 1892, approximately a year after Gley's report. As a professor at Allgemeines Krankenhaus, he performed autografts in cats.

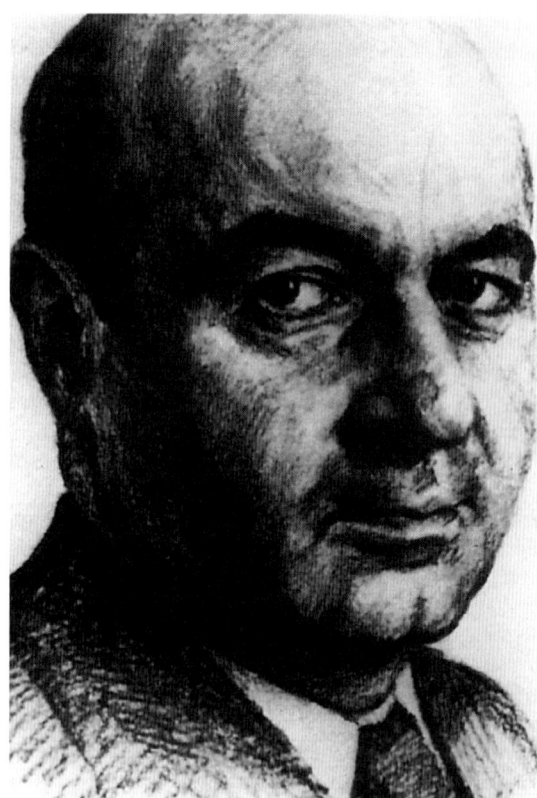

Fig. 1.13 Felix Mandl, Vienna. (From Organ CH Jr. The history of parathyroid surgery, 1850-1996: the Excelsior Surgical Society 1998 Edward D Churchill Lecture. *J Am Coll Surg.* 2000;191[3]:284–299, Fig. 12. Used with permission.)

His technique involved transplantation of half the thyroid and parathyroid glands into the rectus fascia and the peritoneum of animals with tetany.[26] No sign of tetany was observed in these animals 1 month after the procedure.

In 1907 Hermann Pfeiffer and Otto Mayer were the first to achieve clinical success with autografted parathyroid tissue.[4] Halsted proved, in 1909, that even the transplantation of a single parathyroid gland could be lifesaving. He "made the startling and hardly believable observation that the life of a dog could be maintained with a particle of tissue only 0.25 mm in diameter and distinguished by tetany after its removal."[55] He advocated for the prevention of parathyroid gland injury during thyroidectomy and experimentally injected intravenous calcium gluconate to treat tetany in postthyroidectomy animals.[56] As understanding was established of the relationship between tetany and parathyroid glands, many surgeons eventually attempted parathyroid autotransplantation during thyroidectomy. Lahey described human parathyroid autotransplantation into the sternocleidomastoid muscle in 1926. It was not until 1976 that Sam Wells developed autotransplantation after parathyroidectomy. Instead of performing a subtotal parathyroidectomy, Wells excised all glands and autografted gland sections within the muscle of the forearm. These parathyroid gland sections then could be excised later if hyperparathyroidism recurred.[57]

HISTORICAL VIGNETTE OF ENDOCRINE SURGERY AT THE MASSACHUSETTS GENERAL HOSPITAL

MGH, as a teaching hospital of the Harvard Medical School, has a long tradition of excellence in the surgical care of patients with endocrine diseases. MGH has had a rare combination of surgeons and endocrinologists with a special interest in hyperparathyroidism and thyroid diseases as well as the institutional and departmental support for dedicated thyroid and calcium metabolism laboratories, endocrine clinical research units, and clinical assignments that have singled out specific problems, questions, and treatment issues. Some of the major thyroid and parathyroid contributions include the following: the 1934 description of parathyroid clear cell hyperplasia by Fuller Albright, the 1958 recognition of chief cell hyperplasia by Cope, the 1963 development of human PTH immunoassay by John Potts, and the first two-site PTH immunoassay in 1987 and the first intraoperative PTH measurements in 1988 by Samuel Nussbaum. Other significant discoveries were the use of selective venous catheterization for PTH (Potts); intraoperative parathyroid biopsy fat stains (Roth); amino acid sequence for human PTH (Keutman); DNA sequence for human PTH (Kronenberg); detailed *New England Journal of Medicine* (NEJM) report of ectopic PTH production by ovarian carcinoma (Gaz); confocal laser microscopy analysis of parathyroids (White); PTH pulse therapy for osteoporosis (Neer); identification of the PRAD oncogene, monoclonality of adenoma, polyclonality of hyperplasia (Arnold); thyroid lobar ablation (Daniels); and neural monitoring.

The story of (Randolph) hyperparathyroidism and parathyroid physiology is a relatively short one beginning in the early 1900s. Joseph C. Aub began the MGH tradition with studies on lead poisoning and bone metabolism in 1925. Then Fuller Albright (1900-1969) concentrated on the clinical and laboratory study of parathyroid function. He wrote the first significant compendium on parathyroid physiology and pathophysiology. The dissemination of parathyroid knowledge from MGH publications attracted many of the first patients diagnosed with bone disease (osteitis fibrosa cystica) related to parathyroid dysfunction. MGH acquired the first large series of parathyroidectomy patients treated by Oliver Cope (1902-1995) and his associates. The ensuing publications included the story of the famous maritime captain Charles Martell (Figure 1.14): In 1926 Eugene DuBois, in New York, diagnosed Captain Martell with hyperparathyroidism. Martell was transferred for additional study to Joseph Aub, Fuller Albright, and, ultimately, Benjamin Castleman. He underwent the first of two unsuccessful neck explorations in 1927 at the hospital under the care of then chief of surgery Edward Richardson. It was not until the seventh operation by Edward Churchill and Oliver Cope that a 3 × 3-cm mediastinal adenoma was resected. Interestingly, it was Martell himself who insisted on a mediastinal exploration after reading extensively at the Harvard Medical School library about the wide variation of parathyroid gland locations. Sadly, despite the success of this final operation, Martell died 6 weeks later as a result of laryngospasm after a procedure to relieve an impacted ureter stone.

By 1936 Churchill and Cope undertook a series of 30 operations with excellent results. Churchill's experience led to an appreciation that "the success of parathyroid surgery must lie in the ability of the surgeon to know a parathyroid when he sees one, to know the distribution of the glands, where they hide, and also be delicate enough in technique to be able to use this knowledge."[37,38]

The name "Delphian node" was born at the MGH. The Delphian node, also known as the "prelaryngeal node," was named after the Delphic Oracle for its perceived ability to predict advanced disease in thyroid cancer. The name was first suggested to Oliver Cope in 1948 by Raymond V. Randall, a fourth-year student from Harvard Medical School.[58,59]

Chiu-an Wang (1914-1996), the director of endocrine surgery at the MGH for many years, was a remarkable individual. He came from Canton, China, where he studied parasitology and began a brilliant career. After completing his medical education at Harvard Medical School in 1943, he was a general surgery resident at MGH. Then,

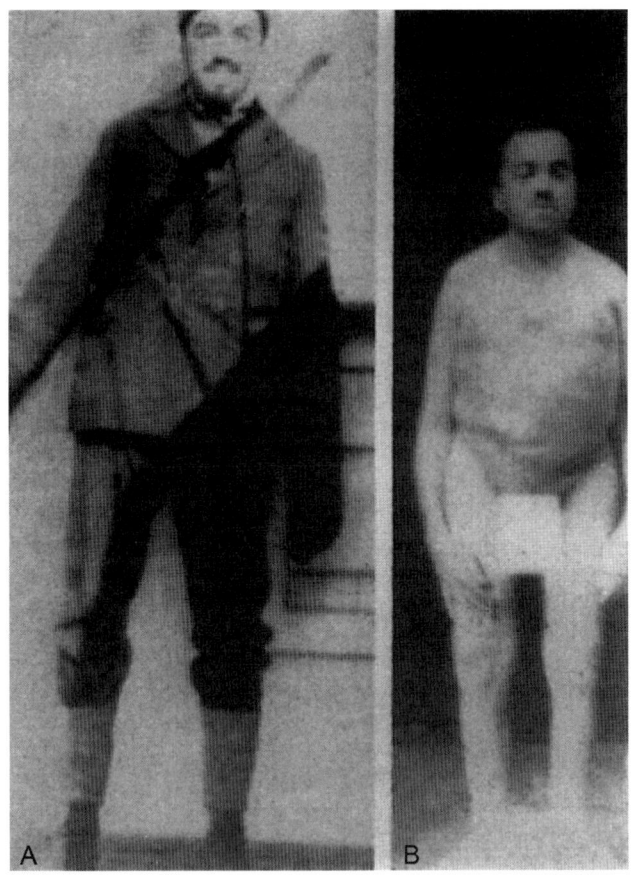

Fig. 1.14 Sea captain Charles Martell **(A)** as a young man, subsequent to the development of severe bone disease **(B)**. (From Organ CH Jr. The history of parathyroid surgery, 1850-1996: the Excelsior Surgical Society 1998 Edward D Churchill Lecture. *J Am Coll Surg.* 2000;191[3]:284–299, Fig. 14. Used with permission.)

returning to China, he practiced in Canton and then Hong Kong, returning to MGH in 1960. Cope assigned him to focus on parathyroid and thyroid surgery. He spent years in the pathology laboratory, dissecting cadavers to write a fundamental treatise on the anatomy of parathyroid glands that continues to be a standard reference for surgeons seeking an understanding of the embryologic relations and locations of these diminutive and elusive structures. Another major contribution was his description of a technique for thyroid needle biopsy. This included a movie showing his use of the 14-gauge Vim-Silverman needle to obtain a copious tissue sample from large thyroid nodules for pathologic diagnosis. Thyroid needle biopsies were rarely performed in the United States during the 1960s, so his descriptions helped spread the use of this diagnostic procedure. Wang was one of the early champions of minimally invasive parathyroidectomy. He performed ultrasound-directed unilateral parathyroid neck explorations (1981), removing the enlarged adenoma and a small snippet biopsy of the ipsilateral second gland and performed an on-the-table sterile Mannitol density test (1978) comparing the two glands. If there was a marked difference in density based on the disparate fat content of the two glands, he was confident of the diagnosis of adenoma and terminated the procedure. If the two glands were similar in density, then he explored the contralateral side, anticipating four-gland hyperplasia. With this methodology he rarely encountered recurrence, with only 1% to 2% of cases requiring reoperation.

Another contribution was the technique of visual anatomic identification of the RLN using the inferior cornu of the thyroid cartilage as a landmark. Wang trained hundreds of surgical students, residents, and fellows in his style of meticulous, function-preserving, and successful operative technique.

Advances in endocrine surgery have come from prepared minds that have analyzed previous knowledge, noted new findings, and tested innovative hypotheses. MGH has brought together gifted surgical scientists, high volumes of patients with endocrine diseases, dedicated clinical research units, basic science laboratories, and teams of ancillary services who have concentrated their efforts. The result has been a continuing high standard of patient care and ongoing new discoveries in the field of endocrine surgery.

SUMMARY

By comprehending the past, we are able to understand the present and push the boundaries of what is possible in the future. Surgeons around the world continue to expand on these surgical techniques advancing the evolution of thyroid and parathyroid surgery. Ultimately, they build on the original work of those who have come before them, while laying the foundation for those that will come after of them, in this ever-evolving field of surgery.

REFERENCES

For a complete list of references, go to expertconsult.com.

Applied Embryology of the Thyroid and Parathyroid Glands

Roma Pradhan, Amit Agarwal, Celestino P. Lombardi, Marco Raffaelli

 This chapter contains additional online-only content available on expertconsult.com.

The modern thyroid or endocrine surgeon should have a complete understanding of the embryonic development of the thyroid and parathyroid glands as well as knowledge of the possible congenital abnormalities associated with these glands, because they may affect the completeness of surgery and cause complications during surgery. The surgeon comes to a more intuitive understanding of surgical anatomy through the comprehensive appreciation of the underlying formative embryology.

THE THYROID GLAND

Normal Development of the Thyroid

The thyroid gland has a double origin: the primitive pharynx and the neural crest (Figure 2.1). The primitive pharynx is responsible for the origin of medial thyroid anlage, whereas the lateral thyroid anlage originates from the neural crest, the source of parafollicular cells, or C cells, that secrete calcitonin. These cells derive from the ultimobranchial bodies.[1] An understanding of the ultimobranchial origin of C cells has come from the studies of patients with DiGeorge syndrome, which causes a complete or partial absence of the caudal pharyngeal complex. Less than one-third of these patients have C cells within their thyroid.[2]

The primitive pharynx is the origin of the main central portion of the thyroid which appears during the second and third week of fetal life (Figure 2.2). This medial thyroid anlage arises on the ventral pharyngeal wall (the *tuberculum impar*) at the level of the second branchial arch, appearing as a single or paired diverticulum. The median anlage forms the bulk of the thyroid gland. Division of the gland into lateral lobes, if not present from the beginning, occurs so early that it is impossible to determine whether the thyroid arises singly or as a paired organ. The median stalk usually has a lumen (the thyroglossal duct) that does not extend into lateral lobes. This diverticulum follows the primitive heart as it descends caudally. It becomes a solid cord of cells that will form the follicular elements. Then it breaks in two: the proximal part retracts and disappears; however, its pharyngeal connection results in a permanent pit, the *foramen cecum* at the apex of the V-shaped *sulcus terminalis* on the dorsum of the tongue. Early during the fifth week, the attenuated duct loses its lumen and shortly afterward breaks into fragments. The caudal end develops as bilobed encapsulated thyroid gland proper, reaches its final adult orthotopic position at the level of the developing trachea by the seventh week, and undergoes histologic differentiation into the typical follicles during weeks 10 and 11, which acquire colloid by the third month.

Please see the Expert Consult website for more discussion of this topic.

The lateral thyroid anlage develops from proliferation of pharyngeal endoderm. The ventral portion of the fourth pharyngeal pouch becomes attached to the posterior surface of the thyroid during the fifth week and contributes up to 30% of the thyroid weight. The right and left lobes of the thyroid grow caudally with the growth of the fetus, taking up their final position at either side of the second to fourth tracheal rings. The line of normal embryologic thyroid descent of the medial anlagen is called a *thyroglossal tract*. The determinants of fusion of the median and lateral anlages are unknown. The site of the fusion of these two structures is stated to occur at the tubercle of Zuckerkandl (TZ).[3,4] Sugiyama speculated that the migration of the ultimobranchial body controls the growth of median anlage.[5] The C cells from the ultimobranchial body of the lateral anlagen are not scattered throughout the entire thyroid but are restricted to a zone deep within the middle to upper thirds of the lateral lobes along a hypothetical central lobar axis.[6] The extreme upper and lower poles, as well as the isthmic regions, are generally devoid of C cells.

Please see the Expert Consult website for more discussion of this topic.

The thyroglossal duct is an epithelial tube that connects the gland and the foramen cecum (see Chapter 5, Thyroglossal Duct Cysts and Ectopic Thyroid Tissue). Early during the fifth week, the attenuated duct loses its lumen and shortly afterward breaks into fragments. During the fifth through the seventh weeks of gestation, the hyoid bone is formed by condensation of mesoderm with subsequent chondrification from the second and third branchial arches; this grows from behind forward, dividing the thyroglossal tract into suprahyoid and infrahyoid portions.[7] The attenuated thyroglossal duct tract usually atrophies and disappears by the end of the eighth week. The tract may persist as a fibrous cord or a minute epithelial tube.

Genetic Control

Please see the Expert Consult website for more discussion of this topic.

Anomalous Development of the Thyroid

Various anomalies of the development of the thyroid gland involving the median or the lateral anlage (or both) have been described (Table 2.1) (see Chapter 5, Thyroglossal Duct Cysts and Ectopic Thyroid Tissue, and Chapter 9, Reoperation for Benign Disease). Developmental variations involving the thyroid can be categorized under the following groups:
1. *Anomalies of median thyroid anlage*
   a. Thyroid ectopias: thyroid rests, lingual thyroid, midline ectopic thyroid
   b. Thyroglossal duct cysts (TDCs) and fistulae
   c. Pyramidal lobe
   d. Agenesis/hemiagenesis

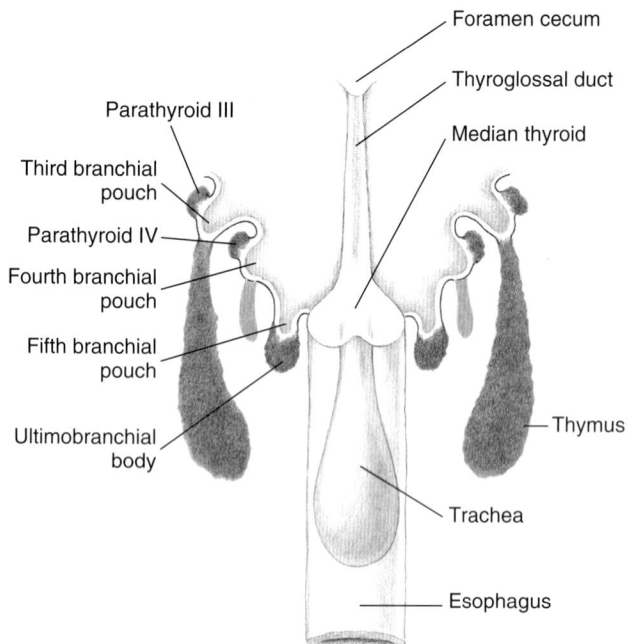

Fig. 2.1 Schematic view of the primitive pharynx of an 8- to 10-mm embryo.

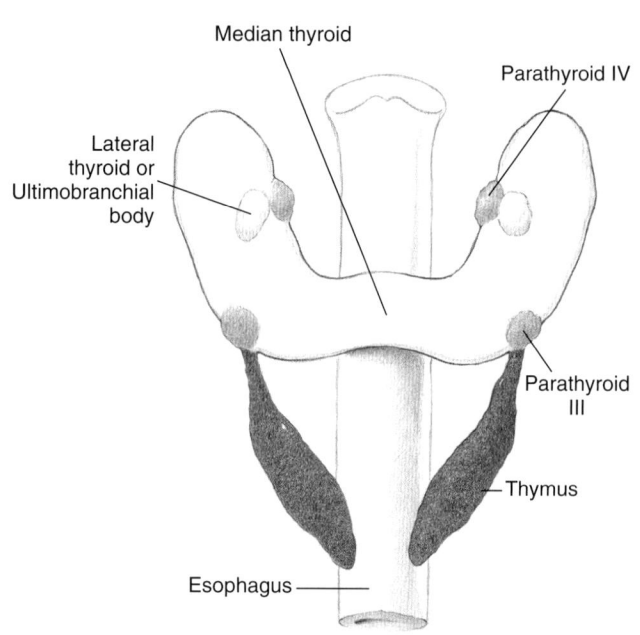

Fig. 2.2 Schematic view of the locations of thyroid, lateral thyroid, thymic, and parathyroid tissue. At the 13- to 14-mm stage, the parathyroid III and the parathyroid IV migrate together with the thymus and ultimobranchial bodies, respectively.

TABLE 2.1 Embryologic Anomalies associated with the Median and Lateral Thyroid Anlages

Both Median and Lateral Anlages	Median Anlage	Lateral Anlage	Neither Anlage

• Variable shape, weight, and symmetry
• Hemiagenesis
	• Agenesis
	  • Isthmus: thick, thin, and absent
	  • Pyramidal lobe
	  • Thyroglossal duct
	• Anomalies of descent along the thyroid line
	  • Lingual
	  • Sublingual
	  • Prelaryngeal
	• Accessory ectopic (i.e., outside the pathway of descent)
	  • Mediastinal
	  • Intratracheal
	  • Lateral to jugular
	  • Ovarian
	  • Sella turcica
	  • Retrotracheal
	  • Preaortic
	  • Pericardial
	  • Cardiac
	  • Porta hepatis
	  • Gallbladder
	  • Groin
	  • Intralaryngeal
	  • Intraesophageal
	• Lateral aberrant thyroid within the capsule of medially located lymph nodes
		• Nonfusion with median anlage
		• Cysts with squamous epithelial lining
		• Solid cell rests; C cells
		• Agenesis: DiGeorge syndrome
		• Pharyngeal pouch remnants
		  • Thymic
		  • Parathyroid
		  • Ultimobranchial body
		• Lateral aberrant thyroid within the capsule of medially located lymph nodes
			• Vessels
			  • Artery
			  • Vein
			  • Lymph
			• Muscles
			• Nerves

2. *Anomalies of lateral thyroid anlage*
   a. Tubercle of Zuckerkandl
3. *Anomalies of abnormal/continued descent*

Thyroid Ectopias

Although ectopic thyroid tissue can be found between the foramen cecum and the normal position of the thyroid gland, the two most common sites of undescended thyroid glands are the lingual thyroid (90%) and the anterior neck (10%) (Figure 2.3, A and B). Most of them are detected during childhood and are often associated with hypothyroidism. Under the influence of continued thyroid-stimulating hormone (TSH) stimulation, they may enlarge and produce local symptoms. The ectopic thyroid tissue in the anterior neck may present as a midline mass and may be misdiagnosed as a thyroglossal cyst.[11] It is important to differentiate ectopic thyroid tissue from the TDC because it frequently represents the only source of thyroid tissue.

Thyroid Rests

Thyroid rests are isolated rests of normal thyroid tissue lying below the lower pole of the thyroid within the line of the thyrothymic tract, or even within the upper anterior mediastinum (see Chapter 6, Surgery of Cervical and Substernal Goiter, and Chapter 9, Reoperation for Benign Disease). They may also have an extension or prolongation of the thyroid tissue attached to the lower pole of the thyroid by a narrow pedicle or even just a fibrovascular band. These rests are presumably an extension of the normal embryologic descent of the thyroid after separation into right and left lobes and are present in over 50% of patients (Figure 2.3, C). Awareness of variable projections or extensions of thyroid parenchyma is critical to ensure complete removal of all thyroid tissue. Thyroid rests can be located within the anterior mediastinum, and they may sometimes be mistaken for small lymph nodes or even parathyroid glands. The development of nodular change within such a rest might be recognized as a thyroid nodule completely separate from and caudal to the lower pole of the thyroid gland. If such a nodule lies even further caudal, within the anterior mediastinum, following the descent of the heart and the great vessels, it might well give rise to the "isolated" mediastinal or "primary" intrathoracic goiter (see Chapter 6, Surgery of Cervical and Substernal Goiter). The blood supply for these intrathoracic rests is usually from intrathoracic vessels. This explains why primary intrathoracic goiters may require a thoracic surgical approach (i.e., sternotomy) to achieve vascular control.

Sackett et al.[12] have suggested a classification for thyroid rests in relation to the thyroid gland (see Figure 2.3, C).

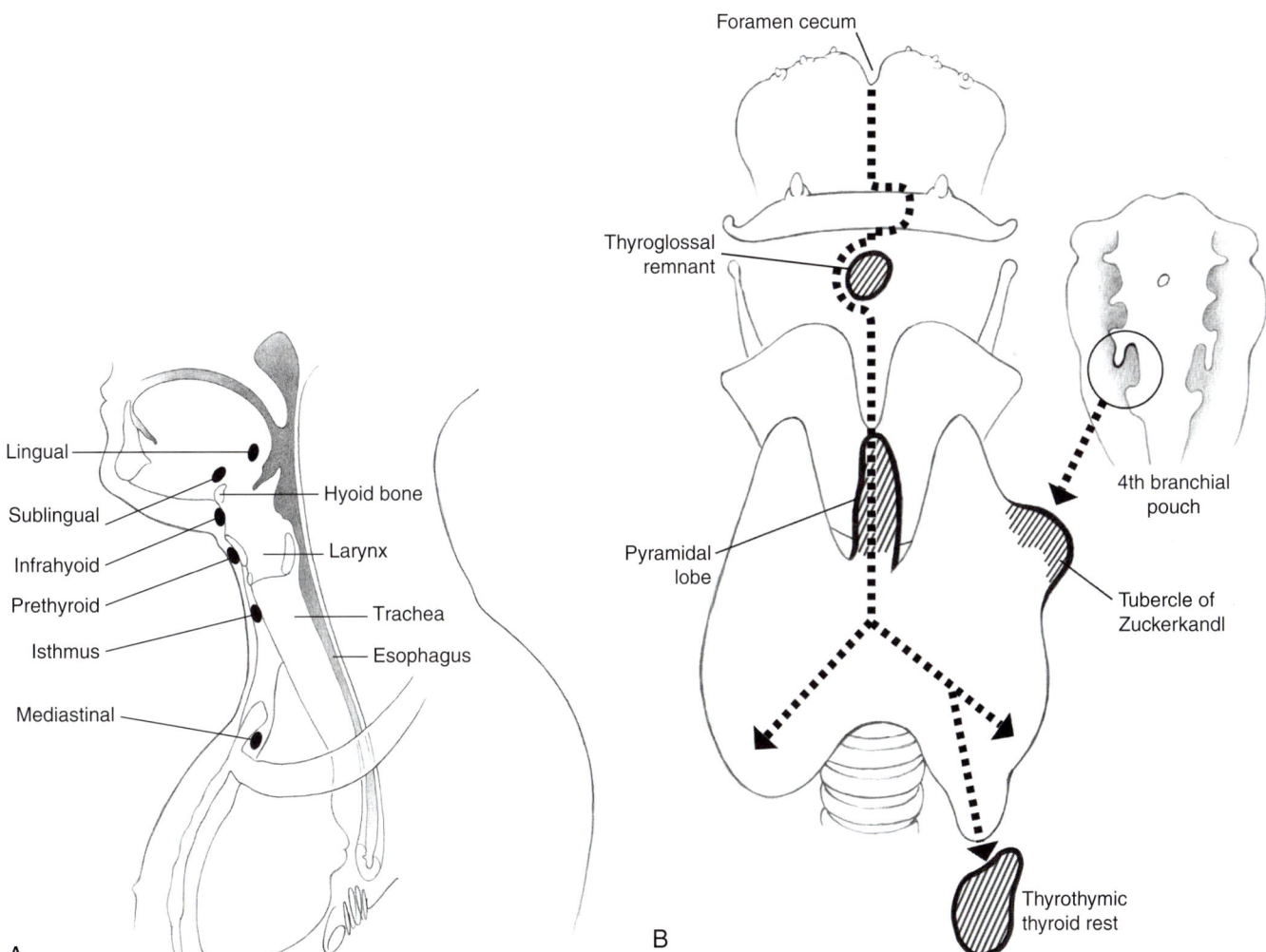

Fig. 2.3 A, Schema illustrating some common sites for midline ectopic thyroid masses. **B,** A summary of the major medial and lateral embryologic elements of the thyroid gland and their potential adult anatomic consequences.

(Continued)

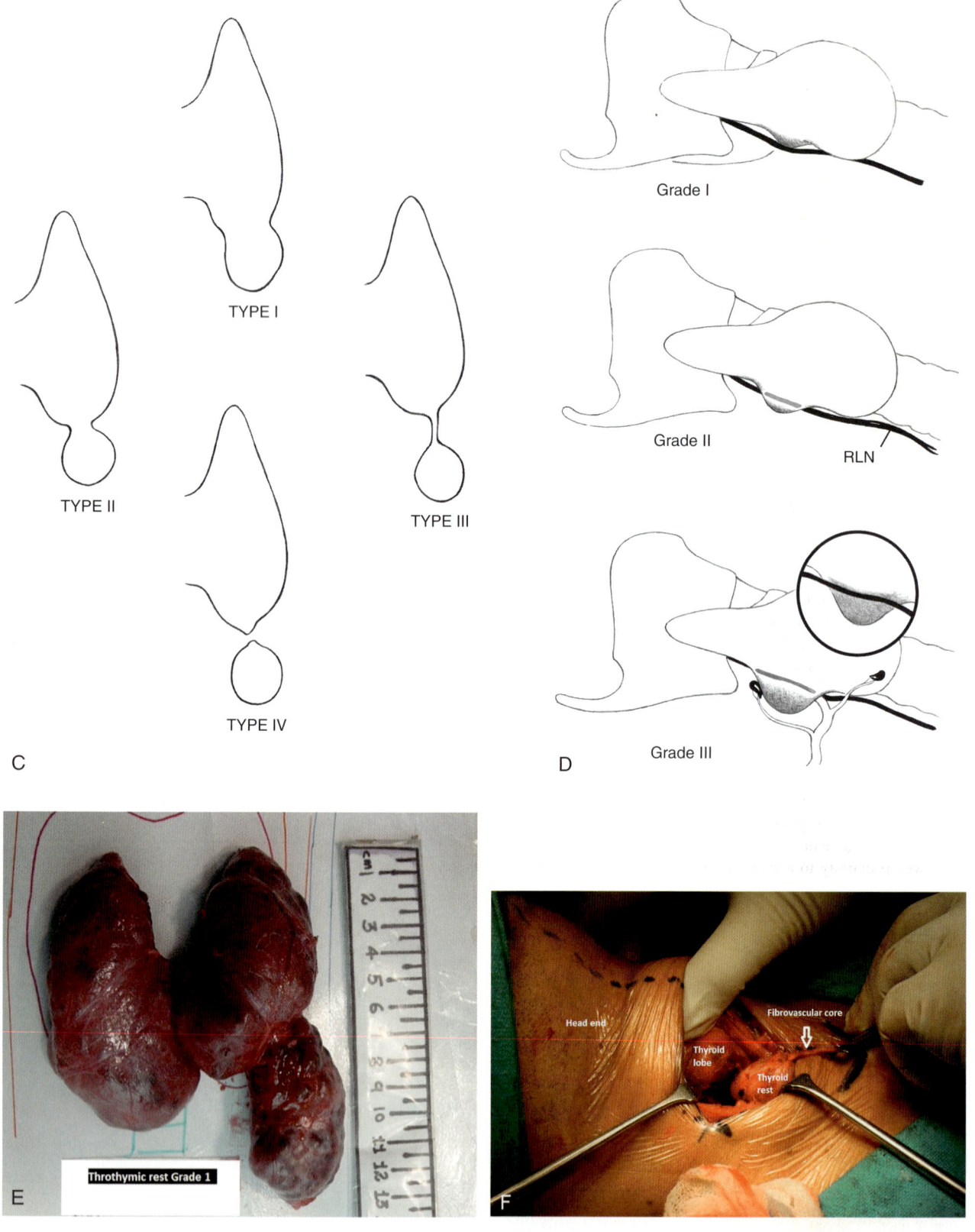

Fig. 2.3, cont'd **C,** Thyroid rests grades I through IV. **D,** Three grades of tubercle of Zuckerkandl (TZ) development. Note also the potential of injury for a ventrally placed recurrent laryngeal nerve (RLN) with a posteriorly situated tubercle. **E,** Thyrothymic rest grade I arising from inferior aspect of thyroid. **F,** Thyrothymic rest grade III attached with fibrovascular core.

CHAPTER 2 Applied Embryology of the Thyroid and Parathyroid Glands

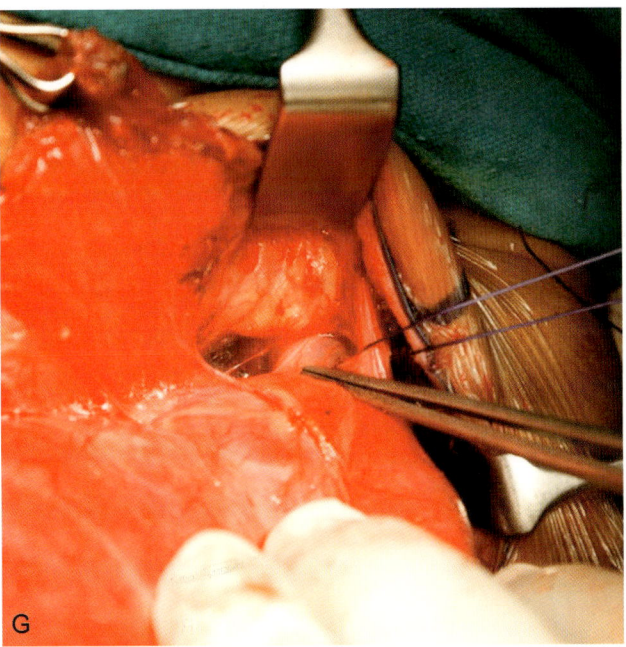

Fig. 2.3, cont'd **G**, RLN passing anterior to TZ.

Grade I. Thyroid rests consist of a protrusion of thyroid tissue arising from the inferior aspect of the thyroid gland in the region of the thyrothymic ligament, which is recognizably distinct from the line of the lower border of the thyroid lobe (Figure 2.3, *E*).

Grade II. Thyroid rests include thyroid tissue lying within the thyrothymic tract and attached to the thyroid proper only by a narrow pedicle of thyroid tissue.

Grade III. Thyroid rests are similar to grade II but are attached to the thyroid gland only by a fibrovascular core (Figure 2.3, *F*).

Grade IV. Thyroid rests have no connection to the thyroid gland.

The thyroid rests sometimes lead to intraoperative difficulty in mobilizing the inferior thyroid pole because of its attachment to the thyrothymic ligament. A parathyroid gland is occasionally found in close proximity to a thyroid rest and adjacent thyrothymic ligament. The inferior parathyroid gland migrates caudally with the thymus gland.[13]

Thyroid rests have clinical significance because they may be the source of recurrent goiters and may lead to compressive symptoms later (see Chapter 9, Reoperation for Benign Disease). They may also be a source of radioactive iodine uptake after total thyroidectomy done for carcinoma. Hence the knowledge of thyroid test anatomy is important to ensure complete removal of all gross thyroid tissue during total thyroidectomy.

Please see the Expert Consult website for more discussion of this topic.

Lingual Thyroid

Failure of the descent of the thyroid gland anlage early in the course of embryogenesis results in a lingual thyroid near the foramen cecum (see Chapter 5, Thyroglossal Duct Cysts and Ectopic Thyroid Tissue). The applied importance of lingual thyroid is as follows:

1. In the majority of cases, the lingual thyroid may be the only functioning thyroid tissue.
2. An enlarging lingual thyroid located at the base of the tongue (Figure 2.4, *A*) may present with symptoms of dysphagia, upper airway obstruction, or even hemorrhage.
3. Although rare (43 reported cases),[15] malignant transformation of the lingual thyroid tissue may occur.

The diagnosis of a lingual thyroid may be confirmed by a radioiodine scan (Figure 2.4, *B*), which would typically reveal an increased uptake focus at the base of the tongue with no apparent activity in the normal pretracheal location of the thyroid gland in the neck. Regarding treatment, in children or young adults who are euthyroid and whose sole thyroid tissue is the lingual thyroid, no treatment would be necessary. However, more commonly these patients develop obstructive symptoms secondary to hypertrophy of the lingual thyroid because of continuous TSH stimulation as a result of hypothyroidism. In such a situation, thyroxine supplementation or sometimes suppression helps shrink the lingual thyroid, and surgical therapy may not be required. Rarely, in situations of continued growth and obstructive symptoms or hemorrhage, surgical removal of the lingual thyroid may be necessary. Ablative radioiodine therapy is an alternative approach recommended in older patients or patients who are not fit for surgery. The surgical approaches include transoral and external approaches.

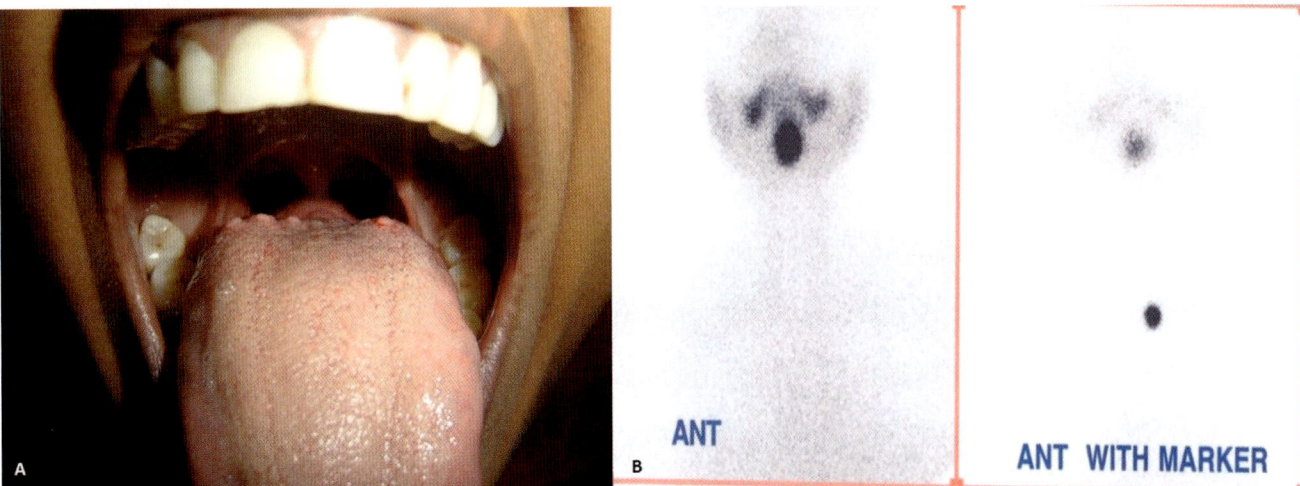

Fig. 2.4 A, An enlarged lingual thyroid located at the base of the tongue. **B,** Radioiodine scan with an increased uptake focus at the base of the tongue with no apparent activity in the normal pretracheal location of the thyroid gland in the neck.

Thyroglossal Duct Cyst

Early during the fifth week, the attenuated duct loses its lumen and shortly afterward breaks into fragments (see Chapter 5, Thyroglossal Duct Cysts and Ectopic Thyroid Tissue). During the fifth through the seventh weeks of gestation, the hyoid bone is formed by condensation of mesoderm with subsequent chondrification from the second and third branchial arches, which as noted previously, grow from behind forward, dividing the thyroglossal duct tract into suprahyoid and infrahyoid portions.[16,17] The attenuated thyroglossal duct tract usually atrophies and disappears by the end of the eighth week. This tract may persist as a fibrous cord or a minute epithelial tube, and this persisting tube/duct/cord is called a *thyroglossal duct,* which connects the gland and the foramen cecum. The thyroid gland may reach its normal position, leaving rests of cells anywhere along this embryonic path, and give rise to postnatal development of cysts; or it may leave rests at any level along the midline developmental pathway (sublingual, prelaryngeal, or rarely, the suprasternal). A TDC does not have a primary external opening, which is characteristic of some branchial cleft cysts, as the embryologic course of the tract never reaches the surface of the neck.

TDCs are the most common congenital cervical abnormalities, three times more common than branchial cleft remnants. Cysts usually present as a painless, asymptomatic midline swelling below the hyoid bone (Figure 2.5) and may be observed at any age. TDCs are present at birth in approximately 25% of cases, most are noted during childhood, and the final third become apparent after age 30. The gender incidence is equal. They can be found anywhere in the midline, from the submental region to the suprasternal notch, but are most commonly located halfway between these extremes, near the hyoid bone. Ward et al.[18] noted that 80% were juxtaposed to the hyoid bone (25% located in the submental region), 2% lingual, and 7% in a suprasternal location. Only 1% of TDCs were lateral to the midline.[18] On examination, cysts are round with a smooth surface and are well defined. With swallowing or protrusion of the tongue, they typically rise in the neck as a result of being anchored to the hyoid bone and the muscles of the tongue. They are usually 1 to 2 cm in diameter, slightly mobile, and nontender unless there is a superimposed infection. Oral bacteria may be transmitted through the foramen cecum. Thyroglossal duct sinuses are secondary to infection of the cysts as a result of spontaneous or surgical drainage and are associated with some degree of low-grade inflammation of the surrounding skin. The cutaneous opening is usually 1 to 3 mm in diameter and may intermittently express small droplets of thin mucoid fluid, which is usually clear or yellowish.

Preoperative thyroid imaging and thyroid function assessment should be done in all patients with TDCs to see the normal thyroid gland. Thyroid scintigraphy can be performed in patients with presumed TDCs to document the presence of a normal thyroid and to exclude the possibility of an ectopic thyroid. Preoperative high-resolution sonography can also identify a normal thyroid gland and exclude ectopic thyroid tissue.

Please see the Expert Consult website for more discussion of this topic.

Pyramidal Lobe

The pyramidal lobe is the embryologic remnant of the thyroglossal tract. It is a variable extension of thyroid tissue from the thyroid isthmus toward the hyoid bone. The frequency of presence of pyramidal lobe varies from 55% to 76% in operative specimens.[22] When present it is more commonly associated with the left side of the isthmus. The pyramidal lobe contains thyroid follicular cells and must be adequately identified and excised along with any fibrous remnant. If overlooked during surgery it may cause recurrent benign nodular goiters or recurrent hyperthyroidism or malignant disease, developing as either a midline or a left-sided neck swelling.

Tubercle of Zuckerkandl

The TZ is believed to represent the remnants of the lateral thyroid processes (ultimobranchial bodies). These bilateral structures arise as a proliferation of pharyngeal endoderm from the ventral portion of the fourth pharyngeal pouch and the vestigial fifth pouch. The ultimobranchial bodies bring to the thyroid gland the superior parathyroid gland and the parafollicular cells.

Eventually the lateral ultimobranchial bodies fuse with the median thyroid process, usually in the fifth week, and become detached from the pharynx. The residual posterolateral projection toward the pharynx, when present, constitutes the TZ. The TZ is a posterolateral projection from the thyroid lobe, located at the point where the lateral and medial components fuse (Figure 2.3, *D*).[4,23,24] Although the incidence of TZ is higher on the right side, it is commonly present bilaterally.[25]

Applied importance. TZ is classified into three grades according to size: grade I, <0.5 cm; grade II, 0.5 to 1.0 cm; and grade III, >1 cm. Most common is the grade II tubercle, found in 60% to 70% of cases.

1. A grade III tubercle can be associated with significant pressure symptoms and may be the cause of persistent symptoms after subtotal thyroidectomy.
2. TZ is intimately associated with recurrent laryngeal nerve (RLN) and the superior parathyroid. Enlargement of the tubercle usually occurs lateral to the RLN—the nerve appears to pass into a cleft medial to the enlarged tubercle. An uncommon but high-risk variant is where the RLN runs ventral to an enlarged tubercle (Figure 2.3, *G*).

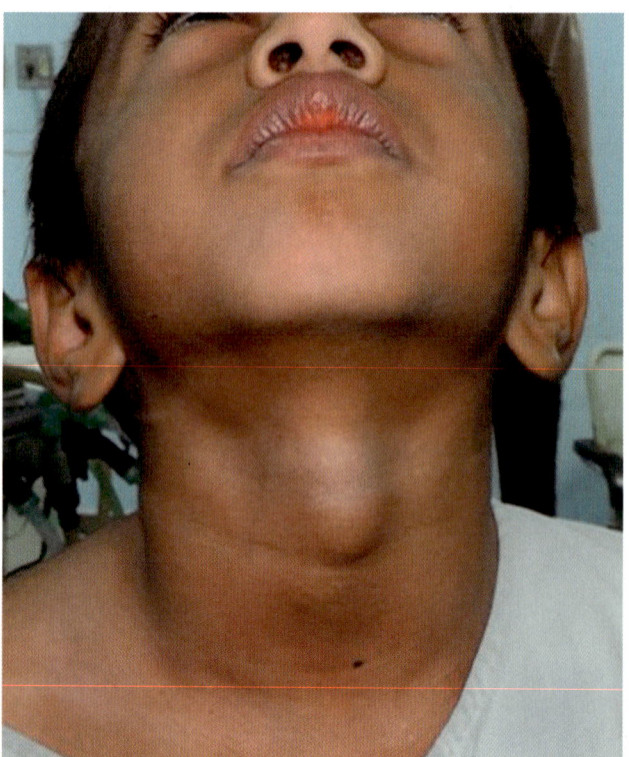

Fig. 2.5 Thyroglossal duct cyst.

3. Elevation of the TZ allows safe dissection of recurrent nerve as it passes medially.
4. The widened prevertebral space, as seen on plain lateral x-rays of the neck, could suggest the presence of an enlarged (grade II/III) TZ.[26]

THE RECURRENT LARYNGEAL NERVE

The anatomic course of the RLN is widely variable. In most cases, variability is related to the relationship between thyroid nodules and the inferior thyroid artery, as well as to precocious and variable branching. These variations are the topic of Chapter 36, Surgical Anatomy and Monitoring of the Recurrent Laryngeal Nerve. It is important for thyroid surgeons to be aware of the possibility of the presence of nonrecurrent inferior laryngeal nerve (NRILN), because it may become damaged inadvertently during a thyroidectomy, causing permanent vocal cord palsy. Several published reports have described the incidence of NRILN at 0.21% to 1.6% on the right side and only very rarely on the left side.[25,27-29]

Normal Embryology of RLN

The inferior laryngeal nerves are derived from the VI branchial arch. These originate from the vagus nerves under the VI aortic arch. Subsequently, the V and the distal portion of the VI aortic arch regress, on both the right and left side, and the two laryngeal nerves remain anchored to the structures that develop from the IV arch (i.e., the right subclavian artery and the aortic arch on the left side). When the heart descends into the thorax, these arteries take with them the nerves, which then assume their normal recurrent course (Figure 2.6).

Anomalous Development of the RLN

When the segment of the fourth right aortic arch between the origin of the right common carotid artery and the right subclavian artery disappears, the resulting break in the primitive arterial ring leads to a left-sided aortic arch, with the right subclavian artery being the last collateral (Figure 2.7). In this case the right subclavian is formed at the expense of the dorsal aorta and the seventh intersegmental artery and runs in an oblique direction (lusoria course) to the right axillary region. This atresia has two other consequences on the vascular system: the absence of the innominate artery and absence of the arterial segment under which the right RLN normally forms a loop. As a result, during the embryonic lengthening of the neck, the nerve branch is not attached at the thorax level and the right RLN arises from the vagus nerve at the cervical level (Figure 2.8). Therefore nonrecurrence of the RLN always results from this vascular anomaly during embryonic development of the aortic arches.[27,30]

Implications of Anomalous Development

Please see the Expert Consult website for more discussion of this topic.

SUPERIOR LARYNGEAL NERVE

The superior laryngeal nerve branches from the vagus nerve near the inferior half of the nodose ganglion. It divides into the internal and external branches. The internal branch, which pierces the thyrohyoid membrane, provides sensory innervation to the supraglottic larynx, whereas the external branch, carrying motor innervation, travels to and innervates the cricothyroid muscle, which functions to tilt the thyroid cartilage and tense the vocal cord. The external branch is the nerve

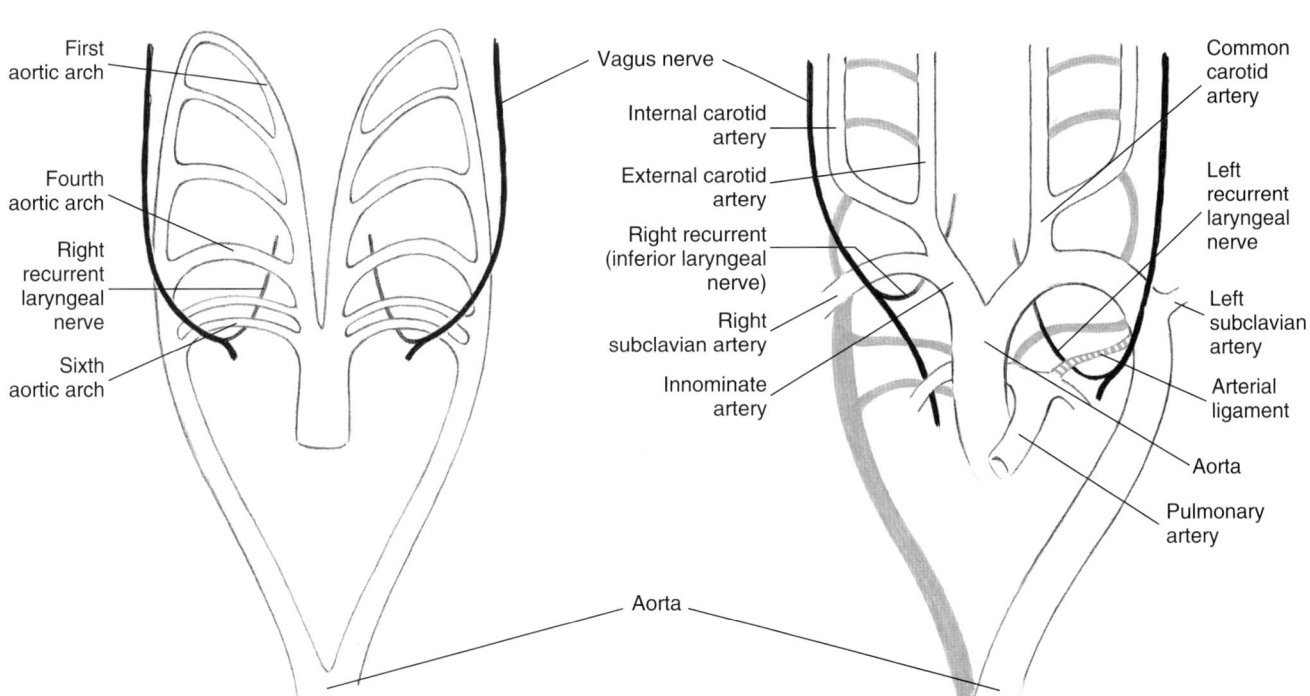

Fig. 2.6 Normal embryonic development of the aortic arches. The inferior laryngeal nerves are dragged down by the lowest persisting aortic arches. On the right side the inferior laryngeal nerve recurs around the fourth arch, which is the subclavian artery. On the left side the inferior laryngeal nerve recurs around the sixth arch, which is the arterial ligament.

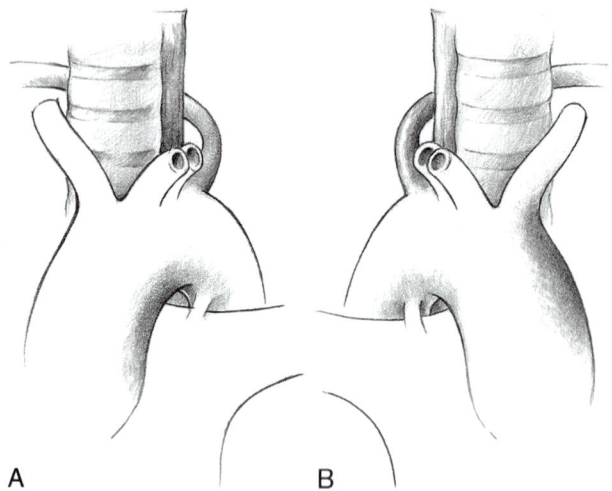

Fig. 2.7 Vascular anomalies required to observe a nonrecurrent inferior laryngeal nerve. **A,** On the right side the right retroesophageal subclavian artery arises as the fourth branch of the aortic arch, after the right and left common carotid arteries and the left subclavian artery. No innominate artery is present. **B,** On the left side, (1) right aortic arch, (2) the left retroesophageal subclavian artery arises as the fourth branch of the aortic arch after the left and right common carotid arteries and the right subclavian artery, and (3) the arterial ligament is on the right.

which we encounter during surgery. Its variation within the course of the nerve, specifically with relation to the superior thyroid vessels, was originally described by Cernea (see Chapter 35 Surgical Anatomy of the Superior Laryngeal Nerve).[29]

APPLIED EMBRYOLOGY OF THE PARATHYROID GLANDS

The parathyroid glands vary considerably in size, shape, number, and location. This wide variability represents a unique challenge for surgeons dealing with parathyroid diseases. Information as to their adult location resides in their embryologic development. Indeed, the developmental embryology and surgical anatomy of the parathyroids are intimately linked. For this reason, a detailed understanding and knowledge of the embryologic development, and consequently, of possible anatomic variations of the parathyroid glands, are prerequisites for devising a successful surgical strategy for patients with hyperparathyroidism and preserving parathyroid glands during thyroid surgical procedures.

Generalities

The parathyroid glands develop from the third and fourth pharyngeal pouches in humans between the fifth and the 12th weeks of gestation.[36]

The *inferior parathyroid glands* originate from the third pharyngeal pouches (see Figure 2.1) and are named *parathyroid III* (PIII) to

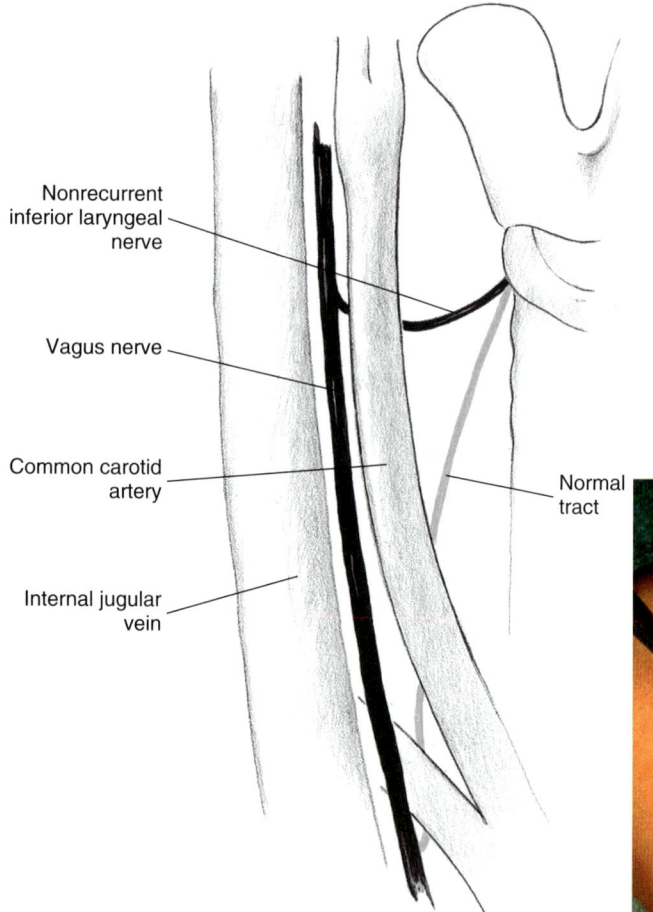

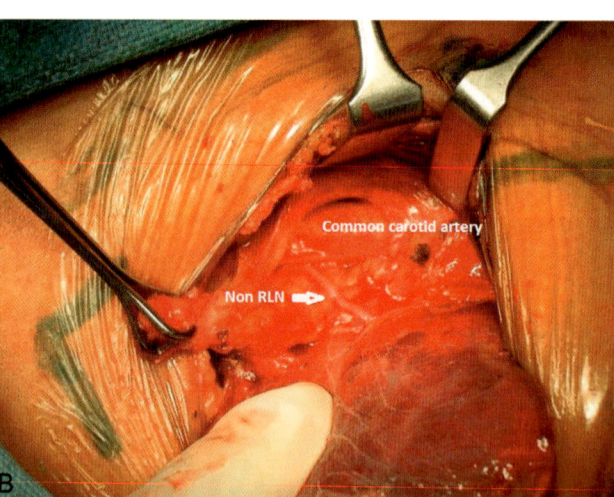

Fig. 2.8 A, Right nonrecurrent inferior laryngeal nerve. The nerve passes behind the common carotid artery, crosses the jugulocarotid groove, making a downward curve, and enters the larynx at the usual level. **B,** Right nonrecurrent laryngeal nerve. *RLN,* Recurrent laryngeal nerve.

understand their origin.[37] The thymus originates from the ventral portion of the same branchial pouch. This common origin justifies indicating the PIII as the *thymic parathyroid*.[38] The PIII and thymus complex has also been termed the *parathymus*.[37] The *parathymus complex* has a relatively long caudal descent to reach the final anatomic position.

The superior parathyroid glands arise from the dorsal portion of the fourth branchial pouches (see Figure 2.1) and are thus named *parathyroid IV* (PIV).[37] The fate of the PIV and of the derivatives of the fourth pharyngeal pouches are related to those of the fifth pouches.[37] The fifth pouch is usually rudimentary or vestigial, is incorporated in the fourth pharyngeal pouch, and contributes to the formation of the ultimobranchial bodies (lateral thyroid). The fourth and the rudimentary fifth pharyngeal pouches together are sometimes indicated as the *caudal pharyngeal complex*. This includes the primordium of PIV (dorsal portion), a *ventral diverticulum* (which corresponds in position to the thymus portion of the third pouch), and an ultimobranchial body derived mainly from the fifth pouch. Although the ultimate fate of the *ventral diverticulum* is not certain in humans, it could give rise to a small amount of thymus tissue (rudimentary thymus IV), which, soon after its formation, disappears.[39,40] Fatty lobules, which are seldom encountered in conjunction with the PIV at their normal site, could constitute the vestigial remnants of this thymic tissue that have not completely disappeared.[41] Because of the common origin with the lateral thyroid, the PIVs are sometimes indicated as *thyroid parathyroids,* analogous to the thymic parathyroid of PIII.[42]

Please see the Expert Consult website for more discussion of this topic.

Genetic Control and Evolutionary Model

Please see the Expert Consult website for more discussion of this topic.

Histogenesis

The epithelium of the dorsal portion of the third and fourth pharyngeal pouches proliferates during the fifth week and produces small nodules dorsally to each pouch. In these nodules, the proliferation of the vascular mesoderm begins and produces a network of capillaries.

Chief cells differentiate during embryonic development first. It is commonly thought that they become functionally active for the regulation of the calcium homeostasis during the fetal life. Oxyphilic cells differentiate at 5 to 7 years of life (see Chapter 65, Surgical Pathology of the Parathyroid Glands).[56]

Please see the Expert Consult website for more discussion of this topic.

Development Process

Please see the Expert Consult website for more discussion of this topic.

Position of Normal Parathyroid Glands, Anomalies of the Embryologic Migration, and Congenital Ectopias

Because of the limited embryologic migration, the PIVs are relatively constant in their position. In more than 80% of the cases, the PIVs are located on the posterior aspect of the thyroid lobe, in an area 2 cm in diameter and centered 1 cm above the intersection of the inferior thyroid artery and the RLN,[60-62] in strict proximity with the cricothyroid junction (i.e., the junction of the cricoid and thyroid cartilage)[63] (Figure 2.9). The PIV often has a surrounding halo of fat and is freely mobile on the thyroid capsule. The surrounding fat may represent atrophic thymic tissue originating from the ventral diverticulum.[39,40] Occasionally, the PIVs are closely associated to the thyroid capsule.[62] In about 15% of the cases, the PIVs are located on the posterolateral surface of the superior thyroid pole,[41,61-64] hidden between the layers of perithyroidal fascia. In such cases it is bound on the posterolateral aspect of the thyroid lobe and is therefore less mobile.[63] The PIV can also be located further in a caudal position, sometimes partially obscured by the RLN, inferior thyroid artery, or TZ,[62] and it may be found even further down, at a considerable distance posterior to the lower thyroid pole.[62]

In less than 1% of the cases, PIVs may be located higher, above the upper thyroid pole.[62] Rarely (up to 3% to 4% of the cases), normal PIVs are found more posterior in the neck in a retropharyngeal or retroesophageal location,[61,62] whereas pathologically enlarged parathyroid glands may be found in a retropharyngeal of retroesophageal position in up to one-third of the cases; this is the result of migration related to the parathyroid weight[64] (see the discussion about acquired ectopic localization presented later). Major ectopic locations of PIV are rare. They may result from descent failure or laterally directed descent and may lead to a superior parathyroid gland adjacent to the common carotid artery.[63] An exceptional superior parathyroid adenoma located in the scalene fat pad lateral to the carotid has been described.[64] These locations account for less than 1% of the cases.[63] Superior parathyroid glands are sometimes found in a subcapsular position or hidden by a cleft of thyroid capsule. True intrathyroidal superior glands are rare and less frequent than PIII, even if the PIV may become included within the thyroid at the time of fusion of the ultimobranchial bodies with the median thyroid rudiment (see the discussion about intrathyroidal parathyroid glands presented later).[61,63,64] If the superior parathyroid primordium fails to separate from the remaining endoderm of the fourth pharyngeal pouch, it may migrate to a retropharyngeal location with the pyriform sinus primordium.[65] A few cases of pathologic parathyroid glands localized in the pyriform sinus have been described.[66]

Because of the longer embryologic migration, the territory of normally located PIIIs is much more widely distributed, and they are more likely to be ectopic than PIVs (Figure 2.10). In about half of the cases (42% to 61%), they are located at the level of the inferior pole of the

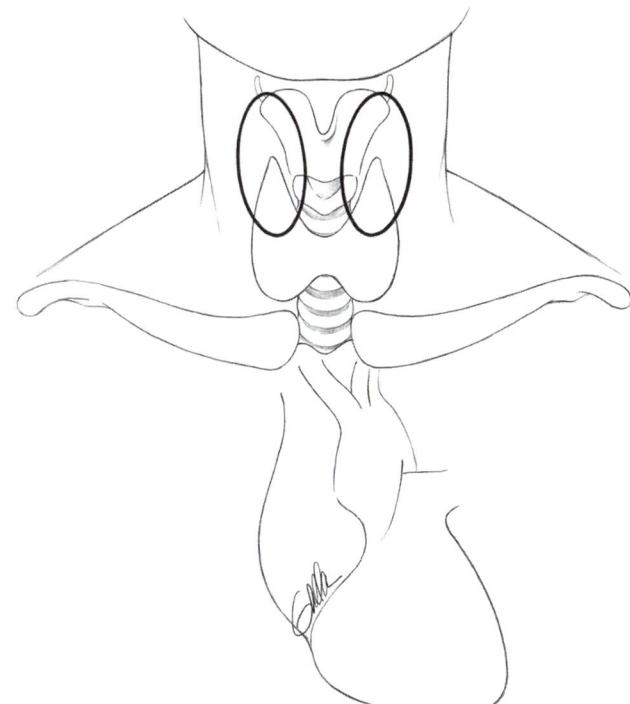

Fig. 2.9 The area of dispersal of the parathyroid IVs is limited by their short embryonic course.

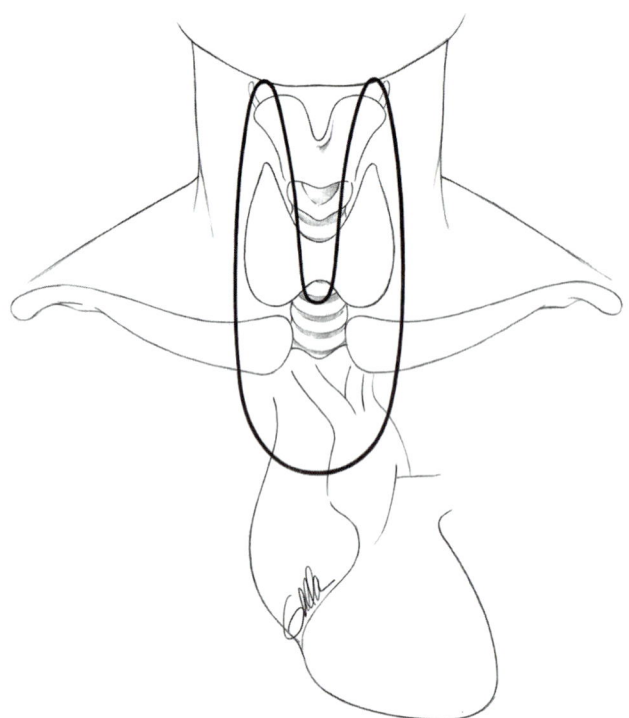

Fig. 2.10 The area of dispersal of the parathyroid III extends from the angle of the mandible to the pericardium.

thyroid lobe, on the anterior, lateral, or posterior aspect.[62,67] The gland typically rests in a fat lobule on or adjacent to the inferior pole. In some cases, PIIIs are located high on the posterior surface of the thyroid lobe, closely attached to the thyroid capsule. In such a position, they can be confused with PIVs.[38,41] A few glands are more deeply hidden in a crease of the thyroid lobe, mimicking an intrathyroidal gland.[61,62] In about one-quarter of the cases, the PIII is located in the thyrothymic ligament or in the cervical portion of the thymus.[62]

As the pathway of embryologic descent of the thymus extends from the angle of mandible to the pericardium, anomalies of migration of the *parathymus complex,* whether excessive or deficient, are responsible for high or low ectopias of PIIIs.[38,41] When the *parathymus complex* fails to descend fully, the inferior parathyroid may become stranded high in the neck, typically along the carotid sheath. Thus during parathyroid exploration if the inferior gland is missing, it is usually found with a fragment of thymic tissue above the thyroid gland and superior to the PIV.[62,67] Often the gland is situated adjacent to the carotid bifurcation, approximately 2 to 3 cm lateral to the thyroid superior pole.[61,63] The undescended PIII can be found even higher in the neck, above the carotid bifurcation, adjacent to the angle of the mandible, near the hyoid bone. In all these cases, the superior thyroid vessels provide vascularization. The incidence of this high ectopia resulting from defective embryologic descent of the parathymus does not seem to exceed 1% to 2%.[41,61,67] On the other hand if the separation from the thymus is delayed, the PIII may be pulled down in the anterior mediastinum to a varying degree (see Figure 2.10). In approximately 4% to 5% of cases, the inferior parathyroid gland is situated in the chest, within the retrosternal thymus, or at the posterior aspect of its capsule or in contact with the great mediastinal vessels (the innominate vein and ascending aorta). Only a few are located outside the thymus adjacent to the aortic arch and the origin of the great vessels. An even lower position results in the inferior parathyroid being in contact with the pleura or pericardium.[68] Most of the ectopic PIIIs, which descend below the level of the innominate vein and aortic arch, develop an ectopic arterial blood supply. Generally this is derived from the internal mammary artery. Occasionally the blood supply may come from a thymic artery or a direct branch from the aorta.[69]

The inferior parathyroid gland is truly intrathyroidal within the lower pole of thyroid in 1% to 3% of individuals (see the discussion about intrathyroid parathyroid glands presented later).

Parathyroid Symmetry

Although the location of individual glands can vary considerably, there is often marked symmetry of the parathyroid glands.[66] Symmetry of the PIV is found in approximately 80% of the cases, whereas only 70% of the inferior glands are symmetric. Relative symmetry of both PIV and PIII glands is reported in about 60% of the cases.[62] Symmetry is less marked when glands are located in an unusual site. The awareness of parathyroid symmetry may facilitate parathyroid gland identification during surgical neck exploration, and the surgeon should keep this in mind when performing thyroid and parathyroid procedures.

The most common asymmetric location is one in which only one of the PIIIs is located in the thymus. Another asymmetric position is when both glands on one side are located above or below the intersection of the RLN and the inferior thyroid artery.[62] Indeed, the PIVs are crossed by the PIII during their descent. This embryologic crossing explains why the PIII and PIV can be very closely associated at the level of the inferior thyroid artery, at the junction of the middle and inferior thirds of the thyroid lobe, depending on the extent of migration of the PIII. Because of this crossing, in some cases both homolateral parathyroids may be at the same level, corresponding to the parathyroids in the midposition of Grisoli.[38,41] In such cases, it is sometimes virtually impossible to distinguish the PIII and PIV.[38,41,62] In rare cases, the two glands are adherent to each other and appear to be fused.[38,41,59] This condition is known as *kissing pairs*.[59,61] It is possible to differentiate this condition from a bilobated gland because of the presence of a cleavage line and a separate vascular pedicle in the kissing pair, and it is essential to carefully identify these pedicles during parathyroid procedures so as not to confuse a bilobar gland with adjacent parathyroids. Such confusion may be a source of error in assessing the findings of a surgical exploration because surgeons may erroneously conclude that they have identified all four glands.

Intrathyroidal Parathyroid Glands

Parathyroid glands may have an intrathyroidal location. A true intrathyroidal parathyroid is defined as a gland that is completely surrounded by thyroid tissue and should be differentiated by subcapsular parathyroid glands and those that are buried in a crease of thyroid capsule.[61,62,64]

The incidence of intrathyroidal parathyroid glands is between 0.5% and 4%,[61,62,66,70] and their frequency seems to be higher in cases of hyperfunctioning glands. Recent reports have shown their prevalence to be on the right side and the inferior portion of the thyroid lobe.[71]

The origin of this entity has not been completely elucidated yet. Indeed, based on parathyroid embryology, one should expect that the intrathyroidal gland would be represented by PIV glands included within the thyroid when the ultimobranchial bodies fuse with the median thyroid rudiment.[61] However, several authors have found that intrathyroidal glands are primarily inferior parathyroid glands.[64,70,72] In particular, Thompson et al.[64] carefully sliced all thyroid lobectomy specimens during a one-decade period and found truly intrathyroidal glands in 3% of the cases. Because all of these glands were located in the lower third of the thyroid lobe, they were considered inferior parathyroid glands, even though recent findings have questioned whether parathyroids located in the lower third of the thyroid lobe should always be considered PIII glands by definition, but could, however, also represent excessively migrated PIVs.[71] According to Gilmour,[39] the intrathyroidal inclusion of parathyroid tissue originating from the third pharyngeal pouch may be found with the same incidence as inclusions of thymic tissue. Indeed, although the main portion of the thymus moves rapidly to its definitive position in the thorax, its tail portion becomes thin and eventually breaks into small fragments that sometimes persist embedded in the thyroid gland.

It is now accepted that intrathyroidal parathyroid glands can be either PIII or PIV and even supernumerary glands.[71-73] Preoperative[71] or even intraoperative ultrasonography[41] may be helpful in intrathyroidal gland identification when it is pathologic. Intraoperative PTH measurements after careful thyroid lobe palpation may reveal a rise in PTH levels and thus indicate a pathologic intrathyroidal gland. Generally subcapsular parathyroid adenomas, hidden just beneath the thyroid capsule, may be revealed by a localized discoloration of the surface of the thyroid parenchyma. Simple incision of the thyroid capsule at this site, which darkens progressively during the dissection, allows dislodgment of the adenoma. True intrathyroidal hyperfunctioning parathyroid glands require thyroidotomy. A plane of cleavage always exists between the thyroid and the parathyroid, so it is usually possible to enucleate the gland. Even if recent reports have indicated a lower incidence of the recurrence of hyperparathyroidism in patients undergoing thyroid lobectomy,[71] one should be reluctant to perform a blind thyroid lobectomy.[41,63,64] Nevertheless, when suspicion remains high and incision has failed to locate the lesion, thyroid lobectomy on the appropriate side is indicated.

Anomalies in Parathyroid Number: Infranumerary and Supernumerary Glands

Please see the Expert Consult website for more discussion of this topic.

Acquired Ectopic Localization

Please see the Expert Consult website for more discussion of this topic.

ACKNOWLEDGMENT

The authors would like to acknowledge and thank Dr. Anand K. Mishra for contributions to the previous edition of this chapter.

REFERENCES

For a complete list of references, go to expertconsult.com.

3

Thyroid Physiology and Thyroid Function Testing

Angela M. Leung, Gregory A. Brent

THYROID PHYSIOLOGY

Thyroid Hormone Synthesis and Regulation

The basic functional unit of the thyroid gland is the thyroid follicle. The thyroid follicle contains a single layer of thyroid follicular cells that form a sphere with a follicular lumen, which is filled with a colloid protein aggregate. Thyroid follicular cells are polar; the apical membrane is adjacent to the follicular lumen, and the basolateral membrane is the one in contact with capillaries and the circulatory system (Figure 3.1).[1] Thyroid hormone synthesis is activated by the binding of thyroid-stimulating hormone (TSH) to the TSH receptor on the basolateral membrane, which activates adenylate cyclase and increases intracellular cyclic adenosine monophosphate (cAMP). This initiates the cascade that results in thyroid hormone synthesis and secretion, which includes iodide transport, synthesis of thyroglobulin, iodination of thyroglobulin, and secretion of the thyroid hormones (see Figure 3.1).[1,2]

After the binding of TSH, the initial step in the thyroid hormone synthesis pathway is iodide transport across the basolateral membrane, mediated by the Na$^+$/I (NIS) symporter.[3] NIS is a sodium-dependent transporter, so iodine is only transported with an inward sodium gradient, which is in turn maintained by the action of the Na-K-ATPase. The transported iodide ion becomes covalently attached to the precursor thyroid hormone glycoprotein, thyroglobulin, at the interface between the apical membrane and the follicular lumen by the enzyme, thyroperoxidase (TPO). Tyrosine molecules in the thyroglobulin molecule are then iodinated to form monoiodotyrosines (MITs) and diiodotyrosines (DITs) (Figure 3.2). Incorporation of iodide into protein is referred to as *organification*. The bioactive thyroid hormones, L-thyroxine (T4) and triiodothyronine (T3), are formed by the coupling of two DITs or one DIT with one MIT, respectively, by TPO (see Figure 3.2). T4 and T3 remain attached to thyroglobulin and are stored as colloid within the follicular lumen, where they remain available for release through TSH stimulation. In healthy and iodine-sufficient individuals, the majority of thyroid hormone in colloid is stored as T4 with a small amount (~20%) stored as T3. Upon stimulation of the TSH receptor, a cytoplasmic vesicle is formed for uptake of colloid into the follicular cell through pinocytosis (see Figure 3.2). The cytoplasmic vesicles fuse with lysosomes, from which proteases hydrolyze the peptide bonds of thyroglobulin to release T4 and T3 into the cytoplasm. The thyroid hormone transporter, monocarboxylate transporter 8 (MCT8), is expressed in the thyroid gland and is important for transport of T4 and T3 out of the thyroid gland and into the circulation.[4] Production of thyroid hormone varies widely between 75 and 250 mcg daily.[5]

In the blood, approximately 99.97% of T4 and 99.7% of T3 are bound to the binding proteins, thyroxine binding globulin (TBG), transthyretin (also known as *prealbumin*), and albumin.[6] Of these, TBG has the highest affinity to bind thyroid hormone (binding approximately 75% of both T4 and T3 in circulation)[6] and is the most clinically relevant among the binding proteins. Transthyretin, previously referred to as *prealbumin*, binds approximately 20% of the circulating T4 and <5% of T3.[6] Albumin has the lowest affinity for thyroid hormone, but is the most abundant of the proteins and binds 5% of the T4 and 20% of the T3.[5] In total, most of the thyroid hormones in circulation are in the bound state and biologically inactive. The unbound thyroid hormones, free T4 and free T3, enter the target cells. In some tissues, such as those from the brain and pituitary, specific thyroid hormone membrane transporters are required for thyroid hormone uptake, principally MCT8. T3 binds with a much greater affinity to the thyroid hormone receptors and for a longer period of time, compared with T4, and is regarded as the primary active thyroid hormone.

T4 is synthesized exclusively by the thyroid gland, whereas T3 is produced primarily in peripheral tissues from the deiodination of circulating T4. Only about 20% of the daily T3 requirement is synthesized directly by the thyroid gland.[7] The activation of T4 to T3 requires the 5′-deiodinase enzymes type 1 (Dio1) and type 2 (Dio2). These enzymes are differentially expressed, with Dio1 predominantly in the liver and Dio2 in tissues that require local T3 production, such as the brain, pituitary, muscle, and brown fat. In the setting of fluctuating T4 levels, deiodinase activity is modulated to maintain normal circulating and target tissue T3 levels (Figure 3.3).[8] When serum T4 levels fall, as in hypothyroidism, Dio2 is activated locally by a deubiquitination process that reduces Dio2 degradation, increases Dio2 activity, and promotes greater conversion of T4 to the bioactive T3. Normal serum T3 levels are maintained until the serum T4 becomes very low.

Thyroid metabolism is influenced by illness and drugs. The activity of Dio1 and the resulting T3 level is reduced in malnutrition, critical illness, and by the action of certain medications (e.g., beta-blockers, ipodate, amiodarone, dexamethasone, propylthiouracil). During starvation and acute illness, expression of the 5 deiodinase type 3 (Dio3) is increased and converts the bioactive T4 and T3 to two biologically inactive molecules, reverse T3 (rT3) and 3,3′-diiodothyronine (T2).[9]

The available free T3 binds to a nuclear thyroid hormone receptor at the target tissue, alters gene expression, and regulates cellular function (Figure 3.4). The thyroid hormone nuclear receptor (THR) is a protein within a superfamily of receptors that bind steroid and steroid-like hormones such as retinoic acid, vitamin D, and estrogen. The THRs mediate the majority of biologic activities of T3. Two *THR genes*, alpha and beta, encode four THR isoforms (alpha 1, beta 1, beta 2, and beta 3). The transcriptional activity of THRs is regulated by the binding of T3, the type of thyroid hormone response elements located on the promoters of the T3 regulated gene, by the developmental- and tissue-dependent

CHAPTER 3 Thyroid Physiology and Thyroid Function Testing

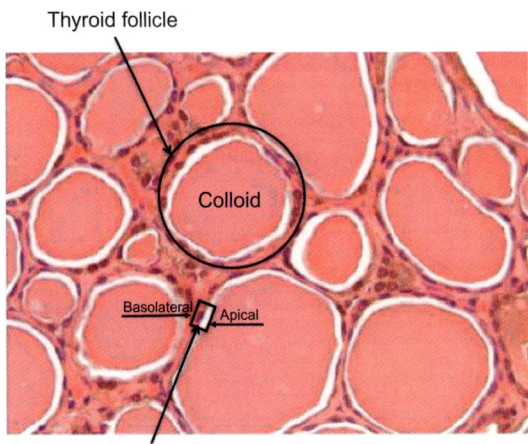

Fig. 3.1 Diagram of a Thyroid Follicular Cell. The follicular cells line the thyroid follicle, which contains colloid, consisting of thyroglobulin substrate for thyroid hormone synthesis. The follicular cell is polar, with the apical membrane in contact with colloid in the follicular lumen, and the basolateral membrane is in contact with the circulation.

expression of THR isoforms and by nuclear cofactors or coregulatory proteins.

There are also nongenomic actions of iodothyronine (T4) that are not mediated by intranuclear THR. Action at the plasma membrane is mediated by the integrin alpha-v beta 3 receptor that binds T4, and activates ERK1/2, which leads to changes in membrane ion transport, such as the $Na^{(+)}/H^{(+)}$ exchanger, and is also involved in other important cellular events such as cell proliferation.[10,11]

Thyroid Physiology During Pregnancy

Significant changes in thyroid physiology occur during pregnancy and can make the interpretation of serum thyroid function tests challenging.[12] During the first trimester of pregnancy, serum TBG concentrations increase by up to 50% as a result of altered estrogen induced glycosylation, which prolongs TBG half-life.[13] The elevated TBG levels increase the quantities of protein-bound T4 and T3, which results in an increase in total serum T4 and T3 concentrations; however, in euthyroid individuals, the active or free levels of T4 and T3 remain normal.

In addition, during the first trimester of pregnancy, levels of placental human chorionic gonadotropin (hCG) steadily increase. Because hCG is a weak TSH receptor agonist, this results in a small increase

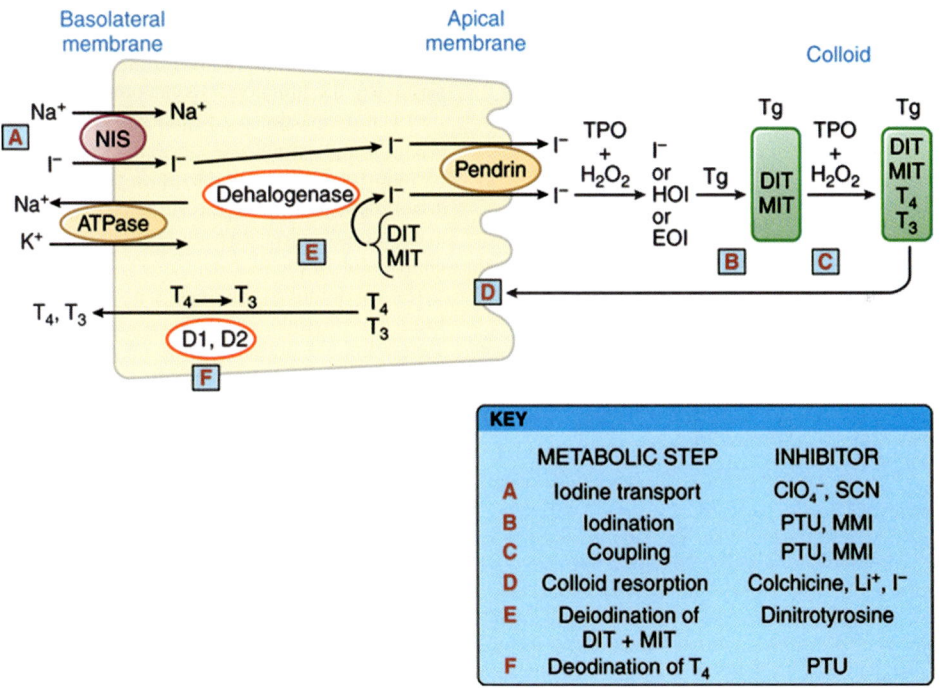

Fig. 3.2 Thyroid Hormone Synthesis in the Thyroid Follicular Cell. Thyroid hormone synthesis and secretion are activated when Thyroid stimulating hormone (TSH) binds to the TSH receptor on the basolateral membrane. Iodide is transported into the cell via the Na^+/I^- (NIS) symporter and flows down an electrical gradient, maintained by the sodium-potassium ATPase. Iodide becomes covalently attached to the tyrosyl residues of the precursor thyroid hormone glycoprotein, thyroglobulin, by thyroperoxidase (TPO) to form monoiodotyrosine (MIT) and diiodotyrosine (DIT). These are subsequently coupled by the action of TPO to form the iodothyronine hormones, tetraiodothyronine (T4) and triiodothyronine (T3). In the process of thyroid hormone secretion, Tg enters the cell by pinocytosis, forming colloid droplets. These fuse with lysosomes, forming phagolysosomes in which Tg is broken down by proteolysis, and then T4 and T3 are released and diffuse into circulation. MIT and DIT are formed by the iodination of tyrosyl amino acids on the thyroglobulin molecule. In a subsequent step, two DITs are coupled to form T4, or one DIT and one MIT are coupled to form T3. (From Brent GA, Koenig RJ. Thyroid and antithyroid drugs. In: Brunton L [ed]. *Goodman and Gilman's The Pharmacological Basis of Therapeutics*. 13th ed. New York: McGraw-Hill; 2017.)

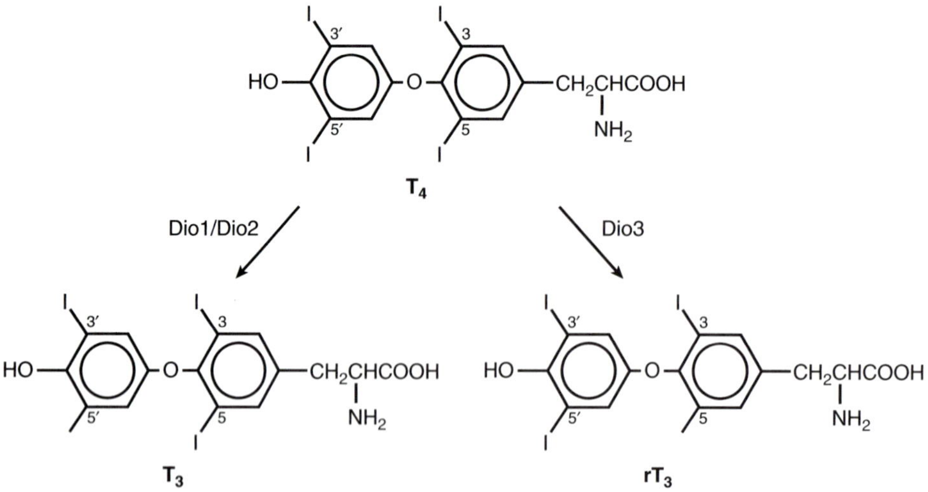

Fig. 3.3 Deiodinases. 5'deiodinases Type 1 and 2 (Dio1 and Dio2) catalyzes the removal of the 5' iodine from the outer ring of thyroxine (T4) to create the metabolically active triiodothyronine (T3). 5 deiodinase type 3 (Dio3) catalyzes the removal of iodine from the inner ring, converting T4 and T3 to metabolically inactive reverse T3.

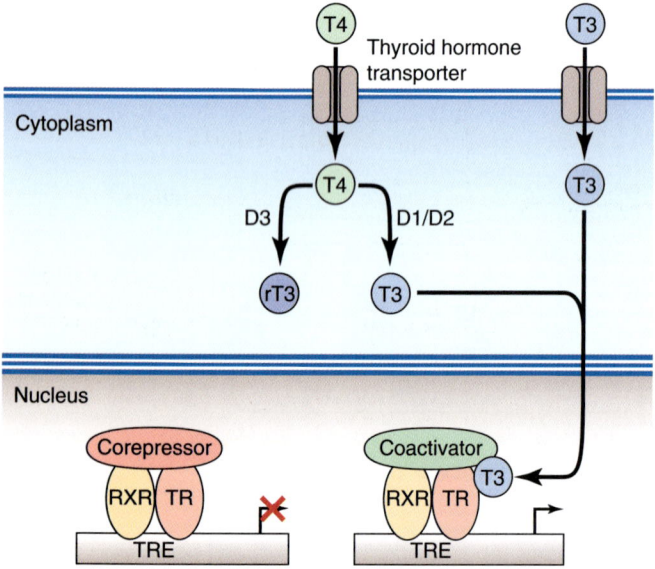

Fig. 3.4 Intracellular Action of T3. After transport of T4 and T3 into cells, T4 is converted by 5' deiodinase to the bioactive T3. After entering the nucleus, T3 binds to thyroid hormone receptors (TRs), which form dimers with the retinoid X receptor (RXR). The dimers interact with thyroid hormone response elements (TREs) in the promoter region of thyroid hormone responsive genes, initiating or inhibiting transcription and altering the production of messenger RNA (mRNA) and protein synthesis. (Redrawn from Brent GA. Mechanisms of thyroid hormone action. *J Clin Invest.* 2012;122[9]:3035–3043.)

of free T4 (although still within the normal range) and a concomitant decrease in TSH, below the lower reference range in up to 15% of normal women in the first trimester.[14] Serum TSH concentrations should thus be assessed using trimester-specific ranges during pregnancy.[15] The changes of reduced TSH and elevated FT4 are more pronounced in pregnancies associated with higher levels of hCG, such as multiple gestations and hyperemesis gravidarum, and are most extreme in hydatidiform moles.[16] The physiologic suppression of TSH does not require medical intervention and usually normalizes after the first trimester of pregnancy.

Thyroid Physiology in Nonthyroidal Illness (Euthyroid Sick Syndrome)

The evaluation of a chronically ill or hospitalized patient with abnormal serum thyroid function tests can often be challenging. Nonthyroidal illness is not considered a primary thyroid disorder, and its pathophysiology is not completely understood, although it is known that the elevation of cytokines and hypoxia plays a significant role. It is generally recommended to avoid measuring serum thyroid function tests during acute illness, unless thyroid dysfunction is thought to be a significant contributor to the illness.

Severe nonthyroidal illness is accompanied by significant alterations in thyroid physiology.[17,18] Due to the decreased availability in all of the thyroid binding proteins, serum total T4 and total T3 levels are reduced, whereas free levels are usually normal or slightly low (Figure 3.5).[19] Total T3 levels are further decreased due to reduced Dio1 activity, which converts T4 to T3. A relatively greater amount of T4 is metabolized to the inactive metabolite, reverse T3 (rT3), by Dio3, although measurement of rT3 does not reliably distinguish nonthyroidal illness from primary hypothyroidism.[20] The degree of serum rT3 elevation,[21] depressed T3/rT3 ratio,[21] and decreased FT3 and FT4 concentrations[22] have been associated with higher mortality among patients in the intensive care unit (ICU). Treatment with T4 or T3, however, does not consistently improve outcome. Whether other T4 metabolites, including 3,3'-diiodothyronine (3,3'-T2); 3,5-diiodothyronine (3,5-T2); and 3-iodothyronamine (3-T1AM), have functional roles in nonthyroidal illness remains unclear.[23]

It is important that the diagnosis of primary thyroid dysfunction is not established during severe illness based solely on an abnormal serum TSH. In nonthyroidal illness, serum TSH concentrations may be low, normal, or high,[18,24] due to the TSH-lowering effects of commonly used medications (glucocorticoids, dopamine) in patients managed for a nonthyroidal illness or from a reversible form of acquired central hypothyroidism in severe nonthyroidal illness.[25,26] During the recovery phase, the TSH may briefly rise above the upper reference range, as suppression of TSH lessens, before it normalizes.[18] When possible, thyroid evaluation after recovery from an acute illness is recommended in patients suspected of having intrinsic thyroid disease.

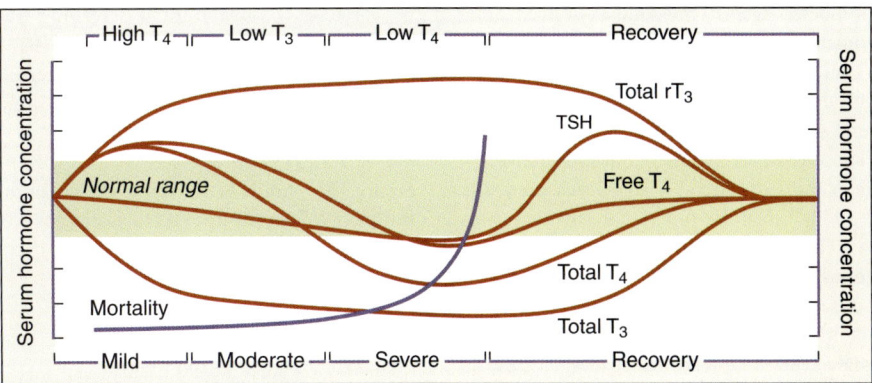

Fig. 3.5 Alternations in Serum Thyroid Hormone Concentrations During Acute Nonthyroidal Illness and Recovery. The degree of change in hormone concentrations relates to the severity and duration of the illness. Thyroid-stimulating hormone (TSH) may also be suppressed during severe illness and transiently rise moderately above the reference range before returning to normal with recovery. Mortality correlates inversely with the degree of reduction in total T4 concentration. (From Farwell AF. Sick euthyroid syndrome in the intensive care unit. In: Irwin RS, Rippe JM, eds. *Intensive Care Medicine*. 5th ed. Philadelphia: Lippincott Williams & Wilkins; 2003.)

DIAGNOSTIC THYROID TESTING

Serum TSH

TSH is produced from the pituitary after stimulation by thyrotropin-releasing hormone (TRH), a modified three-amino acid peptide produced by neurons of the paraventricular nucleus in the hypothalamus. TRH signaling from the hypothalamus is achieved through a portal venous system located in the infundibulum of the pituitary stalk, which allows communication to the pituitary. Both TRH and TSH gene expression are decreased by excess thyroid hormone levels via negative feedback mechanisms (Figure 3.6). Both the hypothalamus and pituitary have high levels of Dio2, so T4 levels are the primary feedback. T4 is converted locally to T3, which suppresses TRH and TSH gene expression.

Pituitary TSH is secreted in a pulsatile manner—higher levels at night and lower levels during the day, the inverse of the cortisol cycle.[27] Although pulse frequency is increased nocturnally to result in a diurnal variation of TSH concentrations, levels remain within the reference range.[28] Generally, laboratory testing of serum TSH concentrations during daylight hours is not substantially affected by the diurnal variation of TSH secretion, but results outside the reference range may occur in euthyroid individuals when drawn outside of these times.

TSH stimulates the synthesis and release of thyroid hormone from the thyroid gland. TSH production from the anterior pituitary is inverse log-linearly regulated by serum thyroid hormone concentrations; when there are small decreases in thyroid hormone levels in circulation, large increases in serum TSH stimulate thyroid hormone production by the thyroid gland. This negative feedback loop between serum TSH and the serum-free thyroid hormones is able to maintain circulating thyroid levels within a tight range.

Serum TSH is the preferred screening test in the evaluation of thyroid function in the ambulatory patient, regardless of whether the patient is taking thyroid hormone replacement medication.[29,30] For the healthy patient in an ambulatory setting, the diagnosis of hypothyroidism or hyperthyroidism may be determined with approximately 98% sensitivity and 92% specificity using serum TSH.[31] In addition, TSH has a narrow intraindividual variability of ± 0.5 mIU/L,[32] such that thyroid dysfunction may be present if there are significant changes in TSH values over time in an individual, even if they remain within the reference range. In certain situations, however, such as known or suspected pituitary or hypothalamic dysfunction, recent hyperthyroidism,

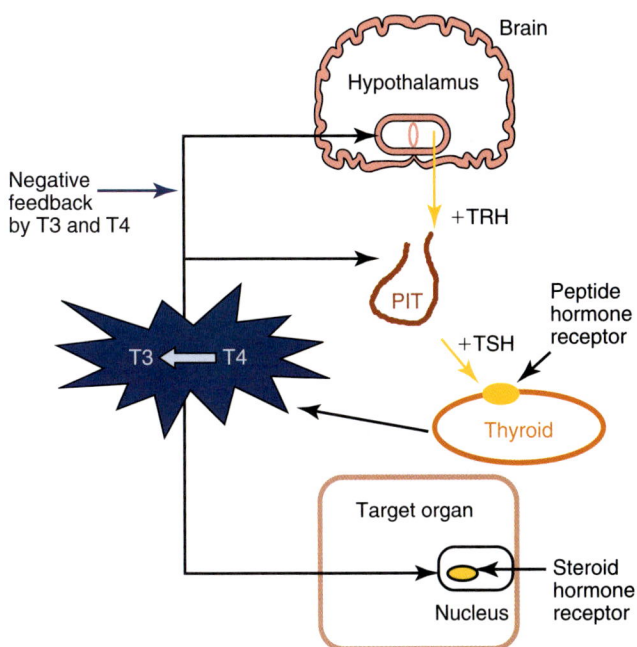

Fig. 3.6 Schematic Representation of Control of Thyroid-Stimulating Hormone (TSH) Secretion by the Thyrotroph Cells in the Anterior Pituitary. High concentrations of T3 suppress TSH release, and low concentrations enhance the expression of TSH. Thyrotropin-releasing hormone (TRH) also stimulates TSH release, and its absence results in failure of the thyrotroph to release TSH, resulting in hypothyroidism. TRH is secreted by cells in the paraventricular nuclei in the hypothalamus and reaches the anterior pituitary via the hypothalamic hypophyseal portal venous system. TSH travels through the circulatory system to stimulate the thyroid and to produce thyroid hormones T4 and T3. By negative feedback inhibition, the circulating thyroid hormones suppress the production and excretion of TRH and TSH to bring the system back into equilibrium to maintain tight control over circulating thyroid hormone levels.

critical illness, starvation, use of certain medications (dopamine or high-dose glucocorticoids), interference with serum thyroid autoantibodies, and thyroid hormone resistance syndromes, the TSH level is inaccurate for the thyroidal status and should not be used in isolation to determine thyroid function.[33] In addition, the presence of interfering heterophile antibodies (antibodies against the animal-derived antibodies used in the immunometric assay) may rarely cause abnormally high or low TSH levels.[34] These conditions should be suspected when the pattern of the TSH levels does not correlate to the clinical presentation or when the peripheral serum hormone levels do not change as expected with elevated or suppressed serum TSH concentrations.

Serum TSH assays have evolved considerably since measurements were first described in the 1960s, when the functional sensitivity was between 1 and 2 mIU/L.[35] The commonly used second-generation TSH assays have an improved functional lower limit of 0.10 to 0.20 mIU/L,[36] which is able to differentiate between euthyroid and hyperthyroid states but does not indicate the degree of hyperthyroidism. In contrast, a third-generation TSH assay can detect levels as low as 0.01 to 0.02 mIU/L and is helpful when there is a challenging pattern of serum thyroid function tests that include an extremely suppressed TSH. In the rare instance they are needed, fourth-generation immuno-chemiluminometric assays are capable of detecting TSH levels in the range of 0.01 to 0.001 mIU/L.[37]

A serum TSH level measured in an ambulatory population that lies within the reference range is generally considered evidence of normal thyroid function and requires no additional testing[29] (Figures 3.7 and 3.8). Reference ranges for serum TSH can vary slightly from one commercial laboratory to another. It should be noted that normal ranges, which are based on the epidemiologic distribution of serum TSH concentrations in healthy populations, from which serum thyroid autoantibody positivity and iodine status (both of which can affect TSH), may

be variable. If an abnormal screening TSH result is encountered, the circulating thyroid hormone levels should be assessed (see Figures 3.7 and 3.8). The specific pattern of tests will allow further insight into whether clinical thyroid dysfunction should be suspected.

Serum Thyroid Hormones

Serum TSH should be the initial choice for the screening of thyroid dysfunction. When the TSH alone is not believed to be sufficient for diagnosis, as in the examples proposed earlier, serum thyroid hormone levels should be assessed.[29]

Serum Total T4 and Total T3

Serum total T4 (TT4) and total T3 (TT3) concentrations are a measure of both the bound and free hormone levels of these two hormones. TT4 or TT3 levels should be interpreted in the context of the clinical situation, because many clinical conditions and medications alter the concentrations of thyroid hormone binding proteins and/or compete with the binding of thyroid hormones to the binding proteins. As such, measured TT4 and TT3 levels may be affected, even though the bioactive free levels and thus, the thyroidal status, remain unchanged.

T3 is the active thyroid hormone and is primarily useful in the diagnosis and management of patients with hyperthyroidism[38] and occasionally, to differentiate Graves' disease (TT3/TT4 ratio >20) from subacute thyroiditis (TT3/TT4 ratio <12).[39,40] Measurement of serum TT3 is not usually helpful if hypothyroidism is suspected because the activity of Dio2, which converts T4 to the biologically active T3,

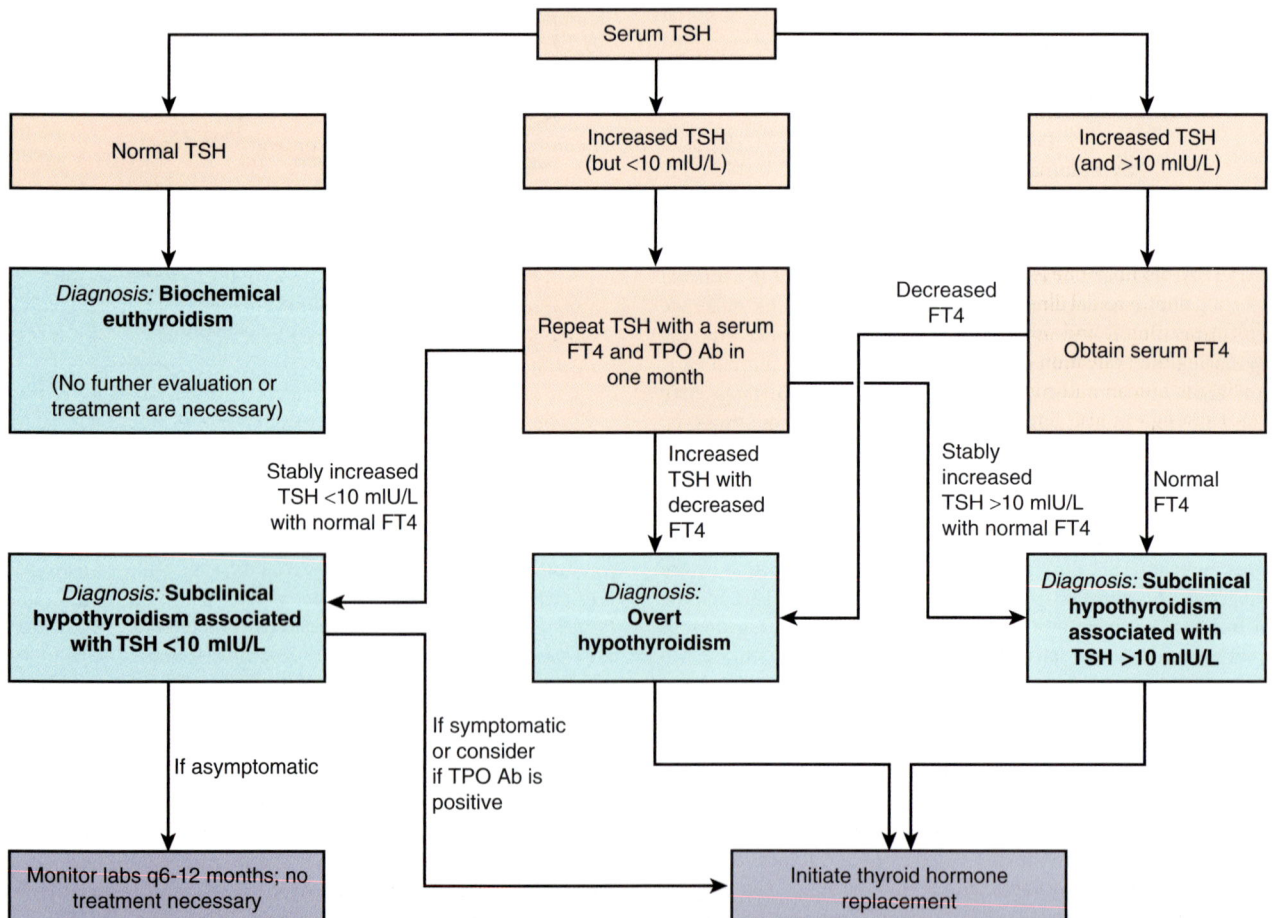

Fig. 3.7 Evaluation and Management of Hypothyroidism in Individuals With Corresponding Signs and Symptoms.

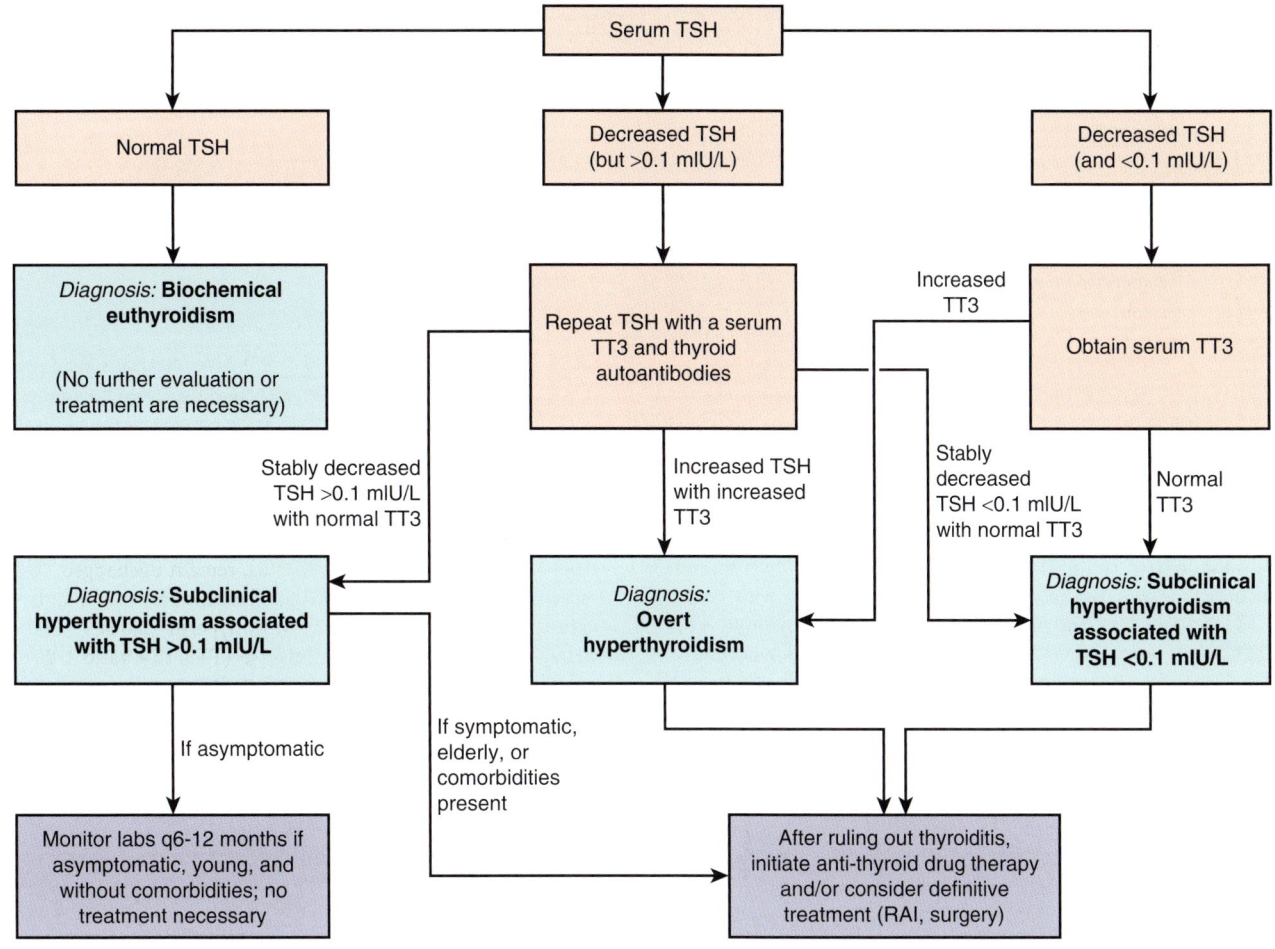

Fig. 3.8 Evaluation and Management of Hyperthyroidism in Individuals with Corresponding Signs and Symptoms.

increases while serum T4 falls, thus maintaining normal T3 levels until the overall thyroid hormone levels are very low. rT3, which may be elevated during nonthyroidal illness, is not biologically active. As such, the utility of measuring it and other forms of inactive iodothyronine are limited during the evaluation of thyroid status.

Finally, the human anti-mouse antibodies (HAMAs) that interfere with TSH testing can also interfere with the thyroid hormone assays. HAMA positivity may result in artificially elevated or reduced TT4, TT3, FT4, and FT3 levels.[41] Patients who have received therapeutic monoclonal antibody treatment may be at increased risk of develop interfering positive HAMA titers.[42]

Serum Free T4

Bioactive free T4 concentrations can be estimated using a variety of indirect (analog, immunometric, and two-step labeled hormone assays) or direct methods (equilibrium dialysis, ultrafiltration), and are the most commonly used measurements of circulating thyroid hormone levels.[43]

Generally, most laboratories estimate free T4 by either the analog immunoassay or a calculated FT4I corrected to thyroid hormone binding capacity. The former is readily available and provides quick results; it does not directly measure the free T4 concentration but is a reliable estimate of FT4 levels in most patients, based on one-step, two-step, or labeled antibody approaches.[37] This type of free T4 estimate is especially sensitive to abnormal serum albumin levels and should not be used with conditions such as familial dysalbuminemic hyperthyroxinemia,[44] pregnancy,[45] or severe nonthyroidal illness.[46] For example, it is common to have a free T4 lower than the reference range in a euthyroid pregnant woman due to the high estrogen state of pregnancy greatly increasing serum TBG concentrations, thus resulting in inaccurate FT4 measurements.

The serum FT4I measurement is a calculated value that is the product of the total T4 concentrations and a correction factor related to the number of available thyroid hormone binding sites (Table 3.1). This correction factor may be called a thyroid hormone binding ratio (THBR), T3 resin uptake (T3RU), or T3 uptake (T3U).[30] The T3RU is inversely related to the free thyroid hormone binding sites but is now used in only a few laboratories.

Free T4 by equilibrium dialysis is the gold standard and measures the 0.03% of T4 that is biologically active and unbound to protein. This assay is available only at reference laboratories and is useful to directly determine free T4 levels when other testing does not provide a clear result.

Serum Thyroid Autoantibodies

Hyperthyroidism and hypothyroidism are often the result of autoimmune diseases, in which immunoglobulin G (IgG) antibodies, such as thyroid peroxidase (TPO Ab, previously known as *antimicrosomal antibodies*), thyroglobulin (Tg Ab), and the TSH receptor (TSHR Ab), are formed against thyroid proteins.[47]

More than 90% of patients with autoimmune thyroid disease (Hashimoto's thyroiditis and Graves' disease) will have elevated titers

TABLE 3.1 Serum Thyroid Function Test and Antibody Patterns in Thyroid Disease

Clinical Condition	Free Thyroxine	Free T3	TSH	Thyroid Autoantibodies
Subclinical hypothyroidism	Normal	Normal	Mildly elevated, usual range of 5-10 mIU/L	Can be TPO positive or negative
Hypothyroidism due to Hashimoto's disease	Low	Normal or low	Elevated, usually > 10 mIU/L	Usually TPO positive
Central hypothyroidism	Low	Normal or low	"Inappropriately" normal or low	Negative
Subclinical hyperthyroidism	Normal	Normal	Low	TRAb or TSI may be positive
Hyperthyroidism due to Graves' disease	Elevated	Elevated	Low	TRAb or TSI positive
TSH-secreting pituitary adenoma	Elevated	Elevated	"Inappropriately" normal or elevated	Negative
Thyroid hormone resistance due to mutation of thyroid hormone receptor beta	Elevated	Elevated	"Inappropriately" normal or elevated	Negative

TSH, thyroid-stimulating hormone, TPO-antithyroperoxidase antibody, TRAb-TSH receptor antibody, TSI-thyroid stimulating immunoglobulin

of second-generation assays for TPO Ab and Tg Ab.[48,49] When biochemical hypothyroidism is found, measuring TPO Ab can be helpful, because its result can provide additional information regarding the etiology of the thyroid dysfunction. Median serum TSH concentrations are increased within the reference range among those with serum TPO Ab and Tg Ab positivity, compared with those without TPO Ab titers,[47] and are a predictor for the development of biochemical thyroid dysfunction in euthyroid individuals.[2,50] In individuals with subclinical hypothyroidism, both serum TPO Ab positivity and sonographic characteristics suggestive of chronic thyroiditis are associated with an increased likelihood of progression to overt hypothyroidism.[51,52]

The TSHR Abs are a group of immunoglobulins that produce Graves' hyperthyroidism, measured as TSH receptor binding, TRAB (TSH-receptor antibody) or in a functional bioassay, thyroid stimulating immunoglobulin (TSI). TSH receptor antibodies are being increasingly recommended for monitoring activity of disease to assess response to therapy in Graves' patients. Less commonly, TSH receptor binding antibodies can block the TSH receptor and produce hypothyroidism. In the setting of normal serum thyroid function, thyroid antibodies should generally not be measured except in special circumstances, such as a history of hyperthyroidism during pregnancy or recurrent miscarriages.[15] In these situations, both the stimulating and inhibiting TSHR Abs can cross the placenta to affect fetal thyroid function and potentially induce fetal goiter. Although serum thyroid antibody positivity during pregnancy is associated with a higher risk of postpartum subacute thyroiditis, antibody screening in pregnant women is not currently recommended.[15]

Serum Thyroglobulin

Thyroglobulin (Tg) is a large glycoprotein that is stored as colloid, the primary storage form of thyroid hormone, in the lumen of thyroid follicles. It is continuously secreted into circulation from the thyroid gland, thereby reflecting the mass of normal and malignant thyroid tissue. Higher serum concentrations result from TSH stimulation and/or injury of thyroid tissue. However, for the individual with an intact thyroid gland, its clinical value for evaluating thyroid dysfunction or goiter is limited in the era of modern serum thyroid function testing and imaging. However, the demonstration of a suppressed serum Tg level in such a patient can be useful in differentiating factitious thyrotoxicosis (from exogenous thyroid hormone ingestion) from excessive endogenous thyroid hormone release of any etiology.[53] In this situation, when thyrotoxicosis is due to ingestion of exogenous thyroid hormone, normal thyroid hormone production is suppressed and serum Tg levels are decreased. In contrast, if excess thyroid hormone is produced from the thyroid, serum Tg levels are elevated.

In current clinical practice, the primary use of serum Tg concentrations is as a tumor marker in patients with differentiated thyroid cancer that is obtained to detect persistent and/or recurrent disease after a total thyroidectomy and radioactive iodine (^{131}I) ablation.[54] Most Tg assays have only first-generation functional sensitivity between 0.5 and 1 ng/mL, but the second generation Tg assays are rapidly becoming the standard and have an improved functional sensitivity of 0.05 to 0.1 ng/mL.[55] The Tg assay can be made more sensitive to detect persistent or recurrent tumor after stimulation by TSH, either endogenously by withholding thyroxine treatment in an athyreotic patient or with administration of recombinant human TSH (rhTSH), the latter of which results in an approximate tenfold increase in basal serum Tg concentrations.[56]

Detection of persistent and/or recurrent disease in thyroid cancer depends on the performance of Tg immunometric assays, which currently have suboptimal sensitivity and high interassay variability. Virtually all immunometric methods will report an undetectable Tg level in euthyroid Tg Ab positive controls,[57] and approximately 25% of patients with differentiated thyroid cancer have a positive serum TgAb titer.[58] Thus when a suspicious lymph node or neck mass is detected in an individual who has undergone a total thyroidectomy, an unmeasurable basal or rhTSH-stimulated Tg in the setting of a positive serum TgAb level does not necessarily exclude thyroid cancer recurrence.[55] It is reasonable in this relatively uncommon situation to measure Tg instead by Tg Ab-resistant radioimmunoassay (RIA)[59] or liquid chromatography tandem mass spectrometry, which are available at some specialty endocrine laboratories.

When the serum Tg Ab titer is positive, it may also be used as a surrogate marker of tumor persistence/recurrence.[58] In one study, a >50% decrease of Tg Ab levels within the first year after a total thyroidectomy was associated with the absence of tumor recurrence/persistence in all patients studied, and tumor recurrence/persistence was present in 37% of patients who had any rise of serum Tg Ab within the same period.[60] Thus thyroid cancer patients with rising Tg antibody levels are at high risk for disease persistence/recurrence and should be evaluated promptly. In addition, the sensitivities and absolute values reported by different methods of measuring Tg and TgAb are highly variable. It is essential to always use the same Tg and TgAb method when following an individual over time for tumor persistence/recurrence.[58]

Finally, the presence of interfering heterophile antibodies (antibodies against the animal-derived antibodies used in the immunometric assay) may rarely result in abnormally high or low serum Tg levels.[61] The most common interfering antibodies are HAMAs, which were discussed earlier. Clinically, this should be suspected when an elevated serum Tg level is inappropriate for the clinical situation and does not increase with rhTSH stimulation. When heterophile antibody is suspected, the clinician should repeat the test using a commercially available heterophile-blocking tube (HBT) or measure Tg with an RIA assay.[61]

Thyroid Imaging

Thyroid gland imaging studies with radionuclides provide both structural and functional information and can be very useful in determining the etiology of biochemical hyperthyroidism. In contrast, thyroidal nuclear imaging is not recommended in the evaluation of a patient with hypothyroidism. For nuclear imaging, scans using radioactive iodine isotopes are most preferred, because these directly reflect the active accumulation (trapping) of iodine by the thyroid follicular cell and covalent attachment (organification) of iodine to thyroglobulin.

The preferred radionuclide for diagnostic nonthyroid cancer imaging is ^{123}I, because this isotope emits only gamma rays that pass through tissue without significant cellular damage. In contrast, ^{131}I emits both gamma rays for imaging, as well as damaging beta particles, and is thus used for the treatment of hyperthyroidism and thyroid cancer to destroy iodine-avid thyroid tissue. For diagnostic imaging, ^{123}I is administered orally with the measurement of iodine uptake and gamma scintigraphy images obtained 4 and/or 24 hours later. Measured thyroidal uptake depends on the activity of NIS and overall iodine status as determined by the amount of circulating nonradioactive iodine. When there is an excess of nonradioactive iodine, the measured radioactive iodine uptake is reduced due to the competition between radioactive and nonradioactive iodine uptake by the thyroid follicular cells. Sources of excess nonradioactive iodine include kelp, seaweed, seafood, iodine-rich medications and agents (amiodarone, saturated solution of potassium iodide [SSKI], Lugol's solution, povidone iodine, tincture of iodine, iodoform gauze), and radiographic contrast media used commonly in computed tomography (CT) scans and gallbladder studies.

An alternate radionuclide is technetium^{99m} pertechnetate (^{99m}Tc), which is administered intravenously. Images are obtained much more rapidly than ^{123}I, usually on the order of 30 to 60 minutes after the administration of the radionuclide tracer. Although ^{99m}Tc will be trapped by the thyroid follicular cells, there is no iodine moiety for attachment to thyroglobulin, and therefore does not as accurately mimic the thyroidal uptake of iodine as radioiodine nuclides. Thus ^{123}I thyroid scans have 5% to 8% fewer false negative results than ^{99m}Tc scans.[62,63] However, because ^{99m}Tc scans are easier, faster, more readily available and less expensive to perform, they have largely replaced ^{123}I scans at some institutions. Studies of direct comparison of radioiodine and ^{99m}Tc thyroid scans have been highly concordant in patients without nodules and in those with cold nodules. One study reported that of 273 patients with thyroid nodules, only two had increased uptake with pertechnetate and no uptake with radioiodine.[63] However, if the results of the ^{99m}Tc scan are not in agreement with the clinical picture, an ^{123}I scan should be performed.

Although nuclear scans are useful in the differential diagnosis of biochemical hyperthyroidism, other radiologic modalities (e.g., ultrasonography, CT, and magnetic resonance imaging [MRI]) provide information regarding structural anatomy of the thyroid and provide no functional data. The primary role of thyroid ultrasound is in the initial evaluation of thyroid nodules, as recommended by the American Thyroid Association[54] and the American Association of Clinical Endocrinologists.[64] Although thyroid ultrasound does not have a role in the initial evaluation of biochemical thyroid dysfunction, it may demonstrate changes that are consistent but are not necessarily diagnostic of chronic lymphocytic thyroiditis, subacute granulomatous thyroiditis, and postpartum thyroiditis.[65-67] Some individuals with subclinical hypothyroidism and sonographic features suggestive of chronic thyroiditis are at significant risk for developing overt hypothyroidism requiring thyroid hormone replacement therapy.[52]

EVALUATION OF HYPOTHYROIDISM

Signs and Symptoms of Hypothyroidism

Commons signs and symptoms of hypothyroidism (Box 3.1) are mostly nonspecific, and some patients may not display any signs or symptoms. Symptoms may be insidious, and in the elderly and middle-aged women, nonspecific complaints may be interpreted as signs of normal aging or depression. Symptoms of hypothyroidism depend on the degree and duration of the disease but most frequently include weight gain, fatigue, constipation, and menstrual irregularities/infertility.

Etiologies of Hypothyroidism

The most common etiologies of decreased serum thyroid hormone concentrations are those associated with primary hypothyroidism, which is defined as underproduction of thyroid hormone at the thyroid gland (Box 3.2). Excluding postsurgical and postablative hypothyroidism, the most common cause of adult hypothyroidism worldwide is Hashimoto's thyroiditis. Causes of hypothyroidism associated with secondary and tertiary disease (when hypothyroidism arises from pituitary and hypothalamic insults, respectively) are much less common.

It is important that hypothyroidism arising from Hashimoto's thyroiditis be distinguished from transient forms of hypothyroidism, such as excess iodine exposure and the hypothyroid phase of subacute thyroiditis. Hypothyroidism arising from Hashimoto's thyroiditis is an indication for lifelong thyroid hormone replacement, but the transient forms of hypothyroidism may not necessarily require this. The most common forms of subacute thyroiditis are postpartum thyroiditis, painful subacute thyroiditis, and painless subacute or silent thyroiditis. All forms of subacute thyroiditis are characterized by the triphasic

---

BOX 3.1 Signs and Symptoms of Hypothyroidism

General
Weight gain
Fatigue
Cold intolerance
Hyponatremia
Hypothermia

Skin
Dry and coarse skin
Dry and coarse hair
Pretibial myxedema (nonpitting edema)
Hair loss

Head and Neck
Hoarse voice
Enlarged tongue
Periorbital edema
Goiter

Gastrointestinal
Constipation

Musculoskeletal
Myalgia

Muscle cramps
Carpal tunnel syndrome
Elevation of serum creatine phosphokinase

Nervous System
Depression
Impaired concentration
Dementia

Cardiovascular
Bradycardia
Diastolic hypertension
Hyperlipidemia
Pericardial effusion
Congestive heart failure

Reproductive
Irregular menstrual periods
Amenorrhea
Galactorrhea if accompanied by elevated serum prolactin levels
Infertility
Miscarriage

> **BOX 3.2 Etiologies of Hypothyroidism**
>
> Hashimoto's thyroiditis (also known as chronic lymphocytic thyroiditis)
> Hypothyroid phase of painful subacute thyroiditis (also known as pseudogranulomatous or De Quervain's thyroiditis)
> Hypothyroid phase of painless lymphocytic thyroiditis
> Hypothyroid phase of postpartum thyroiditis
> Radioactive iodine ablation
> Thyroidectomy
> Head and neck radiation
> Drugs: lithium, amiodarone, interleukin, interferon, propylthiouracil/methimazole, iodine excess in patients with thyroiditis
> Iodine deficiency
> Biosynthetic defects (rare and would usually present in childhood)
> Congenital hypothyroidism (rare and would usually present in childhood)
> Pituitary dysfunction (pituitary damage from tumor, surgery, and/or radiation)
> Hypothalamic damage from tumor or radiation

pattern of transient thyrotoxicosis (i.e., 1 to 3 months), followed by transient hypothyroidism (i.e., lasting up to 6 months), with the eventual return to the euthyroid state, although not all patients will experience all phases.[68] Postpartum thyroiditis occurs in the few months after a miscarriage, therapeutic abortion, or delivery. Subacute painful thyroiditis is associated with an enlarged and tender thyroid gland and variably presents with flulike symptoms, high fever, myalgia, and a high serum erythrocyte sedimentation rate (ESR). Painless or silent lymphocytic subacute thyroiditis is associated with an enlarged thyroid gland. All three types of subacute thyroiditis can be diagnosed by a very low radioactive iodine uptake (see section on Thyroid Imaging in Hyperthyroidism). In most cases, the hypothyroid phase of subacute thyroiditis does not require treatment with thyroid hormone replacement unless the patient is symptomatic or the hypothyroidism is biochemically severe.

Thyroid Function Testing in Hypothyroidism

The initial test recommended in the evaluation of hypothyroidism is a serum TSH concentration if the patient has any of the signs or symptoms shown in Box 3.1 or any of the risk factors shown in Box 3.3. The measurement of a TSH is a very sensitive and specific method to diagnose hypothyroidism. It is almost always elevated in primary hypothyroidism, and the TSH rise occurs before the decreases of serum T4 and/or T3 levels. However, measurement of TSH is not a good initial test for secondary hypothyroidism and thus should not be used to assess the thyroid status of a patient with known or suspected hypothalamic or pituitary disease, or in severe nonthyroidal illness. Serum TSH is also difficult to use when thyroid hormone levels are in flux. If thyroid hormone replacement is not initiated after thyroidectomy, TSH rises to >30 mIU/L within 22 days in 95% of individuals.[69]

An algorithm for the evaluation of hypothyroidism in an individual with signs and/or symptoms suggestive of the disease is presented in Figure 3.7. If the serum TSH is within the normal range, the patient is biochemically euthyroid and no further evaluation is necessary. If the TSH is >10 mIU/L, thyroid hormone replacement should be initiated. An exception is during recovery from an acute illness or in subacute thyroiditis, when the TSH may be transiently elevated before its normalization. If the TSH is elevated above the reference range but still <10 mIU/L, it is recommended that the TSH with an estimate of free T4 and a serum TPO Ab level be repeated in 1 month. If the TSH is elevated on repeat assessment and the free T4 (or FT4I) is decreased, it is recommended to start thyroid hormone replacement therapy for the treatment of overt hypothyroidism. Measurement of total or free T3 levels is not indicated in the evaluation of hypothyroidism, because T3 levels are maintained within the reference range in mild to moderate hypothyroidism due to increased conversion of T4 to T3 via the increased activity of 5'deiodinase.

Subclinical Hypothyroidism

Subclinical hypothyroidism is defined as an elevated serum TSH concentration with a normal measure of free T4 (either as FT4 or FT4I). Of the U.S. population over age 80 years, approximately 15% have a serum TSH level >4.5 mIU/L, particularly among those with serum thyroid antibody positivity.[70] The optimal management of subclinical hypothyroidism has been a matter of controversy.[71] Because the TSH will normalize in approximately one-third of adults over a 3- to 4-year period,[52] it is important to identify those who will have persistent disease and/or those who may benefit from thyroid hormone replacement.

Some small, well-controlled studies have suggested a benefit toward improved well-being and a reduction in cholesterol levels in subclinically hypothyroid individuals treated with thyroid hormone.[72] The benefit of reducing cardiovascular risk is primarily seen in middle-aged patients, with less improvement among older patients. In general, the decision to treat patients with subclinical hypothyroidism depends on the presence of signs or symptoms of hypothyroidism, or the increased risk of progression to overt hypothyroidism, as indicated by a positive risk factor, such as sonographic evidence of thyroiditis, elevated serum antithyroid antibody titers, and the presence of other high-risk conditions such as cardiovascular disease, pregnancy, or infertility.

If the individual is asymptomatic, the most conservative approach is to follow the patient clinically and repeat the TSH in 6 to 12 months or earlier as directed by signs or symptoms (see Figure 3.7). It would also be reasonable to obtain additional data to determine the risk of progression to overt hypothyroidism, including inquiring about a family history of autoimmune thyroid disease, performing a thyroid ultrasound to assess for thyroiditis, and obtaining a serum TPO Ab titer. In one study, women with mild subclinical hypothyroidism and serum thyroid autoimmunity followed for 4 years had a 5%/year risk of developing biochemical hypothyroidism.[73]

Serum Thyroid Antibodies in Hypothyroidism

Measurement of serum antithyroid antibodies in the differential diagnosis of primary hypothyroidism should be interpreted in the context of the clinical findings. TPO Ab or TgAb is positive in most patients with autoimmune thyroiditis (Hashimoto's thyroiditis), and is not required but confirms the diagnosis, and those with high titers are likely to progress more rapidly to overt hypothyroidism. Elevated serum TPO Ab and TgAb can be detected after the release of thyroid antigens in patients with silent subacute thyroiditis, such as postpartum thyroiditis.

> **BOX 3.3 Risk Factors for Hypothyroidism**
>
> Older age
> Family history of autoimmune disease, including thyroiditis
> Infertility and miscarriage
> History of thyroid disease
> Goiter
> Other autoimmune disease (type 1 diabetes mellitus, rheumatoid arthritis, vitiligo, Addison's disease, pernicious anemia)
> History of head and neck radiation
> Drugs: lithium, amiodarone, kelp supplements, iodine-containing expectorants

Thyroid Imaging in Hypothyroidism

Thyroid ultrasound in Hashimoto's demonstrates a characteristic irregular texture and is often associated with diffuse enlargement. Blood flow, as assessed by Doppler, is reduced in subacute thyroiditis, but it is difficult to distinguish reduced flow from normal.[74] Radionuclide imaging of the thyroid is almost never helpful for the diagnosis of hypothyroidism. Thus thyroid ultrasound and/or radionuclide imaging should be performed only to evaluate suspicious structural abnormalities, such as a palpable thyroid nodule in the hypothyroid patient. Although controversial, there is an epidemiologic association of concurrently elevated serum TSH concentrations in thyroiditis with an increased risk of thyroid malignancy. It has been suggested that clinicians use sonography to evaluate patients with thyroiditis, Hashimoto's thyroiditis, and Graves' disease to detect thyroid nodules, which would then require biopsy based on ultrasound features.[75,76]

Treatment of Hypothyroidism

Hypothyroidism is treated with thyroid hormone replacement, usually in the form of oral T4 (levothyroxine). In individuals with little or no endogenous thyroid hormone production, the usual requirement is 1.6 mcg/kg/day.[77] Because 80% of circulating T3 is derived from T4, T4 monotherapy is adequate in most patients for thyroid hormone replacement. Some patients, however, have persistent symptoms of hypothyroidism while on biochemically adequate levothyroxine replacement and prefer the use of T4/T3 combined products, such as desiccated thyroid.[78] The American Thyroid Association guidelines state that there is a lack of high-quality controlled long-term outcome data to routinely support the use of desiccated thyroid extract, combination synthetic T4/T3, or T3 monotherapy over levothyroxine therapy.[79]

In patients with primary hypothyroidism, levothyroxine dose adjustments should be done based on a serum TSH measured 4 to 6 weeks after initiating the medication, due to the long half-life of levothyroxine, which is 7 to 10 days. The goal of treatment is a serum TSH level around the middle of the normal range for otherwise healthy individuals with primary hypothyroidism, and a suppressed TSH or a TSH level at the low end of the normal range is targeted for most patients with differentiated thyroid cancer.[54]

EVALUATION OF HYPERTHYROIDISM

Signs and Symptoms of Hyperthyroidism

Common signs and symptoms of hyperthyroidism include weight loss, heat intolerance, tremors, palpitations, anxiety, menstrual abnormalities, and atrial fibrillation (Box 3.4). Older patients with hyperthyroidism may have more cardiac symptoms but less systemic manifestations of hyperthyroidism.

Etiologies of Hyperthyroidism

Elevated levels of bioactive free thyroid hormones (hyperthyroidism) are almost always associated with suppressed serum TSH concentrations. In iodine-sufficient regions, the most common cause of hyperthyroidism is Graves' disease,[4] an autoimmune disease resulting from elevated serum thyroid-stimulating antibodies. Other common causes of hyperthyroidism include toxic multinodular goiter (MNG), toxic adenoma, and the thyrotoxic phase of subacute thyroiditis (Box 3.5). Because the diagnosis and management of hyperthyroidism is relatively more complex than for hypothyroidism, it would be beneficial to refer patients with hyperthyroidism to an endocrinologist.

If biochemical hyperthyroidism is confirmed, the etiology of the hyperthyroidism should be determined before initiating treatment.

BOX 3.4 Signs and Symptoms of Hyperthyroidism

General
Weight loss
Heat intolerance
Anxiety/nervousness
Insomnia
Muscle weakness

Cardiovascular
Tachycardia
Palpitations
Dyspnea on exertion
Bounding pulses
Atrial fibrillation

Head and Neck
Ophthalmopathy (in Graves' disease only)
Goiter

Skin
Excess perspiration
Palmer erythema

Nervous System
Tremor
Anxiety/nervousness
Hyperkinesis

Gastrointestinal
Frequent stools/diarrhea

Reproductive
Irregular menstrual periods/amenorrhea
Light menstrual flow
Infertility
Gynecomastia (males)

BOX 3.5 Etiologies of Hyperthyroidism

Graves' disease
Toxic multinodular goiter
Toxic adenoma
Thyrotoxic phase of painful subacute thyroiditis (also known as pseudogranulomatous or De Quervain's thyroiditis)
Thyrotoxic phase of painless lymphocytic thyroiditis
Thyrotoxic phase of postpartum thyroiditis
Excessive ingestion of thyroid hormone
Metastatic thyroid carcinoma
Struma ovarii
Iodine-induced thyrotoxicosis
TSH-producing pituitary adenoma
Thyroid hormone resistance syndromes

Clinical data may suffice to distinguish between Graves' disease and other etiologies of hyperthyroidism, because a patient with a diffuse goiter, exophthalmos, and biochemical hyperthyroidism requires no further laboratory studies for the diagnosis of Graves' disease. Often, however, exophthalmos is not present and the goiter may not be evident, especially in older patients who may not have classic symptoms. If the etiology of the hyperthyroidism is unclear, a radionuclide thyroid scan and uptake will be helpful in making the diagnosis. In addition, measurement of serum Tg may help differentiate factitious thyrotoxicosis from hyperthyroidism of other etiologies, because thyrotoxicosis from ingestion of exogenous thyroid hormone will suppress the function of the normal thyroid gland and result in very low levels of circulating Tg.[53]

Thyroid Function Testing in Hyperthyroidism

Biochemical evaluation for hyperthyroidism should be considered in patients with relevant signs and symptoms. Testing should also be routinely performed in those at an increased risk of hyperthyroidism, including those with a strong family history of thyroid dysfunction (hypothyroidism or hyperthyroidism), those with other autoimmune conditions, and those with a goiter who receive iodinated contrast administration or amiodarone therapy. Routine screening of asymptomatic patients and of those without risk factors for hyperthyroidism is not recommended.

The measurement of serum TSH is the most sensitive measure to screen for hyperthyroidism, because it will be suppressed in primary hyperthyroidism (defined as when the source of excess thyroid hormone production is the thyroid gland). However, as certain medical conditions (e.g., severe nonthyroidal illness, acute starvation, first-trimester pregnancy) and medications (e.g., glucocorticoids, dopamine) can also result in a low serum TSH, additional workup is needed once an abnormally suppressed TSH is found. In addition, secondary hyperthyroidism from a TSH-secreting pituitary adenoma is extremely rare but should be suspected when the patient has symptoms suggestive of hyperthyroidism with an inappropriately normal or discordant serum TSH.

A suggested algorithm of thyroid function testing for the evaluation of hyperthyroidism in the ambulatory setting is shown in Figure 3.8. If the serum TSH is within normal limits, the patient is euthyroid and no further workup is indicated. Thyroid function tests should be repeated as clinically indicated. If the TSH is decreased, peripheral serum thyroid hormone levels should be obtained, in addition to a repeat measurement of TSH. Small increases of serum T3 and T4 levels will result in a disproportionate suppression of TSH due to the inverse log-linear relationship between these parameters. As such, the degree of hyperthyroidism cannot be assessed by a second-generation TSH assay because even very mild hyperthyroidism will suppress the TSH to very low levels. Although a third-generation assay can better differentiate between the degrees of hyperthyroidism, routine laboratory measurements of the serum FT4 estimate and total T3 concentrations can also easily and accurately assess the degree of hyperthyroidism. Measurement of total T3 is suggested in the evaluation of hyperthyroidism, because Graves' disease results in a relatively higher ratio of T3 to T4 than for subacute thyroiditis[80] or other etiologies of hyperthyroidism (T3 predominance of Graves' disease).[81] The algorithm also recommends that if the serum TSH is less than the lower limit and serum FT4I and total T3 concentrations are low, secondary (e.g., hypothalamic or pituitary) disease should be considered.

Total T4 and/or total T3 concentrations are not routinely measured at most centers, but they can be elevated due to increased thyroid hormone binding proteins even though the free T4 and TSH levels are normal. Individuals with this clinical entity of hyperthyroxinemia are clinically and biochemically euthyroid.

Subclinical Hyperthyroidism

The combination of a decreased serum TSH with reference range T3 and T4 concentrations is referred to as *subclinical hyperthyroidism*. Patients with subclinical hyperthyroidism may be asymptomatic. The condition must be distinguished from other factors that can suppress TSH (including the use of supplements and medications) by assessing a review of systems and performing a physical examination.

The clinical importance of subclinical hyperthyroidism relates to the potentially adverse effects of even mild thyroid hormone excess on the bone and heart.[82] Subclinical thyroid hormone excess is associated with cortical bone loss,[83] atrial fibrillation,[84] and excess cardiovascular-specific mortality.[84] A practical approach has been to treat subclinical hyperthyroidism in a patient with hyperthyroid symptoms, osteoporosis, heart disease, atrial tachyarrhythmias, and enlarged nodular goiter, especially in older adults, ages greater than 65 years. In one study of 102 older women, those with a baseline serum TSH between 0.2 and 0.4 mIU/L only rarely progressed to overt hyperthyroidism (1%/year) over a median of 41 months; some returned to normal TSH level but most remained subclinically hyperthyroid.[85]

Serum Thyroid Antibodies in Hyperthyroidism

Measurement of serum TSH receptor antibodies is helpful in the evaluation of hyperthyroidism, but is not required for the diagnosis, particularly if a thyroid uptake and scan is consistent with Graves' disease.[47] TSH receptor antibody (TRAB) and the functional measurement, thyroid stimulating immunoglobulin (TSI) levels, correlate with the severity of the disease, and are increasingly recommended to assess disease activity during treatment.[86] TPO Ab is positive in over 80% of patients with Graves' disease but is also present in Hashimoto's thyroiditis, so it is not specific diagnostically.[87]

Thyroid Imaging in Hyperthyroidism

The etiology of thyrotoxicosis is often determined after a detailed medical and family history and physical examination are performed. If the etiology remains unclear, thyroid sonography to confirm thyroiditis or a radionuclide thyroid uptake and scan can be used to confirm Graves' disease. The ^{123}I scan with uptake and the ^{99m}Tc thyroid scintigraphy scan with trapping are the preferred diagnostic studies to determine the etiology of biochemical hyperthyroidism (Table 3.2). However, it is

TABLE 3.2 Diagnostic Findings in the Evaluation of Hyperthyroidism

Thyroid Condition	Severity of Biochemical Hyperthyroidism	Serum TPO Ab Titer	Radioactive Iodine Uptake*	Thyroid Scintigraphy
Graves' disease	++++	+++	++++	Enlarged thyroid with high uptake
Toxic multinodular goiter	+/++	−	Normal/+	Enlarged thyroid with nodules with increased (hot) and decreased (cold) uptake
Thyrotoxic phase of subacute thyroiditis	++++	−/+	<1% at 4 or 24 hours	No uptake in the thyroid
Toxic adenoma	+/++/+++	−	Normal/+	"Hot" nodule with low or absent uptake in the surrounding normal gland
Metastatic thyroid carcinoma	+/++	−	Low	No uptake in the thyroid but increased uptake in metastatic foci of thyroid carcinoma

*Decreased or absent uptake in the thyroid will be seen with excess exogenous administration of thyroid hormone, ectopic thyroid hormone synthesis by a *struma ovarii*, metastatic thyroid carcinoma, or exposure to excess nonradioactive iodine.
TPO Ab, thyroid peroxidase.

important to remember that the nuclear uptake depends not only on thyroid gland autonomy but also on the nonradioactive iodine stores of the patient. These stores of nonradioactive iodine can compete with the radioactive iodine tracer, resulting in a reduced radioactive iodine uptake. Thus in patients with a very high dietary iodine intake or iodine exposure, the radioactive thyroidal iodine uptake may be normal or even low despite hyperthyroidism. A spot urinary iodine concentration may be used to confirm excess iodine status. Thyroid nuclear uptakes and scans are contraindicated during pregnancy and lactation.

Treatment of Hyperthyroidism

It is recommended that the hyperthyroid patient be comanaged in consultation with an endocrinologist. Treatment options for primary hyperthyroidism are antithyroid medications, radioactive iodine ablation, and thyroid surgery.[86] Methimazole and propylthiouracil are both oral medications that block thyroid hormone synthesis and are approved in the United States for the treatment of hyperthyroidism. In 2009 the U.S. Food and Drug Administration (FDA) issued a black box warning of severe liver toxicity associated with propylthiouracil, which has resulted in the limitation of its use to selected hyperthyroid patients during the first trimester of pregnancy and/or with thyroid storm.[88] Beta-blockers can also be used initially to ameliorate the cardiovascular and neuromuscular symptoms of hyperthyroidism. During antithyroidal medical therapy, serum thyroid hormone levels tend to fluctuate frequently due to the effect of the medication and inherent variability of the thyroid disease. Monitoring of thyroid status during medical therapy is done by measurement of serum TSH, total T4 and/or an estimated free T4, and T3 concentrations every 1 to 2 months until euthyroid to adjust the dose of the antithyroid medication. Although serum TSH can remain subnormal for 4 to 6 weeks after serum T4 and T3 have been normalized, antithyroidal medical therapy is insufficient to provide definitive treatment of an autonomous thyroid nodule.

For individuals with autonomous thyroid nodule, or if remission is not achieved after 18 to 24 months of antithyroidal medical therapy in patients with Graves' disease, radioactive ablation or thyroid surgery should be considered to provide definitive treatment of the hyperthyroidism.[86] If surgery is to be considered, a total thyroidectomy would be recommended in patients with Graves' disease, and a lobectomy or resection of the affected part of the thyroid lobe would be sufficient in patients with a solitary toxic thyroid nodule.

THYROID FUNCTION TESTING IN PREGNANCY

Pregnancy and Hypothyroidism

An elevated serum TSH in pregnant women ranges from 2% to 3%.[89,90] Because hypothyroidism is associated with menstrual irregularities and infertility, a new diagnosis of severe overt hypothyroidism during pregnancy is uncommon. When diagnosed, hypothyroidism is thus almost always mild. It is very important to make the diagnosis early, because maternal hypothyroidism is associated with adverse obstetric outcomes and fetal morbidity.[91] Routine screening for hypothyroidism in pregnancy is not recommended by most guidelines,[92] although it is recommended to obtain a serum TSH in those with risk factors that include a history of thyroid dysfunction or pregnancy loss, older age (e.g., >30 years), and known thyroid autoimmunity (see Box 3.3).[15,93]

For women with preexisting hypothyroidism managed with thyroid hormone replacement, dosing requirements increase up to 50% during pregnancy due to multiple factors. Particularly during the first half of pregnancy, TBG levels increase due to rising estradiol levels, thereby resulting in a corresponding increased need for maternal thyroid hormone.[94] There is also increased degradation of T4 and T3 by the type 3 inner ring deiodinase abundantly expressed in the placenta, chorion, and amnion; the volume of T4 distribution is increased during pregnancy, and there is an additional minimal transfer of T4 from the mother to the fetus via the placenta.[94] To meet the increased thyroid hormone requirements, one practical approach has been to increase the daily oral levothyroxine dose by two additional tablets of the usual prepregnancy dose, per week.[95]

In women treated with thyroid hormone replacement, monitoring of serum TSH once monthly until midgestation, then at least once near 30 weeks' gestation, is recommended.[15] The American Thyroid Association recommends that the dose of thyroid hormone should be adjusted throughout pregnancy to maintain a TSH within the local laboratory's pregnancy trimester-specific reference range, or if this is not available, to <2.5 mIU/L.[15]

Serum thyroid antibody positivity in euthyroid pregnant women has been independently associated with an increased risk for miscarriage.[96] Because TPO Ab titers are associated with a higher risk for hypothyroidism, women with Hashimoto's thyroiditis are recommended to have serum TSH tested at the time of pregnancy confirmation and every 4 weeks throughout gestation;[15] elevated TSH levels should be treated in accordance with the targets summarized earlier. However, it is not recommended to routinely screen for serum antithyroid antibody positivity in women without risk factors during pregnancy.[15]

Pregnancy and Hyperthyroidism

Hyperthyroidism during pregnancy ranges from 0.2% to 0.7%.[97] Like in nonpregnant individuals, the differential diagnoses of thyrotoxicosis during pregnancy include Graves' disease, toxic multinodular goiter, toxic adenoma, thyroiditis, and exogenous thyroid hormone use, but can also include trophoblastic disease.[12] As a result of the mild thyroidal stimulatory effect of beta human chorionic gonadotropin (bHCG), women with gestational thyrotoxicosis should have serum thyroid function testing repeated every 4 weeks until normalization of the TSH is confirmed, likely by the beginning of the second trimester. If, however, the serum free thyroid hormone concentrations remain significantly elevated after the first trimester of pregnancy, this is consistent with endogenous hyperthyroidism and treatment should be considered. Radionuclide imaging with any isotope is contraindicated in pregnancy.

It is recommended that women who are thinking about becoming pregnant be rendered euthyroid, either with antithyroidal medications, radioactive iodine, or thyroid surgery, before conceiving.[15] If hyperthyroidism is diagnosed after pregnancy is confirmed or the pregnant woman remains hyperthyroid from a prior diagnosis, there are special considerations for the treatment of hyperthyroidism during pregnancy. Radioactive active iodine is contraindicated, and thyroid surgery should be reserved for the second trimester if that is the desired option. If antithyroidal medications are to be used during pregnancy, propylthiouracil is preferred until 16 weeks' gestation, given the relatively greater risks of birth defects with methimazole therapy; after 16 weeks, it is unclear whether propylthiouracil or methimazole would be the preferred antithyroidal drug.[15] The lowest possible dose of both medications should be used during pregnancy. Because overtreatment of the mother with antithyroid drugs is associated with fetal hypothyroidism, the target is a free T4 in the upper reference range, and the TSH should remain suppressed below normal. Serum thyroid function tests should be monitored every 4 weeks during the entire course of gestation with the aim of maintaining serum FT4 and/or TT4 concentrations at the upper end of their normal ranges.

CONCLUSIONS

In this chapter, the critical aspects of thyroid physiology and tests for assessing thyroid dysfunction have been reviewed. Based on the understanding of thyroid physiology in healthy individuals and in the special situations of pregnancy and nonthyroidal illness, a systematic approach will allow for the appropriate testing and treatment of hypothyroidism and hyperthyroidism.

REFERENCES

 For a complete list of references, go to expertconsult.com.

SECTION 2

Benign Thyroid Disease

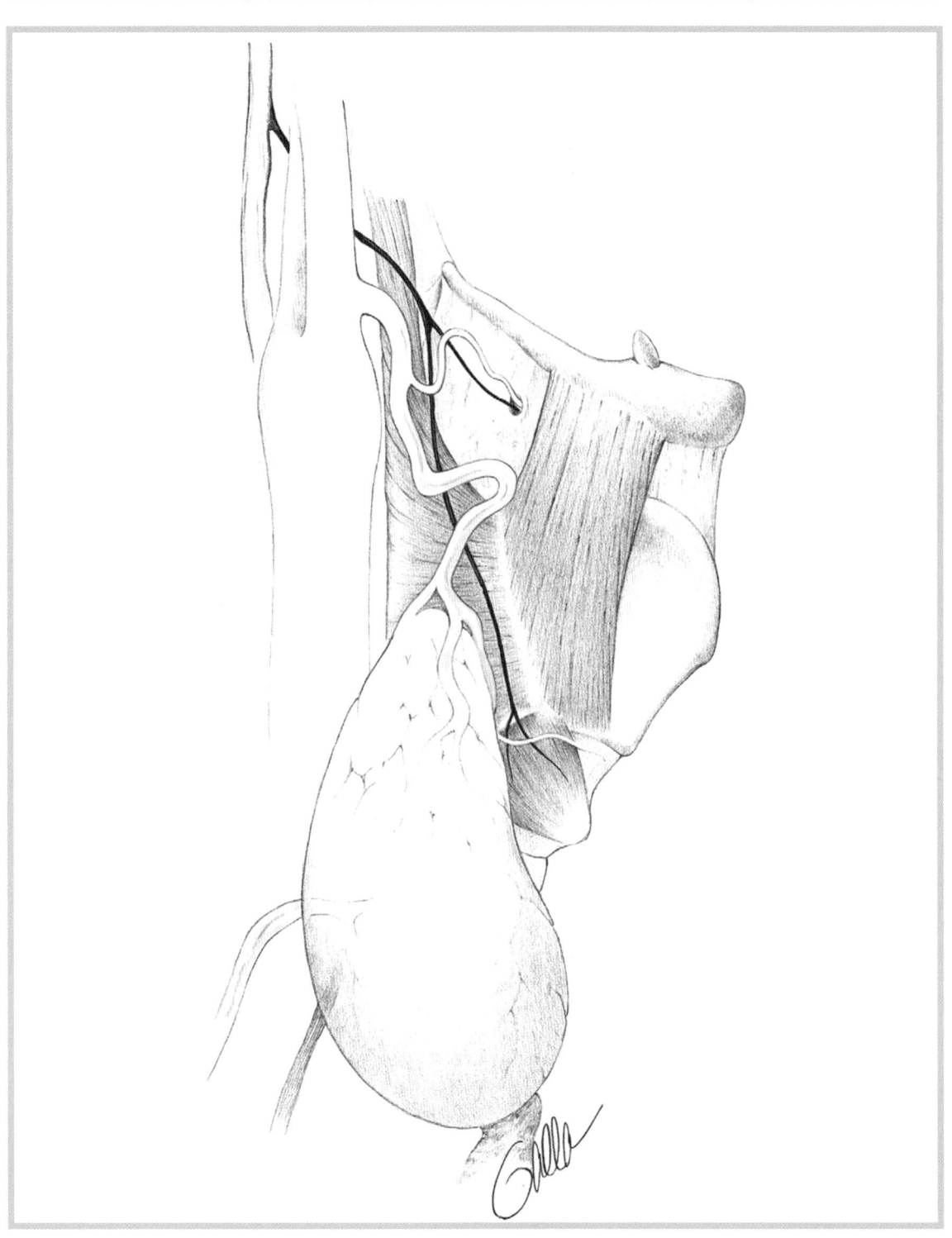

4

Thyroiditis

Trevor E. Angell, Matthew I. Kim, Victor J. Bernet

INTRODUCTION

Thyroiditis consists of a varied assortment of disorders and is fairly commonly encountered in clinical practice. The term *thyroiditis* implies an inflammatory response, and although inflammation of the thyroid may be present in some forms of thyroiditis, in reality some etiologies of thyroiditis are not actually an inflammatory response per se. Forms of thyroiditis may share some features but may have distinct underlying etiologies (Box 4.1), including autoimmune, infectious, drug or radiation related, induced by trauma, or related to invasive fibrotic thyroiditis (Riedel's thyroiditis). The clinical course of thyroiditis can vary in duration from chronic to sudden in onset, and range in severity of symptoms from mild to life threatening. It is important to employ a methodical and thoughtful approach to the evaluation and management of patients with thyroiditis. The clinician will need to integrate a thorough history, medication list, and an insightful physical examination aimed at detecting key findings (Table 4.1). This should be augmented by using a combination of diagnostic tools, including laboratory results, thyroid imaging with ultrasound or scintigraphic agents, and possibly fine-needle aspiration (FNA) cytology. This thorough assessment contributes to the correct identification of a specific thyroiditis, which in turn facilitates implementation of correct management. This chapter provides the critical elements to consider for thyroiditis, and for each etiology of thyroiditis, reviews the essential aspects of pathogenesis, evaluation, and management.

HASHIMOTO'S THYROIDITIS (CHRONIC LYMPHOCYTIC THYROIDITIS)

Of all autoimmune disorders, chronic lymphocytic thyroiditis, also known as *Hashimoto's thyroiditis*, is by far the most prevalent.[1] The eponym Hashimoto's thyroiditis (HT) relates to Dr. Hashimoto, from Japan, who, in 1912, first reported a connection between goiter and intrathyroidal lymphocytic inflammation, referring to it as "struma lymphomatosa"[2] HT is understood to be an autoimmune condition in which activation of the immune system against the thyroid leads to increased presentation of thyroid antigens and a rise in Th-1 T-cell cytotoxic action mediated by ICAM-1-mediated CD8+ cells, thereby causing the disruption of thyroid follicles and cell apoptosis.[3,4] Typically, thyroid peroxidase antibodies (TPOAb) and/or thyroglobulin antibodies (TgAb) can be measured in the serum of patients with active HT.[5] In the general population, up to 20% of adults may have measurable thyroid antibody titers, which occur more often in the elderly and women.[6]

Pathogenesis

A genetic predisposition for HT is evident in about 75% of cases. Certain HLA class II antigens (such as ARG74 in DR3) carry an increased risk for the development of several autoimmune disorders that include HT, with cytotoxic T-lymphocytes antigen-4 (CTLA-4) also playing a role.[7] A growing number of environmental factors have been implicated in the etiology of HT as well.[8] Interestingly, iodine supplementation programs in areas of iodine deficiency have been associated with rising rates of HT and associated hypothyroidism.[9] The element selenium (Se^{++}) is an integral component of the selenoprotein deiodinase enzymes. Deiodinases are present in the thyroid as well as various peripheral tissues regulating deiodination of thyroxine (T4) and triiodothyronine (T3). Reduced serum Se^{++} levels have been noted with cases of HT. Although some reports indicate benefits of selenium replacement therapy to reduce the occurrence of HT and the development of hypothyroidism, this has not yet been fully proven.[10] However, it should be noted that at the time of this writing, a clinical trial is underway assessing if the combination of selenium and levothyroxine (LT4) therapy improves quality of life and/or reduces levels of immune activity markers in patients with autoimmune driven thyroiditis.[11] Remarkably, tobacco and moderate alcohol use, which have other negative effects, appear to be associated with a reduced risk of autoimmune related hypothyroidism.[7,12] Although the development of some autoimmune conditions has been reportedly related to previous infectious exposures, no such association has been noted with HT. Although radiation exposure potentially increases the risk of developing thyroid malignancy, it remains to be proven if this predisposes to the development of thyroid autoimmunity.[13] Other studies have reported a connection between vitamin D deficiency and increased risk of autoimmunity as well as vitamin D supplementation reducing TPOAb titers in patients with HT on LT4 replacement therapy.[14] In other autoimmune conditions such as Graves' disease, stress has been identified as a potential promoting factor, albeit available data has not proven any effect on TPOAb production or development of hypothyroidism. Endogenous factors contributing to the risk for HT include female sex (7:1 female:male ratio), sex hormones such as estrogen, postpartum thyroiditis (PPT), pregnancy, and the presence of fetal microchimerism.[7,15] Patients with Down's and Turner's syndromes also display an increased propensity toward development of autoimmune hypothyroidism.[16,17]

Clinical Manifestations

Patients with HT may present in a euthyroid state with normal thyroid-stimulating hormone (TSH) and free thyroxine (FT4) levels, subclinical hypothyroidism with mild TSH elevations (5 to 10 uIU/mL), and a paucity of symptoms or more significant hypothyroidism with TSH >10 uIU/mL. Although a goiter may be noted during a physical examination, thyroid morphology associated with HT varies widely and ranges from atrophic, barely palpable glands to slightly enlarged glands to very large goiters. The gland texture may be

> **BOX 4.1 Cause of Thyroiditis**
>
> Chronic lymphocytic thyroiditis (Hashimoto's thyroiditis)
> Subacute granulomatous thyroiditis (de Quervain's thyroiditis)
> Silent sporadic thyroiditis
> Postpartum thyroiditis
> Acute suppurative/infectious thyroiditis
> Drug-induced thyroiditis
> Radiation-induced thyroiditis
> Riedel's thyroiditis
> Other forms of thyroiditis: traumatic/palpation thyroiditis, chronic infectious thyroiditis, infiltrative (amyloidosis, sarcoidosis)

smooth as in "simple" goiters or contain numerous nodules as seen with multinodular goiters. Although the euthyroid state may persist for many years, about 4% to 5% of initially euthyroid patients with HT will develop hypothyroidism each year.[18] The rate of progression is somewhat dependent on the intensity of the inflammatory reaction and the concomitant rate of induced thyroid follicle destruction. HT is usually not associated with any neck discomfort, but there are instances where individuals will present with anterior neck pain or tenderness, so HT should be considered in the differential diagnosis of patients with neck discomfort. Episodes of more acute thyroiditis with the development of transient thyrotoxicosis have been reported and been referred to as *Hashitoxicosis*.

Changes from HT noted by thyroid ultrasound, such as heterogeneous parenchyma, may become evident before the ability to measure thyroid antibody titers in the patient's serum.[19] Although thyroid nodules certainly can be present in the context of HT, focal inflammatory changes due to HT may give the false impression of thyroid nodules. The term *pseudonodule* refers to instances where there is the appearance of a thyroid nodule in at least one ultrasound view, but it cannot be reproduced on the additional complementary views.[20] Such lesions may not be evident upon future imaging at a later point in time. Therefore in patients with HT, the possibility of a pseudonodule should be considered before proceeding with FNA sampling.

Thyroid enlargement associated with HT may regress with LT4 therapy, particularly if TSH elevation is present at the time of diagnosis. However, some goiters associated with HT will persist or even grow whether or not LT4 suppression is used. If such patients exhibit progressive goiter growth or develop compressive type symptoms, thyroidectomy may need to be considered. If the goiter is large and especially if tracheal deviation or substernal extension is present, then preoperative imaging with computed tomography (CT) of the neck is warranted to better define the anatomy and help plan the surgical approach.[21] Histopathology is typically notable for prominent lymphocytic infiltration, foci of lymphoid germinal centers, and follicle destruction.[22] Controversy exists if HT patients have an increased risk for thyroid cancer and, if so, whether or not HT is associated with a more aggressive disease pattern.[23-25]

Management

Euthyroid patients with positive thyroid antibody titers can typically be monitored without the institution of thyroid hormone replacement therapy.[26] However, there are some data that pregnant patients with positive thyroid antibody titers may have improved pregnancy outcomes and reduced complications with the institution of LT4 replacement therapy. In non-pregnant patients with hypothyroidism, there are standard recommendations for treatment and monitoring.[27] This usually consist of LT4 therapy and TSH and FT4 monitoring every 6 weeks with adjustments in LT4 dosing until the TSH is within the goal range (typically 1 to 3 uIU/mL) although a higher target range is considered acceptable in the elderly.[28,29]

SUBACUTE THYROIDITIS (DE QUERVAIN'S THYROIDITIS)

Subacute thyroiditis (SAT) is an inflammatory condition of the thyroid. Unlike HT, the typical course is characterized by more rapid thyroid cell destruction over days to months that leads to transient thyroid hormone release followed by hypothyroidism that resolves in most patients (Figure 4.1). Many other names have been used to describe SAT, including painful thyroiditis, giant cell thyroiditis, de Quervain's thyroiditis, subacute granulomatous thyroiditis, migratory thyroiditis,

TABLE 4.1 Comparisons of Features Between Types of Thyroiditis

	THYROIDITIS TYPE				
	Hashimoto's	**Subacute**	**Silent/Postpartum**	**Acute Suppurative**	**Riedel's**
Peak age of onset	30-50 years	20-60 years	30-40 years (Painless)	Children, 20-40 years	30-60 years
Sex ratio (F:M)	8-9:1	5:1	2:1	1:1	3-4:1
Incidence	Very common	Common	Common	Rare	Extremely rare
Etiology	Autoimmune	Viral (?)	Autoimmune	Infectious	Unknown
Pathology	Lymphocytic infiltration, germinal lefts, fibrosis	Giant cells, granulomas	Lymphocytic infiltration	Abscess formation	Dense fibrosis
Goiter	Variable	Yes	No	No	Yes
Thyroid pain	No	Yes	No	Yes	No
Fever and malaise	No	Yes	No	Yes	No
ESR	Normal	High	Normal	High	Normal
Transient thyrotoxicosis	Maybe	Yes	Yes	Usually no	No
Thyroid antibodies	Yes	Maybe (Low, transient)	Yes	No	Yes
24-hour RAIU	Variable	Very low	Very low	Normal	Low/Normal
Permanent hypothyroidism	Frequent	Occasional	Common	Rare	Occasional

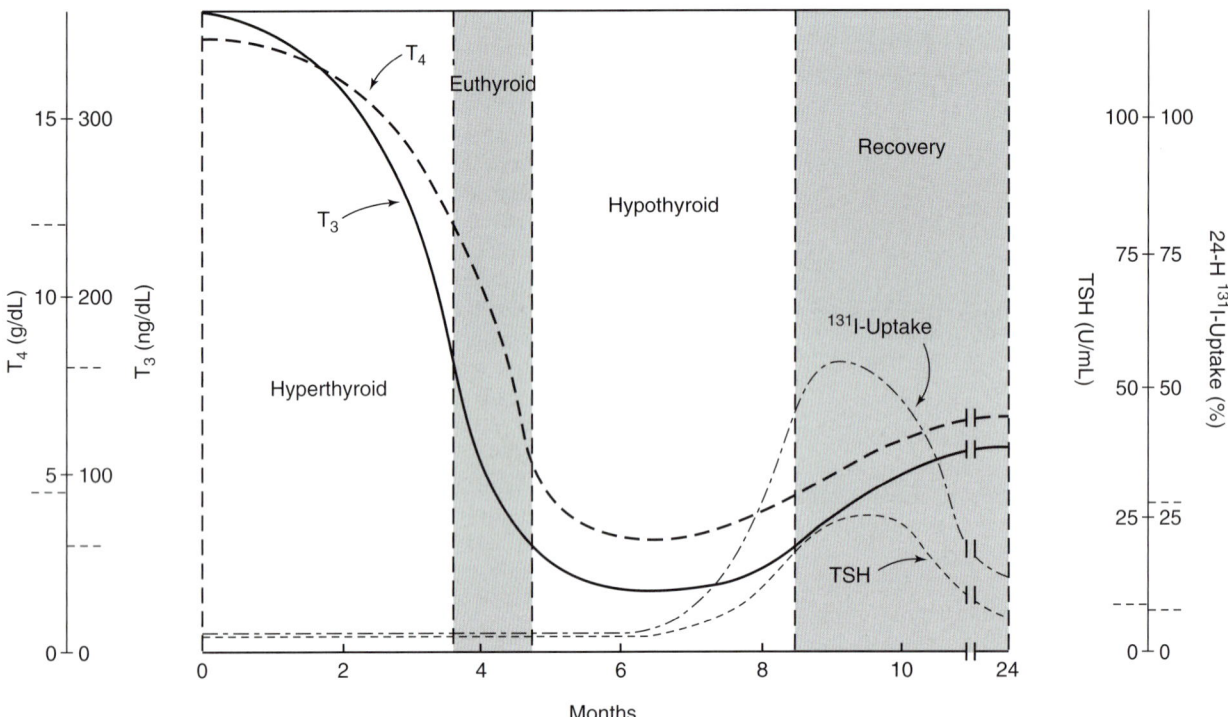

Fig. 4.1 Clinical progression of destruction-induced thyroiditis. (Modified from Woolf OD. Transient painless thyroiditis with hyperthyroidism: a variant of lymphocytic thyroiditis? *Endocr Rev.* 1980;1[4]:411–420.)

viral thyroiditis, and noninfectious thyroiditis.[30] The presence of giant cells and granulomatous changes in the thyroid, originally described by Fritz de Quervain in 1904, are specific to SAT, but such histological confirmation of the diagnosis is rarely if ever needed owing to the typical clinical findings. As in many thyroid disorders, women are more likely to get SAT than men, and it occurs most often in adults in the fifth and sixth decades of life. The differential diagnosis of neck pain should include SAT, recognizing that thyroid pain can be from a number of potential causes (Box 4.2). SAT should be included in the assessment of fever of unknown origin[31,32] and should be considered in anyone with abnormal thyroid hormone testing results because SAT may account for up to 5% of clinical thyroid abnormalities.[33]

Pathogenesis

Many potential causes have been implicated in the pathogenesis of SAT. Predisposing genetic susceptibility loci, autoimmunity, and viral etiologies may interact to ultimately cause this condition. An increased risk of SAT has been noted for specific human leukocyte antigen (HLA) haplotypes (e.g., HLA-Bw35, HLA-B15/62, HLA-DRw8), though the relative risks attributable to these are not well defined.[30,34,35] The occurrence of SAT is not clearly associated with thyroid autoimmunity. Thyroid autoantibodies such as TPOAb or TgAb may be identified during recovery from SAT, but these are most typically not elevated. In contrast, TSH receptor antibodies (TRAb) have been detected in patients with SAT.[36,37] Decreasing titers or complete resolution of TRAb have been noted during follow-up. Whether or not this can be considered pathophysiologically relevant or predictive of risk or natural history is unknown, but generation of TRAb by the immune system in the setting of SAT may be a response to the release of thyroid antigens after initial thyrocyte damage.[37,38]

In contrast to the limited association with genetic and autoimmune factors, there is more evidence linking the pathogenesis of SAT to a direct or indirect sequelae of a viral infection.[39-41] Observational evidence in support of this includes a peak incidence in the earth's temperate zones and during summer months when certain viral infections are at their peak.[41] The condition appears to coincide with prodromal symptoms such as malaise, myalgia, and/or low-grade fever suggestive of a viral etiology and has been associated with numerous viral agents.[39] SAT has also been associated with other noninfectious etiologies.[42-44]

Clinical Manifestations

The development of neck pain in the region of the thyroid raises the possibility of SAT. Neck pain is typically moderate to severe and may diffusely involve the entire thyroid or follow a more gradual and progressive course in which the condition initially occurs in one lobe of the thyroid and later manifests in the other. Pain may be

---

BOX 4.2 Differential Diagnosis of Thyroid Pain

Subacute thyroiditis
Acute suppurative thyroiditis
Acute hemorrhage into a thyroid cyst or nodule (benign or malignant)
Rapidly growing thyroid carcinoma
Painful Hashimoto's thyroiditis
Radiation thyroiditis
Infected thyroglossal duct cyst
Globus hystericus

localized to the thyroid or radiate superiorly to the ear, either unilaterally or bilaterally. A preceding history of viral prodrome (e.g., low-grade fever, malaise, myalgias, upper respiratory track symptoms) may or may not be present. Along with this presentation, many patients will present with classical symptoms of thyrotoxicosis,[33] such as heat intolerance, tremors, palpitations, weight loss, hyperdefecation, anxiety, insomnia, or dyspnea. Proptosis or other signs of ophthalmopathy, thyroid bruit, or pretibial myxedema, which are features specific to Graves' disease, are absent. The presence of higher fever is a notable feature of SAT, potentially reaching 40° C (104° F). Rarely is thyroid pain the only finding present. Pain and thyrotoxicosis are self-resolving over a typical period of 4 to 6 weeks. These and other features help distinguish it from other forms of thyroiditis (see Table 4.1). The recovery after the thyrotoxic phase of SAT typically involves biochemical hypothyroidism, though patients may remain asymptomatic. A minority of patients will acquire permanent hypothyroidism after SAT.

On physical examination, patients may manifest nonspecific signs of thyrotoxicosis. Careful examination of the thyroid is often more revealing of the underlying diagnosis. Palpation of the thyroid is often described as "exquisitely" tender, may provoke the patient to withdraw when severe, and may be associated with referred pain to the ear. Again, tenderness may be diffuse or localized. A hard, focal accumulation of inflammation in SAT may be mistaken for a solitary thyroid nodule, raising concern for possible thyroid malignancy. In contrast to invasive thyroid cancer, suspicious cervical lymphadenopathy is not present in SAT. In such cases, ultrasonographic assessment should be performed to show findings more consistent with SAT (Figure 4.2).

There are no laboratory results that are specific for SAT, though some may be helpful in equivocal cases in which the diagnosis is uncertain. Erythrocyte sedimentation rate (ESR) and C-reactive protein (CRP) levels are markedly elevated. Conversely, active SAT should be considered very unlikely in the setting of a normal ESR or CRP result. Other inflammatory markers such as total white blood cell count and ferritin are frequently elevated. Assessment of thyroid hormone status should be performed to evaluate the presence and degree of thyrotoxicosis during the active phase of the condition. TSH is suppressed to low levels but may still be detectable early in the course. Determination of total T4 and T3 concentration facilitates calculation of the total T3/T4 ratio. Because T3 production is increased under TSH receptor stimulation, T3 levels are expected to be higher in states of endogenous hyperfunction such as Graves' disease, whereas thyroid hormone release found in destruction-mediated thyroiditis is expected to have relatively lower T3. A total T3/T4 ratio <20 suggests thyroiditis though the precise accuracy of this cut-off is uncertain.[45] Similar assessment of the free T3/T4 ratio has been reported but requires further study.[46]

Imaging modalities may also be informative in the assessment of SAT but are not always necessary when the diagnosis is clinically apparent. Ultrasonographic assessment may reveal characteristic diffuse enlargement and hypoechogenicity or may demonstrate an asymmetric or focal pattern (see Figure 4.2).[47] Radioactive iodine uptake using [123]I

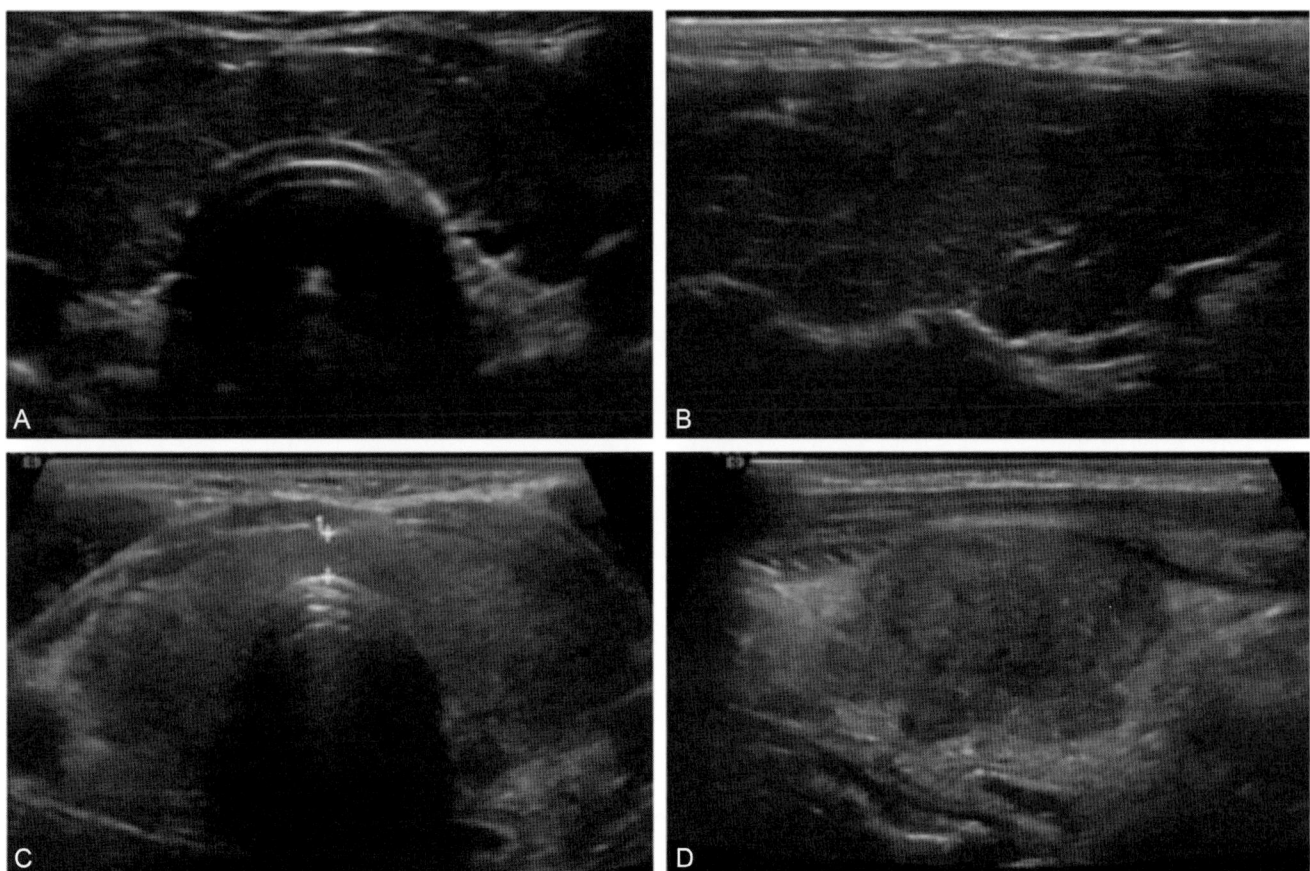

Fig. 4.2 Ultrasonographic findings in subacute thyroiditis. (**A**) Transverse and (**B**) sagittal two-dimensional gray-scale images of the thyroid showing diffuse hypoechogenicity. (**C**) Transverse and (**D**) sagittal two-dimensional gray-scale images of the thyroid showing pseudonodular focal area of asymmetric hypoechogenicity.

distinguishes thyroiditis from hyperfunctioning states by demonstrating very low iodine uptake during the thyrotoxic phase, which are typically <2% to 5% and often undetectable. The absence of uptake using technetium 99m also suggests thyroiditis and may be obtained more rapidly and in patients with recent iodine exposure. Careful attention should be paid to the timing of assessment because uptake can be elevated when obtained during the recovery phase of SAT when TSH may be elevated.

Management

Therapy for SAT is primarily supportive and involves treatment of pain and the symptoms of thyrotoxicosis when present. Specific measures to reduce thyroid hormone levels are most often not required except in cases complicated by thyroid storm. As noted previously, the thyrotoxicosis of SAT is due to a destructive process within the thyroid that causes leakage of thyroid hormone into the circulation. Because of this, antithyroid drugs, methimazole, or propylthiouracil (PTU), which reduce production of thyroid hormones by the thyroid, have no role in management.[45] Thyrotoxicosis can be managed with beta-adrenergic receptor blockers (such as propranolol, metoprolol, or others) for the self-limited duration of these symptoms. Improvement in symptoms can be seen shortly after initiation of treatment, but these medications do not affect the underlying inflammatory condition.

Thyroidal pain may be ameliorated by antiinflammatory medications. In mild to moderate cases, nonsteroidal antiinflammatory drugs (NSAIDs) may be effective, though use at effective doses may be limited by gastrointestinal or renal side effects. Salicylates may cause an increase in free thyroid hormone concentrations and are not favored.[48] For those with severe pain or who are refractory to NSAIDs, oral prednisone can be employed, with initial dosing usually at 20 to 40 mg per day for the first week. This is expected to provide dramatic relief of pain and swelling. Indeed, if pain fails to completely or nearly resolve after 24 to 48 hours of prednisone therapy, the diagnosis of SAT should be reconsidered. Slow tapering of prednisone is done over 4 to 6 weeks because recurrence of neck pain can occur if tapering is done too rapidly. In rare cases in which the course of SAT is prolonged or recurrent, a thyroidectomy or radioactive iodine ablation may be necessary.

After the initial symptoms, thyroid destruction leads to a fall in thyroid hormone production. A typical period of subsequent hypothyroidism lasts from 4 to 6 weeks but can last as long as 6 to 9 months before thyroid function recovers. Some patients will have a period of hypothyroidism that is mild and asymptomatic for which LT4 supplementation may not be necessary. However, for patients with symptomatic or protracted courses of hypothyroidism, replacement LT4 is likely needed. Later withdrawal of LT4 to assess for restored thyroid function is reasonable since only a small minority of patients will have permanent hypothyroidism after SAT.

SPORADIC SILENT AND POSTPARTUM THYROIDITIS

Sporadic silent thyroiditis (ST) and PPT are considered related conditions of destructive thyroiditis, bearing the hallmark pattern of initially high thyroid hormone levels and low radioactive iodine uptake followed by hypothyroidism and usual recovery of function.[49,50] Although they arise from apparent damage to the thyroid gland and the release of preformed thyroid hormone, these conditions do not result in the thyroidal pain seen in SAT (see Table 4.1). PPT is distinguished by its specific incidence after pregnancy and is the most common cause of thyrotoxicosis in the postpartum setting.[51] The reported incidence of PPT varies widely, described in as low as 2% of women but occurring as frequently as 33% to 50% in postpartum women who are TPOAb-positive.[52] By comparison, ST is estimated to occur in <1% of patients diagnosed with thyrotoxicosis, though its true incidence is difficult to assess.[53] Although the natural history and clinical manifestations can be similar, the underlying etiology and epidemiology of ST and PPT differ from SAT, as do the treatments considerations.

Pathogenesis

Both sporadic ST and PPT are considered autoimmune in nature. The evidence of this in PPT includes its association with other autoimmune conditions, particularly type 1 diabetes mellitus and autoimmune thyroid disease.[54,55] Further, PPT is associated with elevated levels of TPOAb, and women with the highest TPOAb levels are at greatest risk.[49,51,52] Positive TPOAb is also associated with ST. Smoking is an additional risk factor and is also associated with immunologic effects. Genetic susceptibility for major histocompatibility complex class II haplotypes has been described.[56] Although the reversal of underlying mechanisms of immune system tolerance during pregnancy may play a role in PPT, the relevance to sporadic ST is unclear. Additionally, excess iodine levels and lower selenium levels both have been correlated with a higher incidence of PPT.[57-59]

Clinical Manifestations

The timing of PPT after pregnancy is variable but most often occurs from 2 to 6 months after delivery. ST, although more common in women than in men, still occurs sporadically. In both conditions, there is spontaneous resolution of thyrotoxicosis, which may be followed by transient or permanent hypothyroidism. In PPT, this occurs 3 to 12 months postpartum, and one study has indicated that as many as 50% of women with PPT may continue to suffer from hypothyroidism 1 year after delivery.[60,61] The clinical manifestations of ST and PPT resemble those of SAT, with the presence of mild to severe symptoms and biochemical evidence of thyrotoxicosis, but they differ in that they present with a nontender goiter or nonpalpable thyroid. Mild symptoms of thyrotoxicosis or hypothyroidism, such as fatigue, anxiety, depression, weight changes, or hair loss, may be confused with nonpathologic symptoms common in the postpartum period. Thus it is important to maintain vigilance to the possibility of PPT.

Biochemically, TSH and thyroid hormone concentrations show thyroid hormone excess but do not reveal any particular cause. A lower total T3 to total T4 ratio (<20) may help distinguish ST and PPT from Graves' disease. PPT may be difficult to distinguish from Graves' disease, which also has an increased incidence after pregnancy. Additionally, radioiodine uptake assessment is contraindicated in the nursing mother, limiting its use. Measurement of thyroid-stimulating immunoglobulin (TSI) may be helpful, given the high sensitivity and specify to detect or exclude Graves' disease.[45,62] Ultrasonographic assessment may show diffuse or more focal hypoechogenicity,[63] although it is not necessary to obtain such testing in most cases. Identification of sporadic thyroiditis would also be performed for individuals not in the postpartum period by using a radioactive iodine uptake assessment. A very low uptake of radioiodine is expected during the thyrotoxic phase of thyroiditis in contrast to states of thyroid hyperfunction. It is important to measure serum TSH at the time the radioisotope test is performed because the radioactive iodine uptake may be normal or elevated as the patient recovers from the acute thyrotoxic phase. It is notable that in rare circumstances painless thyrotoxicosis and a low-undetectable radioactive iodine thyroid uptake can be seen in other conditions, including exogenous thyroid hormone excess (e.g., thyrotoxicosis factitia), metastatic thyroid cancer, and *struma ovarii*.[64]

Management

Patients with ST or PPT should be treated with beta-adrenergic blocking drugs when presenting with moderate to severe symptoms of thyrotoxicosis. As is the case with SAT, antithyroid drugs, methimazole, or PTU, which reduce production of thyroid hormones by the thyroid, have no role in management because the thyroid is not hyperfunctioning. Antiinflammatory medications, used to reduce swelling and pain in SAT, are also not used for patients with PPT or ST.

During the subsequent hypothyroid phase, the need for thyroid hormone supplementation with LT4 depends on the severity of symptoms and other clinical factors. If hypothyroid symptoms are moderate to severe or the reduction of thyroid function is prolonged, LT4 supplementation is needed; however, asymptomatic patients with resolving biochemical hypothyroidism, even if pronounced, may be observed. An exception to this is women with persistent TSH elevation attempting to become pregnant again, for whom restoring adequate thyroid hormone levels may be beneficial for fertility and/or pregnancy outcomes.[65] When LT4 therapy is instituted, withdrawal after 6 to 12 months may be attempted to determine whether thyroid function has normalized. However, up to 20% of women will have permanent hypothyroidism after PPT,[53,54,65,66] and those exhibiting higher TPOAb titers often will have more severe cases of hypothyroidism.

Recurrence of PPT and ST is common. For women with a history of PPT, there is recurrence after a subsequent pregnancy over 50% of the time. Patients who have had sporadic ST may suffer a recurrence though this may not be detected depending on severity. Patients and their providers should remain attentive to this possibility. Additionally, patients with previous thyroiditis are at risk for future hypothyroidism and iodine-induced hypothyroidism if exposed to an acute iodine load.[67,68]

DRUG-INDUCED THYROIDITIS

A growing list of medications have been reported to be associated with drug-induced thyroiditis (Table 4.2), including interferon-alpha, interleukin-2, amiodarone, lithium, tyrosine kinase inhibitors, checkpoint inhibitors, thalidomide, and minocycline. Typically, patients with drug-induced thyroiditis will exhibit a course similar to that of painless thyroiditis.

The antiarrhythmic agent amiodarone has a prominent iodine content (37%) and is known to affect thyroid function in multiple ways.[69] Type 1 amiodarone-induced thyrotoxicosis (AIT) is associated with overproduction of thyroid hormone, and type 2 AIT consists of destructive thyroiditis with thyrotoxicosis from unregulated T4 and T3 release.[70] Clinical differentiation between the two forms can be challenging. It is more common for patients with type 1 to have evidence of a preexisting thyroid condition, whereas patients developing type 2 tend to lack a previous history of thyroid issues.[71] AIT can present relatively soon after exposure to amiodarone or, with a half-life of 100 days, many months after withdrawal.[72] Radioactive iodine uptake results, many times, do not allow for accurate categorization between the two types of AIT. Color flow Doppler ultrasound imaging has been somewhat more useful exhibiting a quiescent vascular pattern with type 2 AIT in contrast to more prominent flow typically noted with type 1 AIT. Type 1 AIT can be successfully treated with antithyroid medication, whereas high-dose prednisone, up to ~60 mg daily, can be used in type 2 AIT.[73-75] However, some patients appear to exhibit a mixed form of AIT, acting as a hybrid between types 1 and 2, and these patients may require combination treatment with both antithyroid medications, such as methimazole, and prednisone for successful control of their thyrotoxicosis.[76] Because many patients on amiodarone have significant underlying cardiac diseases, it is imperative to provide aggressive management to promptly achieve control of thyrotoxicosis.[77]

Lithium can also affect thyroid function in various ways, causing the development of either hypothyroidism or thyrotoxicosis.[78] Patients receiving lithium therapy appear to have an increased risk for development of thyrotoxicosis in comparison to the general population. Additionally, older individuals and those with underlying chronic autoimmune thyroiditis are at increased risk of developing hypothyroidism while on lithium.[79] Lithium appears to potentially amplify the activity of underlying autoimmune thyroid disease as well.[80] Case reports indicate lithium-related thyrotoxicosis can occur in the form of Graves' disease, toxic nodule/multinodular goiter, or as an occurrence of painless thyroiditis.[81,82] The clinical course of thyroiditis encountered with lithium is similar to the other forms of destructive thyroiditis.[82] Glucocorticoid therapy can be considered in cases of lithium-induced thyroiditis accompanied by severe thyrotoxicosis, and beta-blocker therapy can help mitigate any associated tachycardia.[83]

The immune modulating agent interferon-alpha (IFN-α) is prescribed for a variety of clinical conditions. Treatment with IFN-α has been found to be associated with a 6% prevalence of thyroid dysfunction and up to a 70% risk of developing positive thyroid antibody concentrations in patients lacking any previous history of thyroid autoimmunity.[84,85] Two forms of interferon-induced thyrotoxicosis are encountered clinically, the first being a thyrotoxicosis similar to Graves' disease and the other being consistent with destructive thyroiditis.[86] Because IFN-α therapy is usually restricted to a limited period of time and because the course of thyrotoxicosis may be mild, IFN-α treatment can typically be completed while providing symptomatic therapy for thyrotoxicosis. Upon discontinuation of therapy, thyroid function testing tends to return to baseline although such patients are thought to be at an increased risk for development of autoimmune thyroid dysfunction in the future. Cytokine aldesleukin (interleukin-2 [IL-2]), a stimulator of natural killer cell and T-cell activity, causes activation of autoreactive lymphocytes which can then precipitate the development of autoimmune thyroiditis. Thyroid disorders appear to occur in ~10% to 50% of individuals receiving IL-2,[87,88] and cases of hypothyroidism, hyperthyroidism, and thyroiditis have been documented.

TABLE 4.2 Causes of Drug-Induced Thyroiditis

Medication Type	Medication Name
Immune modulating agents	Interferon-alpha
	Interleukin-2 (Cytokine aldesleukin)
	Thalidomide
	Lenalidomide
Iodine containing agents	Amiodarone
	Iodinated contrast media
Alkali metal	Lithium salts
Tyrosine kinase inhibitors	Cabozantinib
	Dasatinib
	Nilotininb
	Sorefanib
	Sunitinib
Checkpoint inhibitors (CTLA-4 and PD-1)	Ipilimumab
	Nivolumab
	Pembrolizumab
Antibiotics	Minocycline

The use of tyrosine kinase inhibitors (TKIs) has become increasingly prevalent, particularly for the treatment of a growing list of malignancies that include renal cell carcinoma, gastrointestinal stromal tumors, and advanced medullary and differentiated thyroid cancer. The occurrence of hypothyroidism in patients receiving these agents is reported to be up to 50% to 70%. The following TKIs have all been associated with cases of destructive thyroiditis: cabozantinib, dasatinib, nilotinib, sorafenib, and most commonly, sunitinib.[89-91] The checkpoint inhibitors, cytotoxic T lymphocyte-associated antigen 4 (CTLA-4) and program cell death-1 (PD-1) receptor agents, are another class of medications which are being more frequently used for the treatment of malignancy and have been associated with adverse endocrine side effects, including hypophysitis, autoimmune diabetes, adrenal insufficiency, and destructive thyroiditis.[92,93] Risk for the development of endocrinopathies appears to be increased with combination therapy such as ipilimumab combined with nivolumab.

The immune modulating agents, thalidomide and its molecular analog, lenalidomide, have also been associated with episodes of drug-induced thyroiditis.[94,95] The thyroid is a vascular gland, and it is believed that these medications induce a destructive thyroiditis by reduced blood flow stemming from the antiangiogenic effects of these agents. Thalidomide has also been associated with thyrotoxicosis, and concomitant radiation exposure may play a role in the occurrence of autoimmune thyroid disease.[96]

Management

It is recommended that before initiation of any of the previously mentioned medications patients should be screened for a family history of thyroid disease, undergo examination of the thyroid, and complete thyroid function testing with TSH and free T4. If there is a family history of, or suspicion for, underlying autoimmune thyroid disease, then measurement of thyroid antibody titers (TPOAb and TgAb) is reasonable because the risk for development of drug-induced thyroid dysfunction appears more likely in patients with positive titers. Importantly, patients taking the offending drugs may also develop subacute, sporadic, or suppurative thyroiditis, so these diagnoses need to also be considered before ascribing an episode of thyroiditis to any drug. Supportive care such as beta-blocker therapy should be used in the presence of cardiac symptoms related to thyrotoxicosis. Drug-induced thyroid abnormalities usually resolve with discontinuation of the offending drug over time.

ACUTE SUPPURATIVE/INFECTIOUS THYROIDITIS

The thyroid gland is invested with properties that make it generally resistant to contiguous and hematogenous spread of infection. These include isolation from other structures in the neck with separation by fascial planes, encasement by a fibrous capsule, drainage into a dense network of blood vessels and lymphatic channels, and storage of concentrated deposits of iodine that may be bactericidal. As a consequence, infection of the thyroid leading to acute suppurative thyroiditis is an uncommon event with reports documenting only about 300 cases in adults and 100 cases in children.[97] Although mortality from this disorder approached 20% to 25% when it was first identified in the early 20th century, at present, it is rarely fatal due to more expedient diagnoses and treatment facilitated by the use of modern imaging modalities and empiric broad-spectrum antibiotics.

Pathogenesis

In the majority of adult cases and almost all pediatric cases, specific anatomic factors appear to predispose to bacterial infection of the thyroid. Fistulas that extend from the left pyriform sinus to the thyroid have been identified as the most common route of transmission, although infections also appear to have spread from branchial pouch and thyroglossal duct cysts, and along tracts introduced by needles used to perform thyroid nodule biopsies.[98,99] Many cases have been preceded by upper respiratory tract infections that appear to have caused inflammation of fistulas with resultant infiltration by pathogenic bacteria. Preexisting neoplastic and autoimmune thyroid disorders also appear to increase susceptibility to bacterial infection. *Staphylococcus aureus* and *Streptococcus pyogenes* have been identified as the sole or predominant pathogen in most adult cases of acute suppurative thyroiditis. Children appear to be more prone to infection by alpha- and beta-hemolytic *Streptococcus* species and anaerobes. Although a range of other pathogens, including parasitic, fungal, and mycobacterial infections,[30] have been identified in specific circumstances, initial empiric antibiotic treatment of suspected cases typically should target these bacterial organisms.

Clinical Manifestations

Most cases of acute suppurative thyroiditis present with pain and tenderness originating from the site of infection that may radiate outward to other structures in the neck including the jaw and ear on the involved side. Swelling caused by abscess formation may be pronounced enough to lead to compression of the esophagus or recurrent laryngeal nerve with resultant dysphagia or dysphonia. With progression, most patients develop systemic symptoms characteristic of an acute bacterial infection, including fevers, chills, and malaise.

It may be challenging to distinguish acute suppurative thyroiditis from SAT because both disorders may initially present with pain and tenderness emanating from a focal mass in the thyroid that developed after a recent respiratory tract infection. Physical examination may provide the most informative clues. Bacterial infection of the thyroid is more likely to present with erythema and warmth overlying the site of identified discomfort and is also more likely to be associated with palpable cervical lymphadenopathy. On serial examination, the infected site may be noted to become more fluctuant to palpation over the course of 2 to 3 days as it starts to transform into an abscess.

Laboratory testing may reveal an elevated white blood cell count with a pronounced left shift that distinguishes it from the milder leukocytosis that may be detected in the setting of SAT. Inflammatory markers, including the ESR and CRP level, may be significantly elevated in both conditions. Thyroid hormone levels are usually normal in patients without any preexisting thyroid disorders.

Ultrasound imaging focused on the site of localized pain and tenderness may reveal a hypoechoic mass extending into the affected lobe.[100] With unchecked progression, this change may spread into adjacent soft tissue to surround the lobe. Although radionuclide imaging may demonstrate normal function of the uninvolved region of the thyroid, it is usually not indicated because ultrasound provides more informative views that can be used to guide sampling and intervention. In cases of severe infection or recurrent infection that may warrant surgical correction of predisposing abnormalities, MRI and CT scanning may help localize pyriform sinus fistulas and branchial pouch cysts. The presence of gas bubbles on any type of imaging may raise concern for infection with anaerobic bacteria.

Definitive confirmation of bacterial infection of the thyroid relies on obtaining samples by FNA for cytologic examination, Gram stain, and culture. Ultrasound guidance can help identify sites most likely to yield discriminant results.[101] Cytology results should always be reviewed because acute hemorrhage into a cystic malignant neoplasm may present with similar clinical manifestations.

Management

If a Gram stain of aspirate material does not identify a predominant bacterial organism, empiric antibiotic treatment should be started. Adult patients can be treated with a penicillinase-resistant penicillin and β-lactamase inhibitor with the addition of vancomycin if methicillin-resistant *Staphylococcus aureus* is suspected.[102] Pediatric patients should be started on treatment with a second-generation cephalosporin or clindamycin. Antibiotic coverage can be narrowed when definitive culture and sensitivity results are returned. Incision and drainage may be required if the infection does not respond to antibiotic therapy or starts to transform into an abscess. In particularly severe cases or in cases of recurrent infection associated with a risk of bacteremia, surgical intervention with a hemithyroidectomy may be required, but most patients who require surgery recover without complication.

INVASIVE FIBROUS THYROIDITIS (RIEDEL'S THYROIDITIS)

Riedel's thyroiditis (RT) is a fibroinflammatory condition affecting the thyroid that is infrequently encountered in clinic practice.[103] It appears to have been first reported in 1864 by Semple, then again in 1888 by A.A. Bowlby, and most famously by Bernhard Riedel in 1894 at the International Congress of Surgery.[104-106] The fibrotic inflammatory response leads not only to destruction of the thyroid but also infiltrates perithyroidal tissues in the neck. Riedel's thyroiditis has been known by several different names over the years, including chronic invasive fibrous or chronic sclerosing thyroiditis, *struma fibrosa*, and Riedel's struma.[107] In 1985, the Mayo Clinic published a case series of 37 cases of fibrotic invasive thyroiditis diagnosed over a 64-year span.[108] The calculated incidence was reported as ∼1.06 cases per every 100,000 individuals. The peak of diagnosis for RT appears to fall between the third and fifth decades of life and, like many thyroid disorders, appears to occur more often in females (approximately 3:1 female:male ratio).[107,109] To date, no specific genetic predisposition has been discovered. Although unproven, previous exposure to the Epstein-Barr virus may be a potential stimulus for the development of RT.[110] In contradistinction to other forms of thyroiditis, medication-induced RT has not been reported.[103]

Pathogenesis

The fibrotic inflammatory process seen with RT may be restricted to the thyroid gland or can involve adjacent cervical structures such as skeletal muscles, blood vessels, nerves, parathyroid glands, and the trachea, with the process resulting in a rigid, white-colored, adherent mass that lacks tissue planes.[111,112] Under microscopic evaluation, a mix of inflammatory cells, including eosinophils, lymphocytes, and plasma cells, is noted. The pathologic changes noted in RT can appear consistent with a severe granulomatous process or malignancy, including a paucicellular type of anaplastic cancer of the thyroid.

Although the exact origin of RT remains undefined, there are several hypotheses on its etiology. It may represent a more extreme form of Hashimoto thyroiditis (HT) or a progressive SAT.[113] The presence of inflammatory cells (eosinophils and monocytes) seems to point to a possible autoimmune process.[114] Although potentially reactive in nature, the finding of antithyroid antibodies in at least some RT cases strengthens the hypothesis that RT is autoimmune related, as does the reported association with other autoimmune disorders, such as diabetes mellitus type 1, Addison's disease, and pernicious anemia.[115] A more recent hypothesis is a purported link between HT and IgG4-related systemic fibrosis and development of RT, which is supported by immunostaining showing high concentrations of IgG4+ plasma cells within the areas of RT-related infiltrative inflammation.[116-118] IgG4-related systemic disease is known to be associated with an obliterative phlebitis-type reaction. Elevated serum levels of IgG4 have been used to confirm the presence of IgG4-related systemic disease and may have a potential, albeit unproven, diagnostic use for RT because some patients display elevated levels but others do not. This may be related to the fact that the quantity of IgG4+ cells in RT appears to be inversely correlated with the duration of the disease.[119] Additional areas of destructive fibrosis may well occur outside the neck in conjunction with RT, whereas it is rare for patients with retroperitoneal fibrosis to later be diagnosed with RT.[107,120,121]

Clinical Management

Patient's with RT commonly present with fibrotic-related compressive symptoms that include hoarseness, aphonia, dysphagia, and/or dyspnea.[122,123] Physical examination many times reveals a fixed and firm thyroid suspicious for the presence of malignancy. If neck surgery is pursued, the surgeon will encounter a large fibrotic mass involving the thyroid and perithyroidal tissue without evident tissue planes.

As the fibroinflammatory reaction progresses, it can affect the thyroid and parathyroid glands, leading to hypothyroidism and/or hypoparathyroidism.[124] Data collected over time indicates that RT-associated hypothyroidism occurs in anywhere from 25% to 80% of patients. Development of hypothyroidism appears to be related to the extent of fibrosis occurring within the thyroid and whether or not background HT exists. In a Mayo Clinic series, 74% of patients with RT had hypothyroidism and a very high rate of antithyroid antibody positivity.[123] If the parathyroid glands are included within the area of invasive fibrosis, hypoparathyroidism can develop. The clinical severity of disease can span from mild hypocalcemia to very low calcium concentrations, low parathyroid hormone levels, and severe symptoms including tetany.[125] Hypoparathyroidism can occur after neck surgery for RT but can also occur spontaneously, typically with hypothyroidism having been diagnosed first.[126] In the Mayo Clinic series, 14% of patients not having undergone a surgical procedure developed hypoparathyroidism.[123] Other laboratory tests that can be altered in relation to RT include a rise in the ESR and sometimes an elevation of white blood cells.[127]

Ultrasound of the thyroid usually reveals a diffusely hypoechoic thyroid that appears hypovascular on color flow Doppler. Encasement of the carotid vessels, not typically seen with other forms of thyroiditis, may be noted in cases of RT.[128] Due to the associated fibrosis with RT, significant tissue stiffness will be noted by elastographic assessment. CT imaging may display cervical enlargement from a dense neck mass with the involved tissue appearing hypodense and lacking enhancement with an iodinated contrast agent,[129] and as with ultrasound, carotid and jugular vessels may be found to be surrounded by the fibrous tissue mass as well as evidence for invasion of perithyroidal tissue. T1- and T2-weighted MRI images tend to reveal a hypointense mass that may or may not enhance with gadolinium contrast.[130] In contradistinction, fibrotic areas involved with RT may demonstrate prominent uptake on fluorine-18 fluorodeoxyglucose positron emission tomography (PET) imaging and may identify affected areas beyond the neck region.[131] Although infrequently used in evaluation of cases of RT, technetium (Tc-99) and iodine (^{123}I or ^{131}I) based scintigraphic imaging is reported to reveal a heterogenous pattern with low avidity for radioactive iodine.[132] More intense uptake can be noted in those patients who have persistent areas of thyroid overactivity related to underlying Graves' disease or toxic nodular goiter.

Because RT can present as a thyroid mass, FNA may be performed. Cytologic results can span from being of nondiagnostic yield to having evidence of inflammatory changes, and can have a fibrous-type pattern with spindle-shaped cells and sometimes even appear as a follicular neoplasm.[133] Because FNA cytology is usually not definitive, tissue obtained during a decompression procedure or open biopsy can provide a histologic diagnosis. Histopathologic criteria for RT include: (1) presence of inflammation extending into neighboring cervical tissue; (2) lack of giant cells, granulomas, oncocytes, and lymphoid follicles; (3) presence of occlusive phlebitis; and (4) no sign of cancerous cells.[134,135] At present, the criteria do not yet include any provision for assessing IgG-4 status by immunohistochemical staining or plasma levels. When considering the diagnosis of RT, it is particularly important to rule out the presence of thyroid lymphoma, anaplastic thyroid cancer, and sarcoma of the thyroid as well as considering the possibility of the fibrosing variant of HT, which may occur in up to 10% of individuals with HT predominantly in older patients.[136-139]

Reports indicate that patients with RT go unrecognized for ~1 to 2 years after presenting with initial complaints such as neck/thyroid enlargement.[123] Individuals may be only mildly symptomatic, whereas others can display progressive and prominent symptoms during their course of disease, and although the disease process may appear to stabilize, patients may note increasing cervical tightness and pressure as well as a choking sensation and even stridor. On physical examination, patients may exhibit evidence of hoarseness from recurrent laryngeal nerve involvement, Horner's syndrome, or Tolosa-Hunt syndrome.[126,140] Extraocular muscle dysfunction or exophthalmos, comparable to Graves' orbitopathy-type changes, may also be found.[141] Fibroinflammatory changes in the parotids have been reported as have fibrotic lesions within the head and neck region.[142] Should the fibroinflammatory process extend inferiorly into the mediastinal region, there are reports of tracheoesophageal fistulas or superior vena cava syndrome occurring.[143] Cardiac problems are also possible and may include the development of pericardial effusions or coronary narrowing and occlusion.[123] Sclerosing cholangitis can develop should the liver become involved.[144] The fibrosis may also affect the retroperitoneal space resulting in renal failure related to hydroureteronephrosis or cholestasis from pancreatic involvement.[145]

Management

Although a total thyroidectomy may be achieved in some cases, the surgical option may be limited to an isthmusectomy, which can at least result in decompression of neck structures and alleviate related symptoms.[33] Surgical removal of a thyroid in a patient with RT carries significant risk because tissue planes cannot be identified and hypoparathyroidism and/or hoarseness from recurrent laryngeal nerve injury can occur at a higher rate than in patients without this process. Even when using more conservative surgical approaches, one study reported a 39% (7/18 patients) complication rate.[123] Based on such data and general experience, it is recommended to avoid attempts at extensive thyroid resection in individuals with RT.

In light of the suboptimal outcomes with surgery, medical treatment has been a focus of pursuit. Treatment with glucocorticoids and tamoxifen have both been proposed as potential treatment options, albeit lacking validation by prospective controlled trials given the rarity of the diagnosis. Glucocorticoid therapy can be associated with significant improvement in compression symptoms, such as hoarseness and upper airway complaints, apparently from shrinkage of the mass as well as a change in tumor consistency. Thyroid histology from a patient with RT who underwent a two-stage thyroidectomy, with a 2-year interval between the procedures, initially revealed extensive fibrosis with an infiltrate consisting of lymphocytes and prominently IgG4+ plasma cells with eosinophils. The later specimen, following a course of glucocorticoid therapy, was noted to be without evidence of a significant inflammatory response appearing hyalinized and acellular without IgG4+ cells.[146] Glucocorticoid dosing for RT treatment is empiric in nature because there are no systematic dosing comparisons available and reports note positive clinical response from prednisone doses ranging between as low as 15 mg daily to up to an initial dose of 100 mg.[147,148] Response to therapy varies from no apparent change to significant improvement in symptoms. Although some responses have been reported to persist long after the weaning of steroids, there are also instances of prompt recurrence even after lengthy rounds of glucocorticoid treatment.[149] Data in one study indicated that RT in nonsmokers may be more apt to respond to steroid therapy than in those who actively smoke tobacco.[123]

Tamoxifen has also been advocated as an option for the treatment of RT.[150] It has shown some efficacy in other conditions that exhibit multifocal fibrosis,[151] potentially through transforming growth factor (TGF)-β1-mediated inhibition of fibroblastic activity.[152] Recommended tamoxifen dosing is ~10-20 mg daily and may be used alone or in conjunction with glucocorticoid therapy.[153,154] As with prednisone, therapeutic response can vary, but reports indicate that at least some patients respond with a reduction in both mass size and associated symptoms.[126] The duration of response after discontinuation of tamoxifen therapy remains an unanswered question.

There are additional potential therapies, though they have been perhaps less well studied. There are a few reports regarding the use of low-dose radiation for treatment of RT, but no systematic evaluation of this therapy exists to date.[112] There is some sparsely published data that indicate at least a modest response to radiation in patients with other non-Riedel's inflammatory fibrotic conditions. With the extremely limited data, it is difficult to recommend radiation as a therapeutic option and especially not as a first-line option. The immune suppressant agent mycophenolate mofetil can be used in conjunction with glucocorticoid therapy. Mycophenolic acid, the active metabolite of mycophenolate, leads to inhibition of T and B lymphocyte production thereby reducing propagation of antibody levels. One example in the literature by Levy et al. describes a patient who did not respond to a combination of tamoxifen and prednisone but then responded to mycophenolate (1 g twice daily) and prednisone (100 mg daily) with significant improvement in compressive symptoms and subsequent successful subtotal thyroidectomy.[155] Rituximab, a monoclonal antibody which destroys B cells by mean of interaction with CD20 protein on the cell surface, has been reported to have favorable effects in IgG4-related systemic disorders and some cases of RT.[156] Two independent case reports describe significant symptomatic response to rituximab therapy (1 g intravenously monthly for 3 months either with 100 mg methylprednisolone or tamoxifen) after failing treatment with glucocorticoids and tamoxifen. The duration of reported responses was 14 and 30 months respectively at the time of the reports. Elevated activin A, a marker of active inflammation, was noted to drop from 218 pg/mL to 122 pg/mL after 10 months of rituximab initiation.

CHRONIC INFECTIOUS THYROIDITIS

Patients who are immunocompromised due to the human immunodeficiency virus (HIV), immunosuppression after organ transplantation, or treatment with myelosuppressive chemotherapy may be susceptible to chronic infection of the thyroid gland resulting from hematogenous spread of pathogenic fungi, mycobacterial organisms, and parasites. Disseminated fungal infections with invasive *Aspergillus* species may spread to involve the thyroid.[157] Acid-fast bacilli have been retrieved from granulomas present in thyroid tissue in patients with a disseminated or miliary mycobacterium tuberculosis infection.[158] Disseminated roundworm infections with *Strongyloides stercoralis* that spread to involve the thyroid may be associated with significant morbidity and mortality.[159] Chronic infections of the thyroid usually present with less severe clinical manifestations, and most cases respond to appropriate systemic treatment without the need for incision and drainage or surgical intervention.

RADIATION-ASSOCIATED THYROIDITIS

Treatment with therapeutic doses of radioactive iodine administered to control hyperthyroidism ascribed to Graves' disease or to ablate residual deposits of tissue after surgery to resect differentiated thyroid cancer may be associated with a low but definable risk of radiation-associated thyroiditis.[160] Up to 5% of patients with Graves' disease who receive targeted doses of ^{131}I may show biochemical evidence of thyroiditis marked by transient increased thyrotoxicosis. Although this condition is usually painless, a small number of patients may report associated pain and tenderness emanating from the thyroid that usually becomes noticeable within 2 to 10 days after administration of a dose of ^{131}I. The risk of developing painful radiation-associated thyroiditis in the setting of Graves' disease may be correlated with the level of the absorbed radiation dose, with a higher risk having been identified in patients with smaller volumes of hyperfunctioning thyroid tissue.[161] In patients who receive radioactive iodine for treatment of differentiated thyroid cancer, the risk of developing painful radiation-associated thyroiditis appears to correlate with the level of uptake in remnant tissue. Higher levels of uptake have been identified in patients who have large amounts of normal thyroid tissue left in place after surgery and in those who have received higher therapeutic doses of ^{131}I.[162] Development of radiation-associated thyroiditis does not appear to impact the effectiveness of postsurgical ablation.

If ultrasound has been performed before administration of radioactive iodine for treatment of Graves' disease, comparative imaging performed after the onset of symptoms may reveal enlargement of the thyroid with diffuse increased echogenicity and blurring of the borders between the thyroid and surrounding tissue.[163] Mild discomfort can be treated with NSAIDs. More severe pain and tenderness may require a treatment with prednisone that can be started at a dose of 20 to 40 mg daily and tapered as warranted for sustained relief. Treatment with a cardioselective beta-blocker may be considered if concomitant thyrotoxic symptoms become disruptive.

PALPATION THYROIDITIS

Initially characterized as an incidental histologic finding noted on pathologic examination, inflammation caused by direct palpation or instrumentation of the thyroid has come to be recognized as a clinically significant condition that may precipitate symptomatic thyrotoxicosis severe enough to trigger atrial arrhythmias.[164] Although the incidence of palpation thyroiditis is unknown, prospective evaluation of patients undergoing parathyroid exploration has shown that postoperative thyrotoxicosis occurred in 31% of patients, half of whom reported concurrent referable symptoms.[165] Similar presentations have been identified in patients undergoing laryngectomy and neck dissection procedures for treatment of head and neck cancer and melanoma.[166]

Immediate recognition of palpation thyroiditis in the proper context may only be possible when there has been preoperative documentation of a normal TSH level. In cases where TSH levels have not been checked before surgery, it may be necessary to expectantly monitor profiles of thyroid hormone levels over time to ensure that identified thyrotoxicosis is a transient condition that does not reflect hyperthyroidism due to underlying Graves' disease or autonomous thyroid nodules. If indicated, disruptive thyrotoxic symptoms may be treated with a cardioselective beta-blocker until thyroid hormone levels normalize.

REFERENCES

For a complete list of references, go to expertconsult.com.

5

Thyroglossal Duct Cysts and Ectopic Thyroid Tissue

Christopher Fundakowski, Erin Felger, Ellie Maghami

EMBRYOLOGY

The median anlage of the thyroid originates from the endodermal segment in the floor of the primitive pharynx at the foramen cecum located in the midline at the junction of the anterior two-thirds of the tongue (first branchial arch derivative) and posterior one-third (third branchial arch derivative) (see Chapter 2, Applied Embryology of the Thyroid and Parathyroid Glands). Between 5 and 7 weeks of gestation, this central element of what will become the thyroid gland migrates caudally from the foramen cecum to its normal position below the thyroid cartilage. The path of descent is closely associated with the hyoid bone and is usually anterior to it but can also be seen posteriorly or within the bone. The lateral thyroid anlage is derived from the ultimobranchial body, a descending diverticulum of the fourth to fifth pharyngeal pouch. The ultimobranchial body ultimately derives from the neural crest and brings C cells to the thyroid gland. Between 7 and 10 weeks of gestation, the thyroglossal epithelial tract obliterates. Failure of the thyroglossal duct tract to obliterate can result in formation of thyroglossal duct cysts (TGDCs).

THYROGLOSSAL DUCT CYSTS

In autopsy series, thyroglossal tract remnants are found in approximately 7% of the normal population.[1] They represent the most common congenital midline mass. TGDCs are found mostly in children and adolescents, but they are also found in patients over 20 years old in one-third of all cases (Figures 5.1 and 5.2). Most TGDCs are found between the hyoid and thyroid cartilage (approximately two-thirds),[2,3] at or above the hyoid/suprahyoid[2,3] (nearly one-third), followed by less common suprasternal[3] and base of tongue locations.

The standard surgical treatment for TGDCs is the Sistrunk procedure. The procedure involves excising the cyst, removing the thyroglossal duct tract along with the central portion of the hyoid bone, and excising a central core of the base of the tongue at the foramen cecum. This procedure has been shown to be associated with very low (<4%) recurrence rates.[2-4]

Minimally Invasive Surgical Approaches

There has been growing experience with minimally invasive surgical techniques applied to TGDCs over the past decade. Different minimally invasive and remote access approaches have been described and include endoscopic, endoscopic with robotic assist, small cervical incision with endoscopic adjunct, modified facelift approach, and bilateral axillo-breast approach (BABA).[5-8] Complications include bleeding, infection, nerve damage, tethering of the tongue by scar tissue, dysphagia, and dysarthria.[5,6] Dysphagia and dysarthria are frequently transient and effectively remedied by the speech and language therapist. For the majority of these procedures, operative times are equivalent to the open Sistrunk procedure.[7,9] Recurrence rates are low with this type of procedure and outcomes are comparable across age groups.[5,9-12]

Endoscopic approaches are done through the floor of the mouth. These surgical procedures are appealing because there is often no visible scar, and most studies suggest there is reasonable visualization of the pathology.[8,9] Because of endoscopic magnification, branching of the TGDC and extension to the base of the tongue are easier to identify; therefore a more complete resection may be achieved. In the pediatric population with smaller pharyngeal work space, conversion to open procedure is more common.[10-12]

It is important to check thyroid function tests before and after surgery to confirm thyroid function is preserved after surgery. Postoperatively, patients are managed similarly to those who have had open procedures for TGDC and are subsequently monitored for recurrence. Overall, minimally invasive surgery for TGDC is well tolerated with comparable results and excellent patient satisfaction.[5,9,11]

TGDC Carcinoma

Management decisions are complicated by the incidental discovery of malignancy within an excised TGDC. The incidence of malignancy in TGDCs is approximately 1%.[13,14] TGDC malignancies are clinically difficult to distinguish from benign TGDCs, and thus, are rarely suspected preoperatively. Ultrasound suggestion of local invasion, metastatic lymphadenopathy, or the presence of microcalcifications should raise suspicion for malignancy. The majority (~90%) are TGDC malignancies; squamous cell carcinoma is rare.[13,15] Local soft tissue invasion may be present in 30% of TGDC malignancies.

With TGDC carcinoma concomitant, PTC in the orthotopic thyroid gland may be present in 11% to 56% of patients.[16-19] Most (80%) thyroid tumors in these patients will be microcarcinomas, with approximately 50% being multifocal. In addition, patients with synchronous cancer in both the thyroid and TGDC tend to be older than those with cancer solely located in the TGDC (44.9 vs. 32 years, p 0.006) and more likely to have metastasis.[20] In a series of 26 patients with TGDC carcinoma by Pellegriti et al., the central compartment did not contain any metastatic nodes when the PTC was confined to the TGDC, as opposed to those patients who had synchronous PTC identified in their orthotopic thyroid glands. Thus in a patient with isolated TGDC PTC, central compartment disease is unlikely. An additional retrospective review of 28 cases of TGDC by Zizic et al. addressed the issue of nomenclature heterogeneity and noted that true TGDC is commonly difficult to differentiate from pyramidal lobe PTC, prelaryngeal (Delphian) nodal PTC metastasis, and indeterminate origin, thus leading to further controversy in management. Consequently they proposed a new terminology of upper neck papillary thyroid carcinoma (UPTC) to group these entities. The authors note that although clinical preoperative diagnosis

CHAPTER 5 Thyroglossal Duct Cysts and Ectopic Thyroid Tissue

adjuvant radioactive iodine, thyroid suppression therapy, and thyroglobulin follow-up assessment.[18,24]

TGDC PTC may be adequately managed with the Sistrunk procedure alone in the following circumstances: young patient (<55 years), no prior radiation, small tumor (<1 to 1.5 cm), normal thyroid gland ultrasound, no evidence of central/lateral adenopathy, and no evidence of soft tissue extension.[25] Surgery is extended to include total thyroidectomy with or without central neck dissection when the tumor is larger than 1 to 1.5 cm, when there is concern for soft tissue invasion, and when there is the presence of concurrent suspicious thyroid nodules or adenopathy.[18] The algorithm by Zizic et al. suggests that in true TGDC, additional orthotopic thyroid surgery is typically not necessary when there is an unremarkable thyroid ultrasound.[21]

In patients with low-risk diseases who are treated with the Sistrunk procedure, there are no data supporting the role of thyroid suppression therapy. The prognosis of PTC arising in TGDC is excellent, with an overall survival rate of 95.6% at 10 years.[13,16] The postsurgical follow-up of patients is limited to an annual clinical and sonographic cervical examination in low-risk patients treated with the Sistrunk procedure. In those who have also undergone total thyroidectomy, serum thyroglobulin levels can also be measured for cancer surveillance, provided the patient does not have antibodies to thyroglobulin.

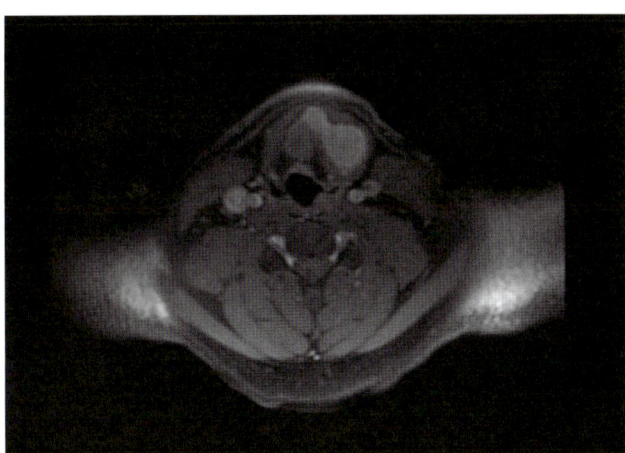

Fig. 5.1 Prelaryngeal ETT in a 37-year-old male with dysphagia and upper neck mass. Magnetic resonance imaging (MRI) image showing solid component with contrast enhancement along the left side of the larynx deep to the strap muscle with a nonenhancing cystic component in the preepiglottic fatty space.

ECTOPIC THYROID TISSUE

Ectopic thyroid tissue (ETT) refers to any thyroid tissue in unusual locations and is a form of thyroid dysgenesis. Thyroid dysgenesis is mostly sporadic and likely caused by epigenetic factors; however, several mutations in genes playing a role during thyroid morphogenesis, such as *NKX2-1 (TTF-1), PAX8, FOXE1 (TTF-2), NKX2-5, HHEX, TSHR,* and *JAG1,* have been implicated.[26,27] The incidence is not yet correlated with any environmental factors.

Autopsy series report an ETT prevalence of approximately 10%, with the majority of cases in women. ETT has been reported on two or even three locations.[28,29] Of the people with ETT, 70% lack a normally located anterior neck pretracheal thyroid gland. Most cases of ETT are diagnosed early in life at times of increased metabolic demand, such as during puberty or pregnancy, when there may be an increase in thyroid-stimulating hormone due to less than normal ETT hormone production, leading to enlargement of the ETT with symptomatic clinical expression.[30] Nuclear imaging with Technetium 99m pertechnetate or ^{123}I is useful when an orthotopic thyroid gland is not identified by ultrasound.[31] Planar scintigraphy is sufficient for diagnosis of ETT, although three-dimensional (3D) SPECT/CT will add useful in situ spatial definition.

ETT is most commonly present in midline body locations from the base of the tongue down into the mediastinum but can occur anywhere (Table 5.1). Approximately 90% of ETT is found in the base of the tongue as a lingual thyroid.[30,32-34] Sublingual ETT is rare. Subdiaphragmatic ETT is even rarer. Ma et al. reported a case of

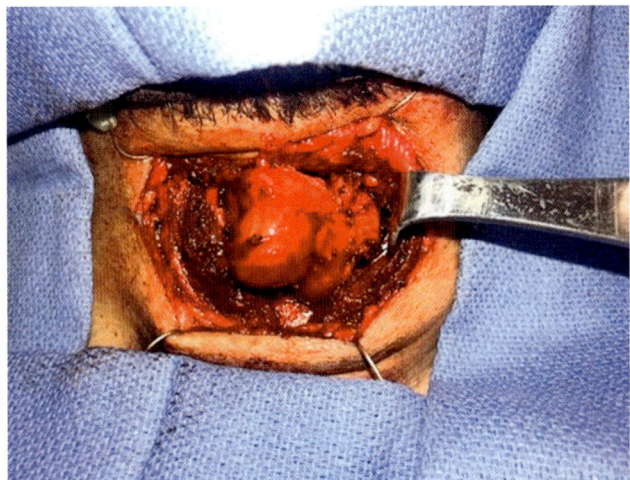

Fig. 5.2 Intraoperative exposure of the prelaryngeal mass deep to the strap musculature.

is difficult, proper pathologic review will allow subcategorization of UPTC in the majority of cases, because true TGDC cancer was diagnosed in only 14% of their series on final review. This subcategorization is clinically relevant, given that it will dictate whether further orthotopic thyroid surgery is warranted.[21]

Most authors believe that incidentally discovered TGDC PTC can be adequately resected by the Sistrunk procedure alone,[13,14,21,22] provided there is no clinical or sonographic suspicion of orthotopic thyroid lesion or cervical adenopathy. This procedure is associated with a cure rate of 95% in reported series.[13,14,22] Others advocate a more aggressive approach—total thyroidectomy along with the Sistrunk procedure.[17,23,24] The argument for a more aggressive surgical approach involves the potential for occult, and likely multifocal, PTC in the thyroid gland and increased likelihood of central compartment metastasis. In the scenario of TGDC with concurrent multifocal orthotopic PTC, nodal metastasis may be present in up to 75% of patients, with 40% of metastases in the central neck and 60% in the lateral neck.[9] In these circumstances concurrent total thyroidectomy will allow for potential

TABLE 5.1	Sites of Ectopic Thyroid
Rare sites	Pituitary, tonsil, iris
Base of tongue	Lingual thyroid
Anterior neck	Sublingual, infrahyoid, prelaryngeal, larynx, trachea
Lateral neck	Lymph nodes, soft tissues, carotid bifurcation, submandibular space, parapharyngeal space
Mediastinum	Thymus, aortic wall, pericardium, heart
Abdomen	Adrenal, gallbladder, liver, pancreas, duodenum
Pelvis	Struma ovarii, fallopian tube, uterus, vagina

pancreatic ETT and reviewed 34 cases of intraabdominal ETT in the literature between 2006 and 2017, the majority of them being in the adrenal gland.[35]

Approximately 10% of ETT is found in the lateral neck and historically referred to as "lateral aberrant thyroid."[36] Lateral aberrant thyroid can occur within jugular chain nodes or exist outside of lymphatic structures, usually in conjunction with an orthotopic thyroid in a euthyroid patient.[37-39] There is ongoing debate regarding the benign or malignant nature of these rare and small lateral neck ETT deposits. Through autopsy studies and surgical case series, some argue that a small amount of normal-appearing thyroid tissue found in a subcapsular location within a lateral neck node may represent embryologic ectopic rest within the node rather than metastasis from an occult thyroid primary.[40,41] Similarly some suggest ETT devoid of lymph node architecture may derive from abnormal growth and separation of tissue from the main thyroid anlage during embryogenesis rather than metastasis from an orthotopic thyroid primary.[42] Some have advocated for at least homolateral thyroidectomy and close clinical follow-up even if the lateral aberrant thyroid tissue was judged benign histologically.[43] Today, immunohistochemical panels and oncogene profiling (*BRAF V600 E* mutation) may help distinguish benign from malignant ETT in the lateral neck compartment.[44]

Clinical presentation of ETT varies depending on the patient's thyroid hormone status, ETT body location, size, and histopathology. In a euthyroid asymptomatic patient, ETT may be an incidental discovery found during imaging or a physical examination. ETT enlargement may lead to various symptoms depending on body location. ETT within the trachea can cause progressive dyspnea, hemoptysis, and stridor. Pelvic ETT can present with abdominal pain or vaginal bleeding. Enlargement in cases of lingual thyroids may cause globus, cough, dysphagia, dysphonia, hemorrhage, pain, dyspnea, and sleep apnea.[39,45] Kansal et al. recommended that patients with a lingual thyroid, even if the lingual thyroid is small, be placed on lifelong thyroxine replacement to prevent subsequent enlargement.[46]

Any thyroid disease may be expressed in ETT, including Hashimoto's thyroiditis, Graves' disease, and cancer. The lingual thyroid is typically benign and can rarely harbor malignancy. ETT can occur in struma ovarii, which is a germ cell tumor of the ovary with thyroid tissue comprising more than 50% of the tissue.[47,48] Struma ovarii represents ETT not through embryologic fragmentation or abnormal migration but from direct thyroid tissue differentiation from primary ovarian embryologic sources. Approximately 5% of struma ovarii are malignant.[47-50] In general, the most common histopathological subtype of malignant ETT is papillary carcinoma followed by follicular carcinoma.[51-53]

Regardless of body location, a thyroid laboratory panel is obtained and a fine-needle aspiration biopsy is frequently employed to guide management. For euthyroid patients with an asymptomatic ETT and benign histopathology, close observation may be advised. Hypothyroidism is corrected with hormone replacement therapy. Thyroid hormone replacement is also useful in suppressing thyroid-stimulating hormone in symptomatic patients with functional and/or cosmetic concerns. Patients with compressive symptoms, ulceration and bleeding, or suspected malignancy need to be treated with either excision surgery or targeted ablative therapies.[54,55] The majority of patients will become hypothyroid after treatment, requiring lifelong hormone replacement therapy. In 75% of patients with a lingual thyroid, it is the only thyroid tissue present and the sole source of thyroid hormone production.[34]

Minimally invasive surgical techniques using carbon dioxide (CO_2) laser and/or robotic technology are frequently employed for surgical resection of symptomatic ETT and when there is concern for malignancy and/or potential for growth and impingement on critical structures.[56,57] For larger tumors, a more traditional open approach for resection of ETT may be necessary. For larger lingual thyroid tissue, a lateral or suprahyoid pharyngotomy may be necessary, and a mandibulotomy may help with exposure. A tracheostomy may be temporarily needed for airway support. Peng et al. reported on 36 cases of intrapericardial ETT, mostly involving the right interventricular septum. The majority underwent surgical excision for diagnosis and to relieve obstruction of the right ventricular inflow and outflow tracts.[58]

REFERENCES

For a complete list of references, go to expertconsult.com.

Surgery of Cervical and Substernal Goiter

Whitney Liddy, James L. Netterville, Gregory W. Randolph

"Guttur homini tantum et suibus intumescit aquarum quae potantur plerumque vitio." (Translation: Swelling of the throat occurs only in men and swine, caused mostly by the water they drink.)

—*Pliny the Elder, 1st century* AD[1]

> Please go to expertconsult.com to view related video:
> **Video 6.1** Surgery for Cervical and Substernal Goiter.
> This chapter contains additional online-only content, including an exclusive video, *Surgery for Cervical and Substernal Goiter* available on expertconsult.com.

The word *goiter* is derived from "guttur," the Latin term for throat.[2] Surgery for goiter is as complex as it is rewarding. With goiter, the normally complex neck base anatomy is distorted in sometimes predictable and often unpredictable patterns. Size, goiter vascularity, distortion of anatomy, substernal extension, and restrictions imposed by the bony confines of the thoracic inlets can make recurrent laryngeal nerve (RLN) and parathyroid gland identification and preservation challenging. William Halsted wrote that "the extirpation of the thyroid gland for goiter better typifies perhaps than other operations, the supreme triumph of the surgeon's art."[3]

Please see the Expert Consult website for more discussion of this topic.

This chapter reviews the patterns of anatomic distortion presented by both cervical and substernal goiter. Substernal goiter represents a distinct subtype of cervical goiter and is discussed separately where appropriate, given its unique challenges. After reviewing key points regarding goiter's definition and clinical evaluation, we shall discuss treatment options, with an emphasis on the surgical approach. The chapter highlights the evaluation of upper airway compromise in patients with goiter, the relationship between the extent of surgery and the likelihood of goiter recurrence, and the predictive risk factors for surgical complications. See also Chapter 7, Approach to the Mediastinum: Transcervical, Transsternal, and Video-Assisted; Chapter 8, The Surgical Management of Hyperthyroidism; and Chapter 9, Reoperation for Benign Thyroid Disease.

GENERAL CONSIDERATIONS

Goiter Definition

First, it is important to come to an understanding regarding what a "goiter" is and to define "big." This is not easy when one looks critically at the literature. Both greatest diameter and goiter weight have been used to define thyroid enlargement. In the studies, methods for determining goiter size range from physical examination measured in centimeters, to physical examination estimated in grams, to surgical specimen measured in centimeters or grams. Preoperative imaging diameters may also be used.

The definition of goiter varies substantially among reports. McHenry suggested 80 g and Russell 100 g, whereas Clark proposed 200 g as the threshold value.[5-9] Studies investigating radioiodine treatment for multinodular goiter often define *significant goiter* as greater than 100 g. Hegedus, Nygaard, and Hansen found that goiter surgical specimens averaged 30 g for unilateral resection and 64 g for bilateral resection.[10] In the study by Katlic, Grillo, and Wang, the average weight of substernal goiter was 104 g (range 25 to 357 g), with the greatest diameter averaging 9 cm (range 5 to 19 cm).[11] In a series of more than 200 cervical and substernal goiters treated at Massachusetts Eye and Ear Infirmary and Massachusetts General Hospital, the mean weight was 143 g and the mean goiter size was 10.5 cm.[12]

Please see the Expert Consult website for more discussion of this topic.

Substernal Goiter Definition

Substernal goiter and its subtypes have been variously termed *retrosternal, subclavicular, intrathoracic, mediastinal, aberrant, wandering,* and *spring goiter,* as well as *goiter mobile* and *goiter plongeant.* Numerous definitions and classification schemes have been proposed for substernal goiter.

Please see the Expert Consult website for more discussion of this topic.
A classification system for substernal goiters is most useful when it takes into account the features of substernal goiters that must be appreciated to extract these goiters safely. We define *substernal goiter* simply as a goiter that is associated with substernal extension such that the thoracic component requires mediastinal dissection to facilitate extraction. We believe that all substernal goiters require axial computed tomography (CT) scanning to differentiate between the various subtypes. Such differentiation provides tremendously useful surgical information. We propose the following substernal goiter classification scheme (Table 6.1).

ANTERIOR MEDIASTINAL GOITER (SUBSTERNAL GOITER TYPE I)

Most surgical and radiographic series suggest that substernal goiters affect the anterior mediastinum in approximately 85% of patients and the posterior mediastinum in approximately 15% (see Table 6.1).[26-29] Extension into the anterior mediastinum brings the mass anterior to the subclavian and innominate vessels and anterior to the RLN. The relationship of the anterior mediastinal goiter to the RLN is the same as the normal cervical gland—that is, the nerve is deep.

POSTERIOR MEDIASTINAL GOITER (SUBSTERNAL GOITER TYPE II)

When substernal goiter expands to the posterior mediastinum, it excavates the region posterior to the trachea, pushing the trachea

TABLE 6.1 Substernal Goiter Classification

Type	Location	Anatomy	Prevalence	Approach, Comment
I	Anterior mediastinum	Anterior to great vessels, trachea, RLN	85%	Transcervical (sternotomy only if intrathoracic goiter diameter > thoracic inlet diameter)
II	Posterior mediastinum	Posterior to great vessels, trachea, RLN	15%	As above; also consider sternotomy or right posterolateral thoracotomy if type IIB
IIA	Ipsilateral extension			
IIB	Contralateral extension			
B1	Extension posterior to both trachea and esophagus			
B2	Extension between trachea and esophagus			
III	Isolated mediastinal goiter	No connection to orthotopic gland; may have mediastinal blood supply	<1%	Transcervical or sternotomy

RLN, recurrent laryngeal nerve.

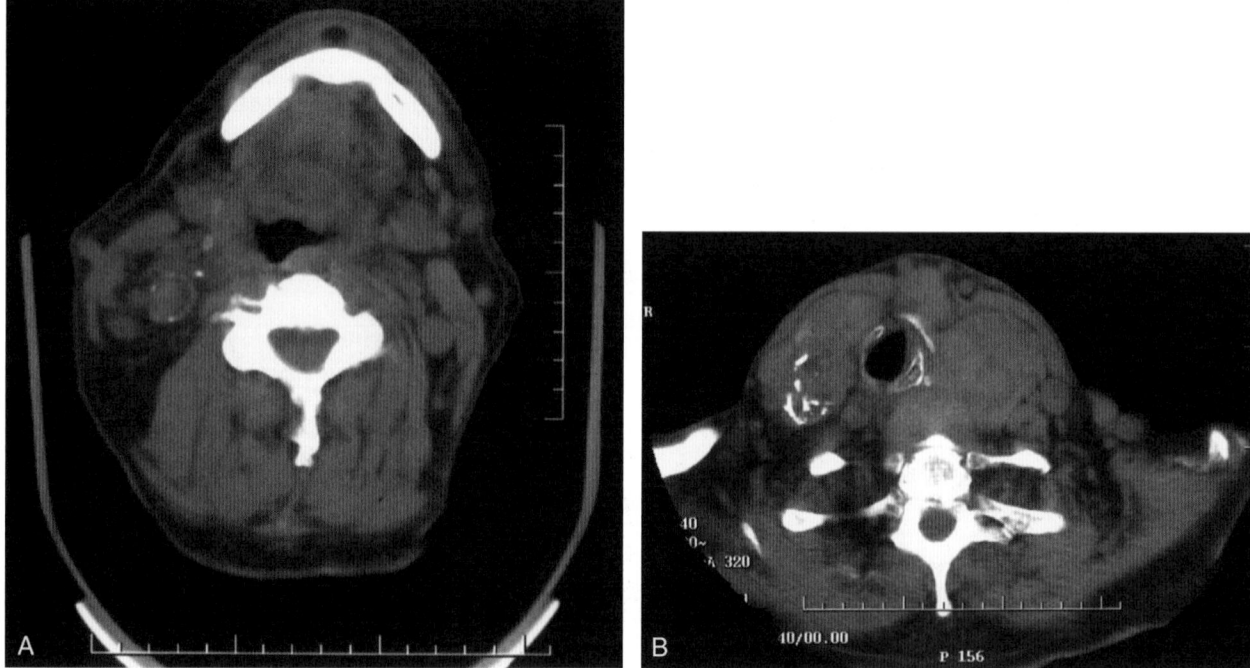

Fig. 6.1 Patient with a large cervical and substernal goiter. Substernal goiter extends into the left chest and then crosses retrotracheally into the right chest, extending between the trachea and esophagus (substernal goiter type IIB2). **A,** Right superior pole extends beneath the sternocleidomastoid muscle to the level of the mandible. **B,** At the level of the cricoid cartilage, goiter is present bilaterally in the neck.

anteriorly and splaying the great vessels anteriorly. The mass then comes to rest in a space posterior to the innominate vein, carotid sheath contents, innominate and subclavian arteries, RLN, and inferior thyroid artery.[26,27,30] It is important to know that the relationship of the mass and the RLN is reversed compared with the normal cervical orthotopic gland-RLN relationship. The RLN is ventral to the inferior component of the mass and, if not recognized early on, can be stretched or cut by even the most meticulous thyroid surgeon. The nerve can also be entrapped between components of the posterior mediastinal goiter; even in these circumstances, a portion of the goiter will be deep to the RLN. Such posterior mediastinal goiters can come to rest in a space bounded inferiorly by the azygous vein; posteriorly by the vertebral column; laterally by the first rib; medially by the trachea and esophagus; and anteriorly by the carotid sheath, subclavian and innominate vessels, superior vena cava (SVC), and phrenic and RLNs.[26,27]

Posterior mediastinal goiter (type IIA) can occur ipsilateral to the cervical gland of origin or may come to rest through retrotracheal extension in the contralateral thorax (substernal goiter type IIB; see Table 6.1). Extension to the right thorax is more commonly seen as a result of aortic arch and is associated branch vessels obstructing the left posterior mediastinal descent pathway.[31,32] Contralateral thoracic extension in the posterior mediastinum may occur either behind the trachea and esophagus (IIB1) or between the trachea and esophagus (IIB2). Axial CT scanning and barium swallow help determine this pattern. Generally, the right thoracic caudal extension is limited at the level of the azygous arch (Figure 6.1).[33]

ISOLATED MEDIASTINAL GOITER (SUBSTERNAL GOITER TYPE III)

Although rare, thyroid masses within the mediastinum may exist without connection to the normal cervical orthotopic gland. Such purely isolated mediastinal goiters represent only 0.2% to 3% of all goiters requiring surgical treatment.[11,24,34,35] Such lesions are important to recognize because unlike all other types of substernal goiters, the blood supply of the isolated mediastinal goiter may be provided through

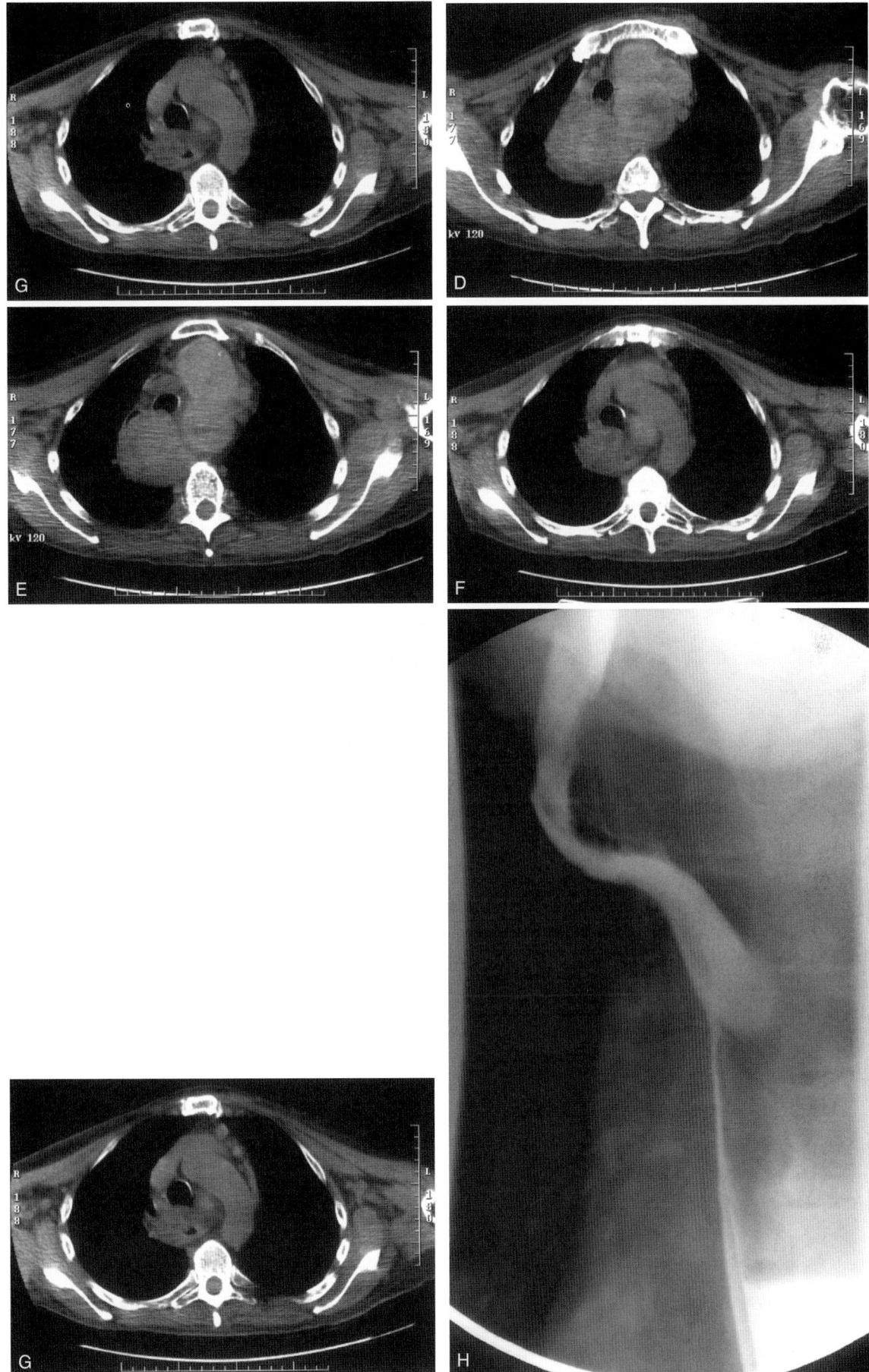

Fig. 6.1, cont'd See legend on next page.

purely mediastinal arteries (including the aorta, subclavian, internal mammary, thyrocervical trunk, and innominate) and veins. This is extremely important when planning surgical resection.[11,24,36-40] This entity is best termed *isolated mediastinal goiter*. Other terms have been used, including *aberrant mediastinal* and *ectopic mediastinal goiter*.

 Please see the Expert Consult website for more discussion of this topic.

PREVALENCE, PATHOGENESIS, AND NATURAL HISTORY

Prevalence

Multinodular goiter affects 4% of the United States' population and up to 10% of the British population.[45,46] New thyroid nodular disease occurs in 0.1% to 1.5% of the general population per year.[47,48] Globally, iodine deficiency contributes to the vast majority of cases of multinodular goiter and was estimated to affect 1.5 billion people, or nearly 30% of the world's population in 1990.[49] Further, it is estimated that approximately 655 million people in 118 countries are affected by endemic goiter. Endemic goiter regions are defined as iodine-deficient regions in which at least 5% to 10% of the population is affected by goiter. In certain iodine-deficient regions, higher goiter rates occur. In 1994 in Bangladesh, approximately 47% of the population was affected by endemic goiter.[50] The majority of the natural iodine supply exists as iodide in the world's oceans. It is therefore mainly noncoastal mountainous and lowland regions—where iodine is leached from the soil by flooding, heavy rainfall, and deforestation—that are at risk for endemic goiter. Sporadic forms of multinodular goiter do occur in iodine-replete regions with lesser prevalence.[16,49] Prevalence estimates of sporadic goiters vary between authors, ranging from less than 4% (clinical evaluation series) and between 16% and 67% (ultrasound series).[51,52]

 Please see the Expert Consult website for more discussion of this topic.

Pathogenesis

Please see the Expert Consult website for more discussion of this topic.

Natural History

The natural history of untreated, sporadic, nontoxic goiter is not completely understood, but slow growth appears to be the general predictable pattern. Berghout et al. suggested a steady volume increase of up to 10% to 20% per year.[75] Pregnancy, iodine deficiency, consumption of goitrogens, and alteration in suppressive or antithyroid medical regimens can result in goiter progression. Hemorrhage into a preexisting nodule can also result in the development of acute, regional, and airway symptoms.[76] In patients presenting with diffuse goiter, there is a general tendency toward nodule formation and progressive autonomy, with hyperthyroidism ultimately developing in up to 10% of patients (see Chapter 8, The Surgical Management of Hyperthyroidism).[77]

 Please see the Expert Consult website for more discussion of this topic.

CLINICAL PRESENTATION

Cervical Goiter

History

The history of goitrous growth and associated symptoms is critical for determining surgical candidacy. This history should be obtained not only from the patient but also from the patient's family. Regional symptoms should be addressed relating to respiration, phonation, swallowing, and the presence of globus (lump sensation). As Pemberton emphasized in 1921, symptoms associated with goiter may be positionally induced.[38] Positions that may provoke goiter regional symptomatology include being supine, arms raised (as when reaching for an upper cabinet), extreme neck extension, extreme neck flexion (as with reading a book in bed), and turning the head to the extreme left or right. Patients thus need to be questioned about positional provocation of regional symptoms. In addition, the family needs to be questioned about nocturnal symptoms, because symptoms may manifest initially in the setting of recumbency and upper airway relaxation during sleep. Symptoms may also be associated with exercise and increased oxygen demands. A history of preceding upper respiratory tract infection may produce dyspnea in a patient with long-standing tracheal obstruction secondary to goiter through new laryngotracheal mucosal edema. Patients with cervical or substernal goiter may present with cough, dyspnea, foreign-body sensation, neck tightness, change in collar size, or wheezing and may come to the head and neck surgeon with a misdiagnosis of asthma or chronic obstructive pulmonary disease (COPD). In our series of patients with large cervical and substernal goiter, we found that 25% of patients were preoperatively asymptomatic.[12]

Symptoms of hypothyroidism and hyperthyroidism should be reviewed. Hyperthyroidism may slowly evolve in patients with multinodular goiter or may develop acutely in response to significant iodine load such as with a CT scan contrast (Jod-Basedow phenomenon) or with the introduction of iodized salt in endemic goiter regions.[82] A history of migration from an area of endemic goiter should be obtained, as well as a history of exposure to known goitrogens, notably iodine and lithium. A family history of thyroid disease should also be obtained.

Physical Examination

After documentation of thyroid size, the examiner should note the consistency and fixation of the mass, especially with respect to the larynx and trachea. Estimation of goiter size by physical examination is clearly an inaccurate method of assessment. Jarlov et al. found substantial errors in the clinical assessment of thyroid size compared with ultrasonographic assessment.[83] Estimated weight based on the physical examination generally underestimates multinodular goiter weight by 25 to 50 g.[47] The larynx (landmarks include thyroid notch and cricoid anterior arch) and trachea should be examined for deviation from the midline. Typically, cervical goiter will deviate the larynx and trachea to the contralateral side. Inability to palpate the lower thyroid lobe edge should raise suspicion for substernal extension and prompt additional evaluation. The neck must also be examined for adenopathy as well as scarring from past thyroid and other neck surgery. Jugular distention

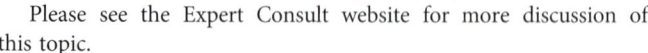

Fig. 6.1, cont'd   C, At the level of the thoracic inlet, the left lobe expands and extends into the left chest and retrotracheally into the right thorax. **D,** The mass extends substernally along the left lateral trachea and retrotracheally, abutting both left and right lung fields, splaying the great vessels. **E,** The distal segment of the substernal mass has several lobulations. The innominate artery is seen anterior to the trachea. A bronchus abuts the lateral aspect of the inferior-most goiter segment. The goiter posteriorly abuts the vertebral column. **F,** The inferior-most extent of the goiter extends retrotracheally deep to the level of the aortic arch. The mass can be seen infiltrating the region between the trachea anteriorly and the esophagus posteriorly. **G,** The mass extends between the trachea and esophagus, ending just above the azygous vein and right mainstem bronchus. **H,** Barium swallow showing substantial cervical and mediastinal esophageal deviation. The mass was resected transcervically without sternotomy, with recurrent laryngeal nerve and vagal monitoring with normal cord motion postoperatively. The specimen weighed 450 g and was 15 cm in greatest diameter.

and subcutaneous venous redistribution should be noted. Although both of these may be present with large benign cervical or substernal goiter, true SVC syndrome is generally due to malignant thyroid disease and warrants careful scanning and evaluation.[11]

It is imperative in all patients with goiter that the larynx be examined. In our series, we have found that 2% of patients with goiter presented with vocal cord paralysis in the setting of benign disease and no prior neck surgery, and 3.5% of preoperative patients presented with goiter overall.[12] Vocal cord paralysis without a history of past thyroid surgery implies invasive thyroid malignancy until proven otherwise. It should be noted, however, that benign goiter may also be associated with vocal cord paralysis, presumably through stretching of the nerve, which may recover postoperatively (see Chapter 36, Surgical Anatomy and Monitoring of the Recurrent Laryngeal Nerve).[84] Certainly, such a preoperative finding focuses the surgeon's attention on the extreme importance of preserving the contralateral RLN. The laryngeal examination in patients with large cervical goiter can be difficult if there is edematous or redundant supraglottic mucosa, laryngeal compression and deviation, and hypopharyngeal crowding resulting from goitrous extrinsic compression. Symptomatic assessment of the voice, like symptomatic assessment of the airway, does not predict objective findings in patients with goiter and should not replace the laryngeal examination. In our patient series, voice change was reported preoperatively in 12.8%, but vocal cord paralysis was present in only 3.5%, consistent with the work of Michel, emphasizing that glottic function cannot be predicted by voice assessment.[85,86] Michel, in his series of substernal goiters, noted that although hoarseness was described in 26%, vocal cord paralysis was only found in 3%.[87] Thus, we reiterate our recommendation that all patients with goiter undergo preoperative laryngeal examination.

Substernal Goiter

Please see the Expert Consult website for more discussion of this topic.

GOITER WORKUP

During the workup of patients presenting with a goiter, the clinician should address the following three important issues: (1) the existence or the potential development of airway compression, (2) the risk of malignancy, and (3) the presence of hyperthyroidism (Boxes 6.1 and 6.2).

Airway Assessment in Thyroid Disease

Foremost in goiter assessment is airway evaluation. The fundamental components of airway evaluation include determination of the rate and pattern of respiration, presence of sound with breathing (i.e., stridor), and voice quality. In patients with significant airway obstruction from thyroid disease, the initial assessment requires integration of a targeted but complete history and physical examination to expeditiously identify the site and magnitude of obstruction. One must always remember to keep in mind the overall global status of the patient with respect to his or her respiratory effort and signs of distress. Fatigue, restlessness, or apprehension can occur in the setting of hypoxia. The patient who is lethargic may be hypercapnic. Body position as an indicator of respiratory comfort, peripheral signs of oxygenation, and cyanosis should be carefully evaluated. Included in this assessment is the taking of vital signs and the use of pulse oximetry. One must be vigilant that a patient with a good pulse oximeter reading—or, for that matter, good arterial blood gas levels—may, a moment later, experience complete respiratory obstruction. The sound of respiration (i.e., the presence of stridor) gives an important clue as to the magnitude and location of airway obstruction. Stridor implies turbulent airflow through a stenotic airway segment. Significant extrathoracic obstruction (most commonly laryngeal, subglottic, or upper cervical tracheal) typically presents with inspiratory stridor and is seen as a variable extrathoracic obstruction on flow volume loop analysis with inspiratory phase flattening. Isolated expiratory stridor is seen in intrathoracic (lower tracheal) obstruction. Here, inspiration is silent and the voice is normal.

Acute Airway Compromise

Please see the Expert Consult website for more discussion of this topic, including Figure 6.2.

EVALUATION OF UPPER AIRWAY COMPROMISE AND OTHER REGIONAL SYMPTOMS

Regional Symptomatic Assessment

Upper airway obstruction is a common finding in patients with goiter, highlighting the importance of optimal airway evaluation. Common presenting symptoms in our series of patients with goiter included shortness of breath (approximately 50%) and dysphagia (approximately 50%), emphasizing the effect of cervical and substernal goiter on the adjacent cervical viscera. Although earnest symptomatic assessment at presentation is crucial in patients with goiter, clinical experience suggests subjective symptomatic assessment of the upper

---

BOX 6.1 Airway Imaging, Flow Volume Loops, and Goiter Symptoms: Summary

- The presence of preoperative shortness of breath correlates with goiter size, but it is of limited value as a screening tool for tracheal abnormalities.
- Dysphagia correlates with radiographic findings of esophageal deviation and compression. In the absence of dysphagia, patients do not require further esophageal imaging.
- Symptomatic assessment of voice does not predict objective findings in patients with goiter and should not replace the laryngeal examination.
- Flow volume loop studies most accurately document airway obstruction in the setting of significant airway compression. However, they correlate poorly with goiter weight and upper airway symptoms. We do not recommend flow volume loop studies as part of the routine workup for patients with goiter.
- Axial computed tomography (CT) scanning is recommended for large cervical and substernal goiters, because it provides a more sensitive airway assessment than patient symptomatic, flow volume loop, and plain film analysis. The finding of tracheal compression on axial CT scanning correlates significantly with the presence of shortness of breath; therefore we consider the finding of CT scan tracheal compression to be an appropriate surgical indication given its symptomatic respiratory correlate.

BOX 6.2 Workup for Benign Goiter

History and physical examination
Symptomatic*
Massive goiter*
Bilateral circumferential goiter*
Suspect substernal goiter*
Suspect cancer (vocal cord paralysis, lymphadenopathy)*
Ultrasound to evaluate for suspicious nodules
Thyroid function tests

*Obtain CT or MRI.
CT, computed tomography; MRI, magnetic resonance imaging.

aerodigestive tract compressive symptoms in patients with goiter can be quite problematic. Although we found that the presence of shortness of breath correlates with goiter size, shortness of breath as a screening tool for tracheal deviation or compression is of limited value. This is despite the fact that the presence of shortness of breath is significantly related to the imaging finding of tracheal compression, consistent with the work of Mackle.[108] Stang et al. also reported a strong association between positional dyspnea and substernal goiter (75.5%), with significant correlation with tracheal compression on axial CT imaging.[109] However, for the airway, symptomatic assessment alone may be inadequate overall in goiter patients. In the setting of large cervical or substernal goiter, one cannot purely rely on the presence or absence of shortness of breath to assess true tracheal compromise without routine axial CT scanning assessment for tracheal compression. In our series there was no significant difference in the percentage of patients with airway symptoms between patients with purely cervical goiter and patients with substernal goiter. However, in our series, substernal goiter was highly associated with tracheal deviation and compression.[12]

Our series also demonstrated a positive correlation between thyroid size, globus sensation, and symptoms of hyperthyroidism. No correlation was established between goiter size and presence of dysphagia, local discomfort, change in voice, hemoptysis, or symptoms of hypothyroidism. There was a significant positive correlation between preoperative dysphagia and the presence of esophageal compression and deviation.[12] Hedayati and McHenry reported that about one-third of 116 patients undergoing surgery for substernal goiter complained of dysphagia on initial presentation.[110]

Flow Volume Loop Analysis
Please see the Expert Consult website for more discussion of this topic.

Imaging
Radiographic Evaluation and Regional Symptomatology
A number of studies question the strength of the correlation between regional symptoms and imaging study findings. In particular, the functional effect of airway narrowing diagnosed via CT scan remains controversial. Alfonso et al. found that two-thirds of surgical goiter patients had preoperative radiographic evidence of compression. Almost half of those patients with evidence of compression had no symptoms. Those patients with airway symptoms who had old radiographs available for comparison were found to have compression up to 3 to 4 months before the onset of airway symptoms.[102] Jauregui found in a series of asymptomatic euthyroid goiter patients that 25% had radiographic evidence of tracheal obstruction and 60% had evidence of airway obstruction by flow volume loops.[114] Cooper et al. found that tracheal diameter and airway symptoms are weakly related.[115] Melissant and others have found little correlation between lung function and the CT scan–defined degree of tracheal obstruction.[111,116]

Conclusions from our series stand in contrast with the previously mentioned literature. As noted earlier, we found a significant correlation between the presence of shortness of breath and the objective CT scan radiographic finding of tracheal compression.[12] Stang et al. found a high correlation of tracheal compression on imaging with positional dyspnea and further showed postsurgical improvement of symptoms in 82.4% of cases.[109] Barker et al. similarly noted that if the CT scan showed greater than or equal to 50% tracheal diameter narrowing, symptoms should be expected.[117] We therefore consider tracheal compression to be an important radiographic finding and an appropriate surgical indication in these patients (see Boxes 6.1 and 6.2).

Please see the Expert Consult website for more discussion of this topic.

Chest Radiography and Barium Swallow Study
Please see the Expert Consult website for more discussion of this topic.

Axial CT Scanning
We have found routine CT scanning to be very helpful in preoperative assessment of patients with large cervical or substernal goiters.[12,121] CT with iodinated contrast may be performed safely (i.e., without the Jod-Basedow phenomenon) in patients with thyroid disease if thyroid-stimulating hormone (TSH) is not found to be suppressed. CT scanning shows the margin of benign goiter to be smooth and may often delineate gross calcification (which may be punctate, linear, eggshell, amorphous, or nodular) versus the fine stippled microcalcification that may be present in papillary or medullary carcinoma (see Chapter 13, Ultrasound of the Thyroid and Parathyroid Glands). In patients with substernal goiter, continuity of the mediastinal mass and cervical orthotopic gland can be identified. Precontrast attenuation of thyroid tissue exceeds adjacent neck musculature by at least 15 Hounsfield units or greater and by more than 25 Hounsfield units after contrast enhancement. In patients with substernal goiter, this high attenuation, which is uncharacteristic in other types of mediastinal disease such as lymphoma or thymoma, can be helpful diagnostically.[33,122] With CT scanning, the extent of cervical and substernal extension can be accurately defined, and the exact relationship of the goiter to the trachea, esophagus, and great vessels can be determined. The presence of nodal disease can also be established through axial scanning. Generally, benign goiter shows heterogeneous density with discrete nonenhancing low-density areas. Malignancy may be considered in the setting of radiographic findings of irregular/infiltrative margins, vocal cord paralysis, and nodal enlargement, especially if the nodes are calcified, cystic, or enhancing.[123-125] Contrary to McHenry's view that preoperative radiographic evaluation does not alter intraoperative management, we believe that CT scanning is essential for all patients with large cervical and substernal goiters.[7] We are more likely to obtain CT scanning if the clinical examination suggests that the goiter is large, symptomatic, bilateral, or substernal or if malignancy is suspected based on vocal cord paralysis or regional lymphadenopathy (see Box 6.2). CT scanning ideally shows the relationship of the goiter to surrounding cervical viscera, including the airway. These relationships can affect not only surgery but also the approach to intubation. Axial CT provides objective, reproducible measures of tracheal caliber. A patient's surgical candidacy may derive from information obtained from axial CT scanning, especially given a lack of sensitivity of symptoms, flow volume loop analysis, and plain radiographic assessment. At our institutions, documentation of substernal extension or tracheal compression on CT is an appropriate surgical indication.[12] CT scanning also provides helpful information to exclude invasive malignancy. It is true that CT scanning does not differentiate well between fibrosis and tumor, although this distinction is generally not a significant clinical issue for routine goiter patients. Finally, enhanced CT scanning is essential in determining the mediastinal relationships to allow safe operative management for large posterior mediastinal goiters. Identification of significant retrotracheal extension of either cervical or substernal goiter helps in predicting preoperatively that the RLN is displaced to a ventral position. Preoperative information of ventral nerve displacement is tremendously helpful in the offering of safe cervical and substernal goiter surgery (Box 6.3).

MRI Scanning
Please see the Expert Consult website for more discussion of this topic.

Sonography and Scintigraphy
Please see the Expert Consult website for more discussion of this topic.

Thyroid Function Tests and Fine-Needle Aspiration

Thyroid function tests must be checked in all patients presenting with goiter. In our series, only 8% of patients had noniatrogenic causes of abnormal thyroid function testing, reaffirming that the majority of patients with goiter, if not on suppressive therapy, are euthyroid.[12] Nevertheless, rates of thyroid dysfunction in patients with goiter are not negligible, and it is imperative that the clinician evaluates for any abnormality. Hyperthyroidism is the foremost concern in patients with goiter. Florid hyperthyroidism has been reported in up to 30% of patients with multinodular goiter.[77,128] Rates of hyperthyroidism in patients with substernal goiter range from 1.3% to 7%, although rates as high as 44% have been described.[11,57,129] Autonomous nodules may elicit a slowly progressive increase in thyroid hormone production independent of TSH levels.[130] Alternatively, hyperthyroidism may manifest acutely in patients with goiter exposed to high iodine, such as in CT scan contrast material or in amiodarone.[131,132] Elderly patients notoriously do not exhibit the typical overt signs and symptoms of hyperthyroidism and are also more prone to cardiac complications. Screening for subclinical hyperthyroidism (TSH low, T3 and T4 normal) is particularly crucial in the elderly population because of the increased risks of atrial fibrillation and accelerated bone demineralization. Subclinical hyperthyroidism may also inform the issue of extent of surgery and may lead more toward total thyroidectomy if present. Iatrogenic iodine exposure should be avoided in elderly patients with subclinical hyperthyroidism to avert the increased risk for the development of overt hyperthyroidism.[133,134] Finally, hypothyroidism (typically Hashimoto's disease) must also be excluded in patients with goiter. A fibrotic variant of Hashimoto's disease can result in a massive firm goiter.

We believe that if the history, physical examination, and CT scan evaluation of the patient with thyromegaly suggest benign goiter requiring surgery and surgical candidacy is established on that basis, then fine-needle aspiration (FNA) is not essential.[2] Certainly, if there is any suspicion on history, physical examination, or radiographic evaluation of malignancy, then FNA should be considered. The 2015 American Thyroid Association guidelines suggest consideration for FNA of nodules ≥1 cm on an individual basis if they show moderate or high suspicion sonographic pattern; FNA may be deferred for low suspicion nodules and should be avoided for hot nodules.[135] Hemorrhage into a nodule after FNA may convert a stable but compromised airway into emergency airway obstruction. FNA information infrequently contributes substantially to preoperative workup in patients with large cervical and substernal goiters.

TREATMENT OPTIONS

Suppressive Therapy
Please see the Expert Consult website for more discussion of this topic.

Radioiodine
Please see the Expert Consult website for more discussion of this topic.

Surgery
Rationale and Indications
Surgery represents a rational treatment option for many patients with cervical goiter and most patients with substernal goiter. Regional compressive symptoms resolve postoperatively and faster than with suppressive or radioiodine therapy. Complication rates are low, subclinical hyperthyroidism remits, airway complications are avoided, and a pathology report is provided. Goiter surgery is most safely offered when it is not offered with undue delay. Waiting until a goiter is massive will likely increase operative complication rates. Surgery brings no risk of radioiodine-induced immediate airway complications, malignancies, or Graves' disease. Surgery also brings no risk of thyroid hormone-induced atrial fibrillation or osteoporosis. A patient cannot be a "nonresponder" to surgery (Box 6.4). Surgery is recommended in patients with multinodular goiter who present with hyperthyroidism, because they do not generally respond well to antithyroid drugs, including perchlorate and iopanoic acid.[164] Furthermore, surgery may be preferred over radioactive iodine treatment in elderly patients with goiter and subclinical or frank hyperthyroidism, to forestall the risk of radioiodine-induced Graves' disease in this cardiac-frail population (see Box 6.4).

Based on our experience, patients can be reasonably considered for cervical goiter surgery in the following situations: (1) if a patient has clear-cut regional upper aerodigestive tract symptoms without other cause, often first manifesting with positional provocation or nocturnally; (2) if radiographic evaluation through axial CT scanning shows evidence of tracheal compression; (3) for masses causing significant

---

BOX 6.3 Imaging: Summary

- Plain chest radiography may detect macronodular metastatic disease but generally offers limited information about the tracheal air column. Airway compression is underestimated and bilateral goiter with circumferential tracheal compression may not be well seen on plain radiographs.
- We recommend computed tomography (CT) scanning in all patients with large cervical and substernal goiters. Axial CT scanning has the advantage of being readily available and easily interpreted by the surgeon. CT scanning is used to judge a patient's surgical candidacy by accurately defining the degree of tracheal impact. In patients with substernal goiter, CT scanning informs surgical planning regarding sternotomy and potential thoracic surgical involvement. CT scanning is helpful in identifying the radiographic correlates of malignancy. It is also of tremendous importance in accurately defining the anatomic relationships, especially in predicting when a recurrent laryngeal nerve (RLN) will be ventral through retrotracheal and posterior mediastinal extension. Contrast should be avoided if the patient's thyroid functional status is unknown or if the patient is subclinically hyperthyroid.
- Advantages of magnetic resonance imaging (MRI) scanning are excellent soft-tissue delineation, excellent definition of the goiter's relationship to mediastinal vessels, and sagittal and coronal display. Disadvantages of MRI scanning include cost, patient claustrophobia in nonopen MRI scanning suites, and poor definition of calcification patterns.

BOX 6.4 Cervical and Substernal Surgery Rationale

- Natural history of goiter is of progressive growth
- Treats existent regional/compressive symptoms
- Avoids rapid and unpredictable increase in size and airway compression
- Provides pathology report; rules out malignancy
- Treats hyperthyroidism and subclinical hyperthyroidism
- Has low operative morbidity
- Thyroid hormone (suppressive) treatment is associated with a high nonresponse rate, requires lifetime treatment, cannot be offered if TSH is <1, risks atrial fibrillation and osteoporosis, and is less likely to be effective with large nodular goiters.
- Radioactive iodine treatment of goiter risks acute radiation thyroiditis and airway compression and, in approximately 10% of patients, induces Graves' disease.

TSH, thyroid-stimulating hormone.

> BOX 6.5 Surgical Indications for Multinodular Goiter
>
> 1. Clear-cut significant regional aerodigestive tract symptom without other cause
> 2. Computed tomography (CT) with tracheal compression
> 3. Masses greater than 5 cm
> 4. Goiter with subclinical or frank hyperthyroidism
> 5. All patients with malignancy suspected or proved
> 6. All patients with substernal goiter

cosmetic concern or those greater than 5 cm, given the increased risk of regional symptoms at or above this size and the decreased accuracy of FNA for excluding malignancy; (4) goiter patients with subclinical hyperthyroidism; (5) patients in whom carcinoma is suspected or proven; and (6) all patients with substernal extension. In our practice, in general, the presence of substernal goiter is a surgical indication because of the strong association of tracheal compression and substernal growth and because the mediastinal component is difficult to follow on physical examination or with fine-needle biopsy (Box 6.5).[12] In our series, substernal extent was the surgical indication in the majority of cases (78%), because this factor is sufficient to warrant excision at our institutions. Additional surgical indications are as follows: compressive symptoms (49.5%), concern for cancer (17%), patient's desire/cosmesis (3%), nonthyroid local neoplasm (1%), and other/nonspecified (1%).[85]

Goiter: Risk of Malignancy

Please see the Expert Consult website for more discussion of this topic.

Surgery for Substernal Goiter

Please see the Expert Consult website for more discussion of this topic.

INTUBATION OF THE GOITER PATIENT AND LARYNGEAL EDEMA

Intubation generally proceeds well in patients with large cervical and substernal goiters, but it can occasionally be difficult. When difficult, anesthesia induction and intubation can represent a dramatic and life-threatening process, given the fact that emergent or "under local" tracheotomies generally are not options because of the mass of the overlying goiter. In patients with goiter, there may be evidence of substantial laryngeal deviation and perhaps vocal cord paralysis at intubation. The surgeon who performs the preoperative laryngoscopy should convey all information regarding the appearance of the larynx, presence of deviation, and vocal cord paralysis to the anesthesia staff, and both the surgeon and the anesthesiologist should review the preoperative CT scans and examine the patient together before induction. Cervical goiter with significant superior pole expansion can indent the supraglottic hypopharynx and lead to difficult laryngeal examination and difficult intubation.

The method of intubation and the size of the tube and contingency plans can be discussed and decided upon through these discussions. Typically, a straightforward induction with transoral intubation can be performed. Laryngeal deviation generally does not represent a problem, and tracheal compression generally yields to a reasonably sized endotracheal tube. An alternative and safe method that we favor is an awake, sitting up, fiberoptic transnasal intubation. This is an especially reasonable course of action if there is any doubt as to the adequacy of a sedated mask anesthesia airway, particularly if the larynx is significantly deviated by the cervical component of the goiter. Video laryngoscopes are also an excellent adjunct for intubation in such patients. Maximum tracheal compression in cervical and substernal goiter usually occurs at the thoracic inlet but may be present further distally.[33] As previously noted, tracheal compression by benign goiter typically yields to a reasonably sized endotracheal tube. One exception is when there is malignant infiltration of the trachea, especially if there is intraluminal disease. In these circumstances, transoral bronchoscopic intubation with bronchoscopic core-out can lead to satisfactory airway. Once again, preoperative CT scanning empowers the surgeon. Vigilance and recognition of nonthyroid factors, such as jaw and tongue size, anteriorly positioned larynx, and available degree of head extension, are also important determinants of difficult intubation.

Our experience has shown that a significant problem in patients with large cervical or substernal goiters, especially with bilateral circumferential goiters, is the development of laryngeal edema with initial intubation attempts by anesthesia. The larynx, which represents the extreme distal end of the airway projected into the hypopharynx, likely has chronically reduced venous and lymphatic drainage as a result of a large, constricting bilateral goiter. Such a larynx is easily made edematous with multiple unsuccessful intubation attempts. This edema can last for weeks postoperatively, sometimes requiring tracheotomy, which usually can be removed after edema resolves. It is therefore best to intubate once correctly. Intubation problems, although rare, can quickly spell disaster. The propensity for laryngeal edema from intubation attempts with goiter has been emphasized in the case reports of Hassard.[172] In our series of 200 patients with goiter, we encountered difficult intubation in only four cases (2%). There were no significant predictors of difficult intubation, including size, substernal extension, preoperative compressive symptoms, or radiographic presence of tracheal deviation or compression. Tracheotomy was performed in only 3% of patients and was done electively at the time of thyroidectomy. Tracheotomy was performed either because of concern about laryngeal edema from multiple intubation attempts or in cases where neural monitoring was not used and the question of vocal cord dysfunction was raised, especially if one vocal cord was known to be paralyzed preoperatively. With neural monitoring, greater certainty exists as to the functional status of both nerves during surgery (see Chapter 36, Surgical Anatomy and Monitoring of the Recurrent Laryngeal Nerve).[85]

GOITER SURGERY

Extent of Surgery

Decisions regarding the extent of surgery relate to the balance between operative complications and the risk of recurrence. Some suggest total thyroidectomy for goiter,[173-175] while others recommend a more conservative initial surgical plan,[11] and some, such as Kraimps, support a selectively aggressive surgical treatment plan based on extent of disease.[176] A 2015 Cochrane database systematic review on total or near-total thyroidectomy versus subtotal thyroidectomy showed decreased recurrence rates with total thyroidectomy (although evidence was limited) and recommended additional long-term randomized controlled trials (RCTs) to address questions of reoperation rates, adverse events, and thyroid cancer incidence rates.[177] Complication rates must be kept extremely low in the setting of treatment of benign thyroid disease. Therefore we suggest a conservative philosophy, tailoring the extent of surgery to the initial disease with the minimum procedure being a total unilateral lobar resection, reserving bilateral surgery for significant bilateral goiter. In our series, this surgical philosophy resulted in unilateral surgery in 63% of patients and bilateral surgery in 37%. Patients undergoing initial surgery at our center experienced a 1.5% recurrence rate.[85]

BOX 6.6 Extent of Surgery for Goiter: Summary

- We believe that complication rates must be low in the setting of surgery for benign thyroid disease.
- Less than unilateral lobectomy leads to extremely high recurrence rates and difficult reoperations and is to be condemned.
- The extent of surgery should be rationally tailored to the extent of initial disease. Dominant goitrous enlargement should be treated with total lobectomy on that side. Preoperative assessment with imaging will help document the extent of surgery necessary on the contralateral side.
- With clear-cut unilateral disease, total lobectomy is appropriate.
- With clear-cut evidence of bilateral goiter, bilateral surgery is appropriate.
- Consideration should be given for more aggressive surgery in young females and in patients with a positive family history of thyroid disease who may have a higher recurrence rate.
- In patients who have required multiple thyroid surgeries for benign recurrence and still have some remnant tissue remaining after the last revision surgery, radioactive iodine ablation can be considered.

Please see the Expert Consult website for more discussion of this topic.

Our experience, similar to the work of Berghout et al., has suggested a greater likelihood of recurrence in females and in patients with a positive family history of thyroid disease.[85,184] Overall, females were found to be three times more likely to require revision surgery, and those with a positive family history of thyroid disease were six times more likely to require revision surgery.[85] Others have found no such increased risk in these populations.[176] We now tend to be more aggressive in females and in those with a positive family history, especially if they are young. Furthermore, we have treated many patients with recurrent disease and appreciate the difficulty of these cases and of the occasional need to leave at least a small thyroid tissue remnant in such revision cases. However, contrary to most reports in the literature, revision cases in our series of patients with goiter, whether unilateral or bilateral, second, third, or fourth revisions, were not more likely to be associated with postoperative complications.[85] We have used radioactive iodine postoperatively after complex multiple revision cases to avoid the need for additional reoperation in these circumstances (Box 6.6).

Hashimoto's Thyroiditis

Please see the Expert Consult website for more discussion of this topic.

SURGICAL TECHNIQUE FOR GOITER

Patient positioning is important. We prefer a thyroid inflatable bag under the shoulders. The surgeon and anesthesiology staff must be comfortable with the degree of head support. The patient is placed into a semisitting position to reduce venous pressure.

Incision

A generous collar incision is mandatory. Endoscopic or minimal access approaches are not appropriate here. When unilateral glandular enlargement has resulted in significant deformity of the anterior neck, that side of the incision can be curved slightly higher because after resection the skin will come to fall caudally to some extent. The incision for a large bilateral cervical goiter extends to the lateral edge of the sternocleidomastoid (SCM) muscle to allow for exposure of the bilateral carotid sheath contents. A subplatysmal upper flap is developed. A lower flap is typically not necessary. Flaps can be sutured in place or several Gelpi retractors, or Beckman goiter retractors, can be used.

Strap Muscles

It has frequently been recommended to routinely section the strap muscles during goiter surgery. Certainly, if there is any question that strap division would help exposure, it should be done without hesitation. This is most often necessary in revision surgery where strap muscle division had been performed during the initial surgery. The muscles in this circumstance are significantly scarred to the surface of the goiter. In first-time surgery in which superior pole exposure is limited, we recommend a "mini strap section" by an isolated incision of the cranial head of the sternothyroid muscle. Although subtle and transient voice changes may arguably accompany strap division, they are of little consequence overall compared with potential division of the RLN or external branch of the superior laryngeal nerve (SLN) through poor exposure. In some massive cervical goiters, the SCM muscle can be sectioned as well as the strap muscles, although this is uncommon. It, like the strap muscles, can be sutured at the completion of surgery with little ill effect. If the strap muscles are sectioned, it is important during surgery to either suture or place a clamp on the divided edges, which have a tendency to retract, with a resultant loss of the perithyroidal plane they define. If the strap muscles are completely sectioned, it is best first to define their lateral edge, which can blend with tissue adjacent to the jugular vein and other carotid sheath contents. In most of the goiter surgeries that we have performed, strap muscles are preserved and retracted. This preserves a perithyroidal plane better than sectioning the muscles in some circumstances, and it helps to preserve anatomic organization to the neck base that can be substantially altered by goitrous change.

Importance of Carotid Sheath

The carotid sheath (including the carotid artery, jugular vein, and vagus nerve) is to the initial steps in goiter surgery what the lateral thyroid region (with RLN and inferior thyroid artery) is to surgery of a normal-sized thyroid gland (Figure 6.3). It is extremely helpful to dissect the carotid artery, jugular vein, and identify the vagus nerve early on during the case. A lateral or inferior approach to the nerve may be used initially, with a superior approach reserved for use only when the goiter size and position prevent the more standard technique (Figure 6.4). A large cervical goiter frequently extends to the carotid sheath, necessitating this dissection, which allows reflection of the jugular vein, and sometimes the carotid artery and vagus, off the lateral surface of the goiter. Identification of the vagus nerve allows intermittent vagal stimulation, a very helpful technique during substernal goiter surgery (see the discussion of vagal monitoring during goiter surgery later in this chapter). The identification and dissection of the carotid artery, as it extends in the neck and more importantly as it extends into the mediastinum, are essential for the surgeon to understand the substernal goiter's relationship to the mediastinum and aortic arch (see Figure 6.3). Once the strap muscles and carotid sheath are dealt with, the procedure continues with the steps typical of routine thyroidectomy, including middle thyroid vein division, inferior thyroid vein division, and identification of the inferior thyroid artery. Because of the size of the goiter, the inferior thyroid artery may not be able to be identified during this segment of the surgery but can be identified later after goiter delivery. The branches of the inferior thyroid artery are taken directly on the thyroid capsule to preserve parathyroid tissue and vascularization.

Goiter and Recurrent Laryngeal Nerve

Approaches to the RLN can be made laterally, inferiorly, or superiorly (see Chapter 36, Surgical Anatomy and Monitoring of the Recurrent

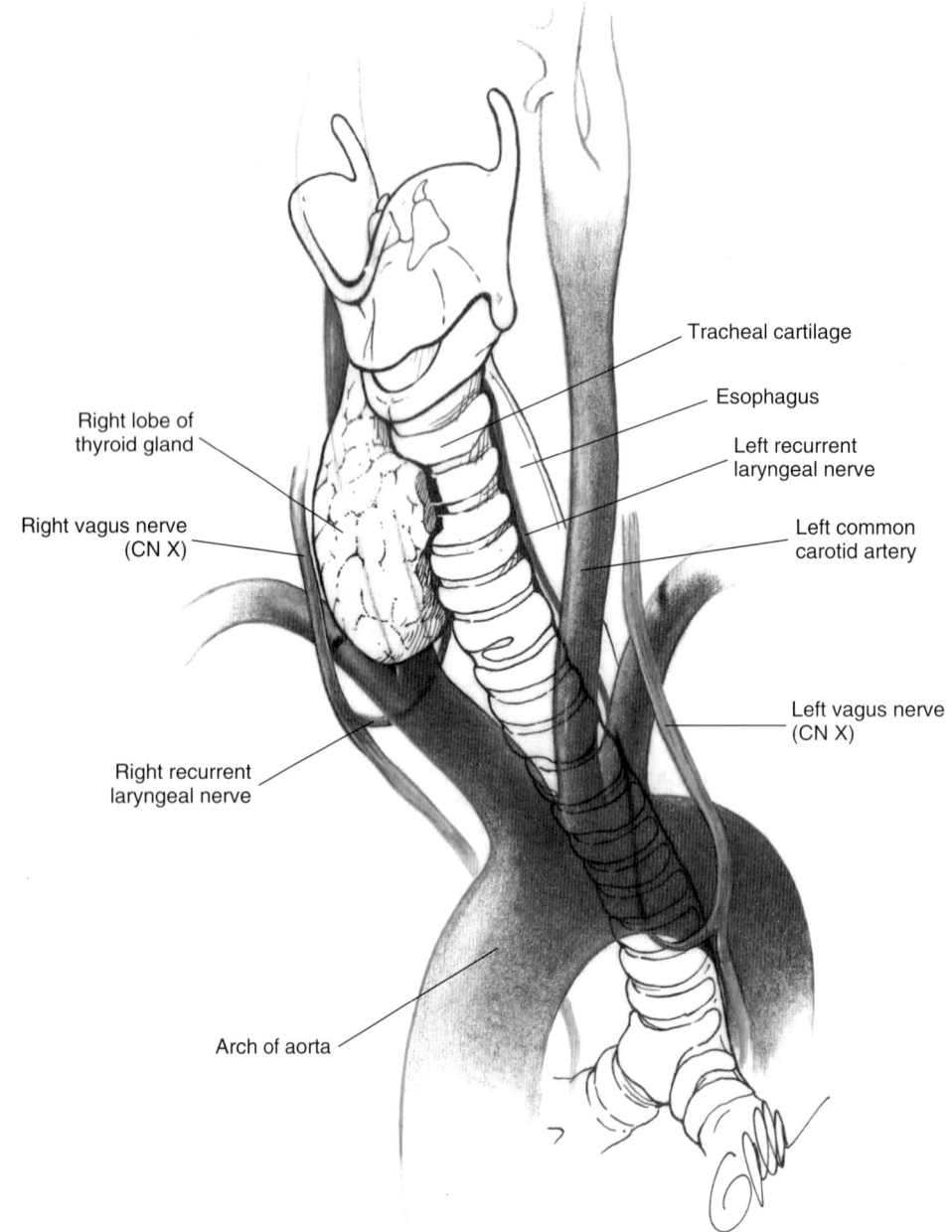

Fig. 6.3 Neural and vascular anatomy of the neck base. (From Janfaza P, et al, eds. *Surgical Anatomy of the Head and Neck*. Philadelphia: Lippincott Williams & Wilkins; 2001. With permission.)

Laryngeal Nerve). Goiter may significantly distort the position of the RLN. In our experience with large cervical and substernal goiters, we have found that in nearly 16% of cases the RLN was entrapped on the surface through fascial band fixation or splayed over the surface of the goiter in such a way that significant traction or goiter delivery without RLN identification would have definitively injured (stretched or avulsed) the nerve (Figure 6.5).[85] We found that left and right lobes were equally affected. Cases of fixation and nerve splaying were more likely with increased goiter size, substernal extension, significant tracheal compression, and intubation difficulties. In our unpublished series of 184 cases of thyroidectomy not involving goiter, we found no such cases of fixation or splaying other than in cases of malignant infiltration. It is interesting to note that Sinclair's work demonstrates that postoperative RLN paralysis in patients with substernal goiter in whom the RLN was not specifically identified during blind digital goiter delivery was 17.5%. Sinclair wrote in several cases that the nerve was associated with the thyroid gland and

> was at serious risk when the retrosternal mass was mobilized into the neck [during] a maneuver usually achieved by dislocating the mass with a finger from below and behind. I believe that this hazard must be recognized by all thyroid surgeons and that every strand of tissue stretched over the retrosternal component of the goiter should be presumed to be nerve until anatomically proved otherwise.[192]

Sinclair's rate of paralysis and our rate of nerves at risk are similar.

We believe that, because of the possibility of nerve fixation and splaying on the undersurface of the goiter, blunt dissection without nerve identification risks stretch injury. Identification of the RLN in such cases is a necessary initial step. The nerve that is fixed to or splayed on the undersurface of the goiter should be dissected before delivery of the gland. The nerve can be identified through a superior approach and can be dissected retrograde off the goiter before digital delivery of the goiter (see Figure 6.4). This dissection is coupled with dissection of the vagus nerve in the carotid sheath laterally and allows the pathway of the vagus and RLNs to be predicted in the mediastinum. After goiter resection the RLN so dissected can appear significantly redundant but will stimulate normally and function postoperatively, despite the intraoperative appearance of laxity (see Figure 6.6, available on expertconsult.com). In some circumstances if the goiter is soft and compressible, the inferior pole can be retracted cranially without delivering it out of the neck, and the RLN, despite impressive goiter size, can be identified through a normal inferior approach.

The Special Case of Retrotracheal Cervical and Posterior Mediastinal Goiter: The Ventral Recurrent Laryngeal Nerve

Retrotracheal cervical goiter and posterior mediastinal goiters (substernal goiter type IIA, B) represent especially unique surgical challenges (Figure 6.7). Approximately 9% to 15% of all substernal goiters extend into the posterior mediastinum.[11,22,29,30,86] The chief difficulty is that in these cases, thyroid tissue has excavated posteriorly and deeply to the RLN. This causes displacement of the RLN ventral to the thyroid lobar tissue, defined as an L2b (left) or R2b (right) RLN, according to the International RLN Anatomic Classification System.[193] As the posterior mediastinal goiter descends, it pushes the trachea anteriorly and splays the great vessels.[26,27,194] For the surgeon the ventral RLN is a disorienting and high-risk RLN position. The RLN in all other cases of thyroidectomy is always deep to the thyroid gland. The most complex posterior mediastinal goiters are those that descend from the left lobe and then cross, being pushed by the aortic arch and its branches to the right thorax (substernal goiter type IIB). These crossings may occur either behind both the trachea and esophagus (type IIB1) or between the trachea and esophagus (type IIB2; see Table 6.1 and Figure 6.1, A-H).[26,27,30] Some have recommended sternotomy,[30,194] and some advocate posterolateral right thoracotomy[22,195,196] along with a cervical approach. Right thoracotomy, when necessary, is performed through the right fourth and fifth intercostal space. The lung is retracted, and the goiter is identified posterior to the SVC, superior to the azygous vein, and anterior to the vertebral column. The pleura over the goiter is incised, and the goiter is manipulated into the thoracic inlet with the help of traction from above.[60] Katlic, Grillo, and Wang found 7 of 80 patients with substernal goiter extended into the posterior mediastinum that could typically be removed through a cervical approach.[11] DeAndrade's extensive experience with posterior mediastinal goiter

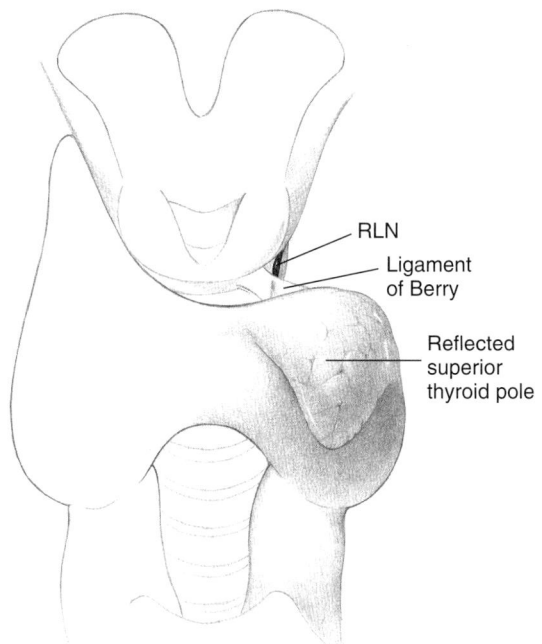

Fig. 6.4 Superior approach to the recurrent laryngeal nerve (RLN).

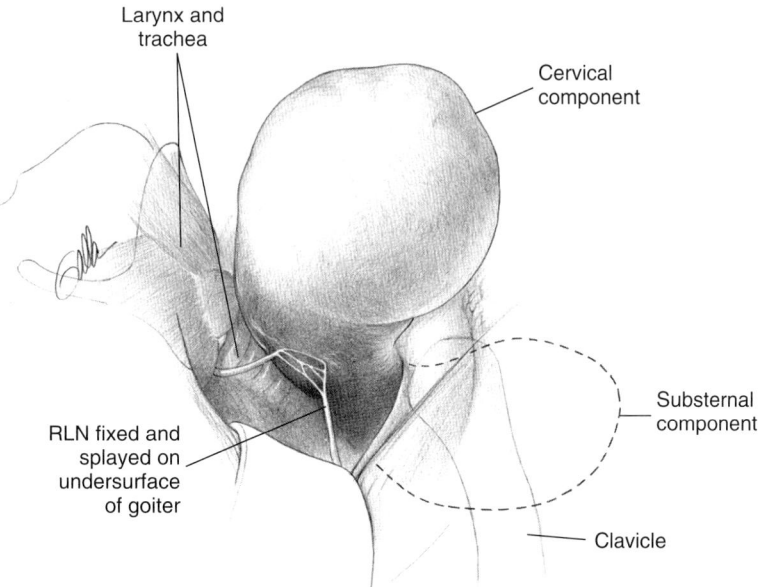

Fig. 6.5 Demonstration of fixation and splaying of the RLN in patients with substernal goiter. RLN, recurrent laryngeal nerve.

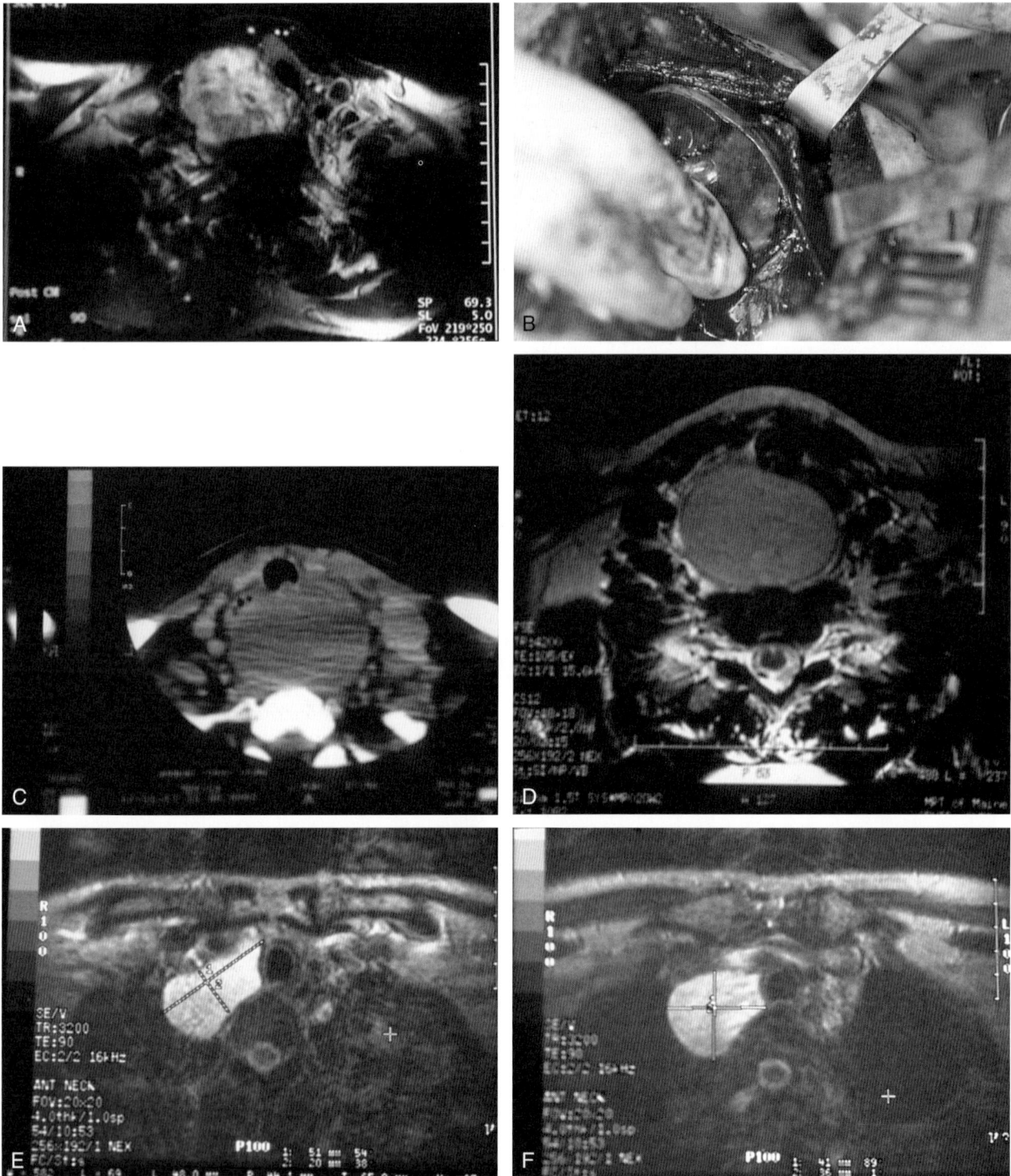

Fig. 6.7 Retrotracheal masses excavate the region posterior to the trachea, bringing the nerve ventral to the lesion. **A,** A cervical goiter with some retrotracheal extent. **B,** At surgery, the recurrent laryngeal nerve (RLN) was found to be displaced anteriorly and was adherent to the ventral surface of the mass. The nerve was identified through neural monitoring, dissected away, and functioned normally postoperatively. **C,** Female with large retrotracheal mass shown on computed tomography (CT). **D,** The RLN was ventral to this mass seen here on magnetic resonance imaging (MRI) and was identified with neural monitoring, dissected away, and functioned normally postoperatively. **E** and **F,** Lymphangioma arising from the inferior pole of the thyroid, extending inferiorly into the mediastinum approximately 13 cm. **E** and **F,** Axial cuts in the neck base and upper chest. The mass was excised completely and was deep to the RLN, which was closely associated with it. The nerve was identified through neural monitoring, dissected away, and functioned normally postoperatively. The lymphangioma was resected completely.

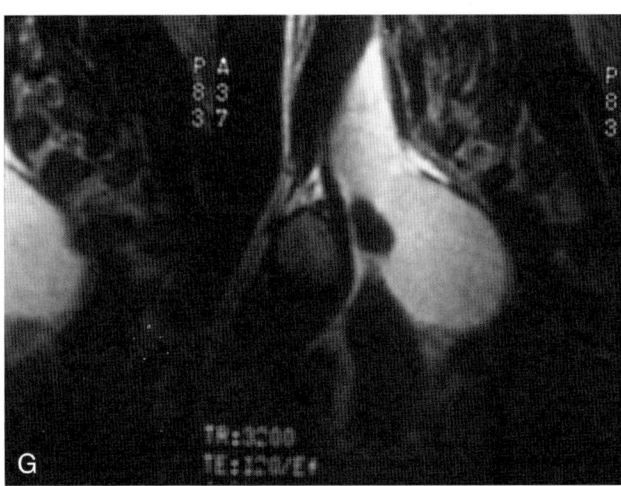
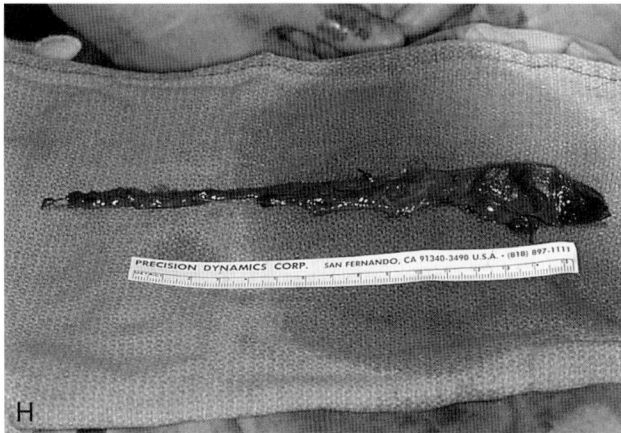

Fig. 6.7, cont'd G, Asymmetric goiter that caused rotation of the larynx. The RLN entry point was rotated because of the laryngeal rotation such that the nerve entered the larynx in the midline. **H,** Cervical goiter that had a tightly adherent RLN through crossing vessels on the undersurface of the left smaller side. This RLN was dissected away and preserved. Such vessels can be seen and predicted on preoperative CT as shown here.

found that virtually all could be extracted through a cervical incision and were vascularized by the inferior thyroid artery.[29] Certainly, these cases make clear the need for preoperative imaging and should be handled by experienced surgical teams (see Chapter 7, Approach to the Mediastinum: Transcervical, Transsternal, and Video-Assisted).

Superior Goiter Extent

Please see the Expert Consult website for more discussion of this topic, including Figure 6.8.

Parathyroid Preservation During Goiter Surgery

The distal inferior thyroid artery is taken after the RLN is identified and either before or after goiter delivery. The artery is taken directly on the thyroid capsule to reduce the risk of parathyroid ischemia. The superior parathyroid glands are more constant in position and are more frequently seen at thyroidectomy for goiter; therefore they are more readily preserved. In their series of 80 substernal goiters, Katlic, Grillo, and Wang noted that upper glands were seen twice as often as lower glands.[11] The inferior parathyroid gland is more widely distributed and more likely to be significantly displaced by inferior pole goitrous change. Therefore our real emphasis during goiter surgery should be on superior parathyroid preservation. Inferiorly, we must strictly adhere to capsular dissection so as to preserve displaced inferior parathyroid glands. It is important to emphasize that with goiter surgery, as with all thyroid surgery, any resected thyroid specimen must be meticulously examined for capsular parathyroid glands before being sent to pathology. Any capsular parathyroid glands that are found should be dissected off, biopsied to confirm parathyroid tissue, and then autotransplanted. These glands may be found within folds and crevices of the goiter surface.

Substernal Goiter Techniques for Delivery

As previously described, after the RLN is identified and completely dissected away from the goiter (typically allowing it to fall away posterolaterally), finger dissection in a strictly capsular plane, with an understanding of the specific goiter/mediastinal anatomy, can allow for safe goiter delivery (Figures 6.9 and 6.10)—one finger on a strictly capsular location medially adjacent to the trachea and one finger laterally adjacent to the carotid sheath. The goiter is slowly incrementally mobilized upward. Thin, fascial band attachments drawn up with the finger are stimulated with the nerve stimulator and cauterized or clamped. Slow, step-by-step incremental goiter delivery is achieved from the mediastinum with substernal goiter or out of the thyroid bed for cervical goiter. RLN identification and dissection before delivery are mandatory, as previously noted. The vagus may be intermittently stimulated as the goiter is mobilized, or continuous vagal monitoring can be used (see Chapter 36, Surgical Anatomy and Monitoring of the Recurrent Laryngeal Nerve). In patients with large substernal goiters with a contralateral cervical component, performing surgery on the contralateral side first may be necessary to increase the mobility of the laryngotracheal complex and to allow for substernal goiter delivery. If all these maneuvers are not effective, sternotomy may be considered. Despite nearly 80% of patients having substernal extension, the sternotomy rate was only 1% in our series of patients with goiter,[85] which is consistent with that seen in the literature.[197-199] It is important that any surgeon who does not routinely perform sternotomy himself or herself review preoperative CT scans of patients with substernal goiters with thoracic surgical colleagues and arrange the surgical date when a thoracic surgeon is available, if needed.

Substernal goiter is a product of the neck. The blood supply to substernal goiters is almost always cervical (i.e., the inferior thyroid artery). One must keep in mind that although cervical goiters' and the majority of substernal goiters' blood supplies are through the inferior thyroid artery, there are rare cases of substernal and even cervical goiter with aberrant intrathoracic blood supply.[22,82] Substernal goiters thus infrequently obtain significant blood supply from mediastinal vessels such as the thyroid ima, subclavian, or internal mammary artery or aorta.[25,34,36,86] In our series of 200 thyroidectomies for goiter, we found only two cases where the blood supply to the thyroid mass was provided by vessels of intrathoracic origin.[85] With this in mind it is best that fascial bands produced during digital dissection of the substernal goiter be cauterized only if transparent. Thicker pedicles of tissue should be clamped and securely tied only after the RLN and vagus locations are completely understood along their full course.

Morselization is a technique that has been performed in the past to help reduce goiter size and provide for delivery. It was first described by Kocher in 1889, popularized by Lahey in 1945, and has its more recent proponents.[20,78,188,200] We believe that this technique should be abandoned because it risks significant and perhaps uncontrollable hemorrhage as well as the spread of carcinoma if ultimately found to be

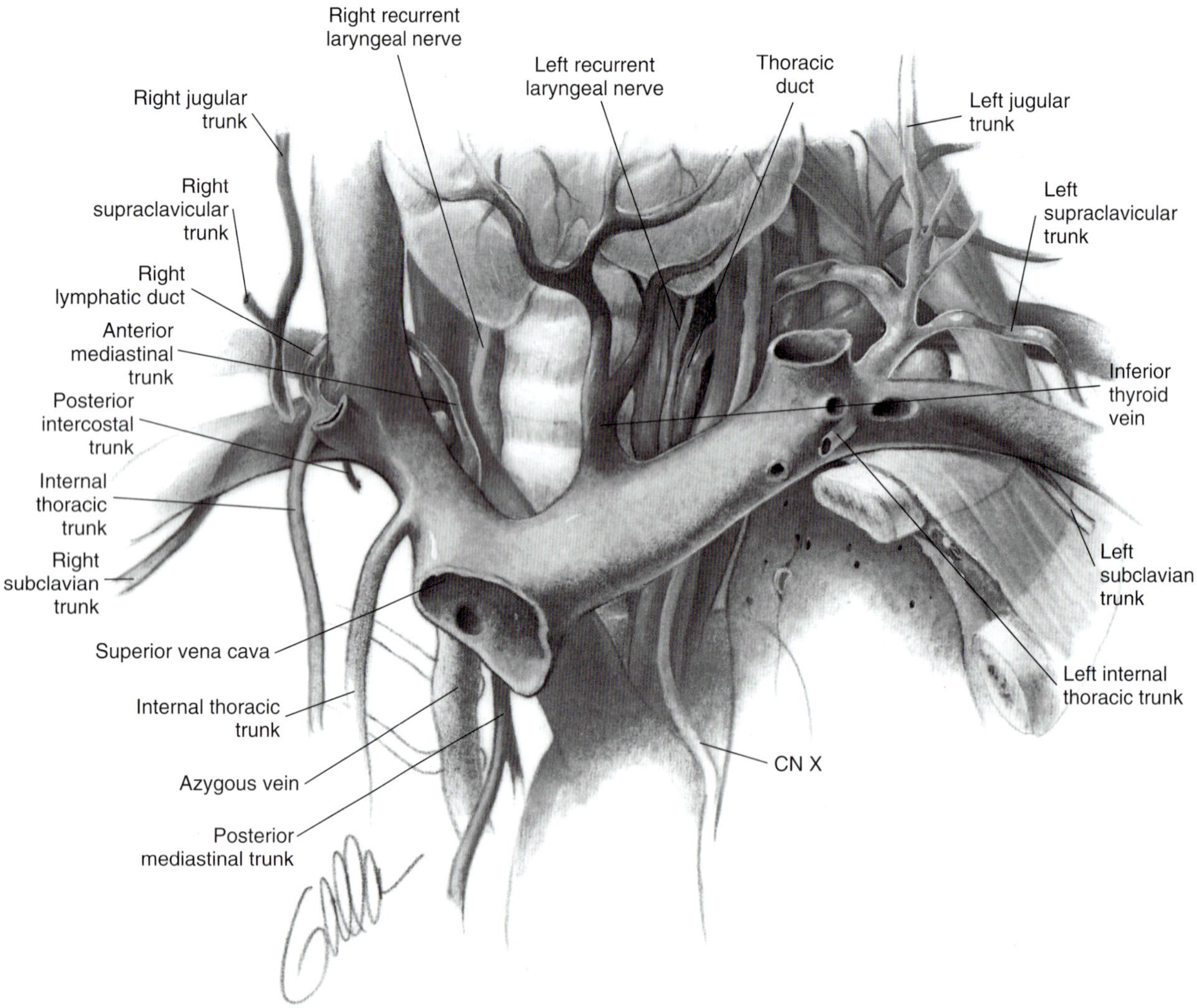

Fig. 6.9 Vascular anatomy of the neck base and upper mediastinum. (From Janfaza P, et al, eds. *Surgical Anatomy of the Head and Neck*. Philadelphia: Lippincott Williams & Wilkins; 2001. With permission.)

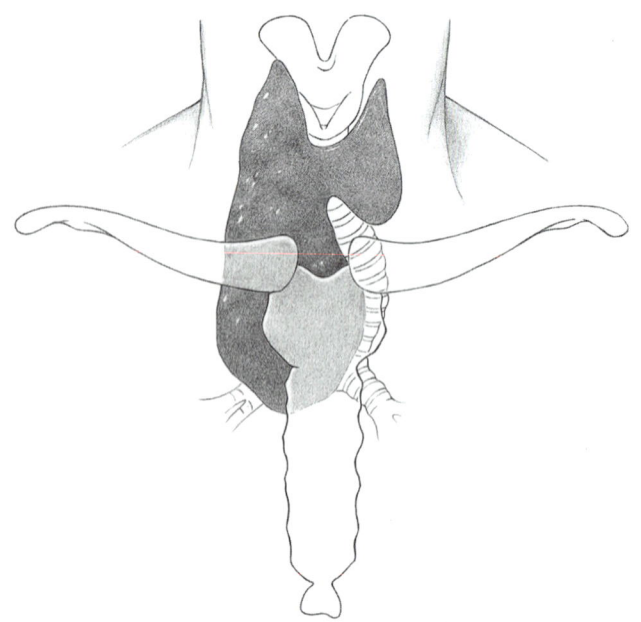

Fig. 6.10 Substernal goiter extension on the right, with tracheal deviation in the upper mediastinum.

present.[11] Johnson and Swente have reported a case of mediastinal hematoma and death after morselization of a large posterior mediastinal goiter.[22] Allo and Thompson described a form of morselization with thyroid capsular incision and insertion of a suction.[56] Recently, a powered endoscopic debrider instrument initially designed for cartilage ablation during endoscopic knee surgery and later modified for endoscopic sinus surgery was used for goiter morselization. This new technology makes morselization no more appealing, given the risks of bleeding and cancer dissemination.[201] Cysts within the thyroid, if benign, can be decompressed with a needle, although such a technique is rarely necessary. A variety of instruments have been used to facilitate substernal goiter delivery. Kocher introduced a mediastinal goiter spoon to facilitate substernal goiter delivery. The use of this blunt instrument breaks negative intrathoracic pressure and occupies less space than the surgeon's finger.[188,202] Sanders has used a Foley catheter placed into the mediastinum and inflated it to assist in the delivery of substernal goiter without sternum split.[20]

Sternotomy for Substernal Goiter

Multiple substernal goiter series show sternotomy rates of between 1% and 8% (see Chapter 7, Approach to the Mediastinum: Transcervical, Transsternal, and Video-Assisted).[11,20,56,58,86,90,91,101,203,204] Resection of the medial one-third of the clavicle can also be used to increase the bony confines of the thoracic inlet (see Figure 6.10).[205] Sternotomy must, in all cases, be discussed preoperatively with the patient and thoracic surgical colleagues. Clearly, there is increased morbidity associated with the addition of a transthoracic approach. In a National Surgical Quality Improvement Program (NSQIP) database review of 2716 patients with substernal goiter, Khan et al. showed increased rates of unplanned intubation, need for transfusion, and length of hospital stay.[206] The decision to perform sternotomy should be considered carefully and may be needed in the following circumstances:

- Known or suspected malignancy extending into the mediastinum
- Posterior mediastinal goiter if associated with contralateral extension (substernal goiter type IIB)
- Cases in which goiter blood supply is mediastinal. This information may not always be available preoperatively. Patients with isolated mediastinal goiter (substernal goiter type III) are at higher risk for having noncervical blood supply.
- Cases associated with true SVC syndrome identified preoperatively, which suggests substantial neck base/mediastinal venous obstruction. True SVC syndrome should raise the specter of mediastinal malignancy rather than benign substernal goiter.
- Recurrent large substernal goiters
- Any case in which delivery maneuvers reveal an immobile substernal component or where goitrous adhesions to surrounding mediastinal vessels and pleura are identified. Increased fibrosis or scarring may be seen with prior radiation or surgery of the neck or chest.
- Cases in which substernal goiter delivery is associated with substantial mediastinal hemorrhage
- Cases in which the diameter of the intrathoracic component of the goiter is substantially greater than the diameter of the thoracic inlet
- Cases where there is a long thin stalk from the cervical to the substernal component. Such stalks may fragment with significant retraction, especially if the mediastinal component is wide and bulbous.

Sternotomy or thoracotomy, as an isolated approach to substernal goiter, is not appropriate because of the greater risk to the RLN during such a procedure and the inability to effectively control the inferior thyroid artery.[91,96]

Vagal Monitoring During Goiter Surgery

We have used intermittent vagal stimulation to help preserve the vagus and RLNs during surgery of large cervical and substernal goiters. Initially, the vagus nerve can be identified during carotid sheath dissection. Vagal stimulation can be used intermittently during goiter surgery to test the entire "circuit" (i.e., the entire ipsilateral vagus and RLN) and ensure that it is intact during maneuvers that, because of goiter size or substernal extent, risk neural stretch. Such maneuvers are performed slowly with progressive incremental goiter delivery during ongoing passive neural vagal monitoring and intermittent vagal stimulation. If any change in stimulation is detected, the vagal and RLN course and surgical maneuver are reevaluated to ensure that neural stretch is not occurring.

We have seen no adverse neural, cardiopulmonary, neurologic, or cardiovascular effects with stimulation of either the left or right vagus despite repetitive, constant current pulse stimulation in the 1 to 2 mA range, 4 pulses per second, 100 μs stimulation duration. The latency is longer (average 6 to 8 ms), as one would expect, compared with RLN stimulation during thyroidectomy (see Chapter 36, Surgical Anatomy and Monitoring of the Recurrent Laryngeal Nerve; Figure 6.11). The safety of vagal stimulation is in agreement with the works of Friedman et al., Leonetti et al., and Eisele.[207-209] Satoh, using penetrating electrodes, transcutaneously stimulated the human vagus nerve in the lower neck and found that ipsilateral thyroarytenoid electromyographic (EMG) activity was biphasic or triphasic, with latency of 6 to 8 ms (2 to 3 ms shorter on the right), amplitude of 0.4 to 0.7 mV, and response duration of 4 to 5 ms.[210] Friedman et al. documented the cardiac safety of vagal stimulation in dogs with stimulation in the 1 to 10 mA range, with 0.4 ms duration at 10 to 100 Hz.[207] Intermittent vagal stimulation through an implanted vagal coil electrode was introduced in 1990 as treatment for some forms of refractive epilepsy. Such stimulation has been shown to be well tolerated and safe.[211,212] Lundy studied the laryngeal effects of vagal stimulation for epilepsy in humans. The induced position of the vocal cord is felt to depend on the amplitude and frequency of electrical stimulation (see Chapter 36, Surgical Anatomy and Monitoring of the Recurrent Laryngeal Nerve). No adverse cardiopulmonary effects were seen with a

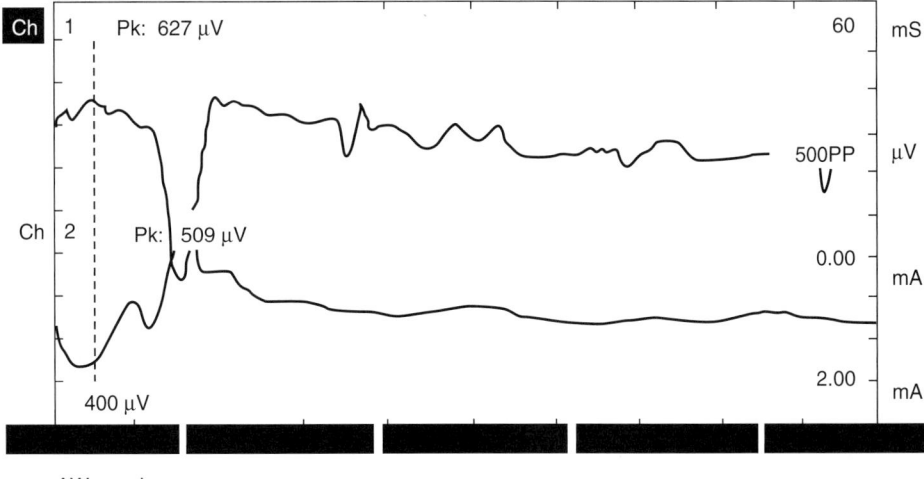

Fig. 6.11 Electromyographic activity recorded in the thyroarytenoid/vocalis muscle of the larynx during ipsilateral vagal nerve stimulation at 2 mA. Note the increased latency of the evoked response from stimulation artifact compared with recurrent laryngeal nerve stimulation (stimulation artifact represented by the *dotted line* on the left).

frequency of stimulation less than 40 Hz. At 3 mA, stimulation of less than 10 Hz resulted in oscillation of the vocal cord at the rate of stimulation. Stimulation from 10 to 30 Hz resulted in vocal cord *ab*duction. Stimulation at 40 Hz or greater resulted in *ad*duction, with progression to tetany. Others have documented vagal stimulation safety in humans.[203,213-215]

Vagal stimulation can also be used to diagnose cases of nonrecurrent RLN. In such cases, vagal stimulation high in the neck results in laryngeal EMG activity, but stimulation low in the neck below the larynx and below the RLN branch point does not. We have used such stimulation to diagnose nonrecurrence of the right RLN before the nerve is directly visualized.

POSTOPERATIVE COMPLICATIONS OF GOITER SURGERY

Recurrent Laryngeal Nerve

RLN paralysis rates vary significantly from study to study, but in general, they are consistently higher when surgery is performed for goiter as compared with routine thyroidectomy. It is encouraging to note that in highly skilled hands, even recurrent substernal goiter can be surgically removed with very low complication rates, as noted by Australian workers.[180] In our series, the rate of RLN permanent paralysis was zero, and the rate of transient paralysis was 2.5% of procedures and 1.8% of nerves at risk, all resolving within 7 months.[85] Sinclair, while noting a 1.1% permanent RLN paralysis rate overall in his series of 767 thyroid surgeries, described a 17.5% rate with substernal goiter, associated with a policy of not identifying the RLN before goiter delivery.[192] Hockauf and Saylor, in treating 1713 patients with goiter, noted a 6.8% rate of permanent RLN paralysis for goiter overall and a 27% rate of RLN paralysis with substernal goiter.[216] MacIntosh described a 10% rate of RLN paralysis with substernal goiter.[217] In a German multicenter study of 7266 patients with benign goiter, Thomusch found transient RLN paralysis occurred in 2.1% of patients and permanent RLN paralysis in 1.1%. Bilateral RLN transient paralysis occurred in 0.002% and bilateral RLN permanent paralysis in 0.001%.[218] Shen, in a surgical series of 60 patients with substernal goiter, found 12% had airway complications postoperatively but did not provide information regarding postoperative laryngeal examination in these patients.[219] Rios-Zambudio, in 301 patients with goiter operated on by experienced endocrine surgeons, found RLN injury occurred in 8.6% of patients and was more likely in patients with hyperthyroidism and in those with larger and substernal goiters. Again, routine laryngoscopy was not performed.[220] In our series, laryngeal nerve monitoring was associated with a significant decreased risk of RLN paralysis by 87%. Analysis of risk factors in our series revealed that RLN paralysis during goiter surgery found that increased RLN risk was predicted by the presence of bilateral cervical goiter, but not by size, presence of revision surgery, substernal extension, or preoperative compressive symptoms. We also confirmed that retrotracheal goiter and posterior mediastinal goiter, when identified on preoperative CT scan, can help predict a ventrally displaced RLN, which is at extremely high risk during surgery.[85]

Parathyroid Glands

Rates of hypoparathyroidism vary significantly between series in goiter surgery. Rates in expert hands as low as 1% to 1.5% have been reported.[88,218] Thomusch found that transient parathyroid hypofunction occurred in 6.4% of patients, and permanent parathyroid dysfunction occurred in 1.5% of patients in his multicenter study on benign goiter. There was a correlation between long-term hypoparathyroidism and extent of thyroid resection.[218] We found permanent hypoparathyroidism in 8% of patients undergoing bilateral surgery and in 3% of patients overall, including patients with revision surgery.[85] Hypothyroidism can be expected based on degree of thyroid resection, dietary iodine status, and presence of autoimmune thyroid antibodies.

Risk Factors for Complications During Goiter Surgery

Several series suggest an increased risk of both RLN and parathyroid complications for substernal versus cervical goiter.[192,216] Lo, Kwok, and Yuen found increased RLN risk during goiter surgery with longer operative procedures and those associated with increased blood loss.[221] Torre et al. found increased risk if substernal goiter had a "complex endothoracic" relationship or if total thyroidectomy was performed.[8] Agerback et al. found increased RLN risk with increasing goiter size.[209] Calik et al. found increased risk to both the RLN and parathyroids with recurrent goiter, cases associated with thyroid cancer with nodal resection, and thyroiditis.[222] Judd, Beahrs, and Bowes found an increased overall complication rate in patients requiring sternotomy.[96] In our series, we identified a number of other factors that are important in the conduct of surgery, including degree of capsular blood vessel engorgement and friability, goiter consistency, and compressibility.[85]

Thomusch, in a German multicenter study, provided a multivariate analysis of complications that occurred during benign goiter surgery in 7266 patients.[218] Using logistical regression analysis, RLN injury was found to be associated with (1) extent of surgery, (2) recurrent goiters, and (3) failure to identify the RLN. It is of interest that failure to identify the nerve resulted in a 9.9-fold increase of nerve paralysis for patients undergoing total thyroidectomy. Hypoparathyroid complications were found to be associated with (1) extent of resection, (2) recurrent goiters, (3) age, (4) gender (female more than male), (5) volume of thyroid surgery done in the hospital, and (6) presence of Graves' disease. Also interesting was Thomusch's finding that, unlike RLN identification, the identification of at least one parathyroid gland during the goiter surgery did not affect the rate of postoperative hypoparathyroidism.[218]

Other Complications

Please see the Expert Consult website for more discussion of this topic.

Tracheomalacia

Tracheomalacia is poorly understood, extremely rare, and apparently reversible. Geelhoed and Green et al. have reported tracheomalacia after goiter surgery.[230,231] The incidence of tracheomalacia has previously been estimated to be between 0.001% and 1.5%.[95,231,232] Of note, Sitges-Serra and Sancho, in reviewing six major studies, found two cases of what they believed was tracheomalacia.[95] In 72 patients with substernal goiters, Rodriguez noted no cases of tracheomalacia.[88] McHenry and Protrowski, Mellière et al., Shaha et al., and Wade found no cases of tracheomalacia in their series.[5,56,105,233] In our combined series of 200 large cervical and substernal goiters treated at Massachusetts Eye and Ear Infirmary and Massachusetts General Hospital, we did not come across a single case of tracheomalacia from benign goiter, even in the setting of chronic significant tracheal deviation, compression, and remodeling with massive and recurrent goiters. Tracheotomy was performed in only 3% of patients, and in none of these cases was it performed for tracheomalacia.[85] In all cases the trachea can be evaluated directly through the wound to determine whether there is evidence of poor tracheal integrity or dynamic change with the respiratory cycle. We have seen cases that were referred with a presumptive diagnosis of tracheomalacia that ultimately were found to have bilateral vocal cord paralysis that had not been recognized. It is our strong clinical impression that tracheomalacia from goiter is rare and likely has arisen as a diagnostic error for underlying bilateral vocal cord paralysis. We do not advocate routine postsurgical bronchoscopy or prophylactic tracheotomy. If tracheomalacia exists as a diagnostic entity from chronic goiter compression, it is unclear how a trachea that has been rendered significantly structurally insufficient (i.e., floppy) by chronic goiter compression would become structurally intact by a short-term intubation. A variety of recommendations have been made regarding the treatment of tracheomalacia, including intubation, tracheotomy, Marlex mesh of the trachea, tracheopexy, and various types of tracheal grafting.

RECURRENT GOITER: PREVENTION AND TREATMENT

Please see the Expert Consult website for more discussion of this topic.

REFERENCES

For a complete list of references, go to expertconsult.com.

Approach to the Mediastinum: Transcervical, Transsternal, and Video-Assisted

Uma M. Sachdeva, Cameron D. Wright, Douglas J. Mathisen

It is not uncommon that resection of thyroid or parathyroid pathology requires entry into and exploration of the mediastinum. Although resection can often be achieved through a transcervical approach, surgeons treating thyroid and parathyroid diseases must be familiar with thoracic approaches to the mediastinum and the circumstances under which it might benefit to seek the involvement of a cardiothoracic surgeon either preoperatively or intraoperatively. In this chapter, the indications for an extracervical approach to the mediastinum will be reviewed as well as an overview of the various types of thoracic incisions and their uses (see Chapter 6, Surgery of Cervical and Substernal Goiter).

INDICATIONS

A thoracic approach to the mediastinum may be necessary to treat either benign or malignant conditions. Several groups have published their experiences with resection of mediastinal pathology due to thyroid or parathyroid disease. Monchik et al. reported that 29% of patients who underwent resection of a mediastinal thyroid mass required a thoracic approach, including full sternotomy, partial sternotomy, or posterolateral thoracotomy, whereas the remainder underwent successful transcervical resection.[1] Our own experience would suggest that this is a high estimate, with well under 10% needing a thoracic approach. Indications for surgery included benign goiter, aberrant thyroid tissue, papillary carcinoma, substernal goiter, follicular carcinoma, or reoperation for either benign or malignant disease.[1]

Substernal Goiter

The most common indication for mediastinal exposure for thyroid disease is the presence of a substernal goiter (Figure 7.1). Substernal, retrosternal, or intrathoracic goiters are commonly defined as having at least 50% of their mass below the thoracic inlet. Alternate definitions that have been used in the literature include a gland extending 3 cm below the sternal notch or extending below the fourth thoracic vertebra.[2-5] The incidence of substernal goiter is reported to range between 0.2% and 0.5% of the general population and 0.2% and 45% of all patients undergoing thyroidectomy.[6] This tissue may arise as an extension of the cervical thyroid, sharing its vascular supply with the main thyroid gland (secondary mediastinal thyroid goiters), or it may arise independently of the cervical thyroid gland, as a result of ectopic thyroid tissue that migrated to a mediastinal location during embryogenesis (primary mediastinal thyroid goiters). In the latter case, the arterial supply can be separate from that of the cervical thyroid gland and arises from the internal thoracic vessels. Primary thyroid goiters comprise roughly 1% of mediastinal goiters, with the vast majority being secondary in nature. The majority of secondary goiters lie in the anterior mediastinum, with only 10% to 15% located in the posterior mediastinum.[7]

Substernal goiter can be suspected if the inferior border of the thyroid gland cannot be palpated in the neck on physical examination. Alternatively, it may be found on workup of associated symptoms resulting from compression of adjacent structures by the substernal mass, including dyspnea, dysphagia, insomnia, hoarseness, and facial swelling from superior vena cava syndrome. Workup of suspected substernal goiter should include imaging by computed tomography (CT; see Figure 7.1). This imaging provides essential information regarding the location of the substernal mass and its relationship to critical mediastinal structures, including the aortic arch, superior vena cava, innominate vein, esophagus, and mediastinal trachea. Magnetic resonance imaging (MRI) may be obtained to provide further information about the relationships between soft tissue structures, but it is often not required preoperatively. Although final determination of whether a thoracic surgical approach is necessary is often not possible until intraoperative evaluation, close examination of the CT scan should provide a reasonable assessment of whether an extracervical approach to the mediastinum may be required for complete resection. The most commonly reported factor to suggest successful transcervical approach for resection of a substernal goiter is maintenance of intact fascial planes surrounding the gland on preoperative CT scan, which suggests that the gland may be gently lifted out of the thoracic inlet and dissected free from the inferior parathyroid glands and the bilateral recurrent laryngeal nerves through a standard collar incision. However, blind substernal dissection of a gland that is fixed or does not lift out of the mediastinum with only gentle traction predisposes to hemorrhage or damage to the recurrent laryngeal nerves and other adjacent structures, and should not be performed in favor of a thoracic approach. Additional tools that may assist with preserving a transcervical approach include the use of a spoon,[8] a Foley balloon catheter,[9] and, rarely, morselization.[10]

Several factors have been reported to increase the likelihood of needing a thoracic approach and include: size larger than the thoracic inlet; location within the posterior mediastinum; proximity to the tracheal bifurcation or aortic arch; compression of the superior vena cava, trachea, or esophagus; recurrent goiter; reoperative surgery; or malignancy with suspicion of involvement of adjacent structures.[7] In our institutional experience, 3% of patients undergoing resection of a substernal goiter required a partial or full sternotomy.[11,12] The only case requiring a full sternotomy in our series was a patient who had undergone previous resection of a goiter through a posterolateral thoracotomy. In that case full sternotomy was required to safely remove the recurrent goiter because of the massive size, location, and previous operation.

Thyroid Malignancy

Malignant thyroid masses extending into the mediastinum are much less common than benign goiters but can require a thoracic approach for

CHAPTER 7 Approach to the Mediastinum: Transcervical, Transsternal, and Video-Assisted

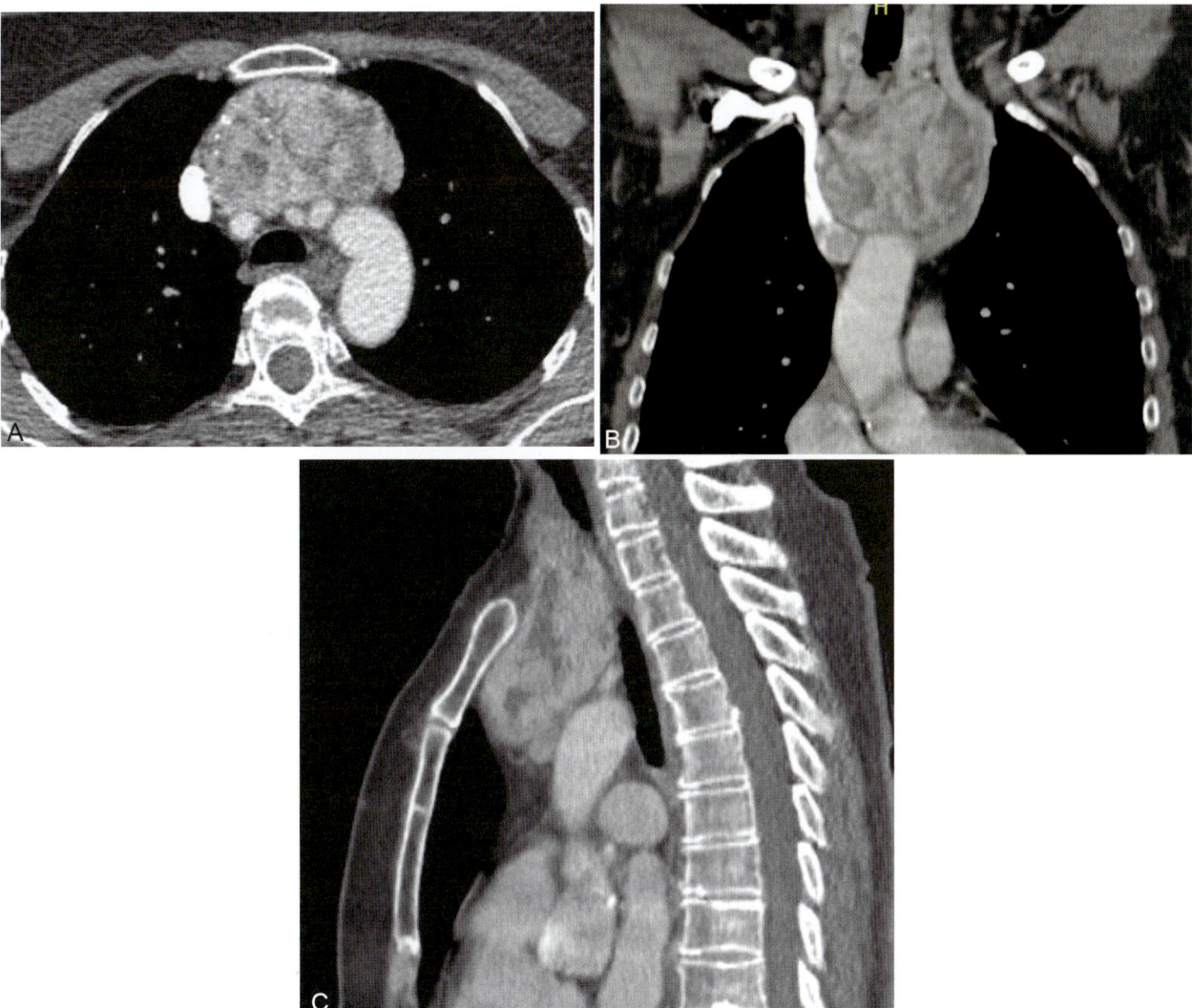

Fig. 7.1 CT scan of the chest with axial (**A**), coronal (**B**), and sagittal (**C**) views showing an intrathoracic substernal goiter, lying deep to the manubrium but superficial to the aorta. This was resected through a cervical incision with extension to partial sternotomy.

resection due to adherence or local invasion into adjacent structures. Indications that a thoracic approach may be necessary from preoperative imaging are similar to those for substernal goiter, and include size, proximity to or compression of critical mediastinal structures, and obliteration of encapsulating fascial planes. Monchik et al. reported that 56% of their cases requiring a thoracic approach for thyroid pathology had a malignant neoplasm,[1] whereas Nervi et al. reported only 20% of their cases that required mediastinal exposure had malignant disease.[13] Although any thyroid malignancy may extend into the chest, the most common pathologies mirror those affecting the thyroid gland, including papillary and follicular carcinoma.

Posterior Mediastinal Thyroid

Posterior mediastinal goiters represent roughly 10% of all substernal goiters and are more common in women and in patients over 50 years of age. Posterior mediastinal goiters result in complex vascular and especially neural relationships that must be clearly understood regardless of the surgical approach; these will be reviewed in detail elsewhere in this text (see Chapter 6, Surgery of Cervical and Substernal Goiter). Although benign goiters in the posterior mediastinum are less likely,

they are more likely to be symptomatic than anterior intrathoracic goiters. Patients may present with a palpable or visible cervical mass on physical examination and report symptoms resulting from compression of adjacent structures, including the trachea and esophagus. These symptoms include dyspnea on exertion or when supine, stridor, hoarseness, and dysphagia. Migration of the mass into the thoracic inlet can cause Pemberton's sign, with facial flushing or a choking sensation with arms raised and may occur also when the patient is supine. Patients may develop Horner's syndrome due to compression of the sympathetic chain, or jugular venous distention, thrombosis, cerebrovascular steal syndrome, or superior vena cava syndrome if the mass compresses mediastinal venous structures. When identified, these masses should routinely be resected, even in the absence of symptoms, given the risk for development of compressive symptoms with continued growth. They are often continuous with the cervical thyroid gland and can usually be excised through a cervical incision. In the largest published series to date, DeAndrade et al. reported that out of a total of 9100 patients with goiters, 1300 (14.2%) had intrathoracic lesions, with only 128 located within the posterior mediastinum.[10] In this series, all of these goiters were removed through a transcervical approach and did not require thoracic exposure. Nevertheless, familiarity with thoracic approaches is beneficial should the need arise for enhanced exposure intraoperatively, either for complete dissection, or in the case of inadvertent injury to adjacent vessels, nerves, or to the aerodigestive structures.

Mediastinal Nodal Extension

Mediastinal lymph node metastasis is exceedingly rare in the setting of thyroid and parathyroid carcinomas, which more frequently metastasize to the nodes of the central or lateral neck compartments. In the series by Zhang et al., out 17,745 patients undergoing thyroidectomy for cancer, only 73 underwent mediastinal lymph node dissection through either a cervical or thoracic approach.[14] The majority of these patients underwent transcervical dissection, with only three requiring sternotomy. Of these patients, 82.2% had papillary thyroid cancer, 16.4% had medullary thyroid cancer, and 1.4% had anaplastic thyroid carcinoma. The vast majority of these patients also had positive central or lateral nodes, with only 2.7% having positive nodes solely in the mediastinum. Patients requiring thoracic access for resection underwent full sternotomy for complete lymph node dissection, which is consistent with other reported series, where full or partial sternotomy seem to be the favored approaches for resection of metastatic mediastinal nodes in the setting of thyroid carcinoma.[14] Predictive factors for mediastinal lymph node involvement remain controversial but include poorly differentiated tumors, bilateral cervical metastases, and distant metastases.

Thoracic access may also be required to completely access enlarged level IV lymph nodes that extend below the level of the clavicle and may involve the jugular, subclavian, or innominate veins (Figure 7.2). This can be accomplished through partial sternotomy, with or without resection of the clavicular head, or through a trapdoor incision with elevation of the clavicle and first and second ribs away from the remainder of the chest wall. Potential need for a thoracic approach for mediastinal exposure is often suggested from preoperative CT or positron emission tomography (PET) imaging, although intraoperative evaluation remains the final determinant.

Mediastinal Parathyroid Gland

Mediastinal parathyroid glands occur due to aberrant migration of the parathyroid during embryogenesis in a similar mechanism to that

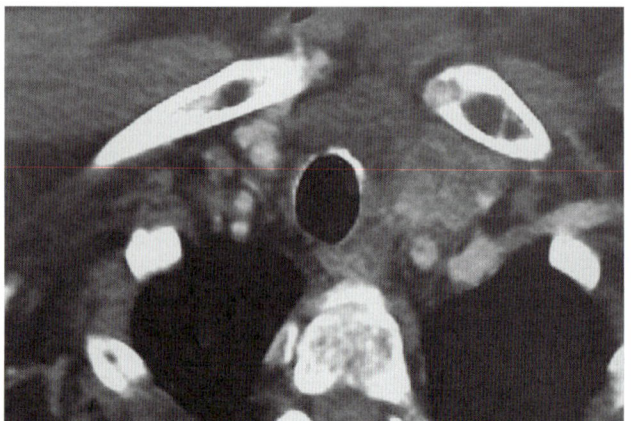

Fig. 7.2 Computed tomography (CT) scan of the chest showing lymph node extension from metastatic papillary thyroid carcinoma involving the anterior mediastinal nodes. The mass can be seen extending behind the left clavicular head and adjacent to the internal jugular vein. This was resected by cervical collar incision with partial sternotomy and trapdoor extension.

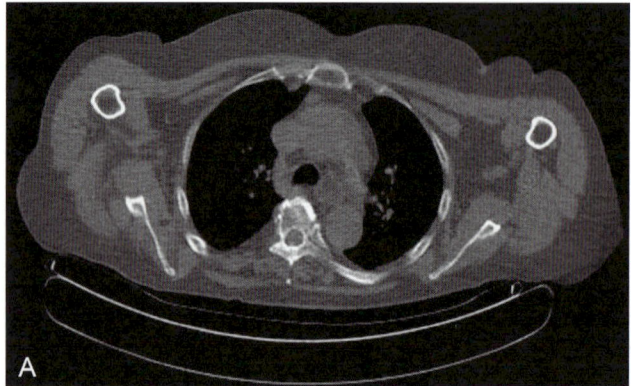

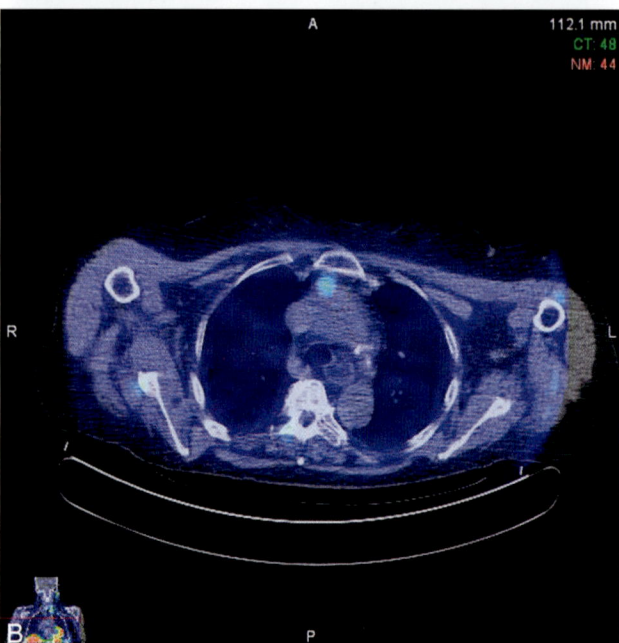

Fig. 7.3 Computed tomography (CT) scan of the chest (**A**) with intravenous Technetium 99m sestamibi injection (**B**) showing an ectopic parathyroid adenoma located in the anterior mediastinum. The mass can be seen anterior to the superior vena cava and aortic arch in the right anterior mediastinum. This was resected via VATS approach with en bloc total thymectomy to ensure complete resection.

of primary substernal goiters (see Chapter 2, Applied Embryology of the Thyroid and Parathyroid Glands). This more commonly occurs with the inferior glands rather than the superior parathyroid glands. The most common location for mediastinal inferior parathyroid glands is within the thymus (Figure 7.3), whereas the most common location for ectopic superior glands is within the tracheoesophageal groove. Other ectopic mediastinal locations include the aortopulmonary window and along the pericardium. The most common indication for resection of these glands is hyperparathyroidism associated with parathyroid adenoma. These ectopic glands are often resected by transcervical approach, with thoracic access required in roughly 1% to 2% of the cases.[15] The need for a thoracic approach is often predictable by location of the ectopic parathyroid at or below the level of the aortic arch. In this case, mediastinal glands can be resected via sternotomy, thoracotomy, mediastinoscopy, video-assisted thoracoscopic, or robot-assisted thoracoscopic surgical approaches, all of which will be discussed later in this chapter. The best approach for resection can be determined preoperatively in collaboration with a thoracic surgeon and is dictated by localization on preoperative imaging studies, including CT, MRI, PET, or technetium 99m sestamibi scans.

SURGICAL APPROACHES TO THE MEDIASTINUM

Partial Sternotomy (Sternal Split)

Partial sternotomy is a useful approach for resection of anterior mediastinal masses that extend to the level of the aortic arch but do not extend significantly below the level of the carina. If anticipated, patients should be positioned with an inflatable thyroid bag or axillary shoulder roll behind the scapulae to extend the neck and bring the carina to the level of the angle of Louis. Division of the manubrium to just beyond the angle of Louis exposes the upper mediastinum and is often sufficient for resection of anterior substernal goiters or mediastinal parathyroid glands. The standard collar incision is extended inferiorly at the midpoint to just below the angle of Louis (Figure 7.4). The location of this incision in the midline can be ensured by using a free silk suture to imprint a linear template onto the skin from the middle of the sternal notch to the xiphoid process. Once the skin and subcutaneous fat and soft tissue have been dissected down to the level of the sternum and the bone is exposed, the sternal notch is dissected free from posterior fascial attachments using electrocautery until the surgeon can hook his or her finger around the notch posteriorly and clear any residual attachments. This ensures that the bone is free, that the innominate vein and pleura are displaced from the posterior aspect of the manubrium, and that there is sufficient room behind the bone to engage the sternal saw. The sternum is then scored down the midline until the inferior extent of the intended sternal split has been reached, often to the inferior aspect of the manubrium, to delineate the path for sternal division. The sternum is then divided with either a bone saw or a Lebsche knife (Figure 7.5). Once the manubrium has been divided, a pediatric sternal spreader is placed to expose the mediastinum (Figure 7.6, *A*). Through a manubrial split incision, the surgeon can now access the upper mediastinal trachea, esophagus, innominate vein, and innominate artery (Figure 7.6, *B*). Access to the tracheoesophageal groove and into the angle formed by the arch of the aorta and the innominate artery is also possible. Mediastinal exposure can be further enhanced with inferior extension of the partial sternotomy. Once the mediastinal lesion has been resected, the manubrium and sternum are reapproximated with sternal wires placed through the bone on either side of the split.

Complications of partial sternotomy include division of the innominate vein; pneumothorax resulting from pleural entry; and bleeding from soft tissues, the divided bone, or exposed marrow. The development of the free space under the sternal notch using blunt finger dissection is important to prevent inadvertent division of the innominate vein during creation of the partial sternotomy. Should this occur, hemorrhage can be temporarily controlled with direct pressure by compressing the vessel against the posterior aspect of the sternum until definitive repair can be undertaken. This often requires completion of a full sternotomy or trapdoor extension to gain clear and direct access to the vessel. If proximal and distal control of the vessel can be obtained, small tears can be repaired using a 5-0 Prolene suture in either figure-of-eight or running fashion, depending on the size of the defect. If the vein has been completely sheared or is unable to be repaired, complete ligation of the innominate vein is well tolerated. Close communication with the anesthesia team is essential in the setting of innominate vein injury, because any intravenous infusions running through the left arm should be discontinued and transferred to the right arm or to a lower extremity, and clear instructions to avoid intravenous access in the left upper extremity should be given to all caregivers postoperatively. The primary complication of innominate vein ligation is left upper extremity swelling, which can improve with postural maneuvers such as arm elevation.

Pneumothorax may develop if the pleural space on either side is entered inadvertently during creation of the partial sternotomy. To minimize the risk of pleural entry, ventilation is held during creation of the sternotomy with the saw or Lebsche knife. Pleural entry is often apparent during the procedure. In this case the pleural space can be evacuated intraoperatively using a suction catheter, or a small chest tube can be placed externally. Evacuation using a temporary suction catheter is achieved by placing a purse-string suture around the site of pleural entry, with the suction catheter placed through this opening into the pleural space. With the lungs held inflated by the anesthesiologist, suction is applied to the intrapleural catheter, and the catheter is removed while the purse-string suture is tied down by the assistant to close the pleural space.

All patients who undergo sternal split should have a chest x-ray performed in the recovery unit to evaluate the pleural space for either effusion or pneumothorax. Small volumes of intrapleural air or fluid can be followed, but moderate-sized pneumothoraces or effusions should be drained with a thoracostomy tube. The presence of a significant effusion raises concern for postoperative hemorrhage, and complete blood count and coagulation studies should be obtained in addition to drainage of the pleural space with a chest tube. A large volume of bloody output from the chest tube should raise concern for ongoing hemorrhage, and immediate return to the operating room for exploration should be considered.

Sources of hemorrhage after partial or full sternotomy include injury to the innominate vein, tearing of small venous branches during dissection, inadvertent injury to the internal mammary arteries during the sternotomy or during placement of sternal wires for closure, or oozing from the bone surface or marrow. Close inspection of the mediastinal space, the posterior aspect of the chest wall, and the bony edges of the sternotomy to ensure hemostasis is essential before closure. Most bleeding from the bone marrow stops once the bone has been reapproximated with wires.

Full Sternotomy

A complete sternotomy, extending from the sternal notch to the tip of the xiphoid, may be required if complete exposure of the anterior mediastinum is necessary for resection, such as may be the case for very large

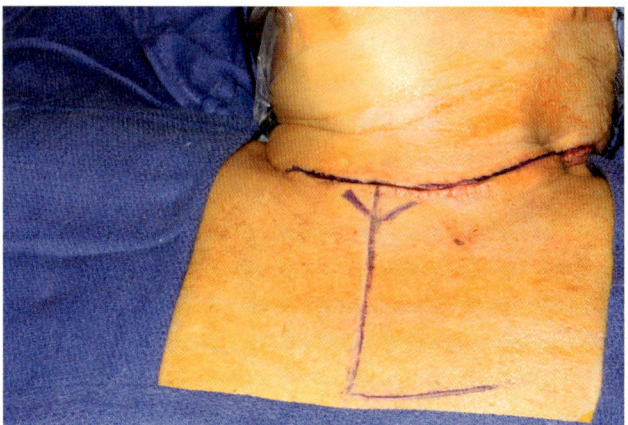

Fig. 7.4 Cervical collar incision with preoperative planning for sternal split with left-sided trapdoor extension through the second intercostal space. This patient had metastatic papillary thyroid carcinoma, previously resected via collar incision, but required reoperation with trapdoor incision to resect metastatic nodal disease extending into the left infraclavicular space.

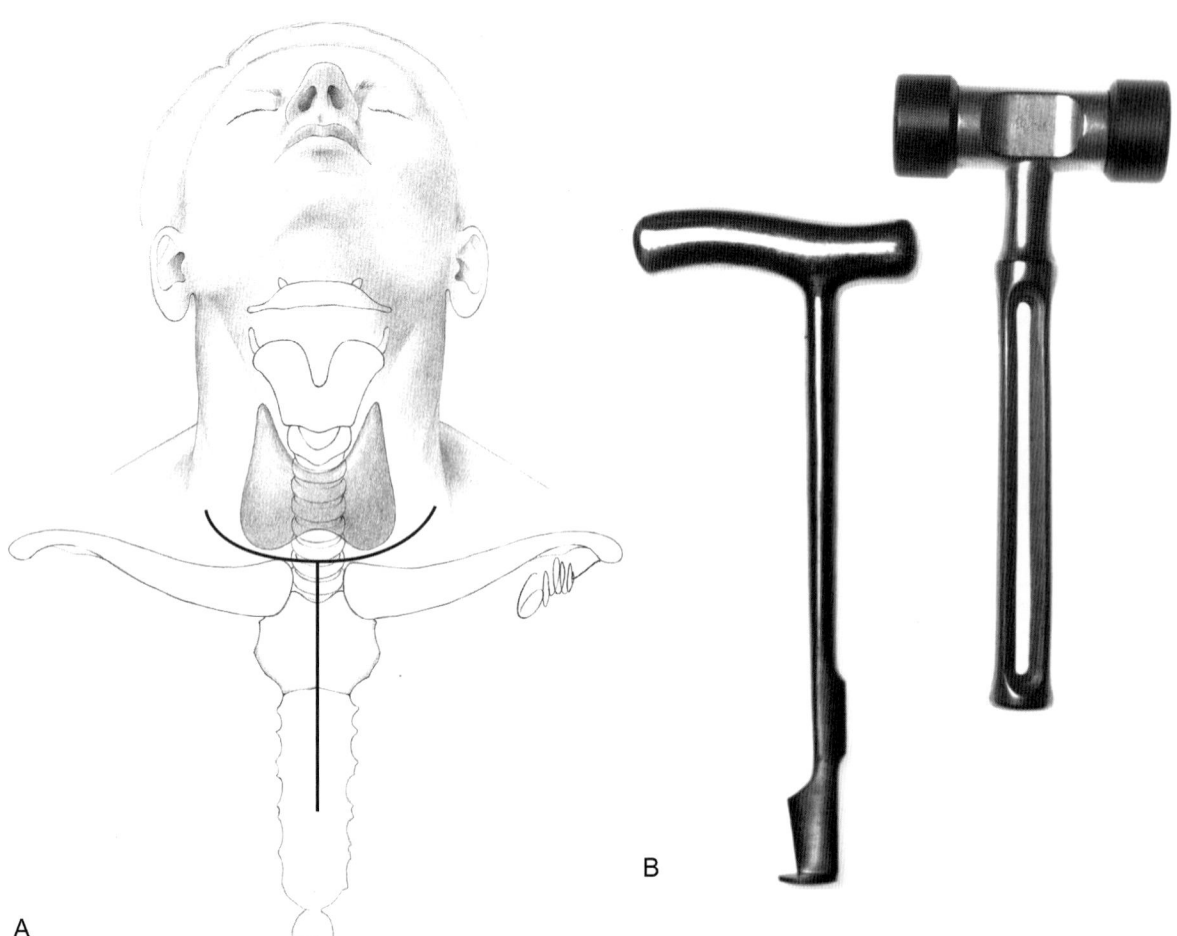

Fig. 7.5 Positioning for the partial sternotomy includes placement of an axillary roll behind the scapula to extend the neck and bring the carina to the level of the angle of Louis (**A**). The solid line indicates the midline location of intended partial sternotomy. The Lebsche knife (**B,** *left*) and mallet (**B,** *right*) are used to make the partial sternotomy. The handle at the top is used to hold the knife, which hooks behind the sternum to elevate it. The footplate seen at the bottom is inserted under the sternal notch. The mallet strikes the knife on the flat surface just above and posterior to the footplate.

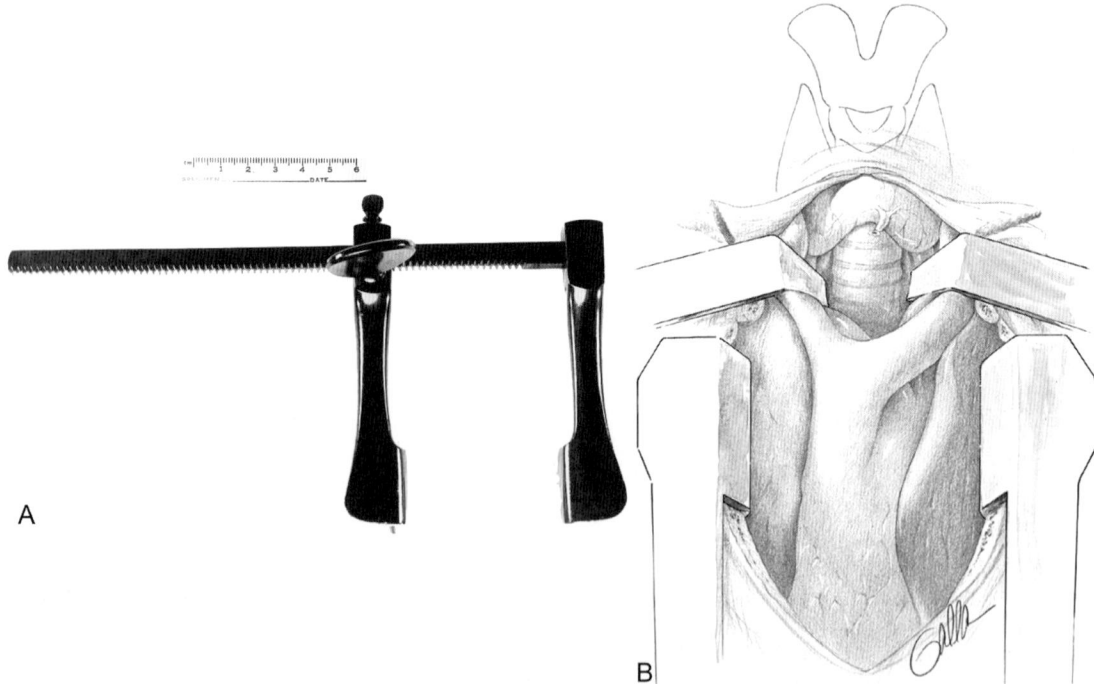

Fig. 7.6 A small pediatric sternal spreader (**A**) can be inserted in the divided manubrium to give wide exposure to the mediastinum (**B**).

goiters, tumors adjacent or adherent to major mediastinal structures, extensive nodal involvement, or ectopic parathyroid glands in the aortopulmonary window along the pericardium or the diaphragm. The patient is positioned as described for the partial sternotomy. The skin incision again extends inferiorly from the midline of the collar incision, this time to the xiphoid process. As for the partial sternotomy, the skin and subcutaneous fat and soft tissue are dissected down to the level of the bone, and the sternal notch is freed posteriorly, with the innominate vein and pleura swept away using blunt finger dissection. The tip of the xiphoid is dissected in a similar fashion, sweeping the diaphragmatic fibers and pericardial attachments posteriorly and inferiorly, away from the xiphoid process. The midline of the sternum is scored from sternal notch to tip of the xiphoid with electrocautery, and the sternum is opened with the electric handheld sternal saw. It is essential to divide the sternum in the midline to ensure proper healing and stability of the sternum, and to minimize the risk of postoperative dehiscence and resulting mediastinitis. The lungs are again deflated when creating the sternotomy to avoid injury to the pleura or to the lungs themselves. The xiphoid can be divided either with the sternal saw or with heavy scissors. The edges of the cut bone are cauterized for hemostasis, and the marrow can be treated with bone wax or other hemostatic agents as needed. Risks of sternotomy are identical to those of the partial sternotomy, with the added risk of injury to the pericardium or heart itself. This is unusual in virgin chests but can be more common and life threatening in the setting of reoperative surgery. In these cases, the sternum is opened using an electric oscillating saw rather than the standard sternal saw. Closure is again performed with sternal wires, placing two or three wires through the manubrium and five additional wires in the intercostal spaces around the sternum. It is important to close the abdominal fascia inferior to the diaphragm to prevent herniation of abdominal contents into the space. At least one mediastinal or pleural drain is placed within the chest before closure of the sternum to evacuate any air or fluid and to prevent accumulation of mediastinal hematoma that can exert pressure on the heart and mediastinal structures. Additional postoperative complications are as discussed for partial sternotomy and include bleeding due to injury to venous structures or the internal mammary arteries, wound infection, sternal dehiscence, and mediastinitis.

Trapdoor Incision

A trapdoor incision is the extension of a partial sternotomy laterally through the second intercostal space to expose the area beneath the clavicle (Figure 7.7). The head of the clavicle can be removed for better exposure of the subclavian vessels, although this step is often not necessary. This incision may be required to resect masses involving the subclavian or jugular vessels, often due to extension of a substernal goiter or metastatic nodal involvement extending into this space. After completing the partial sternotomy, the sternum is then transected on the side of the pathology, and the internal thoracic vessels are ligated and divided. The incision is then extended into the second interspace. The pleural cavity is intentionally entered to allow access behind the clavicle. A self-retaining retractor can be placed at an angle to spread the chest wall laterally and anteriorly away from the sternum, or a Rultract retractor can be used to elevate the chest wall away from the sternum. The Rultract retractor provides excellent exposure through adjustable traction both laterally and anteriorly while using minimal space within the operative field (Figure 7.8). Using this incision, the jugular and subclavian veins can be circumferentially dissected and even ligated if necessary, depending on the extent of vascular involvement (Figure 7.9). The ribs are reapproximated with number 2 Vicryl pericostal sutures after placement of a pleural drain, and the sternum is reapproximated with wires, as previously described. One additional

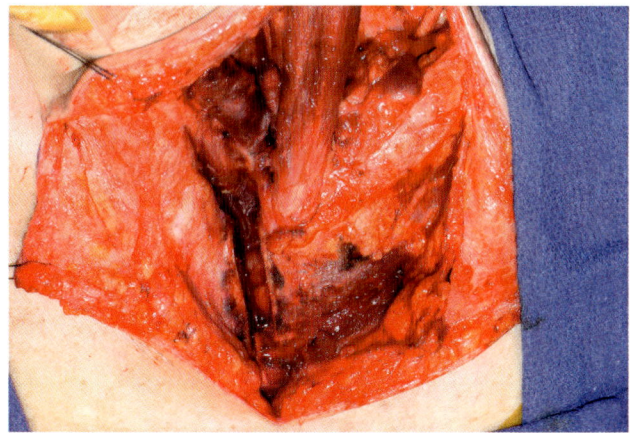

Fig. 7.7 Partial sternotomy with left sided trapdoor extension into the left second intercostal space for resection of metastatic nodes from papillary thyroid cancer.

wire is placed diagonally across the point of hemitransection of the sternum. Postoperative complications are similar to those previously described.

Thoracotomy

A posterolateral thoracotomy is not often required in the setting of thyroid or parathyroid disease but may occasionally be used for resection of posterior mediastinal masses, most commonly substernal goiters located in this position. It is rare to have an ectopic parathyroid gland within the posterior mediastinum, because they are usually located in the anterior mediastinum and accessible by an open or minimally invasive anterior approach. However, 10% to 15% of mediastinal goiters are located in the posterior mediastinum, and this approach has been described for removal of goiters by several groups.[1,13,16,17] The patient is intubated with a double lumen endotracheal tube and selectively ventilated on the nonoperative side. The patient is then placed in the lateral decubitus position with the operative side facing up. This positioning will be discussed further during the discussion of minimally invasive approaches. A posterolateral incision is then made roughly 2 cm below the scapula, with the length determined by extent of exposure required for excision of the mass. The incision can extend as far posterior as the paraspinous muscles and as anteriorly as needed, although the usual length of the incision is roughly 15 cm. The latissimus dorsi muscle is divided and the serratus anterior is retracted anteriorly. A scapula retractor is positioned to elevate the scapula and expose the chest wall, and the chest cavity is entered at an appropriately selected interspace, most commonly the fifth or sixth interspace, entering the chest above the rib to avoid injury to the neurovascular bundle that runs along the inferior aspect. Chest wall retractors are then placed for intrathoracic exposure. If necessary, a small subcentimeter segment of the inferior rib can be resected posteriorly to allow the chest wall to be spread further. With the lung deflated, the posterior mediastinal lesion is identified, mobilized, and resected. The ribs are reapproximated with number 2 Vicryl pericostal sutures after placement of a pleural drain, and the serratus anterior is reattached to adjacent fascia. The cut edges of the latissimus dorsi are reapproximated in one or two layers, and the subcutaneous fat and soft tissues are closed in layers, followed by skin closure. Although this approach provides excellent exposure to the posterior mediastinum, postoperative pain control is essential given the large incision size and division of the latissimus muscle. It is important to pursue aggressive pain management to promote optimal respiratory mechanics postoperatively, and a thoracic epidural is often placed

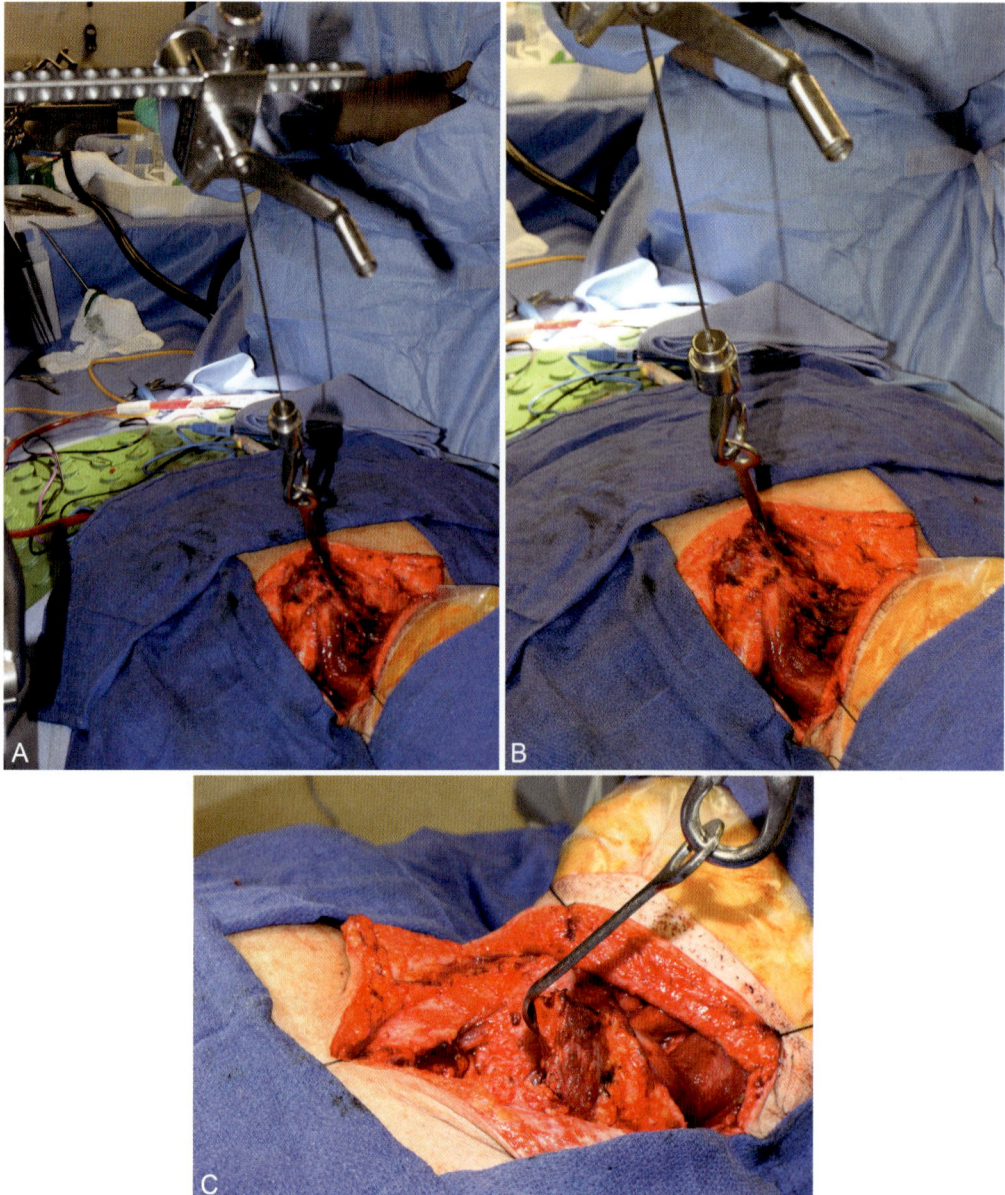

Fig. 7.8 The Rultract retractor is affixed to the operating room (OR) table (**A**) and can be used to hook under the divided second rib to elevate the upper chest wall (**B**) after trapdoor incision. Elevation of the upper portion of the chest wall and retraction anteriorly and laterally can expose the anterior mediastinum and the subclavian and jugular vessels under the clavicle without requiring division and removal of the clavicular head (**C**).

preoperatively if this approach is planned. Aggressive chest physiotherapy is critical to preventing postoperative pneumonia. Patients can experience urinary retention with epidural analgesia and may require a Foley catheter for the duration. Minimally invasive approaches are usually preferred to open thoracotomy for resection of substernal goiters when possible due to less pain and a faster recovery process.

Minimally Invasive Approaches

Over the past several years, minimally invasive approaches to the mediastinum have become standard techniques for resection of both anterior and posterior mediastinal masses. These approaches allow visualization and dissection of mediastinal structures with less pain, faster recovery, and superior cosmesis relative to standard open approaches. However, it is important to carefully assess whether a mass is amenable to minimally invasive resection, which does not provide ready access to major blood vessels in the event of injury during dissection. For this reason, lesions that are more suited to minimally invasive resection include well-circumscribed lesions with intact fascial planes that are easily separable from the surrounding tissues but are located below the level of the aortic arch and not easily accessible through a transcervical approach. Preoperative imaging with CT scan is essential to evaluate the location and appearance of the lesion within the chest. Lesions that involve major vessels, the phrenic nerve, or other critical structures are often best approached through open sternotomy, with either partial, full, or trapdoor incisions, as previously described.

Mediastinoscopy

Mediastinoscopy provides access to the anterior mediastinum using a mediastinoscope that is inserted into the chest in the pretracheal plane. The patient is placed in the supine position with the neck extended, and an inflatable thyroid bag or axillary roll is placed between the scapulae. A small collar incision is created 1 to 2 cm superior to the sternal notch.

CHAPTER 7 Approach to the Mediastinum: Transcervical, Transsternal, and Video-Assisted

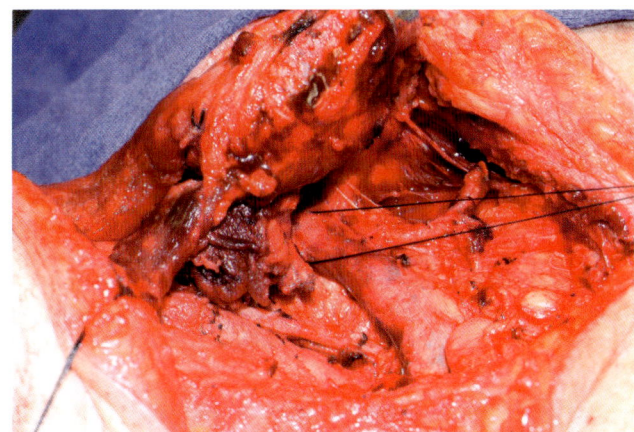

Fig. 7.9 Exposure of the innominate vein via trapdoor incision, with silk suture placed around the left internal jugular vein at its confluence with the left subclavian vein. This was performed in the setting of papillary thyroid cancer with metastatic nodes adherent to the wall of the left internal jugular vein. In this case the internal jugular vein was sacrificed and removed en bloc with the metastatic nodal disease.

The platysma is divided, and the strap muscles are separated at the midline. For isolated mediastinoscopy, division of the thyroid isthmus is often not necessary, although this may already be resected in the setting of mediastinoscopy performed for removal of substernal goiter or nodal involvement for thyroid carcinoma. The pretracheal fascia is dissected bluntly in the midline until the pretracheal space is entered. This space is then opened in an inferior direction using blunt finger dissection by sliding the finger along the anterior surface of the trachea. The pretracheal space is opened in this way to just below the level of the innominate artery. The mediastinoscope is then inserted into this space to expose the anterior mediastinum to just beyond the level of the carina. Video mediastinoscopy allows projection of the view onto a monitor so that both the surgeon and the assistant can see the image projected from the scope. Instruments including electrocautery, biopsy forceps, suction, and other dissectors can be inserted through the scope to allow for resection of the target lesion. Through this approach, metastatic lymph nodes and anterior ectopic thyroid tissue or substernal goiter can be resected. Ectopic parathyroid glands in the anterior mediastinum can also be resected using the mediastinoscope. This approach has been used to resect parathyroid glands located above the aortic arch,[18] within the tracheobronchial angle,[19] and within the thymus.[20] Venissac et al. reported their experience using video-assisted mediastinoscopy for therapeutic procedures in 23 patients and found that this technique was effective for mediastinal lymphadenectomy in the setting of thyroid cancer and resection of ectopic hyperfunctioning parathyroid glands as well as resection of a mediastinal cyst, mediastinal hematoma evacuation, and closure of a bronchopleural fistula.[20]

VIDEO-ASSISTED THORACOSCOPY

Video-assisted thoracoscopic surgery (VATS) represents a very common thoracic surgical approach to access the anterior or posterior mediastinum in a minimally invasive fashion. It is particularly useful in the case of ectopic mediastinal parathyroid glands or for substernal goiters extending below the level of the aortic arch. Primary advantages for a VATS approach relative to open techniques include decreased postoperative pain, shorter length of stay, improved postoperative pulmonary function, and enhanced cosmesis. Through a VATS approach the mediastinum can be approached from either the right side or the left side or occasionally bilaterally. Three ports are usually employed; one port is used for either a 5-mm or 10-mm VATS camera, with two additional working ports for dissection. For this reason, preoperative imaging for precise localization of the target lesion is critical for operative planning to determine the side of entry. When operating on intrathoracic ectopic parathyroid adenomas, preoperative localization with Technetium 99m sestamibi or 4D CT scanning is also helpful.

Once the operative side has been confirmed, a double lumen endotracheal tube is placed upon induction of general anesthesia to selectively ventilate the lung on the nonoperative side. For this reason, preoperative pulmonary function testing should be obtained in smokers and in patients with known pulmonary conditions or significant cardiovascular comorbidities to predict their tolerance for intraoperative single lung ventilation. The patient can be positioned in a lazy lateral position with a pillow placed underneath the chest on the operative side, but most often the lateral decubitus position is used. Once the patient is turned on his or her side, the bed is flexed to widen the intercostal spaces to make room for the thoracoscopic trocars. For midline lesions, laterality of surgical approach may depend not only on the location of the disease, but also on surgeon preference. In performing VATS thymectomy, advocates of a right-sided approach assert that operating from the right chest is ergonomically easier on the operator, allows greater maneuverability in the wider right pleural space, and makes identification of the innominate vein easier because the superior vena cava serves as a landmark.[21] The proponents of a left-sided approach advocate that the dissection maneuvers are safer because the superior vena cava lies outside the surgical field, thus reducing the risk of iatrogenic injury, and it provides access to the left cardiophrenic angle and the aortopulmonary window.[22] Alternatively, the patient can be placed in the supine position, which allows a simultaneous bilateral approach if needed.

A 30-degree thoracoscope is most commonly used, placed through a 5- to 10-mm incision at the midaxillary line, with the other two trocar sites triangulated with respect to the lesion. A utility incision is then made anteriorly between the midaxillary line and the sternum and can range in size but is often a few centimeters in length. This incision is used for dissection, often inserting multiple instruments simultaneously through the same port, and for extraction of the specimen. A third access port is made posterior to the camera port to assist with retraction and dissection. Although a VATS approach can provide excellent visualization of the mediastinum, it can be more challenging for central lesions due to the lateral approach, for very anterior or high mediastinal lesions or very posterior and inferior lesions due to the angles required for dissection, or for lesions adherent to adjacent vascular or nervous structures. If there is suspicion for local adherence or invasion into vessels, nerves, or other adjacent structures, then conversion to an open approach should be undertaken to ensure safety and completeness of resection. At the conclusion of the VATS procedure, a chest tube is placed into the pleural space and connected to a 3-chamber closed suction system, such as a Pleur-evac, to evacuate air and fluid from the space and assist with reexpansion of the lung. This tube is often removed, and the patient is discharged on the first postoperative day.

Robot-Assisted Thoracoscopy

Within the past decade, the use of the operating robot has become increasingly common in thoracic surgery. Lesions amenable to robot-assisted surgery are similar to those accessible by VATS, with the added advantage of greater instrument range of motion due to more degrees of freedom afforded by the robotic arms. Additional advantages of the robot include enhanced optics with three-dimensional (3D) visualization, and the ability of the operating surgeon to be in control of driving the camera, which is performed by the assistant in VATS cases.

The surgeon or surgical assistant places the ports and docks the robot at the patient's bedside; the surgeon then moves away from the bedside and sits at the robotic console while the surgical assistant remains sterile at the operating table. As for VATS approaches, preoperative localization is critical to determine the laterality of the procedure. The procedure is again performed using single lung ventilation through placement of a double lumen endotracheal tube or bronchial blocker. A robot-assisted approach can be used for primary resection or to assist resection through a transcervical approach. Podgaetz et al. described a combined cervical-mediastinal robotic approach for resection of a posterior mediastinal goiter as early as 2009.[23] The blood supply of this mass originated from the internal mammary artery, which was dissected free from surrounding structures through the right chest using the operating robot. Once it was completely mobilized within the mediastinum, the mass was then extracted through a cervical incision. Robot assistance has been shown to be particularly helpful in accessing lesions located in the inferior and posterior mediastinum, which are difficult to access using traditional VATS approaches. Cerfolio et al. reviewed their experience using robot assistance for resection of mediastinal masses and found that out of 153 cases performed over a 30-month period, 75 of these patients had masses in the inferior or posterior mediastinum, and 78 had lesions in the anterior mediastinum.[24] Of the patients with posterior or inferior lesions, 41 of these were metastatic lymph nodes. Advantages to a robotic approach, in terms of improved postoperative pain control and shorter length of stay, are similar to VATS, with seven patients being able to be discharged home the day of surgery in the Cerfolio series.

As for the VATS approach, patients are positioned in the lateral decubitus position with the operative table flexed. Four ports are most commonly used for the robotic arms. Again, preoperative localization is critical, both for laterality and to determine the optimal port placement and positioning of the robot itself relative to the patient and the operating table. If the target lesion is located inferior to the inferior pulmonary vein or posterior and inferior, it has been suggested that all trocars should be placed anterior to or at the midaxillary line, with the robot positioned at the patient's back.[24] For anterior mediastinal pathology, the robot is usually positioned cephalad, with the arms docked over the patient's head.[25] Carbon dioxide insufflation is often used to enhance lung deflation and improve visualization.

There is a significant learning curve associated with robot-assisted thoracic surgery, but outcomes are equivalent to VATS approaches. Postoperative care is similar, with similar postoperative pain scores and lengths of stay. As with VATS, a chest tube is placed at the end of the case and removed before discharge, typically on the first postoperative day.

SUMMARY

Overall, the need for a thoracic approach to the mediastinum for resection of thyroid or parathyroid pathology is rare. Preoperative imaging can often indicate whether a transthoracic approach may be required, though intraoperative assessment may find that enhanced exposure to the mediastinum may be beneficial even in cases that appear resectable through a transcervical approach on imaging. Transthoracic approaches to the mediastinum can include partial or full sternotomy, trapdoor incision, posterolateral thoracotomy, or minimally invasive VATS or robot-assisted approaches. Through careful preoperative planning and a collaborative multidisciplinary surgical approach, complete resection of the mediastinal pathology with low morbidity, good functional outcomes, and optimal cosmesis can be achieved.

REFERENCES

For a complete list of references, go to expertconsult.com.

Surgical Management of Hyperthyroidism

Lisa A. Orloff, Maisie L. Shindo

INTRODUCTION

Primary hyperthyroidism is a condition in which the thyroid gland synthesizes and secretes inappropriately high levels of thyroid hormone(s), causing signs and symptoms of hypermetabolism and excess sympathetic nervous system activity. The term *hyperthyroidism* is distinct from thyrotoxicosis, a clinical state in which there is an inappropriately high thyroid hormone action in tissues. Thyrotoxicosis can result from hyperthyroidism as well as from other etiologies. Patients with subacute, painless, or radiation-induced thyroiditis, excess thyroid hormone ingestion, struma ovarii, and functional metastatic thyroid cancer are examples of those who have thyrotoxicosis that is not attributed to hyperthyroidism. The causes of hyperthyroidism include Graves' disease, toxic multinodular goiter, a solitary toxic adenomatous nodule, viral infections, autoimmune (Hashimoto's) thyroiditis, autoimmune-(Hashimoto's), amiodarone-induced thyrotoxicosis, and very rarely, a thyroid-stimulating hormone(TSH)–producing pituitary tumor. The overall prevalence of hyperthyroidism is 1.3% in the U.S. population. It occurs in 2% of women and 0.5% of men, and its prevalence can be as high as 5% in older women.[1] This chapter focuses on the clinical presentation, diagnosis, and surgical management of hyperthyroidism.

The excess synthesis and secretion of thyroid hormone that occur in patients with hyperthyroidism may produce a variety of clinical manifestations and findings on physical examination (Figures 8.1 and 8.2). Elderly patients are more likely to present with subtle symptoms of thyrotoxicosis such as asthenia, fatigue, and weakness, and a syndrome referred to as *apathetic hyperthyroidism*. Elderly patients are also more likely to present with cardiovascular manifestations of hyperthyroidism such as atrial fibrillation, ischemic heart disease, and congestive heart failure.

The best initial screening test for suspected thyrotoxicosis is a serum TSH level (see Chapter 3, Thyroid Physiology and Thyroid Function Testing). With the rare exception of a TSH-secreting pituitary tumor, patients with hyperthyroidism will have a low serum TSH level. In patients whose serum TSH level is found to be low, a free T4 (FT4) and a free T3 (FT3) level should be measured to help determine the severity of hyperthyroidism. Patients with a low serum TSH level and normal FT4 and FT3 levels are defined as having subclinical hyperthyroidism. A FT3 level is important to make a diagnosis of "T3 thyrotoxicosis" in a patient with a suppressed serum TSH level and a normal FT4 level. In most patients, T3 thyrotoxicosis is an early manifestation of Graves' disease.

Once the diagnosis of primary thyroid-mediated hyperthyroidism is confirmed biochemically (low TSH with normal or elevated T4, T3), the etiology of hyperthyroidism should be determined.[2] If clinical examination does not readily reveal the etiology, such as ophthalmopathy associated with Graves' disease, thyroid uptake scintigraphy with iodine-123 (^{123}I) or technetium-99m (^{99m}Tc) can be helpful in determining the cause of hyperthyroidism. Thyroid uptake is elevated in patients with Graves' disease and may be elevated or normal in patients with toxic multinodular goiter or a solitary toxic nodule.[2] It is low or undetectable in patients with thyrotoxicosis from thyroiditis. Thyroid scintigraphy typically demonstrates diffuse symmetrical uptake in patients with Graves' disease, heterogeneous uptake in patients with toxic multinodular goiter (the scintigraphic regions on functional scanning may not necessarily correspond to the areas of gross nodularity on ultrasound), and a single area of hyperfunction with a variable degree of suppression of the remainder of the thyroid gland in patients with a solitary toxic nodule (Figure 8.3). Measurement of thyroid-stimulating immunoglobulin (TSI) or TSH receptor antibody (TRAb) may help establish a diagnosis of Graves' disease when radioiodine scanning is contraindicated or cannot be obtained in patients who have recently received iodinated contrast for a computed tomography (CT) scan or who are on antithyroid medications to treat the hyperthyroidism. Measurement of thyroid peroxidase antibody (TPOAb) may support a diagnosis of thyrotoxicosis due to Hashimoto's thyroiditis.

GRAVES' DISEASE

Pathogenesis

Graves' disease is an autoimmune disorder with familial predisposition. It is clinically characterized by hyperthyroidism associated with ophthalmopathy or dermopathy with anti-TSH receptor antibodies (TRAb) directed against the TSH receptor with receptor stimulation.[3] TRAb activates TSH receptors in the membrane of the follicular epithelial cells of the thyroid gland, resulting in excess synthesis and secretion of thyroid hormone and growth of the thyroid gland.

Epidemiology

The most common cause of hyperthyroidism in iodine-replete regions is Graves' disease with an annual incidence estimated to be 30 to 38 per 100,000 population, occurring more frequently in women than men.[4,5] Its peak incidence is usually between the ages of 30 and 60 years, with an increased incidence in African Americans.[6] It can be associated with other autoimmune diseases such as rheumatoid arthritis, systemic lupus erythematosus, chronic lymphocytic thyroiditis, Sjögren's syndrome, vitiligo, pernicious anemia, type 1 diabetes mellitus, Addison's disease, myasthenia gravis, and idiopathic thrombocytopenic purpura. It is important to be aware of such associated disorders and potential comorbidities when surgery is being considered.

Clinical Presentation

The clinical manifestations of Graves' disease include symptoms and signs of thyrotoxicosis (Boxes 8.1 and 8.2), a diffuse symmetrical goiter,

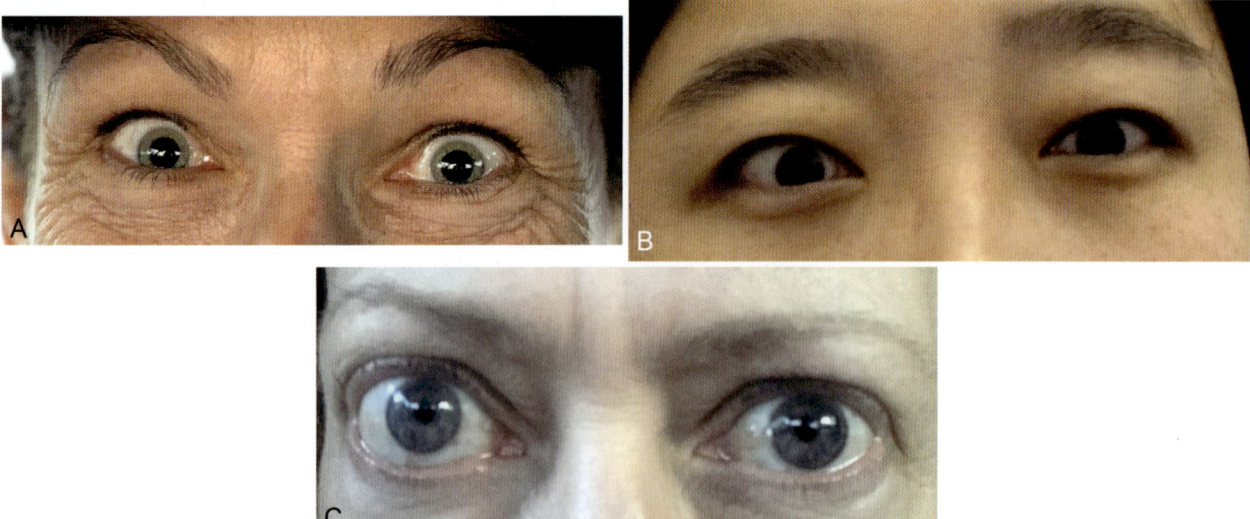

Fig. 8.1 Thyroid Eye Disease. Patients may present with lid retraction (**A**) or unilateral (**B, C**) or bilateral proptosis/ophthalmopathy.

often with a palpable thrill or an audible bruit, a variable degree of presence of extrathyroidal manifestations such as ophthalmopathy (see Figure 8.1), dermopathy such as pretibial myxedema, and acropachy. Extrathyroidal manifestations occur as a result of cellular infiltration and glycosaminoglycan deposition in the soft tissues, such as extraocular muscles and retroorbital fat, in response to antibody reactions to tissue antigens, which crossreact with the TSH receptor in the thyroid gland.

Clinically relevant ophthalmopathy occurs in 20% to 30% of patients with Graves' disease and is vision-threatening in 3% to 5%.[7] It is more common in cigarette smokers and patients with higher levels of TRAb. Ophthalmopathy results from antibody-mediated inflammation of the extraocular muscles, retroorbital fat and connective tissue, and the optic nerve.[8] Stare, lid lag, and eyelid retraction are manifestations of excess sympathetic nervous system stimulation of the levator palpebrae superioris muscles (see Figure 8.1) and may occur in patients with hyperthyroidism due to all causes, but only patients with Graves' disease have ophthalmopathy. Periorbital edema, chemosis, exophthalmos, and extraocular muscle weakness are more specific manifestations of Graves' ophthalmopathy. Patients may experience a gritty feeling in the eyes, eye pain, photophobia, tearing, diplopia, and decreased visual acuity. These symptoms should be queried during the patient history. Corneal ulcerations may result from proptosis and lid retraction, and severe proptosis can cause optic neuropathy and blindness.

Pretibial myxedema occurs in 0.5% to 4.3% of patients with Graves' disease.[9] It is an infiltrative dermopathy most often involving the skin of the legs. It is manifested by painful, pruritic, raised plaque-like violaceous and hyperpigmented lesions that have the texture of an orange peel. Acropachy occurs in less than 1% of patients with Graves' disease and is manifested by clubbing and periosteal new bone formation of the metacarpal bones and the phalanges.

Diagnosis and Evaluation

The diagnosis of Graves' disease is established by the association of hyperthyroidism, a diffuse symmetrical goiter, and presence of ophthalmopathy or dermopathy as described earlier. In the absence of ophthalmopathy or dermopathy, abnormal levels of TRAb or TSI levels will confirm the diagnosis; however, they may not always be elevated. Thyroid scintigraphy is also helpful in confirming the diagnosis (Fig. 8.3) but not always necessary if a clinical or laboratory diagnosis can be made. If obtained it will demonstrate diffuse increased uptake. Measurement of thyroid uptake and thyroid scintigraphy are primarily of value in helping differentiate thyrotoxicosis caused by Graves' disease from toxic multinodular goiter, a solitary toxic adenoma, or thyroiditis. Differentiating the etiology of hyperthyroidism is necessary in management, especially surgical planning. Thyroid ultrasonography should be performed to further elucidate the etiology, with recognition that patients with Graves' disease can also harbor thyroid malignancy.

Treatment

The goals of therapy for Graves' disease are rapid amelioration of symptoms and prevention of recurrent hyperthyroidism. There are three therapeutic alternatives for Graves' disease: antithyroid drugs (ATDs), radioactive iodine (RAI) ablation, and thyroidectomy. Each modality has its own advantages and disadvantages. Patient, physician, institutional, or geographical preferences often influence the choice of therapy. In the United States, radioiodine ablation has traditionally been

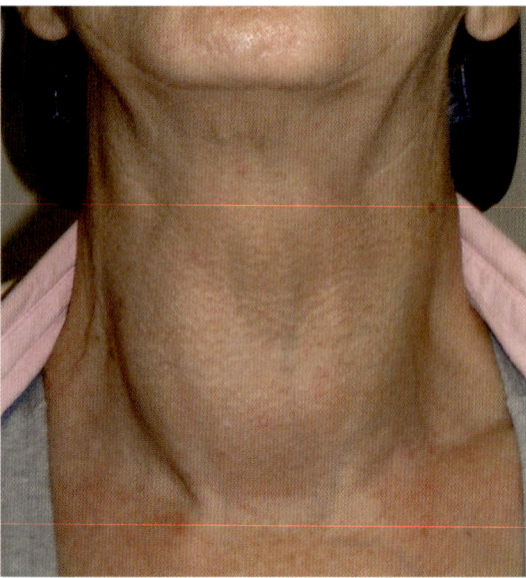

Fig. 8.2 Visible and palpable diffuse goiter, characteristic of Graves' disease.

the primary treatment used; however, a 2011 survey indicates that there has been a trend toward increasing the long-term use of ATD in lieu of RAI.[10] In Europe, Japan, and South America, prolonged ATD therapy is a preferred option.[11-13]

Antithyroid Drugs

The initial treatment of overt hyperthyroidism from Graves' disease involves immediate initiation of an ATD. The ATDs that are used are the thionamide agents, propylthiouracil and methimazole. Both agents decrease thyroid hormone synthesis and reestablish a euthyroid state in 3 to 8 weeks. A beta-blocker is often added for the rapid amelioration of symptoms attributable to excess sympathetic nervous system activity such as palpitations, tachycardia, tremor, heat intolerance, diaphoresis, and anxiety. Permanent remission of Graves' disease occurs in 20% to 50% of patients after 12 to 18 months of therapy, typically in patients with smaller goiters and with less severe hyperthyroidism.[14] The relapse rate has been reported to be 48%, with the risk of relapse increasing with disease severity.[15]

Graves' disease patients who relapse after discontinuation of ATD can be retreated if the goal is long-term ATD therapy. However, in the United States, lifelong administration of ATDs is seldom used as the definitive therapy for Graves' disease. ATDs are routinely used for

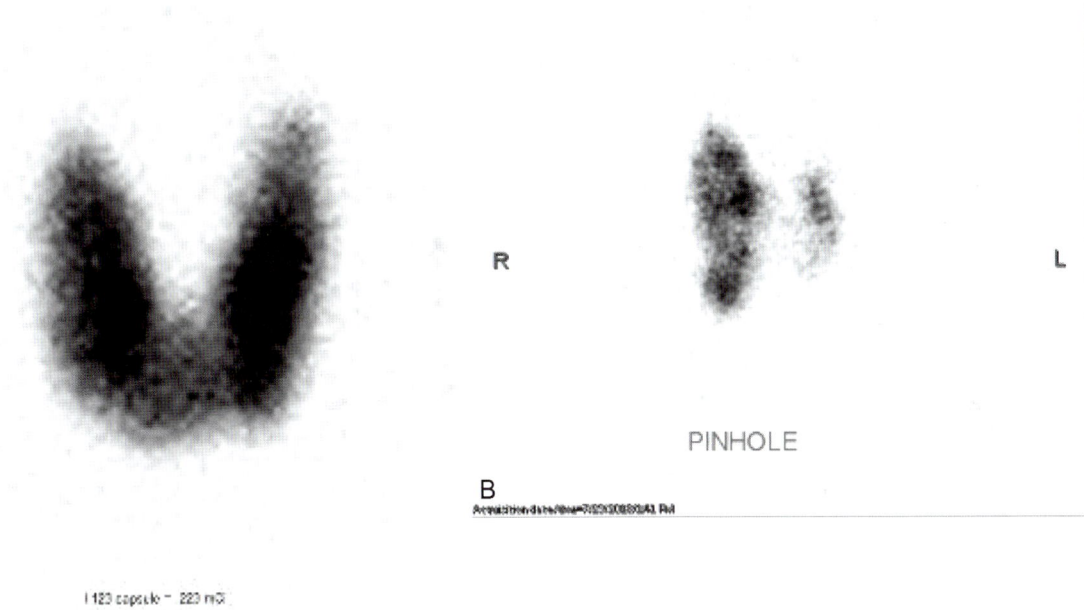

Fig. 8.3 Thyroid Uptake Scintigraphy. **A,** Homogeneous increased uptake typically seen with Graves' disease. **B,** Heterogeneous but overall increased uptake in a toxic multinodular goiter. **C,** Unilateral focal increased uptake in a "hot" (toxic) adenomatous nodule. **D,** Overall diffuse increased uptake in a patient with Graves' disease (65%, with normal 10% to 30%), yet with a large cold nodule in the right inferior lobe.

(Continued)

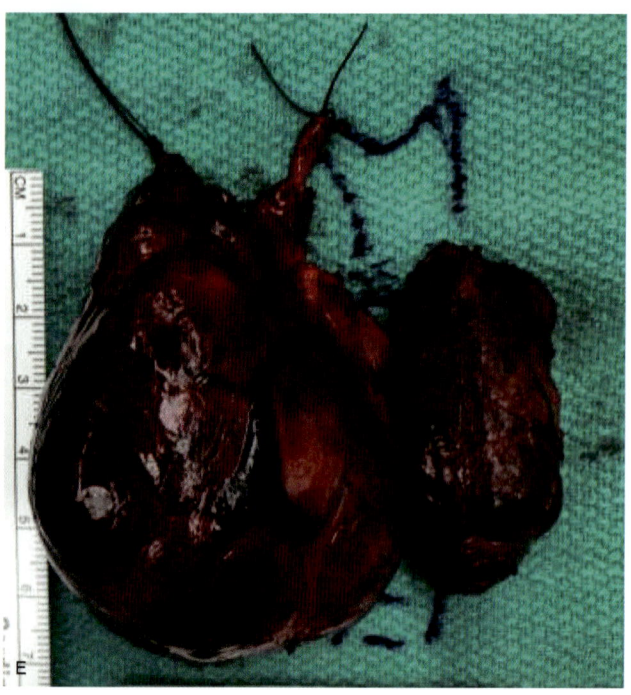

Fig. 8.3, cont'd E, Total thyroidectomy surgical specimen of patient in **(D)** with dominant nodule in right inferior pole that was benign.

preoperative preparation.[2,16] Minor adverse reactions to ATDs occur in approximately 5% of patients and include rash, urticaria, arthralgia, fever, anorexia, nausea, and abnormalities of taste and smell. Major adverse effects include agranulocytosis, which occurs in approximately 0.1% to 0.3% of patients, and hepatotoxicity, an even rarer complication, which may be fatal. Methimazole is the preferred drug due to more convenient dosing but also because of the higher incidence of hepatotoxicity and risk of fatal hepatic necrosis with liver failure associated with propylthiouracil.[17-19] However, propylthiouracil is preferred for the management of Graves' disease during pregnancy because methimazole has been associated with birth defects.[20,21]

Radioactive Iodine (RAI)

RAI was introduced for treatment of hyperthyroidism in the 1940s.[22] Before the 1940s, subtotal thyroidectomy was the standard therapy for Graves' disease. Iodine-131 (^{131}I) gradually became the first-line treatment for Graves' disease in the United States. ^{131}I emits beta particles, which destroy the follicular cells of the thyroid gland. At most centers, the goal of RAI therapy is to induce hypothyroidism to prevent recurrence of Graves' disease, which is achieved in approximately 80% of patients with either a calculated or fixed dosage regimen.[23]

RAI ablation therapy takes a median of 3 months and sometimes multiple doses before hyperthyroidism is corrected.[24] RAI therapy is contraindicated in women who are currently or soon planning to become pregnant or who are breastfeeding.[2,12] A pregnancy test should be obtained before radioiodine administration in all women of reproductive age. RAI is excreted in the urine, exposing the pelvic viscera to radiation. Radioiodine also crosses the placenta, where it can be taken up by the fetal thyroid gland. It is generally recommended that women do not become pregnant for 6 to 12 months after RAI treatment.[2,12] Side effects of RAI ablation include neck pain and tenderness from radiation-induced thyroiditis, transient increase in thyroid hormone levels, and worsening of Graves' ophthalmopathy.[2,12]

Surgery

Surgical treatment of Graves' disease is indicated for (1) patients with a concomitant thyroid nodule that is malignant or suspicious for malignancy, (2) failure of RAI therapy, (3) massive thyroid enlargement (see Figure 8.2) with compressive symptoms, (4) severe ophthalmopathy, (5) patient preference, and (6) pregnant patients requiring high doses of an ATD or who are intolerant to the drugs. Patient preference is often related to the desire for the most rapid amelioration of symptoms (RAI take several months to render a patient hypothyroid), a reluctance to receive RAI because of having young children, a desire to become pregnant, and a fear of exposure to radiation. The advantages of surgical therapy are that patients experience immediate symptomatic improvement; and with total thyroidectomy, the risk of recurrent hyperthyroidism is eliminated. It also allows for treatment of concomitant thyroid nodules and incidental thyroid carcinoma. The incidence of concurrent thyroid nodules and carcinoma in Graves' disease has been reported to be 44% and 6%, respectively.[25,26] In addition, total thyroidectomy has been associated with improvement in eye manifestations attributable to excess adrenergic activity.[27]

BOX 8.1 Symptoms and Manifestations of Hyperthyroidism

Palpitations
Nervousness
Restlessness
Weight loss
Increased appetite
Anxiety
Irritability
Emotional lability
Heat intolerance
Increased sweating
Fatigue
Muscle weakness
Insomnia
Thinning of the hair and hair loss
Brittle nails
Increased bowel movements
Irregular menses
Impaired fertility
Osteoporosis and increased fracture risk
Atrial fibrillation or other supraventricular arrhythmias
Congestive heart failure
Male gynecomastia and erectile dysfunction

BOX 8.2 Signs of Hyperthyroidism

Stare
Lid lag
Tachycardia
Irregularly irregular pulse
Systolic hypertension
Proximal muscle weakness
Hyperreflexia
Resting tremor
Warm, moist skin
Thin, fine hair
Onycholysis

The disadvantage of surgical treatment of Graves' disease is the risk of complications from thyroidectomy, which include recurrent and/or superior laryngeal nerve injury, hypoparathyroidism, hematoma, and thyroid storm. Hypothyroidism is an intended consequence of total thyroidectomy and requires lifelong thyroid hormone replacement. When total thyroidectomy is performed by a skilled surgeon, the incidence of recurrent laryngeal nerve injury and hypoparathyroidism is approximately 1% to 2%, and neck hematoma is 1% or less.[28-32]

Thyroid storm is a life-threatening condition that can be precipitated by surgery in a patient with poorly treated hyperthyroidism. It is characterized by severe manifestations of hyperthyroidism along with fever, nausea, vomiting, diarrhea, tachyarrhythmias, congestive heart failure, agitation, and delirium. The risk of thyroid storm can be eliminated by adequate preoperative preparation.[33-35] An ATD is used to normalize FT4 and FT3 levels before the operation. A beta-blocker is used for symptomatic treatment of adrenergic symptoms and tachycardia. Once the patient's FT4 and FT3 levels are normalized or near normal, a saturated solution of potassium iodide [SSKI] or Lugol's solution is administered for 5 to 10 days before surgery (Box 8-3). One must keep in mind that TSH suppression may be long-lasting even after FT4 and FT3 levels are normalized. Preoperative iodide treatment has been shown to decrease the rate of thyroid blood flow and vascularity, which makes identification of the laryngeal nerves and parathyroid glands less difficult, and reduces overall blood loss during thyroidectomy for Graves' disease.[34-35] The American Thyroid Association and European Thyroid Association recommend presurgical treatment with iodine;[2,12] however, the need for this has recently been challenged.[36] In patients who are noncompliant or intolerant to ATDs, thyroidectomy can still be performed by reducing T4 and T3 using glucocorticoids and, in some instances, cholestyramine along with potassium iodide. In those who are hyperthyroid before surgery due to intolerance of ATDs or are symptomatic, ensuring adequate beta-blockade preoperatively and during surgery with propranolol (20 to 40 mg every 6 hours) or longer acting beta-blockers (e.g., atenolol) is essential.[2,12,37] High-dose propranolol has the added advantage of blocking peripheral T4 to T3 conversion; however, because it is a non-selective beta-blocker, it should not be used in patients with asthma. Preoperatively, the vitamin D level should be checked and optimized to reduce risk of hypoparathyroidism.

The extent of thyroidectomy for the treatment of Graves' disease has been controversial in the past, but current trends strongly emphasize the offering of a total thyroidectomy to most patients. The goal of surgery should be to avoid complications, such as laryngeal nerve injury and hypoparathyroidism, but at the same time to minimize the risk of persistent or recurrent hyperthyroidism. Some surgeons have, in the past, advocated subtotal thyroidectomy leaving bilateral or unilateral thyroid remnants, approximately 6 to 7 g total. The problem with subtotal thyroidectomy is that it is difficult to standardize remnant sizes and to establish a reproducible relationship between remnant size and a

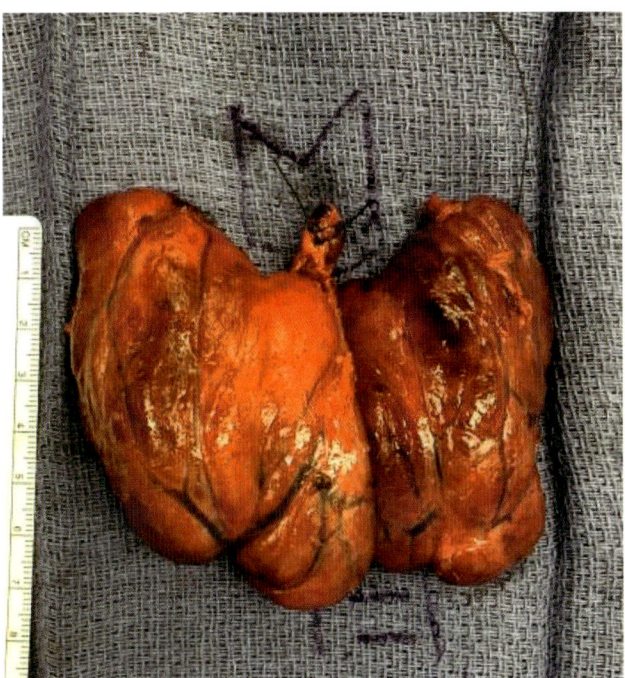

Fig. 8.4 Total thyroidectomy specimen for Graves' disease.

euthyroid state postoperatively.[38] Forty percent to 60% of patients with Graves' disease treated with bilateral subtotal thyroidectomy become hypothyroid within 20 years of operation.[39] As a result, diligent long-term follow-up is necessary to prevent delay in diagnosis and treatment of hypothyroidism and development of untoward sequelae. Bilateral subtotal thyroidectomy is also associated with an approximate 8% to 28% rate of persistent or recurrent hyperthyroidism depending on the size of thyroid remnants.[40,41] Total thyroidectomy has been shown to achieve better long-term outcomes than subtotal thyroidectomy for Graves' disease[31] (Figure 8.4). Thus total thyroidectomy is the preferred surgical option for treatment of Graves' disease when thyroid hormone replacement therapy is readily available. Removal of essentially all thyroid tissue eliminates the potential for persistent or recurrent hyperthyroidism, which is a particularly undesirable outcome because it then subjects patients to RAI therapy, which they may have initially declined, or reoperative surgery, which has an increased risk of morbidity. Total thyroidectomy, if the patient has access to a surgeon experienced in Graves' disease surgery with low complication rates, simplifies the postoperative follow-up because all patients are started on a replacement dose of thyroid hormone. In addition, total thyroidectomy eliminates the antigen that is the source for the TSH receptor antibodies and other antibodies that crossreact with antigens in the extraocular muscles, the retroorbital connective tissue, and the optic nerve.[42]

TOXIC NODULAR GOITER

Toxic nodular goiter (TNG), also known as *Plummer's disease*, refers to hyperthyroidism resulting from autonomously functioning thyroid nodules independent of TSH regulation. Autonomous nodules are the second most common overall cause of thyrotoxicosis, accounting for 5% to 15% of all causes of hyperthyroidism.[43] The prevalence of TNG increases with age,[44-47] making it the most common cause of thyrotoxicosis in the elderly,[48] whereas solitary toxic adenomas are more often found in younger individuals.

BOX 8.3 Two Options for Preoperative Preparation for Graves' Surgery

1. Saturated solution of potassium iodide (SSKI) 50 mg iodide/gtt
   1 to 2 gtts (0.05 to 0.1 mL)
   – tid in water or juice for 5 to 10 days preop
2. Lugol's solution
   8 mg iodide/gtt
   5 to 7 gtts (0.25 to 0.35 mL)
   – tid in water or juice for 5 to 10 days preop

TOXIC MULTINODULAR GOITER

Pathogenesis

The etiological factors involved in the formation of a multinodular goiter include an inherent functional heterogeneity of thyroid follicles, the effect of growth factors and goitrogens, the presence or absence of iodine, and genetic abnormalities that include somatic activating mutations of genes that regulate thyroid growth and hormone synthesis.[44,45,49] In contrast to Graves' disease, in which the thyroid follicular cells become hyperfunctional as a result of antithyroid immunoglobulins that bind to and activate the TSH receptor, autonomous thyroid nodules develop hyperfunction through replication and increased growth of thyroid follicular cells. It is postulated that in iodine-deficient cases, chronic TSH stimulation increases the replication of follicular cells and results in the appearance and expression of mutations in the TSH receptor gene.[50,51]

Nodular goiter results from hyperplasia of clusters of follicular cells with abnormal growth potential at scattered sites in the thyroid gland. The final phase in the evolution of a goiter is when nodules become autonomous, progressing from a nontoxic to a toxic state with loss of TSH regulation and nonsuppressibility with thyroxine administration. Despite a suppressed TSH level, FT4 and FT3 levels become elevated. Hyperfunctioning nodules can be identified as "hot" with increased uptake on ^{123}I thyroid scintigraphy. A nontoxic multinodular goiter is present for an average of 17 years before becoming toxic.[52] During this evolution, patients with nontoxic multinodular goiter have a high prevalence of subclinical hyperthyroidism (i.e., suppressed TSH with normal thyroid hormone levels).[53-55]

The prevalence of toxic multinodular goiter is significantly higher in areas of iodine deficiency. As previously noted, toxic multinodular goiter generally affects older individuals with a history of a long-standing nontoxic multinodular goiter.[56] Acute iodine-induced thyrotoxicosis or the Jod-Basedow phenomenon can be precipitated in patients with nontoxic multinodular goiter by iodine-containing drugs or iodinated contrast.[57] Iodine-induced thyrotoxicosis is a self-limited condition but indicates that toxic multinodular goiter may develop in the future, if not already present.[49]

Clinical Presentation

Toxic multinodular goiter typically occurs in individuals over 50 years of age, with a female predominance, and in those who have a preexisting history of a long-standing nontoxic multinodular goiter.[43,58] Patients present with symptoms and signs of hyperthyroidism (see Boxes 8-1 and 8-2), and on physical examination, the thyroid gland is enlarged with multiple nodules but the infiltrative ophthalmopathy and dermopathy of Graves' disease are absent.[57,58] The hyperthyroidism is usually less severe than in Graves' disease, but the degree depends on the stage of the goiter's development of autonomous activity. The onset of hyperthyroidism is insidious and is often preceded by a long period of subclinical hyperthyroidism. Overt manifestations of thyrotoxicosis are often masked in older patients, whereas cardiac manifestations, such as atrial fibrillation, tachycardia, congestive heart failure, and accelerated angina, are more common. Unexplained weight loss, anxiety, insomnia, and muscle wasting are also more likely to occur in the elderly patient with hyperthyroidism.

As with other types of goiter, patients with marked thyroid enlargement may present with compressive symptoms attributable to mass effect (Figure 8.5), particularly when there is substernal extension.

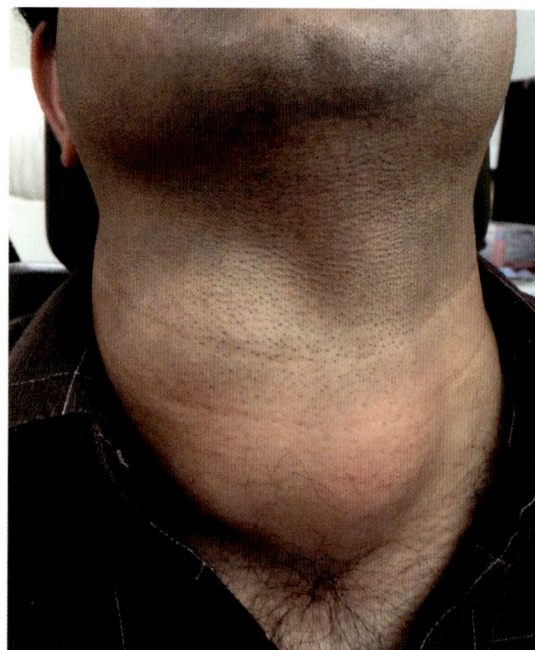

Fig. 8.5 Markedly enlarged thyroid in a patient with a toxic multinodular goiter.

Patients may complain of dysphagia (Figure 8.6), dyspnea, decreased exercise tolerance, cough, and a choking sensation (Figure 8.7). Hoarseness and other voice changes may occur as a result of compression or stretch of the recurrent and/or superior laryngeal nerves.

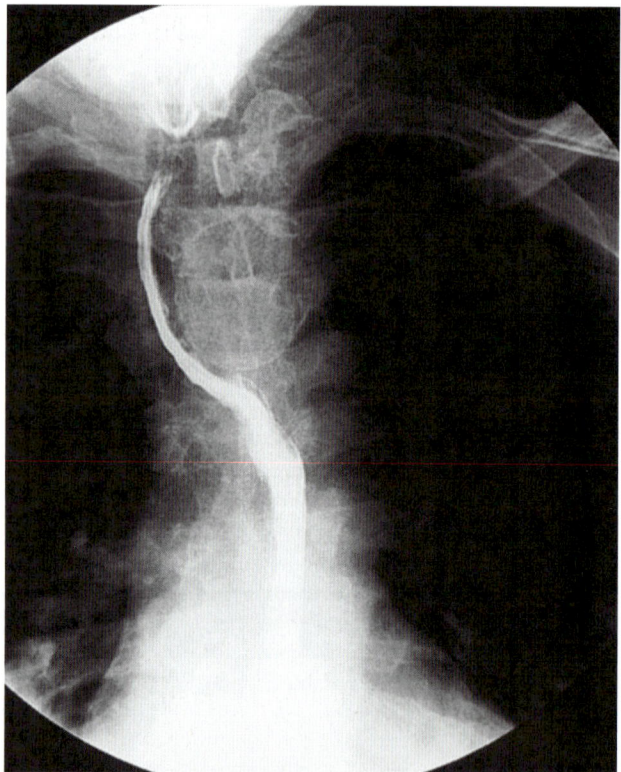

Fig. 8.6 Esophageal displacement and compression from a substernal nodular goiter.

CHAPTER 8 Surgical Management of Hyperthyroidism

Diagnosis and Evaluation

The diagnosis of toxic multinodular goiter is usually made based on symptoms of hyperthyroidism; signs of an enlarged nodular goiter on physical examination; and laboratory values, including a low serum TSH level with or without elevated FT4 and FT3 levels. However, a significant percentage of toxic multinodular goiters are not palpable, especially in older patients and those with kyphosis or substernal thyroid extension (Figure 8.8). Ultrasonography and the measurement of radioiodine uptake and thyroid uptake and scanning are not routinely necessary to make a diagnosis but are often helpful in identifying the cause of thyrotoxicosis. Ultrasound demonstrates multiple coalescent benign-appearing nodules of varying size and number (Figure 8.9). Fine-needle aspiration (FNA) cytology is not required unless there is a sonographically suspicious or dominant nodule. Thyroid scintigraphy reveals a heterogenous pattern of iodine uptake, with focal areas of increased uptake corresponding to the hyperfunctioning nodules[58] (see Figure 8.3) but overall only a slight elevation or high-normal iodine uptake. A CT scan may be necessary to assess for substernal extension, but iodine contrast should only be administered with caution.

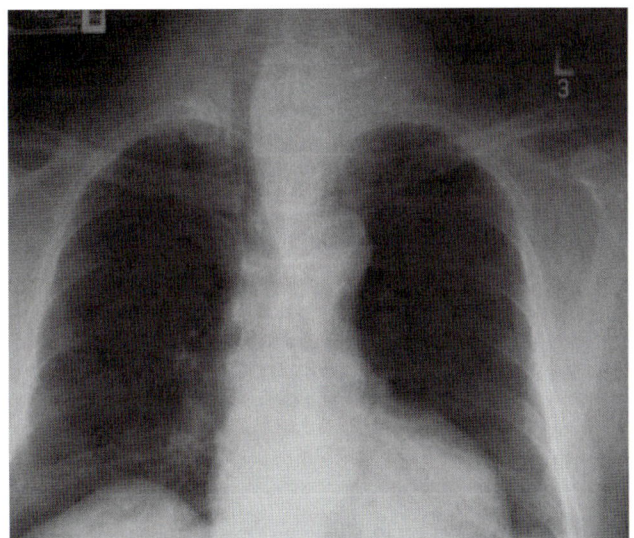

Fig. 8.7 A large toxic multinodular goiter with retrosternal extension causing tracheal narrowing and deviation to the right seen on plain chest x-ray.

Treatment

The goals of treatment in patients with toxic multinodular goiter are to eradicate all autonomously functioning thyroid tissue and to alleviate compressive symptoms. The definitive treatment options are radioiodine ablation or thyroidectomy.[2,43,49,58] Treatment with ATDs (propylthiouracil or methimazole) is only temporizing and not definitive. Relapse has been seen to occur in 95% of patients with TNG compared with 34% of patients with Graves' disease after restoring biochemical euthyroidism, treating with ATDs for at least 1 year and following for a minimum of 2 years.[59,60]

Radioactive Iodine (RAI)

RAI treatment of toxic multinodular goiter may be preferred in elderly patients with medical comorbidities that increase their risk for surgery. The goal of RAI therapy is complete thyroid ablation to prevent recurrence, and as a result, permanent hypothyroidism is an accepted consequence.[58] The usual dose of ^{131}I varies between 15 and 30 mCi, depending on the size and RAI uptake of the gland. Higher (>50 mCi) and several repeated doses of ^{131}I are often required to control hyperthyroidism because of the typical large goiter size and lower ^{131}I uptake compared with patients with Graves' disease. Patients typically become euthyroid within 8 weeks after the administration of ^{131}I, although it may take longer,[43] or they usually go on to become hypothyroid and require levothyroxine replacement. The recurrence rate after ^{131}I treatment is approximately 20%.[43,58,61] Because toxic multinodular goiter contains nonfunctioning nodules and areas of fibrosis and calcification, ^{131}I treatment is only variably effective in reducing goiter size and in relieving compressive symptoms. However, a reduction in thyroid volume and an increase in the cross-sectional area of the tracheal lumen have been demonstrated by magnetic resonance imaging (MRI) after treatment of toxic and nontoxic multinodular goiter with ^{131}I.[62,63]

Surgery

Surgical resection is the preferred method of treatment for most patients with toxic multinodular goiter because of the typically large goiter size and presence of compressive symptoms, unless there are contraindications (Figure 8.10).[59] The presence of substernal thyroid extension or airway obstruction is a relative contraindication for ^{131}I because of the potential for transient increase in size of the goiter

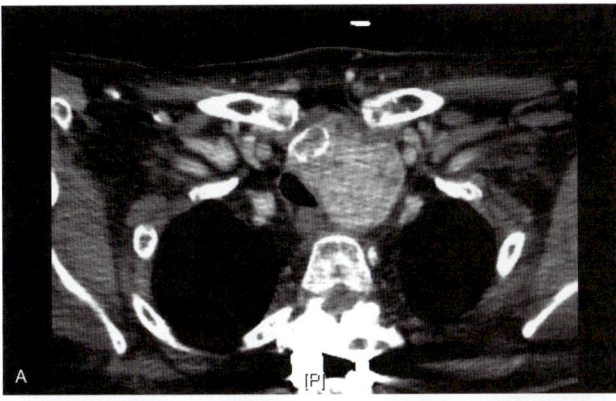

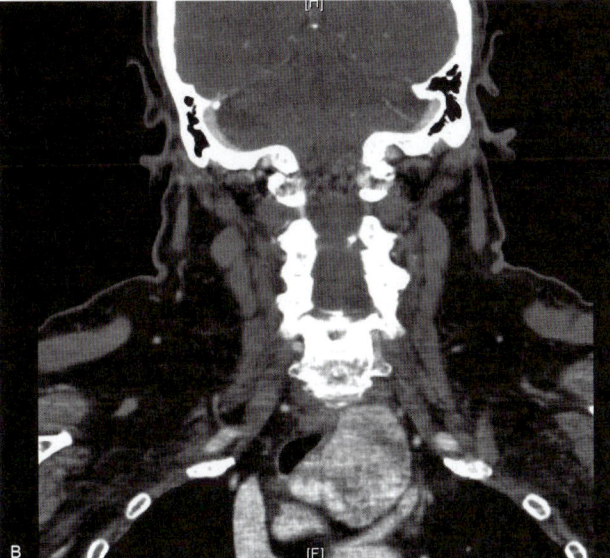

Fig. 8.8 Toxic multinodular goiter is often asymmetrical, and substernal extension may make it less apparent on physical examination (**A,** axial and **B,** coronal neck computed tomography [CT]).

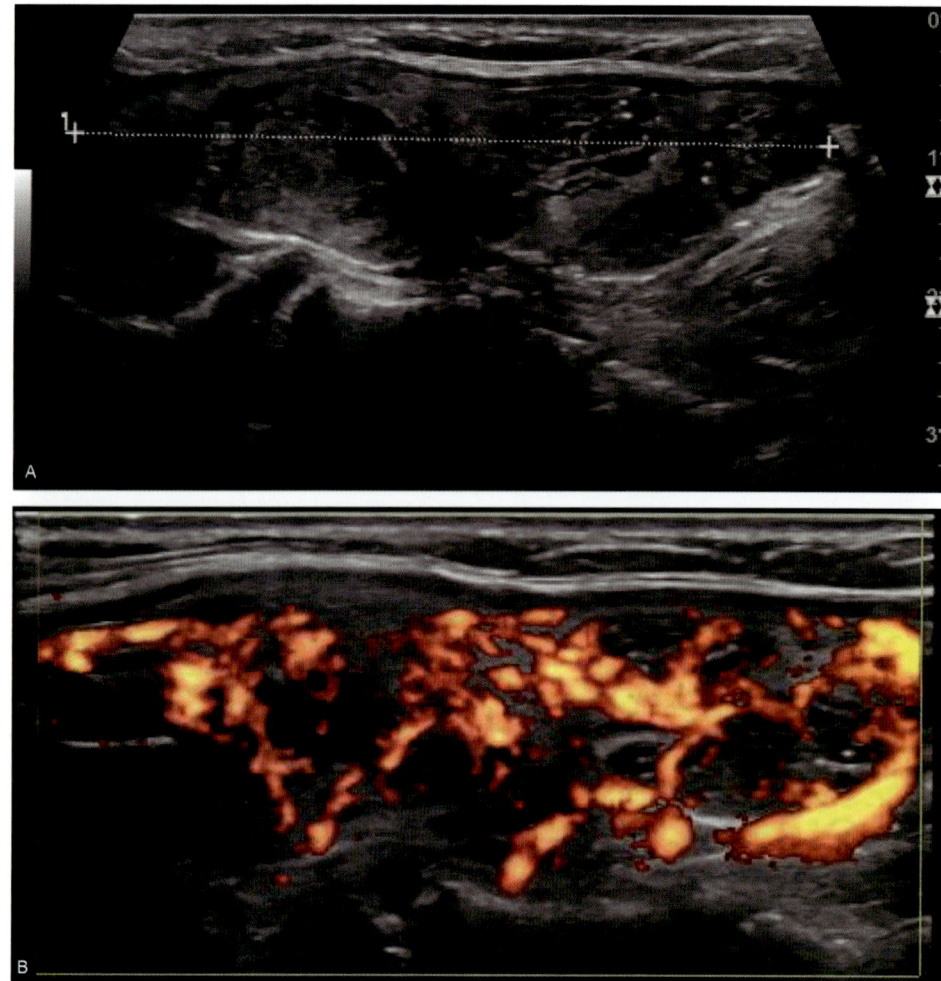

Fig. 8.9 Sagittal Ultrasound Image of Toxic Multinodular Goiter. B-mode (**A**) and Doppler mode (**B**).

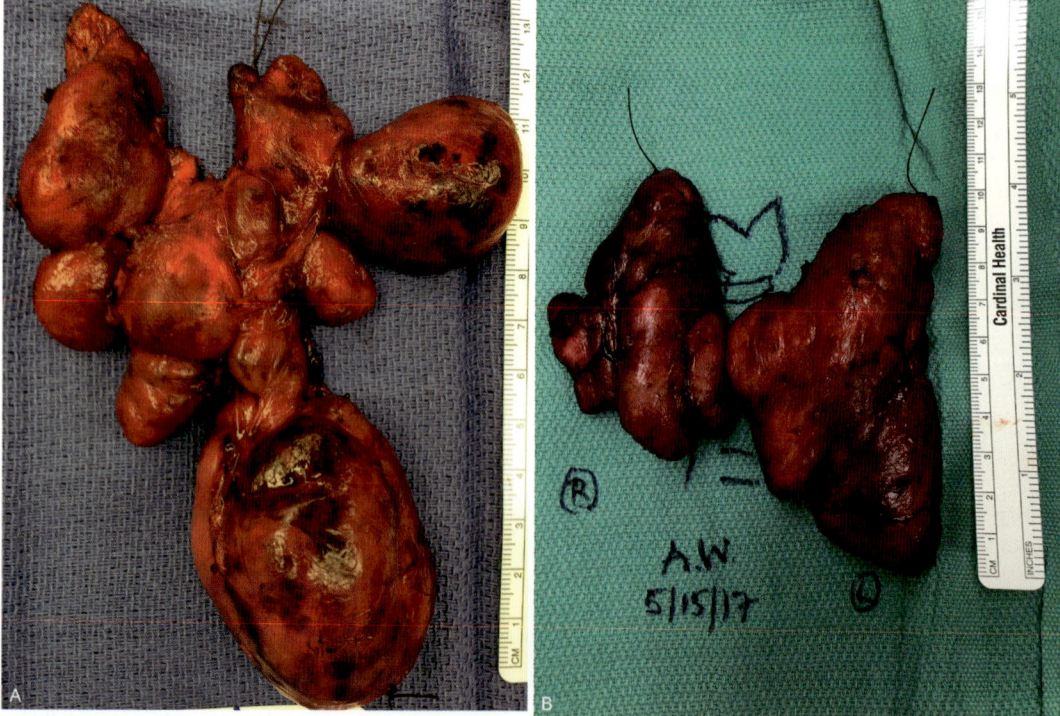

Fig. 8.10 Total Thyroidectomy Specimen for Toxic Multinodular Goiter. **A,** Specimen with substernal extension. **B,** Multinodular goiter with background of Hashimoto's thyroiditis.

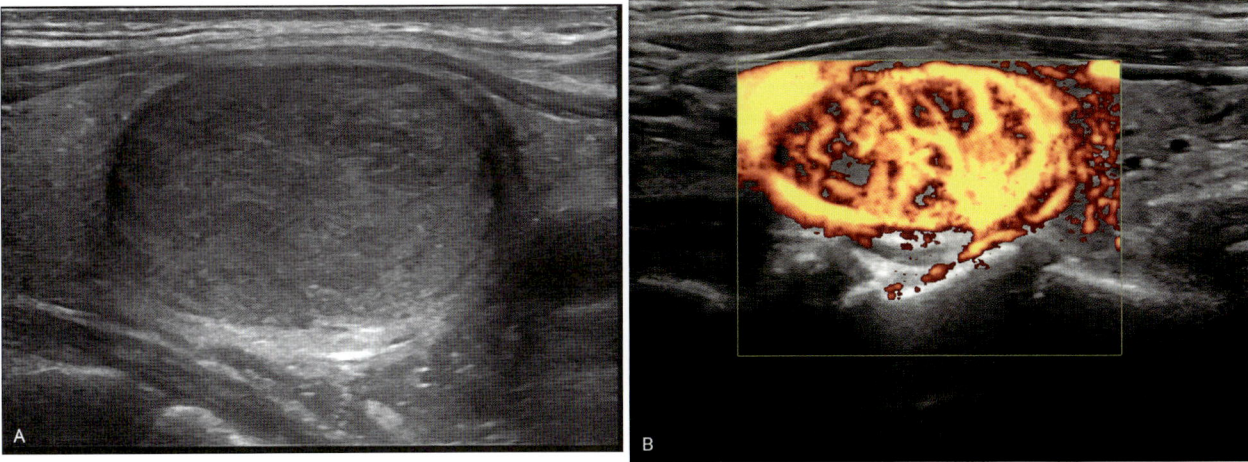

Fig. 8.11 Ultrasound Images of Toxic Nodules. **A,** B-mode, sagittal view. **B,** Doppler ultrasound of a different toxic nodule showing intense vascularity, sagittal view.

and worsening of airway compromise through RAI-induced transient radiation thyroiditis. Surgical resection should consist of removal of all abnormal thyroid tissue, and this is usually best accomplished by performing a near-total or total thyroidectomy. Subtotal thyroidectomy is an option and may actually prove to be prudent if there is loss of signal (LOS) on monitoring of the recurrent laryngeal nerve on the first (dominant) lobe dissected. A potential advantage of subtotal thyroidectomy is avoidance of hypothyroidism. Should less than a total thyroidectomy be performed, one must be aware that the areas of scinitigraphic activity may not necessarily overlie the gross nodular disease evidenced on ultrasound. However, recurrence of thyrotoxicosis after incomplete surgery for multinodular goiter can be as high as 50% to 78%.[64-66] Total thyroidectomy, when it is performed by an experienced surgeon, is preferable because it eliminates the risk of recurrence with a minimal risk of permanent hypoparathyroidism or recurrent nerve injury.[67] SSKI is not given preoperatively because it may actually worsen the hyperthyroidism. Fortunately, the thyroid gland in patients with toxic multinodular goiter is less vascular than in patients with Graves' disease. Although it is difficult to compare, a model that explores the lifetime cost of surgery versus ^{131}I therapy and that measures outcomes in quality-adjusted life years found that for patients less than 62 years of age, surgery, when performed by experienced surgeons, is more cost effective than ^{131}I therapy.[68] Surgery has the added advantage of obtaining thyroid nodules for histological assessment and potentially curing incidental concomitant thyroid carcinoma, which occurs in 3% to 9% of patients with multinodular goiter.[69-71] Older age (>50 years) and cold nodules are significant risk factors for malignancy.[71]

SOLITARY TOXIC NODULE

Pathogenesis

A solitary toxic nodule is an autonomously hyperfunctioning nodule present in an otherwise normal thyroid gland that causes hyperthyroidism. Five percent to 15% of all thyroid nodules are "hot" or hyperfunctioning (a nodule that takes up greater RAI than the surrounding thyroid tissue). Only 25% of hyperfunctioning nodules are true toxic nodules that cause hyperthyroidism. Still, the risk of toxicity increases with size and with patient age, and approximately 20% of patients with a hyperfunctioning nodule ≥3 cm in diameter will develop thyrotoxicosis compared with 2% to 5% of patients with nodules <3 cm in diameter.[72]

The majority of solitary toxic nodules are functioning follicular adenomas, and a minority are adenomatous nodules. These follicular adenomas represent monoclonal expansion of thyroid follicular cells with a high prevalence of activating mutations in the gene for the TSH receptor.[49,50] Development of a solitary toxic nodule parallels the development of a toxic multinodular goiter. In its early phase of development, as a solitary nontoxic hyperfunctioning nodule gradually increases in size and function, it escapes the regulatory control of TSH and becomes autonomous. The low serum TSH level can suppress the RAI uptake of the remainder of the thyroid gland. In this situation, thyroid scans show a hot nodule within a cold background of reduced or absent uptake in the remaining thyroid tissue.

Hyperthyroidism typically does not occur until a hyperfunctioning nodule is ≥3.0 cm in diameter. In a study of patients with nontoxic autonomous nodules larger than 3 cm, 20% developed thyrotoxicosis within 6 years of observation.[72] Thyroid hormone secretion may increase acutely, and patients may become thyrotoxic after receiving an iodine load. Spontaneous remission of thyrotoxicosis can occur from hemorrhage or cystic degeneration within a nodule, resulting in the loss of autonomy and a decrease in the size of the nodule.[73]

Clinical Presentation and Evaluation

A solitary toxic nodule can occur at any age but is most often seen in younger patients ranging from 30 to 50 years of age. The signs and symptoms of hyperthyroidism (see Boxes 8-1 and 8-2) are milder than in patients with Graves' disease. Most patients present with a palpable thyroid nodule. Hyperfunctioning nodules grow to a relatively large size before the onset of hyperthyroidism; as a result, patients usually come to medical attention because of a neck mass rather than symptoms of thyrotoxicity. Serum TSH levels are low and serum FT4 and FT3 are normal to high. Occasionally, the serum FT3 level is elevated with a normal FT4 level (T3 thyrotoxicosis). Although FNA biopsy is routinely performed for sizeable solitary nontoxic thyroid nodules, the presence of a low serum TSH level should change the diagnostic algorithm, with radionuclide imaging as the next diagnostic test.[43,49,58,74] In patients with a thyroid nodule and a low serum TSH level, thyroid scintigraphy can distinguish a hyperfunctioning nodule from a hypofunctioning nodule in a patient with Graves' disease. A solitary toxic nodule may appear "warm" or "hot" on an ^{123}I or technetium 99m-pertechnetate thyroid scintigraphy.[2] Overall RAI uptake is normal to high but is concentrated in the nodule, with a variable degree of suppression of the surrounding thyroid tissue depending on the stage of development (see Figure 8.3). In reality, ultrasonography is often performed on patients with palpable thyroid nodules before results of laboratory studies are available and usually shows a solid, well-defined nodule within a homogeneous background of thyroid parenchyma (Figure 8.11). Doppler ultrasonography can be used to measure thyroidal blood flow, and thyroid hyperactivity (increased flow) can be distinguished from destructive thyroiditis (decreased flow).[75] FNA of a toxic nodule is rarely necessary, but if suspicious sonographic features are present, then a biopsy is generally indicated. Otherwise, when FNA is performed it is often indeterminate, showing characteristics of a follicular neoplasm with varying degrees of nuclear atypia and hypercellularity.[76] In an autonomous functioning nodule that is not toxic, the risk of malignancy varies between 2% to 6%, and in toxic nodules the risk is less than 1%.[77]

Treatment of Solitary Toxic Nodule
Surgery

Patients with a hyperfunctioning nodule who are asymptomatic and not thyrotoxic can be followed by history, physical examination, and serum TSH monitoring without intervention. A solitary toxic nodule should be treated either with RAI or with partial thyroidectomy surgery. ATD therapy is not curative and is therefore not considered a primary therapeutic alternative. Treatment with a thionamide drug does not cause nodule regression, and hyperthyroidism recurs when the therapy is discontinued. Because an autonomous nodule usually continues to grow and secrete thyroid hormone, it is generally recommended that a patient undergo definitive therapy.

Surgical therapy for a solitary toxic nodule is generally preferred and consists of a unilateral thyroid lobectomy (Figure 8.12). The advantages of surgery are removal of the nodule; immediate resolution of symptoms of hyperthyroidism and the presence of a mass; avoidance of radiation exposure to the normal thyroid tissue; confirmation of tissue diagnosis in rare cases of suspected carcinoma; and preservation of thyroid function in the remaining lobe, potentially avoiding levothyroxine supplementation after surgery. Persistent or recurrent hyperthyroidism is uncommon (^{99m}Tc).[68,78,79] The incidence of hypothyroidism is low with a reported rate of 14% with hemithyroidectomy compared with 22% for RAI therapy.[63,68,78-80] The potential morbidity associated with unilateral thyroid lobectomy is generally fairly minimal and includes bleeding and recurrent laryngeal nerve injury.

The preoperative preparation of the patient with a toxic solitary nodule is similar to that for the patient with a toxic multinodular goiter. To reduce the risk of thyroid storm, patients are treated with a thionamide agent to normalize the FT4 and FT3 levels before operation. Beta-blockers for 1 to 2 weeks are an alternative for preoperative preparation in patients who are unable to take a thionamide agent. Preoperative iodine therapy is not indicated.

Radioactive Iodine (RAI)

^{131}I administration is also effective but is a less targeted therapy for a solitary toxic nodule. RAI treatment usually requires higher doses of ^{131}I (25 to 40 mCi) than are used for the treatment of Graves' disease. Although Ross reported a cure rate of 90% with a mean dose of 10 mCi of ^{131}I,[81] Eyre-Brook and Talbot found a relapse rate of 73% in patients treated with doses of 1.2 to 15 mCi.[82] Using a median dose of 29 mCi, O'Brien found a 4.4% incidence of persistent hyperthyroidism and 0% incidence of recurrence.[83] Higher doses of ^{131}I are associated with lower rates of persistent and recurrent hyperthyroidism but an increased risk of hypothyroidism. Complete nodule regression occurs in 2.2% to 56.3% of cases, in a dose-dependent manner.[81,83] Persistent nodules require careful follow-up.[49] The disadvantages of RAI therapy are the persistence of the nodule, delay in symptomatic relief, and exposure of the normal adjacent thyroid tissue to radiation with the potential development of hypothyroidism in up to 36% of patients.[81]

Ethanol Injection

Percutaneous ethanol injection is another, newer option for treating a solitary toxic nodule (see Chapter 16, Laser and Radiofrequency Treatment of Thyroid Nodules and Parathyroid Adenoma). Using real-time ultrasound guidance, sterile 95% ethanol is injected into the nodule. Four to eight injections are frequently needed for satisfactory treatment, and the total amount of ethanol is usually about 50% more than the nodule volume.[84-86] The ultimate goal is to ablate the vascular supply of the nodule. A prospective nonrandomized multicenter Italian study evaluated 429 patients with a solitary toxic or hyperfunctioning nodule treated with 2 to 12 ethanol injections.[87] Reported complications included neck pain (90%), fever (8%), transient dysphonia (4%), neck hematoma (4%), and internal jugular vein thrombosis (0.2%). At 1-year follow-up, 67% and 83% of patients with a toxic or "pretoxic" nodule respectively were successfully treated. Percutaneous ethanol injection is generally considered as a third-line treatment for patients with solitary toxic nodules when patients decline or have contraindications to surgery or ^{131}I therapy. Ethanol injection can be used in combination with RAI therapy for patients with solitary toxic nodules >4 cm when surgery is not an option. A more significant reduction in nodule size and persistent hyperthyroidism can be achieved than with ^{131}I alone.[88]

REFERENCES

For a complete list of references, go to *expertconsult.com*.

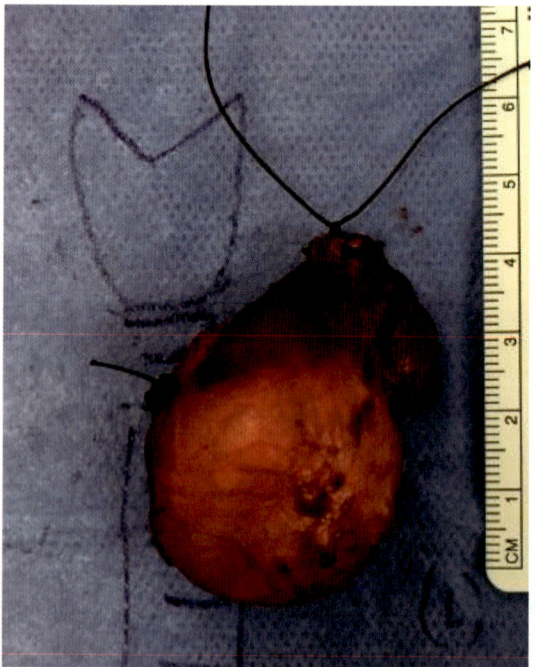

Fig. 8.12 Thyroid lobectomy specimen, toxic nodule (adenoma).

Reoperation for Benign Thyroid Disease

Mark Sywak, Ruth Prichard, Leigh Delbridge

This chapter contains additional online-only content available on expertconsult.com.

INTRODUCTION

Thyroid disease is broadly divided into hypothyroidism, hyperthyroidism, structural abnormalities of the thyroid, and neoplasia of the thyroid gland (see Chapter 6, Surgery of Cervical and Substernal Goiter). Thyroid cancer is a relatively uncommon malignancy in most countries, accounting for just 1% of all cancers in the United Kingdom and representing the 11th most commonly diagnosed cancer in Australia. In contrast, benign thyroid disease, either benign nodular goiter or Graves' disease, is an extremely common endocrine disorder worldwide and affects at least 5% to 7% of the world's population.[1,2] Of these, 10% to 12% will require primary operative intervention.[3] Although the aim is always to treat surgical disorders of the thyroid in a single well-executed procedure, reoperation for recurrent benign disease may be necessary in up to 13% of patients who have had an initial thyroid procedure performed. The surgical management of recurrent benign thyroid disease requires careful preoperative planning and considerable technical expertise to minimize operative complications.

Please see the Expert Consult website for more discussion of this topic.

This chapter describes the clinical presentation, perioperative management, and operative strategies that will help the surgeon achieve success in patients presenting with recurrent benign nodular goiter and Graves' disease.

EPIDEMIOLOGY

Worldwide, it is estimated that at least 2 billion people continue to have iodine deficiency despite major national and international efforts to increase iodine intake. Although the magnitude of the problem has long been recognized in developing countries, iodine deficiency remains an issue in Continental Europe, the United Kingdom, and in areas previously thought to be iodine sufficient such as Australia and New Zealand.[5] Iodine deficiency is closely associated with an increased risk of nontoxic nodular goiter.

Please see the Expert Consult website for more discussion of this topic.

Operative intervention for recurrence accounts for anywhere between 5% to 25% of all thyroid surgeries performed.[9,10] Subtotal thyroidectomy was previously considered the standard in the surgical management of multinodular goiter, with the aim being to reduce injury to the recurrent laryngeal nerve (RLN), avoidance of hypoparathyroidism, and reduction in the need for thyroid hormone replacement. The downside of this more conservative approach is that between 2% to 39% of patients treated in this way develop clinically significant recurrent disease.[11] However, since the early 1990s there has been a shift away from conservative primary operations such as bilateral subtotal thyroidectomy, and this should begin to be mirrored by declining recurrence rates. Not surprisingly, there appears to be a trend toward longer times to recurrence from the initial surgical intervention. The documented rate of recurrence in our unit is 0.32% after a total thyroidectomy as an initial operation.[12]

CLINICAL PRESENTATION OF RECURRENT NODULAR GOITER

The recurrence rate for goiter after less than total thyroidectomy procedures varies from 13% to 60%, according to the extent of initial resection.[13] Recurrent benign goiter can present in the following ways:
- Asymptomatic recurrence detected on imaging
- Palpable neck mass
- Compressive symptoms, dysphagia, airway obstruction, or dysphonia
- Mediastinal mass
- Decreasing requirement for thyroid hormone replacement
- Thyrotoxicosis

The clinical presentation of recurrent benign goiter varies from being asymptomatic to severe compressive symptoms with or without progressive thyroid hyperfunction. Asymptomatic recurrence can be detected on routine physical examination or commonly on imaging performed for another reason. The manner of a patient's presentation with recurrent disease typically depends on the type of follow-up from the original surgery. Patients under regular review tend to present with asymptomatic, impalpable disease detected on ultrasound. This type of recurrence rarely requires surgical intervention.[14] Alternatively, patients lost to follow-up may present with a large palpable cervicothoracic mass causing compressive symptoms and a compartmental syndrome. In our experience a common presentation is a progressively decreasing requirement for thyroid hormone replacement medication, leading to thyrotoxicosis, in a patient who has previously been on stable thyroxine therapy. Figure 9.1 illustrates the case of a 65-year-old female who had total thyroidectomy performed for compressive multinodular goiter some 8 years previously. She presented with dyspnea and was found to have a large mediastinal recurrence of thyroid tissue.

Please see the Expert Consult website for more discussion of this topic.

Clinical Setting of Goiter Recurrence

There are five typical clinical scenarios in which recurrent benign thyroid disease presents itself to the surgeon. These include the following:
1. Previous thyroid lobectomy with recurrent contralateral disease
2. Previous thyroid nodulectomy or enucleation of dominant nodules in a multinodular goiter

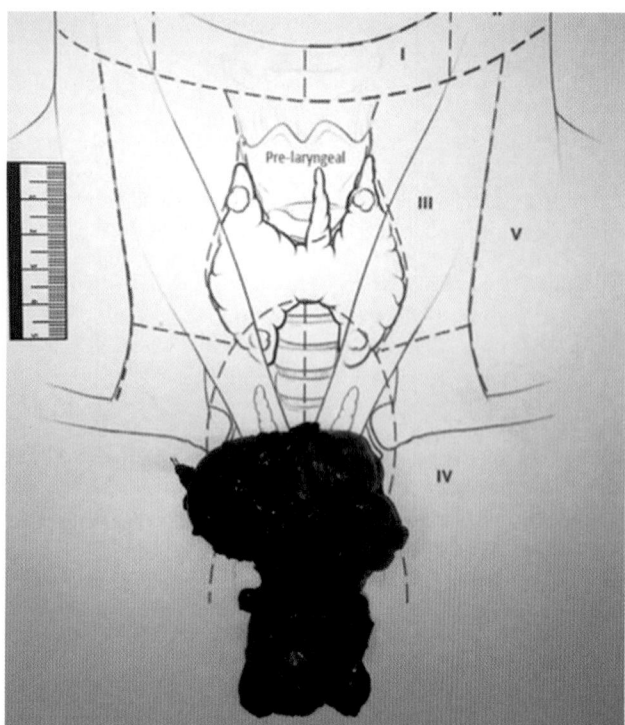

Fig. 9.1 Recurrent benign mediastinal goiter presenting several years after total thyroidectomy.

Please see the Expert Consult website for more discussion of this topic.

When recurrent nodular goiter does occur, it is important to obtain accurate imaging of both sides of the neck with ultrasound and/or computed tomography (CT). Recurrence on the operated side should be very infrequent if the initial procedure is performed expertly and with care. The surgeon must exclude recurrent disease in the operated thyroid bed before any planned contralateral surgery. Fine needle biopsy of suspicious nodules should be incorporated into the workup. Completion thyroidectomy comprising a second thyroid lobectomy on the side with recurrent nodular change has a low risk of complications. However, it is vital for fiberoptic laryngoscopy to be performed in all cases of recurrent nodular goiter preoperatively. An undiagnosed, well-compensated RLN injury from the initial operation could lead to the serious complication of bilateral RLN palsy requiring tracheostomy. It is imperative that a pre-existing RLN palsy is appreciated and the implications of further surgery carefully discussed. Likewise, the approach to the parathyroid glands requires careful consideration and operative technique, and in general we work on the assumption that there is no functioning parathyroid tissue on the operated side. The risk of permanent RLN injury on the reoperative side is typically low in expert hands at 0.77%, with the incidence of permanent hypoparathyroidism being 1.5% and similar to that described in primary surgery.[23]

INITIAL INADEQUATE PARTIAL RESECTION OR ENUCLEATION FOR NODULAR GOITER

Inadequate or partial initial operations, such as isthmusectomy, nodule enucleation, or subtotal lobectomy, have been identified as increasing the likelihood of recurrence, even in the setting of an isolated thyroid nodule.[20,24,25] These incomplete or atypical initial procedures were usually performed several decades ago, at a time when the principal motivation of many surgeons was to avoid complications by avoiding posterior dissection near the RLN or parathyroid glands. In select patients who present with a solitary toxic nodule, which is not positioned posteriorly in the thyroid lobe, we have performed a minimally invasive thyroid nodulectomy and demonstrated reduced rates of postoperative hypothyroidism. These cases require careful selection, and the long-term durability of this approach is yet to be proven.[26]

3. Recurrence after bilateral subtotal thyroidectomy
4. Recurrent disease in an embryologic remnant that was not apparent at initial total thyroidectomy
5. Aggressive benign nodular recurrence after total thyroidectomy

The etiology of recurrent thyroid disease is multifactorial, and the actual pathogenesis remains poorly understood. However, understanding the five clinical scenarios in which recurrence develops is critical if a good outcome is to be achieved. These clinical scenarios will be examined in depth in the following sections.

Please see the Expert Consult website for more discussion of this topic.

DEVELOPMENT OF CONTRALATERAL DISEASE AFTER PREVIOUS LOBECTOMY

In patients who have had a lobectomy for unilateral nontoxic goiter, 7.4% to 12% will ultimately require reoperation for contralateral disease.[20] The most common pathology seen in a clinically solitary nodule is, in fact, a dominant colloid nodule in a multinodular goiter. Other pathologies may include benign follicular adenoma, thyroid cyst, or nodular change in Hashimoto's thyroiditis. For patients with a symptomatic solitary nodule, the standard approach is a formal thyroid lobectomy, leaving the normal contralateral side intact. Careful selection of patients will, of course, minimize recurrence rates. Patients selected should have predominantly unilateral nodularity with minimal disease evident on the contralateral side. Small volume subclinical disease is often present in the contralateral lobe, and this common situation requires a careful discussion with the patient regarding the extent of the initial thyroidectomy. In our experience most patients tend to express a clear personal choice between initial lobectomy and total thyroidectomy.

Please see the Expert Consult website for more discussion of this topic.

INITIAL BILATERAL SUBTOTAL PROCEDURE FOR MULTINODULAR GOITER

Until the early 1990s, the operation of choice for benign bilateral multinodular goiter was a subtotal procedure, either a bilateral subtotal thyroidectomy, leaving two posterior thyroid remnants, or a thyroid lobectomy on one side and subtotal lobectomy on the other, leaving only one posterior remnant. Complete removal of one thyroid lobe with subtotal lobectomy on the contralateral side is referred to as the *Dunhill procedure*.[27] Typically 3 to 5 g of thyroid tissue were retained in the region of the ligament of Berry or superior thyroid pole to approximate the volume of a normal thyroid lobe. The rationale for this approach was to lower the risk of damage to the RLN and the parathyroid glands and to preserve thyroid function. Although the rate of transient hypoparathyroidism appears to be lower in subtotal thyroidectomy, the incidence of recurrent goiter is much greater and there is no difference in the rate of permanent RLN palsy and permanent hypocalcemia compared with total thyroidectomy. In addition, very few patients achieve euthyroidism after subtotal thyroidectomy, with up to 84% of patients becoming hypothyroid and requiring levothyroxine replacement.[28]

This experience has influenced most high-volume centers to abandon subtotal thyroidectomy in the surgical management of benign goiter.

Please see the Expert Consult website for more discussion of this topic.

Revision surgery for bilateral nodular recurrence after previous subtotal thyroidectomy potentially represents one of the most technically challenging procedures for the thyroid surgeon. The degree of difficulty may be even greater if an experienced thyroid surgeon performed the initial procedure. Under these circumstances, it is likely that both RLNs were exposed at least in part of their cervical course and may well be encased in scar. Likewise, previous bilateral subtotal thyroidectomy typically involves dissection of both the upper and lower thyroid poles. Hence it is highly likely that the parathyroid gland blood supply was significantly disturbed, and the glands themselves may be surrounded by scar tissue. The difficulty regarding parathyroids lies in the fact that there is no way of predicting how many parathyroid glands may have been inadvertently removed or devascularized at the initial procedure. The patient may well be maintaining his or her entire parathyroid hormone (PTH) secretion from a single tenuous parathyroid gland located anteriorly in scar tissue on the surface of the residual lobe with recurrent nodular change. It is important to review the previous operative record and histopathology report; however, even this information cannot clarify which parathyroid glands remain viable with certainty. The surgical approach shown in Figure 9.2 illustrates careful capsular dissection preserving branches of the inferior thyroid artery to preserve the right inferior parathyroid gland (**A**) and superior parathyroid gland (**B**) to maintain parathyroid function. Despite these challenges, with care and appropriate technique, bilateral reoperative surgery can be performed safely. Within the University of Sydney Endocrine Surgery Unit, our experience of bilateral reoperative surgery for recurrent goiter demonstrates that low complication rates can be achieved with careful technique. Our data show that a complication rate of permanent RLN damage and permanent hypoparathyroidism of less than 1% can be achieved even in the reoperative setting.[8]

RECURRENT DISEASE IN AN EMBRYOLOGIC REMNANT AFTER TOTAL THYROIDECTOMY

A relatively frequent source of recurrent benign nodular goiter is the growth of thyroid tissue in an embryologic remnant. These remnants of thyroid tissue were either not appreciated at the original procedure or developed into clinically apparent disease from a subclinical or microscopic rest of tissue after total thyroidectomy.

Please see the Expert Consult website for more discussion of this topic, including Figure 9.3.

We believe that the presence of these embryologic remnants has considerable clinical importance, especially in the development of recurrent nodular thyroid disease. There are four common sites of embryologic recurrence or persistence of nodular goiter:
1. Thyroglossal duct tract
2. Pyramidal lobe of thyroid
3. Thyroid tissue rests along the thyrothymic tract
4. Posterior remnants associated with the tubercle of Zuckerkandl.

Please see the Expert Consult website for discussion of the thyroglossal duct tract and pyramidal lobe of the thyroid, including Figure 9.4.

Thyroid rests are deposits of normal thyroid tissue that lie in the line of the thyrothymic tract at or below the lower pole of the thyroid. They are common, with an incidence of over 50% in individuals undergoing thyroid surgery and are found along the course of embryologic thyroid descent. In 57% of patients with thyroid rests, they occur bilaterally.[43] Most thyroid rests are small, with 88% measuring less than 1 cm in maximum diameter. There are four grades of thyroid rest (I to IV), according to their relationship with the thyroid gland. Grade I rests consist of a protrusion of thyroid tissue arising from the inferior aspect of the thyroid gland in the region of the thyrothymic tract. These are distinctly recognizable from the lower border of the thyroid gland itself but retain a direct attachment to the inferior pole of the thyroid gland. Grade II rests include thyroid tissue lying within the thyrothymic tract and are attached to the thyroid by a narrow pedicle of thyroid tissue. Grade III rests are similar but are only attached by a thin fibrovascular core. Grade IV rests have no connection to the thyroid gland and may extend as far down as the anterior mediastinum (Figure 9.5).

Please see the Expert Consult website for more discussion on thyroid rests, including Figure 9.6.

The tubercle of Zuckerkandl is a posterior extension of the thyroid, which may give rise to persistent or recurrent disease. The tubercle of Zuckerkandl was first described by Zuckerkandl in 1902 as the "processus posterior glandulae thyroidea."[44] This is a common anatomic feature of the thyroid that is apparent in more than 50% of thyroidectomies and is more obvious on the right side.[45] Its significance lies in the fact that enlargement and nodular change in the tubercle may be

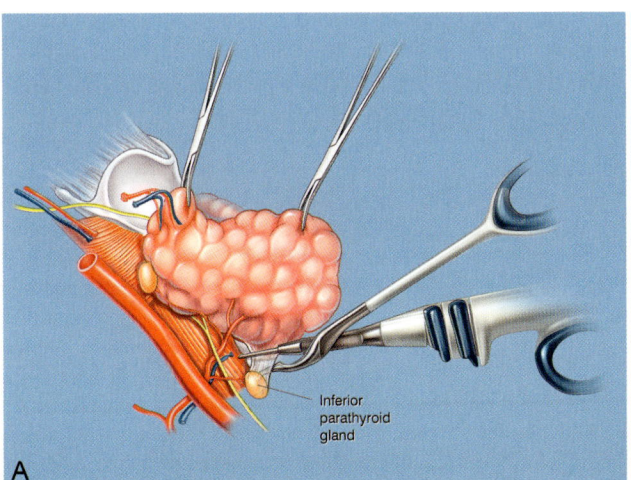
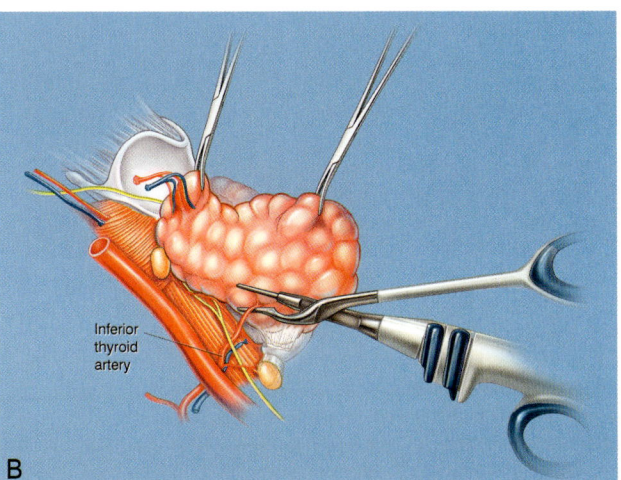

Fig. 9.2 Illustration of Capsular Dissection Technique Preserving Branches of the Inferior Thyroid Artery.
A, Right inferior parathyroid gland preserved. **B**, Right superior parathyroid preserved.

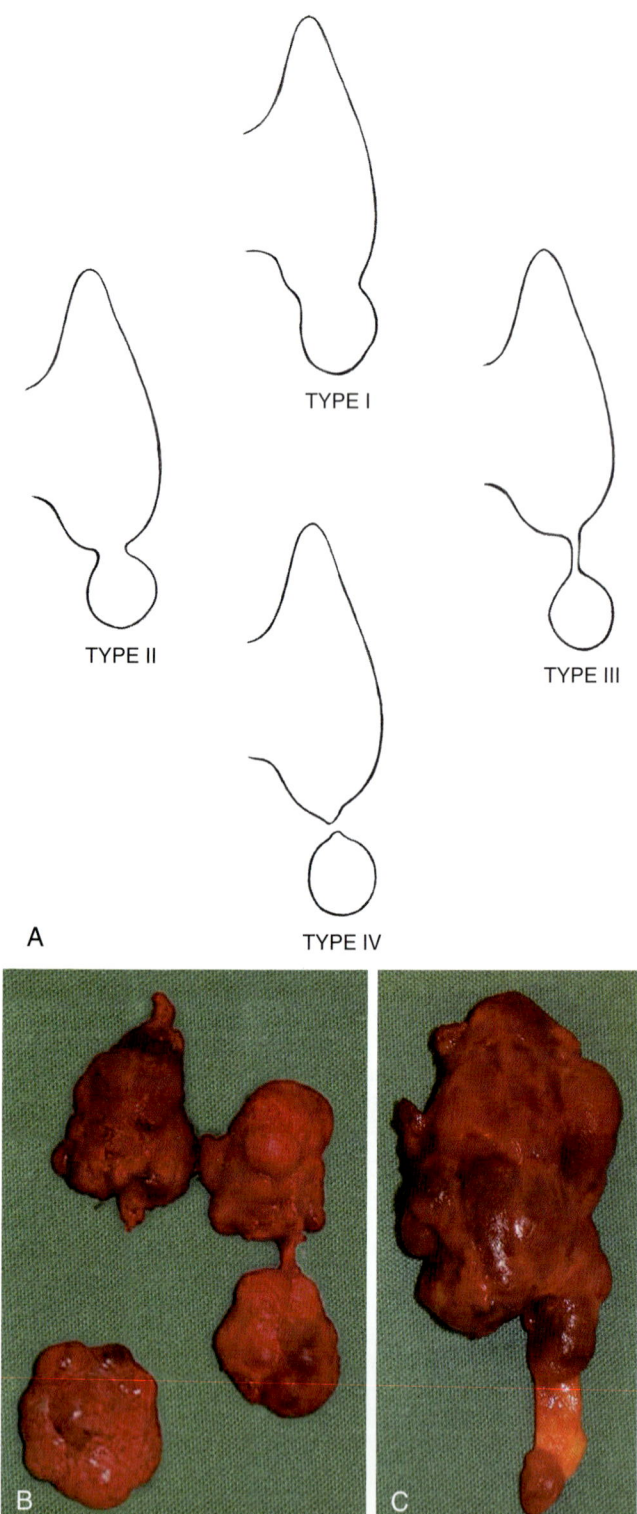

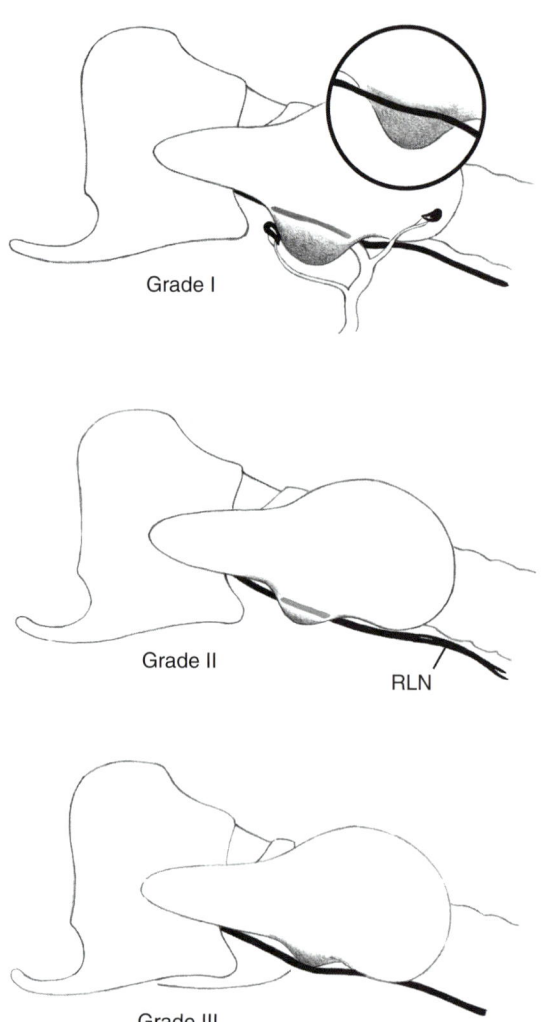

Fig. 9.5 Thyroid Rests. These remnants often lie medial to the thymus and are mistaken at the initial operation for central lymph nodes. They may also present as true retrosternal recurrence. **A,** The classification scheme for thyroid rests. Classification of thyroid rests in the thyrothymic area: grade I—protrusion of thyroid tissue, recognizably distinct from the lower border of the thyroid lobe; grade II—attached to the thyroid proper only by a narrow pedicle of thyroid tissue; grade III—attached to the thyroid gland by a fibrovascular core; grade IV—no connection to the thyroid gland. **B,** Below the right thyroid *(left)*, a type 4 thyroid rest and, associated with the left thyroid lobe *(right)*, a type 3 thyroid rest. **C,** A type 4 thyroid rest with associated thymus.

Fig 9.6 Recurrence in the posterior element of the tubercle of Zuckerkandl, which may lie behind the esophagus or between trachea and esophagus.

primarily retroesophageal and not observed at initial surgery. As a result, the posterior component may be inadvertently retained at initial thyroidectomy, leading to posterior persistence or recurrence (see Figure 9.6).

Please see the Expert Consult website for more discussion of the tubercle of Zuckerkandl.

UNDERLYING AGGRESSIVE BENIGN NODULAR DISEASE CAUSING RECURRENCE

Occasionally, despite meticulous initial total thyroidectomy, small remnants of residual thyroid tissue can grow and present with clinical recurrence. This occurs most commonly in the setting of a previous "near-total" thyroidectomy where a small remnant, often less than 1 gm of tissue, has been left behind to protect a parathyroid gland or the RLN. Such small thyroid remnants can regrow and present as clinical recurrence despite thyroid hormone supplementation because of an aggressive, albeit benign, process such as dyshormonogenesis.[12] This pathologic process differs from that of a benign multinodular goiter (BMNG). BMNG results from heterogeneity of the thyroid-stimulating hormone (TSH) receptor resulting in nodular change admixed with areas of degeneration. Dyshormonogenetic goiter, on the other hand, results from chronic stimulation of the TSH receptor due to a disturbance in the feedback system of thyroid hormone synthesis.[47] Dyshormonogenetic goiters are characterized by hypercellular nodules that are solid and microfollicular. Nuclei may be enlarged, irregularly shaped, and often bizarre, and can be difficult to distinguish from thyroid carcinoma.[48]

Please see the Expert Consult website for more discussion of this topic.

Risk Factors for Benign Nodular Recurrence

A number of factors may contribute to the development of recurrent nodular goiter, including the patient's age and family history as well as surgeon experience. The factors that may be associated with an increased risk of nodular goiter recurrence include the following:
- Family history of goiter
- Level of experience of surgeon
- Age of patient
- Multinodular or bilobar disease
- Extent of initial surgery

Family History

Performing a meticulous total thyroidectomy should reduce the risk of recurrence to almost zero despite the presence of a family history. Before the introduction of more definitive surgical procedures, a positive family history was thought to increase the risk of recurrence, and indeed some authors recommend treating these patients on suppressive doses of postoperative thyroxine. Berghout et al. demonstrated that recurrent disease was twice as likely to develop if there was a positive family history (65% versus 37%), whereas Kraimps et al. demonstrated no increased risk in recurrent disease with a family history.[8,51] The issue of a positive family history as a risk factor for recurrence remains unresolved; however, our preference is to approach these patients with a more aggressive surgical plan and offer total thyroidectomy in most cases.

Level of Experience of Surgeon

There are a number of studies looking at the association between surgeon experience, hospital volume, and clinical outcomes.[52-54] It has been very clearly shown that in thyroidectomy individual surgeon experience is closely associated with lower complication rates and shorter lengths of hospital stay.[53] However, the relationship between recurrence and experience has not been specifically documented. High-volume surgeons are more likely to perform a total thyroidectomy and leave significantly smaller thyroid remnants with similar complication rates to low-volume surgeons, which may in turn relate to lower rates of recurrence.[52,53]

Age of Patient

Patients presenting at a younger age have a significantly higher risk of goiter recurrence requiring reoperative surgery. In a case-control study performed by Gibelin, patients undergoing reoperative surgery were on average 8 years younger than the control group operated on for nonrecurrent goiter.[7] In a study by Rios et al., they looked at the recurrence rate in patients who were under 30 years of age at their initial surgery compared with those over 30 years.[31] They demonstrated that in younger patients who underwent a partial resection, there was a 40% overall recurrence rate, dependent on the type of procedure performed. At 5 years, 11% of those who had a Dunhill operation, 20% who had bilateral subtotal thyroidectomies, 17% who had hemithyroidectomies, and 50% who had unilateral subtotal thyroidectomies had recurrent disease. At 10 years follow-up, these figures were 25%, 50%, 44%, and 60%, respectively. Given the propensity for recurrent disease in the younger patient, we especially advocate a total thyroidectomy in these cases particularly if the preoperative ultrasound confirms bilateral nodularity. The fact that there is an increasing incidence of recurrence with time tends to guide us toward more extensive thyroidectomy in the younger patient as opposed to the elderly patient with a shorter life expectancy.

Bilobar Multinodular Disease

The presence of multinodular change in the presenting goiter is a strong predictor of future recurrence, particularly if the initial procedure performed was a partial or subtotal thyroidectomy. Whether to offer the patient total thyroidectomy or hemithyroidectomy at the initial procedure depends largely on the volume of disease in the nondominant thyroid lobe. In patients with symptomatic nodular goiter, when the contralateral lobe is small and nodules are <1 cm without any concerning sonographic features, it is reasonable to offer a lobectomy/hemithyroidectomy as the initial procedure. In our experience, this scenario will ultimately result in 12% of patients requiring completion lobectomy at some time in their life. In cases where the nondominant lobe already has significant nodular disease with nodules >1 cm, a total thyroidectomy is advised.

Extent of Initial Surgery

The recurrence rate for benign goiter is very closely associated with the extent of the initial surgery. This observation is best illustrated in a prospective study undertaken by Barczyński, which documented recurrence rates after 5 years of follow-up for total thyroidectomy, Dunhill procedures, and bilateral subtotal resection. The recurrence rates were 0.5% for total thyroidectomy, 5% for Dunhill procedures, and 12% for bilateral subtotal procedures.[55] These data allow an open and informed discussion to take place with each patient regarding their expectations and balancing the risks of surgery against the possibility of recurrence. Given the high rate of recurrence associated with subtotal resections, we believe that subtotal resections should be discontinued and total thyroidectomy procedures replace them as the preferred operative approach.

PREOPERATIVE EVALUATION

The preoperative assessment of patients with recurrent disease follows an investigative pathway, which is similar to that for patients with primary disease with some important additions. These additions include careful review of the previous operative note and pathology, routine fiberoptic laryngoscopy and a thorough discussion of the increased operative risks. A full clinical history, including the type of previous surgery, as well as the time frame from surgery must be documented. When the previous surgery was undertaken and the level of experience of the original surgeon are important to note because this will provide information regarding the extent of the original dissection. Exposure to previous radiation and the presence of a family history are also important aspects to note. The physical examination may be normal or may demonstrate the presence of a firm immobile cervical mass, which, because it is fixed in dense scar tissue, may mimic a carcinoma. Symptomatic nodular recurrence often causes tracheal shift to the contralateral side of the neck. Tracheal position should be carefully noted during examination. In cases where there is a significant retrosternal component, Pemberton's sign may be positive, with facial plethora becoming apparent after the patient has had his or her arms raised for up to 1 minute. Respiratory distress or inspiratory stridor and distension of neck veins may be observed in cases of thoracic inlet obstruction. We have not found percussion of the manubrium to be a reliable sign of retrosternal goiter. If a thyroid lobectomy has been previously undertaken, patients may present with a nodule on the contralateral side. When possible it is important to obtain not only the previous surgical operative notes but also the final pathology report of the previous intervention. In particular it is important to note if any parathyroid tissue was inadvertently removed at the primary surgery.

Thyroid function must be assessed before surgery. Hyperthyroid patients should be treated with appropriate antithyroid medication and when possible rendered euthyroid before surgery. Serum calcium, PTH, and vitamin D levels are routinely measured preoperatively. The majority of patients will, however, be normocalcemic, and, as previously noted, it is notoriously difficult to ascertain the status of all four remaining parathyroid glands before surgical intervention. It is possible that up to three glands may have been inadvertently removed or devascularized at initial surgery with the patient's calcium being maintained by a single remaining gland. Some authors advocate the use of pre- and intraoperative PTH assays, drawn from the lowermost part of both internal jugular veins, to determine whether the parathyroid glands are absent or nonfunctioning on one side.[56,57] There is, however, little evidence to support this practice, and it is not used routinely in our unit. The best and safest practice is to ensure the identification and preservation of all remaining parathyroid glands during the operative procedure. In the future, intraoperative photodynamic detection of normal parathyroid glands during surgery may prove beneficial. 5-Aminolevulinic acid has been shown to be useful in the localization of normal parathyroid glands during surgery; however, this has not yet been incorporated into routine surgical practice.[58] Adequate parathyroid function is best confirmed with a PTH level drawn approximately 4 hours after surgery. We use this protocol to identify and treat patients at risk of postoperative hypocalcemia.[59]

All patients presenting with recurrent disease should have comprehensive imaging studies performed. For example, the operative note indicating that the previous surgeon had performed a "complete thyroid lobectomy" may not reflect the reality of the situation at imaging, and a bilateral recurrent procedure may be required instead of a planned unilateral recurrent procedure. Ultrasound examination of the neck is a very useful initial imaging modality, and in our setting it is now undertaken by the operating surgeon as an office procedure. In reoperative goiter surgery we undertake CT examination in most patients to exclude retrosternal recurrence. A contrast-enhanced CT scan of the neck and chest will allow assessment of the position of the recurrence and the degree of tracheal deviation and compression. This information is of particular importance to the anesthesiologist in planning the technique for intubation. Fine needle aspiration may be performed where there is a suspicion of carcinoma; however, the majority of fine-needle aspiration cytologies (FNACs) will confirm the presence of a benign goiter. Respiratory function should be assessed in patients with recurrent retrosternal goiter to determine the degree of airway compromise. This is best done with a flow-volume loop assessment, which will demonstrate an obstructive pattern in those patients with tracheal compression. In patients who present with thyrotoxicosis, thyroid scintigraphy provides valuable information regarding thyroid function and anatomy, and we undertake this imaging modality in all cases of hyperthyroidism. Our preferred imaging technique is to acquire images using technetium 99m pertechnetate single-photon emission computed tomography (SPECT)/CT. We have also found scintigraphy particularly useful in the evaluation of the mediastinal mass where the nature of the mass is uncertain.

Preoperative fiberoptic laryngoscopy is mandatory for all patients undergoing reoperative thyroid surgery. The presence of a normal voice should not preclude this procedure from being performed, because 32% of individuals with RLN dysfunction will be asymptomatic.[10] Previous vocal cord damage can be concealed by contralateral vocal cord compensation. In primary thyroid surgery, we have found ultrasound to be an accurate modality in the assessment of vocal cord functionality; however, we do not advocate this approach in the reoperative setting.[60] Of patients presenting with recurrent disease, up to 20% may have unidentified preexisting permanent RLN palsy.[61,62]

OPERATIVE STRATEGY

The aims of operative intervention are to relieve patients' compressive symptoms, to prevent future recurrence, to treat hyperthyroidism in the thyrotoxic patient, and to exclude malignancy. The operation of choice in all cases of recurrent nodular goiter should be a completion total thyroidectomy. In recent times, the drive to offer patients scarless surgery has seen the development of transoral endoscopic thyroid surgery and transaxillary robotic thyroidectomy (see Chapter 32, Robotic and Extra Cervical Approaches to the Thyroid and Parathyroid Glands and Chapter 33, Transoral Thyroidectomy).[63-65] In both of these new approaches reoperative surgery is considered a contraindication and conventional open thyroidectomy remains the gold standard for recurrent goiter. In the large majority of cases, we are able to use the existing and usually well-healed neck incision. These patients in most cases have experienced excellent cosmetic outcomes following the first procedure and are generally happy to proceed with conventional open surgery for the subsequent procedure. Surgeons performing reoperative surgery should be experienced with primary thyroid operations and need to be able to adjust their operative technique if scar tissue prevents them from making progress in one particular area. The surgeon needs to recognize and prevent potential hazards and to balance the risk of recurrent nerve injury and hypoparathyroidism with the need for complete resection. In some reoperative situations it may be preferable to retain a small volume of benign thyroid tissue and preserve RLN rather than achieve a complete anatomic resection with nerve injury. Some authors advocate the use of a staged resection for bilateral recurrence, with commencement of the operation on the symptomatic side.[19] The main reason for a staged approach is to avoid a bilateral RLN palsy, which may require tracheostomy. Certainly it is our practice, if any RLN injury occurs on the initial side, to halt the procedure once that side has been completed and delay contralateral surgery. The use of intraoperative neuromonitoring (IONM) is very helpful in this setting, and it is our practice to use intermittent IONM in all reoperative procedures.

The surgical approach is dependent on the extent of the initial operation and the size and location of the recurrent goiter, as previously detailed. Where previous conservative surgery has taken place, such as simple excision of the isthmus or nodulectomy, reoperative surgery is similar to an initial primary procedure in a preserved surgical field because the posterolateral aspects of the thyroid will have been left largely undisturbed. In patients who have previously undergone a thyroid lobectomy, the contralateral lobe in most cases has not been mobilized and thus the RLN should not be at increased risk. These procedures can be undertaken with a similar approach to primary surgery after excision of the original cervical incision. The strap muscles are adherent to the thyroid capsule anteriorly, and once these are carefully dissected free the lateral and posterior dissection continues as normal.

Reoperation after a subtotal or total thyroidectomy is more hazardous and requires a methodical and standardized operative approach. Although any of the general complications of thyroid surgery can equally occur in reoperative thyroid surgery, the risk of permanent RLN injury and permanent hypoparathyroidism are clearly greater and deserve particular attention.

The key technical steps in undertaking reoperative procedures are as follows:
- Excision of part or all of the previous neck incision and freeing of thyroid remnant from the strap muscles
- Identification of anatomic landmarks outside of the original operative field to facilitate orientation and subsequent dissection
- Identification of the RLN in undissected territory
- Capsular dissection of thyroid remnant to preserve parathyroid function
- Confirmation of RLN function using IONM before progressing to the contralateral side

The first step in reoperative surgery is to excise the scar and raise the skin flaps in a standard fashion. The anterior border of the sternocleidomastoid muscle is exposed, and to enter the field of dissection away from scar tissue it is best to commence mobilization of the strap muscles laterally. The carotid sheath is exposed and retracted laterally.

The ansa cervicalis is preserved and the strap muscles are dissected free from the thyroid remnant, keeping in mind that RLN may be adherent to the posterior aspect of the muscle. In our experience safe surgery is facilitated by transverse division of the strap muscles to improve exposure. The carotid sheath may, however, be displaced medially and lie abutting both fibrous tissue and the thyroid remnant. At this point we confirm RLN function by stimulating the vagus nerve within the carotid sheath. Dissection continues posteriorly to the prevertebral fascia then medially to the region of the esophagus where the lateral aspect of the thyroid lobe will be encountered. It is important to ensure that the RLN is not ventrally displaced and encased within the strap muscles before their division. The next step is to identify the trachea in the midline by direct dissection, which is always a safe maneuver provided it is undertaken with care as it relates to the innominate artery and brachiocephalic vein. This now provides clear anatomic boundaries both medial and lateral to the reoperative field and narrows down the location of the RLN, which in most cases will be found within the tracheoesophageal groove. However, about 1% will lie anterolateral to the trachea, and a further one-third will lie lateral to the trachea.[66,67] Furthermore, although the majority of surgeons consider the planes anterior to the inferior thyroid artery safe, about one-third of the nerves are found anterior or interdigitating with the branches of the artery.[66]

For reoperative surgery, there are three principal approaches to finding the RLN in undissected territory, and each can be used depending on the individual situation encountered. The preferred initial technique is the "lateral" or "backdoor approach," which involves dissecting down the medial border of the sternomastoid muscle as previously described, then across the common carotid to the prevertebral fascia. Dissection continues medially toward the esophagus and tracheoesophageal groove. Careful progressive dissection can be assisted by palpation in the reoperative area to reveal the RLN before it enters the scarred reoperative site (Figure 9.7, A). Once the RLN is exposed, stimulation using intermittent IONM will verify the anatomy. If the nerve cannot be identified because of extensive lateral scar tissue, an alternative strategy is the "inferior approach," where the tracheoesophageal groove is approached anteriorly, dissecting across and lateral to the thymus as low as possible in the neck. The RLN is identified as it emerges from the upper mediastinum having "recurred" around the aortic arch on the left side or the subclavian artery on the right (Figure 9.7, B). Other than where the initial procedure involved removal of a retrosternal goiter, it would be most unusual for this area to have been disturbed, and the RLN can usually be readily identified and dissected superiorly through the scar tissue. Failing that, the last strategy is the "medial superior pole approach." If the upper pole has previously not been dissected, then the avascular plane between the upper pole and cricothyroid muscle is developed, with the upper pole being retracted laterally. Progressive dissection inferiorly along the larynx to the lower edge of the cricoid will lead to the RLN as it passes under the cricopharyngeus muscle (Figure 9.7, C). The nerve can then be progressively dissected inferiorly to free it from any scar tissue. Dissection in the region of the superior thyroid pole should also incorporate identification of the external branch of the superior laryngeal nerve (EBSLN). Demonstrating cricothyroid muscle twitch while stimulating EBSLN is a useful way of confirming integrity of this nerve.[68]

Even though the advantages of intermittent IONM in the primary setting continue to be argued vigorously, most authors would agree that it has a very beneficial role in reoperative thyroid surgery.[67,69-71] Although there can be no technological substitute for experience, routine anatomic nerve exposure, and meticulous surgical technique, the use of routine IONM in reoperative surgery allows the surgeon to distinguish between longitudinal scar tissue and the RLN or to identify the RLN lying beneath a layer of impenetrable scar tissue.[72]

Preservation of any remaining parathyroid glands is best achieved by capsular dissection on the thyroid surface, maintaining a vigilant search for any parathyroid tissue, which can often be difficult to identify within scar tissue. We do not undertake an exhaustive search for parathyroid glands not immediately encountered during the dissection of the thyroid remnant. It needs to be understood that, given the disruption to the previous vascular anatomy from previous surgery, preservation of parathyroid tissue on an intact vascular pedicle is often difficult in reoperative surgery. For that reason we prefer a policy of "ready autotransplantation"—that is, a very low threshold to autotransplant any parathyroid tissue that cannot be assured an intact vascular supply. Placing a small incision on the surface of any parathyroid gland that appears compromised is a useful technique to release venous congestion and confirm arterial flow. Once the operative specimen has been excised, a careful inspection of the capsular surface must be undertaken to avoid inadvertent parathyroid gland removal. Normal parathyroid glands may be easily retained within scar tissue and adherent to the thyroid capsule. Our technique of parathyroid autotransplantation[70] is to mince the parathyroid gland into a 2-mL balanced salt suspension and to inject that into the sternomastoid muscle. This is a safe and effective technique for ensuring the viability of autotransplanted parathyroid cells.

Substernal Goiter

Please see the Expert Consult website for discussion of this topic.

POSTOPERATIVE COMPLICATIONS

Reoperative thyroid surgery can be associated with significant morbidity. This results from the presence of fibrosis and altered anatomy, which make the dissection considerably more challenging. Early published work from Beahrs and Vandertoll evaluated 548 secondary thyroidectomies between 1952 and 1961 and found significantly higher rates of both RLN damage and hypoparathyroidism.[75]

More recently, Moalem et al. published an evidence-based review of this topic.[19] They examined the complication rates after recurrent benign thyroid surgery compared with primary procedures from 10 studies published since the early 1990s. They found that reoperative surgery compared with primary surgery was associated with a higher RLN injury rate, both temporary (0% to 22% versus 0.5% to 18%) and permanent (0% to 13% versus 0% to 4%). In terms of hypoparathyroidism, there was no difference in the rates of temporary hypocalcemia (0% to 25% versus 1% to 27%). However, there was a significant difference in the rates of permanent hypoparathyroidism (0% to 22% versus 0% to 4%), with higher rates for reoperative patients as opposed to those undergoing primary surgery. Postoperative hematoma may occur after repeat thyroid surgery; however, the rate does not seem to be greater than that seen in primary procedures. Rare complications, including tracheal and esophageal injury and chyle leak, are described but occur very infrequently.[76] In general we avoid the use of postoperative drains after revision thyroid surgery unless the goiter is particularly large and a significant dead space exists at the conclusion of the procedure.

The rate of permanent RLN dysfunction after reoperative surgery, in our experience, has been 1.5%, which is higher than our comparable rate for primary procedures (0.3%).[8] The rate of permanent hypoparathyroidism in this unit has fallen from 3.5% to 1.6% over a 20-year period for secondary operations, predominantly as a result of our policy of "ready autotransplantation." Similar results have been achieved in other high-volume units.[23]

POSTOPERATIVE MANAGEMENT AND PREVENTION OF FURTHER RECURRENCE

With the increasing acceptance of total thyroidectomy as the operation of choice for benign thyroid disease, the expected recurrence rate will

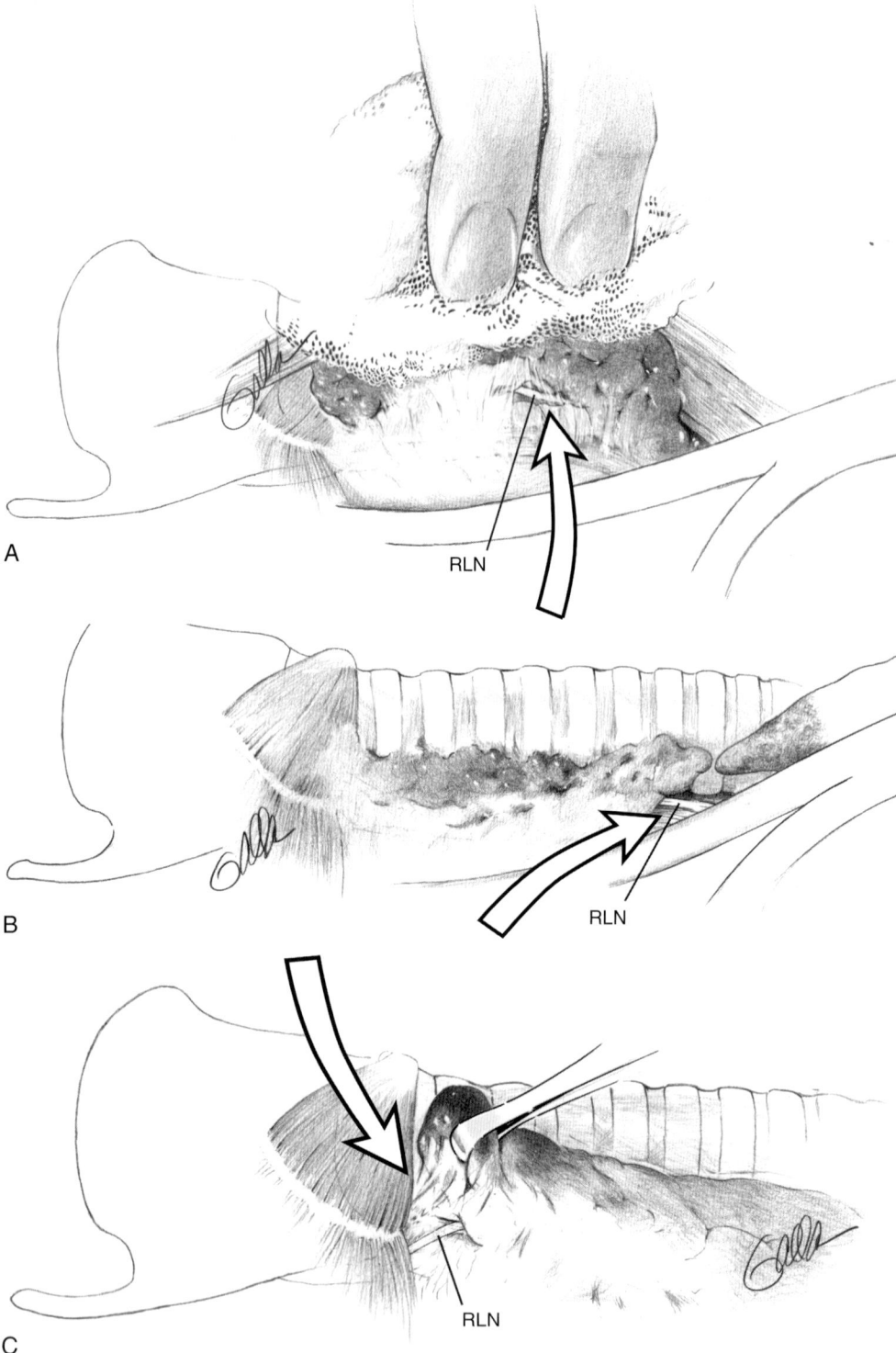

Fig. 9.7 A, Lateral or backdoor approach dissecting along the medial border of the sternomastoid, across the common carotid to the prevertebral fascia, then medially to find the recurrent laryngeal nerve (RLN). **B,** Inferior approach dissecting across the thymus to find the RLN as it appears from out of the mediastinum having "recurred" behind the aortic arch on the left and subclavian on the right. **C,** Superior approach finding the avascular space lateral to the cricothyroid muscle then dissecting inferiorly to the laryngotracheal groove to find the RLN.

fall considerably in the coming years. These patients require replacement doses of levothyroxine to ensure they remain euthyroid, aiming for a TSH of approximately 1.0 mIU/L. We initiate levothyroxine replacement based on a daily dose of 1.6 ug/kg. For those not receiving total thyroidectomy, some have suggested postoperative administration of suppressive doses of either thyroxine alone or in combination with iodine in an attempt to prevent or delay recurrence.

TSH Suppression

Thyroxine has been used in the treatment of nontoxic multinodular goiters since 1896, when early reports on the favorable influence on thyroid size were first published.[77,78] The aim is to minimize TSH release, creating a mild thyrotoxic state, which suppresses the growth of thyroid follicular cells. There is now a significant body of evidence to suggest that this can be an effective preoperative treatment, which can produce a clinically significant decrease of up to 40% in nodule size.[79] The adverse effects of long-term subclinical hyperthyroidism must be borne in mind and may limit its applicability in some patients.

The role of suppressive doses of thyroxine given postoperatively, in an attempt to prevent recurrence, is less clear-cut. Most of the research investigating its role is made up of predominantly small retrospective studies that are heterogeneous, making comparison or meta-analysis impossible. Essentially, half of the available studies support the hypothesis that TSH suppression postoperatively reduces recurrence rates, whereas the other half dispute these findings.[51,79-84] Overall, the combined data are poor: the type of surgery is not standardized; half the studies performed were in endemic areas; the majority of studies had only limited follow-up (with only four studies having longer than 10 years of follow-up); and finally, the method of detection of recurrent disease was highly variable (palpable disease versus ultrasound detection).

Please see the Expert Consult website for more discussion of this topic.

Therefore it seems that suppressive doses of thyroxine do not universally prevent recurrence. The proposed reasoning behind this conclusion is that some thyroid nodules in recurrent disease may become autonomous and are no longer subject to regulation by the hypothalamus-pituitary-thyroid axis. Instead, because of the polyclonal nature of recurrent disease, there may be multiple regulatory pathways, including insulin-like growth factors and their binding proteins.[3,50] Because this unit has a policy of total thyroidectomy for BMNGs, we do not routinely use suppressive doses of thyroxine postoperatively. Indeed, the use of suppressive doses of thyroxine must be balanced against the long-term cardiovascular and skeletal detrimental effects of subclinical hyperthyroidism.

Iodine Supplementation

In iodine-deficient areas, the use of iodine either alone or in combination with thyroxine has been proposed as an alternative to treatment with suppressive doses of thyroxine to prevent recurrence.[82,86,87] In iodine-deficient areas, postoperative normalization of the iodine supply is possible without risk after the adequate elimination of autonomous tissue. The anticipated advantage is to allow a lower dose of thyroxine to be used with less associated TSH suppression, thereby reducing the complications associated with long-term subclinical hyperthyroidism. A study by Carella et al. demonstrated that the combination of levothyroxine and iodized salt showed a statistically significant difference in the reduction of thyroid remnant size compared with levothyroxine alone (39.7% versus 10%).[87] The reduction in size was independent of the degree of TSH suppression. Potassium iodine has also been used as monotherapy to reduce recurrence and has been shown to have results equivalent to standard therapy with thyroxine at 1.5 µg/kg.[88] Although these results are interesting, the follow-up periods studied are too short to make meaningful recommendations. The administration of postoperative iodine is not currently routine practice in this unit or in iodine sufficient areas.

MANAGEMENT OF RECURRENT GRAVES' DISEASE

The primary definitive management of Graves' disease differs significantly around the world (see Chapter 8, Surgical Management of Hyperthyroidism). In some countries, radioiodine ablation is the preferred option, whereas in other countries, such as Japan, surgical resection is the primary modality of definitive management. Surgery is the preferred option over other modalities in cases where there is a desire to avoid the side effects of antithyroid medications or radiation exposure and in patients where rapid correction of thyrotoxicosis is needed. It was the Australian surgeon Dunhill who championed safe surgery and anesthesia for patients with Graves' disease in the early 1900s. He performed subtotal thyroidectomies in patients with Graves' disease under local anesthetic with a mortality rate of less than 2%. The controversy regarding the extent of surgical intervention for Graves' disease centers around the higher rates of complications reported for total thyroidectomy compared with more conservative surgical options. A recent evidence-based review has provided strong support for total thyroidectomy.[89] One meta-analysis and three retrospective case studies examined the risk of complications and also the recurrence risks associated with differing degrees of surgery.[90-92] A meta-analysis performed by Palit examined 6703 patients from 35 different studies, with follow-up varying from 4 to 12 years. Total thyroidectomy was performed in 538 patients, with 6165 patients undergoing a subtotal thyroidectomy. There was no statistically significant difference in the rates of either permanent RLN palsy (0.9% versus 0.7%) or hypoparathyroidism (0.9% versus 1.0%). There was, however, a striking difference between the rates of recurrence with a mean follow-up of 5.6 years. No recurrences were detected after a total thyroidectomy (0%) compared with 7.9% for those patients who had a subtotal thyroidectomy.[90] Similar results were found in three retrospective case series—the recurrence rate for conservative operations was between 5% to 20%, with no reduction in the postoperative complication rates.[90,93,94] We therefore advocate the use of a total thyroidectomy for Graves' disease. Total thyroidectomy is just as safe as lesser surgery, but it is associated with a significant reduction in the rates of recurrence thereby reducing the need for either reoperative surgery or radioactive iodine ablation. It also avoids the risk, with subtotal operation, of leaving incidental carcinomas untreated. This is especially important in patients with Graves' disease, because some authors have reported an increased rate of micropapillary thyroid carcinoma (8%) in association with this condition.[95]

As with the surgical management of BMNG, surgery for Graves' disease may still be associated with recurrent disease. There are a number of situations where surgeons may be faced with the need for reoperation for recurrent Graves' disease:
- The patient underwent a formal bilateral subtotal thyroidectomy, or Dunhill procedure, with total lobectomy and contralateral subtotal lobectomy, but the residual remnant size was excessive and has led to persistent or recurrent disease in the remnant(s).
- The patient has had an initial "total" thyroidectomy but has developed recurrent disease in one of the embryologic thyroid remnants not identified or recognized at the initial operation.
- The patient has had an initial thyroid procedure for euthyroid nodular disease (e.g., lobectomy) and now presents with Graves' disease de novo in the residual lobe.

Patients presenting with recurrent Graves' disease after previous thyroidectomy should first be reassessed for definitive management by radioiodine ablation. Although it is likely that the initial indications that led to the choice of surgery rather than radioactive iodine as definitive therapy are still present, in a number of patients the increased risks of reoperative balance may be sufficient to weight the decision in favor of radioiodine for management of the recurrence. Sometimes in patients treated with radioiodine ablation for recurrence, radioactive iodine fails to control the hyperthyroidism, either because of a large recurrent goiter or an aggressive disease. The combination of scarring from previous surgery and radiation-induced fibrosis can then make further surgery very difficult.

Please see the Expert Consult website for more discussion of this topic.

CONCLUSION

Reoperative surgery for benign recurrent thyroid disease is likely to become less common as total thyroidectomy becomes more widespread as the initial surgical therapy of choice. Reoperative procedures require careful planning and are best performed by experienced thyroid surgeons. Evaluation of laryngeal nerve function is mandatory preoperatively, and patients will benefit from the routine incorporation of neuromonitoring technology.

REFERENCES

For a complete list of references, go to expertconsult.com.

SECTION 3

Preoperative Evaluation

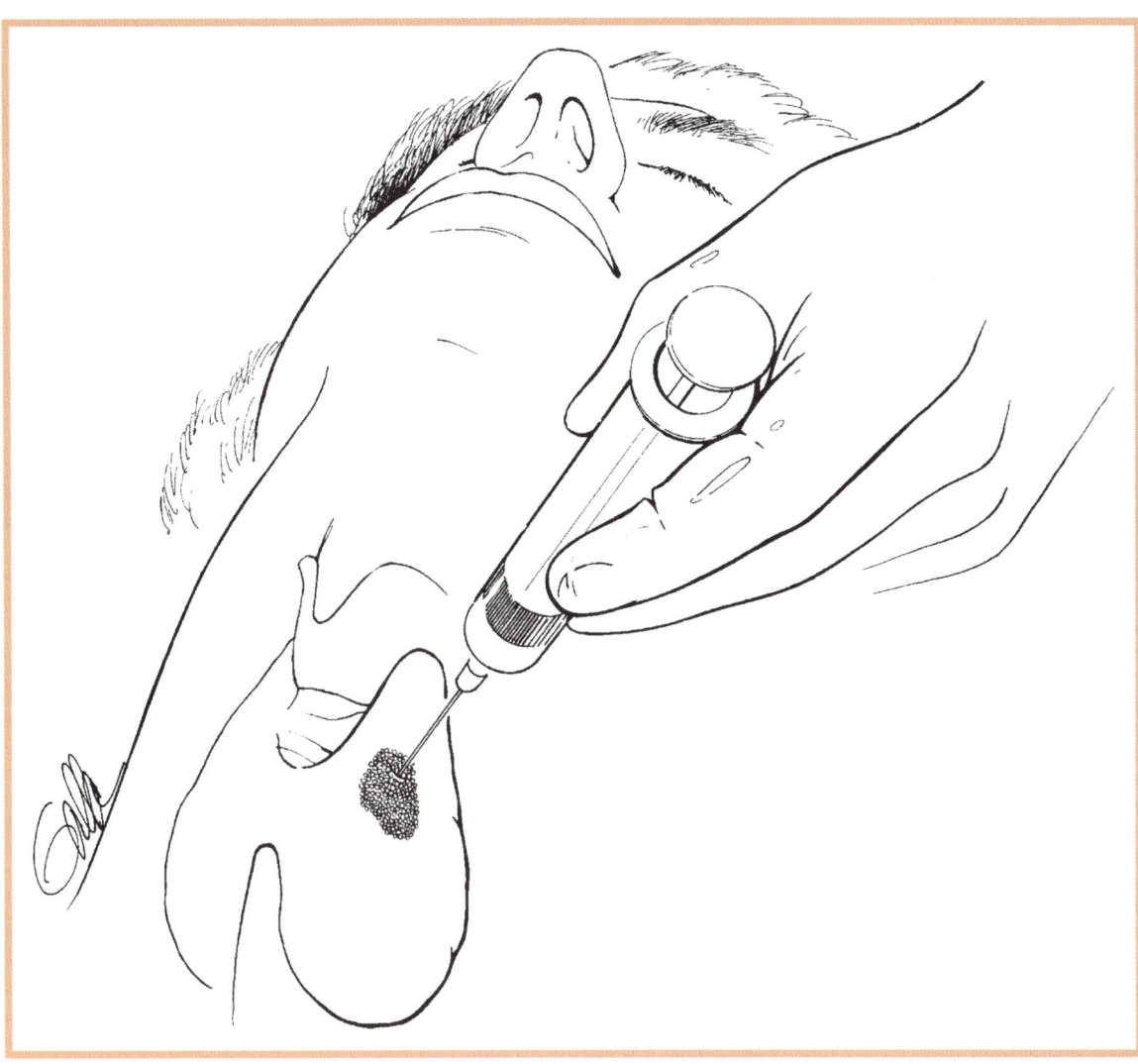

10

The Evaluation and Management of Thyroid Nodules

Kevin J. Kovatch, Elizabeth N. Pearce, Megan R. Haymart

> Please go to expertconsult.com to view related video:
> **Video 10.1** Introduction to Chapter 10, The Evaluation and Management of Thyroid Nodules.

INTRODUCTION

Thyroid nodules are common and may be found in up to two-thirds of the population.[1] By definition, thyroid nodules are discrete lesions contained within, yet radiologically distinct from, the parenchyma of the thyroid gland.[2] A substantial increase in both thyroid nodule detection and thyroid cancer detection has occurred over the past three decades; this is largely attributable to increases in health care access/utilization and the use of medical imaging.[3,4] Despite increased detection of thyroid nodules and malignancies, thyroid cancer mortality has remained low and virtually unchanged.[5]

The initial workup of thyroid nodules includes clinical history, physical examination, assessment of risk factors, thyroid function tests, and neck ultrasound. Subsequent cytologic evaluation by fine needle aspiration (FNA) is guided largely by size, sonographic features, and consideration of other risk factors. Definitive surgical management is recommended based on either symptomatology or high-risk FNA classification. Diagnostic surgery is required in selected cases where cytology is indeterminate; molecular testing is assuming a greater role in guiding such cases. Although many aspects of workup and management of thyroid nodules are well described, there continues to be a high degree of variation in care.

The challenge clinicians face, as increasingly more nodules are being identified, is to determine which nodules are clinically significant, specifically those which will require intervention due to high risk of malignancy or large size with compressive symptoms. Overall, the vast majority (about 90%) of thyroid nodules will not pose any risk to the patient and will not require intervention.[2] Herein, we discuss the evaluation and management of thyroid nodules with a focus on recent literature and updated practice recommendations.

RISK FACTORS FOR NODULES AND MALIGNANCY

Clinical Risk Factors

Thyroid nodule evaluation begins with history and physical examination focused on the thyroid and cervical neck. In general, risk factors for nodules include increased age, female sex, obesity, and iodine deficiency. Nodules may be identified at differing rates depending on survey method (e.g., ultrasound versus palpation). Therefore thresholds to perform these elements or extensions of physical examination should be considered based on symptomatology or risk of malignancy. Malignancy occurs in approximately 8% to 15% of cases, and risk is similarly influenced by clinical variables, such as sex, age, and the presence of unique symptoms or examination findings.[2,6] Elements of patient history that are concerning for thyroid malignancy include history of childhood irradiation to the head and neck, exposure to radioactive fallout, family history of thyroid cancer in a first-degree relative, or family history of hereditary syndromes associated with thyroid cancer (e.g., multiple endocrine neoplasia type 2 [MEN 2] association with hereditary medullary thyroid cancer [MTC]).[2]

Family History and Radiation Exposure

The strongest risk factors for differentiated thyroid cancer (DTC) are family history and prior head and neck radiation exposure. Family history of DTC is a known risk factor for thyroid malignancy. Epidemiologic evidence shows that 5% to 10% of DTCs have a familial occurrence; however, it is often unclear whether diagnosis of DTC in patients with a positive family history represents familial versus sporadic disease. Pedigrees showing one to two family members with thyroid cancer are not uncommon; evidence shows that the chance of nonmedullary DTC being sporadic is much lower when three or more family members are affected (<6% sporadic), compared with two or fewer (62% to 69%).[7] Syndromes associated with DTC in a first-degree relative include phosphatase and tensin homolog (PTEN) hamartoma tumor syndrome (i.e., Cowden's disease), familial adenomatous polyposis (FAP), and Carney complex.[8]

Thyroid exposure to ionizing radiation during childhood imparts significant risk for malignancy, because the thyroid is among the most radiosensitive organs.[9] Importantly, radiation exposure increases thyroid cancer risk predominantly when the exposure occurs during childhood. Risk is most significant when exposure occurs at <5 years of age, and no increased risk is observed when exposure occurs beyond 20 years of age.[10] Further, radiation-induced cancers often harbor mutations that convey more aggressive clinical behavior, including a high prevalence of RET/PTC (rearranged during transfection/papillary thyroid carcinoma) chromosomal rearrangement. Annual thyroid examination by palpation (though not routine ultrasound) has been advocated for survivors of childhood cancer previously treated with neck radiation.[11]

The Chernobyl nuclear power station explosion in 1986 is a notable example of widespread radiation exposure, and the effects of this exposure on thyroid cancer risk have been well studied. It is estimated that this exposure was responsible for >4000 new cases of thyroid cancer between 1986 and 2002 in Belarus, Russia, and Ukraine. A nearly 150-fold increase in incidence between 1986 and 1996 has been recorded in the most heavily-contaminated regions of Belarus (0.085 to 12.6 per 100,000 children/year).[12] A similar trend was seen after the Fukushima Daiichi nuclear power plant accident in 2011.[13]

Age and Sex

Increasing prevalence of nodular disease is observed as patient age increases.[14,15] In a large prospective cohort analysis of more than 6000 patients with more than 12,000 thyroid nodules, Kwong et al. found that the average number of thyroid nodules increased with age (1.6% annual increased risk for multinodularity); however, there was a lower risk of malignancy in newly-identified nodules with advancing age (2.2% annual decrease in relative risk of malignancy between 20 to 60 years of age). Despite the latter finding, older patients were also observed to have higher-risk histologic phenotypes. Although older patients are at increased risk for high-risk cancer, the number of individuals with high-risk cancer is low; older patients with nodular thyroid disease and additional comorbidities, such as other cancers and coronary artery disease, are more likely to die of their comorbidities.[15]

The incidence of thyroid cancer is highest in patients age 65 and older.[3] The balance of treatment risks and benefits is shifted in favor of more conservative care in the older patient population. Advanced age is more associated with higher rates of thyroid-specific surgical complications than historically reported in literature, with hypocalcemia and vocal fold paralysis observed in up to 13.6% and 7.1% to 9.5% of patients >65 years, respectively.[16,17] The increased risk of thyroid cancer recurrence and disease-specific mortality in older patients argues in favor of surgical management, and it is reflected in more advanced staging schema for patients ≥55 years in the updated American Joint Committee on Cancer (AJCC) 8th edition staging system.[18] However, limited life expectancy, significant comorbidities, and risk of surgical complications argue in favor of more conservative treatment or observation. Therefore advanced age is an important factor when considering surgical intervention for thyroid nodules.

Thyroid cancer is three times more common in women, but men evaluated for thyroid nodules are more likely to have a thyroid malignancy.[19] In a retrospective study of nearly 2000 nodule patients with more than 3500 thyroid nodules, the rate of thyroid cancer in men was nearly double that of women.[20] The biological mechanism for this increased risk is unclear; however, this trend is, in part, explained by the much higher incidence of thyroid nodules identified in women overall.

SIGNS, SYMPTOMS, AND PHYSICAL EXAMINATION

When present, symptoms of thyroid nodules are related to location, size, and compression of nearby structures. Common symptoms associated with large or enlarging thyroid nodules include difficult or painful swallowing (dysphagia, odynophagia as seen in nodules in a posterior location with compression of esophagus), foreign body sensation in the throat (globus as seen with large central nodules), dyspnea, hoarseness or other voice complaints, and pain. A very rapidly enlarging nodule is also concerning for hemorrhagic nodule, high-risk malignancy such as anaplastic cancer, thyroid lymphoma, or infection.

Rapid growth of a thyroid nodule, the presence of firm neck adenopathy, or nodule fixation to surrounding structures are all associated with a higher risk of malignancy. Characterization of nodules and/or lymph nodes on examination by neck palpation is limited to rough size estimates and gross localization (e.g., right versus left lobe, superior versus inferior pole), and tactile features (e.g., firm versus soft, mobile versus fixed). Nodules that are small or posteriorly located may not be appreciated on examination. Thus thyroid/neck ultrasound is the gold standard for nodule characterization and provides additional data to drive risk stratification.

LABORATORY TESTING

Serum thyrotropin measurement of thyroid stimulating hormone (TSH) should be included in the initial workup of known or suspected thyroid nodules (Figure 10.1).[2] Suppressed TSH may be indicative of hyperfunctioning nodules, which are associated with an exceedingly low risk of malignancy. Radionucleotide scan should be performed to identify hyperfunctioning nodules when serum TSH is low and nodules are present; this may distinguish between a solitary hot nodule, toxic multinodular goiter, or scintigraphically cold nodule(s) concurrent with Graves' disease.

Thyroglobulin is commonly used to monitor thyroid cancer patients treated with thyroidectomy for recurrence; however, measurement of baseline thyroglobulin is not recommended as part of the workup of thyroid nodules.[2] Likewise, calcitonin is a serum marker useful in the diagnosis and surveillance of MTC of parafollicular C cell origin; this is not routinely evaluated for thyroid nodule workup in the absence of high clinical suspicion for MTC. When there is suspicion for MTC, serum calcitonin levels >100 pg/mL are suggestive of MTC, with higher levels being more suggestive of metastatic disease.[21] Additional laboratory tests, such as serum calcium or 25-OH vitamin D may be included in the preoperative evaluation; however, such tests do not aid in the characterization of thyroid nodules.

SCREENING FOR THYROID NODULES

Routine screening for thyroid nodules has been controversial, given their known high prevalence and the low probability of clinical relevance. The recognized harms of routine screening are related to a propensity toward overdiagnosis and overtreatment when otherwise asymptomatic nodules are identified.[22] Here, overdiagnosis and overtreatment refer to instances where nodules that would not otherwise go on to cause symptoms or death are diagnosed and/or treated, as is the case for roughly 90% of evaluated thyroid nodules.[23] Overdiagnosis is a well-appreciated phenomenon for thyroid cancer at the population level, where there is a large reservoir of clinically insignificant disease and increased detection via directed screening or incidental finding.[23,24] Current estimates suggest that 45% to 80% of thyroid cancers in the United States are overdiagnosed.[25]

For patients who otherwise do not have symptoms or risk factors, routine screening for thyroid nodules by neck palpation, neck ultrasound, or other techniques should not be performed. The US Preventative Services Task Force (USPSTF) makes formal, evidence-based recommendations regarding the efficacy of specific preventative care services for asymptomatic patients. Upon review of the evidence surrounding thyroid cancer screening, the USPSTF released an updated statement in 2017 recommending against routine screening for thyroid cancer in asymptomatic individuals (grade D recommendation, "moderate or high certainty that this services had no net benefit, or that the harms outweigh the benefits").[26,27] This recommendation is largely based on evidence that a minority of thyroid nodules harbor malignancy and that, even when diagnosed, most thyroid cancers are indolent. There is currently no evidence to support reduced mortality or improved quality of life when patients with low-risk thyroid malignancy (most commonly papillary thyroid carcinoma) are treated at an asymptomatic stage. Thus eliminating screening of asymptomatic patients aims to minimize unnecessary workup, biopsies, surgeries, and other therapies for nodules, which are not clinically relevant. Notably, this recommendation is not applicable to patients with symptomatology or clinical risk factors.

The South Korean experience is perhaps the most dramatic example of how thyroid cancer screening practices can lead to overdiagnosis. Rates of thyroid cancer diagnosis increased 15-fold from 1993 to 2011, owing to a national program offering neck ultrasonography as a low-cost addition to a battery of routine screenings for cancer and other common diseases.[28] Subsequently, the Physician Coalition for

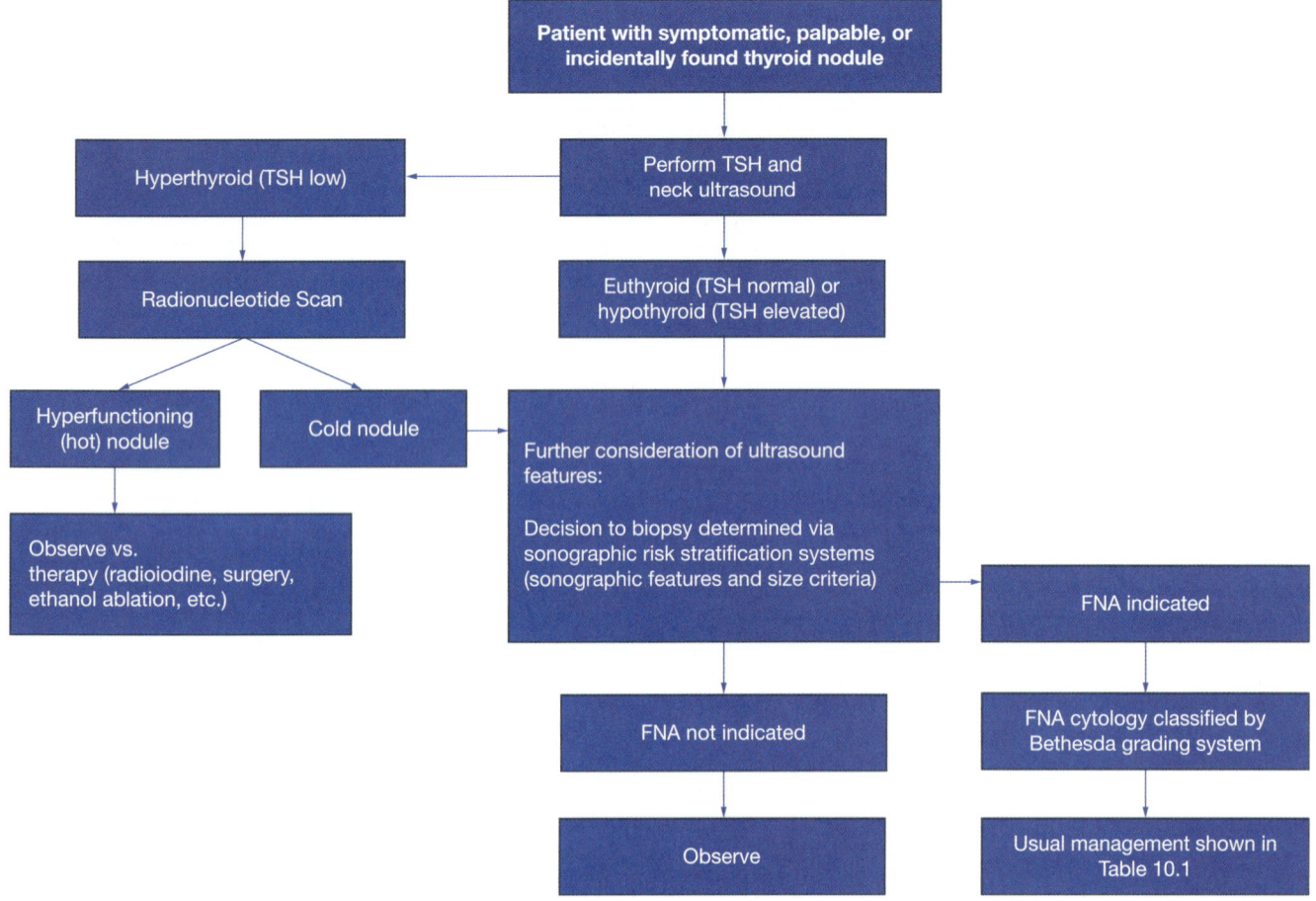

Fig. 10.1 Workup and Management of Known Thyroid Nodule. TSH, thyroid stimulating hormone; FNA, fine needle aspiration.

Prevention of Overdiagnosis of Thyroid Cancer released a statement discouraging ultrasound screening in healthy patients, which ultimately resulted in stabilization of thyroid cancer incidence and a 35% reduction in thyroid cancer surgeries by 2015. This was attributable to a decrease in screening practices, which prompted a formal recommendation from the Korean Committee for National Cancer Screening Guidelines against thyroid ultrasonography in otherwise healthy patients.[29]

INCIDENTALLY FOUND THYROID NODULES

As an extension of the USPSTF recommendation against routine screening, providers must also be wary of nodules identified unintentionally on physical examination or imaging for complaints unrelated to the neck, particularly when these are small and asymptomatic nodules. Incidentally found nodules, often termed thyroid "incidentalomas," are most commonly detected on ultrasound, computed tomography (CT), magnetic resonance imaging (MRI), or positron emission tomography (PET) studies covering the spine, neck, chest, or whole body for indications unrelated to thyroid disease. The reported rate of incidental nodules is highest with ultrasound at 65%, followed by CT and MRI at 25%, and PET between 1% and 2%.[30] A number of risk-stratification systems based on sonographic findings exist. Although CT and MRI may easily detect thyroid nodules, the radiographic features of these tests have not been reliably associated with benign or malignant disease.[31] Conversely, nodules with Fludeoxyglucose (FDG) avidity on PET scan or focal uptake of radiotracers on other nuclear medicine studies have been associated with higher rates of malignancy, with rates as high as 55%.[32-34] Thus FNA is recommended for PET-avid nodules $\geq$1 cm.[2]

The population risk and cost of working up and/or treating incidentally found nodules is substantial.[22] Fear of death from cancer, fear of "missed diagnosis," and discomfort with uncertainty drive the workup and treatment of nodules even in asymptomatic patients, often resulting in unnecessary imaging, biopsies, and surgeries. Up to 41% of patients who undergo FNA for incidental nodules may undergo surgery due to indeterminate pathology; a majority of these cases will show benign pathology.[35] Not all incidentally identified nodules will require dedicated thyroid/neck ultrasound or tissue diagnosis by FNA. Radiologists and referring physicians have a professional and ethical responsibility to make best practice judgments on whether or not evaluation with dedicated ultrasound is warranted.[36]

The American College of Radiology (ACR) has released guidelines suggesting pursuit of dedicated ultrasound for incidentally found nodules only for patients 35 years of older with nodules $\geq$1.5 cm in size, and patients who are younger than 35 years of age with nodules $\geq$1.0 cm in size with an absence of suspicious findings (e.g., local invasion, abnormal or enlarged lymph nodes, focal FDG avidity, or suspicious features such as calcification).[37,38] For incidental nodules, ultimately undergoing ultrasound evaluation, biopsy should be guided by risk stratification based on a combination of size, radiologic features, and clinical risk factors. Education and counseling should be provided to patients with incidental nodules, including cases where no further workup is pursued.

ULTRASOUND EVALUATION FOR KNOWN OR SUSPECTED THYROID NODULES

The workup of known or suspected thyroid nodules includes ultrasound evaluation (see Figure 10.1). Diagnostic ultrasound should include a high-resolution (≥12 MHz) examination of the thyroid gland and the cervical lymph nodes. Diagnostic reports should comment on nodule number, location, size in three dimensions, sonographic features (e.g., composition, echogenicity, margins, calcifications, shape, and vascularity) of thyroid nodules, location and imaging characteristics of cervical lymph nodes (e.g., central and lateral neck compartments), as well as the background thyroid parenchyma, and gland size.[2,39]

The goal of diagnostic thyroid/neck ultrasound is to determine which nodules meet sonographic criteria for FNA. There is an abundance of evidence supporting risk stratification using ultrasound grayscale features. Features with high specificity (>90%) for thyroid cancer notably include the presence of microcalcifications, irregular margins, and taller-than-wide shape.[2] Echogenicity and composition are also predictive of malignancy, with hypoechoic and solid nodules conferring the highest risk. Spongiform nodules, defined as nodules with >50% small multicystic composition, exhibit an extremely low likelihood of harboring malignancy; despite this, microcystic components can resemble microcalcifications, and FNA is recommended at higher size cutoff by some guidelines (e.g., ≥2 cm for American Thyroid Association [ATA] 2015 Guidelines).[2,40] Purely cystic nodules are invariably benign and do not require diagnostic evaluation. Risk stratification systems making use of constellations of sonographic features are used to determine when FNA is indicated and are further discussed in the "Radiologic Risk Assessment" section.

EVOLVING IMAGING MODALITIES

Adjuncts to traditional ultrasound examination have been described. Ultrasound elastography patterns are being studied as predictors of benign versus malignant nodules and may ultimately add another variable to determine which nodules warrant FNA.[41] Radiomics, likewise, is evolving as a modality where prediction models are generated by pattern recognition and imaging data. This has been proposed as a tool for thyroid nodule classification, which may be more sensitive than radiologist visual interpretation alone.[42]

SIZE, GROWTH PATTERN, AND MULTINODULARITY

Generally, only nodules >1 cm will require evaluation due to the greater likelihood of clinical significance. Even when malignant, PTC tumors ≤1 cm, termed "papillary thyroid microcarcinomas" (PTMC) by the World Health Organization, have extremely low locoregional recurrence rates (2% to 6%), and disease-specific mortality <1%.[43] Nodules >2 cm show higher rates of distant metastases for PTC and FTC histologies.[44] A large study of the National Cancer Institute (NCI) Surveillance, Epidemiology, and End Results (SEER) database found a 99.4% 10-year relative survival for patients with thyroid cancers <3 cm.[45] Such evidence regarding nodule size and cancer outcomes contributes to the size thresholds for performing FNA described in the risk stratification systems. Composition and other sonographic features beyond size alone also are predictive of malignancy. Sonographic measurements tend to be greater than those in surgical pathology specimens, which may have implications for preoperative risk assessment as well as clinical versus pathologic staging.[46]

The majority of benign nodules exhibit slow growth.[47] Prior work suggested that benign and malignant nodules often show differential growth rates, with malignant nodules more likely to grow >2 mm per year compared with benign nodules, particularly when malignant nodules exhibit higher-risk phenotypes.[48] This trend is reflected in the current ATA guidelines; when growth of a nodule (>20% in two dimensions and a minimal increase of 2 mm, or ≥50% increase in volume) is detected during ultrasound surveillance, shorter-interval observation, repeat biopsy, or diagnostic lobectomy should be considered.[2] Although growth should be considered, malignancy in nodules that are followed is better predicted by changes in sonographic appearance than in growth pattern.[47]

The presence of two or more thyroid nodules 1 cm or larger occurs in about half of patients with nodular disease, with higher rates related to female sex, obesity, and increased age.[14,15,49,50] The initial evaluation of these patients should proceed similar to the evaluation of those with a single nodule (including TSH and ultrasound), noting that each nodule >1 cm carries an independent risk of malignancy. In contrast to historical suggestions, multinodular goiter does not predict a lower risk for malignancy. Data confirm that the risk of malignancy per patient is similar whether a single nodule or multiple nodules >1 cm are detected.[20]

With this in mind, nodules within a multinodular goiter should be chosen for biopsy based on sonographic appearance and size cutoff. Radionucleotide scan should be performed in patients with suppressed TSH, and only iso- or hypo-functioning nodules should be considered for biopsy.[2] The American College of Radiology Thyroid Imaging Reporting and Data System (ACR TI-RADS) Committee recommends targeting no more than two nodules with the highest suspicion for FNA.[51] Further, the committee discourages use of the term "dominant nodule" (i.e., largest) in reporting because this wording wrongly suggests greater importance of size, rather than nodular architecture. Among patients with multiple thyroid nodules >1 cm in diameter who proved to have thyroid cancer, the malignancy was located in the largest nodule only 72% of the time, and the predictive value of largest-nodule aspiration decreased as the quantity of nodules in the gland increased.[20]

Large multinodular goiter (MNG) may be readily apparent on physical examination and may show an ultrasound pattern with a gland replaced by multiple, confluent nodules of similar appearance. FNA for diagnosis is not necessary before surgical treatment of MNG when no suspicious nodules are observed on sonography. MNG is far more common in iodine deficient regions. Surgery is often sought when cosmetic concerns or compressive symptoms arise.

CERVICAL LYMPH NODES

The presence of radiologically suspicious cervical lymph nodes is a high-risk feature for which biopsy of concurrent thyroid nodules (and suspicious lymph nodes if this would change management) is recommended.[2] Radiographic features suggestive of malignancy in lymph nodes include the absence of an echogenic hilum, round shape, cystic component, irregular borders, hyper-echogenicity, and peripheral vascularity.[52] FNA of cervical lymph nodes showing thyroid cancer is presumed metastatic disease from a thyroid gland primary tumor. Regional spread of thyroid disease most commonly involves the central neck (level IV), followed by the lateral neck (levels II to IV) and posterior neck (level V).[53] (See ultrasound evaluation of thyroid nodules and cervical lymph nodes discussed in Chapter 13, Ultrasound of the Thyroid and Parathyroid Glands and Chapter 14, Preoperative Radiographic Mapping of Nodal Disease for Papillary Thyroid Carcinoma).

THYROID NODULE RISK STRATIFICATION

In the past decade, several guidelines have been proposed for thyroid nodule risk stratification based on sonographic features; the goal of the guidelines is to determine which nodules warrant further evaluation by either biopsy or follow-up. Not all nodules require biopsy or follow-up, and a common goal of these risk stratification systems is to maximize identification of clinically significant malignancies (or those high-risk nodules requiring further evaluation by FNA) while simultaneously minimizing the number of biopsies performed on benign nodules.

The ATA released its most recent iteration of management guidelines for patients with thyroid nodules and DTC in 2015.[2] These guidelines notably include a widely-accepted, pattern-based risk stratification system using sonographic features to determine recommended size cutoffs to perform FNA. Here, FNA is recommended for size cutoffs of ≥ 1.0 cm ("high suspicion" or "intermediate suspicion"), ≥ 1.5 cm ("low suspicion"), and ≥ 2.0 cm ("very low suspicion").

Other professional groups, including the Korean Society of Thyroid Radiology (KSThR, 2016),[54,55] European Thyroid Association (ETA, 2017),[56] and combined American Association of Clinical Endocrinologists (AACE), American College of Endocrinology (ACE), and Associazione Medici Endocrinologi (AME, 2016)[57] have developed and subsequently updated similar classification systems, although with varying size cut-offs and delineation of risk by specific features.

In 2017, the ACR released updated guidelines for sonographic risk stratification in thyroid cancer termed TI-RADS (Thyroid Imaging, Reporting and Data System) modeled on the analogous and widely-accepted Breast Imaging and Reporting Data System (BI-RADS).[51] ACR TI-RADS scores thyroid nodules based on sonographic features including composition, echogenicity, shape, margin, and echogenic foci; nodules are then categorized by point-score as "benign" (TR1), "not suspicious" (TR2), "mildly suspicious" (TR3), "moderately suspicious" (TR4), or "highly suspicious" (TR5). TR1 and TR2 categories do not require FNA or monitoring, whereas TR3-5 nodules should undergo FNA at size cut-offs of ≥ 2.5 cm (TR3), ≥ 1.5 cm (TR4), and ≥ 1.0 cm (TR5). TR3-5 nodules not meeting FNA criteria are also recommended to be followed by ultrasound at more inclusive thresholds of ≥ 1.5 cm, ≥ 1.0 cm, and ≥ 0.5 cm, respectively. Importantly, these additional recommendations for follow-up, rather than immediate FNA, may allow fewer biopsies for patients with likely benign nodules or indolent cancers while allowing significant malignancies to be detected.[58,59]

Middleton et al. compared the performance of the ACR TI-RADS, KSThR TI-RADS, and ATA guidelines in a multi-institutional study of 3422 thyroid nodules with final pathology available.[60] ACR TI-RADS had the highest yield of malignancy at 14.2% for FNA-recommended nodules. Although this system only recommended biopsy for 68.2% of nodules that it ultimately found to be malignant (KSThR TI-RADS 78.7%, ATA 75.9%), the ACR TI-RADS recommended that 89.2% of malignant nodules be *biopsied or followed* and had the lowest percentage of benign nodules recommended for biopsy at 47.1% (KSThR TI-RADS 79.1%, ATA 78.1%). The ACR TI-RADS was also unique in that it was able to classify all nodules, whereas the KSThR TI-RADS and ATA guidelines were unable to classify 3.9% and 14.2%, respectively. A study by Yoon et al. additionally found that the ATA guidelines were unable to classify 3.4% of thyroid nodules, 18.2% of which were subsequently found to be malignant.[61] In such circumstances, the decision of whether or not to biopsy must be based on clinical judgment. These studies are notably biased by inclusion of only those nodules undergoing FNA or surgery.

All of these classification systems share an underlying goal of decreasing unnecessary FNAs and increasing the FNA yield of high-risk cancers. There is currently insufficient evidence or longitudinal follow-up to determine which classification system is best. Due to variation in interpretation, these systems are limited by less-than-perfect interrater reliability; however, the systems tend to provide overall similar determinations of which nodules to biopsy.[62,63] Each system balances resource overutilization and risks of unnecessary biopsy of clinically insignificant nodules while simultaneously attempting to maximize identification of malignancies that require further treatment. Regardless of which sonographic classification schema is used, the ultimate decision to perform FNA should also weigh physician clinical judgment, physician and patient preferences, and additional patient factors including clinical risk factors for malignancy, comorbidities, life expectancy, and goals of care.

FINE NEEDLE ASPIRATION, BETHESDA CLASSIFICATION, AND MOLECULAR TESTING

Fine Needle Aspiration

FNA is the diagnostic test of choice to distinguish benign versus malignant thyroid nodules.[2] FNA is accepted as a safe, cost-effective, and reliable procedure that may be performed by a range of providers in a multidisciplinary care team, including surgeons, endocrinologists, and radiologists. It may be performed in a variety of settings (e.g., simple clinic room, procedure room, or radiology suite) and most commonly requires only local anesthetic. The FNA procedure is typically performed with a simple 5- or 10-cc syringe attached to a 25- to 27-gauge needle (Figure 10.2). After lidocaine administration, the needle is inserted under ultrasound guidance and undulated with the tip of the needle visualized within the thyroid nodule. Between 2 and 5 separate needle samples are combined to constitute an adequate FNA biopsy for one nodule. Risks of FNA are rare and include pain, infection, and localized bruising. When performed by a trained provider under ultrasound guidance, the risk of tracheal, carotid, or jugular puncture is extremely low. A practical discussion of risks and benefits of this procedure include the more likely event that results will return as insufficient (5% to 10%) or indeterminate (20% to 30%), which may require subsequent biopsy or diagnostic surgery.[64]

Ultrasound guidance is recommended for thyroid nodule FNA. Compared with palpation-guided FNA, ultrasound-guided FNA offers lower rates of nondiagnostic samples, lower rates of false negatives, better diagnostic accuracy, and increased cancer yield.[65,66] Nodules with initial nondiagnostic cytology should be repeated with ultrasound guidance and onsite cytologic evaluation, when available.[2] The presence of immediate, onsite microscopic sample analysis allows for immediate assessment of whether samples are adequate for diagnostic classification, which allows the physician to perform more passes at the same visit, if initially deemed inadequate. However, this may not be logistically feasible in all practice settings. Up to 50% of FNAs repeated after nondiagnostic cytology will ultimately produce a diagnostic sample.[67] Repeatedly nondiagnostic nodules may be followed by observation or undergo diagnostic lobectomy. Presence of higher-suspicion sonographic patterns, nodular growth on surveillance, or clinical risk factors favor lobectomy for histopathologic diagnosis.[2]

Therapeutic aspiration of purely cystic nodules may be performed to alleviate symptoms related to size and compression, although recurrence of cystic fluid is common. When 100% cystic, cytologic analysis is not necessary. Recurrent cystic nodules with benign cytology can alternatively be managed by concurrent aspiration with percutaneous ethanol injection, which has been shown to have lower recurrence rates

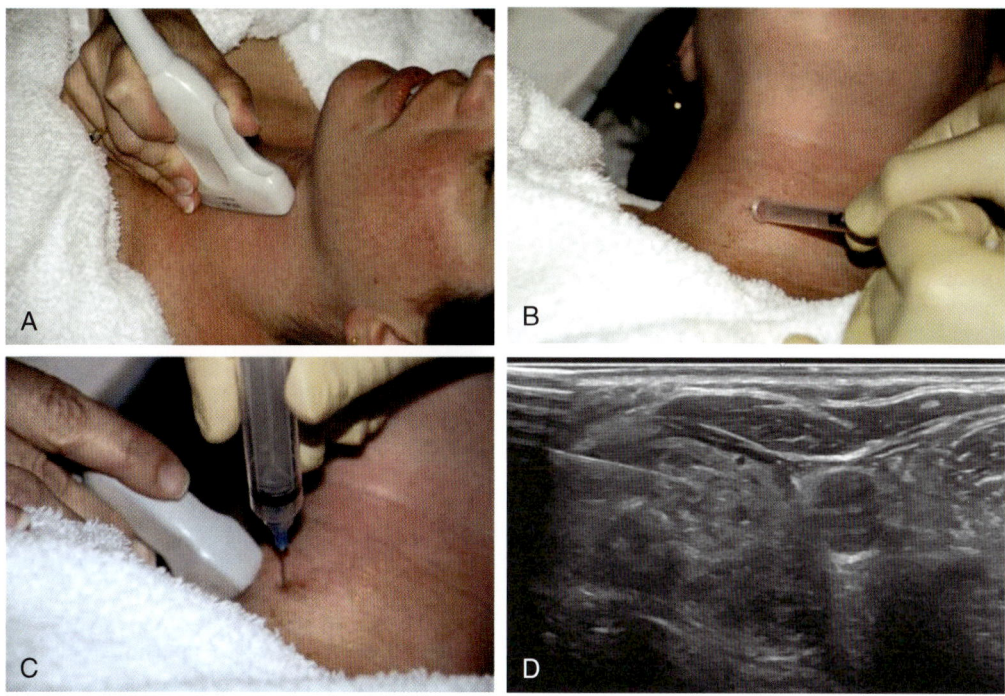

Fig. 10.2 Thyroid Nodule FNA Technique. **A,** Ultrasound identification of thyroid nodule and superficial skin marking. **B,** Subcutaneous lidocaine administered with a 30-g needle. **C,** Fine-needle aspirations performed with 10-cc syringe and 25-g needle. **D,** Sonographic view during procedure with needle in thyroid nodule.

than simple aspiration alone.[63] Image-guided procedures, such as radiofrequency, laser, microwave, and high-intensity focused ultrasound ablation, have more recently emerged as minimally-invasive techniques for the treatment of cystic or solid benign thyroid nodules.

Cytology and Bethesda Classification

The Bethesda System for Reporting Thyroid Cytopathology, updated in 2017, is the most widely accepted classification system for reporting FNA cytology.[64,68] Thyroid nodule cytology is reported in one of six diagnostic categories, each with a determined risk of malignancy (Table 10.1).[69]

Bethesda category 1 (nondiagnostic) is discussed in the previous section and warrants repeat FNA with ultrasound guidance. Category 2 (benign) lesions are typically managed with clinical and/or sonographic follow-up with the specific elements and timing of follow-up determined by sonographic patterns (See Chapter 11, Fine-Needle Aspiration of the Thyroid Gland—The 2017 Bethesda System). Bethesda categories 5 and 6 are generally treated surgically, with extent determined by tumor size, concern for extrathyroidal extension, nodal involvement, clinical risk factors, surgeon/patient presences, and personalized decision making.[2,70] Bethesda category 3 (atypical of undetermined significance [AUS] or follicular lesion of undetermined

TABLE 10.1 The 2017 Bethesda System for Reporting Thyroid Cytopathology and Implied Risk of Malignancy

Diagnostic Category	Risk of Malignancy if NIFTP ≠ CA (%)	Risk of Malignancy if NIFTP = CA (%)	Usual Management*
(I) Nondiagnostic of Unsatisfactory	5–10	5–10	Repeat FNA with ultrasound guidance
(II) Benign	0–3	0–3	Clinical and sonographic follow-up
(III) Atypical of Undetermined Significance (AUS) or Follicular Lesion of Undetermined Significance (FLUS)	6–18	10–30	Repeat FNA, molecular testing, or lobectomy
(IV) Follicular Neoplasm (FN) or Suspicious for Follicular Neoplasm (SFN)	10–40	25–40	Molecular testing, lobectomy
(V) Suspicious for Malignancy	45–60	50–75	Near-total thyroidectomy or lobectomy[†,‡]
(VI) Malignant	94–96	97–99	Near-total thyroidectomy or lobectomy[‡]

*Actual management may depend on other factors (e.g., clinical, sonographic) besides the FNA interpretation.
[†]Some studies have recommended molecular analysis to assess the type of surgical procedure (lobectomy versus total thyroidectomy).
[‡]In the case of "suspicious for metastatic tumor" or a "malignant" interpretation indicating metastatic tumor rather than a primary thyroid malignancy, surgery may not be indicated.
NIFTP, noninvasive follicular thyroid neoplasm with papillary-like nuclear features, CA, carcinoma, FNA, fine-needle aspiration.
Adapted from Ali S, Cibas E. *The Bethesda System for Reporting Thyroid Cytopathology: Definitions, Criteria, and Explanatory Notes.* 2nd ed. New York, NY: Springer; 2018.

significance [FLUS]) and 4 (follicular neoplasm [FN] or suspicious for follicular neoplasm [SFN]) are considered indeterminate cytology. Follicular and Hurthle cell neoplasms (adenoma versus carcinoma) have traditionally required diagnostic lobectomy to assess architecture, capsular invasion, and vascular invasion for confirmatory diagnosis. Furthermore, diagnostic lobectomy is required for diagnosis of the more recently-defined entity of noninvasive follicular tumor with papillary-like features (NIFTP).[71] NIFTP represents new nomenclature for noninvasive encapsulated follicular variant of papillary thyroid carcinoma (EFVPRTC). On long-term follow-up, EFVPRTC has proven to have little or no propensity toward recurrence or metastasis.

The updated Bethesda System for Reporting Thyroid Cytopathology includes recalculated risks of malignancy based on post-2010 data and includes two sets of risk estimates for malignancy to accommodate NIFTP, which may be classified as benign or malignant. Similarly, definitions of PTC and FN/SFN have been revised to reflect that some of these may prove to be NIFTP. Finally, "usual management" of indeterminate categories (3, AUS/FLUS; and 4, FN/SFN) now recognizes the option for molecular testing.

Molecular Testing

Over the past decade, molecular testing has evolved in an effort to reduce unnecessary diagnostic lobectomy for indeterminate nodules.[72] These ancillary tests leverage the fact that thyroid cancers exhibit common pathogenic patterns of gene mutation (e.g., *BRAF* in PTC) or rearrangement (e.g., *RET/PTC* oncogene in radiation-induced PTCs). Logistically, testing involves sending cytologic samples obtained by FNA for further analysis. The cost of molecular testing is substantial, estimated at $3000 to $5000 depending on which test is chosen.[73] The most commonly used testing strategies include mutational analysis (seven-gene mutation panel), gene expression analysis (Afirma GSC), or a combined, comprehensive approach (ThyroSeq, ThyGenX/ThyraMIR). An additional approach to molecular testing includes microRNAs tests (Rosetta GX Reveal), which act as gene regulators and may show differential expression patterns in thyroid cancer.[74]

Mutational analysis involves genetic sequencing of cells isolated by FNA. Mutational analysis is termed a "rule-in" test because it has high positive predictive value (PPV) and specificity; when the commonly tested mutations and fusion genes are positively identified, the likelihood of thyroid cancer is very high.[75] Thus this test is designed to identify nodules that will require surgical intervention and has the potential to decrease the number of patients who require two-stage surgeries (positive diagnostic lobectomy followed by completion thyroidectomy) when an indication for total thyroidectomy can be predicted up front. The latter benefit is of more limited value in the recent era; indications for lobectomy as definitive surgery for low-risk malignancy have expanded.[2] PPV and specificity for "rule-in" testing are reported to be as high as 87% to 88% and 97% to 99%, respectively (seven-gene mutation panel).[76]

Gene expression analysis or genomic sequencing classifier (GSC) testing uses rapid genetic sequencing of a large panel of genes within a propriety algorithm to predict benign versus malignant disease. GSC testing is termed a "rule-out" test; it is designed a priori to have a high negative predictive value (NPV) and high sensitivity. When nodules are classified as "benign" rather than "suspicious," the risk of malignancy is very low.[77,78] The NPV of GSC tests approximates that of a benign cytology finding. Thus the utility of GSC testing is in determining which patients can avoid diagnostic surgery. A decreased number of surgeries and associated complications in cases where GSC is negative argues for cost-effectiveness as a major strength of testing.[79] NPV and sensitivity for molecular testing are reported to be as high as 96% to 97% (ThyroSeq v2.1[80]) and 92% to 94% (Afirma GSC,[77] ThyGenX/ThyraMIR[81]), respectively.

Molecular testing is increasingly entering the decision-making algorithm used by practitioners to guide management of thyroid nodules. Providers wishing to incorporate molecular testing into their clinical practice should do so with a clear understanding of testing goals and limitations, which should also be discussed with the patient. The PPV and NPV of these tests are notably dependent on the prevalence of malignancy, which can vary geographically or by institution. With continued improvement, an attractive prospect of molecular testing includes the potential to provide prognostic information to inform treatment decisions, specifically in determining which cancers allow observation, warrant surgical removal, or would benefit from additional adjuvant radioactive iodine or systemic therapy. Molecular testing is further discussed in Chapter 12, FNA and Molecular Analysis.

MANAGEMENT OF THYROID NODULES

Observation Strategies

Cytologically benign nodules, or those not meeting size criteria for biopsy based on sonographic suspicion pattern, may be observed. Observation strategies are variable and depend on a number of clinical, radiographic, and cytologic factors. According to the 2015 ATA guidelines, cytologically benign nodules with high-suspicion sonographic patterns warrant repeat ultrasound and FNA within 12 months.[2] Benign nodules with intermediate- or low-suspicion sonographic features may have repeat ultrasound or FNA (particularly if growth has occurred). Nodules which have benign cytology results on two ultrasound-guided FNAs have an exceedingly low likelihood of malignancy and do not require continued surveillance.[82] Nodules that have not had FNA should undergo repeat ultrasound evaluation with the interval determined by sonographic pattern. The 2015 ATA guidelines provide recommendations for the timing of repeat ultrasound of high-suspicion nodules (6 to 12 months), intermediate-/low-suspicion nodules (12 to 24 months), and very low–suspicion nodules ($\geq$24 months, if ever).[2] In sonographic follow-up, new suspicious sonographic features or nodular growth (20% in 2 dimensions, 2 mm, or 50% volume increase) warrants consideration of repeat FNA. Durante et al. have proposed a similar algorithm for the follow-up of cytologically benign thyroid nodules or nodules without indication for FNA.[83] Asymptomatic hyperfunctioning nodules may also be observed. Currently, there is no clear consensus on the duration of follow-up for benign nodules. (See management of cytologically benign nodules, as discussed in Chapter 11, Fine-Needle Aspiration of the Thyroid Gland—The 2017 Bethesda System).

Although a mainstay of the management of thyroid nodules in the past, TSH-suppressive dosing of thyroid hormone is no longer recommended due to the potential harms of iatrogenic hyperthyroidism. Despite this recommendation, nearly one fourth of managing physicians were recently reported to continue this practice.[2,57,84]

Treatment for Benign Thyroid Nodules and Role of Diagnostic Lobectomy

Surgery for cytologically benign nodules should be considered when there are compressive symptoms, cosmetic concerns with a very large goiter, hyperfunctioning nodule(s), or for diagnostic purposes in the rare situation were malignancy is strongly suspected despite benign cytology.[2,57]

Hyperfunctioning thyroid nodules in the setting of thyrotoxicosis may represent solitary or multiple toxic nodular disease. Radioiodine therapy (^{131}I) and surgery are the mainstays of treatment for toxic nodules. Radioiodine aims to ablate all autonomously functioning thyroid tissue and is generally preferred for patients who are poor surgical candidates, such as the elderly or those with significant medical comorbidities. Surgical treatment with near-total or total thyroidectomy (e.g., due to toxic nodular goiter) versus thyroid lobectomy (e.g., due to solitary toxic nodule) is more definitive and is favored in cases that are refractory to radioiodine ablation or in cases of substernal/compressive goiter ^{131}I. Such cases may transiently worsen compressive symptoms due to radiation thyroiditis. Solitary toxic nodules may also be managed with percutaneous ethanol injection in cases where contraindications to both surgery and ^{131}I exist, or in combination with ^{131}I when surgery is not an option. Treatment strategies for toxic multinodular goiter and solitary toxic nodule are further discussed in Chapter 8, The Surgical Management of Hyperthyroidism.

Indications for diagnostic lobectomy include repeated nondiagnostic FNA or indeterminate FNA, as described earlier, although such nodules may also be observed depending on level of suspicion and patient-specific risks and benefits. The subsequent decision to perform completion thyroidectomy is determined by final pathology. As a general rule, the final extent of surgery should reflect that which would have been performed if the final pathology was known before diagnostic lobectomy. Compared with total thyroidectomy, thyroid lobectomy carries significantly lower risk of surgical complications.[85]

Management of Malignant Thyroid Nodules

Management of malignant thyroid nodules is complex and beyond the scope of the current chapter. Decision making, active surveillance, and surgical management for thyroid cancer are discussed at length in the following sections of the text: Section 4, Thyroid Neoplasia; Section 5, Thyroid and Neck Surgery; Section 6, Postoperative Considerations; and Section 7, Postoperative Management.

CONCLUSION

Most thyroid nodules are low-risk. Thus thyroid nodule evaluation and management should strive to identify clinically significant nodules that will require treatment while minimizing unnecessary patient risk and optimizing resource utilization. The most effective approach to both evaluation and treatment includes a multidisciplinary care team including primary care, internal medicine, endocrinology, radiology, cytopathology, general/endocrine surgery, and otolaryngology. A guiding principle of nodule evaluation and management is accurate risk stratification; as diagnostic and prognostic tests continue to improve, patient care will benefit from a more personalized approach to medical decision making.

REFERENCES

For a complete list of references, go to expertconsult.com.

Fine-Needle Aspiration of the Thyroid Gland
The 2017 Bethesda System

William C. Faquin, Guido Fadda, Edmund S. Cibas

> Please go to expertconsult.com to view related video:
> **Video 11.1** Thyroid Nodule Fine-Needle Aspiration.
> **Video 11.2** Fine-Needle Aspiration Slide Preparation.

INTRODUCTION

Fine-needle aspiration (FNA) is an essential test in the evaluation of a patient with a thyroid nodule. The result of the FNA determines, in large part, whether a patient can be followed clinically or referred for surgery. Guidelines have been established for selecting a nodule for aspiration.[1] Once the decision has been made to perform an FNA, its value can be enhanced by attention to technical details. In general, smaller needles (25 and 27 G) are superior to larger ones; a shorter "dwell time" (the time the needle is kept in the lesion) is often superior to longer dwell times, which introduce more blood; and rapid oscillations within the nodule (two to five per second) are better than slow excursions with the needle. Communication between the operator (if the FNA is not performed by a pathologist) and the pathologist is essential. The pathologist's interpretation is greatly aided if essential clinical information (e.g., history of hypothyroidism, etc.) is provided on the requisition form. The Bethesda System for Reporting Thyroid Cytopathology (TBSRTC) has standardized the reporting of thyroid cytopathology and consists of six diagnostic categories.[2,3]

INDICATIONS FOR THYROID FNA

Thyroid nodules are discovered either by palpation or by an imaging study. A palpable thyroid nodule should undergo further evaluation to determine whether an FNA is warranted.[1] Before the decision is made, a serum thyroid stimulating hormone level (TSH) and thyroid ultrasound (US) should be obtained. Patients with a normal or elevated serum TSH level should proceed to a thyroid US to determine whether an FNA needs to be performed. Those with a depressed serum TSH should have a radionuclide thyroid scan, the results of which should be correlated with the sonographic findings. Functioning thyroid nodules in the absence of significant clinical findings do not require an FNA because the incidence of malignancy is exceedingly low.[4] A nodule that appears either iso- or hypofunctioning on radionuclide scan should be considered for FNA, based on the US findings.

Incidental thyroid nodules (i.e., incidentalomas) are detected by US,[5] ^{18}F-fluorodeoxyglucose-positron emission tomography (^{18}FDG-PET), sestamibi, computed tomography (CT), and magnetic resonance imaging (MRI) scans. Incidental thyroid nodules detected by US should undergo a dedicated thyroid sonographic evaluation. Lesions with a maximum diameter greater than 1.0 to 1.5 cm should be considered for biopsy unless they are simple cysts or septated cysts with no solid elements. FNA may also occasionally be replaced by periodic follow-up for nodules of borderline size (between 1.0 and 1.5 cm in maximum diameter) if the nodules have sonographic features that are strongly associated with benign cytology.

A nodule of any size with sonographically suspicious features should also be considered for FNA. Sonographically suspicious features include microcalcifications, hypoechoic solid nodules, irregular/lobulated margins, intranodular vascularity, and nodal metastases (or signs of extracapsular spread). The recommendation for FNA is controversial because it includes patients with microcarcinomas, in whom a survival benefit after an FNA diagnosis has not been documented. If the FNA reveals that the nodule is malignant, surgery is generally recommended, but the natural history of papillary microcarcinomas is not well understood. Most remain indolent, as implied by the 13% prevalence of micropapillary cancers in the United States at autopsy examination.[6] A minority of cases follow a more aggressive course; this subgroup might be identified by sonographic evidence of lateral cervical node metastases, tumor multifocality, extrathyroidal invasion, or cytopathologic features that suggest a high-grade malignancy.[7]

Incidentalomas detected by ^{18}FDG-PET (2% to 3% of all PET scans) are unusual but have a substantial risk of cancer of approximately 35%.[1,8-16] A focally ^{18}FDG-PET–avid thyroid nodule is much more likely to represent thyroid cancer than metastatic disease to the thyroid, even in patients with an extrathyroidal malignancy. Therefore a focal nodule that is ^{18}FDG-PET-avid is an indication for FNA. Diffuse increased uptake on ^{18}FDG-PET does not warrant FNA unless thyroid sonography detects a discrete nodule.

Thyroid incidentalomas detected on sestamibi scans have a high risk of cancer that ranges from 22% to 66%.[5,17-20] All focal hot nodules detected on sestamibi scans and confirmed by US to be a discrete nodules should undergo FNA.

Thyroid incidentalomas detected by CT or MRI are seen in at least 16% of patients evaluated by neck CT or MRI.[21] The risk of cancer in one study was predicted at 10%, but it included only a limited number of patients who went on to FNA.[22] CT and MRI features cannot determine the risk of malignancy, except in very advanced cases that are unlikely to be incidental. Until more data are available, incidentalomas seen on CT or MRI should undergo dedicated thyroid sonographic evaluation. Any nodule with sonographically suspicious features (as mentioned previously) should be considered for FNA, especially if the nodule has a maximum diameter greater than 1.0 to 1.5 cm.

FNA TECHNIQUE

The core-needle biopsy (CNB) is a procedure that involves the use of spring-activated large bore needles (18 G to 21 G), which produces a small tissue fragment. The advantage of this technique is a larger amount of cells, which may decrease the rate of inadequate diagnoses and may allow the application of ancillary studies.[23,24] The disadvantages of CNB include the increased rate of complications, such as hemorrhage, local pain, as well as difficulty in performing multiple samplings of the lesion.[25-28] Some organizations have endorsed the use of CNB only in cases of repeated nondiagnostic yields using conventional cytology.[29]

FNA of the thyroid gland can be processed by making conventional smears (CS), either air-dried or ethanol-fixed, or by using the thin-layer or liquid-based cytology (LBC) technique. LBC was originally developed for application to gynecologic cervical smears, and CS was the traditional method for decades. Both CS and LBC are acceptable methods, and some laboratories prefer to use a combination of CS and LBC. In addition, a formalin-fixed cell block can be made in selected cases for the purpose of performing ancillary studies.

The LBC technique is based on a two-step procedure: (1) the fixation of the FNA material in an alcohol-based solution (methanol or ethanol depending on the technique, discussed later), and (2) the automated processing of the material to obtain a thin layer of representative cells. LBC uses an innovative, computer-assisted device that allows the transfer of the fixed and partially disaggregated cells onto a single slide. The two most common methods for processing the cytologic samples use an alcohol-based fixative solution. In the first method (ThinPrep™ system, Hologic Co., Marlborough, Massachusetts), the cells are aspirated from a methanol-based solution (Cytolit™) then filtered and transferred onto a positively charged slide with a gentle positive pressure. In the second method (BD SurePath™ liquid-based technique, Wokingham Berkshire, UK), the cells are collected in an ethanol-based solution (CytoRich™), centrifuged twice, then slowly sedimented onto a poly L-lysinated slide, and then eventually stained with a specific hematoxylin-eosin stain. The final result for both methods is one slide for each lesion where all cells are concentrated in a thin layer on the central area of the slide measuring 20 square mm for ThinPrep and 13 square mm for SurePath.[28,30,31] The LBC method enables the storage of a variable amount of cells in a preservative solution for up to 6 months after the biopsy and the making of a cell block directly from the leftover material.[32]

If pathologists perform the FNA and perform rapid on-site evaluation (ROSE), the adequacy of the sample will likely be higher; however, this requires a significant investment of resources. Treating clinicians, who are more familiar with the clinical picture, more often perform the FNA themselves. The different rates of inadequacy of FNA carried out by treating clinicians suggest that experience is an essential requisite to obtaining an adequate cytologic sample.[33,34] However, regardless of the subspecialty of the operator, the procedure should be carried out with appropriate frequency and information exchange between the clinicians (e.g., pathologists, endocrinologists, and surgeons) who treat the patient.[35,36,37,38]

ACCURACY OF THYROID FNA

Thyroid FNA is widely accepted as a highly cost-effective and accurate means of evaluating a thyroid nodule. For the diagnosis of papillary thyroid carcinoma, FNA is considered by some to be at least as accurate as frozen section, reflecting the importance of nuclear cytology for diagnosing papillary carcinoma.[37,38] False-negative and false-positive thyroid FNA diagnoses occur, but such occurrences are uncommon, averaging less than 5% and 1%, respectively.[39] Errors are a result of both sampling and interpretation. In experienced hands, the diagnostic accuracy of thyroid FNA for technically satisfactory specimens is greater than 95%, with positive predictive values of 89% to 98% and negative predictive values of 94% to 99%.[40,41] However, these values are dependent on how the "atypia of undetermined significance/follicular neoplasm of undetermined significance" and "suspicious for a follicular neoplasm" categories are used in the calculations.[42] The risk of malignancy (ROM) can vary depending on how noninvasive follicular thyroid neoplasm with papillary-like nuclear features (NIFTP) is incorporated into the calculations.[3] Sensitivities for thyroid FNA range from 43% to 98% and specificities range from 72% to 100%.[40,41] These wide ranges, in part, reflect the skill of the person performing the FNA as well as the expertise of the cytopathologist interpreting the specimens. For the evaluation of cystic thyroid lesions, FNA is reported to have a low sensitivity (40%), because cystic aspirates will often yield cyst contents only (e.g., foam cells, hemosiderin-laden macrophages, and acellular debris) with rare epithelial cells. Caution is warranted in interpreting cystic thyroid aspirates because a subset of thyroid cysts represent cystic papillary carcinomas.

REPORTING TERMINOLOGY: THE BETHESDA SYSTEM

For clarity of communication, TBSRTC recommends that each report begin with one of six *general diagnostic categories* (Box 11.1).[2,3] For some categories, TBSRTC offers a choice of two names; a consensus was not reached at the National Cancer Institute (NCI) conference on a single name for these categories. Each of the categories has an implied cancer risk that links it to an evidence-based management guideline (Table 11.1). The term "indeterminate" is not advised for reporting thyroid FNA results because its meaning is not sufficiently specific and its use has been highly variable.

For some of the general categories, subcategorization can be informative and is often appropriate; recommended terminology is shown in Box 11.1. Additional descriptive comments beyond such subcategorization are optional and left to the discretion of the cytopathologist. Each of the six categories is discussed in greater detail in the sections that follow.

NONDIAGNOSTIC THYROID ASPIRATES

In the best interest of the patient, the cytopathologist must receive an adequate FNA specimen to make a meaningful cytopathologic evaluation and a correct diagnosis. The final cytologic specimen must be adequate in terms of cellularity, and the specimen must be satisfactory in terms of quality (e.g., thickness, fixation, and staining).

Both operators and patients should be aware that FNAs are not always effective; patients should also be given detailed information (e.g., informed consent) regarding the complications of the maneuver

> **BOX 11.1 2017 The Bethesda System for Reporting Thyroid Cytopathology**
>
> **I. Nondiagnostic or Unsatisfactory**
> Cyst fluid only
> Virtually acellular specimen
> Other (obscuring blood, clotting artifact, etc.)
>
> **II. Benign**
> Consistent with a benign follicular nodule (includes adenomatoid nodule, colloid nodule, etc.)
> Consistent with lymphocytic (Hashimoto's) thyroiditis in the proper clinical context
> Consistent with granulomatous (subacute) thyroiditis
> Other
>
> **III. Atypia of Undetermined Significance or Follicular Lesion of Undetermined Significance**
>
> **IV. Follicular Neoplasm or Suspicious for a Follicular Neoplasm**
> Specify if Hürthle cell (oncocytic) type
>
> **V. Suspicious for Malignancy**
> Suspicious for papillary thyroid carcinoma
> Suspicious for medullary thyroid carcinoma
> Suspicious for metastatic carcinoma
> Suspicious for lymphoma
> Other
>
> **VI. Malignant**
> Papillary thyroid carcinoma
> Poorly differentiated carcinoma
> Medullary thyroid carcinoma
> Undifferentiated (anaplastic) carcinoma
> Squamous cell carcinoma
> Carcinoma with mixed features (specify)
> Metastatic carcinoma
> Non-Hodgkin's lymphoma
> Other

From Ali SZ, Cibas ES. *The Bethesda System for Thyroid Cytopathology: Definitions, Criteria, and Explanatory Notes.* 2nd ed. New York, NY: Springer; 2018. With kind permission of Springer Science and Business Media.

and the possibility of a nondiagnostic result. Nondiagnostic samples can occur for two reasons: (1) the sampling of the lesion yields material unsatisfactory for a definitive diagnosis or (2) the aspirated material is nonrepresentative. FNAs are defined as nondiagnostic when fixation, smearing, or staining artifacts impair the interpretation of the final slide (Figure 11.1). A slide is nonrepresentative when the cellularity does not represent the true components of the lesion (e.g., insufficient number of follicular cells). In the first instance, the inadequacy of the sampling could be attributed to an incorrect technique or to preparation artifacts.[43] In the latter, the characteristics of the lesion do not allow a definitive cytologic diagnosis.[2,44,45] In both CS and LBC, the adequacy criteria are met when at least 6 clusters of 10 well-preserved cells are observed.[2,46-48]

Even a discrete amount of colloid on a smear may not mean the nodule is a benign nodule unless the amount of the follicular component is appropriate. When the LBC slide does not contain an adequate number of cells, a second slide can be made with the residual material to meet the adequacy criteria.[49]

Among the nondiagnostic FNA cases, cystic lesions are the most frequently encountered.[50] A thyroid cyst frequently represents a cystic or hemorrhagic regression of a follicular nodule, which might be benign or malignant after repeated samplings. Thyroid cysts may be associated with solid areas at the sonographic examination. In this instance, these solid areas should be specifically sampled under sonographic guidance and, if the cytologic report is nondiagnostic (only red blood cells and hemosiderin-laden histiocytes), a careful US follow-up should be planned (6 to 18 months according to different guidelines).[1,2,29,51]

A "nondiagnostic" FNA report does not mean that the result of the FNA is benign, but that the aspiration must be repeated to assess the nature of the lesion. When a thyroid FNA of a cystic nodule with a solid component is repeatedly nonrepresentative, surgical excision of the nodule may be considered to avoid the possibility of a malignant lesion; such instances of malignant lesions occur in 8% to 19% of cases.[35,45,50,52,53]

BENIGN CONDITIONS

Goiter

About 90% of all thyroid diseases are benign and encompass a wide range of pathophysiologic alterations. *Goiter* is a clinical term meaning an increase of the gland size caused by intermittent or persistent

TABLE 11.1 The 2017 Bethesda System for Reporting Thyroid Cytopathology: Implied Risk of Malignancy and Recommended Clinical Management

Diagnostic Category	Risk of Malignancy if NIFTP = CA (%)	Risk of Malignancy if NIFTP ≠ CA (%)	Usual Management*
Nondiagnostic or unsatisfactory	5-10	5-10	Repeat FNA with ultrasound guidance
Benign	0-3	0-3	Clinical and sonographic follow-up
Atypia of undetermined significance or follicular lesion of undetermined significance	~10-30	6-18	Repeat FNA, molecular testing, lobectomy
Follicular neoplasm or suspicious for a follicular neoplasm	25-40	10-40	Molecular testing, lobectomy
Suspicious for malignancy	50-75	45-60	Near-total thyroidectomy or lobectomy
Malignant	97-99	94-96	Near-total thyroidectomy or lobectomy

*Actual management may depend on other factors (e.g., clinical, sonographic) besides the FNA interpretation.
NIFTP, noninvasive follicular thyroid neoplasm with papillary-like nuclear features, CA, carcinoma, FNA, fine-needle aspiration.
Modified from Ali SZ, Cibas ES. *The Bethesda System for Thyroid Cytopathology: Definitions, Criteria, and Explanatory Notes.* 2nd ed. New York, NY: Springer; 2018. With kind permission of Springer Science and Business Media.

CHAPTER 11 Fine-Needle Aspiration of the Thyroid Gland

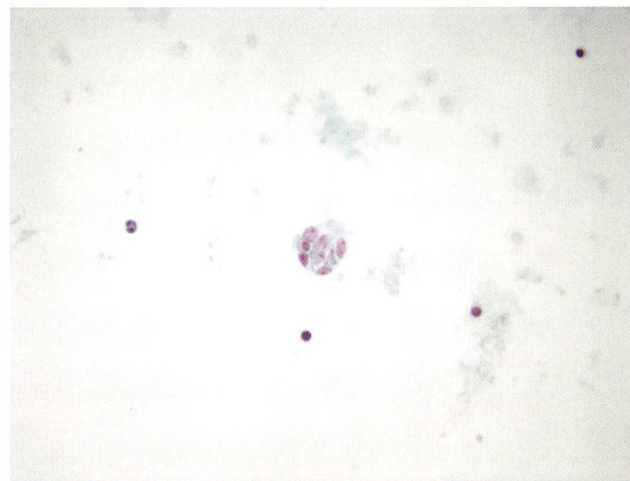

Fig. 11.1 **Nondiagnostic.** A rare cluster of poorly preserved follicular cells showing some nuclear enlargement due to air-drying artifact. Caution is warranted not to overinterpret such artifactual changes as suspicious for a neoplasm. (LBC, Papanicolaou stain.)

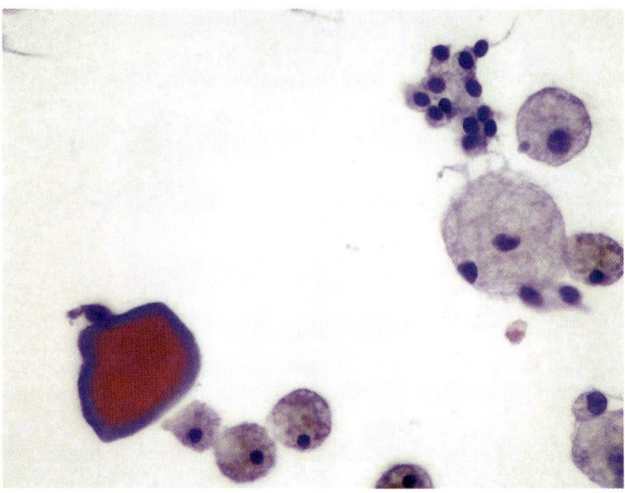

Fig. 11.2 **Benign Goiter.** An adenomatous nodule in a goiter processed by the liquid-based cytology (LBC) technique. The colloid droplet in the right side shows the usual amphophilic staining with the Papanicolaou stain (the center stains orange, the contour blue). The follicular cells with dark regular nuclei and the foamy histiocytes have the same appearance as in conventional smears. (LBC, Papanicolaou stain.)

hyperplasia in response to thyroid-stimulating hormone (TSH). The rise in serum TSH is compensatory to hypothyroxinemia related to different factors (see the following). A goiter may occur as a diffuse enlargement of the thyroid (i.e., diffuse hyperplastic goiter) or may be represented as one or more nodules (i.e., nodular hyperplastic goiter).

Goiter is the most frequent thyroid disease in the world and is often an expression of a decreased ability of the gland to meet the metabolic requirements of the organism. Neoplasms account for a minor portion of thyroid diseases, but the difficulty in segregating hyperplastic from neoplastic disease has led to many studies in the literature.[33,35,38,52-54]

FNAs of nodules in a goiter span a wide spectrum of morphologic changes reflecting different stages of the disease: early follicular hyperplasia, cycles of involution/regeneration, and nodule formation. Secondary changes, such as oxyphilic metaplasia, recent and old hemorrhage, cystic degeneration, necrosis, granulation tissue, fibrosis, and calcification may occur in all of these stages. The most common cytologic picture of "colloid nodule" is characterized by moderate cellularity composed of small thyrocytes, many vacuolated (foamy) histiocytes, and, in the background, abundant colloid, which stains amphophilic with the Papanicolaou stain and deep blue with May-Grünwald Giemsa. Sometimes red blood cells may contaminate the smear, and it is not unusual to find hemosiderin-laden macrophages, which witness a previous hemorrhage. Longstanding goiter may give scanty cellularity composed of fibrovascular tissue with trapped, small epithelial cells. These cases, if colloid and foamy histiocytes are poorly represented, can be easily misdiagnosed as "follicular neoplasms." The nodules in a goiter may reveal a wide range of cytologic components including Hürthle (or oxyphilic) cells, fire-flare (hyperfunctioning) cells and lymphohistiocytes.[35,54]

Cytologically, one of the most important changes occurring in LBC compared with CS slides, is the appearance of the colloid that is fragmented during the filtering procedure (Figure 11.2). Therefore the colloid is observed as small droplets in the background of a benign nodule; the higher the number of these colloid droplets, the higher the likelihood of a benign thyroid nodule.[47,55-57]

A colloid nodule bears a very low risk of malignancy (<5%). Nonetheless, a benign nodule should be followed-up for at least 2 years with US examinations to avoid false-negative results and, if necessary, the FNA could be repeated.[1,2,29,51]

Thyroiditis

A cytologic diagnosis of thyroiditis can, at times, be very challenging diagnostically; the clinical and immunologic findings must be considered.[58,59] A clinical picture of a tender gland with small inconspicuous nodules (the cytology of which shows mature lymphocytes, plasma cells and scattered giant cells) is likely to be a granulomatous thyroiditis (i.e., De Quervain's). An enlargement of the gland, with or without nodules, which exhibits lymphocytes, clusters of histiocytes with tingible body macrophages, and aggregates of oxyphilic cells, favors a diagnosis of chronic lymphocytic thyroiditis (CLT). The latter diagnosis is confirmed by the elevation of serum antibodies against thyroglobulin and/or thyroperoxidase. Different combinations of clinical, serologic, and morphologic profiles may occur. The LBC picture of thyroiditis is similar to CS with one exception: in CLT, the amount of lymphocytes in the background of the slide can be higher than normal because of the concentration of the material before the automated process with LBC. When CLT is suspected, the detection of lymphoepithelial clusters in an inflammatory background is a key to the cytologic diagnosis[47] (Figure 11.3).

A cytologic diagnosis of thyroiditis means a benign lesion in the majority of instances. Oxyphilic hyperplastic nodules in a CLT are not usually surgically removed because they represent the functional replacement of the follicular parenchyma infiltrated by the inflammatory cells. The occurrence of an oxyphilic carcinoma within a CLT is exceedingly uncommon when compared with the frequency of papillary carcinoma, which can readily be detected by cytology.[60,61]

Toxic Goiter

FNA is infrequently used in cases of toxic goiter unless a lesion which is "cold" by scan is detected. However, some cases in which the cytopathologist faces this diagnosis can occur: (1) a preclinical hyperfunctioning nodule, where a decrease of the circulating TSH is the only clinical sign; (2) a "cold" nodule within a toxic goiter, where the sampled lesion can be a hyperplastic nodule inhibited by the surrounding toxic goiter; (3) a rapidly growing toxic nodule during suppressive therapy; and (4) a hyperplastic nodule in a CLT. The cytologic picture of a toxic nodule is, in both CS and LBC, a follicular lesion showing microfollicles layered by medium-sized thyrocytes with distinctive vacuolated cytoplasms

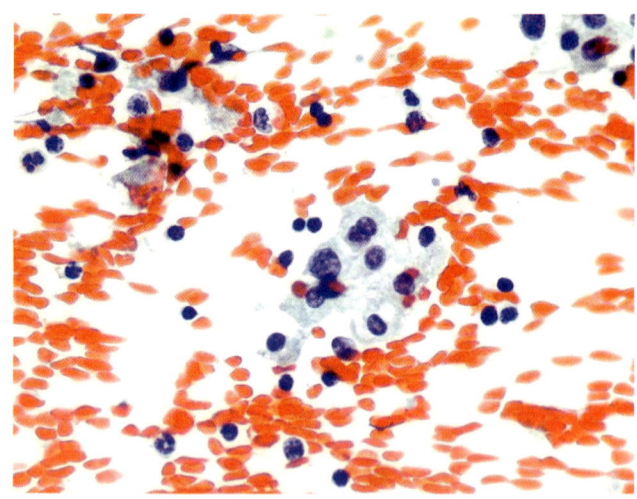

Fig. 11.3 Benign, Chronic Lymphocytic Thyroiditis. This aspirate shows a background of mature lymphohistiocytic elements and a cluster of oxyphilic cells in the center that are characteristic of chronic lymphocytic thyroiditis. (Papanicolaou stain.)

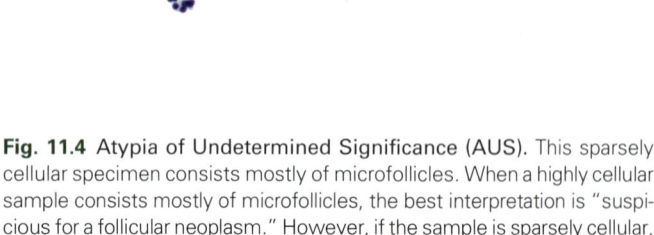

Fig. 11.4 Atypia of Undetermined Significance (AUS). This sparsely cellular specimen consists mostly of microfollicles. When a highly cellular sample consists mostly of microfollicles, the best interpretation is "suspicious for a follicular neoplasm." However, if the sample is sparsely cellular, it is best interpreted as AUS. A repeat fine-needle aspiration in 3 to 6 months will often clarify the uncertainty in diagnosis. (Papanicolaou stain.)

("fire-flare" or "flame cells").[62] The colloid in the background is scant and focal nuclear pleomorphism in a longstanding goiter may be detected. Scattered lymphoid cells may be present in a smear of a toxic goiter, and cells with features of hyperfunction may appear in an otherwise obvious colloid nodule or in thyroiditis.

The hyperfunctioning features described previously are important in the decision for clinical follow-up rather than surgery in a single follicular-patterned thyroid nodule.[63] Because the risk of malignancy in a toxic nodule is low, the detection of hyperfunctioning thyrocytes rules out this possibility, which may help avoid an unnecessary thyroidectomy.

ATYPIA OF UNDETERMINED SIGNIFICANCE OR FOLLICULAR LESION OF UNDETERMINED SIGNIFICANCE

Some thyroid FNAs are not easily classified into the benign, suspicious, or malignant categories. Such cases represent a minority of thyroid FNAs and in TBSRTC are reported as "Atypia of Undetermined Significance (AUS)" or "Follicular Lesion of Undetermined Significance (FLUS)." AUS and FLUS are synonymous, so the laboratory should choose the one it prefers and use it exclusively for this category. The AUS/FLUS category is reserved for specimens "that contain cells (follicular, lymphoid, or other) with architectural and/or nuclear atypia that is not sufficient to be classified as suspicious for a follicular neoplasm, suspicious for malignancy, or malignant. On the other hand, the atypia is more marked than can be ascribed confidently to benign changes."[2] A common contributing factor to the diagnostic uncertainty is the comprised nature of the specimen (e.g., sparse cellularity, obscuring blood, etc.), but these compromising conditions are not sufficient per se to place a specimen in the AUS category.

The heterogeneity of this category precludes outlining all scenarios for which an AUS/FLUS interpretation is appropriate. Two examples are illustrated in Figure 11.4 and Figure 11.5. The most common scenarios are described in the Bethesda System atlas.[2,3]

An AUS/FLUS result is obtained in 1% to 22% of thyroid FNAs.[3,35,38,64] An effort should be made to use this category as a last resort and limit its use to approximately 10% or fewer of all thyroid FNAs. Higher rates likely represent an overuse of this category when other interpretations are more appropriate.

The risk of malignancy for an AUS/FLUS nodule is difficult to ascertain because only a minority of cases in this category have surgical follow-up. Those that are resected represent a selected population of patients with repeated AUS results or worrisome clinical or sonographic findings. In this selected population, up to 50% of patients with AUS/FLUS prove to have cancer after surgery, but this is undoubtedly an overestimate of the risk for all AUS interpretations.[35,38] The true risk of malignancy is estimated at 10% to 30% (6% to 18% if NIFTP is not considered a malignancy).

The recommended management for most patients with an initial AUS/FLUS interpretation is a repeat FNA and/or molecular testing.[1] In most cases, a repeat FNA results in a more definitive interpretation; only about 20% of nodules are repeatedly AUS/FLUS.[38,64,65] In some cases, however, the physician may choose not to repeat the FNA. Instead, the physician may follow the nodule clinically or may refer the patient for surgery because of concerning clinical and/or sonographic features.

SUSPICIOUS FOR A FOLLICULAR NEOPLASM/FOLLICULAR NEOPLASM: FOLLICULAR ADENOMAS AND FOLLICULAR CARCINOMAS

Because FNA cannot detect invasion, the role of FNA in evaluating follicular and oncocytic (Hürthle cell) lesions of the thyroid is to function as a screening test. Thus, although a specific diagnosis may not be given, it is possible to subcategorize these lesions into two groups: (1) those that are almost certainly benign (including most multinodular goiters and some adenomas), and (2) those that are suspicious for a follicular neoplasm and possibly malignant (including all carcinomas and some adenomas). This subcategorization identifies a majority of patients with benign lesions for whom surgical intervention can usually be avoided.

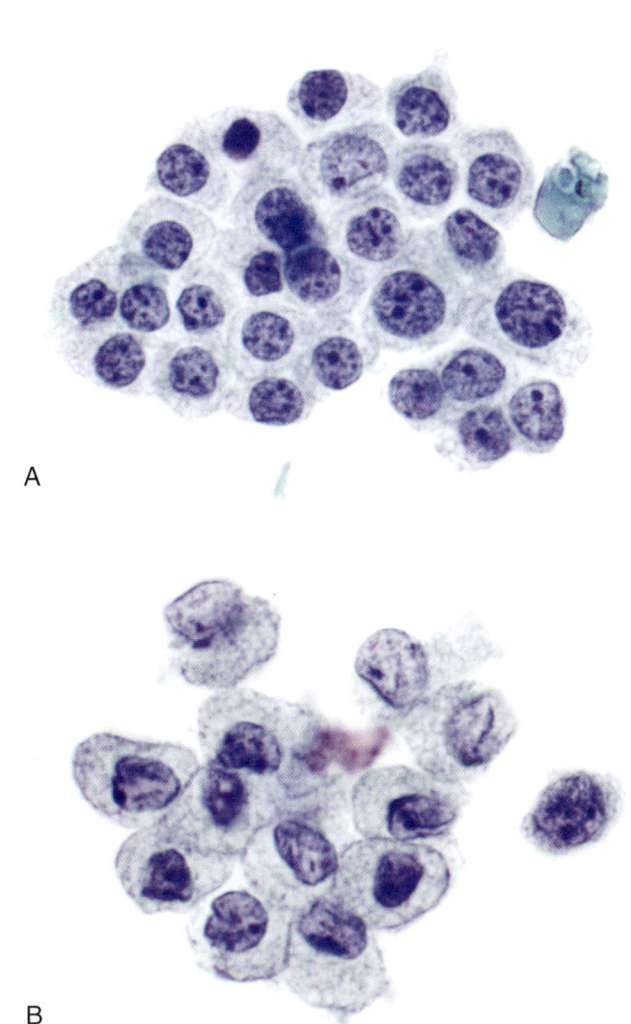

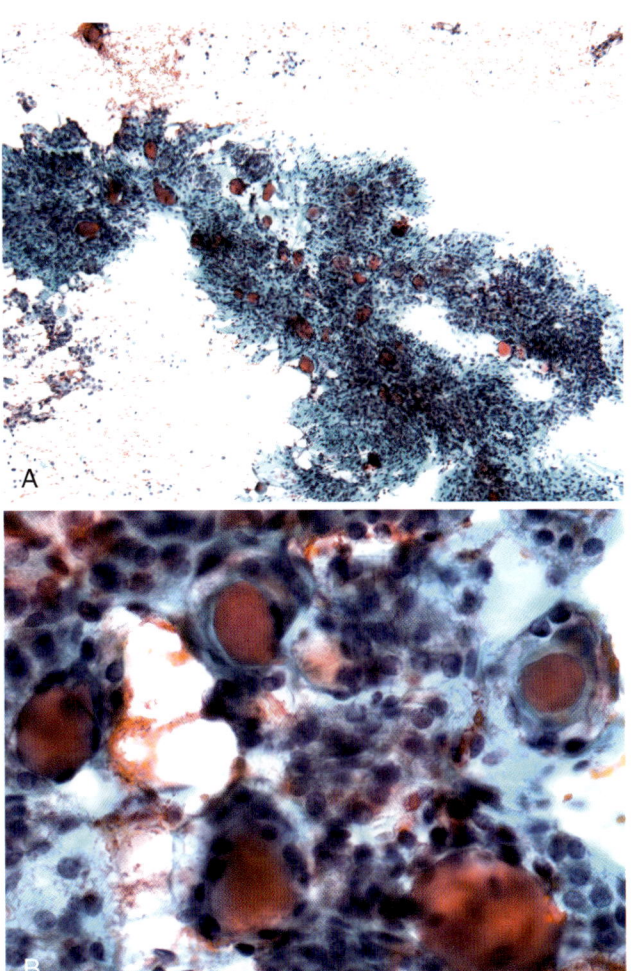

Fig. 11.5 Atypia of Undetermined Significance (AUS). **A,** Most of the follicular cells in this sample are benign-appearing macrofollicle fragments, as seen here. **B,** A very small proportion of cells have pale nuclei and nuclear grooves. When such cells are few in number, an AUS interpretation is more appropriate than "suspicious for malignancy." (**A** and **B,** Papanicolaou stain.)

Fig. 11.6 Suspicious for a Follicular Neoplasm. **A,** The aspirate is cellular and composed of crowded groups of follicular cells and some microfollicles. This cytoarchitectural pattern is suggestive of a follicular neoplasm. **B,** Higher magnification view shows follicular cells arranged in microfollicles, which are small follicular groups with a central droplet of colloid. (Papanicolaou stain.)

The cytologic criteria used to distinguish benign from potentially malignant thyroid lesions include the follicular group architecture, amount of colloid, and cytologic atypia. By far, the most important of these criteria is follicular architecture, specifically whether the lesion is composed predominantly of macrofollicles or microfollicles, trabeculae, and crowded groups (Figure 11.6, *A*). This approach works because follicular carcinomas are virtually never composed of predominantly normal-sized or macrofollicles. In smears of thyroid aspirates, macrofollicles are recognized as numerous follicular cells in flat sheets in a background of colloid. The flat sheets result from fragmentation of macrofollicles with extrusion of colloid. As discussed previously, aspirates with a predominance of macrofollicles and flat, orderly honeycomb sheets of follicular cells are diagnosed as "benign" by FNA. In contrast, thyroid aspirates composed of microfollicles (small follicular groups of 6 to 12 follicular cells with or without a small amount of central colloid) (Figure 11.6, *B*) or crowded trabeculae and 3D groups of overlapping follicular cells are a feature of follicular carcinomas as well as some adenomas.[3,37] These aspirates are diagnosed as "suspicious for a follicular neoplasm" or "follicular neoplasm," and it is this group of patients for whom surgical removal of the lesion is generally considered warranted. American Thyroid Association (ATA) guidelines also recognize ancillary molecular testing as an acceptable method to help consider triage patients for lobectomy versus clinical follow-up for an FNA sample classified as "suspicious for a follicular neoplasm."[1] The majority of follicular lesions diagnosed by FNA as "suspicious for a follicular neoplasm" are adenomas with a microfollicular or trabecular architecture, and a minority are actually follicular carcinomas. With the introduction of the second edition of the TBSRTC, the follicular neoplasm category now includes aspirates of follicular-patterned lesions with mild to moderate nuclear atypia.[3] The latter accommodates for a subset of those thyroid lesions that, on histologic evaluation, are classified as NIFTP.

HÜRTHLE CELL NEOPLASMS

Follicular neoplasms composed of oncocytic cells (oxyphilic cell neoplasms (OCNs or Hürthle cell neoplasms [HCNs]) show histologic patterns overlapping with nononcocytic follicular neoplasms. The cytologic features of an oncocytic lesion[2,29,51] include the following: groups or small follicles made up of cells with medium to large round nuclei, prominent nucleoli, and a large amount of granular cytoplasm (Figure 11.7). Colloid is scant and features of old hemorrhage (hemosiderin-laden histiocytes) may coexist. Sometimes fire-flare cells (detected in hyperfunctioning lesions or in juvenile thyroiditis) and small follicular cells can be detected, which suggests a benign lesion with an oncocytic component. Unlike their nononcocytic follicular counterpart, oncocytic cells may exhibit nuclear enlargement and pleomorphism either in benign neoplasms, carcinomas, or even in hyperplastic lesions. The most common example is represented by hyperplastic oncocytic nodules in CLT, which may show a striking nuclear pleomorphism of the oncocytic component.[54,60,61,66,67] Some authors have attempted to correlate the atypia of the oncocytic cells (and some other features, such as transgressing vessels) with the risk of malignancy, but their results are still debatable.[66,68,69]

A diagnosis of OCN correlates with a 15% to 40% risk of malignancy. Therefore every lesion composed predominantly of Hürthle cells should be diagnosed as OCN, unless an inflammatory background or a clinical/US picture of thyroiditis is detected.[60,69,70] On the other hand, oncocytic nodules in a CLT should usually be regarded as non-neoplastic lesions because the risk of malignancy is similar to goiter.[60]

MALIGNANT TUMORS

Papillary Thyroid Carcinoma

Papillary thyroid carcinoma is, by far, the most common malignant neoplasm of the thyroid, and it accounts for up to 80% of all thyroid malignancies.[71] FNA is highly accurate in the diagnosis of papillary thyroid carcinoma owing to the fact that the classic diagnostic criteria are principally cytologic characteristics. Over 90% of papillary thyroid carcinomas are correctly diagnosed as malignant or suspicious for malignancy on FNA.[72] However, a small proportion of papillary carcinomas may be particularly challenging when encountered in cytologic preparations; these papillary thyroid carcinomas include those with minimal nuclear features for diagnosing papillary carcinoma, as well as certain variants of papillary thyroid carcinoma (e.g., the follicular variant).[68] Complicating the cytologic evaluation of aspirates suspected of being papillary thyroid carcinoma is the recently described entity, NIFTP, which cannot be distinguished by FNA from the follicular variant of papillary thyroid carcinoma.[73]

Aspirates of classical papillary thyroid carcinoma are composed of enlarged epithelial cells in syncytial monolayered sheets, papillary groups, and crowded clusters that have lost the orderly honeycomb arrangement found in benign follicular lesions. The cytoplasm of papillary carcinoma can vary from scant to abundant and densely granular or eosinophilic, but it is the nucleus that holds the cytologic key to diagnosing papillary thyroid carcinoma. The nuclei of classical papillary thyroid carcinoma have the following characteristics: (1) enlarged and oval shape with a small, marginated nucleolus; (2) pale, "powdery" chromatin; (3) longitudinal nuclear grooves; and (4) occasional intranuclear pseudoinclusions (Figure 11.8). The most sensitive, diagnostically important feature of papillary thyroid carcinomas is the presence of extensive well-formed longitudinal nuclear grooves (Figure 11.9); however, nuclear grooves are not entirely specific for papillary carcinoma and can be seen in benign conditions as well as in NIFTP. Nuclear grooves are seen in almost all cases of papillary thyroid carcinoma, although they may be sparse in up to 25% of cases. There are also many other secondary features that can be used in the cytologic diagnosis of papillary carcinoma, such as psammoma bodies, multinucleate giant cells, papillary architecture, and thick hypereosinophilic colloid. Psammoma bodies (laminated round calcifications) in thyroid aspirates, especially in a cystic background, strongly suggest the possibility of classical papillary carcinoma; however, psammoma bodies must be distinguished from nonspecific calcifications as well as laminated inspissated colloid.

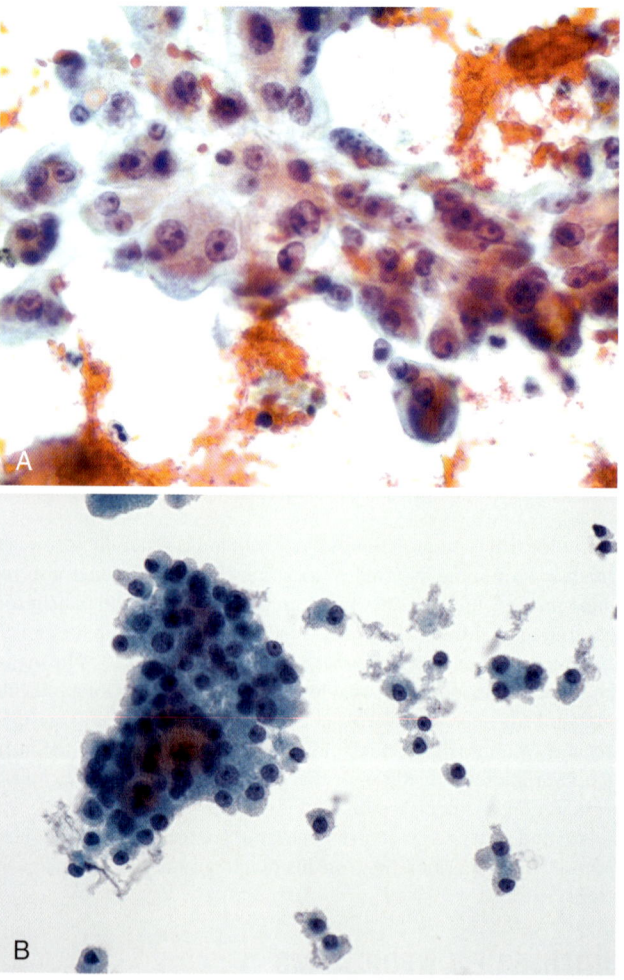

Fig. 11.7 Suspicious for a Follicular Neoplasm with Oncocytic Features. A, A cluster of oxyphilic cells with abundant granular cytoplasm, enlarged round nucleus, and prominent nucleolus is indicative of a Hrthle cell neoplasm. **B,** This thin-layer preparation of a Hürthle cell neoplasm contains Hürthle cells in a large cluster and as isolated cells. (Papanicolaou stain.)

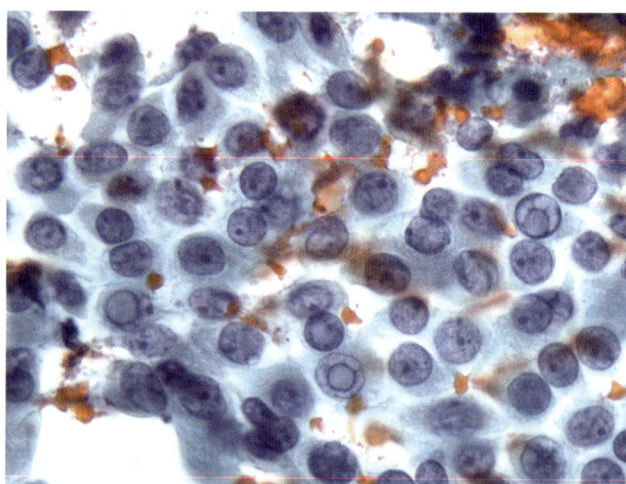

Fig. 11.8 Papillary Thyroid Carcinoma. The cells in this group have oval nuclei with several prominent intranuclear pseudoinclusions. (Papanicolaou stain.)

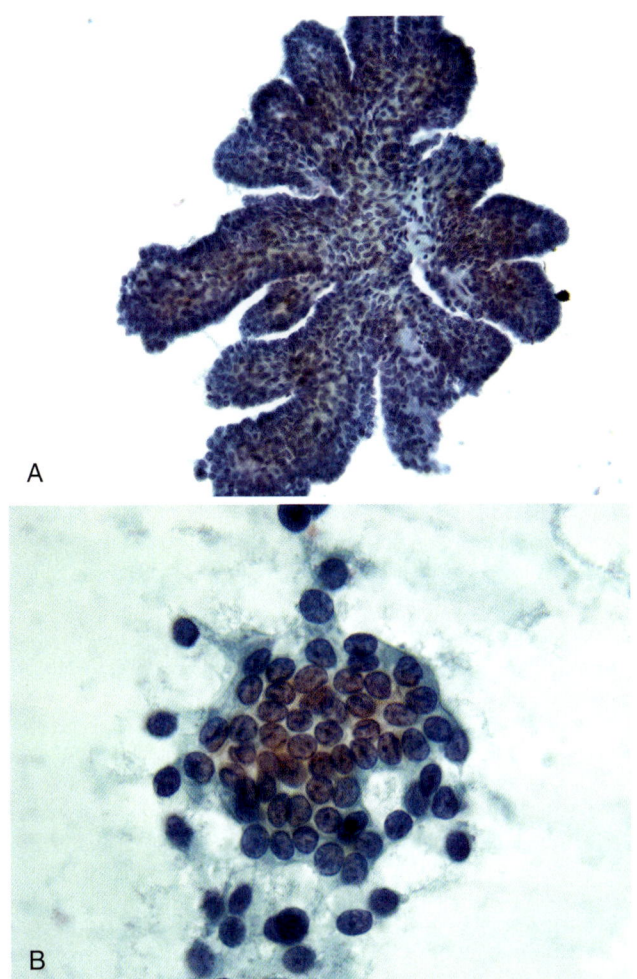

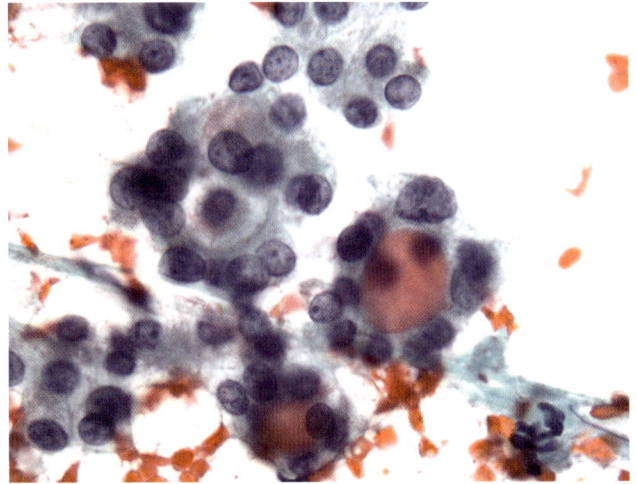

Fig. 11.10 **Follicular Variant of Papillary Thyroid Carcinoma.** Although the cells in this aspirate are arranged in a follicular pattern, the nuclei exhibit characteristic features of papillary carcinoma. Nonetheless, caution is warranted because the differential diagnosis includes noninvasive follicular thyroid neoplasm with papillary-like nuclear features. (Papanicolaou stain.)

Fig. 11.9 **Papillary Thyroid Carcinoma. A,** This aspirate of papillary carcinoma shows crowded cells arranged in fibrovascular cores. **B,** The cells in this syncytial group have oval nuclei with frequent longitudinal nuclear grooves. (Papanicolaou stain.)

In addition to the classic type of papillary carcinoma, there are several variants, such as the follicular variant, macrofollicular, diffuse sclerosing, and oncocytic, Warthin-like, tall cell, cribriform-morular, and columnar cell variants may be detected by FNA. Although identification of a particular variant on FNA may not affect the surgical management of the case, it is important to be aware of the variants that can be encountered, because they may mimic other thyroid lesions and lead to an incorrect cytologic diagnosis. The follicular variant of papillary thyroid carcinoma (FVPTC) represents up to 15% of papillary thyroid carcinomas, and it may pose a diagnostic challenge due to the lack of papillarity and the abundance of microfollicles mimicking a follicular neoplasm (Figure 11.10). NIFTP is cytologically indistinguishable from FVPTC; it is recommended that a "malignant" diagnosis be avoided for those aspirates with nuclear features of PTC that also have a follicular architectural pattern. The latter can be classified as suspicious for malignancy or as follicular neoplasm.[3]

Anaplastic Thyroid Carcinoma

The cytologic appearance of this highly aggressive carcinoma includes a cellular aspirate with malignant-appearing, sometimes bizarre, spindled and multinucleated tumor giant cells in groups and as single cells in a background of tumor diathesis.[74] The cells can be spindled, squamoid, giant cells, or a combination of cell types (Figure 11.11).

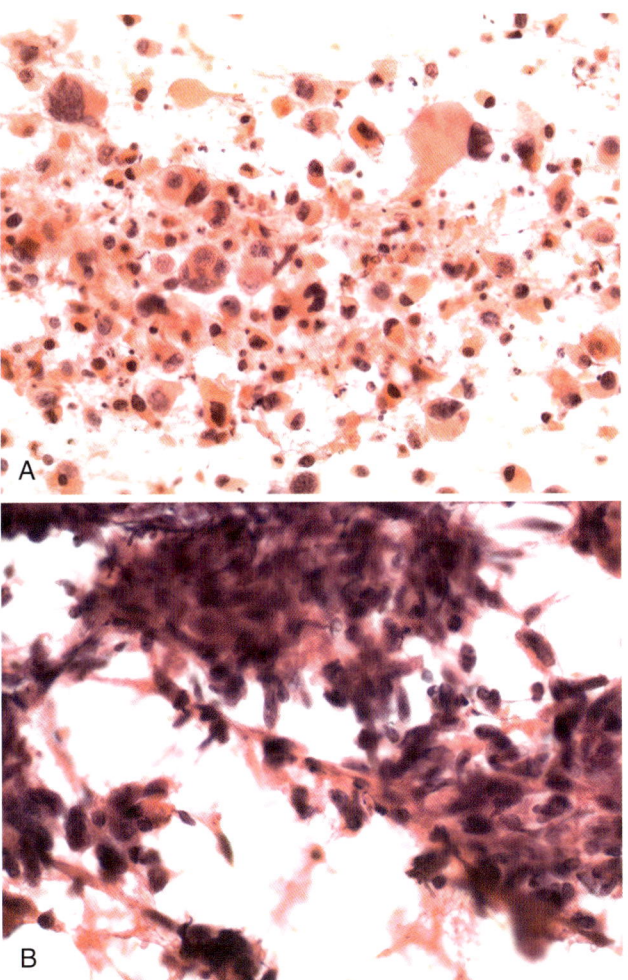

Fig. 11.11 **Undifferentiated (Anaplastic) Carcinoma. A,** The malignant cells are highly pleomorphic with bizarre shapes and hyperchromatic nuclei in a background tumor diathesis. **B,** This spindle cell form of undifferentiated carcinoma resembles a high-grade sarcoma. (Papanicolaou stain.)

The nuclei of anaplastic thyroid carcinoma are highly pleomorphic with dark, irregular chromatin clumping, macronucleoli, and occasional intranuclear pseudoinclusions. Numerous mitoses and atypical mitotic figures are often seen. Immunocytochemically, anaplastic carcinomas are often, but not always, positive for keratins, PAX-8, and p53, but they are usually negative for thyroglobulin, TTF-1, and calcitonin. Clinical and radiologic correlation are usually needed to help exclude metastatic disease from the differential diagnosis.

Medullary Thyroid Carcinoma

Medullary thyroid carcinoma is a neuroendocrine carcinoma arising from the C cell of the thyroid. Cytologically, medullary thyroid carcinoma is characterized by a uniform, predominantly dispersed population of neuroendocrine cells and amyloid (Figure 11.12).[74,75] Depending on the case, a variable combination of any of the following three cell types occurs: plasmacytoid, spindled, and granular. Nuclei are often eccentrically placed, and the chromatin shows a typical neuroendocrine "salt-and-pepper" texture with inconspicuous nucleoli (although occasional cells will exhibit prominent nucleoli). Larger binucleated or multinucleated cells are also commonly encountered, and intranuclear pseudoinclusions identical to those seen in papillary thyroid carcinoma are found in more than 50% of cases.

Medullary carcinoma has a wide range of appearances and variants; thus it can often mimic other neoplasms. Some cases of medullary thyroid carcinoma are predominantly spindled; therefore medullary carcinoma should be considered in the differential diagnosis of any FNA of a spindle cell lesion of the head and neck region. When medullary carcinomas exhibit an oncocytic appearance, Hürthle cell neoplasia should be excluded from the differential diagnosis, and some cases of medullary carcinoma can have bizarre giant cells mimicking anaplastic carcinoma. Fortunately, medullary carcinoma has a distinct immunocytochemical profile (calcitonin +, CEA +, chromogranin +, TTF-1 +, thyroglobulin) that can be used to distinguish it from other thyroid tumors (see Figure 11.12, B).

Malignant Lymphoma

Primary thyroid lymphoma accounts for approximately 1% to 3% of thyroid malignancies, and it characteristically occurs in the setting of Hashimoto's thyroiditis (HT).[76,77] Other primary thyroid lymphoproliferative disorders (e.g., Hodgkin's lymphoma, plasmacytoma, and T-cell lymphomas) have been reported in the thyroid but are very rare. The cytologic diagnosis of malignant lymphoma is usually straightforward owing to the fact that diffuse large B cell lymphomas (DLBCL) account for up to 75% of cases.[76,77] The remainder of primary thyroid lymphomas are mainly extranodal marginal zone lymphomas of mucosa-associated lymphoid tissue (MALT) type. The key to the diagnosis of thyroid lymphomas is demonstration of light chain restriction and immunophenotyping using flow cytometry. Microscopically, aspirates of DLBCL are cellular and composed of large, highly atypical immature B-lymphocytes in a background of scant-to-absent follicular cells. The dispersed large lymphocytes often have irregular nuclear membranes and contain prominent nucleoli (Figure 11.13); lymphoglandular bodies (small cytoplasmic fragments) are identifiable in the smear background. Extranodal marginal zone lymphoma of MALT type is a low-grade lymphoma that may pose a diagnostic challenge due to its resemblance in aspirates to HT. Aspirates of MALT lymphoma contain an increased proportion of intermediate-size lymphocytes resembling centrocytes (Figure 11.14).

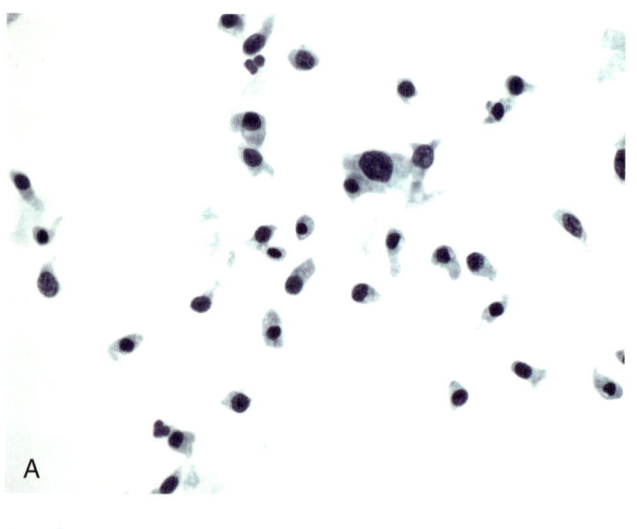

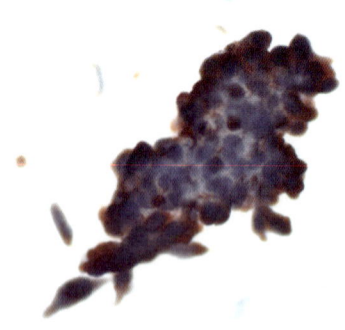

Fig. 11.12 Medullary Thyroid Carcinoma. A, The neoplastic cells are dispersed as single cells and have a bland plasmacytoid appearance. (Papanicolaou stain.) **B,** An immunocytochemical stain for calcitonin is positive.

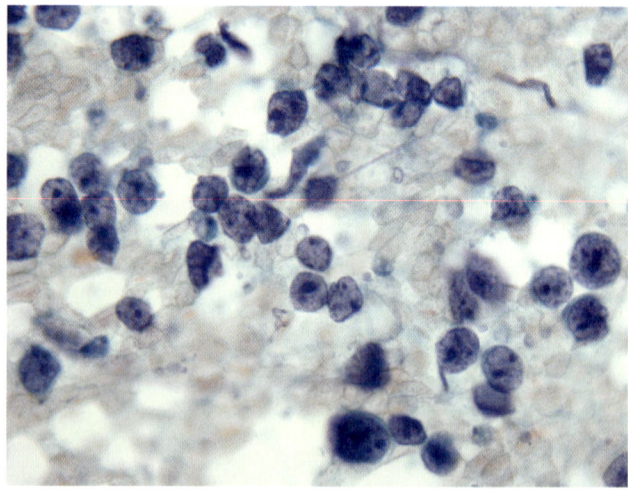

Fig. 11.13 Diffuse Large B Cell Lymphoma. The malignant lymphoid cells are dispersed and have large round nuclei with a prominent nucleolus and high nuclear to cytoplasmic ratio. (Papanicolaou stain.)

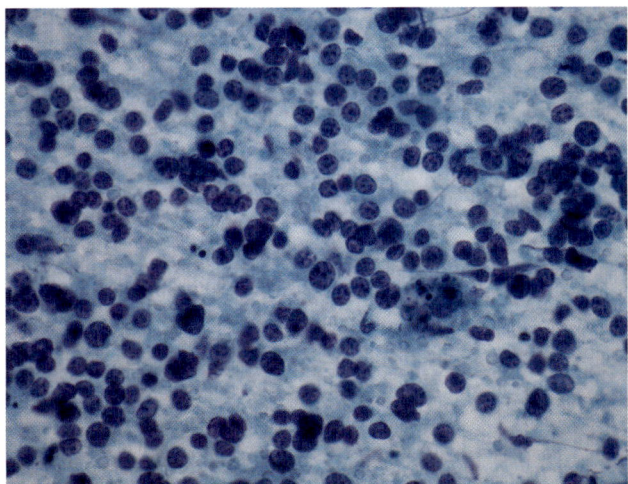

Fig. 11.14 Extranodal marginal zone lymphoma of mucosa-associated lymphoid tissue (MALT) type. Aspirates of MALT type lymphomas consist of lymphoid cells which are small to intermediate in size; flow cytometry is often needed to distinguish this pattern from chronic lymphocytic thyroiditis. The background contains blood and lymphoglandular bodies. (Papanicolaou stain.)

When the possibility of involvement by a lymphoproliferative disorder is suspected in a thyroid FNA, ancillary marker studies, such as flow cytometry or immunocytochemistry (using air-dried cytospins or cell blocks), are indicated.

Secondary Tumors of the Thyroid

Metastatic tumors to the thyroid may present as either multifocal or solitary nodules, but they are uncommonly encountered, being detected in approximately 0.1% of thyroid FNAs.[78,79] The most frequent metastatic tumors to the thyroid include kidney, colorectal, lung, breast, melanoma, lymphoma, and head and neck squamous cell carcinoma.[78,79] The possibility of a metastatic tumor should be considered whenever there is a history of a primary cancer elsewhere in the body, and especially whenever the cytologic features of the malignant cells do not match those of standard thyroid neoplasms (papillary carcinoma, follicular carcinoma, medullary carcinoma, and anaplastic carcinoma). Two other features suggesting the possibility of metastatic disease are an admixture of unremarkable follicular cells with malignant cells and a background tumor diathesis (acute inflammation admixed with necrotic debris). Although infrequent, two of the most difficult thyroid metastases to diagnose are renal cell carcinoma (Figure 11.15) and breast carcinoma because both carcinomas can mimic the cytologic features of a follicular neoplasm. Metastatic melanoma can mimic medullary carcinoma or anaplastic carcinoma. Metastatic papillary lung cancer can be misinterpreted as papillary thyroid carcinoma. Immunocytochemistry for thyroglobulin, TTF-1, PAX-8, and calcitonin can be very helpful in evaluating such challenging cases.

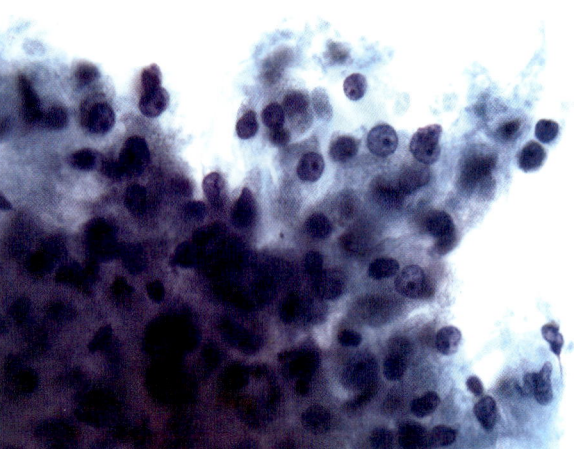

Fig. 11.15 Metastatic Renal Cell Carcinoma to the Thyroid Gland. The cells in this crowded group have abundant delicate cytoplasm and distinct nucleolus resembling a Hürthle cell neoplasm. (Papanicolaou stain.)

THYROID FNA COMPLICATIONS

The most common complication after thyroid FNA is a hematoma secondary to the highly vascular nature of the thyroid gland.[80,81] Because of the latter, a needle track confined to a narrow region, rather than using a "fanning" motion, is recommended. Vasovagal episodes are a second potential complication during thyroid FNA. In such cases, the FNA should be stopped and the patient placed into a supine position with the legs slightly elevated. Vital signs should be obtained and documented and the referring physician notified of the adverse event. Because of the thyroid gland's anatomic location (anterior to the trachea), the needle could potentially pass into the trachea during the procedure. If this occurs, there will usually be a loss of vacuum in the syringe, and the patient may cough or produce a small amount of blood-tinged sputum. Such aspirates may contain ciliated respiratory epithelial cells.

REFERENCES

For a complete list of references, go to expertconsult.com.

12

Fine-Needle Aspiration and Molecular Analysis

Benjamin J. Gigliotti, Marika D. Russell, David Shonka, Nikolaos Stathatos

> Please go to expertconsult.com to view related video:
> **Video 12.1** Introduction to Chapter 12, Fine-Needle Aspiration and Molecular Analysis.

INTRODUCTION

Ultrasound-guided fine-needle aspiration (FNA) biopsy is the gold standard for diagnostic assessment of thyroid nodules, yet cytologic evaluation may be limited, with up to 30% of samples classified as cytologically indeterminate by the widely accepted Bethesda classification scheme (see chapter 11 Fine-Needle Aspiration of the Thyroid Gland–Bethesda II).[1] Nodules characterized as Bethesda III ("atypia of undetermined significance/follicular lesion of undetermined significance" [AUS/FLUS]) or Bethesda IV ("follicular neoplasm/suspicious for follicular neoplasm" [FN/SFN]) are estimated to carry a malignancy risk of 6% to 18% and 10% to 40%, respectively, with rates that have been shown to vary widely across practice settings.[1-4] This is especially notable for the AUS/FLUS category, where reported malignancy rates range from 6% to 40%.[5] Nodules classified as Bethesda V ("suspicious for malignancy" [SFM]) carry a 45% to 60% risk of malignancy.[1]

The diagnostic uncertainty associated with indeterminate cytology (Bethesda III/IV) presents a management challenge. Traditionally, options were limited to repeat biopsy or diagnostic thyroid lobectomy. Although some reports suggest that repeat FNA may yield a more definitive diagnosis the majority of the time, others show that the indeterminate read is likely to persist; the discrepancy is likely due to institutional factors, including local rates of malignancy for each Bethesda category.[6,7] Although conventional wisdom has led to the recommendation of waiting 8 to 12 weeks to avoid FNA-related atypia, one study showed that time between the initial and repeat FNA was not a predictor of diagnostic yield or accuracy.[8] Waiting 4 to 6 weeks or possibly less is likely sufficient, especially if the cytopathologist interpreting the specimen is aware of the timeline.

There are errors possible in both directions with these indeterminate nodules. Most nodules characterized as AUS/FLUS and FN/SFN that undergo surgical resection prove to have benign histology; lobectomy may be retrospectively viewed as "unnecessary." In contrast, for those nodules that prove to be malignant with a size >4 cm or with features that would otherwise lead to a recommendation for total thyroidectomy, lobectomy may be insufficient and completion thyroidectomy is warranted.[9] As such, lobectomy for cytologically indeterminate nodules is not an ideal management strategy, and improved diagnostic methods are needed to guide management decisions.

As a result of advances in next-generation sequencing (NGS) technology and the understanding of thyroid carcinogenesis, molecular diagnostic tools have become widely available for clinical use; understanding their role in the management of cytologically indeterminate thyroid nodules is the subject of this chapter. By identifying benign nodules and improving preoperative detection of malignant nodules, molecular testing has the potential to prevent diagnostic surgeries and guide surgical planning for malignant disease.[10,11] The American Thyroid Association (ATA) guidelines on management of thyroid nodules and differentiated thyroid cancer include molecular testing as an acceptable adjunct to cytologic evaluation of indeterminate nodules and state that informed application of these tools is critical.[9,12]

PRINCIPLES OF MOLECULAR TESTING

Molecular Alterations in Thyroid Cancer

Over the past two decades, research into the molecular pathogenesis of thyroid cancer has elucidated many of the genetic drivers of carcinogenesis.[13] Although thyroid cancers have long been known to exist on a spectrum of clinical severity that parallels the degree of cellular differentiation, the molecular alterations behind these phenotypic changes are increasingly being defined (and are more thoroughly reviewed in Chapter 18, Molecular Pathogenesis of Thyroid Neoplasia). These discoveries, coupled with novel technologies that enable molecular profiling of individual tumors, have led to the burgeoning field of molecular diagnostic pathology. The application of molecular profiling to the evaluation of cytologically indeterminate nodules is a rapidly evolving field that leverages the unique biologic signature of each thyroid cancer subtype compared with normal thyroid tissue and each other.

The most common thyroid cancers are collectively referred to as "differentiated thyroid carcinomas" (DTC) due to their usually indolent nature and close resemblance to the thyroid follicular epithelial cell from which they originate. DTC is subdivided into papillary (PTC) and follicular thyroid carcinomas (FTC), both of which have many subtypes with unique phenotypic features and behaviors.[14] PTC and its variants are by far the most common type of thyroid cancer (80%) and harbor a relatively simple and quiet genome. The majority of mutations are in the mitogen-activated protein kinase (MAPK) pathway, which regulates cell growth and differentiation.[15] *BRAF* V600E is the most prevalent alteration, followed by alterations in the signaling of tyrosine kinase receptors such as *RET* and *NTRK*.[16] FTC, on the other hand, is associated with mutations in *RAS*, *PTEN*, and *PIK3CA*, and the *PAX8-PPARγ* rearrangement.

Molecular diagnostics have shed light on the disparate clinical behavior exhibited by several DTC subtypes and may enhance traditional pathology and lead to revised classification schema. For instance, *RAS* mutations, which are mutually exclusive of *BRAF* V600E, can be found in both FTC and the follicular variant of papillary thyroid cancer (FVPTC, the most common PTC subtype) but almost never in classical

PTC. FVPTCs have long been recognized to be heterogeneous tumors; use of integrated genetics to articulate "BRAF-like" and "RAS-like" tumors has shed light on this diversity in clinical behavior.[15,17] Indeed, *BRAF* V600E mutant tumors are typically locally invasive and behave like classical PTC, whereas *RAS* mutant FVPTCs tend to be encapsulated and behave more like follicular adenomas or carcinomas.[18] Because *RAS* mutant FVPTCs have more in common with follicular tumors than they do classical PTC, they should be managed and perhaps reclassified as such. Another example is Hürthle cell carcinoma (HCC), which has traditionally been classified as a variant of FTC. However, data suggest it has a distinct genomic signature, including chromosomal copy number alterations and novel mutations in mitochondrial DNA.[19,20]

Poorly differentiated and undifferentiated (anaplastic thyroid carcinoma, ATC) thyroid carcinomas are rarer, have more complex and widespread alterations, and behave more aggressively.[21] Increased MAPK pathway output, combined with mutations in the *TERT* promoter, *EIF1AX*, DNA repair genes (*CKEK2, SWI/SNF* complex, etc.), and *P53* have all been implicated in the process of de-differentiation and genomic instability. Clinical consequences of these changes can include loss of thyroglobulin expression and failure to respond to radioactive iodine, along with increasing aggressiveness; ATC carries a dismal prognosis.[22,23] Medullary thyroid carcinoma is a biologically unique malignancy that arises from the neuroendocrine parafollicular "C" cells and, compared with follicular cell tumors, has a higher rate of being hereditary.[24] The most common mutations are in the *RET* gene, although *RAS* mutations are also common in sporadic tumors.

Molecular Techniques

Molecular profiling relies on several different NGS and gene expression technologies, each of which imparts unique characteristics to testing platforms and affects performance as a "rule in" or "rule out" test. Fundamentally, techniques differ in their testing substrate (DNA versus RNA) and whether they employ gene sequencing and/or expression methodologies.[25] All methods rely on some form of nucleic acid extraction and preservation, often using proprietary preservatives, followed by amplification and detection. Sequencing is typically performed using oncogene or fusion-specific primers by polymerase chain reaction (PCR, for DNA), reverse transcription polymerase chain reaction (RT-PCR, for RNA), or using microarrays.

The first genotyping assays were designed to detect point mutations and gene fusions but over time have evolved to also identify insertions/deletions, along with copy number alterations. Notably, whereas *BRAF* V600E, *TERT* promoter, and *P53* mutations have proven highly specific for malignancy, alterations in *RAS, PTEN,* and others may be found in follicular adenomas and other benign lesions, thereby creating challenges in using these signatures to differentiate benign from malignant specimens. Expression analyses using messenger RNA (mRNA) rely on RNA sequencing (RNA-Seq) and microarray technologies to determine differentially expressed genes between benign and malignant tissues. More recently, microRNA, which are small noncoding RNAs that indirectly regulate gene expression through modulation of mRNA, have also been used. Regardless of the RNA substrate, machine learning algorithms are typically used to perform pattern recognition to distinguish a benign from malignant expression signature.

At the time of writing this chapter, there are three commercially available tools, all of which use some combination of the aforementioned methods: ThyroSeq, Afirma, and ThyGeNEXT/ThyraMIR (Table 12.1).

Clinical Utility

To understand the clinical utility of molecular testing, it is worthwhile to briefly review the statistics associated with test performance. In molecular testing for cytologically indeterminate thyroid nodules, the histopathology of the surgically excised nodule serves as the standard for whether the nodule is benign or malignant. Sensitivity and specificity, as determined by validation studies, are immutable characteristics of the test under consideration. Sensitivity represents the proportion of malignant nodules that will test positive (true positives); specificity represents the proportion of benign nodules that will test negative (true negatives). A highly sensitive test is useful as a "rule out" test because a negative result is unlikely to be a false negative (a test with 100% sensitivity will detect all individuals with the condition). A highly specific test is useful as a "rule in" test because a positive result is unlikely to be

TABLE 12.1 Overview of Commercially Available Tests for Indeterminate Cytopathology

Company	Afirma® Veracyte, Inc.	ThyroSeq® UPMC, CBLPath, Inc.	ThyGeNEXT®-ThyraMIR® Interpace Diagnostics, Inc.
Assay Methodology	Gene Sequencing Classifier (2017) Microarray expression analysis (1115 "core" genes); RNA sequencing for SNV (BRAF) and gene fusions (RET-PTC 1-3) loss of heterozygosity Xpression Atlas: RNA sequencing panel includes 511 genes, 761 variants, 130 fusions	ThyroSeq v3 (2017) NGS of 112 genes to detect mutations (12,135 SNVs and indels), gene fusions (>120), gene expression alterations (90 genes) and copy number variations (10 regions for FNA, 27 regions for tissue)	ThyGeNEXT®-ThyraMIR® (2018) ThyGeNEXT®: NGS of 10 genes (42 SNVs) and 28 gene fusions ThyraMIR®: PCR expression of 10 microRNAs
Version History	Gene Expression Classifier (GEC, 2011) – 167 genes (25 screening for MTC/parathyroid/metastases, 142 in main classifier)	ThyroSeq v0 (2007): 7 genes ThyroSeq v1 (2013): 15 genes (NGS introduced) ThyroSeq v2 (2014): 56 genes	ThyGenX (2015): 8 genes - miR*Inform*: 4 genes, 3 fusions
Sample Preparation	2 dedicated FNA passes, collected in FNAprotect™, shipped with frozen "cold bricks" to Veracyte; 2 dedicated passes for cytology to be shipped concurrently*	1 dedicated FNA pass, collected in ThyroSeq*Preserve*; FFPE specimens or cell block can also be used	1 dedicated FNA pass, collected in RNA*Retain*; cytology slides can also be used
Cytopathology	Central cytology review required*	Local review accepted; central review offered	Local review accepted; central review offered

Continued

TABLE 12.1 Overview of Commercially Available Tests for Indeterminate Cytopathology—cont'd

Company	Afirma® Veracyte, Inc.	ThyroSeq® UPMC, CBLPath, Inc.	ThyGeNEXT®-ThyraMIR® Interpace Diagnostics, Inc.
Reporting Paradigm	GSC: Binary ("benign" or "suspicious") Xpression atlas: Specific fusions and SNVs	Specific mutations for risk stratification	ThyGeNEXT: Specific mutations for risk stratification ThyraMIR: Binary "positive" or "negative"
Clinical Validation	Patel et al. *JAMA Surg.* 2018	Steward et al. *JAMA Oncol.* 2018	Labourier et al. *J Clin Endocrinol Metab.* 2015
Cancer Prevalence	24% (45/190)	28% (69/247)	32% (35/109)
Sensitivity	91%	94%	89%
Specificity	68%	82%	85%
PPV	47%	66%	74%
NPV	96%	97%	94%

*Some academic centers excepted
FFPE, formalin-fixed paraffin-embedded, FNA, fine-needle aspiration, GSC, gene sequencing classifier, NGS, next-generation sequencing, SNV, single nucleotide variations, indels insertions/deletions, UPMC, University of Pittsburgh Medical Center.

a false positive (a test with 100% specificity will be negative for all those without the condition).

When applying a test clinically, the true diagnosis is unknown; what clinicians and patients must know for clinical decision making is the positive predictive value (PPV) and negative predictive value (NPV) of the test. For molecular testing of cytologically indeterminate nodules, the PPV indicates the percentage of patients with a positive result that will actually have a malignancy (true positives); the NPV indicates the percentage of patients with a negative result that will truly not have a malignancy (true negatives). It is important to recognize that PPV and NPV are influenced by the sensitivity and specificity of a test, as well as the prevalence of the disease state in question. For a given sensitivity and specificity, as disease prevalence rises, PPV increases and NPV decreases, affecting the clinical utility of the test. Conversely, decreased disease prevalence decreases the PPV and increases the NPV. Given the wide variability in reported rates of malignancy for cytologically indeterminate specimens, it is critical to know local rates of malignancy to understand test performance in a specific population. Clinicians are urged to recognize how the local prevalence of malignancy in each Bethesda category affects a test's reported PPV and NPV when it is applied to their individual clinical setting.[12]

It should be noted that the recent reclassification of noninvasive follicular thyroid neoplasm with papillary-like nuclear features (NIFTP) from malignancy to neoplasm has bearing on the interpretation of molecular testing. The term "NIFTP" was introduced in 2015 to describe encapsulated follicular variant papillary thyroid cancers that harbor no capsular or vascular invasion and exhibit indolent behavior with an excellent prognosis.[26,27] Cytologic specimens from NIFTP lesions are frequently indeterminate (Bethesda III to V); its reclassification as a neoplasm lowers the risk of malignancy in each group.[4,28,29] During the development and validation of first- and second-generation molecular tests, nodules that would now be diagnosed as NIFTP would have been considered malignant. It follows that NIFTP renders a "suspicious" or positive result on molecular tests, thereby lowering the PPV.[30-32] However, although NIFTP is clinically regarded as a low-risk neoplasm, it is a histologic diagnosis and thus requires a surgical excision to be made, and its malignant potential, if left untreated, is unclear. As such, lobectomy directed by a "suspicious" or positive result is in line with current diagnostic and therapeutic recommendations.[9] For this reason, grouping a NIFTP with malignant nodules optimizes test performance and interpretation when results are reported in a binary fashion.

THYROSEQ®

Background

The first version of ThyroSeq was developed for clinical use at the University of Pittsburgh Medical Center in 2007. This panel (ThyroSeq v0) initially evaluated seven genes for mutations (*BRAF, NRAS61, HRAS61, KRAS12/13*) or rearrangements (*RET/PTC1, RET/PTC3, PAX8/PPARγ*). The 7-gene panel had high PPV but low NPV for the detection of malignancy in indeterminate nodules.[33] Since then, there have been multiple iterations of the ThyroSeq test, which have employed the use of NGS of DNA and RNA. Each successive iteration has evaluated a larger number of genes; ThyroSeq v1 was a 15-gene panel and v2 was a 56-gene panel. Although initially developed as a "rule in" test, the sensitivity and NPV have increased with each new version of the test.[34]

The most recent version, ThyroSeq v3, was developed in 2017 and analyzes 112 genes for four classes of genetic abnormalities, including mutations, gene fusions, gene expression alterations, and copy number variations.[35] A proprietary algorithmic analysis of all detected genetic abnormalities is used to generate a genomic classifier (GC) score; each abnormality detected is assigned a value from 0 to 2 commensurate with its association with malignancy, and these individual values are summed. The test is reported as positive if the GC score is ≥1.5 or negative if the GC score is <1.5.[36] Additionally, the test report provides information about the specific genetic abnormalities detected.

Clinical Validation

ThyroSeq v3 has been validated in a prospective, blinded, multicenter study.[37] In this study, 286 FNA samples from nodules with indeterminate cytology (Bethesda III to V) were evaluated with ThyroSeq v3 and compared with histologic findings after thyroidectomy. Ten percent of samples were inadequate for evaluation, due to either low total nucleic acids or insufficient thyroid cells present. Of the remaining 257 samples, 152 (59%) tested negative and 105 (41%) tested positive. One hundred and forty-seven of the 152 nodules that tested negative were benign on final pathology. Of the five nodules with false negative results, four were PTC and one was a minimally invasive FTC; all fell into the ATA low risk category. For the subset of nodules with Bethesda III or IV cytopathology, the disease prevalence (cancer/NIFTP) as determined by histologic evaluation of the thyroidectomy specimen was 28%. In these 247 samples, the sensitivity, specificity, NPV, and PPV were 94%, 82%, 97%, and 66%, respectively.[37]

As previously discussed, test utility is dependent on the prevalence of the disease in a studied population, with NPV decreasing as disease prevalence increases. For ThyroSeq v3, the NPV remains 95% or greater for a disease prevalence of up to 40% for Bethesda III and 60% for Bethesda IV nodules.[37] It has limited applicability as a "rule out" test for Bethesda V lesions (SFM) due to the higher cancer prevalence in patients with this FNA finding. In these patients, a negative test result carries a risk of malignancy of 20%.[38] For nodules with Bethesda III/IV cytopathology, the 3% to 5% cancer risk (at typical rates of disease prevalence) with a negative test is comparable with the cancer risk in nodules diagnosed as Bethesda II by FNA cytology.[37]

The benign call rate (BCR), defined as the percentage of cytologically indeterminate specimens that are subsequently found to be benign on molecular analysis, is an important measure of test utility. In applying a molecular test with a high NPV, the BCR determines the number of patients that can be managed nonoperatively. One study found the BCR of ThyroSeq v3 to be 74.1% for patients with Bethesda III/IV cytopathology.[38]

Studies have demonstrated the validity of ThyroSeq v3 in the evaluation of Hürthle cell thyroid lesions. Notably, all 10 HCCs were correctly identified with positive test results in the initial validation study.[37] In another analysis of the performance of ThyroSeq v3, 39 of 42 (93%) Hürthle cell malignancies were correctly identified; among all oncocytic nodules, sensitivity and specificity were 93% and 69%, respectively.[36] It has been suggested that ThyroSeq v3 can be used to help determine the extent of surgery for Hürthle cell neoplasms.[39]

Regarding NIFTP, the prospective multicenter study for ThyroSeq v3 grouped NIFTP with cancerous nodules.[37] Previous validation studies occurred before the introduction of NIFTP and therefore overestimated cancer prevalence within the Bethesda III/IV groups. A study specifically evaluating the effect of the classification of NIFTP as a benign lesion showed a decrease in the PPV of ThyroSeq v2 when NIFTP was classified as benign.[31]

Practical Considerations

To obtain ThyroSeq v3 testing, sample collection kits can be requested that contain a test requisition form, ThyroSeq*Preserve,* and shipping materials. FNA is performed in the typical fashion, and it is recommended that one pass be placed in ThyroSeq*Preserve* and sent for evaluation. Once the specimen has been placed in ThyroSeq*Preserve,* it can be kept for up to 12 months in a freezer. Cytopathologic evaluation of the FNA specimen can be performed locally or can be requested in addition to the ThyroSeq v3 testing at CBLPath (an additional needle pass is encouraged when requesting cytopathologic interpretation by CBLPath). ThyroSeq v3 testing can also be performed on slides prepared from a cell block as long as the hematoxylin and eosin (H&E) slides are reviewed to verify that >300 cells are present. Similarly, slides prepared from formalin-fixed paraffin-embedded specimens can be tested. A sample report is provided in Figure 12.1.

AFIRMA® EXPRESSION CLASSIFIER

Gene Expression Classifier

The Afirma Gene Expression Classifier (GEC, Veracyte, Inc, South San Francisco, CA) was the first generation of a proprietary molecular classifier that became available for clinical use in 2011. Developed as a "rule out" test to identify benign nodules, it was designed to achieve a high sensitivity and NPV of 95%, commensurate with the false negative rate for benign cytology of ≤5% accepted by National Comprehensive Cancer Network (NCCN) guidelines (NCCN Thyroid Guidelines https://www.nccn.org/professionals/physician_gls/pdf/thyroid.pdf). The tool used microarray analysis of the expression profile for 167 genes differentially expressed in thyroid cancers.[40] Samples submitted for Afirma GEC testing underwent a 25-gene screen for medullary thyroid carcinoma (Afirma MTC), parathyroid tissue, and metastatic tumors; samples that screened negative for these were submitted to the principal 142-gene classifier and were reported as either "benign" or "suspicious."[10] To improve the PPV for GEC-suspicious results, Veracyte also included Afirma BRAF, a GEC trained to detect the expression profile for BRAF V600E to enrich their detection of PTC.

Clinical Validation

The clinical validation study for Afirma GEC performed by Alexander et al. was a prospective double-blind multicenter study evaluating the performance of the GEC on 265 cytologically indeterminate nodules (Bethesda III, IV, and V) with a histopathologic reference standard. The study reported an overall 92% sensitivity, with a specificity of 52%. NPV for AUS/FLUS, SFN/FN, and SFM was 95%, 94%, and 85%, respectively, with a malignancy prevalence of 24%, 25%, and 62%, respectively. PPV was a modest 38% and 37% in AUS/FLUS and SFN/FN, respectively, and 76% in nodules classified as SFM. Of seven false negative results, six were found to be due to insufficient sampling of follicular epithelium rather than a failure of the classifier algorithm itself. The high NPV for AUS/FLUS and SFN/FN affirmed the GEC's utility in risk stratifying nodules in these categories, with a benign result supporting clinical observation.[41]

Postvalidation studies at several institutions evaluated the "real world" performance of the GEC and its effect on clinical decision making with general corroboration of its high NPV.[42-49] Notably, although it is important to understand test performance in these observational settings, studies of this nature are inherently problematic because nodules determined to be benign are not routinely resected. Without a histopathologic reference standard, true negative and false negative rates are difficult to ascertain. Duh et al. conducted a review of studies evaluating the diagnostic accuracy of the GEC for indeterminate nodules using a QUADAS-2 tool customized to evaluate methodological flaws within these studies. The authors found significant methodological heterogeneity among these studies, with the most common methodological flaw being the lack of an assigned diagnostic reference standard for unexcised GEC-benign nodules.[50] Nonetheless, several studies characterized clinical follow-up for GEC-benign nodules that would suggest clinical observation in these cases is appropriate.[51-54]

For nodules with Hürthle cell (oncocytic) features, the diagnostic accuracy of the GEC was noted in several studies to be problematic, with the classifier disproportionately assigning a "suspicious" result to nodules with oncocytic cell types.[41,44,45,49,55] Indeed, the 2012 GEC validation study reported a GEC-benign result in only 19% of Hürthle cell adenomas, compared with a GEC-benign result for 58% of follicular adenomas without Hürthle cell features.[41] In a study of 58 indeterminate nodules submitted for Afirma GEC testing, Harrell et al. reported that 9 of 13 false positives were determined to have benign oncocytic histopathology; in this study, 19 of 21 Hürthle cell nodules were GEC-suspicious.[49] Brauner et al. examined GEC performance in 46 indeterminate (Bethesda III/IV) nodules with Hürthle cell features and noted an overall specificity of just 7.5%.[55] Collectively, these findings raised concerns for the test's accuracy in Hürthle cell samples.

GENE SEQUENCING CLASSIFIER

In 2017, Veracyte released the Afirma Gene Sequencing Classifier (GSC), developed to maintain the high sensitivity and NPV of the GEC and improve its specificity and PPV. The GSC uses NGS technology and enhanced machine learning strategies to evaluate the

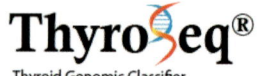

| Patient
DOB/Age/Sex
Client Identifier
Collection Date
Accession Date
Reported Date | Client
Requesting Physician
Ordering Physician
T
F | Accession #:
Client Accession #: |

CLINICAL HISTORY
FNA cytology: AUS/FLUS (Bethesda III)

THYROSEQ® V3 GC RESULTS SUMMARY
RIGHT THYROID FNA

Test Result	Probability of Cancer	Potential Management
POSITIVE	High (>80%)	Surgical consultation * *See interpretation below for details

INTERPRETATION
- RAS mutation was identified in this sample together with copy number alterations and abnormal gene expression profile.
- Co-occurrence of these molecular alterations is associated with ~80% risk of cancer, typically follicular variant of papillary carcinoma. The remaining tumors are expected to be pre-malignant NIFTP or benign follicular adenomas.
- Risk of cancer recurrence associated with the combination of these alterations is expected to be low to intermediate.
- Patient management decisions must be based on the independent medical judgment of the treating physician. Molecular test results should be taken into consideration in conjunction with all relevant imaging and clinical findings, patient and family history, as well as patient preference.

DETAILED RESULTS

Specimen cellularity/adequacy for interpretation: **ADEQUATE**

Marker Type	Marker Result			AF
Gene mutations	HRAS	p.Q61R	c.182A>G	36%
Gene fusions	Negative			
Copy number alterations	Positive			
Gene expression profile	Positive			
Parathyroid	Negative			
Medullary/C-cells	Negative			

AF=Variant Allele Frequency

Page 1 of 3

Fig. 12.1 ThyroSeq® v3 Sample Report. (Molecular and Genomic Pathology, UPMC, Pittsburgh, PA.)
Continued

CHAPTER 12 Fine-Needle Aspiration and Molecular Analysis

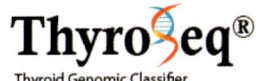

BACKGROUND

Diagnostic use of molecular markers in FNA samples with indeterminate cytology. Thyroid cancer is characterized by common occurrence of various genetic alterations (1). Based on the results of multicenter prospective double-blind study of ThyroSeq v3 (2,3), in the populations with pre-test cancer prevalence of 23-35%, the probability of cancer in thyroid nodules with Bethesda III (AUS/FLUS) and Bethesda IV (FN/SFN) cytology and negative ThyroSeq v3 test result is 2-3%. Based on our validation analysis, the probability of cancer in nodules with suspicious for malignant cells (Bethesda V) cytology and negative ThyroSeq test result is ~20% (data on file).

Patient management. Management of patients with thyroid nodules can be informed by the results of FNA cytology and ThyroSeq test. Importantly, in addition to the test results, clinical features of the nodule, patient history as well as patient preference must be considered when formulating the medical or surgical management approach.

ThyroSeq test result NEGATIVE: According to the National Comprehensive Cancer Network (NCCN) clinical practice guidelines (4), if molecular testing, in conjunction with clinical and ultrasound features, predicts a risk of cancer comparable to the risk of malignancy seen in a benign FNA cytology (approximately 5% or less), observation can be considered. Therefore, in those clinical situations where the pre-test probability of cancer in nodules with Bethesda III and IV cytology is <44%, negative ThyroSeq test results would confer the cancer probability of 5% or less (3), justifying observation in lieu of surgical management in appropriately selected cases. Because the probability of cancer in such nodules is comparable to benign FNA cytology, the management of patients may follow the recommendations for nodules with benign cytology, which, based on the 2015 American Thyroid Association (ATA) guidelines, should be determined based on ultrasound (US) pattern (5): For nodules that have high suspicion US pattern, repeat US and US-guided FNA within 12 months; for nodules with low to intermediate suspicion US pattern, repeat US at 12-24 months and if sonographic evidence of growth or development of new suspicious sonographic features, the FNA could be repeated or observation continued with repeat US, with repeat FNA in case of continued growth (Rec. #23 in ref. 5). In nodules with Bethesda V cytology and negative ThyroSeq result, the residual cancer risk of ~20% does not allow to avoid surgical management; thyroid lobectomy may be sufficient initial treatment for many of these patients as the majority of these nodules are expected to be benign.

ThyroSeq test result: CURRENTLY NEGATIVE: Test results are reported as currently negative when the sample is found positive for a low-risk (LR) gene mutation that alone is not sufficient for full cancer development (eg. PTEN, EIF1AX) and also found in a subpopulation of cells (6). Although at the time of sampling most of these nodules are benign, some of them may undergo clonal expansion and acquire additional mutations. In the absence of high suspicion US pattern or other clinical risk factors, many of these patients are likely to benefit from active surveillance with potential repeat of FNA and molecular testing in 1 year.

ThyroSeq test result POSITIVE: For these nodules, the type and level of mutation(s) provide further refinement of the probability of cancer and allow estimating cancer aggressiveness/risk. According to the ATA risk stratification system for thyroid cancer, the risk of structural disease recurrence can be low (~1-5%), intermediate (~10-20%), and high (30-55%) (5).

ThyroSeq test positive for an isolated RAS or RAS-like mutation (e.g. BRAF K601E, PPARG fusions) predicts a high probability (~80%) of either low-risk cancer (2,3) or a pre-cancerous tumor, NIFTP (7). Many of these nodules may be managed by therapeutic lobectomy, which is currently recommended by the ATA guidelines for low-risk papillary and follicular carcinomas (Rec. #35 in ref. 5) and NIFTP (8).

ThyroSeq test positive for an isolated BRAF V600E or BRAF V600E-like mutation (e.g. RET/PTC, BRAF fusions) confers a very high (>95%) probability of cancer that typically is at intermediate risk for recurrence (9). According to the ATA guidelines (5), BRAF-mutated unifocal intrathyroidal carcinoma is low risk for disease recurrence and therefore may be treated with thyroid lobectomy alone, whereas 1-4 cm intrathyroidal BRAF-positive PTC is an intermediate-risk tumor, where total thyroidectomy or lobectomy should be considered based on clinical and US findings.

ThyroSeq test positive for multiple high-risk (HR) mutations (e.g. BRAF V600E and TERT) is virtually diagnostic of cancer and predicts an elevated risk of disease recurrence by the ATA guidelines (5) and of tumor-related mortality by several studies (10-12). Most of these patients would likely benefit from total thyroidectomy, with possible consideration for regional lymph node dissection if one of the mutations is BRAF V600E (13).

Fig. 1. Potential management of patients with Bethesda III-IV cytology. (LR – low-risk; HR – high-risk; NIFTP – non-invasive follicular thyroid neoplasm with papillary-like nuclear features; LND – lymph node dissection)

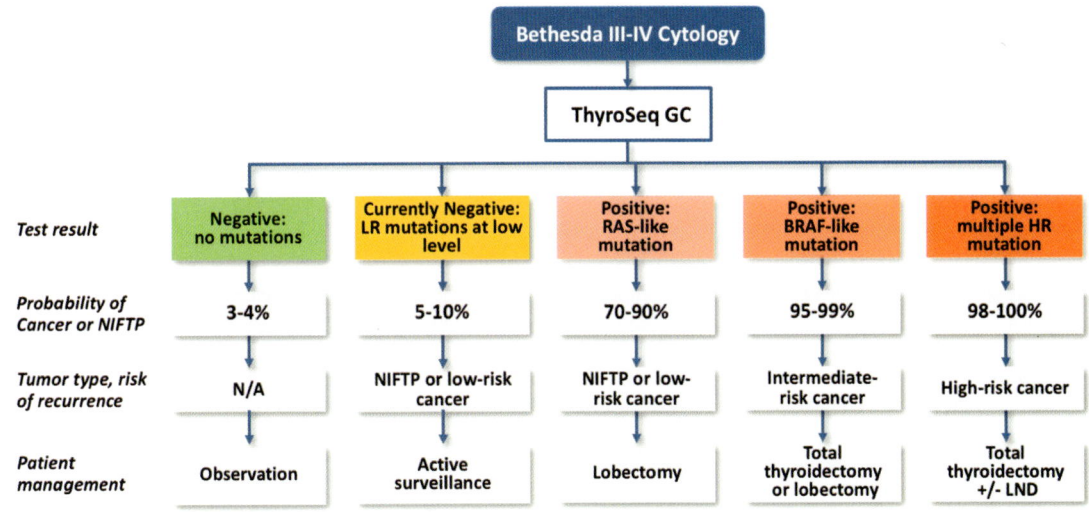

Fig. 12.1, cont'd

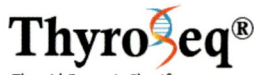

Other applications. In addition to the primary application for indeterminate FNA cytology, ThyroSeq may have clinical utility in a subset of FNA samples with benign (Bethesda II) or malignant (Bethesda VI) cytology. Up to 30% of nodules with benign cytology but suspicious clinical features have detectable mutations, and most of those are found malignant after surgery (14,15). One study showed that testing for BRAF and RAS mutations decreased the false-negative rate of cytology from 4.8% to 0.4%, concluding that molecular testing could be helpful, but only in the presence of clinical suspicion for malignancy (15). In cytology samples with positive for malignancy (Bethesda VI) cytology and in surgically removed cancer samples, ThyroSeq testing may contribute to thyroid cancer risk stratification and optimizing patient management, including decision-making related to the use of radioiodine (16-18). In advanced thyroid cancer, mutational status may impact selection of targeted therapies (19).

References
1. Agrawal N, et al. Cell. 2014;159:676-90; 2. Steward D, et al. Thyroid. 2017;27:A-168; 3. Nikiforova M, et al. Thyroid. 2017;27:A-181; 4. 2016 National Comprehensive Cancer Network (NCCN) clinical practice guidelines for thyroid carcinoma. https://www.nccn.org/ 5. Haugen BR, et al. Thyroid. 2016;26:1-133; 6. Karunamurthy A, et al. Endocr Relat Cancer. 2016;23:295-301; 7. Nikiforov YE, et al. JAMA Oncol. 2016;2:1023-9; 8. Haugen BR, et al. Thyroid. 2017;27:481-483; 9. Yip L, et al. Ann Surg. ;262:519-25; 10. Xing M, et al. J Clin Oncol. 2014;32:2718-26; 11. Song YS, et al. Cancer. 2016;122:1370-9; 12. Melo M, et al. J Clin Endocrinol Metab. 2014;99:E754-65; 13. Howell GM, et al. Ann Surg Oncol. 2013;20:47-52; 14. Nikiforov YE, et al. J Clin Endocrinol Metab. 2009;94:2092-8; 15. Proietti A, et al. Cancer Cytopathol. 2014;122:751-9; 16. Tufano RP, et al. Medicine (Baltimore). 2012;91:274-86; 17. Xing M, et al. Lancet. 2013;381:1058-69; 18. Xing M, et al. J Clin Oncol. 2009;27:2977-82; 19. Bible KC, et al. Nat Rev Clin Oncol. 2016;13:403-16;

METHODOLOGY
Nucleic acids (DNA/mRNA) are isolated from thyroid FNA samples collected in the ThyroseqPreserve solution or from fixed samples. If required, manual microdissection is performed from unstained slides under the microscope with H&E guidance. The NGS analysis is applied to detect SNVs/indels, gene fusions (GF), gene expression alterations (GEA), and copy number alterations (CNAs) in targeted regions of 112 thyroid-cancer related genes (AGGF1, AGK, AKAP13, AKAP9, AKT1, ALK, APC, BANP, BCL2L11, BRAF, C7orf10, CALCA, CCDC149, CCDC30, CCDC6, CCNY, CHEK2, CHGA, CITED1, CREB3L2, CTNNB1, DICER1, EIF1AX, EML4, EP300, ERBB4, ERC1, ETV6, EZH1, EZR, FAM114A2, FAM193A, FARSB, FGFR2, FKBP15, GFPT1, GLIS3, GNAS, GOLGA5, GORASP2, GTF2IRD1, HOOK3, HRAS, IDH1, IDH2, IGF2BP3, IRF2BP2, KIAA1217, KIAA1598, KIF5B, KLK1, KRAS, KRT20, KRT7, KTN1, LOC389473, LTK, MACF1, MEN1, MET, MKRN1, NCOA4, NF2, NRAS, NTRK1, NTRK3, OFD1, PAX8, PCM1, PGK1, PICALM, PIK3CA, POR, PPARG, PRKAR1A, PTEN, PTH, RAF1, RBPMS, RET, RNF213, ROS1, SLC26A11, SLC5A5, SND1, SPECC1L, SQSTM1, SS18, SSBP2, STK11, STRN, SYN2, TBL1XR1, TERT, TFG, THADA, TP53, TPM3, TPR, TRA2A, TRIM24, TRIM27, TRIM33, TRIM61, TSC2, TSHR, UACA, VCL, VHL, WARS, ZBTB8A, ZC3HAV1). The Torrent Suite v5.2.2, Variant Explorer v2 and Genomic Classifier (GC) algorithm is used for data analysis. Test results are reported as Negative (low probability of malignancy) or Positive (high probability of malignancy). Specimen adequacy, mutation type, gene expression and CNA profiles are reported in the Detailed Results section. In FNA samples, GC sensitivity is 93% and specificity is 81% (2). The GC limits of detection (LOD) is 6-12% of thyroid cells (3). Analytical sensitivity (PPA) and analytical specificity (PPV) for SNVs/indels is >99%/99% at 3-5% AF (6-10% of tumor cells), for GF is >99%/99% at >1-3% of tumor cells, for GEA is >99%/99% at 10% of tumor cells, and for CNA is 92%/100% with LOD 20-25% of tumor cells in FNA samples and 40-70% of tumor cells in FFPE samples. The assay minimal required sequencing depth is 500x. Genetic regions that did not meet minimal sequencing coverage requirements are specified in the report as failed.

Additional details of DNA sequence variants

Gene	Transcript	Genomic Position
NRAS	NM_002524.4	chr1:115256529T>C

LOW COVERAGE HOTSPOTS OBSERVED IN THE FOLLOWING GENES
NONE

GROSS DESCRIPTION
1 FNA vial(s) labelled with patient name and identifiers received from CBLPATH, INC.

DISCLAIMER
ThyroSeq is a diagnostic test that was developed and its performance characteristics determined by the UPMC Molecular and Genomic Pathology laboratory. It has not been cleared or approved by the U.S. Food and Drug Administration. The FDA has determined that such clearance or approval is not necessary. This test is used for clinical purposes. It should not be regarded as investigational or for research only. This laboratory is certified under the Clinical Laboratory Improvement Amendments (CLIA) as qualified to perform high complexity clinical laboratory testing. ThyroSeq test does not sequence genes in their entirety and mutations outside of mutation hotspots, some insertions and deletions, some novel gene fusions, and genomic alterations below sensitivity cut offs may not be detected. This test does not provide information on germline or somatic status of detected mutations. Certain sample characteristics may result in reduced sensitivity, including sample heterogeneity, low sample quality, and other causes. The information in this report must be used in conjunction with all relevant clinical information and does not intend to substitute clinical judgement. Decisions on patient care must be based on the independent clinical judgement of the treating physician. A treating physician's decision should not be based solely on this or any other single tests or the information in this report.

Electronically signed out by:

01/05/2018 14:41

Fig. 12,1, cont'd

expression profile of more than 10,000 genes, of which 1115 core genes drive the ensemble classification model. Among these core genes are 140 of the 142 genes that were included in the GEC classifier. The GSC incorporates RNA-Seq to detect point mutations and gene fusions, as well as genomic copy number alterations, including loss of heterozygosity.[56,57] Samples submitted for GSC testing are first screened for parathyroid tissue, as well as MTC, BRAF V600E, and RET-PTC1/3 fusions, genomic alterations linked to PTC. Samples that screen positive for one of these "malignancy classifiers" are reported as such and are not evaluated by the main classifier.

Several features were added to improve performance of the GSC classifier, including upstream analysis of follicular cell content to ensure quality control. To improve specificity for Hürthle cell nodules, the Hürthle cell index and Hürthle cell neoplasm index classifiers were incorporated into the main classifier. The Hürthle cell index classifier uses gene expression and mitochondrial transcript analysis to detect the presence of Hürthle cells. If identified, the Hürthle cell neoplasm index classifier determines whether the nodule is neoplastic, incorporating analysis of copy number alterations and loss of heterozygosity, molecular signatures that are common to Hürthle cell neoplasms.[58] Nodules positive for Hürthle cells that are determined to be neoplastic are submitted to the standard GSC classifier and reported as GSC-benign or GSC-suspicious. Nodules that are positive for Hürthle cells but determined to be nonneoplastic are submitted to the main classifier with an adjusted threshold that allows more samples to be assigned a GSC-benign result.

For GSC-suspicious nodules, the Afirma Xpression Atlas (XA) became available as a supplementary test panel to identify genetic alterations implicated in thyroid carcinogenesis. Also offered for Bethesda V and VI nodules, the XA uses RNA-Seq to detect variants and fusions in more than 500 genes; genetic alterations that are identified may be used to guide clinical decision making but are not assigned risk of malignancy estimates for indeterminate samples. Of note, the XA employs RNA-Seq of transcribed portions of the genome, so genetic alterations that occur in noncoded regions of DNA, such as the TERT promoter, are not assessed with the XA.[57]

Clinical Validation

The GSC was clinically validated in a blinded study using the same cohort of samples with a histopathologic reference standard prospectively collected for the GEC clinical validation study.[41,56] Of the 210 Bethesda III/IV nodules included in the GEC study, 191 (91.0%) retained sufficient RNA for analysis with the GSC. High sensitivity was maintained for the GSC at 91%, and specificity was improved from the GEC's 48% to 68% for Bethesda III/IV samples. At a malignancy prevalence of 24% (Bethesda III/IV), NPV for the GSC was 96% and PPV was 47%. Of the 191 samples, 26 (13.6%) were Hürthle cell neoplasms on histopathology. Among this subgroup, sensitivity of the GSC was 88.9% and specificity was 58.8%, reflecting improved performance compared with the GEC's specificity of 11.8% for this same group of nodules. The overall improved specificity with an increased number of benign results (BCR) suggests an improved ability to triage nodules for clinical observation.[56]

Postvalidation studies have compared the performance of the GEC and GSC in observational settings. Angell et al. retrospectively examined the BCR for indeterminate (Bethesda III/IV) nodules tested with the GEC (N 486) or the GSC (N 114) after it became clinically available. Overall, the GSC had a higher BCR than the GEC (65.8% versus 47.9%, $p < 0.001$).[59] Similarly, Endo et al. retrospectively compared GEC-tested (N 343) and GSC-tested (N 164) Bethesda III/IV nodules and found a higher BCR (76.2% versus 48.1%, $p < 0.001$), specificity (94.3% versus 61.4%, $p < 0.001$), and PPV (60.0% versus 33.3%, $p = 0.01$) for the GSC compared with the GEC when considering all unresected GEC/GSC-benign nodules to be true negatives. These authors reported a 66% relative reduction of indeterminate nodules progressing to surgery with the GSC compared with the GEC, with the majority of the reduction occurring for Bethesda III nodules.[60] Harrell et al. reported a statistically significant improvement in the BCR with the GSC (N 139) versus the GEC (N 481) (61.2% versus 41.6%) and a concomitant 45% relative reduction in surgery with application of the GSC compared with the GEC.[61] Improved performance of the GSC for nodules with Hürthle cell cytology was also consistently demonstrated in these studies with a higher BCR for the GSC compared with the GEC.[59-61]

Practical Considerations

Samples may be collected for Afirma testing with a repeat procedure after an initial FNA renders a cytologically indeterminate result or may be collected at the time of initial biopsy and submitted for testing if cytology proves to be indeterminate. Alternatively, reflex testing may be performed after rapid cytologic interpretation at the time of initial biopsy. Two dedicated FNA passes into a proprietary nucleic acid preservative are required and shipped to Veracyte with frozen "cold bricks" in prepared packaging. Veracyte requires a concurrent cytology specimen be sent for diagnostic verification at a centralized cytopathology laboratory (Thyroid Cytopathology Partners in Austin, TX), though several academic medical centers are excepted from this requirement. A sample report is provided in Figure 12.2.

THYGENEXT®-THYRAMIR®

Background

ThyGeNEXT®-ThyraMIR® (Interpace Diagnostics, Inc, Parsippany, NJ) is a combination NGS panel and microRNA expression classifier. ThyGeNEXT® has undergone multiple iterations over time, although the underlying methods have remained consistent. The test was originally marked as miR*Inform* Thyroid (Asuragen, Inc, Austin, TX) and included analysis of mutations in four genes (*BRAF, KRAS, HRAS, NRAS*) and three fusion transcripts (*RET/PTC1, RET/PTC3, PAX8/PPARγ*) based on multiple published reports of high specificity in indeterminate cytology.[62,63] Addition of the *PIK3CA* gene and migration of the panel to a new platform led to the development of ThyGenX® (Interpace Diagnostics, Inc, Parsippany, NJ). Further panel expansion has led to ThyGeNEXT®, the most recent generation, which includes a total of 10 genes and 38 fusion transcripts, coupled with additional markers for MTC and parathyroid tissue.

ThyraMIR® is a microRNA expression classifier that generates a binary "low risk" or "high risk" reading based on the expression pattern of 10 microRNAs. ThyraMIR® was added to ThyGeNEXT® to improve the clinical sensitivity and NPV, which have been lacking with genotype-based testing. The current combined platform uses sequential testing, starting with the ThyGeNEXT® mutation analysis and if negative, reflex testing to ThyraMIR®. However, samples can be submitted for ThyGeNEXT® only.

Clinical Validation

Clinical validation was performed by Labourier et al. using the previous generation ThyGeNEXT®-ThyraMIR® platform. Testing was performed on a total of 109 Bethesda III/IV nodule aspirates from patients across 12 endocrinology centers with a 32% prevalence of malignancy. The platform carried a clinical sensitivity of 89%, specificity of 85%, NPV of 94%, and PPV of 74%; 61% of the specimens were called benign with a 6% risk of malignancy.[64] Postvalidation studies, along with validation of the newer ThyGeNEXT® panel, are currently planned or ongoing.

SECTION 3 Preoperative Evaluation

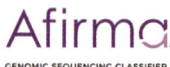

PATIENT REPORT

REPORT STATUS: Final
PAGES: 1 of 1
CLIENT ID:
AFIRMA REQ:

PATIENT INFORMATION

PATIENT:	DOB:	GENDER:	LAB ID:	MRN:
COLLECTION DATE	2019	FACILITY NAME		
RECEIVED DATE	2019	SUBMITTING PHYSICIAN		PHONE
REPORT DATE	2019	TREATING PHYSICIAN/CC		PHONE

CLINICAL HISTORY: No Clinical History Provided
REQUISITION COMMENTS: Suspicious for Hurthle Cell neoplasm

RESULTS SUMMARY

NODULE	CYTOPATHOLOGY	AFIRMA GSC	MALIGNANCY CLASSIFIERS
A	---	Benign (ROM <4%[1])	Negative

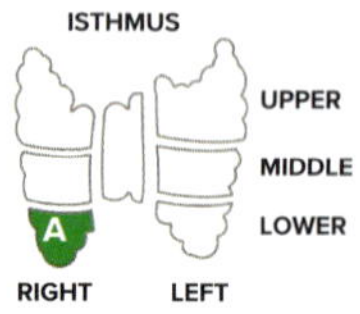

ISTHMUS / UPPER / MIDDLE / LOWER / RIGHT / LEFT

RESULTS DETAILS

NODULE A	SIZE: 1.5 cm	LOCATION: Lower Right
AFIRMA GSC RESULT	Benign	
MALIGNANCY CLASSIFIERS RESULTS	Negative: *BRAF* p. V600E c. 1799T>A, MTC Not Detected: *RET/PTC1*, *RET/PTC3*	
MALIGNANCY CLASSIFIERS COMMENTS	MTC and *BRAF* malignancy classifier results were negative and *RET/PTC1* and *RET/PTC3* were not detected. These results do not change the risk of malignancy (ROM) of the Afirma GSC Benign result.	
GROSS DESCRIPTION	Received one vial of FNAprotect, labeled with the Requisition Form # and patient initials.	

RESULTS INTERPRETATION[1]

Afirma GSC	Cytopathology Diagnosis Indeterminate*		Malignancy Classifiers			
			MTC	*BRAF*[‡]	RET/PTC	Parathyroid
Risk of Malignancy: **Afirma GSC Benign**	<4%	Sensitivity/Specificity	>99% / >99%			>99% / >99%
Risk of Malignancy: **Afirma GSC Suspicious**	~50%	PPA/NPA		>99% / >99%		
Sensitivity:	91%	PPV/NPA			>99% / >99%	
Specificity:	68%	Limit of Detection[†]	25%	5%	10%	15%
Limit of Detection[†]:	5%					

References: 1. Data on file. 2. Haugen BR, et al. *Thyroid* 2016.

* Indeterminate includes Atypia of Undetermined Significance / Follicular Lesion of Undetermined Significance and (suspicious for) Follicular Neoplasm / Hürthle Cell Neoplasm.
[†] Analytical sensitivity studies demonstrated the test's ability to detect malignant cells in a background of benign cells.
[‡] *BRAF* classifier performance is based on a comparison to a castPCR DNA assay for the *BRAF* V600E mutation.

Afirma Thyroid FNA Analysis is a diagnostic service provided by Veracyte, Inc. for the assessment of thyroid nodules that includes cytopathology and gene expression testing. Afirma GSC, *BRAF*, MTC and *RET/PTC* tests and their performance characteristics were determined by Veracyte. MTC is an RNA classifier that identifies the presence of medullary thyroid carcinoma (MTC); *BRAF* is a *BRAF* p. V600E, c. 1799T>A RNA classifier; *RET/PTC* is a gene expression marker of somatic rearrangements of the *RET* protooncogene (*RET/PTC1* and *RET/PTC3*).

E-SIGNED ON 2019 BY:
Veracyte Inc. CLIA # 05D20141206000 Shoreline Ct, Suite 100, South San Francisco, CA 94080

CLIA#05D2014120
CA License CLF340176
Lab Director: Robert J Monroe, MD, PhD

A copy of this form shall be as valid as the original. C758.1.1705 © 2017 Veracyte, Inc. All rights reserved. The Veracyte and Afirma name and logos are trademarks of Veracyte, Inc. Afirma Thyroid FNA Analysis is used for clinical purposes and clinical correlation of its results are recommended. The Veracyte laboratory is certified under the Clinical Laboratory Improvement Amendments of 1988 (CLIA) to perform high-complexity clinical testing. This test has not been cleared or approved by the FDA.

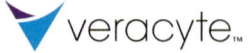

6000 Shoreline Court, Suite 700	T 888.9AFIRMA (888.923.4762)	F 650.243.6388
South San Francisco, CA 94080	T 650.243.6350 (International)	E support@veracyte.com

Fig. 12.2 Afirma® GSC Sample Report. (Courtesy Veracyte, Inc., San Francisco, CA.)

Practical Considerations

Samples are collected for ThyGeNEXT®-ThyraMIR® in a similar fashion to ThyroSeq and Afirma. Testing kits are complimentary and contain a test requisition form, RNA preservative, shipping materials, and prepaid return postage. Samples must contain at least 50 ng of total nucleic acid substrate garnered from one dedicated FNA pass (preserved in RNA*Retain,* a proprietary nucleic acid preservative). Refrigeration is not required for storage or shipping, and specimens are stable at room temperature for up to 6 weeks. Interpace Diagnostics, Inc. also offers cytology review (which requires at least one additional pass in CytoLyt® preservative) with reflex testing to ThyGeNEXT® alone or ThyGeNEXT®-ThyraMIR® if it is indeterminate. Testing is also available using cytology slides via proprietary extraction methods. A sample report is provided in Figure 12.3.

CHOOSING A MOLECULAR TEST

With three commercially available molecular tests and others in the pipeline, not to mention innumerable "home grown" institutional panels, choosing a testing platform may seem daunting. Although selection of a test based on its ability to "rule out" versus "rule in" malignancy has been a standard approach, this is giving way to practical conditions because newer tests use multiple methods or reflex testing to boost both PPV and NPV. The clinical context of the patient, insurance coverage/cost, and local rates of malignancy for each Bethesda category (particularly for III/IV/V) are helpful variables to consider in choosing when and how to judiciously use molecular diagnostics. It bears specific mention that molecular testing has been validated in cytologically indeterminate nodules; application to other Bethesda categories is unfortunately not uncommon despite incurring excessive cost with little benefit.[48] Molecular testing is less useful when clinical factors such as nodule size, suspicious radiographic features of the nodule or surrounding lymph nodes, or presence of compressive symptoms warrant surgery, or when patients have a strong up front opinion regarding surgery versus surveillance.[65] Determining institution- or practice-level malignancy rates can enable clinicians to calculate their own PPV/NPV for each test; this calculation is especially important in settings where malignancy prevalences deviate from those in the validation studies.

Several studies have attempted to compare the performance of available molecular tests. However, comparative and cost-effectiveness analyses are challenging to perform and interpret in the context of the rapid evolution of testing technologies and frequent revision of which alterations are included in the panel. Sciacchitano et al. performed a meta-analysis comparing the Afirma® GEC ± BRAF, ThyGenX®-ThyraMIR®, and Thyroseq® V2, among others, and found that all three had acceptable sensitivity and NPV, although BRAF mutation analysis and ThyroSeq® had the highest specificity/PPV.[66] Livhits et al. demonstrated that ThyroSeq® v2 had higher specificity compared with the Afirma® GEC and led to fewer surgeries.[67] Borowczyk et al. showed that, although the Afirma® GEC had higher sensitivity compared with ThyroSeq® V2 and was a more ideal "rule out" test, the higher specificity and accuracy of ThyroSeq® coupled with an acceptable sensitivity, made it a better "all-around" test.[68] However, these results are likely to be different with Veracyte's recent addition of the Afirma® GSC to increase its specificity and PPV. The authors of this chapter do not recommend one test over any another.

The cost effectiveness of molecular testing remains a topic of research, especially for newer versions of testing platforms. Yip et al. used hypothetical testing scenarios that demonstrated cost savings with molecular testing, predominantly by avoiding the need for completion thyroidectomy.[69] Although one small study has shown cost savings using molecular testing over diagnostic lobectomy, a case-based estimation showed molecular testing has higher costs, largely due to long-term nodule surveillance after testing.[70,71] Further research is underway to determine the effects of molecular testing on health care costs.

ILLUSTRATIVE CASES

Case # 1

A 29-year-old asymptomatic woman presented with a left thyroid nodule identified during a routine physical examination of the neck. The thyroid-stimulating hormone level was normal. On ultrasound, the 2.7 cm nodule was solid and somewhat hypoechoic but was wider than it was tall, had smooth margins, and had no internal echogenic foci (ATA Intermediate Suspicion, TI-RADS 4). An office-based ultrasound-guided FNA was performed. Cytopathologic evaluation showed a follicular lesion with Hürthle cell features (Bethesda III). A lymph node mapping ultrasound wdid not reveal any nodes that were suspicious for malignant involvement. ThyroSeq v3 testing was obtained on a specimen from the cell block prepared from the previously performed FNA biopsy specimen and was found to be positive (see Figure 12.1). Based on these results, a thyroid lobectomy was performed. Final pathology showed completely excised follicular variant PTC with several foci of capsular invasion but no angioinvasion (ATA low risk). Active surveillance was initiated.

Case # 2

A 53-year-old woman presented with a palpable right anterior neck mass. Ultrasound revealed a 3.5 cm well-circumscribed heterogeneous, predominately isoechoic right thyroid nodule and a 1.1 cm hypoechoic left thyroid nodule with internal microcalcifications. An ultrasound-guided fine-needle biopsy of the right thyroid nodule revealed AUS (Bethesda III). Biopsy of the left thyroid nodule revealed PTC. An additional sample from the right thyroid nodule was sent for Afirma GSC testing, which rendered a "suspicious" result with negative "malignancy classifiers." Whereas a "benign" result may have led to a recommendation for left thyroid lobectomy to address only the PTC, the "suspicious result" led to the recommendation of a total thyroidectomy. On histopathology, the right thyroid nodule proved to be a NIFTP, and the PTC was found to be multifocal and positive for a BRAF V600E mutation. The patient elected not to receive radioactive iodine, and active surveillance was initiated.

FUTURE APPLICATIONS

Although molecular testing has undoubtedly proven clinically useful in the assessment of indeterminate cytopathology, there are other applications that hold great promise. Molecular diagnostics may be leveraged to better articulate prognosis, which has potential implications in discussions with patients, determination of surveillance intervals, and therapy selection. It has long been known that RET/PTC rearrangements tend to occur in indolent PTC tumors.[72] Whereas both *BRAF V600E* and *TERT* promoter mutations are associated with a higher rate of tumor recurrence, the combination carries a markedly higher rate of recurrence, suggesting oncogene cooperativity.[73] Identification of these mutations in small cancers that might otherwise undergo active surveillance or conservative management may change management.[74] However, it remains unclear whether molecular markers carry independent prognostic value after adjusting for traditional clinicopathologic risk factors; gene panels or integrated measures of MAPK pathway output may be more robust biomarkers.[15,75]

As the pathways in thyroid carcinogenesis are better defined and molecular alterations become actionable with development of novel

Test Result Report

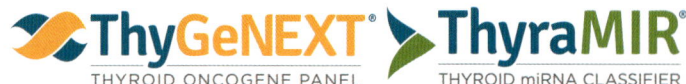

PATIENT INFORMATION

Patient Name: **John Q. Public**	MRN: 12345678
DOB: **5/11/2018** Gender: Male	Accession #: RP18-00000
Date Collected: 5/5/2018	Submitting Physician: Jane P. Smith, MD
Date Received: 5/7/2018	Treating Physician: John T. Smith, MD
Date Accessioned: 5/7/2018	Facility Name: Regional Community Hospital
Specimen Type Received: RNA Retain	Cytology Diagnosis Provided By: Requisition

RESULTS SUMMARY

Nodule	Cytopathology	ThyGeNEXT	ThyraMIR
Thyroid Isthmus FNA	Indeterminate (B-III)	BRAF (V600E) Mutation TERT (C250T) Mutation	Not Required

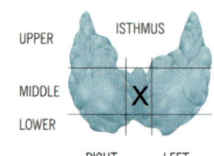

INTERPRETATION AND RISK ASSESSMENT

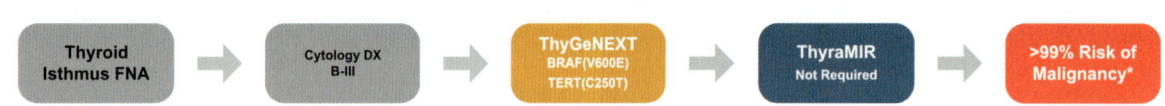

Thyroid Isthmus FNA → Cytology DX B-III → ThyGeNEXT BRAF(V600E) TERT(C250T) → ThyraMIR Not Required → >99% Risk of Malignancy*

* Risk assessment is based on disease prevalence of associated cytology diagnosis, mutational changes, microRNA expression, clinical experience, submitted manuscript and associated poster/platform presentation "The Utility of Combined Mutations and microRNA Expression Profiling in Assessing Cancer Risk in Thyroid Nodules", ATA Annual Meeting, October 2017 in addition to clinical validation[1](See Test Result Interpretation section)

TEST RESULT INTERPRETATION

Thyroid nodules showing both BRAF point mutation and TERT mutation are highly likely to be malignant with an aggressive form of thyroid carcinoma (1).

The BRAF oncogene involves 32% of the DNA copies present in the sample while the TERT mutation involves 54% of the DNA copies in the sample. Although BRAF and TERT separately are highly associated with conventional papillary thyroid carcinoma, coexistence of these mutations is commonly associated with aggressive clinicopathologic characteristics such as extrathyroidal extension or metastases. (2,3,4) Management for aggressive disease including total thyroidectomy and possible lymph node sampling may be considered. Correlation with clinical and radiological findings is recommended.

Although molecular parameters are useful in predicting biological aggressiveness, they can be imperfect hence all decision factors, including ultrasound results, nodule size, cytology and patient history need to be taken into account in diagnosis and determining patient management.

Continued on next page

MUTATIONS ANALYZED with ThyGeNEXT and ThyraMIR

DNA Point Mutation Analysis		Messenger RNA Translocation Analysis		microRNA Classifier Analysis
Gene	**Single Nucleotide Variants**	**Key Gene**	**Fusion Partner**	
ALK	L1198F, G1201E	ALK	STRN, EML4	miR-204-5p
BRAF	V600E, K601E, A598V	BRAF	AGK, AKAP9, SPTLC2	miR-139-5p
GNAS	R201H, L203P, Q227E, R844C	NTRK1	TPM3, TPR, TGF	miR-375
HRAS	G12V, G13R, Q61R, Q61K	NTRK2	TERT	miR-29b-1-5p
KRAS	G12D, G12V, G13D, G13R, Q61K, Q61R, Q61H	NTRK3	ETV6, SLC12A6	miR-155-5p
NRAS	G12D, G13D, G13R, Q61K, Q61R, Q61P	PPRAg	BMS1, PAX8, CREB3L2	miR-551b-3p
PIK3CA	E542K, E545K, H1047L, H1047R	RET	CCDC6, ELKS, GOLGA5, HOOK3, KTN1, NCO4	miR-146b-5p
PTEN	C124F, R130X	RET	NCOA4, PCM1, PRKAR1A, RFG9, TRIM	miR-31-5p
RET	M918T, C630R, D631G, C634W, A883F, E921K	THADA	IGF2BP3, TRA2A, LOC389473	miR-222-3p
TERT	-124C>T, -146C>T, -138_139CC>TT, -161C>T	Housekeeping genes - NKX2.1, PAX8, TBP, USP33		miR-138-1-3p

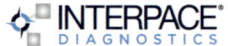

Interpace Diagnostics, 2515 Liberty Avenue, Pittsburgh, PA 15222
www.interpacediagnostics.com | TEL: 800.495.9885 | FAX: 888.674.6894 | labsupport@interpacedx.com

Page 1 of 3

Fig. 12.3 ThyGeNEXT®/ThyraMIR® Sample Report. (Courtesy Interpace Diagnostics, Inc., Parsippany, NJ.)

Continued

CHAPTER 12 Fine-Needle Aspiration and Molecular Analysis

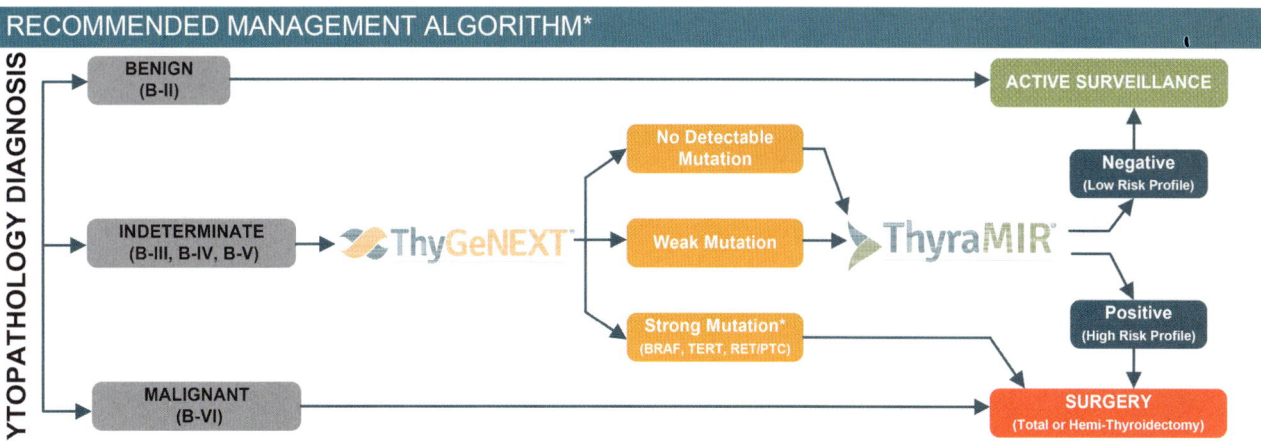

*ThyGeNEXT samples that are positive for BRAF, TERT, ALK and RET/PTC will solely receive a ThyGeNEXT test result. ThyGeNEXT samples that test positive for markers that have a lower risk of malignancy, such as RAS, will also receive a ThyraMIR test result.
**Patient management shown above is based on cytological diagnosis (if available) and molecular findings. However, actual management may differ, since clinical decisions are based on comprehensive evaluation of patient characteristics, sonographic findings, and correlative clinical factors.
***NCCN guidelines for management of nodules with B3 and B4 cytology diagnoses includes consideration of molecular analysis[5].

TEST RESULT INTERPRETATION (Continuation)

1. E. Labourier et al, Multi-categorical testing for miRNA, mRNA and DNA in fine needle aspiration improves the preoperative diagnosis of thyroid nodules with indeterminate cytology, Endocrine Reviews, 86(2), 2015
2. Beaudenon-Huibregtse S, et al, Centralized molecular testing for oncogenic mutation complements the local cytopathology diagnosis of thyroid nodules. Thyroid 2014, 10: 1479-87
3. Liu, R, Xing, M, Diagnostic and Prognostic TERT Promoter Mutations in Thyroid Fine Needle Aspiration Biopsy, Endocrine Related Cancer, 2014, October; 21, 825-830
4. Liu R, Xing M, TERT Promoter Mutations in Thyroid Cancer, Endocrine Related Cancer, 2016; 23, R143-R155
5. NCCN guidelines, Version 1.2018, Thyroid Carcinoma – nodule evaluation, THYR-4

The ThyGenX component of the testing was performed at Interpace Diagnostics, 2515 Liberty Ave, Pittsburgh, PA 15222, USA (CAP# 7186526; CLIA# 39D1024654). The ThyraMIR component of the testing was performed at Interpace Diagnostics, 2515 Liberty Ave, Pittsburgh, PA 15222, USA (CAP# 7186526; CLIA# 39D1024654).

REGULATORY

The ThyGeNEXT™ Thyroid Oncogene Panel provides PCR-based enrichment from fine-needle aspiration biopsies of thyroid nodules and next-generation sequencing (NGS) DNA and RNA analysis. The DNA analysis interrogates 10 genes relevant to thyroid carcinoma, including BRAF, TERT, ALK, RET, PTEN, HRAS, KRAS, NRAS, GNAS, PIK3CA, and 38 RNA fusion transcripts including PAX8/PPARgamma, RET/PTC, and various fusion partners of ALK, RET, BRAF, NTRK, and THADA. Duplicate PCR enrichment was performed using custom oligonucleotide primers with analysis on a MiSeq platform (Illumina).

The analytical sensitivity of this assay is at least 3% for mutant DNA and at least 5% for RNA translocations in a background of wild-type genomic DNA and RNA, respectively. The reporting range is at least 5% for DNA variants, with the exception that the reporting range for BRAF V600E mutation is at least 3%. For the ThyGeNEXT panel, the overall, clinical sensitivity for this analysis is 63% and the specificity is 84% in cases with indeterminant cytology.

The ThyraMIR™ miRNA Classifier is a microRNA (miRNA) based discriminator of benign versus malignant disease using mathematical algorithm of 10 specific microRNAs trained and validated using thyroid nodules with known outcome. For fine needle aspirates in preservative solution, this assay requires a minimum of RNA equivalent to that for ThyGenX (1000 relative fluorescent units of housekeeping RNA genes). Discrimination can be affected by admixture with blood and normal RNA sources and has been shown to be operative within the range of admixture typically encountered in sampling of thyroid nodular disease.

The combined testing platform of ThyGenX with ThyraMIR has a clinical sensitivity of 89% and specificity of 85% for cases with indeterminate cytology diagnosis. (*The Journal of Clinical Endocrinology & Metabolism*, Volume 100, Issue 7, 1 July 2015, Pages 2743–2750) Laboratory analytical validation of ThyGeNEXT confirmed 100% agreement (95% CI: 99.5 to 100%) for the 5 genes (BRAF, HRAS, KRAS, NRAS, PIK3CA) and 6 fusions (PAX8-PPARG and RET-PTC) interrogated by ThyGenX. Based on this comparison, the performance of ThyGeNEXT is expected to be similar to ThyGenX; however, ThyGeNEXT will provide additional information on gene alterations strongly associated with aggressive forms of differentiated thyroid cancer and/or poor outcome.

Testing performed on material created for microscopic evaluation (cytology slide smears, cell block, or thin prep), depending on cellularity and extractable nuclei acid, may have similar or slightly lower test performance characteristics to that stated above.

Interpace Diagnostics, 2515 Liberty Avenue, Pittsburgh, PA 15222
www.interpacediagnostics.com | TEL: 800.495.9885 | FAX: 888.674.6894 | labsupport@interpacedx.com

Fig. 12.3, cont'd

REGULATORY (Continued)

DISCLAIMER:
This test was developed and its performance characteristics determined by Interpace Diagnostics Clinical Laboratory. It has not been cleared or approved by the FDA. The laboratory is regulated under CLIA as qualified to perform high-complexity testing and is used for clinical purposes. A negative result does not indicate a benign result. This test detects only the mutations listed above, which account for >80% of thyroid cancers. Other, rare mutations, that may be indicative of cancer may not be detected by this test. In addition, about 30% of thyroid cancers have no known genetic alterations and/or mutations.

CLIA# 39D1024654, CAP# 7186526 • Sydney D. Finkelstein, MD, Medical Director
Confidentiality of this medical record shall be maintained except when disclosure is required or permitted by law, regulation, or written authorization by the patient.

Interpreted By

Sydney Finkelstein, MD
Medical Director

Report Date

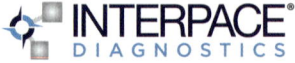

Interpace Diagnostics, 2515 Liberty Avenue, Pittsburgh, PA 15222
www.interpacediagnostics.com | TEL: 800.495.9885 | FAX: 888.674.6894 | labsupport@interpacedx.com

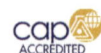

Fig. 12.3, cont'd

therapeutics, it's clear that we are entering an era of "precision medicine."[76] Several multikinase inhibitors have been approved by the Food and Drug Administration for advanced thyroid cancers, including sorafenib and lenvatinib for DTC, along with vandetanib and cabozantinib for MTC.[77,78] The combination of dabrafenib (BRAF V600E inhibitor) and trametinib (MEK inhibitor) has been approved for ATC and is the first approved genotype-specific therapy for thyroid cancer.[79] Molecular testing will likely play a vital role in the selection of patients and optimal therapies, along with the identification of markers of treatment resistance.[80] Lastly, the identification of circulating tumor cells and cell-free tumor DNA in the blood of patients with advanced malignancy has raised the possibility of diagnosing and characterizing cancer through a minimally invasive peripheral blood draw rather than through biopsy.[81] Circulating tumor cells and/or cell-free DNA have been detected in the blood of patients with advanced thyroid cancers and may be a novel source of actionable genetic information.[82,83]

CONCLUSION

An improved understanding of genetic drivers of thyroid cancer, coupled with advancements in molecular diagnostics, have revolutionized the preoperative risk stratification of thyroid nodules with indeterminate FNA cytopathology. Judicious application of these technologies can assist in the triage of patients for active surveillance or surgery and may also inform the extent of surgery, supplement traditional clinicopathologic variables to refine prognosis, and reveal targets for current and evolving molecular therapies.

REFERENCES

For a complete list of references, go to expertconsult.com.

13

Ultrasound of the Thyroid and Parathyroid Glands

Kevin T. Brumund, Susan J. Mandel

> Please go to expertconsult.com to view related video:
> **Video 13.1** Ultrasound of the Thyroid and Parathyroid Glands: Equipment and Techniques.
> This chapter contains additional online-only content, including exclusive video, available on expertconsult.com.

INTRODUCTION

The clinical utilization of ultrasound (US) continues to expand, with increasing applications in the head and neck. US remains the primary imaging tool for the thyroid gland. It is cost effective, rapid in information accrual, well-tolerated by patients, and helps patients avoid unnecessary radiation exposure. The image processing capabilities of current US machines used in tandem with high-frequency transducers can provide unmatched resolution and anatomic detail. Even small, portable systems are now able to provide meaningful imaging information. Thus US has become an indispensable tool of the clinician in the outpatient setting, and it represents an extension of the physical examination. The machines have become more affordable and portable, and there are numerous formal educational opportunities to learn the technology and its applications. In-office point of care US has many advantages for the patient; a single patient's in-office visit may include both diagnostic and interventional US procedures, which can help maximize efficiency and convenience. Specific to the thyroid gland and its associated pathologies, US has become integral to initial assessment and workup, preoperative planning, and long-term follow-up and surveillance.

 Please see the Expert Consult website for a brief discussion of the limitations of US.

PHYSICS AND PRINCIPLES OF ULTRASOUND

The US system has three basic components: (1) the transducer, which delivers and receives sound energy directly to and from the tissues; (2) the console, which among other things contains the sophisticated computer software, conversion algorithms, storage, and Doppler methodology; and (3) the display, which permits the observer to view and select anatomic areas of interest. An understanding of how sound energy and tissues interact has permitted a marriage of theory and technology. Whereas artifacts with other radiologic modalities (e.g., dental restoration production of scatter and degradation of computed tomography [CT] images) present an unwanted problem, artifacts in US enhance clinical information, which can be used to advantage.

 Please see the Expert Consult website for more discussion of this topic.

As a sound wave moves through a medium, the energy of the sound wave creates areas of compression and rarefaction of the molecules. This is displayed mathematically by the sine wave curve. The velocity of the sound wave is equal to the frequency times the wavelength. For any given medium, the velocity of the sound wave is the same regardless of the frequency. The relationship of frequency to wavelength is an inverse one; a lower frequency wave has a longer wavelength and a higher frequency wave has a shorter wavelength. Sound frequency is measured in cycles/second or hertz (Hz). US is defined at frequencies greater the 20 kilohertz (kHz; above audible sound) with medical applications of US within the 3 to 18 megahertz (MHz) range. Sound waves move through different media at different velocities and, generally, the denser the medium the higher the velocity.

As the sound waves enter the skin and deeper tissues, they meet elements of varying density, shape, and reflectivity. Most waves continue to penetrate the tissues and pass on in a linear fashion or scatter oblique to the path of the sound wave. In fact, only 1% of the transmitted sound is reflected back to the transducer.

There are three fundamental principles of sound waves: impedance, attenuation, and resolution. Acoustic impedance is the resistance of a medium to the propagation of a sound wave and is affected by the tissue density. Impedance differences between tissue interfaces results in a reflection. The greater the difference in impedance, the more the sound wave is reflected. A small impedance difference between tissue types (muscle and fat) results in a small reflection and most of the sound wave passing through; however, a large impedance difference may occur with such tissues as muscle and bone. During a large impedance difference, a large reflection and little of the sound wave will pass through as a result.

Sound waves progressively lose amplitude as they pass through tissues. This attenuation results from a combination of scattering and absorption and is dependent on the density of the tissues and depth of a targeted anatomic structure. Attenuation increases with increasing distance from the sound wave source (the transducer). The frequency of emitted sound has differing attenuation characteristics in tissue. Low frequencies in the range of 3 to 5 MHz are not attenuated readily and thus are more suited to demonstrating deeper structures. In contrast, high-frequency sound waves attenuate rapidly and have less depth of penetration. Hence, low frequency transducers are suitable for abdominal US, but higher frequency transducers (in the 10 to 15 MHz range) are ideal for visualizing the relatively superficial structures in the head and neck.

Wave emission from the transducer is not linear but has an hourglass configuration. The optimum point of tissue resolution is at the narrowest portion of this configured wave and designated the focal zone. Stated another way, the reflected waves from adjacent point tissue targets are seen as separated entities rather than combined blurred images when the focal point is properly aligned. The focal zone can be manipulated to a shallow or deeper plane within the region of interest. At the focal zone, tissue properties show the best *lateral resolution*. Similarly, the frequency of the transmitted wave is important. High-frequency waves produce better abilities than low-frequency waves to resolve adjacent tissue elements in the direct path of the sound wave. This property is designated *axial resolution*. Just as a newspaper image with relatively few points of dark ink and luminosity produces a relatively coarse image on magnification, a high megapixel photograph rendered from a digital single-lens reflex camera produces a sharper image with many more of these points per unit area. The example of the newspaper image is analogous to the lateral and axial resolution characteristics of penetrating and resolving sound waves, which combine to produce the ideal image. Where depth of penetration is the most important priority, the lower frequency waves must be utilized with some sacrifice in resolution. In US of the head and neck, where structures of interest are only a few centimeters below the skin surface, higher frequency waves with better axial resolution can be used. In summary, resolution or clarity on the monitor depends on both frequency and, to a lesser degree, alignment of the focal zone relative to the target. Selection of emitted transducer frequency and location of focal zone will depend on whether deep or superficial anatomic structures are to be studied.

Echogenicity is the term used to describe the appearance of an object or anatomic structure when using US. A reference point is used to define echogenicity; in the neck, normal thyroid tissue is typically referenced as the isoechoic structure. Isoechoic structures have nearly the same echogenicity as the surrounding tissue (or reference tissue). Anechoic structures have virtually no echoes with them and appear nearly black on US, which indicates through transmission of sound without reflection. Fluid filled structures, such as a thyroid cyst or the carotid artery, are described as *anechoic*. Hypoechoic structures appear darker, or less echogenic, than the surrounding tissue and hyperechoic structures appear brighter, or more echogenic.

Please see the Expert Consult website for more discussion of this topic.

Artifacts

In ultrasonography, artifacts are images that appear on the display and do not represent real anatomic structures. Rather, they are shadows or enhanced representation of tissue elements that are consistent and can be informative. Pure cysts have a thin discrete capsule and are entirely fluid-filled without significant solid components. Sound enters from a superficial direction and as yet unattenuated waves easily penetrate the anterior capsule. Because the interior of the cyst is fluid without elements that reflect sound, the parallel sound waves strike the posterior capsule. Through the acoustical mismatch, the posterior capsule acts as a reflector. A large proportion of these waves penetrate this capsule and return as bright, high amplitude signals from just beyond. This produces a relatively broad reflected area that is hyperechoic to adjacent tissues and the cyst itself. This artifact is designated "posterior enhancement" and is usually diagnostic of a cyst (Figure 13.1). In contrast, coarse calcifications block transmission of the sound waves to deeper tissue planes, producing a dark rectangular void deep to the densely hyperechoic structure. Known as *posterior shadowing* (Figure 13.2), this particular artifact represents coarse calcifications often seen in portions of a multinodular goiter and to a lesser degree in some cancers. In contrast, microcalcifications (Figure 13.3), generally seen in papillary carcinoma of the thyroid gland, do not produce posterior shadowing artifact as a result of their small size. These microcalcifications are small points of hyperechoic signal and are thought to represent either psammoma bodies defined histologically in papillary carcinoma of either the primary thyroid or metastatic adenopathy, or inspissated colloid. When planning fine-needle aspiration (FNA) cytology, these areas are good sampling targets under US guidance. Other artifacts may be confused with microcalcifications. One such confusion can occur with "comet tail" artifact (Figure 13.4). These are hyperechoic points with a tapering

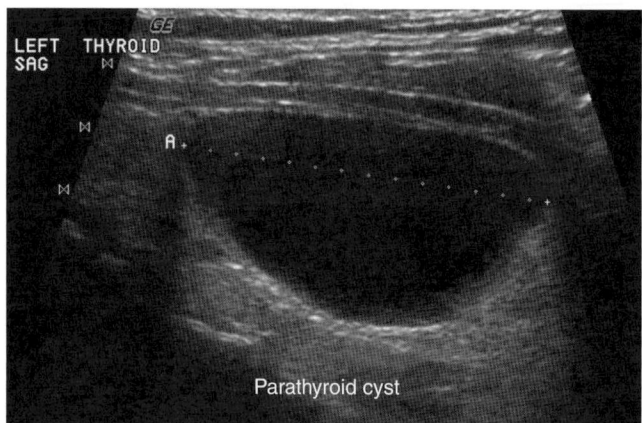

Fig. 13.1 Posterior enhancement deep to a parathyroid cyst.

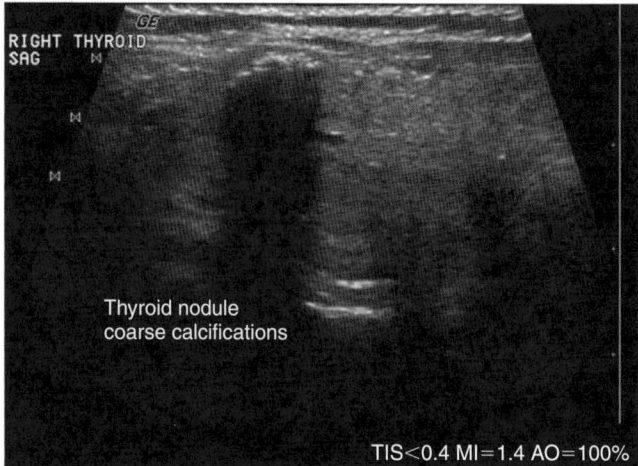

Fig. 13.2 Hyperechoic dense calcification in a thyroid nodule prevents penetration of sound, and a resultant deep shadow is identified.

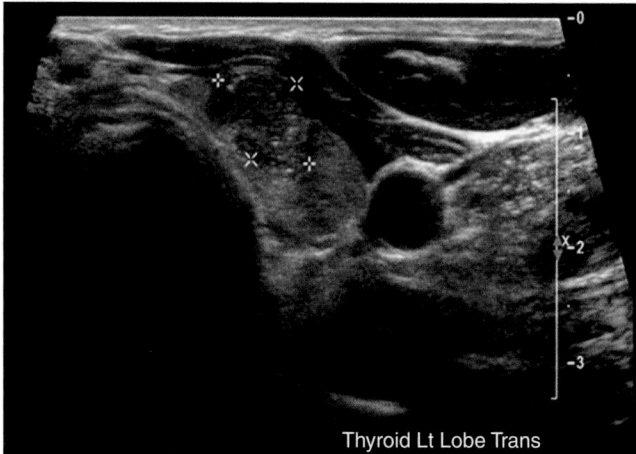

Fig. 13.3 Microcalcifications do not produce posterior shadowing artifact.

core of hyperlucency extending from and deep to the circular dot. When examined more closely, the tail portion is actually a form of reverberation artifact. One accepted explanation is that areas of colloid crystallize and serve both as finite obstructions to transmission and deeper reverberation of the US waves. Ahuja has studied comet tail artifacts in a large number of thyroid conditions. Invariably, he has found

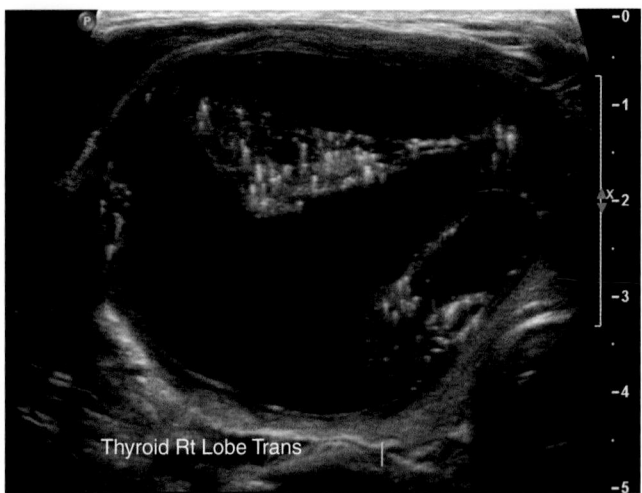

Fig. 13.4 Comet-tail artifact is similar in appearance to microcalcifications, but the comet tail clearly differentiates it from the representations of psammoma bodies.

that the underlying processes are benign.[4] Examples of structures that commonly demonstrate reverberation (Figure 13.5) are the anterior wall of the trachea, the anterior wall of the carotid artery, comet tails from small colloid crystals, and biopsy needles in their long axes.

Doppler

Doppler is a relevant and technically different process than grayscale US in the assessment of vascularity of anatomic and pathologic elements.[5] In simplistic terms, the Doppler shift of sound waves occurs when waves imparted at an angle to a blood vessel strike directionally moving red blood cells and are reflected. If the waves are reflected toward the transducer, the velocity of this reflection is augmented. If the sound waves are reflected away from the transducer, signifying blood flow away from the transducer, the velocity is reduced. This velocity of red cell movement can be calculated, and directional flow given a color designation—that is, flow toward the transducer is red and flow away from it is blue by convention. These Doppler images are superimposed over the corresponding B mode display in a rapidly alternating fashion such that the eye sees a moving color video rendition of this activity. This color Doppler imaging and flow interpolation is highly relevant to the study of carotid and peripheral vascular anatomy and restriction of flow. Power Doppler is a separate technique that ignores these calculations and directional relationships. Power Doppler is more sensitive to and has better resolution for small vessels with low flow, such as those found within a lymph node or parathyroid adenoma (Figure 13.6). In fact, power Doppler can often be used as a differentiating tool between these two structures in the clinical setting. Power Doppler will still reveal large vessels in the head and neck but cannot render actual flow values.

THYROID ULTRASOUND

US is the first-line recommended imaging modality for the thyroid gland and thyroid nodules.[6,7] Its use in thyroid disorders is widely acknowledged, and its benefits and indications continue to expand. Surgeons and endocrinologists in the office-based setting have adopted thyroid US for the evaluation and management of patients with thyroid, parathyroid, and many other head and neck disorders. Its versatility, convenience, safety profile, ability to offer dynamic real-time images, low cost compared with other radiologic modalities, and the outstanding quality of the images produced by high frequency, high-resolution US, have all contributed to its popularity. The relatively superficial location of the thyroid gland in the neck makes evaluation with US easy and practical. The images obtained from high resolution US allows for straightforward detection and description of thyroid gland pathology. Normal thyroid is uniform and homogeneous in appearance and described as *isoechoic*. Box 13.1 lists the principal goals of and indications for thyroid ultrasonography.

Please see the Expert Consult website for more discussion of this topic.

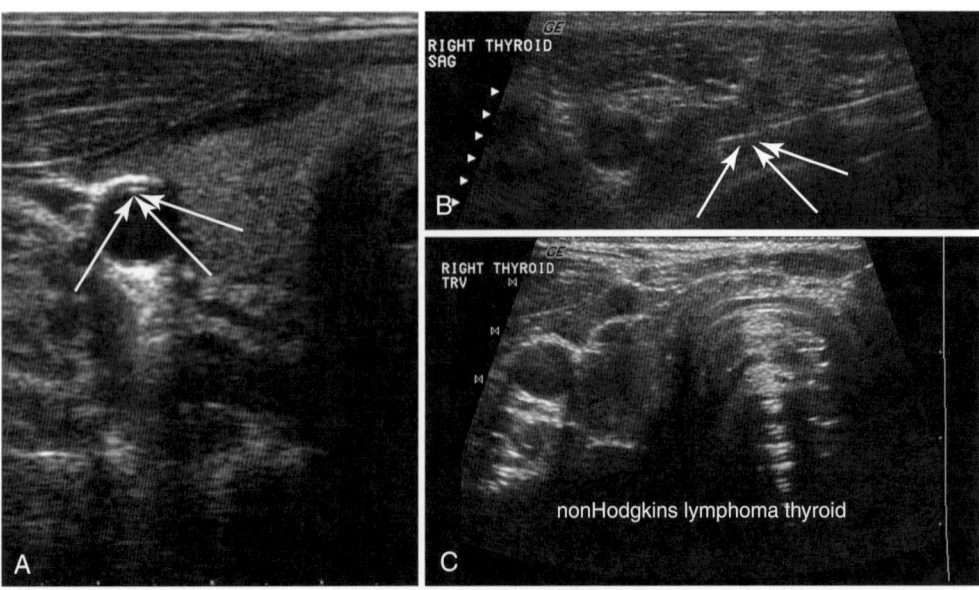

Fig. 13.5 Reverberation artifact can be seen in the following: **A,** anterior wall of the carotid artery; **B,** biopsy needles in the long axis; **C,** anterior tracheal wall. *Arrows* demonstrate the reverberating artifacts.

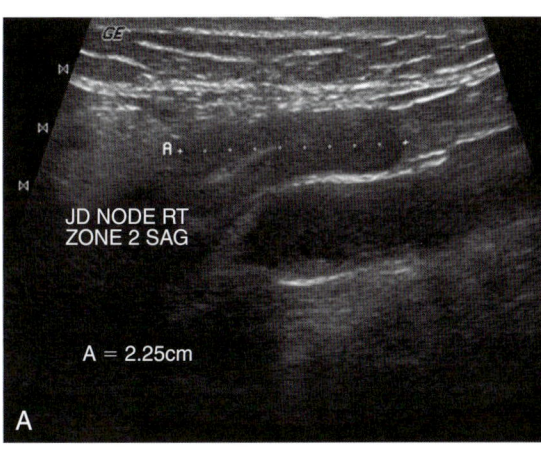 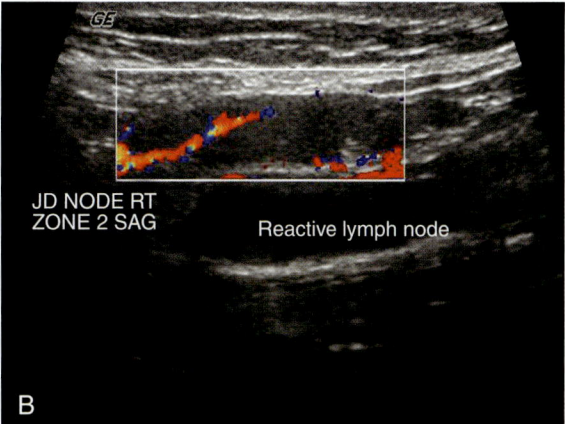

Fig. 13.6 Power Doppler demonstrates small vessels and their pattern in a hyperplastic lymph node (**A**, gray-scale; **B**, power Doppler overlay).

BOX 13.1 Thyroid Ultrasonography: Principal Goals and Indications

Assess palpable thyroid nodules and enlargement
Assess nonpalpable thyroid nodularity generally detected incidentally
Identify characteristics associated with malignancy
Assess the thyroid and extrathyroidal neck in patients with thyroid cancer before treatment
Monitor treated thyroid cancer patients for early evidence of recurrence
Monitor nodules, goiters, or lymph nodes in patients undergoing treatment or observation of thyroid disease
Screen high-risk patients (with familial forms of thyroid cancer, a history of radiation exposure, fluorodeoxyglucose [FDG] avidity on positron emission tomography [PET], etc.)
Screen for thyroid lesions in patients with other diseases in the neck, such as hyperparathyroidism, who are undergoing treatment planning
Guide fine-needle aspiration (FNA) biopsy and other interventions

Role of Ultrasound in the Initial Evaluation of the Thyroid Nodule

Thyroid US is recommended for all patients with suspected thyroid nodules,[6,7] including patients with palpable abnormalities, nodular goiter, and thyroid lesions incidentally found by other imaging studies. Appropriate initial management uses US to characterize any and all thyroid nodules to determine which ones potentially need further evaluation, if at all. A goal of characterizing by US is to recognize patterns that may distinguish benign from malignant nodules and determine which ones warrant further investigation with FNA biopsy.

Please see the Expert Consult website for more discussion of this topic.

The use of US guidance improves the overall sensitivity, specificity, and accuracy of FNA compared with palpation-guided FNA.[17-19] US-guided FNA appears to be most valuable in patients with nonpalpable nodules, small palpable nodules, posterior nodules, multiple nodules, partially cystic nodules, or concomitant glandular disease. US-guided FNA is also beneficial for sampling specific areas of a nodule, such as the solid part of a mixed solid-cystic nodule. Cesur et al. found the rates of inadequate FNA samples to be significantly improved in palpable nodules 1 to 1.5 cm using US- versus palpation-guided FNA (37.6% versus 24.4%, p = 0.009), but not for palpable nodules 1.6 cm or larger.[17]

US-guided FNA is also specifically recommended when repeating FNA for a nodule with an initial nondiagnostic cytology result.[6]

Ultrasonography Technique and Measurements

Please see the Expert Consult website for discussion of this topic, including Figures 13.7 and 13.8.

Ultrasound Characteristics of Thyroid Nodules

US is a powerful tool in the diagnosis and management of thyroid nodules. All patients with a confirmed or suspected thyroid nodule should have a formal US of the entire neck, including the thyroid gland. Many distinctive US characteristics of malignant thyroid nodules have been identified (Table 13.1). Although these US characteristics offer high sensitivity, no single criterion offers sufficient specificity to differentiate benign from malignant lesions.[25] When characteristics are combined into sonographic patterns, specificity improves as well as the ability to stratify nodules based on risk of malignancy. One large prospective, observational study comparing US and FNA results with surgical pathology found that performing FNA on nodules with one of three US criteria—microcalcifications, blurred margins, or hypoechoic pattern—missed only 2% of cancers.[26] Kim et al. prospectively analyzed 155 incidentally discovered, nonpalpable, solid thyroid nodules and found a mean number of 2.6 suspicious US characteristics per malignant nodule and an overall sensitivity and specificity of 94% and 66%, respectively.[27]

Particular US features of thyroid nodules and their ability to suggest benign versus malignant lesions include the following.

TABLE 13.1 Ultrasound Features Associated with Malignancy

Margins	Blurred, ill-defined
Halo/rim	Absent, avascular
Shape	Irregular, spherical, tall
Echo structure	Solid
Echogenicity	Hypoechoic (especially markedly so)
Calcifications	Microcalcifications, internal
Vascular pattern	Intranodular, hypervascular
Elastography	Decreased elasticity
Lymph nodes	Abnormal lymphadenopathy

Size

Nodule size does not predict malignancy, because nodules of all sizes harbor a similar risk of malignancy. The risk of malignancy for palpable thyroid nodules is approximately 10%, and a similar incidence of malignancy is found in nodules smaller than 1 cm.[28-30] Thyroid cancers less than 1 cm in size tend to behave in an indolent manner, and therefore suspicious subcentimeter lesions that are not treated should be followed with periodic US surveillance with the option for further evaluation by FNA if growth is observed. FNA biopsy of subcentimeter nodules can be considered if there is high risk of malignancy (family history of thyroid cancer, history of external beam or ionizing radiation, history of thyroid cancer, or positron emission tomography [PET] positive nodules); if there is a suggestion of extrathyroidal spread on US imaging; or if there is suspicious concomitant lymphadenopathy, in which case FNA of the lymph node should be performed.[6]

Margins and Halo/Rim

Benign lesions are often associated with a hypoechoic circumferential vascular "halo" (Figure 13.9) thought to represent compressed vascularity within thyroid parenchyma adjacent to a nodule.[31] Neoplasms may display a partial or absent halo, and its presence or absence has been found to be suggestive but not diagnostic.[32,33] For malignant lesions, the halo is typically avascular and represents a true capsule that may by invaded by neoplastic cells. The interface between a nodule and the surrounding thyroid parenchyma is typically well-defined; however, the borders of a malignant nodule can be irregular or infiltrative.[26,32,33] Extrathyroidal extension, with part of the nodule extending beyond the thyroid capsule into the surrounding soft tissue of the neck (i.e., strap muscles), should be noted on US and is highly suggestive of malignancy.[6] The mobility of the nodule with respect to surrounding structures can be assessed by dynamic palpation during US. Fixation suggests malignant invasion of the surrounding tissue.

Shape

Nodule shape has been implicated as a prognostic factor. Nodules that are more tall than wide on transverse view (i.e., greater anteroposterior diameter than transverse diameter [Figure 13.10]) are more likely to harbor cancer.[27] This characteristic has been found to predict malignancy in breast US as well.[34] However, one retrospective analysis also found that thyroid nodules with a more spherical shape had a higher incidence of malignancy.[31] Irregular shape and microlobulated borders (Figure 13.11) have also been implicated in malignancy.[27,33]

Echo Structure

Nodule composition varies from purely cystic to completely solid. Many thyroid nodules have cystic components, such as cystic degeneration of a follicular adenoma (Figure 13.12) or are found in the setting of multinodular goiter. Malignancy has been more closely associated with solid nodules than with cystic or mixed nodules.[26,33] Purely cystic nodules are unlikely to be malignant,[35] and those with a spongiform appearance (Figure 13.13), defined as an aggregation of multiple microcystic components in more than 50% of the nodal volume, are more than 99% specific for benign histology.[36,37]

Echogenicity

The echogenicity of a thyroid nodule should be compared with that of surrounding thyroid tissue. In diffuse thyroid disorders, such as thyroiditis, the entire abnormal gland may be hypoechoic, so assessment of any nodule must be relative to the normal thyroid gland, not the surrounding abnormal tissue. Most benign adenomas or adenomatous nodules are slightly hyperechoic to slightly hypoechoic compared with normal thyroid tissue (Figure 13.14), whereas malignant nodules are frequently markedly hypoechoic (Figure 13.15) or more hypoechoic than adjacent muscle.[27,33]

Calcifications

The presence of calcifications has variable significance. Peripheral calcification, also referred to as "eggshell calcification," has traditionally been considered a benign feature representing previous hemorrhage and degenerative change. However, a disruption in a rim calcification with soft tissue extrusion is suggestive of malignancy.[6] Coarse calcifications (measuring >1 mm) demonstrate posterior acoustic shadowing because the sound waves cannot penetrate the calcium deposit and are reflected back to the transducer. Calcifications alone are not associated with cancer, but they are more worrisome for potential malignancy when seen in the center of a solid hypoechoic nodule (see Figure 13.2). Microcalcifications (<1 mm hyperechoic lucencies) are even more

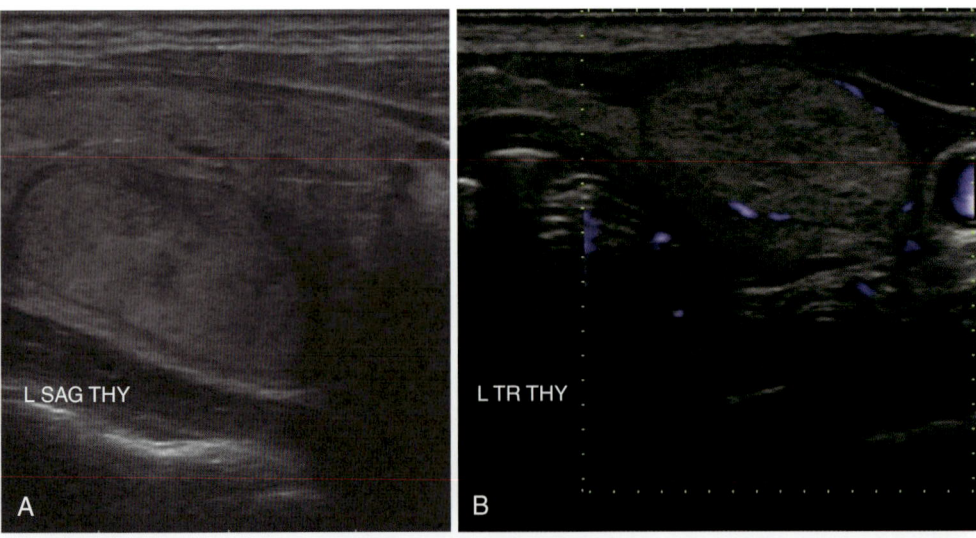

Fig. 13.9 A, Thin hypoechoic circumferential "halo" surrounding a benign thyroid nodule. **B,** Vascularity within the "halo" on Doppler imaging.

CHAPTER 13 Ultrasound of the Thyroid and Parathyroid Glands

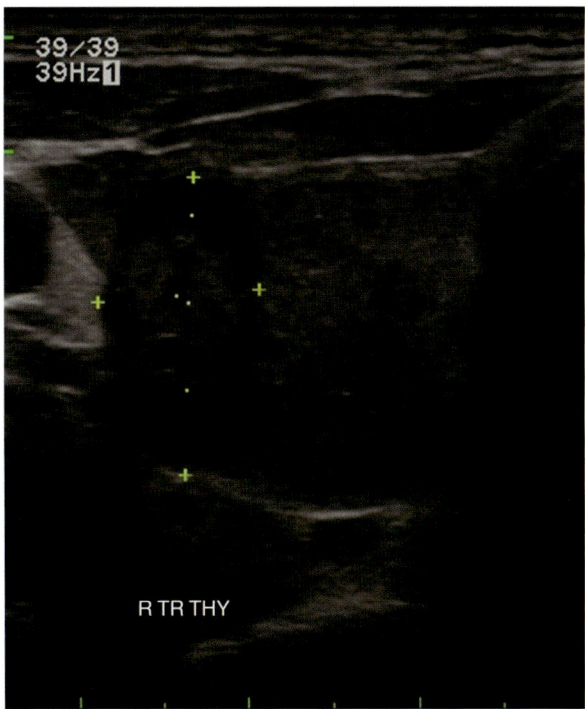

Fig. 13.10 Taller than wide (and markedly hypoechoic) nodule that proved to be malignant on surgical pathology (right transverse view of thyroid).

strongly associated with an increased risk of malignancy.[26] A reported 45% to 60% of malignant nodules demonstrate microcalcifications, as opposed to 7% to 14% of benign nodules.[27,38] Approximately 60% of patients with microcalcifications have malignant disease.[39] Microcalcifications in malignant nodules are often attributed to psammoma bodies in papillary thyroid carcinoma (PTC) (Figure 13.16), but are also frequently seen in medullary thyroid carcinoma (MTC). Although suggestive of malignancy, the overall specificity of microcalcifications for thyroid carcinoma has been reported to range from 71% to 94% with a sensitivity of 35% to 72%.[26,40,41] Therefore microcalcifications should not be solely relied upon to differentiate benign from malignant lesions.

Vascular Pattern

The vascular pattern around or within a nodule may correlate with the probability of malignancy. Chammas et al. classified thyroid nodules according to the pattern of vascularity seen with power Doppler into five types: absent blood flow, perinodular flow only, perinodular flow as great or greater than central blood flow, mainly central nodular flow, and central flow only.[42] Nodules with exclusively central blood flow or central blood flow greater than perinodular flow had a higher incidence of malignancy (Figure 13.17). Follicular carcinomas also tend to show a moderate increase in central vascularity by power Doppler compared with follicular adenomas that favor peripheral flow (Figure 13.18).[43] In general, increased vascularity in the interior of a thyroid nodule suggests malignancy but should not be considered a pathognomonic feature. The evidence correlating vascular pattern with malignancy is inconsistent, such that it is no longer included in the list of criteria used for risk stratification of thyroid nodules.[6,7]

Capsular Contact

The presence of contact between a nodule and the adjacent thyroid capsule is defined when there is no intervening thyroid tissue between the thyroid nodule and the capsule. Capsular contact of greater than 25% by US has been found to be a useful marker for predicting extrathyroidal extension of cancer[44] (Figure 13.19).

Elastography

Please see the Expert Consult website for discussion of this topic.

Ultrasound Characteristics of Benign Thyroid Nodules

Overall, the most common types of nodules are benign hyperplastic (colloid) nodules and benign follicular adenomas (Figure 13.20, available on ExpertConsult.com). Colloid nodules consist of colloid and benign follicular cells and are associated with small, hyperechoic, internal lucencies on US, known as the "comet tail" sign (see Figure 13.4).[45] Follicular adenomas are the most common type of thyroid neoplasm and are, with few exceptions, not considered a forerunner of carcinoma.[46] They are typically round, well-encapsulated lesions with a clear margin or "halo" that distinguishes them from the surrounding normal thyroid tissue. Spontaneous or traumatic hemorrhage may occur into the nodule (Figure 13.21, available on ExpertConsult.com).

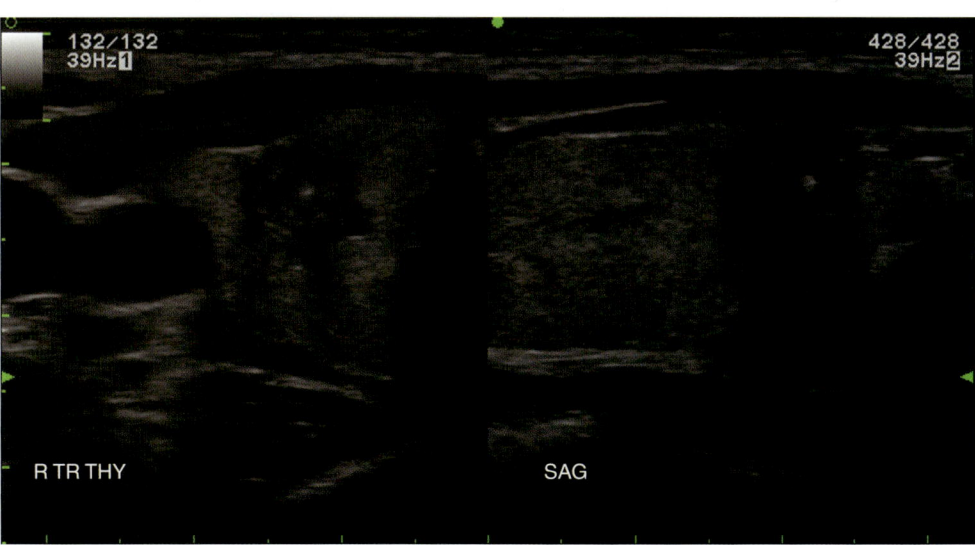

Fig. 13.11 Irregularly shaped nodule with microlobulated borders, confirmed to be a papillary carcinoma.

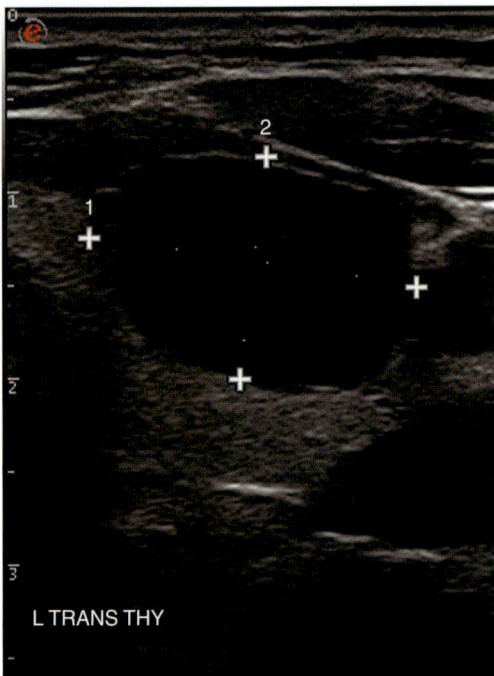

Fig. 13.12 Cystic degeneration of a benign thyroid nodule.

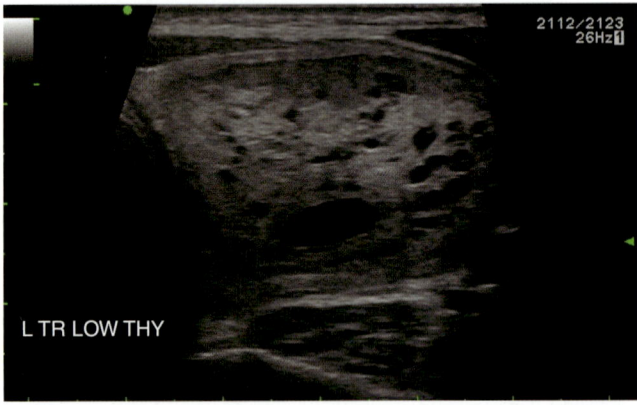

Fig. 13.13 Benign, spongiform thyroid nodule, with multiple microcystic components.

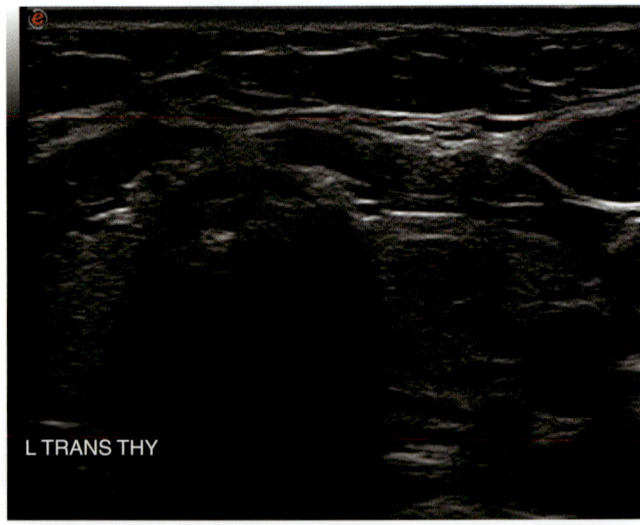

Fig. 13.14 Slightly hypoechoic benign adenomatous nodule.

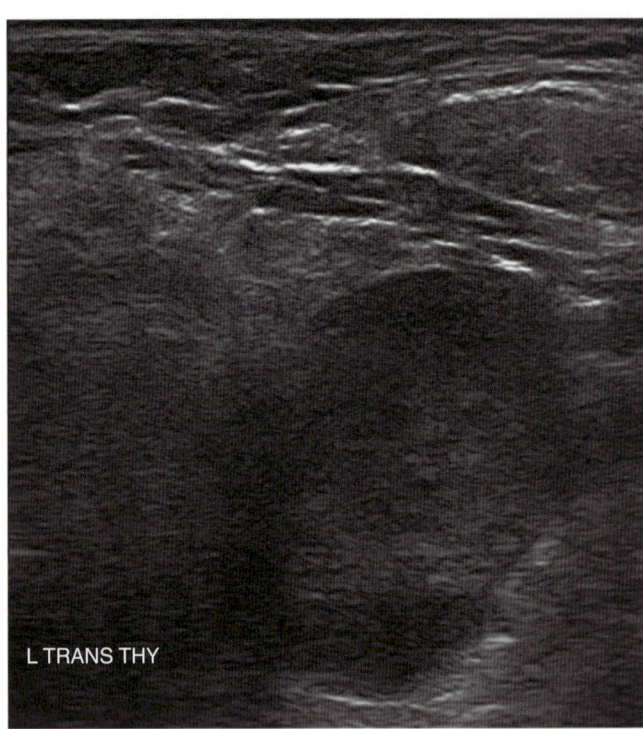

Fig. 13.15 Moderately hypoechoic and elongated nodule that proved to be a follicular carcinoma.

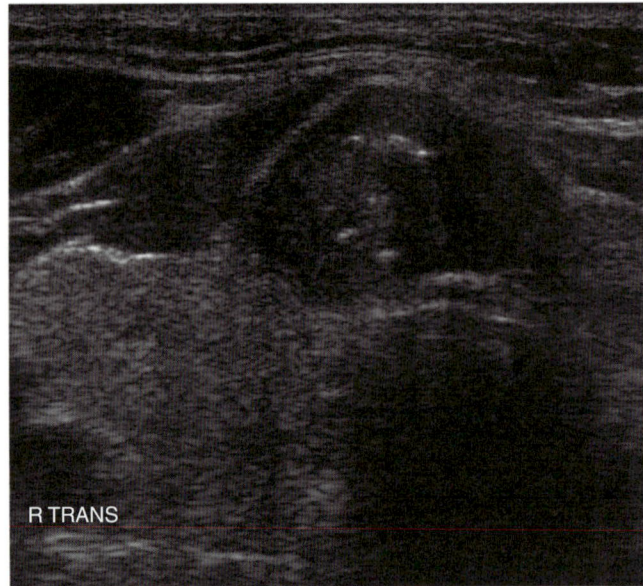

Fig. 13.16 Microcalcifications in a papillary thyroid carcinoma.

Thyroid Cysts

Mixed cystic solid nodules represent approximately 20% of all thyroid nodules.[25] Purely cystic lesions are nearly uniformly benign; however, these comprise only 2% of all cystic lesions.[35] Approximately 15% of partially cystic nodules represent necrotic papillary cancers, and 30% represent hemorrhagic adenomas.[13] Rates of nondiagnostic FNA are higher with cystic lesions than with solid nodules. Therefore US-guided FNA is recommended to ensure sampling of the solid cellular component.[6]

CHAPTER 13 Ultrasound of the Thyroid and Parathyroid Glands   139

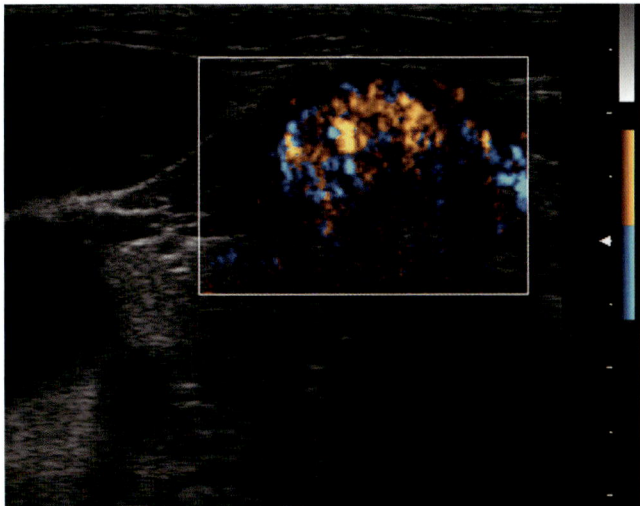

Fig. 13.17 Increased central blood flow in a papillary carcinoma.

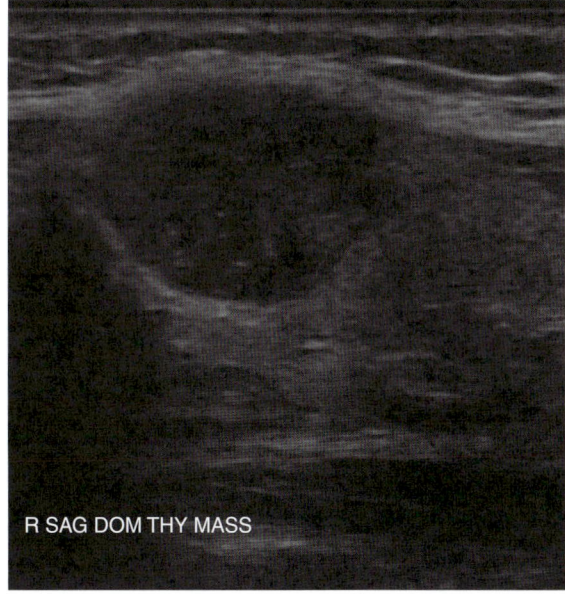

Fig. 13.19 Thyroid nodule with greater than 25% capsular contact, confirmed to be papillary carcinoma with extrathyroidal extension.

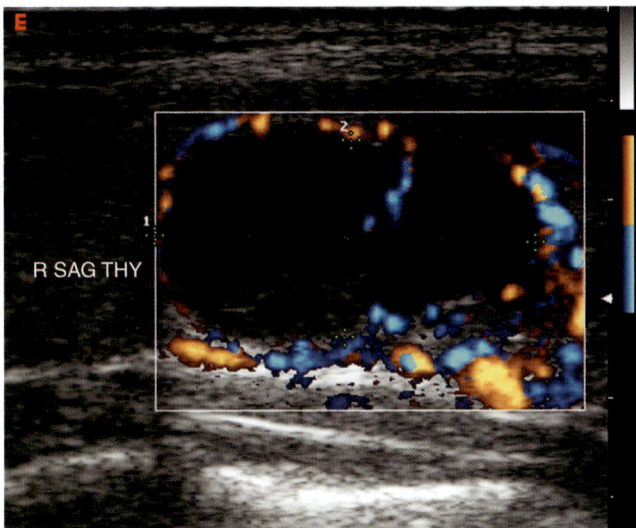

Fig. 13.18 Follicular adenoma with peripheral blood flow.

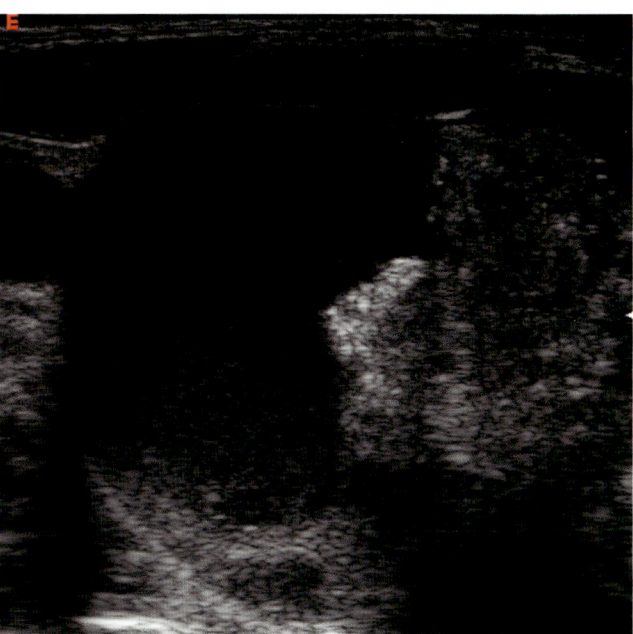

Fig. 13.22 Cystic papillary carcinoma. Note aggregated microcalcifications.

ULTRASOUND CHARACTERISTICS OF MALIGNANT LESIONS

Although the majority of thyroid nodules are benign, a top priority in the management of thyroid nodules is to identify the approximately 10% of nodules that harbor malignancy.[47] Most thyroid cancers are of follicular cell origin, including papillary, follicular, and Hürthle cell carcinoma (collectively known as *well-differentiated thyroid cancers*). Other malignancies, including MTC, anaplastic carcinoma, lymphoma, and metastatic disease, are less common. Although US characteristics of thyroid nodules do not offer sufficient specificity to diagnose malignancy, US represents an invaluable tool for identifying thyroid lesions and determining which lesions should undergo further evaluation through biopsy or other investigations.

Papillary Thyroid Carcinoma

PTC represents at least 80% of all thyroid cancers. Multifocal lesions and regional nodal metastases are common in PTC, whereas distant metastases to bone or lung are less common. Local invasion of the larynx, trachea, esophagus, spine, or soft tissues of the neck is seen in only the most aggressive forms of PTC.

US features typical of PTC, especially the classic variant, include a solid, hypoechoic lesion with microcalcifications. Cystic components may be present within a solid lesion (Figure 13.22), and although an incomplete halo may be seen, ill-defined margins are more common. Doppler examination may also reveal disorganized hypervascularity. Of these features, microcalcifications may be the most specific for PTC because psammoma bodies are a histopathologic feature considered pathognomonic for PTC. Psammoma bodies are composed of tiny laminated, spherical collections of calcium that reflect sound waves and appear as tiny bright foci.

Follicular Carcinoma

Follicular carcinoma accounts for approximately 10% of thyroid malignancies.[48] Unlike PTC, follicular carcinoma is more likely to spread via hematogenous than lymphatic routes, accounting for less frequent metastatic lymphadenopathy but a higher incidence of distant metastases than PTC. Follicular carcinoma has a poorer prognosis than PTC.

Follicular neoplasms, both benign and malignant, typically appear as solid, iso/hyperechoic, and homogeneous lesions (Figure 13.23, available on ExpertConsult.com). Cystic components and calcifications are rare, and a halo may or may not be seen. An avascular halo is a more worrisome indication of follicular carcinoma. Internal hypervascularity is common, and FNA samples are often bloody. The most important prognostic histologic feature is whether vascular, extracapsular, or local invasion is present. Because follicular adenoma cannot be distinguished from follicular carcinoma on cytology, molecular testing may prove beneficial in these patients to differentiate benign from malignant disease. In the absence of conclusive genetic mutational analysis, diagnostic lobectomy may be required to obtain a definitive histopathologic diagnosis.

Hürthle Cell Carcinoma

Hürthle cell tumors are a subtype of follicular cell neoplasm. Approximately 20% of Hürthle cell lesions are malignant, and these account for only 3% of all thyroid cancers. These tumors may behave more aggressively than either PTC or follicular carcinoma and may have with a higher risk of regional lymph node, distant metastasis, and poor iodine avidity.

On US, Hürthle cell tumors are solid with both hypoechoic and hyperechoic components with an irregular border (Figure 13.24, available on ExpertConsult.com). Most do not have calcifications or a halo.

Medullary Thyroid Carcinoma

MTCs account for 5% of thyroid cancers. They arise from parafollicular C cells that are primarily concentrated in the superior poles.[48] MTC occurring in the setting of a multiple endocrine neoplasia (MEN) syndrome is usually multifocal and bilateral. Spread to regional lymph nodes in the neck or mediastinum and hematogenous spread are common.

MTC appears solid and hypoechoic on US, yet it frequently has hyperechoic foci representing both amyloid deposition and calcification (Figure 13.25, available on ExpertConsult.com). These foci may also appear within affected lymph nodes. As with PTC, Doppler examination may reveal disorganized hypervascularity.[4]

Anaplastic Carcinoma

Anaplastic carcinoma is the most aggressive type of thyroid cancer and is often seen in the elderly.[49] Although rare, it is the most lethal type of thyroid cancer. Most anaplastic carcinomas develop in the setting of a preexisting or coexisting thyroid cancer or goiter and may represent malignant transformation of a previously well-differentiated carcinoma. The majority of patients have lymph node involvement at the time of diagnosis. Patients may present with a rapidly enlarging neck mass and associated symptomatology such as pain, dyspnea, dysphagia, or dysphonia.

US demonstrates a diffusely hypoechoic, irregularly shaped lesion often infiltrating the entire thyroid lobe with areas of necrosis or ill-defined calcifications (Figure 13.26, available on ExpertConsult.com). Involved lymph nodes may also have necrotic changes. Invasion into surrounding vessels or soft tissue is often seen.

Lymphoma

Lymphoma involving the thyroid gland is rare and is usually associated with a history of Hashimoto's thyroiditis.[49] In fact, the cytologic diagnosis can be easily mistaken for chronic lymphocytic thyroiditis. Patients may present with an enlarging neck mass that is concerning for an aggressive primary thyroid malignancy. Local soft tissue and vascular invasion are both common.

On US, lymphoma may appear as a focal lesion within a lobe or as a diffuse abnormality involving the entire gland (see Figure 13.5, C), which is often with associated regional lymph node enlargement. The involved tissue is usually heterogeneous and hypoechoic and may be mistaken for anaplastic carcinoma. "Pseudocysts" with posterior enhancement are sometimes seen.

Thyroid as a Site of Cancer Metastases

Metastases to the thyroid gland are uncommon and usually arise from a primary melanoma, breast, lung, or renal cell carcinoma.[4,48] Thyroid metastases usually involve the inferior poles and are homogeneous, hypoechoic, and noncalcified.

Role of Ultrasound in Other Thyroid Gland Diseases

Goiter

Goiter is a general term used to describe an enlarged thyroid gland. It may occur in the setting of multinodular goiter, thyroiditis, thyrotoxicosis, or iodine deficiency. When evaluating a patient with a goiter using US, it is important to note the following: whether the gland is diffusely enlarged or if one lobe predominates; whether nodularity is present; and whether vascularity is increased, decreased, or average. Cross-sectional imaging (CT or MRI) will often provide better information on the overall extent of a goiter, especially into regions that are inaccessible to US evaluation, such as the retrosternal and retropharyngeal areas.

Graves' Disease

Graves' disease is the most common cause of thyrotoxicosis. It is an autoimmune disorder that includes such symptoms as hyperthyroidism, diffuse thyroid enlargement, infiltrative ophthalmopathy with exophthalmos, and skin changes from myxedema. Palpable thyroid nodules are found three times as frequently in patients with Graves' disease compared with the general population; approximately 17% of the nodules harbor malignancy.[50] US examination of all patients with Graves' disease is advisable.

US features of Graves' disease include heterogeneous thyroid tissue with diffuse hypoechogenicity and hypervascularity. The velocity of flow in the inferior thyroid artery is typically increased. Color flow mapping may be useful in selecting the optimal dose of antithyroid medication to achieve a euthyroid state[51] and may also predict the likelihood of relapse after the withdrawal of antithyroid medications.[52,53]

Multinodular Goiter

The risk of malignancy is similar in patients with multiple nodules compared with those with solitary nodules.[12] The number of nodules present has not been demonstrated to correlate with risk of malignancy.[42] Each nodule should be evaluated independently and FNA should be guided by US characteristics suspicious for malignancy rather than size alone.[6,7] If multiple enlarged nodules are present, and no nodule displays suspicious findings on US, only the largest nodules should be measured to facilitate surveillance with serial US examinations.[6]

Thyroiditis

The most common type of thyroiditis is chronic lymphocytic thyroiditis or Hashimoto's disease (see Chapter 4, Thyroiditis). The rate of malignancy in nodules in patients with Hashimoto's thyroiditis is equal to or greater than those in normal thyroid glands.[54,55] The ATA recommends that all patients with an increased thyroid-stimulating hormone

(TSH), usually the result of thyroiditis, undergo diagnostic US.[6] US findings of Hashimoto's thyroiditis include ill-defined hypoechoic areas separated by echogenic septa, with increased (early) or decreased (late) vascularity (Figure 13.27, available on ExpertConsult.com). Intrathyroid lymphoid tissue accumulates because of the autoimmune process in association with thyroid peroxidase antibodies,[56] and patients with Hashimoto's thyroiditis have up to a 60-fold increase in risk of developing lymphoma.[57,58] Chronic lymphocytic thyroiditis is also often associated with central compartment inflammatory lymphadenopathy that may be difficult to distinguish from small malignant lymphadenopathy.

Subacute or de Quervain's thyroiditis is characterized by an acute period of neck pain, fever, and lethargy after an upper respiratory illness; the symptoms are generally accompanied by thyrotoxicosis that resolves in approximately 6 weeks. Sometimes this is followed by a 3- to 6-month period of hypothyroidism. During the acute phase, patients present with a tender, palpable thyroid, which may be asymmetric and be identified as a thyroid nodule. However, this can be sonographically distinguished from an adenomatous nodule by the lack of calcification or halo; the surrounding thyroid tissue is generally heterogeneous. In the subacute period, the affected lobe or sometimes the entire gland is hypoechoic and enlarged. Once the disease has been resolved, the thyroid returns to normal.[4]

Acute suppurative thyroiditis is a rare condition affecting children. Because the thyroid gland has a thick, fibrous capsule, it is relatively resistant to infection.[4] The presence of an abscess can be confirmed on US as a hypoechoic fluid-filled collection that may contain pockets of gas.

ULTRASOUND-GUIDED THYROID PROCEDURES

FNA biopsy improves the selection of patients with thyroid nodules for surgery and extent of surgery. US-guided FNA, with visualization of needle placement directly into the target, is more accurate than palpation-guided FNA and reduces the number of passes required to obtain a diagnostic specimen from thyroid nodules.[59-61] The needle may be introduced at the end of the long axis of the transducer (parallel technique) or at the midpoint of the transducer opposing its short axis (perpendicular technique) and its tip visualized within the lesion during collection of the specimen. Transducer orientation should optimize the lesion by locating the maximal dimension of the nodule, which allows for the shortest needle path and helps avoid vital structures. Smaller needle size (24 to 27 gauge) and the use of capillary action can decrease the rate of nondiagnostic specimens and increase yield.[62] The presence of an onsite cytopathologist may reduce the number of samples required for a diagnostic result but is not necessary. For most nodules, three samples or passes are adequate.[63] Nondiagnostic findings can be the result of many factors, including poor targeting, poor slide preparation or fixation, and dilution from excessive blood.

Please see the Expert Consult website for more discussion of this topic.

Thyroid Elastography

Elasticity imaging, or elastography, is a rapidly developing field that images tissue elasticity or stiffness properties to characterize pathologic processes. Ultrasonographic elastography is a technique that combines the diagnostic advantages of high-frequency US examination with the assessment of a tissue's or lesion's stiffness to distinguish benign from malignant masses. There are two kinds of elastography: strain elastography and shear wave elastography (SWE). Strain elastography requires external palpation with the transducer, which results in tissue displacement by mechanical stress. Tissue deformation from the stress is measured and used to construct an elastogram. The elastic image is superimposed on the B-mode image, and tissue stiffness is displayed along a continuum. SWE provides quantitative elastic information of tissues and produces a real-time elastogram. Shear waves are the transverse components of particle displacement that are rapidly attenuated by the tissue. SWE is more operator-independent, reproducible, and quantitative. Because tissue firmness or hardness is more likely associated with malignancy, the goal of clinical application of elastography to conventional head and neck US is to improve diagnostic capabilities. Different elastography, or tissue-stiffness, scales have been described and applied clinically.[65] Elastography is meant to be used as an adjunct to conventional US and not as an independent test. The hope is that adding an objective assessment of tissue firmness to already used US parameters would improve the diagnostic ability to differentiate between benign and malignant disease. The addition of elastography to B-mode US appears to hold the greatest promise in the assessment of thyroid nodules and cervical lymph nodes, although further experience and refinement are necessary.[66-68]

Please see the Expert Consult website for more discussion of this topic, including Figures 13.28 and 13.29.

SONOGRAPHY OF NECK NODES

Metastasis to cervical and paratracheal lymph nodes is common in thyroid carcinomas, so it is vitally important to examine the entire neck when performing a standard preoperative US examination. Although no single sonographic feature can distinguish a benign from a metastatic lymph node, characterization by US can determine need for further assessment. Lymph nodes should be assessed for size, shape, number, echogenicity, composition, capsule border, hilum structure, and ancillary features. The addition of Doppler helps to further assess and characterize hilar structure and blood flow. On US, benign lymph nodes are oblong or kidney bean shaped, have a well-defined capsule, and appear hypoechoic with a hyperechoic hilar line within the node. Benign, reactive lymph nodes may be enlarged or even rounded; however, benign, reactive lymph nodes typically maintain a normal vascular hilum.

Features that are characteristic of malignancy in the primary thyroid neoplasm are also seen in the involved lymph nodes.[72] Microcalcifications, cystic degeneration, peripheral vascularity, enlargement, a rounded shape, irregular or indistinct margins, or extracapsular extension may be present. Other findings that should be considered include thrombus within the internal jugular vein, or evidence of extrathyroidal invasion of the strap muscles, esophagus, or trachea[72] (Figure 13.30).

After surgical management of thyroid carcinoma, it is invaluable to perform US of the neck to monitor for recurrence in the thyroid bed and the entire central and lateral cervical lymph node compartments and soft tissues. US is increasingly replacing radioactive iodine scanning in the ongoing surveillance of the thyroid cancer patient because of its superior anatomic resolution, ease of performance, low cost, avoidance of radiation exposure, lack of need for preparation, and its reduced morbidity associated with thyroid hormone withdrawal, recombinant TSH injection, and low-iodine diet limitations.

The superficial location of neck nodes and the use of high-resolution transducers make it possible to accurately evaluate the nodes and perform guided biopsies under US control.

Sonographic examination of neck nodes consists of two essential parts:
Grayscale sonography evaluates nodal morphology and features such as size, shape, internal architecture (cystic change/necrosis), nodal margins, and the presence or absence of echogenic hilus and intranodal calcification.

Doppler US evaluates the presence and distribution of intranodal vessels.

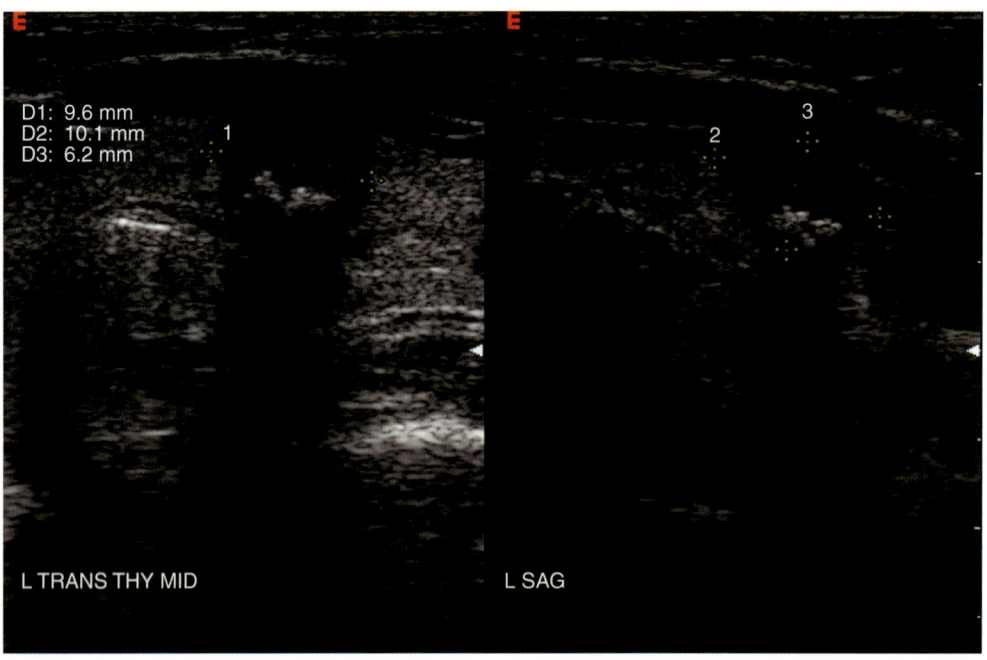

Fig. 13.30 Extrathyroidal spread: papillary thyroid carcinoma with extrathyroidal spread to the strap muscles (left transverse and sagittal views).

It is important to remember that no single sonographic criterion will accurately differentiate a benign from a malignant node. The probability of malignancy is higher if many of the sonographic criteria (grayscale and Doppler) are present within the same node.[73] Once a suspicious node has been identified, US is readily combined with FNA biopsy, and these together yield a sensitivity of 89% to 98%, specificity of 95% to 98%, and an overall accuracy of 95% to 97%.[74,75]

Equipment and Technique

Each side of the neck is scanned with the chin turned toward the opposite side. One typical examination sequence begins in the midline submental region. Subsequently, the scanning proceeds through the submandibular region, intraparotid area, along the jugular cervical chain, followed by the central neck paratracheal regions (including the sternal notch), and then the accessory chain or posterior neck. The contralateral neck is then scanned in a similar way. The order of compartment scanning is immaterial, but a detailed and consistent approach ensures a high-quality and complete examination of neck nodes.

Although the paratracheal nodes are often involved in metastatic nodes from thyroid cancer, their sonographic examination is difficult and suboptimal in the presence of the thyroid because of the shadowing from the thyroid and adjacent air containing structures, including larynx and trachea.

Please see the Expert Consult website for more discussion of this topic.

Ultrasound Features of Malignant Nodes (Table 13.2)
Nodal Distribution

Please see the Expert Consult website for more discussion of this topic, including Figure 13.31.

TABLE 13.2	Sonographic Features of Benign and Malignant Lymph Nodes	
Lymph Node Sonographic Features	**Benign Lymph Node**	**Malignant Lymph Node**
Nodal shape	Elliptical	Round

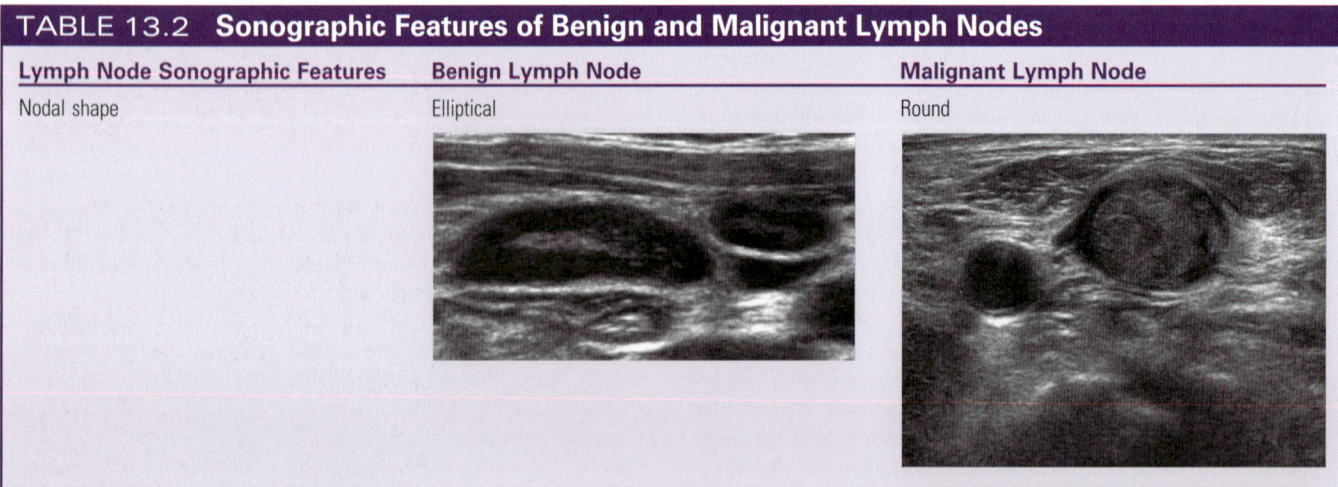

Lymph Node Sonographic Features	Benign Lymph Node	Malignant Lymph Node
Intranodal echogenic hilus	Present	Absent
Echogenicity	Hypoechoic, elliptical in shape	Hypoechoic, round in shape
		Hypoechoic in papillary carcinoma
Intranodal necrosis	Absent	Present
Intranodal calcification	Absent	Punctate calcification in papillary carcinoma

TABLE 13.2 Sonographic Features of Benign and Malignant Lymph Nodes—cont'd

Continued

TABLE 13.2 Sonographic Features of Benign and Malignant Lymph Nodes—cont'd

Lymph Node Sonographic Features	Benign Lymph Node	Malignant Lymph Node
Nodal border	Ill-defined	Well-defined unless extranodal extension
Nodal vascularity	Hilar 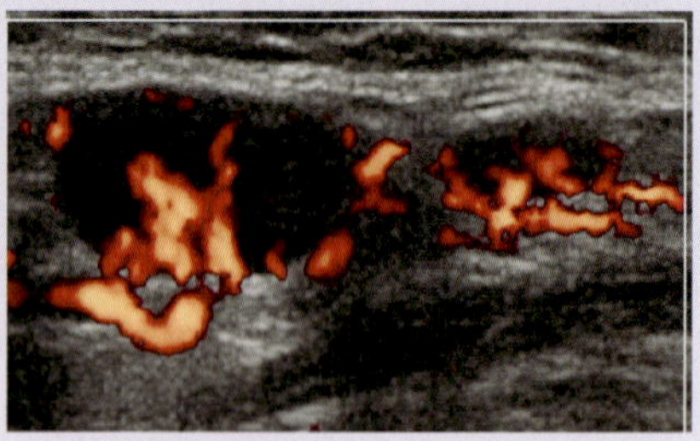	Peripheral 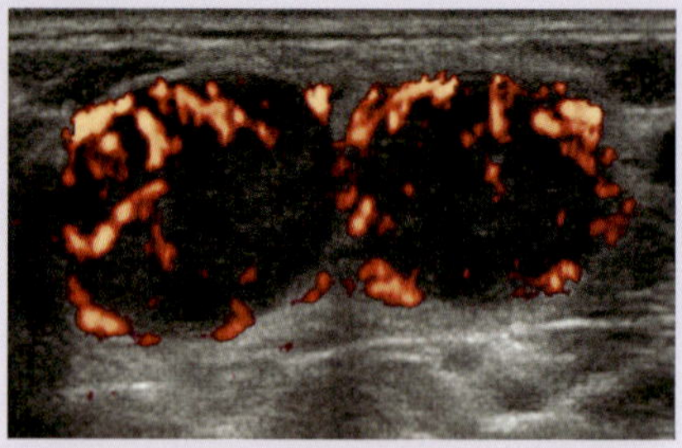 Chaotic 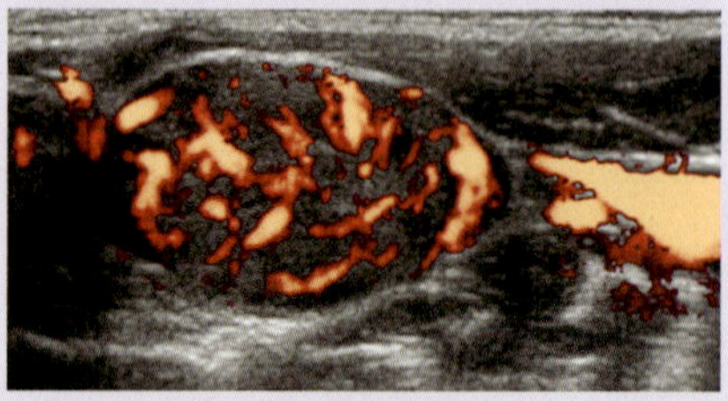
Elastography	Soft 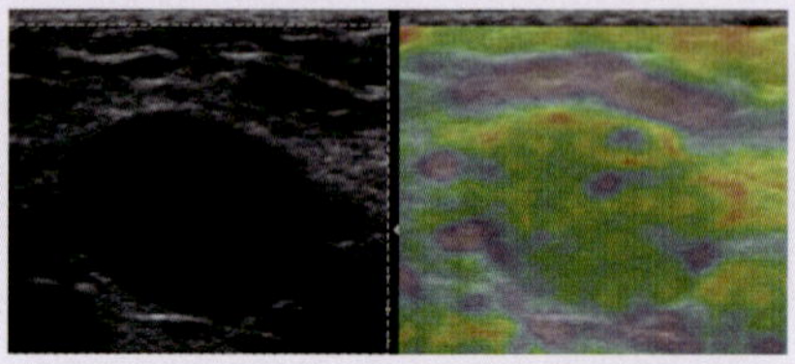	Hard 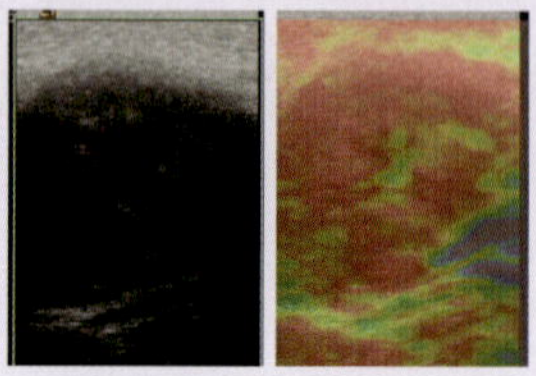

Nodal Size

Size alone cannot be used as a reliable indicator of malignancy because metastatic nodes may be small and reactive nodes may be large. The minimal axial diameter of the node is the most accurate dimension for predicting malignancy.[79,80] A minimal axial diameter of 9 mm for subdigastric nodes and 8 mm for all other neck nodes has an overall accuracy of 75%.[81] However, in patients with a known head and neck primary, with nodes in the known draining sites, the size threshold is reduced to 4 mm.[82] This is well within the resolution of US. In a patient with a known head and neck cancer, increasing size of nodes on serial examination is highly suspicious for metastases. US is valuable in monitoring the change of size of nodes to assess treatment response.[83,84]

Nodal Shape

Benign nodes tend to be elliptical in shape and malignant nodes round in shape (Figure 13.32).[78,85-87] However, one must note that normal intraparotid and submandibular nodes are usually round. A short-to-long axis ratio (S/L) less than 0.5 indicates a fusiform node, whereas an S/L ratio greater than 0.5 indicates a round node.[88,89]

Intranodal Echogenic Hilus

The medullary sinuses within the node produce multiple acoustic surfaces reflecting sound and appearing bright on US, producing the echogenic hilus (or hilum) that is invariably continuous with surrounding soft tissue fat.[90-92] The deposition of intranodal fat further makes the hilus more conspicuous.[86] It was previously believed that the presence of an echogenic hilus suggested benignity[86] because most malignant nodes do not show an echogenic hilus (see Figure 13.32). However, with modern high-resolution transducers, one may see an echogenic hilus

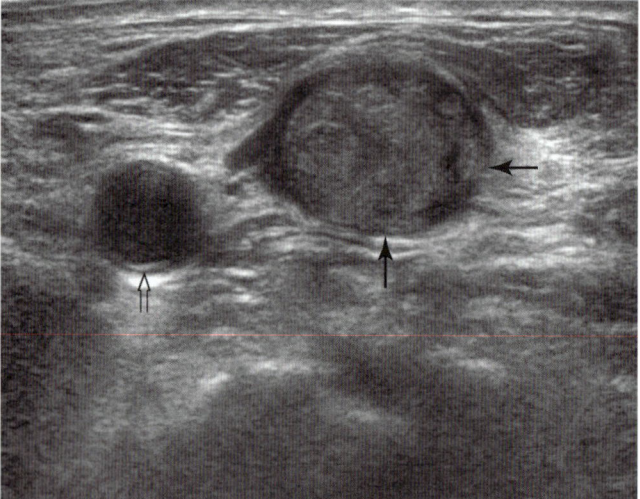

Fig. 13.32 Transverse grayscale ultrasound showing a metastatic node *(arrows)*. Note it is solid, round, well-defined, and it does not demonstrate a normal echogenic hilus. The open arrow identifies the common carotid artery.

even in malignant nodes, because the medullary sinuses may not be completely disrupted in early metastatic infiltration.[91]

Nodal Echogenicity

Metastatic nodes are usually hypoechoic compared with adjacent muscle.[76,79,87] The only exceptions in the head and neck are metastatic nodes from PTC, because these are often hyperechoic (see Figure 13.32) compared with muscle.[93,94] This sonographic feature is a good clue for predicting metastatic nodes from a PTC.

Intranodal Calcification

Metastatic nodes from PTC and MTC may demonstrate intranodal calcification.[93-95] The calcification in metastatic nodes from PTC are typically fine, bright echogenic foci (Figure 13.33) and demonstrate fine shadowing only when the transducer frequency is increased (>10 MHz). The calcification (representing calcium deposits within amyloid) in metastatic nodes from MTC is usually coarse with dense shadowing.

Nodal Border

On US, inflammatory nodes tend to have unsharp borders because of periadenitis, and malignant nodes have a sharp border (see Figure 13.31, available on the Expert Consult website) because of the sharp attenuating interface between the node and the adjacent soft tissues. However, if a node has all the other features of a malignant node but has unsharp borders, one must suspect extracapsular spread. Larger nodes have a higher likelihood of extracapsular spread compared with smaller nodes.[96] Sonographic invasion of adjacent soft tissues is a good indicator of extracapsular spread (Figure 13.34).

Intranodal Necrosis

Intranodal necrosis can be either cystic or coagulation necrosis, and both signify nodal abnormality, irrespective of nodal size (see Figure 13.34). Cystic necrosis is more common and is seen as a cystic/anechoic area within a node. Coagulation necrosis is seen as an echogenic region within the node and is not continuous with surrounding soft tissue fat; this distinguishes it from the echogenic hilus. Intranodal necrosis, particularly cystic necrosis, is common in metastatic

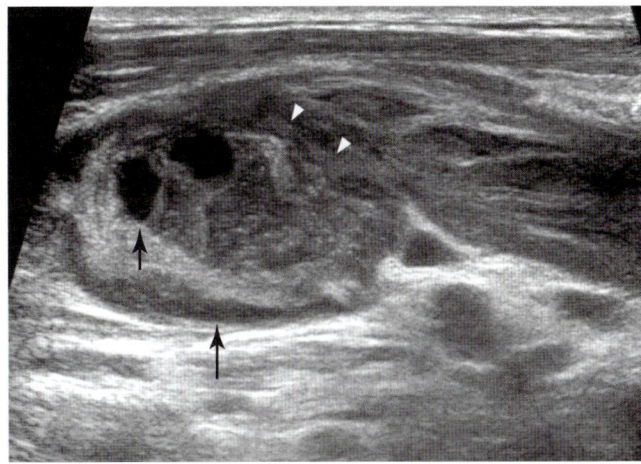

Fig. 13.34 Longitudinal grayscale ultrasound showing a metastatic node (large arrow) with extracapsular spread (arrowheads). Note anteriorly the node is inseparable from adjacent soft tissues and muscle. Also note the intranodal cystic necrosis (small arrow).

nodes from PTC and oropharyngeal squamous cell carcinoma[93,96,97] and in tuberculous neck nodes.

Nodal Vascularity

Malignant nodes tend to demonstrate peripheral vascularity ([Figure 13.35, A and B] related to angiogenesis leading to recruitment of peripheral vessels within lymph nodes), whereas benign nodes show hilar vascularity.[98-101] Metastatic nodes may also show mixed vascularity (hilar + peripheral). The presence of peripheral vascularity combined with round shape, intranodal necrosis, and absent hilus has been reported to have a specificity of 100%.[102]

Contrast Enhancement

Please see the Expert Consult website for more discussion of this topic.

Elastography of Thyroid Lymph Node Metastases

Please see the Expert Consult website for more discussion of this topic.

PARATHYROID ULTRASOUND

In patients with known hyperparathyroidism, US is very useful for detecting enlarged parathyroid glands, especially in the detection of solitary adenomas in primary hyperparathyroidism. Knowledge of the embryology, anatomy, and vascular supply of the parathyroid glands helps the sonographer/clinician differentiate lymphadenopathy and thyroid pathology from true parathyroid lesions. Furthermore, the history and laboratory data will influence the clinician's degree of concern as to whether one or more glands are enlarged. For example, patients with renal failure or those with MEN syndromes are likely to demonstrate multiple gland enlargement. Office-based ultrasonography by a skilled operator can localize parathyroid adenomas to the correct side and location (right versus left and superior versus inferior) with greater sensitivity than sestamibi scanning (90% for US compared with 70% for sestamibi[108]), especially when detecting subcentimeter adenomas. US can safely be used as the initial, and often the sole, localization study before parathyroidectomy. An advantage of using US for parathyroid localization is the detection of coexistent thyroid disease. As indicated, appropriate workup of any concurrent thyroid pathology can be completed before contemplating surgery in the central neck and likely addressed at the same sitting.

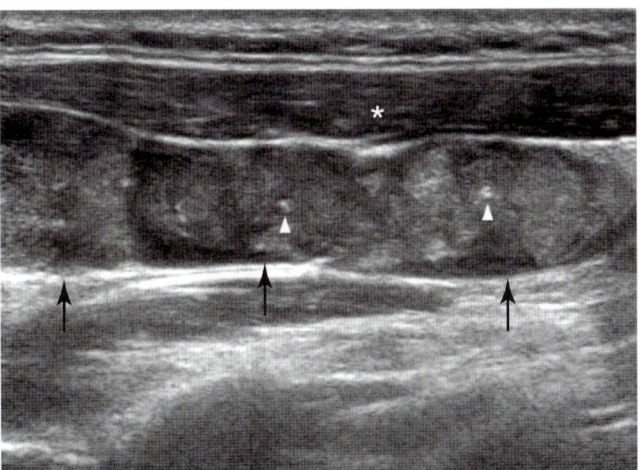

Fig. 13.33 Longitudinal grayscale ultrasound showing a chain of metastatic nodes (arrows) from thyroid papillary carcinoma. Note they are brighter/hyperechoic compared with adjacent muscle (asterisk). Also note the small echogenic foci (arrowheads) representing microcalcifications/psammoma bodies within the nodes.

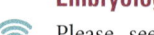

Fig. 13.35 **A,** Longitudinal grayscale ultrasound shows multiple, metastatic nodes *(black arrows)*. Note they are predominantly solid, hypoechoic, round, well-defined, and do not show the normal echogenic hilus. One of the nodes shows a focal area of intranodal necrosis *(white arrow)*. **B,** Corresponding power Doppler ultrasound shows multiple, abnormal peripheral vessels, typically seen in metastatic nodes. They represent angiogenesis with recruitment of adjacent vessels. Note the peripheral vessels do not originate from any hilar vessels.

Embryology

Please see the Expert Consult website for more discussion of this topic.

Normal Anatomy

Please see the Expert Consult website for more discussion of this topic, including Figure 13.36.

Ectopic Position

Please see the Expert Consult website for more discussion of this topic.

Vascular Pattern

The parathyroid glands have a distinct and often dual blood supply. The inferior thyroid artery is the principal contribution to both the superior and inferior parathyroid glands. However, the superior parathyroid may have its sole vascular supply from the superior thyroid artery. Regardless, each parathyroid gland has a dominant single vessel. It is important to emphasize that there is a limited vascular contribution to the parathyroid gland from the adjacent thyroid capsule or parenchyma. The venous outflow accompanies the main artery.

Technical Considerations

Generally, normal parathyroid glands cannot be visualized even with high resolution US. Enlarged, hypercellular parathyroid glands have a distinct appearance on grayscale imaging. The typical parathyroid adenoma is hypoechoic, oblong or ovoid-shaped, has a uniform echogenicity, and is at least two to three times the size of a normal gland.[109] The addition of Doppler can help confirm that the structure in question is an enlarged parathyroid gland. A polar vessel will be seen entering the adenoma and will bluntly terminate a few millimeters after entering the gland parenchyma.

Although the initial focus of the US examination is in the central neck, parathyroid adenoma localization with US requires a meticulous and methodical examination of the entire neck. Careful scanning in both planes and on both sides of the neck may help identify enlarged parathyroid glands, even in ectopic locations.

The inferior adenoma is usually immediately adjacent to the posterolateral thyroid capsule (Figure 13.37). The superior adenoma in the cardinal position is ovoid in shape, similarly enlarged, and resides posterior to the superior thyroid capsule (Figure 13.38). In each of

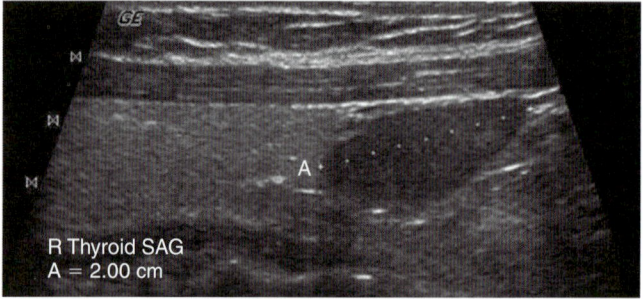

Fig. 13.37 Typical inferior parathyroid adenoma sagittal plane.

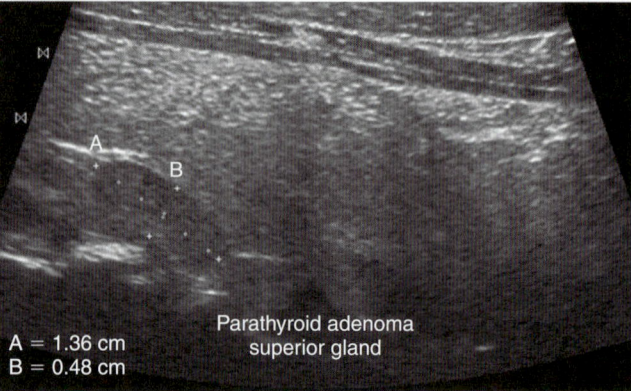

Fig. 13.38 Typical superior parathyroid adenoma sagittal plane.

these circumstances, the adenoma capsule is distinct and hyperechoic relative to its parenchyma. The single arterial supply to the adenoma is usually identified immediately adjacent and generally anterior to the enlarged gland. In some instances, the superior parathyroid may actually be below the level of the enlarged inferior parathyroid gland (Figure 13.39). Ectopic superior parathyroids are difficult to visualize or identify with US when they are posterior to the esophagus or within the chest. In Gilmore's autopsy studies,[110] 6% of individuals have only three parathyroid glands. In 6% of the individuals, there are five or more parathyroid glands. US may identify more than the usual four glands in hyperplasia when Tc sestamibi cannot be relied upon to provide preoperative imaging information. When an inferior parathyroid

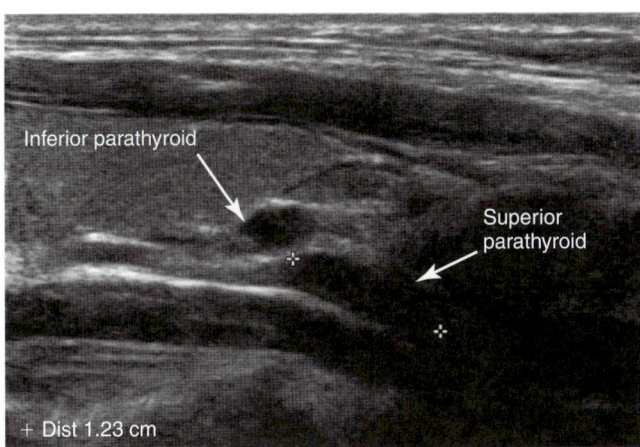

Fig. 13.39 Parathyroid hyperplasia in multiple endocrine neoplasia I syndrome. Note that the enlarged superior parathyroid gland is actually inferior to the inferior gland in this patient in this sagittal view.

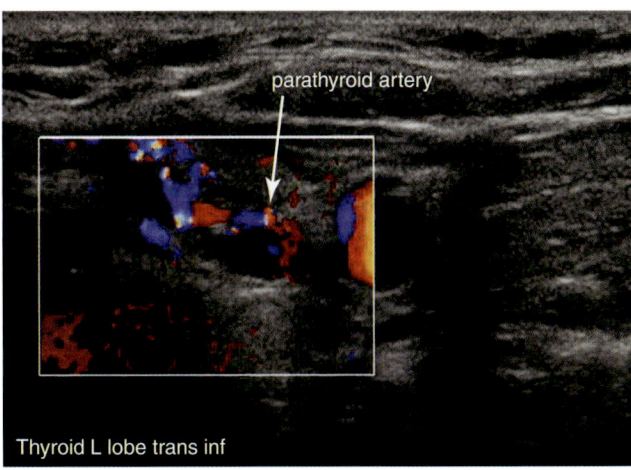

Fig. 13.41 View of the inferior thyroid artery giving rise to the parathyroid artery with power Doppler.

adenoma is ectopic in the anterior mediastinum, it may be properly imaged with the transducer in the transverse orientation and angled in a downward position. In certain circumstances, a lower frequency setting is helpful and can allow deeper penetration for improved imaging. A true intrathyroidal adenoma may be impossible to differentiate from a thyroid adenoma in grayscale alone. The power Doppler demonstration of a discrete vascular hilum can be helpful for differentiating a thyroid nodule from an intrathyroidal parathyroid adenoma. To qualify as a true intrathyroidal adenoma, the entire adenoma must be completely surrounded by thyroid (Figure 13.40). When a parathyroid adenoma cannot be imaged in the usual locations, a complete US survey must then ensue. The entire neck must be examined systematically with specific inspection of the full carotid sheath, upper neck, paraesophageal regions, and as much of the mediastinum as the anatomy will allow.

Please see the Expert Consult website for more discussion of this topic.

Power Doppler

Ultrasonographic display of the vascular supply of a parathyroid adenoma is a little recognized advantage.[111] There is always a large vessel in close proximity to the lesion,[112] usually contributing to the end artery, which enters the adenoma typically from an anterior and superior position (Figure 13.41). The most important characteristic on power Doppler is a reproducible blunt termination of the vessel a few millimeters after it enters the parenchyma of the adenoma[111] (Figure 13.42). In contrast, the vascular supply of a lymph node within its parenchyma is quite different in distribution. The primary vessel in a lymph node arborizes into smaller arteries, which may be properly demonstrated with appropriate manipulation of the Doppler gain. This issue is particularly important when an adenoma is ectopic to the anterior mediastinum and the clinician must differentiate adenoma from lymph node, especially when the sestamibi scan is negative. Smaller adenomas may not demonstrate sestamibi uptake, making US often the only imaging study that defines the proper preoperative location of the offending gland.[113]

Aspiration Parathyroid Hormone Rinsing

US-guided FNA is a fundamental element of assessment of thyroid nodules. In circumstances where a patient with primary hyperparathyroidism has an undetected adenoma in the usual expected position and an

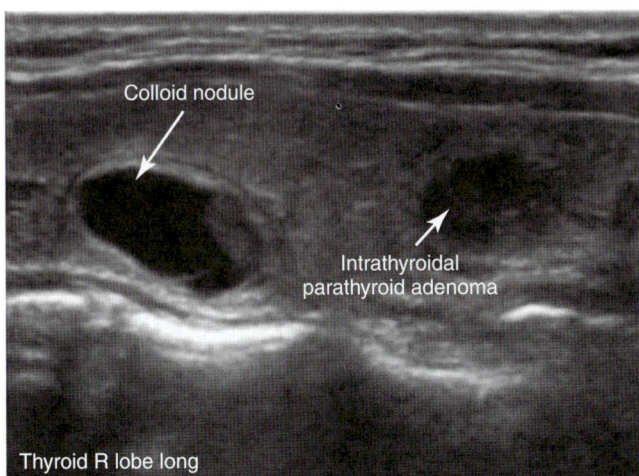

Fig. 13.40 Patient with primary hyperparathyroidism and two masses within the thyroid gland. The superior mass is a colloid cyst. The inferior solid lesion is an intrathyroidal parathyroid adenoma, proved with aspiration for parathyroid hormone.

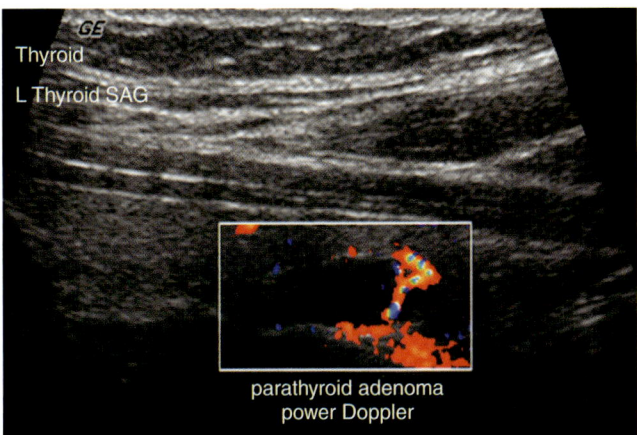

Fig. 13.42 Power Doppler demonstrates the blunt entry of the terminal parathyroid artery into the parenchyma of a parathyroid adenoma. This vascular pattern is often a distinguishing feature.

ipsilateral thyroid nodule demonstrated, an intrathyroidal parathyroid adenoma is to be considered.[114] This is the perfect scenario for US-guided aspiration for PTH and needle rinse with 0.5 cc of saline. Even moderate elevation of PTH from the aspirate is supportive of an intrathyroidal parathyroid adenoma. Often, the values are excessive and measured in the thousands. Similarly, a hypoechoic nodule parathyroid adenoma candidate elsewhere in the neck can be aspirated for PTH. The cytology is less likely to be definitive; in this circumstance, the chemical value is all-important.

Other Issues

Please see the Expert Consult website for more discussion of this topic, including Figure 13.43.

SUMMARY

US has many uses in the head and neck, but perhaps none more frequent and standardized as the inspection of the thyroid gland, lymph nodes, and enlarged parathyroid glands. This technology is relevant to both initial diagnosis and follow-up of both benign and malignant conditions. There are clearly limitations to viewing static images, but US can provide maximal diagnostic information obtained through real-time or via preservation of video clips. In US, areas of interest can be inspected methodically, repetitively, interactively, and in a multiplanar manner. In spite of the limitations outlined earlier in this chapter, there are many more advantages than disadvantages to the incorporation of US into the endocrine surgical practice.

REFERENCES

For a complete list of references, go to expertconsult.com.

Preoperative Radiographic Mapping of Nodal Disease for Papillary Thyroid Carcinoma

Sara L. Richer, Dipti Kamani, Robert Levine, Zaid Al-Qurayshi, Gregory W. Randolph

Papillary thyroid carcinoma (PTC) is the most common histologic type of thyroid carcinoma worldwide. Microscopic lymph node (LN) metastases occur in the majority of patients presenting with PTC.[1] LN metastases are associated with an increased risk of local or regional recurrence of cancer, and they can be a negative prognostic indicator relative to survival in certain groups such as papillary thyroid cancer.[2-4] LN metastases may necessitate a need for more extensive surgery, and they are linked to increased use of radioactive iodine, postoperatively. To develop an appropriate plan to clear all clinically apparent macroscopic disease during the initial surgery, a thorough examination of LNs with preoperative radiographic mapping is essential.

MACROSCOPICALLY POSITIVE VERSUS MICROSCOPICALLY POSITIVE METASTASIS

An important issue in the discussion of PTC nodal metastasis is the segregation of LNs into macrometastasis (or clinically apparent metastasis) and micrometastasis. Studies of patients with PTC demonstrate that macroscopic cervical nodal metastasis (as determined by detection through preoperative physical examination [PE], ultrasound [US], or intraoperative detection) will occur in 21% to 35% of patients at presentation.[1,2,5] Microscopically positive nodes are far more prevalent, occurring in 23% to 81% of patients with clinically negative preoperative nodal assessments on whom prophylactic LN dissection is performed.[1,6-13] Therapeutic nodal dissections target macroscopically positive nodes, whereas prophylactic neck dissections target normal or microscopically positive LNs.[14]

Macroscopic LN metastases are associated with increased rates of recurrence-free survival (RFS), unlike micrometastases.[5,15] In fact, several studies have shown that patients with microscopically positive nodes have recurrence rates similar to those of patients with pathologically negative nodes.[16,17] Although some authors have shown an intermediate outcome in patients with microscopic LNs, radiographically identified macroscopic nodes in the lateral neck have been shown to be associated with significantly lower RFS rates compared with pathologically positive and US-negative nodes (i.e., microscopically positive nodes).[15,18]

Therefore not all nodes are created equal in terms of actual prognostic downside; it is only macroscopically identified nodes (i.e., clinically apparent nodes) that require detection and resection.

IMPORTANCE OF RADIOGRAPHIC DETECTION OF MACROSCOPICALLY POSITIVE NODES PREOPERATIVELY

Nodal surgery for macroscopically positive nodes is required in approximately one third of patients who have PTC. If doctors do not recognize this task preoperatively, then persistence or recurrence of nodal disease is certain. Revision surgery is recognized to be more difficult than primary surgery due to scarring from the initial surgery. Therefore to save the patient from additional surgery and increased risk, removal of all macroscopic metastatic disease at the time of the initial surgery is desired. A surgeon cannot ascertain involvement of LNs from tumor characteristics alone, even though extrathyroidal extension and tumor size have shown correlation with positive macroscopic LNs.[19] Therefore it is essential to use high resolution radiographic analysis before surgery to detect macroscopically positive nodes to plan an operation appropriate for each patient's individual disease extent.

CENTRAL NECK NODES

Despite the high prevalence of cervical LN metastases, controversy exists regarding the extent of neck dissection needed for patients with PTC. Some surgeons perform prophylactic central neck dissection (pCND), but this additional surgery across all surgical settings will undoubtedly increase complications, such as hypoparathyroidism and recurrent laryngeal nerve injury. This procedure (pCND) harvests normal or at best microscopically positive nodes. In light of what we know about microscopically positive nodes as stated earlier, it is not surprising that pCND has been shown to have no effect on survival or recurrence.[20,21]

Intraoperative palpation to detect nodal disease also demonstrates a low degree of sensitivity and reliability. Studies have shown experienced surgeons can identify fewer than 50% of grossly positive nodes through intraoperative palpation.[22,23]

Societies worldwide have various recommendations for central neck dissection in thyroid cancer surgery. The 2015 guidelines from the American Thyroid Association recommend a therapeutic central compartment neck dissection in patients with clinically involved central nodes and a pCND in those with advanced papillary tumors or clinically involved lateral nodes.[24] The National Comprehensive Cancer Network's expert panel and the European Society of Endocrine Surgeons recommend pCND in advanced or high-risk tumors, especially at specialized centers.[25] The British Thyroid Association states that the benefit of pCND for high-risk patients is unclear; and recommends personalized care on a case by case basis with an understanding of the expertise of the given surgical team. In contrast, the Japanese Society of Thyroid Surgeons and the Japanese Association of Endocrine Surgeons recommend routine pCND; the two groups state that it is helpful in preventing LN recurrence.[25] Although opinions differ on prophylactic neck dissection, therapeutic neck dissection is recommended for clinically involved central nodes. Therefore objective radiographic data obtained preoperatively are required before surgery.

LATERAL NECK NODES

In the lateral neck, PTC spreads in a pattern that primarily encompasses anatomic levels II, III, and IV; typically in level IV initially.[24] However, PTC does not necessarily spread uniformly or sequentially to all these levels—the so-called skip-metastases may also. Ectopic nodes occur in various locations, most commonly in the retropharynx. Ectopic nodes appear in up to 9% of nodal recurrences.[19]

Patients generally tolerate lateral neck dissection well, but the operation is not without risk. Risks include hematoma, neck pain, chyle leak, increase in incision size, damage to great vessels, shoulder dysfunction and damage to cranial nerves VII, X, and/or XII. Prophylactic lateral neck dissection is not recommended in PTC.[24] The lateral neck is not exposed in a routine thyroidectomy approach; hence, it is imperative to search for metastatic disease in the lateral neck before surgery.

PREOPERATIVE RADIOGRAPHIC EVALUATIONS: ULTRASOUNDS AND CAT SCANS

Methods to evaluate patients for LN metastases after surgery can include US, iodine-131 (^{131}I) whole-body scans, and thyroglobulin measurement. Because ^{131}I whole-body scanning and thyroglobulin measurements are not useful screening tools in the preoperative period, methods to detect nodal metastases preoperatively are US, PE, and axial imaging, including computed tomography (CT) scanning.

PHYSICAL EXAMINATION

Both endocrinologists and endocrine surgeons routinely palpate patients' necks. Unfortunately, palpation is a unreliable detection method for small LN metastases. Generally, PE detects only large LNs, and even intraoperative palpation only detects 64% of LN metastases. Neck palpation has been associated with a sensitivity of 9% in the central neck and 24% in the lateral neck in the detection of positive papillary nodes.[26] Given the accuracy limitations of palpation, surgeons must rely on preoperative radiographic studies to assess LN involvement accurately.

ULTRASOUND

The 2015 American Thyroid Association Management Guidelines recommend performing a preoperative neck US of cervical LNs on all patients undergoing surgery for malignant or suspicious cytologic or molecular findings.[24] The advantages of US include low cost, point-of-care availability, and lack of radiation exposure. US characteristics of LNs with thyroid carcinoma metastases include an absent central hilum; hyperechogenicity; a rounded shape (increased short or long axis); calcification; disordered or peripheral vascularity on Doppler; cystic degeneration; and size[27-31] (Figures 14.1 and 14.2). Although size, shape, and loss of the central hilum are very sensitive findings, they lack adequate specificity for prediction of metastatic involvement. The most specific findings are calcification and cystic degeneration, with both approaching 100% specificity; however, these both lack sensitivity at 46% and 11%, respectively. Disordered or peripheral vascularity may offer the best combination of sensitivity and specificity at 86% and 82%, respectively.[30] When cervical LNs are considered suspicious because of US findings, fine-needle aspiration (FNA) biopsy with US guidance can be performed for both cytology and thyroglobulin. The ability to perform an LN biopsy at the time of detection of the abnormal node is another advantage of US as a primary diagnostic tool. In addition to assessing LNs, a comprehensive preoperative cervical US may identify high-risk features of the primary thyroid malignancy, such as extrathyroidal extension, multifocality, or abutment of the tumor against the trachea or the location of the recurrent laryngeal nerve.

Disadvantages of US for assessing cervical LNs include operator variability and insensitivity for imaging the central neck (i.e., region VI), as well as an inability to image retropharyngeal and mediastinal LNs, which can be involved in PTC. The central compartment is a

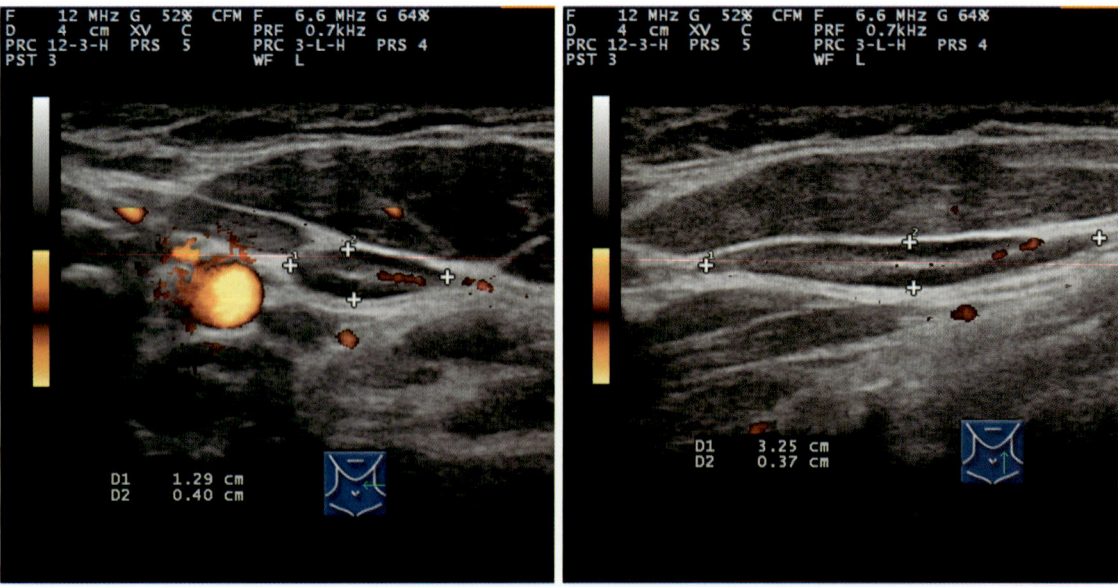

Fig. 14.1 Benign lymph node on ultrasound demonstrating normal echotexture, elongated shape (short/long ratio <0.5), a clear central hilar line, and Doppler vascularity limited to the central hilum.

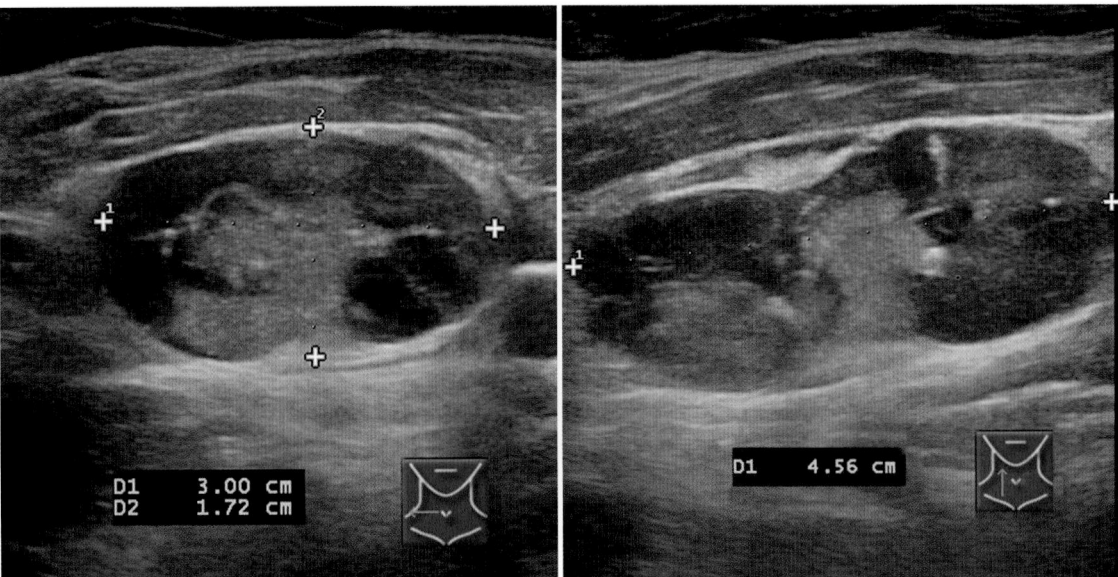

Fig. 14.2 **Malignant Lymph Node With Metastatic Papillary Carcinoma.** It is enlarged, heterogeneous, with cystic degeneration and calcifications.

frequent site of metastases; however, the sternum, clavicles, and echo shadows of the laryngeal, tracheal skeleton, and the thyroid cartilage limit the amount of information that can be gathered from US. Preoperatively, the thyroid gland can limit visualization of the central neck; thus when the thyroid gland is intact, a preoperative US of the central neck has a very low sensitivity for detecting metastatic nodes. Studies have found that the sensitivity of US for detecting central neck metastases is only 10% to 27%.[15,32] Likewise, preoperative FNA of such nodes can be contaminated by thyroid tissue and therefore should be interpreted with caution. Physicians should keep in mind that a negative preoperative central neck US before a thyroidectomy does not rule out metastatic central LNs. A CT scan of the neck complements US; it is especially helpful when the thyroid gland is *in situ*. Additionally, US does not deliver the detailed anatomic information and relationship of LNs to important neck structures useful for surgical planning and ultimately surgical localization. Despite its downsides, the advantages and widespread use of US in detecting metastases of thyroid nodules and cervical LNs have made it an important first-line tool in the detection of metastatic thyroid disease.[30,33]

Office-Based Ultrasound

Radiologists traditionally performed ultrasonography of the head and neck, but recent advances in technology and the availability of training courses have resulted in a marked increase in the use of office-based, or point-of-care, US. Many endocrinologists and thyroid surgeons now perform diagnostic and interventional thyroid procedures. The advantages of office-based US include correlating PE findings with US, limiting the waiting period to get a US, and procuring an immediate opportunity to perform US-guided fine-needle aspiration (USgFNA) to obtain cytologic diagnosis of suspicious lesions. However, it can be time consuming, and equipment can be expensive. It is essential that the clinician performing the study be extremely knowledgeable about normal and abnormal head and neck anatomy as well as corresponding ultrasonographic appearances. A certification or accreditation to perform office-based US is highly recommended.[34]

CT SCANNING WITH CONTRAST

Contrast-enhanced CT imaging is a common tool used to evaluate nodal metastases in the head and neck. The procedure does not depend on operator ability; and is performed with 1.5 mm axial cuts. Surgeons are familiar with CT scans, which can provide detailed anatomic information. Additionally, CT is the tool of choice for the evaluation of laryngeal or tracheal cartilage invasion in advanced thyroid cancer. CT performs better than magnetic resonance imaging (MRI) in the determination of metastatic LNs and shows higher sensitivity than positron emission tomography-computed tomography (PET-CT).[28,35] Characteristics of LN metastases shown on a CT scan include rounded shape, loss of hilar anatomy, cystic change, enhancement, calcification, and enlarged size. In patients with large volume disease and/or extranodal extension, it may be difficult to fully characterize these LNs via US, and CT scans are imperative to define the extent of disease.[31] A CT scan has also been recommended when US expertise is not available.[33] When the CT is performed with iodinated contrast, the patient will need to wait approximately 2 months before receiving radioactive iodine. Recent data have shown, however, that such delays in radioactive iodine do not have an adverse effect.[36-38] Generally, patients do not receive radioactive iodine treatments until 6 to 8 weeks after surgery; therefore the delay in radio active iodine treatment caused by the CT contrast imaging is minimal. The benefits of contrast for localizing LN metastases outweigh the short wait for radioactive iodine while the patient recovers from surgery.

COMBINATION OF CT SCAN AND ULTRASOUND

Evidence has emerged that the combination of CT and US gives the highest yield in preoperative nodal planning (Figures 14.3 to 14.5). The US-CT combination has been found to be superior to US alone.[39] Kim and others found that the combination approach increases the sensitivity of detection of central LN metastases compared with US alone.

In a study examining the efficacy of LN detection by PE, US, and contrast-enhanced CT, a combination of CT and US showed the greatest sensitivity in imaging.[26] The sensitivity of CT scanning was found to

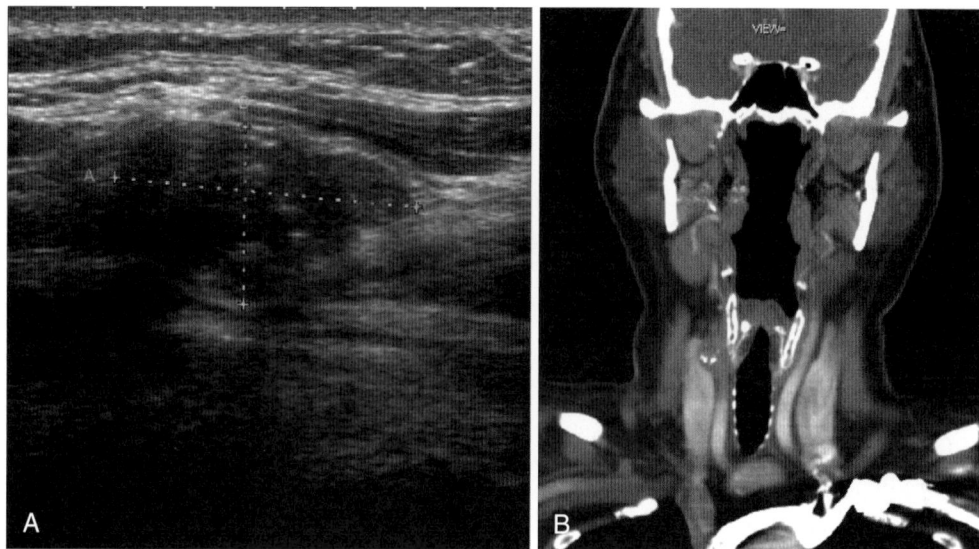

Fig. 14.3 A, Neck ultrasound of a patient with a history of total thyroidectomy for papillary thyroid carcinoma and increasing thyroglobulin levels. The ultrasound was able to detect a lymph node metastasis in the right neck. **B,** Computed tomography (CT) scan of the same patient preoperatively demonstrates the lymph node metastasis with calcification. The precise localization of the node was important because of the location of the recurrence on the right vagus nerve. The patient had a left vocal cord paralysis from her initial thyroidectomy done elsewhere. A focused directed dissection in the carotid sheath was performed with the CT images displayed in the operating room. Vocal cord function was unchanged postoperatively.

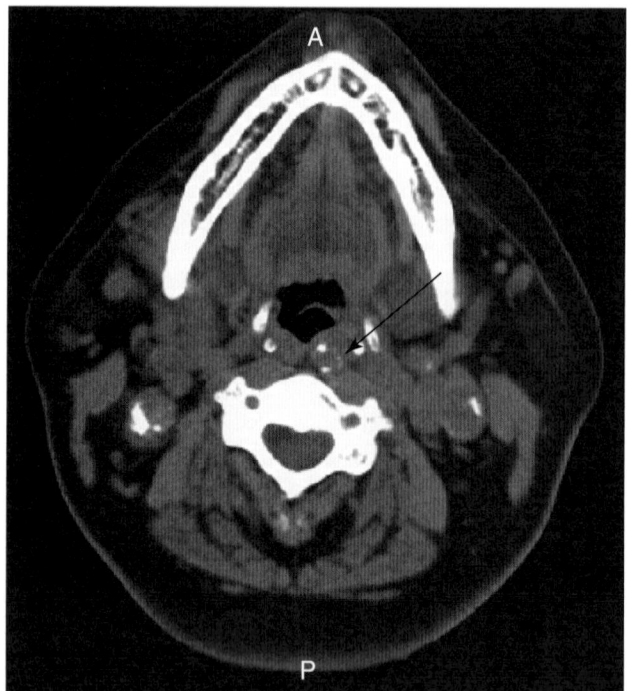

Fig. 14.4 Node of Rouvière *(Arrow)* in a Patient With Papillary Thyroid Carcinoma. The node was identified on a preoperative computed tomography scan but could not be detected by ultrasound. The node was removed intraorally during the initial operation. The patient had lung metastases and subsequently received radioactive iodine treatment.

be superior to US for imaging the central neck of patients undergoing primary surgery for thyroid cancer (50% versus 26%). Adding CT scan gave valuable information about macroscopic disease in the central neck that would have been missed by using US alone. This study showed that a importantly, in 25% of patients undergoing primary surgery and 27% of patients undergoing revision surgery had LNs removed because of CT findings that would not have been removed based on US alone.[26] These findings represent a significant number of patients who may have been spared further surgeries. Smaller studies have reached a similar conclusion: the sensitivity of CT and US in combination is superior in nodal detection for PTC.[39,40] Other authors have used a fusion of CT and US, which they found to be superior in LN detection. A real-time neck CT-guided US demonstrated a statistically significant better sensitivity than US alone.[41] The combination approach of US and CT ensures that all compartments are viewed adequately before surgery; the two modalities complement each other. US gives specific information about the LNs, including hilar anatomy, length-to-width ratio, calcifications, and cystic change. CT imaging provides localization of the LNs in relation to surrounding viscera—information that the surgeon can easily use. It also images the LN regions that are less accessible or less accurately seen by US, such as the central neck, mediastinum, and retropharynx. During surgery, the CT scan, with its full image of the neck and anatomic landmarks, can guide the surgeon to the precise location of the previously mapped LNs (Figures 14.6 and 14.7).

Cunnane et al. have proposed a radiographic cervical nodal classification for differentiating thyroid carcinoma. It uses anatomic boundaries identifiable radiographically as well as intraoperatively. It employs simple and uniform nomenclature to facilitate interdisciplinary communication and helps create a reproducible radiographic nodal map for optimum surgery as well as for follow-up surveillance[42] (Table 14.1).

With more thorough initial surgery, it is reasonable to predict lower posttreatment thyroglobulin levels, fewer investigative tests for recurrent disease, and a decreased number of reoperations and repeated radioactive iodine treatments. The clinical and psychological benefits to the patient can be significant. It is essential that all patients undergoing thyroid cancer surgery have comprehensive imaging of the central and lateral neck performed before surgery. US has been the

CHAPTER 14 Preoperative Radiographic Mapping of Nodal Disease for Papillary Thyroid Carcinoma

workhorse in the detection of thyroid disease, and CT scanning has been the workhorse in the detection of nodal metastases in the head and neck. It is natural for these complementary radiographic approaches to be used preoperatively to detect nodal thyroid disease. Current guidelines from the American Thyroid Association and American College of Endocrinology recommend that all patients undergoing thyroidectomy for suspected or documented thyroid malignancy have a preoperative neck US. They further recommend CT with contrast for patients with clinical suspicion for advanced disease, including invasive primary tumors or clinically apparent LN involvement that is multiple, bulky, or widely distributed.[24,33] The individualized preoperative radiographic mapping with combined CT and US data identifies the macroscopic nodal disease, which then directs the nodal dissection, so that each thyroid cancer patient undergoes an appropriate therapeutic dissection.

REFERENCES

For a complete list of references, go to expertconsult.com.

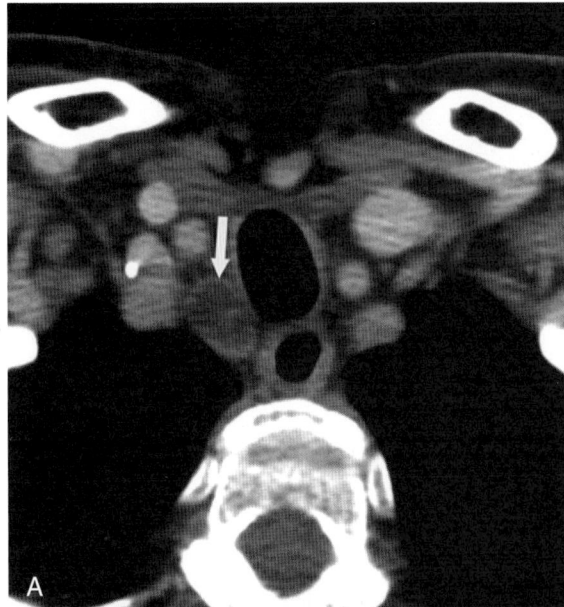
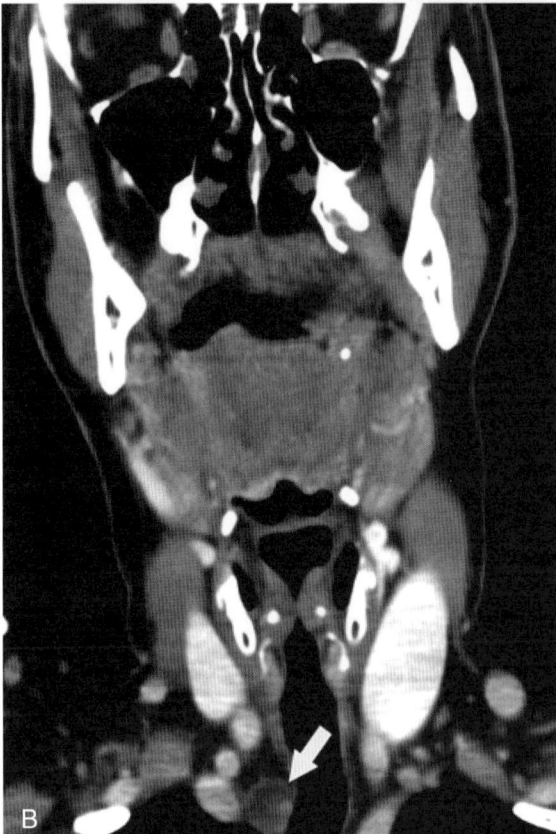

Fig. 14.5 Central neck lymph node seen only on computed tomography (axial and coronal) (**A**), not seen on ultrasound (**B**).

154 SECTION 3 Preoperative Evaluation

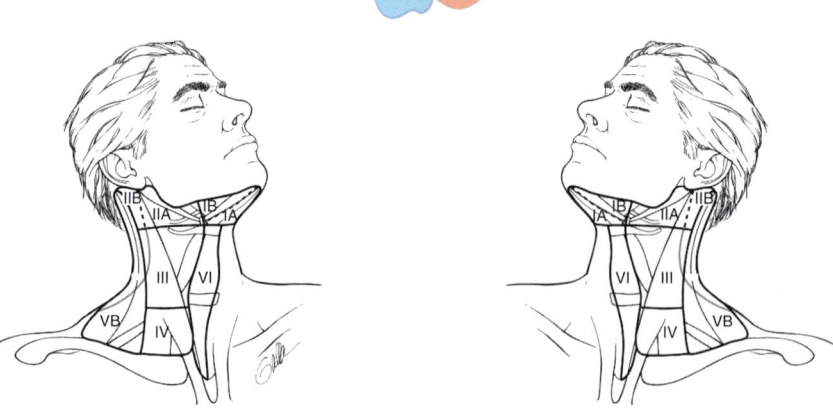

Fig. 14.6 Ultrasound and computed tomography combined information is drawn on a preoperative map; the map is discussed with the patient during the preoperative visit and is brought to the operating room on the day of surgery. A, right lateral neck; B, left lateral neck; C, right central neck; D, left central neck; T, pretracheal; L, prelaryngeal; E, ectopic.

CHAPTER 14 Preoperative Radiographic Mapping of Nodal Disease for Papillary Thyroid Carcinoma

CERVICAL LYMPH NODE MAP PRE-OP

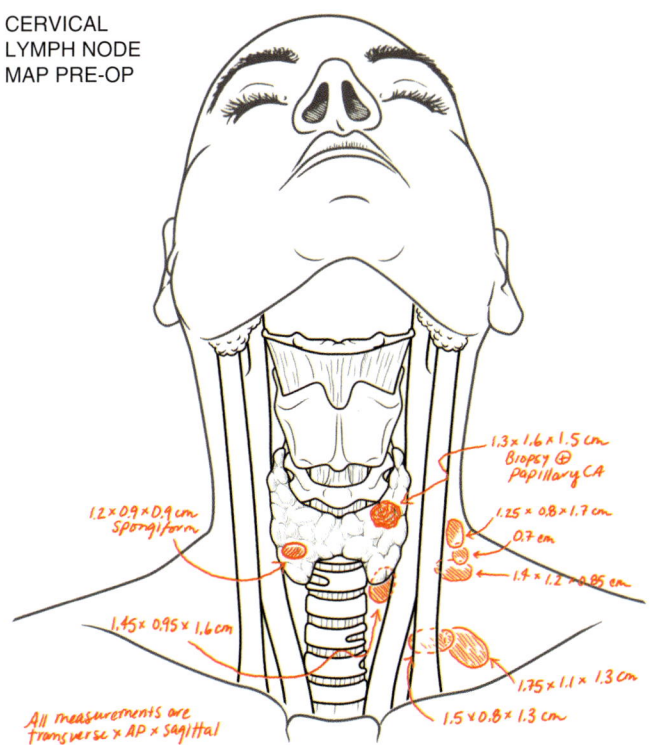

Fig. 14.7 An example of a preoperative map prepared from computed tomography and ultrasound images, provided to assist in surgical planning.

TABLE 14.1 The Imaging-Based Cervical Node Classification Derived Specifically for Differentiated Thyroid Cancer

MEEI Symbols	Lymph Node Groups	Description
A	Right lateral neck	Inferior to the digastric muscle, posterior to submandibular gland, deep to the sternocleidomastoid muscle. This includes nodes that lie either anterior or posterior to the common carotid artery.
B	Left lateral neck	Inferior to the digastric muscle, posterior to submandibular gland, deep to the sternocleidomastoid muscle. This includes nodes that are located either anterior or posterior to the common carotid artery.
C	Right central neck	Nodes located medial to the common carotid artery, between it and the trachea.
D	Left central neck	Nodes located medial to the common carotid artery, between it and the trachea.
T	Pretracheal	Nodes located anterior to the trachea.
L	Prelaryngeal	Nodes located anterior to the thyroid cartilage or the hyoid bone.
E	Ectopic	Nodes located in sites outside of typical neck regions. These ectopic sites include retropharyngeal, mediastinal, and axillary regions.

From Cunnane M, Kyriazidis N, Kamani D, et al. A novel thyroid cancer nodal map classification system to facilitate nodal localization and surgical management: the A to D map. *Laryngoscope*. 2017;127(10):2429–2436.

15

Laryngeal Examination in Thyroid and Parathyroid Surgery

Neil Tolley, Ian Witterick, Gregory W. Randolph

> Please go to expertconsult.com to view related video:
> **Video 15.1** Fiberoptic Laryngeal Exam: Laryngeal Anatomy and Function.

INTRODUCTION

Thyroid and parathyroid surgery is undertaken by surgeons from a variety of surgical disciplines and backgrounds. The implications of this type of surgery on the voice are a frequent patient concern and a major determinant of surgical quality outcomes. Although several neural and non-neural factors can influence voice outcomes, injury to the recurrent laryngeal nerve (RLN) has the greatest effect.

Incidence vocal cord paralysis (VCP) is a key performance indicator of surgical quality that requires gold-standard presurgical and postsurgical laryngeal examination to assess paralysis rate. After the recommendation by Randolph in 2010,[3] many national guidelines and consensus documents included a recommendation for all patients to undergo an examination of the vocal cords both before and after surgery.[1,2]

In a 2003 study, Saunders et al. found that 50% of thyroidectomies in the United States are performed by surgeons operating on fewer than five cases annually.[4] There is overwhelming evidence that shows a correlation between volume and surgical outcomes in thyroidectomy.[5,6] VCP and other complications have shown an inverse relationship with increased volume. An annual thyroid volume of higher than 50 has been shown to be protective.[7] The literature reports a further decrease in complications when volumes exceed 100.[8] This figure has been supported by the 5th BAETS (British Association of Endocrine and Thyroid Surgeons) National Audit, which is the largest endocrine surgical database in the world, containing in excess of 115,000 operations.[9]

A preoperative knowledge of vocal cord function is vital for surgical planning and is imperative when obtaining informed consent from patients. Operations performed on patients with only one functioning cord involve a very different conversation with the patient. Patients are increasingly forward in asking surgeons about what their operative volume and outcomes will be. In the absence of a preoperative laryngeal examination given national and international guidelines, a patient-turned-litigant's complaint may be likely to be supported in a court of law in the event of injury.

A change in voice is the most common complication after thyroid surgery. Although VCP rates in the extant literature have quoted low paralysis rates, there has been an increasing focus on patient outcomes in recent years. Often, these reports derive from high-volume surgeons and centers and may not have routine laryngeal examination postoperative evaluations. Paralysis rates after surgery have been shown to be significantly underreported. The variable, inconsistent adoption of presurgical and postsurgical laryngeal examination are primarily responsible.

RLN injury is the most common cause of litigation in endocrine surgery.[10] A study by Abadin et al. revealed that RLN injury contributed to 46% of thyroidectomy malpractice litigation between 1989 and 2009.[11] In a 2003 study, Lydiatt found that 67% of unilateral VCP lawsuits had a favorable outcome for the plaintiff with a deficiency in informed consent responsible in 78% of cases.[10]

Having a better understanding of the implications of VCP from a patient's perspective is valuable; a useful reading on the subject can be found in Munch and DeKryger's article from 2001.[12]

ANATOMY AND THE VOICE

Voice is unique to the individual; it serves as an indicator of emotion, background, education, and many other personal qualities. The voice, speech, and language have been developed only in the human. The generation of voice is complicated and relies on the integration and coordination of designated areas within the cerebral cortex that direct the laryngeal muscles and resonance of air through the upper airway.[13] Airflow through the cords leads to subtle movements of the inner epithelial cover of the vocal cords referred to as the *mucosal wave*. This process is attributed to the interplay of several factors (Table 15.1, Figure 15.1).

The larynx has a shield-shaped thyroid cartilage composed of a left and right lamina, which sits posteriorly on the inferior ring-like cricoid cartilage through the cartilaginous cricothyroid joints. The true vocal cords consist of a lining of squamous unciliated, nonkeratinized epithelium draping the fine laryngeal musculature. The cords project into the laryngeal lumen that is located halfway down the thyroid cartilage. The posteriorly placed arytenoid cartilages rest on the posterior cricoid lamina and contribute to the posterior cartilaginous third of the true cord. The cords insert anteriorly into the inner surface of the midline thyroid cartilage at Broyles' ligament. The movements of the arytenoids are rotational, but they also glide subtly along the face of the cricoid. Abduction is caused by a rotation of the arytenoid laterally, whereas medial rotation leads to adduction of the cords. The laryngeal musculature can be divided into intrinsic or extrinsic muscles. They are of 4th and 6th branchial arch derivation and are innervated by the external branch of the superior laryngeal nerve (EBSLN) (4th arch) and the RLN (6th arch). Sensory supply of the supraglottis derives from the superior laryngeal nerve (SLN), whereas the infraglottic sensory supply is via the RLN. The cricothyroid muscle is the only external laryngeal muscle situated on the outer surface of the larynx; as a consequence, it is within the thyroidectomy field and is easily and frequently injured.

CHAPTER 15 Laryngeal Examination in Thyroid and Parathyroid Surgery

TABLE 15.1 Factors Contributing to Production of Normal Voice

Cartilages	Thyroid cartilage	Represents the anterior insertion of the VC
		Forward tilting of the thyroid cartilage onto the cricoid cartilage under the action of the cricothyroid muscle leads to increased tension of the VCs, allowing for higher vocal registries and voice projection
	Cricoid cartilage	The posterior lamina offers support to the arytenoid cartilages
	Arytenoid cartilages	Represent the posterior insertion of the VC
		When they rotate laterally, they cause abduction of VC
		Medial rotation leads to adduction of VC
Muscles	Thyroarytenoid muscle (vocalis muscle)	Represents the main muscular component of the VC and acts as an adductor
	Adductors of VC	All intrinsic muscles of the larynx
	Abductors of VC	Posterior cricoarytenoid muscle
	Strap muscles	Sternohyoid, sternothyroid
Nerves	RLN	Carries motor fibers to all intrinsic laryngeal muscles with the exception of cricothyroid muscle
	EBSLN	Innervates the cricothyroid muscle

VC, vocal cord, RLN, recurrent laryngeal nerve, EBSLN, external branch of the superior laryngeal nerve.

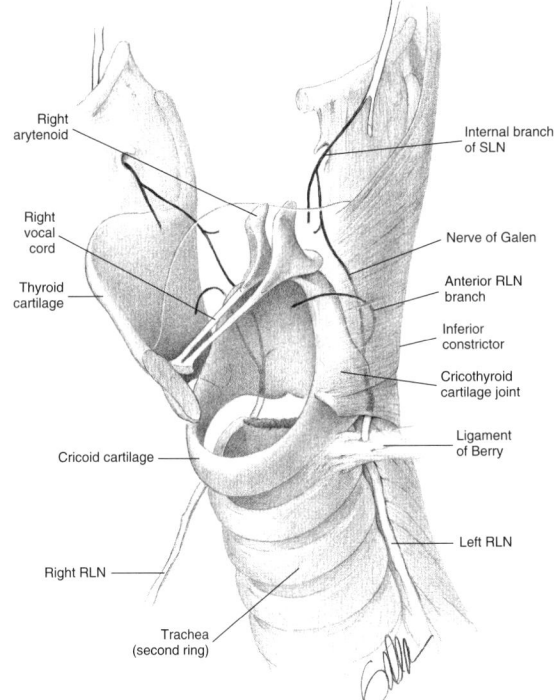

Fig. 15.1 Isolated Laryngeal Anatomy. Three-dimensional view of bilateral recurrent laryngeal nerve (RLN) entry into the larynx underneath the lower edge of the inferior constrictor. This shows both the anterior and posterior branches of the RLN within the larynx. The left thyroid lamina is not shown.

The cricothyroid muscle tilts the thyroid cartilage forward, which lengthens and tenses the cords facilitating a higher vocal register and voice projection. The cricothyroid muscle is extremely important for singing and vocal projection; significant injury may be career-ending for the professional singer (see Chapter 35, Surgical Anatomy of the Superior Laryngeal Nerve).

The RLN is a mixed nerve that carries motor, sensory, and autonomic fibers. It innervates all intrinsic muscles of the larynx except the cricothyroid muscle, which is innervated by the EBSLN. The RLN also innervates the inferior constrictor muscle of the pharynx and cricopharyngeus muscle carrying sensory fibers from the larynx, upper esophagus, and trachea. These RLN sensory fibers may be injured during thyroidectomy; this is why swallowing problems can be a postoperative complication with or without a VCP (see Chapter 36, Surgical Anatomy and Monitoring of the Recurrent Laryngeal Nerve).

Trauma to the epithelial lining of the vocal cords is invariable after insertion of an endotracheal tube and may influence the subtle mucosal wave movements; this may result in a change in voice quality generically described as *hoarseness*. Voice change from a VCP usually has a more distinctive character more accurately termed *breathiness*. This is a weak voice and cough caused by glottic incompetence during phonation because of the lateral resting position of the cord, which is typical for most paralyzed vocal cords (see Chapter 42, Pathophysiology of Recurrent Laryngeal Nerve Injury, and Chapter 43, Management of Recurrent Laryngeal Nerve Paralysis).

Iatrogenic RLN injury is most commonly mechanical (compression and stretching) or thermal (diathermy and energy devices). Minimal injury of the myelin sheath of the RLN causes temporary blockage (i.e., neuropraxia) of nerve conduction, which usually recovers fully after 6 to 8 weeks (see Chapter 36, Surgical Anatomy and Monitoring of the Recurrent Laryngeal Nerve). More severe trauma to the RLN, particularly from thermal injury, may damage the myelin sheath neural fibers (axonotmesis). Recovery is still possible, but with a greater delay, and is often suboptimal manifested by reduced mobility and dysfunctional reinnervation known as synkinesis; the manifestation of these symptoms have a negative effect on the voice. Greater RLN injury (neurotmesis) leads to interruption of endoneurial, perineurial, or epineurial sheaths. This type of injury is associated with incomplete or absent nerve regrowth and connectivity.[14]

Unilateral vocal fold paralysis can be well tolerated, particularly if the cord remains in a paramedian position. Factors that control the final resting position of the cord after RLN injury are not understood. This and intubation edema can often allow for a near-normal voice in the initial days after surgery. Patients may not, therefore, complain of a change in voice until weeks have passed after their surgery. In more severe injuries, symptoms usually appear as a consequence of laryngeal muscle and cord atrophy. Patients complain of a weak, breathy, and hoarse voice. Laryngeal examination often reveals an immobile cord in a lateralized position. Injuries to the EBSLN can be extremely difficult or impossible to diagnose by laryngeal examination, even by expert laryngologists using stroboscopy. In pure SLN injuries, the cord can be apparently thinner and shorter, and the posterior glottis may "point" to the injured side. Injury to the cricothyroid muscle as a gold-standard test can only be confirmed by electromyography (EMG) (see Chapter 35, Surgical Anatomy of the Superior Laryngeal Nerve).

Lateral displacement of the paralyzed vocal cord leads to a glottic gap that lets air escape during phonation (breathy voice). Cord level can be also be different compared with the normally moving side, which further contributes to poor voice quality. Because of impaired glottic competence, the patient can complain of swallowing difficulties, which may predispose them to coughing spasms secondary to aspiration. Recent big data studies revealed associated morbidity and long-term mortality associated with VCP. VCP is significantly associated with emergency admission within 12 months after surgery, the development of pneumonia, and a ten-fold increase in the risk of gastrostomy for feeding issues. Furthermore, there was a long-term increase in mortality associated with VCP from bronchopneumonia.[15]

As discussed previously, the EBSLN innervates the cricothyroid muscle. Injury to the muscle causes a problem when projecting the voice because it is a tenser of the cords important in attaining higher registers; this injury is especially significant to the singing voice. The cricothyroid muscle has two components: the oblique and transverse bellies. The external nerve inserts between the two bellies and lies in the normal position 2 mm below the insertion of the superior head of the sternothyroid muscle along the oblique line of the thyroid cartilage lamina.[15a] An attempt should always be made, where possible, to identify the nerve. Division of the superior aspect of the sternothyroid muscle often assists by improving exposure to the superior thyroid pole.

The SLN has also been known as the *nerve of Amelita Galli-Curci*, named after the famous soprano whose career was brought to a ruinous end in 1935 because of thyroid surgery performed under local anesthesia. Newspapers at the time wrote that after thyroid surgery, "the surprising voice is gone forever. The sad spectre of a ghost replaces the velvety softness."[16]

Bilateral VCP usually, but not always, presents acutely at extubation. If it is not recognized immediately after surgery, respiratory arrest can occur (in several hours or in the early days after surgery), which makes this even more dangerous. In cases of severe injury, both cords are usually in a paramedian position causing variable airway obstruction. In cases of patients with a bilateral VCP, 50% of patients will require some form of airway surgery; half of these surgeries will entail tracheostomy. The patient may have biphasic stridor and be in frank respiratory distress. As mentioned previously, patients do not necessarily have airway symptoms in the immediate postoperative period. The recently intubated glottis may be stented open for some period of time, so the glottis may narrow progressively in the ensuing hours and days postoperatively. The patient may, therefore, present at outpatient follow-up complaining of shortness of breath or stridor on exertion.

REPORTED PREVALENCE OF RECURRENT LARYNGEAL NERVE PARALYSIS

The true incidence of VCP is unknown due to a failure of long-term consistency in adoption of the gold-standard of performing both a pre- and postoperative laryngeal examination in all patients undergoing thyroid and parathyroid surgery. What is known is that the true incidence is considerably underestimated and underreported.

A bedside assessment of the voice has poor sensitivity and specificity for vocal cord palsy.[17,18] Validated thyroid voice questionnaires have been developed, but they fail to meet the accuracy of a laryngeal examination and cannot be recommended as an alternative.[19]

A systematic review in 2009 by Jeannon et al. of 27 articles and 25,000 patients showed a wide variation in cord palsy based on the laryngeal examination method used. An average initial paralysis rate of 9.8% (range 2.3% to 26%) was found in their study.[20]

The goal of the review was that anonymous reporting in national audit databases might provide a more accurate picture of palsy. In Sweden, the Scandinavian Quality Register (SQR) of 2008 reviewed 3660 thyroidectomies performed during a 12-month period. This analyzed data from 26 specialist endocrine surgical units from Sweden and Denmark and revealed an immediate 4.3% paralysis rate.[21,22] Furthermore, this rate doubled when patients were submitted to routine laryngeal examination (as opposed to postoperative laryngoscopy performed only in patients with persistent and severe voice changes). The 2009 3rd BAETS National Audit report of 10,814 thyroidectomies reported a permanent palsy rate of 2.5% with 4.9% of patients reporting a change in voice. For first-time surgery, the reported incidence of a cord paralysis was 1.4% after lobectomy and 3.7% after total thyroidectomy. A significant increase in cord palsy was associated with revision surgery with rates of 5.4% for lobectomy and 6.9% for total thyroidectomy. This was from self-reported and unvalidated data entry from surgeons focusing on thyroid surgery; the surgeons in question did not uniformly conform to the gold-standard practice of laryngeal examination in all operations. As a result, these data are likely significant underestimations of true paralysis rates. Only a minority (21.5%) of patients in this 2009 audit underwent a postoperative laryngeal examination.[22a]

The 2012 4th BAETS National Audit reported a preoperative laryngeal examination rate of 60.9% in primary and 86.7% in revision surgery, respectively.[22b] Postoperative laryngeal examination occurred in less than 20% of patients with a higher than 20% rate of missing field data. As one might expect, postoperative paralysis rates were shown to increase with increasing laryngoscopy rates. When the postoperative laryngeal examination rate was less than 30%, 30% to 80%, and >80%, respectively, which correlates with the rates revealed in the SQR 1.7%, 2.5%, and 4.2% paralysis rates were reported. Finally, the 2017 5th BAETS National Audit showed an increase in the preoperative laryngeal examination rate to 73% and 86% in primary and revision surgery, respectively; however, a postoperative laryngeal examination was performed in only 40% of patients, and there was more than 20% of missing field data. Therefore the true incidence of vocal cord palsy in the UK registry report of 2017 that analyzed 47,493 thyroidectomies remains unknown and could not be accurately reported.

The early diagnosis of cord paralysis is important because there is evidence that treatment within 3 months of surgery leads to significantly better patient outcome.[23,24] There have been advances in the management of the paralyzed vocal cord with the proven safety and effectiveness of transcutaneous in-office injection.[25-29]

Vocal cord injection is one of a number of techniques available to manage cord paralysis (see Chapter 42, Pathophysiology of the Recurrent Laryngeal Nerve Injury, and 43, Management of Recurrent Laryngeal Nerve Paralysis).

An open thyroplasty method involves a skin incision and partial thyroid cartilage removal with placement of an implant or spacer material lateral to cord in the paraglottic space. This procedure may be combined with the arytenoid adduction, a technically difficult operation, where the arytenoid cartilage is repositioned through suture placement to reposition the cord; this is indicated where injection thyroplasty may be less suitable in patients with a large posterior glottic gap and, in particular, if the cord is at a different level than the opposite normal non paralyzed cord.

GLOTTIC EXAMINATION AND THE VOICE

Preoperative VCP can be caused by benign and malignant thyroid disease. It can also be present in the absence of any voice symptoms. This knowledge supports the recommendation for a preoperative laryngeal examination of all patients to help deliver and uniform gold-standard care for patients. The discrepancies between cord function on laryngeal examination and voice symptoms are due to many variables. Whether paralysis or paresis exist, the variability of contralateral cord compensation and other mechanisms are at play. Commonly in known cases of VCP, symptoms improve over time. This may be due to either a resumption of normal function or an evolution of cord position into a more favorable medial position. Only laryngeal examination will make a distinction between these two scenarios of "apparent or true" functional vocal cord recovery.

VOICE SYMPTOMS WITH NORMAL VOCAL FOLD MOBILITY

Voice symptoms after thyroidectomy are common without apparent laryngeal nerve injury.[30] In addition, some patients complain of difficulty swallowing and a pulling sensation with neck extension.

The postoperative subjective and objective voice changes commonly occur in patients with intact vocal fold mobility. Usually, the symptoms are transient and consist of vocal fatigue during phonation, difficulty reaching higher pitches, and a reduction in vocal range.[31] The speech may be more monotone, and the vocal pitch can be more than two semitones lower. Reported series vary on the rate of postoperative subjective voice complaints after various forms of thyroid or parathyroid surgery; however, they are in the range of 30% to 87%.[22,32-36]

In a prospective study of 42 patients with node-negative papillary carcinoma undergoing total thyroidectomy, impaired communication was the primary theme derived from patient interviews after surgery. Among 42 patients, voice symptoms persisted for 21 patients (50%) for at least 1 year of follow-up.[37]

In a prospective multicenter observational study from France, 203 patients (who had a total thyroidectomy and no preoperative voice problems) were followed for 6 months using a self-administered questionnaire (Voice Handicap Index). Patients with postoperative RLN paralysis were excluded from analysis. Twenty percent of patients had initial voice impairment at 2 months with progressive recovery to preoperative levels; however, 6% of patients had persistent voice complaints.[38]

Objective early voice changes are common in the majority of patients undergoing thyroidectomy but do not necessarily correlate with objective findings. In one prospective series with two control groups undergoing endotracheal intubation for other reasons (one neck surgery and one non-neck surgery), the acoustic and aerodynamic parameters were similar in all groups at 1 week. At 8 weeks, patients aged 40 and older in the thyroidectomy group showed persistent objective changes but did not report vocal abnormalities; their perceptual evaluation was similar to their preoperative evaluation.[39] Another recent study also found an age-related association with age ≥50 years was independently associated with the development of voice or swallowing problems postthyroidectomy with intact RLN function.[40]

In a systematic review and meta-analysis on acoustic voice parameters after uncomplicated thyroidectomy, five acoustic voice parameters were measured at less than 3 months and greater than 3 months postoperatively. The fundamental frequency, shimmer, and maximum phonation time significantly worsened in the early (<3 months) but not in the late postoperative period (>3 months). The fundamental frequency impairment was perceptually significant; males undergoing total thyroidectomy experienced greater voice impairment in the early (<3 months) period.[41]

Voice change after thyroidectomy has been associated with local wound adhesion and impairment of laryngeal vertical movement.[42] Radioactive iodine has not been found to affect voice quality subjectively or objectively.[43]

The proposed mechanisms for voice alteration despite normal RLN function are insufficiently understood (Table 15.2). Direct cricothyroid muscle dysfunction by direct injury or transient wound fluid-related myositis may play a role. Regional soft tissue changes may affect the larynx, including edema, strap muscle retraction and denervation, and ultimately perilaryngeal scarring. Although strap muscle management during surgery could affect laryngeal function (and therefore conceivably affect postoperative voice), one study found no relationship between strap muscle division and postoperative voice outcome.[44]

Strap muscles are known to activate during lower pitch vocalization.[45] Certainly, intubation-related[46] vocal cord changes, including short-term edema, vocal cord laceration, arytenoid dislocation, or more long-term vocal cord granuloma formation,[47] are all possible sources of vocal changes despite grossly normal neurologic function (see Table 15.2). Echternach et al. reported that a surprisingly high 42% of their patients

TABLE 15.2 Factors Causing Postoperative Voice Change

Injury	Functional Consequence	Effect on Voice Character
Neural		
RLN injury (complete or partial, transient or permanent)	Immobile and laterally displaced cord	Breathy voice
	Inadequate closure of vocal cords with phonation and swallowing	Vocal fatigue
		Hoarseness
	Loss of VC bulk and tone	
	Bowing atrophy of vocal cord	
External branch of the superior laryngeal nerve (EBSLN) injury (complete or partial, transient or permanent)	Posterior glottic rotation toward the paretic side	Easy voice fatigue
	Bowing of the vocal fold on the weak side	Decreased pitch
	Inferior displacement of the affected cord	Inability to project voice
Non-Neural		
Direct cricothyroid muscle injury—transient myositis or direct injury	As for EBSLN	As for ESBLN
Regional soft tissue injury (in the presence of intact neurologic function)	Laryngotracheal regional scar with fixation	Voice fatigue
	Strap muscles denervation or trauma	Decrease in vocal range
	Local hematoma or edema	Vocal pitch can be lower
Intubation-related injuries	VC trauma (i.e., edema, hematoma, and laceration)	Hoarseness
	VC granuloma	Odynophagia
	Arytenoid dislocation	
Voice change from unrelated intercurrent URTI	Typically, viral-related laryngitis unrelated to surgery, rarely associated with VCP	Hoarseness, breathy voice if VCP

RLN, recurrent laryngeal nerve, VC, vocal cord, EBSLN, external branch of the superior laryngeal nerve, URTI, Upper respiratory tract infection, VCP, vocal cord paralysis.

undergoing thyroid surgery had laryngeal complications from intubation when an experienced otolaryngologist performed a laryngeal examination 3 to 4 days after surgery.[48] Most studies suggest lower rates of laryngeal trauma from intubation, ranging from 6% to 13%.[46,49] Laryngeal trauma from intubation usually only affects voice quality for less than 1 week postoperatively.[50]

The extent of surgical trauma and incidence of voice problems may vary depending on thyroidectomy approach and the experience and technique of the surgeon. There are differences in reported outcomes; some conclude that the incidence and severity of voice and swallowing complaints are less common in patients undergoing video-assisted thyroidectomy.[51] However, in a Korean study with functioning RLNs, there were no significant differences in postoperative voice change or swallowing difficulty between open, endoscopic, and robotic approaches.[52]

There have also been rare reports of endotracheal intubations independently causing VCP, even though the setting of surgeries did not involve the vagus or RLN. It has been suggested that the cuff pressure on the more distal course of the anterior branch may result in such RLN paralysis.[53,54] However, VCP from endotracheal intubation exclusively is extremely rare and only affects 0.04% of patients.[55,56] A patient may also occasionally present with hoarseness postoperatively after thyroidectomy from intercurrent upper respiratory tract infection. This typically results in transient upper respiratory tract-related laryngitis. Such viral upper respiratory tract infections may rarely be associated with VCP (see Table 15.2).

Injury to the EBSLN can result in diminished vocal projection and inability to attain a higher vocal pitch. Injury to the RLN can cause paresis or paralysis of the nerve and thereby affect vocal quality. Non-neural etiologies include direct cricothyroid muscle dysfunction as well as stiffness and/or fibrosis of the regional soft tissues.

VOCAL CORD PARALYSIS WITHOUT VOICE SYMPTOMS

In the setting of postoperative VCP, it is common to have initial symptoms offset by early postoperative vocal cord edema. During later phases of the postoperative period, VCP can be asymptomatic because of a variety of mechanisms, such as remaining partial neural function, variability in paralytic cord position, and variability in contralateral cord compensation. It is common with permanent VCP that symptoms improve over time because of contralateral cord compensation. This can falsely suggest that the VCP has resolved.[17,57] In a study of 98 patients with VCP, voice was judged to be normal in 20% and improved to normal in an additional 8%. Therefore nearly one-third of patients with VCP were or became asymptomatic.[58] The incidence of an asymptomatic patient can still be a significant and potential source of learning for the surgeon who seeks to relate the surgical conduct of that case to its postoperative outcome. There is also the significance of asymptomatic VCP in terms of swallowing safety and the potential for increased respiratory morbidity if the contralateral nerve is operated on in a future surgery.

RATIONALE FOR PREOPERATIVE LARYNGEAL EXAMINATION

Selective laryngeal examination is recommended by some guidelines (see Laryngeal Examination Guidelines section) for patients undergoing thyroid or parathyroid surgery. Some groups argue that the incidence of asymptomatic vocal cord paresis/paralysis is low in previously unoperated patients; therefore routine preoperative laryngoscopic examination should be reserved for those with previous thyroidectomy and/or voice/swallowing symptoms.[59] The routine use of perioperative laryngoscopy in patients undergoing parathyroid surgery has also been questioned.[60] Some arguments, which use decision tree modeling, claim that preoperative routine laryngoscopy in the surgical treatment of sonographically low-risk differentiated thyroid cancer is not cost-effective.[61]

These studies, recommending "selective" application of laryngeal examination, suggest reliance on self-reported voice symptoms or physician identified voice symptoms as major criteria to examine the larynx preoperatively.[59,60,61] However, VCP, as noted earlier, can be present without significant vocal symptoms; a lack of such symptoms is not a reliable indicator of RLN function. Two studies investigating preoperative voice changes and VCP found the sensitivity of voice change in predicting VCP ranged between 33% and 68%.[17,18] In addition, whatever caused the patient's VCP preoperatively often will have happened many years earlier. The patient and their family may have adapted to the voice sound and quality, so they may not perceive any abnormality. Furthermore, the sensitivity of thyroid surgeons to screen and detect voice abnormalities preoperatively was tested by Al-Yahya et al.; however, the study did not reach the desired sensitivity as a screening tool for patients with underlying VCP.[62]

Preoperative recognition of VCP is essential in planning the procedure because management of the RLN found to be invaded at surgery is based on knowledge of its preoperative function.[17] It has been reported that the presence of RLN palsy has an excellent predictive value for invasive thyroid disease (sensitivity 76%, specificity 100%).[17] Preoperative knowledge of invasive disease may allow for more appropriate preoperative imaging and patient counseling. For example, in a patient with a unilateral malignancy and a paralyzed vocal cord on the contralateral side, the conversation with the patient should include the possibility of the requirement for a tracheostomy with all the associated sequelae and potential morbidities. In this scenario, many surgeons would also opt to include continuous intraoperative nerve monitoring during the operation, or the physician may defer contralateral surgery. Without the knowledge of the paralyzed vocal cord preoperatively, the surgeon may be unaware of the potentially devastating consequences of the surgery; such consequences may lead to a second and bilateral RLN paralysis.

There are important quality-assurance and medicolegal considerations because knowledge of preoperative vocal cord function is necessary before assuming responsibility for any postoperative VCP.

LARYNGEAL EXAMINATION GUIDELINES

Increasing awareness of the importance of vocal outcomes after thyroid surgery has led to a number of guidelines from national organizations devoted to the care and management of patients with thyroid disorders. The guidelines are primarily for thyroid surgery but are also applicable to parathyroid surgery.

The 2011 BAETS consensus statement advises both a pre- and postoperative vocal cord examination in all cases of parathyroid and thyroid surgery. The 2013 American Academy of Otolaryngology Head and Neck Surgery (AAO/HNS) clinical practice guidelines for improving voice outcomes after thyroid surgery recommend preoperative laryngoscopy in all patients undergoing thyroid surgery for the following indications: (1) abnormal voice; and (2) normal voice and the patient has (a) thyroid cancer with suspected extrathyroidal extension, (b) prior neck surgery that increases the risk of laryngeal nerve injury (carotid endarterectomy, anterior approach to the cervical spine, cervical esophagectomy, and prior thyroid or parathyroid surgery), or (c) both.[63]

The 2013 German Association of Endocrine Surgeons recommended preoperative laryngoscopy after previous neck surgery and when the voice is deemed abnormal; vocal cord dysfunction can significantly influence treatment decisions, especially when thyroid surgery is an option and surgical procedures need to be planned.[64]

The 2014 British Thyroid Association (BTA) Guidelines for the Management of Thyroid Cancer recommended endoscopic examination to assess vocal cord function and to search for evidence of direct involvement of the larynx and upper trachea (if disease appears localized and amenable to surgery).[65]

The 2015 American Thyroid Association (ATA) guidelines for thyroid nodules and differentiated thyroid cancer recommends laryngeal examination similar to the 2013 American Academy of Otolaryngology-Head and Neck Surgery (AAO/HNS) guidelines for all patients at high-risk for nerve injury who are undergoing thyroid surgery. Examples include preoperative voice abnormalities, a history of previous neck or upper chest surgery, extension of the primary thyroid carcinoma posteriorly, and extensive neck nodal metastases.[66] Subsequent suggestions related to the ATA guidelines recommend endocrinologists and surgeons ensure that voice and laryngeal evaluations are completed before surgery.[67]

The 2016 American Head and Neck Society (AHNS) consensus statement recommends preoperative laryngeal examination in all patients undergoing thyroid surgery, especially those who are at high risk for nerve injury similar to the previous recommendations.[1,63,64,66,67]

The 2018 National Comprehensive Cancer Network (NCCN) clinical practice guidelines for management of thyroid carcinoma recommend considering the evaluation of vocal cord mobility (ultrasound, mirror indirect laryngoscopy, or fiberoptic laryngoscopy) in patients with abnormal voice, surgical history involving the RLN or vagus nerves, invasive disease, or bulky disease of the central neck.

RATIONALE FOR POSTOPERATIVE LARYNGEAL EXAMINATION

The 2014 BTA recommended that patients with a voice change after thyroidectomy undergo laryngoscopy. The BTA also promoted routine postoperative laryngoscopy in patients who have undergone thyroidectomy.[65] The AAO/HNS and ATA guidelines recommend laryngeal examination if postoperative voice abnormalities are detected.[63,66] Lang et al., in a decision-analytic model, estimated the cost-effectiveness of both a routine postoperative laryngeal examination and a selective laryngeal examination. From their institution's perspective, they found a routine laryngeal examination was not cost-effective, and they suggested that a 3-month examination was a reasonable and acceptable strategy.[68] The 2016 AHNS guidelines recommended that all patients should be considered for postoperative laryngeal examination.[1]

The timing of postoperative laryngoscopy is influenced by many factors. The earlier the vocal cord function is assessed, the higher the incidence of abnormalities observed. In one large Italian study of 825 nerves at risk, the VCP rate was 6.4% (on the day of surgery), 6.7% (on day 1), 4.8% (on day 2), 2.5% (on day 14), and 0.8% (at 6 weeks).[69] This knowledge could also have important implications for a patient's ability to swallow safely, especially in the early postoperative period.

Postoperative laryngoscopy is the only reliable way of knowing the real incidence of VCP after surgery. Given the clear-cut divergence between voice symptoms and objective vocal cord function, it would seem that routine postoperative laryngeal examination is required in all patients undergoing thyroid surgery; this would help surgeons have accurate information regarding their surgical outcomes.

FLEXIBLE LARYNGOSCOPY: A STANDARD TECHNIQUE TO BE MASTERED BY ALL THYROID SURGEONS

The arguments presented support routine laryngeal examination in all patients undergoing thyroid surgery (Box 15.1). Because the professional background/training of thyroid surgeons is variable, some might be reluctant to adopt the technique and might feel it necessary to refer patients to a specialized otolaryngology-head & neck surgery clinic. Instead, all surgeons should become confident with the technique and proceed to examine their own patients routinely.

Laryngeal examination techniques include mirror examination, flexible transnasal fiberoptic laryngoscopy, laryngeal stroboscopy, laryngeal ultrasound, cross-sectional imaging, and EMG. Ideally, surgeons want to know about function of the RLNs and SLNs, the laryngeal musculature, mobility of the cricoarytenoid joints, and laryngeal phonatory function. However, for widespread use, any examination technique should be relatively low cost, noninvasive, reproducible, easy to perform and teach, and well tolerated by patients. For the vast majority of patients undergoing thyroid or parathyroid surgery, the primary goal and most important piece of information to gain from any laryngeal examination is the mobility of both vocal cords.

Indirect mirror laryngoscopy is still practiced; however, it takes many months to learn proper technique and to gain the ability to adequately visualize the larynx. In addition, there are some patients for whom it is impossible to see the vocal cords adequately because of local anatomy, a strong gag reflex (despite topical anesthesia as well as patient apprehension), and intolerance of the procedure. Some of these issues are still present with flexible transnasal fiberoptic laryngoscopy. Generally speaking, however, it is a much easier skill to master and to be able to correctly identify vocal cord mobility. Research on the learning curve suggests that only six attempts on average are required for a novice to become competent in performing flexible laryngoscopy.[70] Figure 15.2 shows

---

BOX 15.1 Rationale for Routine Laryngoscopy in Thyroid Surgery

Preoperative Laryngoscopy
- VC palsy can be present in the absence of voice complaints.
- VC palsy suggests invasive malignancy preoperative planning and radiographic analysis can be robust.
- Management of invaded RLN found at surgery is, in part, affected by knowledge of preoperative functional status.
- Responsibility for postoperative VC palsy can be wrongly attributed if one fails to demonstrate its preoperative existence.
- Preoperative laryngoscopy provides a preoperative baseline for postoperative laryngeal assessment.

Postoperative Laryngoscopy
- Glottic examination is the only existent accurate postoperative RLN outcome measure; voice changes occur in the majority of patients in the absence of RLN injury, hence it is important for the functional and psychological recovery of the patients to be informed that no RLN injury has taken place.
- Postoperative functional information allows for maximum interpretation of intraoperative EMG data from neural monitoring.
- VCP has implications for safety of swallowing and of future contralateral surgery.
- Early detection of VCP allows for earlier treatment and better vocal outcomes long term.

VC, vocal cord, RLN, recurrent laryngeal nerve, EMG, electromyography, VCP, vocal cord paralysis.

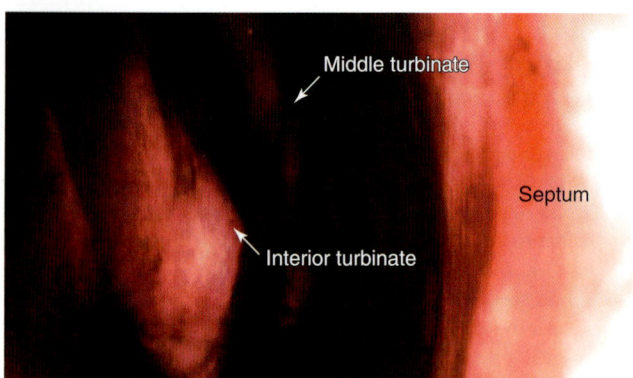

Fig 15.2 Key nasal anatomic landmarks Seen During Flexible Laryngoscopy.

important nasal anatomic landmarks seen when performing flexible laryngoscopy. Skilled examiners, who may or may not require topical anesthesia, generally try to avoid mucosal contact as much as possible. Patients should be positioned comfortably on a chair, with the back supported and the head in slight extension. Once the scope is in the pharynx, the epiglottis is easily apparent. The scope is flexed so that it can advance in front of the epiglottis. The patient is asked to say "e," and the adduction movement of the vocal cord is easily apparent. The "e" is alternated with a "sniff in" maneuver, and abduction will be apparent.

There are a number of aspects of the examination that can be evaluated in a short period of time, including vocal cord mobility, laryngeal elevation, evidence of laryngopharyngeal reflux, cricoid and/or upper tracheal invasion, as well as any other laryngeal pathology. If available, photo or video documentation of any abnormality helps for comparison purposes postoperatively. Flexible transnasal laryngoscopy is considered the optimal method for pre- and postoperative examination of the larynx on the basis of widespread availability, patient tolerance, and the assessment of both the RLN and the EBSLN.[1] Unilateral lack of vocal cord movement or asymmetric movements are diagnostic of RLN paralysis or paresis. Signs of EBSLN paralysis are difficult to routinely observe. Typically, the affected vocal cord is somewhat bowed, lower, and may be rotated toward the affected side.

Laryngeal stroboscopy is an excellent examination technique to slow down the motion of the mucosal wave and vocal fold vibrations and is usually performed with a rigid transoral laryngoscope with the patient upright and in a forward leaning position. Stroboscopy is not required to identify an obviously immobile or paralyzed vocal cord, but it does help in the identification of subtle degrees of hypomobility or paresis. It can also be helpful in identifying a unilateral SLN paralysis or paresis.[71] The interpretation of stroboscopy findings is subjective with no established measurement tools. In addition, if the mucosal wave is not periodic, synchronization of the strobe light may be technically difficult; this may limit the diagnostic ability of this technique.

Transcutaneous laryngeal ultrasound has been used to evaluate vocal cord motion, vocal cord lesions, invasion of the thyroid cartilage, and perioperative investigation of stridor and other upper airway problems.[72,73] It is a relatively straightforward procedure to perform with a linear transducer set at 7 to 10 MHz. The true vocal cords are usually seen as hypoechoic with a fine hyperechoic line. Subtle vocal cord abnormalities cannot be reliably identified. Downsides of the technique include the cost of the ultrasound machine, considerable interobserver variability, and thyroid cartilage calcification. In older male patients, thyroid cartilage calcification may not allow transmission of the ultrasound signal.[73]

In patients with VCP, cross-sectional imaging with computed tomography (CT) or magnetic resonance imaging (MRI) may show dilation of the ipsilateral piriform fossa, atrophy of muscle (thyroarytenoid and/or cricoarytenoid), and vocal fold bowing. These imaging modalities are best suited for evaluating laryngeal, tracheal, or esophageal invasion and should not be reliably used in the detection of vocal cord motion abnormalities.

Laryngeal EMG is another tool that can be used to assess function of the RLN and EB SLN. It is usually performed percutaneously to sample the thyroarytenoid and cricoarytenoid muscles. This method of laryngeal evaluation is not in widespread use and requires skilled clinicians for needle insertion and interpretation of the findings. It is a qualitative and not quantitative examination of laryngeal muscle firing. The EMG signal can vary significantly depending on the position in the muscle, the degree of effort made by the patient, the timing from nerve injury and the impedance of the electrode.[74] This form of laryngeal examination is usually only available in specialized laryngology centers.

SUMMARY

Low rates of laryngeal nerve injury have traditionally been reported in the peer reviewed literature; however, it is clear that true nerve injury rates are significantly underreported. The factors responsible for this have been highlighted and are consistent with guideline and consensus statements from both national and international professional organizations; the rationale for both a pre- and postoperative examination of the vocal cords has been emphasized.

A normal voice both presurgery and postsurgery does not exclude a significant laryngeal nerve injury. Discovering this preoperatively is important for surgical planning and informed consent. Postoperatively, it permits early rehabilitation and treatment of both voice and swallowing. Finally, it allows the surgeon to record and reflect upon the results as a key performance indicator of surgical quality. This is an important adjunct to appraisal, revalidation, and credentialing for all surgeons.

REFERENCES

For a complete list of references, go to expertconsult.com.

16

Radiofrequency and Laser Ablation of Thyroid Nodules and Parathyroid Adenoma

Jung Hwan Baek, Auh Whan Park

> Please go to expertconsult.com to view related video:
> **Video 16.1** Laser and Radiofrequency Treatment of Thyroid Nodules and Parathyroid Adenoma.
> **Video 16.2** RFA of a Thyroid Nodule Using the Trans-isthmic Approach and the Moving Shot Technique.
> **Video 16.3** RFA of a Recurrent Tumor in the Subcutaneous Location with Hydrodissection and the Moving Shot Technique.
> This chapter contains additional online-only content, including figures and exclusive video, available on expertconsult.com.

INTRODUCTION

Historically, surgery, radioiodine therapy, and levothyroxine medication have been the main treatment options for benign thyroid nodules; however, each of these has particular drawbacks. Surgery results in a scar, requires general anesthesia, and places patients at risk for hypothyroidism, bleeding, and voice change.[1-4] Radioiodine therapy can pose logistical difficulties for patients and results in the need for lifelong thyroid hormone supplementation. Image-guided ablation techniques, such as ethanol ablation (EA), laser ablation (LA), radiofrequency ablation (RFA), microwave ablation (MWA), and high intensity focused ultrasound ablation (HIFU), have been developed to treat benign thyroid nodules and recurrent thyroid cancers.[5-11] As clinical applications of EA and RFA increase, RFA guidelines have been published by Korean and Italian groups.[3,4,12] This chapter reviews the physics of ablation, ablative techniques, clinical applications, society guidelines, and the results of thyroid RFA and LA studies, with a brief review of the other modalities.

RADIOFREQUENCY ABLATION

Mechanism of Action

 Please see the Expert Consult website for Figure 16.1.

Radiofrequency ablation (RFA) uses an alternating electric current oscillating between 200 and 1200 kHz.[13] The general set up and mechanism of action of RFA is depicted in Figure 16.1 (available on expertconsult.com). The radiofrequency (RF) electrode is not the source of heat; instead, it acts as the cathode of an electric circuit that is closed by the application of dispersing pads on the patient's thighs (see Figure 16.1, *A*). The ions adjacent to the tip of the RF electrode vibrate rapidly in response to the alternating current. This kinetic energy is transformed into heat due to local resistance to the motion of the ions around the electrode (see Figure 16.1, *B*). Energy deposition and temperature drop exponentially away from the probe as the heat is transmitted relative to the tissue's thermal conductivity (see Figure 16.1, *C*).[13,15] At a high temperature, coagulative necrosis of tissue occurs immediately. Significantly, coagulative necrosis of tissue occurs only a few millimeters adjacent to the probe.

Several factors determine the efficacy of RFA. The first consideration is the temperature around the electrode tip.[13,16,17] Irreversible cellular damage occurs when temperatures are increased to 46° C. Near-immediate tissue coagulation is induced between 60° C and 100° C, and temperatures >100° C result in tissue vaporization and carbonization.[13,14,16] Vaporization and carbonization retard optimal ablation. When the tissue around the probe becomes desiccated or charred, it acts as an insulating sleeve around the probe; this limits the transmission of further electrical or thermal energy. When tissue vaporization occurs, a large amount of gas, primarily nitrogen, is released from the cells. The gas that is formed around the electrode acts as an insulator, preventing the production and spread of heat. By maintaining a temperature between 50° C and 100° C, these negative effects can be prevented. The second consideration is the heterogeneity of the target tissue. Fibrosis and calcification can alter the electrical and thermal conductivity of the tissue adjacent to the RF probe; this decreases the predictability of the ablation zone size and shape.

The third consideration is blood flow within or around the tumor. Hypervascularity results in perfusion-mediated tissue cooling due to a heat-sink effect and reduces the extent of thermal ablation. This effect can be used to protect adjacent critical structures from thermal injury by artificially injecting fluid around the ablation target; this process is called *hydrodissection*.

Inclusion Criteria

As evidence supporting thyroid RFA increased, the Korean Society of Thyroid Radiology (KSThR) introduced its first guidelines in 2012 with subsequent revisions in 2018.[3,4] According to the newly revised KSThR guidelines published in 2018, the inclusion criteria for treating benign thyroid nodules are as follows:

1. Patients with benign thyroid nodules producing symptoms or of cosmetic concern
2. Autonomous functioning thyroid nodules (AFTN), either toxic or pretoxic

Thyroid nodules should be confirmed as benign with at least two ultrasound (US)-guided fine-needle aspirations (FNA) or core needle biopsies (CNB) before RFA.

A single benign diagnosis on FNA or CNB is sufficient when the nodule has US features highly specific for benignity or for AFTN. In addition, caution should be taken in the use of RFA in pregnant women, patients with serious heart problems, and those with preexisting contralateral vocal cord palsy.[4]

The exclusion criteria are as follows:
1. Follicular neoplasm or malignancy on FNA or CNB
2. A nodule with US criteria suggesting malignancy, despite FNA or CNB results[1,2,17,18]
3. Cystic and predominantly cystic thyroid nodules, in which EA has been suggested as a first-line treatment.[19,20]

 Please see the Expert Consult website for more discussion on this topic.

Preprocedural Workup

 Please see the Expert Consult website for discussion of this topic, including Table 16.1 and Box 16.1.

Equipment

An RF generator system is shown in Figure 16.2. The RF generator supplies RF power to the tissue through an electrode (see Figure 16.2, *A*). A straight, internally cooled electrode is the mainstay of thyroid RFA.[11] A modified straight internally cooled electrode has been designed with a short shaft length (7 cm) and a small diameter (18- or 19-gauge [G]) to allow for ease of use and reduced trauma to the traversed normal thyroid tissue.[7] Probes with different active tip length are available, including 3.8 mm, 5 mm, 7 mm, and 10 mm lengths (see Figure 16.2, *B*). Small active tips, such as 3.8 mm or 5 mm (both 19-G), have been used to treat small recurrent thyroid cancers.[34,38,39]

Patient Preparation

Before each procedure, the patient is placed in the supine position with a mild neck extension (Figure 16.3). Two grounding pads are firmly

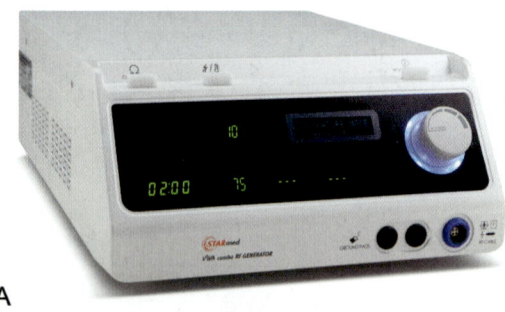

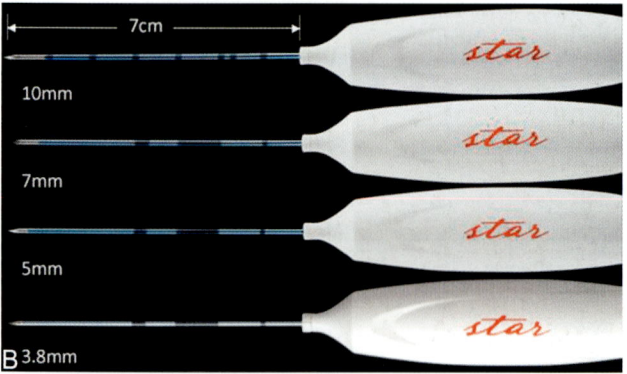

Fig. 16.2 Radiofrequency (RF) Generator System. **A**, VIVA combo RF System from STARMed Co., Ltd (Goyang, South Korea). **B**, Internally cooled electrodes with different active tip lengths. A short shaft length (7 cm) allows operators to easily handle the probe during the moving shot technique because of the superficial location of the thyroid gland. Depending on the size of a thyroid nodule or recurrent cancer, an appropriate length of active tip can be selected to improve the efficacy of tumor ablation and reduce the thermal injury of nontargeted structures. (Images courtesy STARMed Co., Ltd., Goyang, South Korea.)

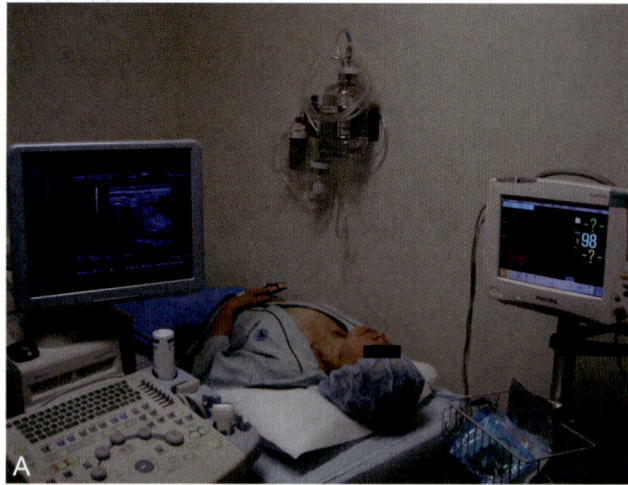

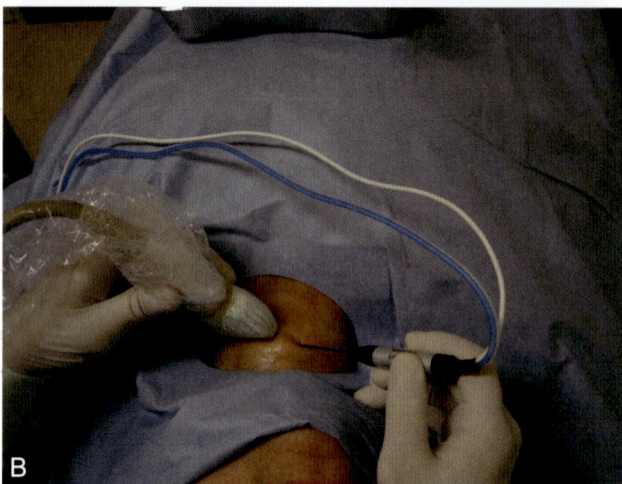

Fig. 16.3 Patient Preparation for Radiofrequency Ablation Procedure. **A**, The patient is placed in the supine position with a mild neck extension and an operator stands close to the patient's head. **B**, The operator's left-hand holds ultrasound probe and the right-hand grips the handle of an electrode.

attached to both thighs to prevent skin burn. An intravenous line should be established in an antecubital vein for intraprocedural medications (e.g., for control of pain or hypertension).

Procedure and Techniques

Most operators use local anesthesia during the procedure rather than deep sedation or general anesthesia, which are actions recommended by the 2012 and 2018 KSThR guidelines.[5,22,28,40,41] Deep sedation or general anesthesia may delay detection of pain as an early warning sign of thermal injury to the perithyroidal critical structures, which can result in serious complications.[42] When providing local anesthesia, injecting sufficient lidocaine at the skin puncture site and around the thyroid capsule is important to alleviate pain during RFA (Figure 16.4).

Two key techniques have been proposed and developed by Dr. J.H. Baek: (1) the "transisthmic approach method" and (2) the "moving shot technique" under local anesthesia (see videos).[5,7,22,43-45] In the transisthmic approach method, an electrode is inserted through the isthmus from medial to lateral and then into the targeted nodule under US guidance. This method has several advantages.[8,40,46] First, because the probe is stabilized by the length of the parenchymal track, it prevents a change in the position of the electrode tip caused by the

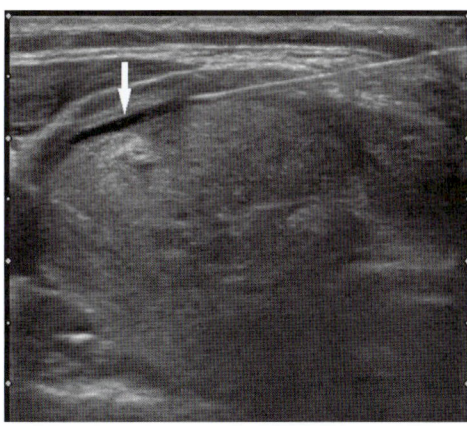

Fig. 16.4 Perithyroidal Lidocaine Injection. Injected lidocaine appears as an anechoic band *(arrow)* separating the thyroid gland and strap muscle.

patient swallowing or talking. It also allows for clear US visualization and monitoring of the target nodule, the electrode tip, and their relation to adjacent perithyroidal structures. Injury to the recurrent laryngeal or vagus nerves can be prevented or minimized by continuous US monitoring.

In the moving shot technique, a targeted thyroid nodule is divided into multiple conceptual ablation units, and ablation is performed unit by unit by moving the electrode tip. These conceptual ablation units are smaller in the periphery of the nodule to reduce the risk of thermal injury to the adjacent critical structures, such as the recurrent laryngeal nerve, vagus nerve, esophagus, and trachea (Figure 16.5).

The electrode tip is positioned in the deepest part of a nodule first because the resulting microbubbles will obscure the sonographic window as ablation proceeds. Ablation starts at either 20 W (7 mm active tip) or 50 W (10 mm active tip) of RF power. When a transient echogenic area appears at the targeted ablation unit, the electrode tip is moved to an untreated area proximally. Ablation is performed continuously from deep to superficial distal-to-proximal and deep-to-superficial conceptual units of the nodule by repeated distal-to-proximal movements of the electrode. The extent of the ablated area is determined by increased echogenicity around the electrode. If a transient hyperechoic zone is not formed at the electrode tip within 5 and 10 seconds, RF power is increased in 10 W increments to a maximum of 80 W. If the patient cannot tolerate the pain associated with ablation, the power is reduced or turned off until the pain subsides. The RF ablation is terminated when all conceptual units of the targeted nodule are ablated with transient hyperechoic zones (Figure 16.6). The area close to the danger triangle could remain untreated because of its close approximation to the recurrent laryngeal nerve, trachea, or esophagus (see Figure 16.5).

The "hydro-dissection technique" also has been used to achieve a complete ablation of the tumor margin for more peripheral lesions (Figure 16.7).[39,47-49] This technique was originally developed for treating the liver to avoid thermal injury to adjacent critical structures. Before the insertion of the electrode, 5% dextrose in water (D_5W) solution is injected into the tissue plane between the target tumor and the adjacent critical structure to be protected. However, in the neck, the injected fluid may spread rapidly along the longitudinally arranged neck muscle plane.[39] To achieve a sufficient safety margin by hydro-dissection, the fluid should be infused continuously throughout the procedure, with an injection needle remaining in place. A solution of D_5W is recommended rather than normal saline.[49] Due to its iso-osmolarity (252 mOsmol/L) and nonionic composition, D_5W does not conduct electricity and provides a thermal barrier to the adjacent structures when it surrounds the target organ.[49]

Please see the Expert Consult website for more discussion on this topic, including Figure 16.8.

Immediate Postprocedure Care

Please see the Expert Consult website for discussion of this topic.

FOLLOW-UP EVALUATION

Please see the Expert Consult website for discussion of this topic.

Clinical Results

Benign Nonfunctioning Thyroid Nodules

There is mounting evidence to support the use of RFA for benign thyroid nodules. In 2008, Jeong et al. reported their experience with RFA performed in 236 patients with 302 benign thyroid nodules.[22] Eighty-six percent of the patients had a solitary nodule. About 70% of the nodules were treated in a single session of RFA. The volume reduction at 1, 3, and 6 months after ablation was 58%, 74%, and 85%, respectively. A volume reduction greater than 50% (definition of therapeutic success) was observed in 91% of lesions, and 28% of index nodules had disappeared on the follow-up US.

According to a prospective randomized study at a 6-month follow-up, the RFA group (n = 15) showed a significant volume reduction, with a mean volume reduction of 49% at 1 month and 80% at 6 months, in comparison with the control group (n = 15).[5] Another prospective multicenter study was performed in 276 patients with 276 nodules by a trained and experienced group of physicians using similar techniques and devices.[50] The primary outcome of mean volume reduction was 80% at 12 months. The study revealed a 95% volume reduction at a 5-year follow-up.

Please see the Expert Consult website for more discussion on this topic.

Cystic and Predominantly Cystic Thyroid Nodules

In cystic thyroid nodules (cystic component >90%), EA has been suggested as a first-line treatment modality. Two published studies compared the efficacy of EA with RFA in treating benign cystic thyroid nodules.[20,25]

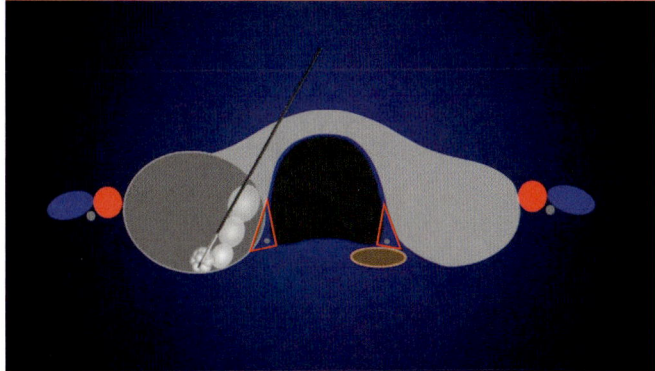

Fig. 16.5 Transisthmic Approach Method and Moving Shot Technique for Radiofrequency Ablation (RFA). A thyroid nodule is divided into multiple small conceptual ablation units, and RFA is performed unit by unit by moving the electrode. The conceptual ablation units are smaller at the periphery of the nodule and larger in the center of the nodule, which protects critical structures from a potential thermal injury. The recurrent laryngeal nerve *(gray color)* is within the danger triangle *(red color)*. The carotid artery *(red color)*, internal jugular vein *(blue color)*, and vagus nerve *(gray color)* are located lateral to each thyroid lobe.

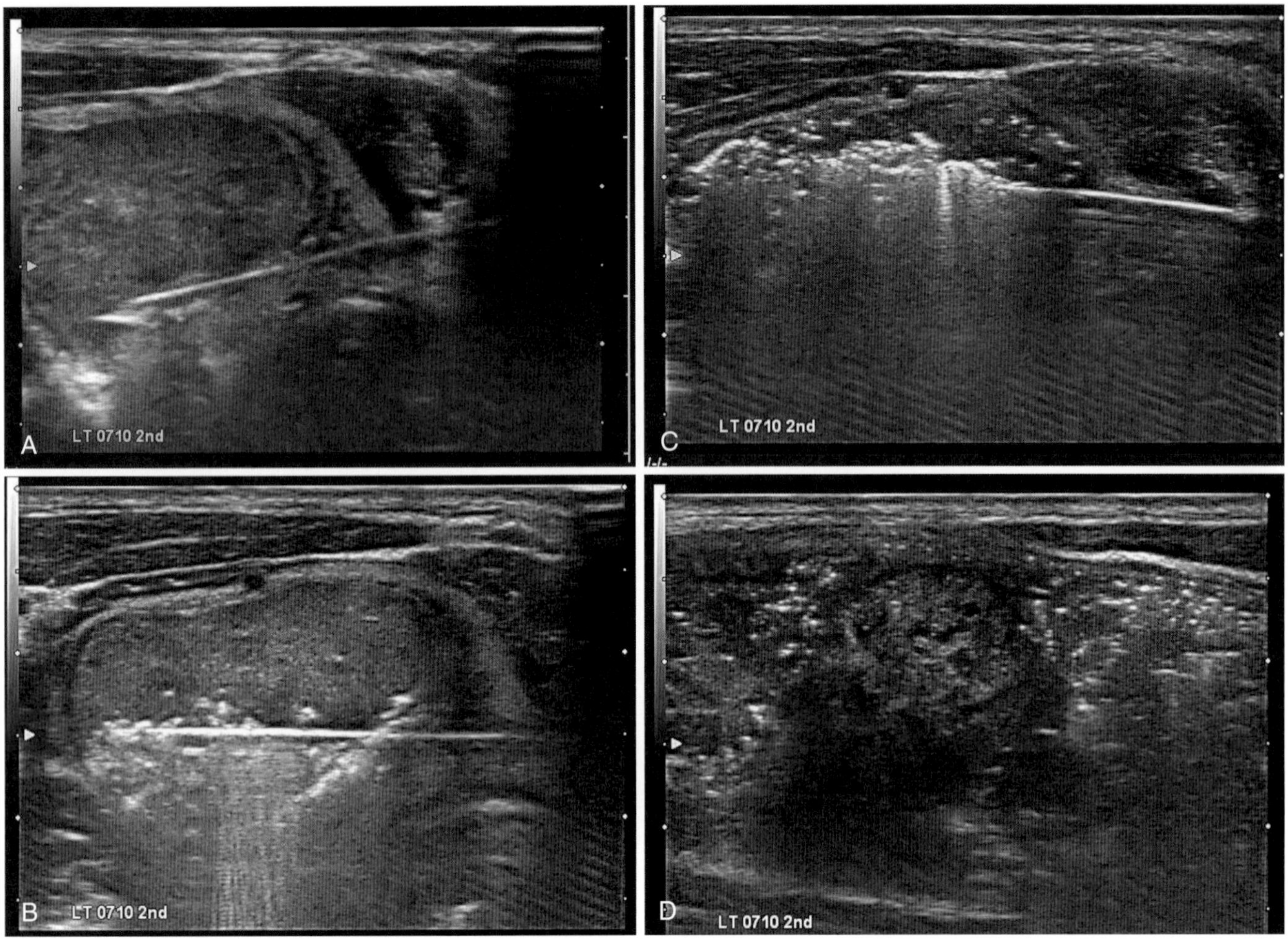

Fig. 16.6 Axial Ultrasound (US) Images of the Moving Shot Technique. The nodule is divided into multiple conceptual ablation units, and radiofrequency ablation is performed unit by unit. **A,** Insertion of the electrode. **B** and **C,** The electrode is moved within the thyroid nodule in distal-to-proximal and seep-to-superficial sequences. **D,** Final US feature after ablation.

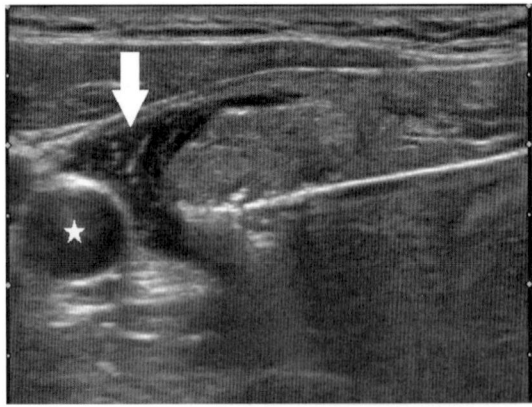

Fig. 16.7 Hydrodissection Technique. Before radiofrequency ablation, dextrose 5% in water (D_5W) is injected into the tissue plane between a target nodule and an adjacent critical structure to be protected. The injected D_5W *(arrow)* is seen between the thyroid nodule and the right carotid artery *(star)*.

There was no difference in the efficacy between EA and RFA including mean volume reduction, therapeutic success rate, and improvement of clinical symptoms. No major complication occurred in either EA or RFA.[25] However, the number of treatment sessions was fewer in EA. A similar result was reported with a single session treatment in a randomized noninferiority trial.[20] Both studies demonstrated that EA is superior to RFA in terms of volume reduction and cost-effectiveness; fewer treatment sessions are necessary for EA. In summary, EA can be considered the first-line treatment for cystic thyroid nodules.

In predominantly cystic thyroid nodules (90% with a cystic component >50%), EA was also suggested as the first-line treatment through a randomized controlled trial in comparison with RFA.[19] Nevertheless, there is ongoing debate; it was reported that predominantly cystic nodules showed a higher recurrence rate than purely cystic nodules because the solid component was the main causes of recurrence.[53] Treatment of the solid component in the predominantly cystic thyroid nodule has been proposed to reduce the recurrence rate.

Lee et al.[43] suggested a step-by-step management strategy that included EA first, followed by RFA. Among 137 patients who underwent EA, 27 patients had additional RFA. After the secondary RFA, there was further improvement of clinical symptoms, and the mean volumes were all significantly reduced from those measured before RFA. Jang et al.[10] prospectively reported that RFA is effective in the treatment of benign, predominantly cystic thyroid nodules in patients whose clinical problems were incompletely resolved after EA. Park et al.[38] suggested a simultaneous combination technique of EA and RFA for predominantly cystic thyroid nodules.

Please see the Expert Consult website for more discussion on this topic.

Autonomously Functioning Thyroid Nodules

The first study of RFA for the treatment of AFTN was reported by Baek et al.[7,28] RFA was effective in reducing the volume of treated nodules and improved nodule-related symptoms, cosmetic issues, and hyperthyroidism. Volume reduction was 36% at 1 month and 71% at 6 months. The reduction in volume is slightly lower than that of cold thyroid nodules.

Recently, a Korean multicenter study using RFA achieved substantial volume reduction of AFTN and control of hyperthyroidism without major complications.[55] The study included 44 patients (with 23 toxic and 21 pretoxic nodules) who were not suitable for surgery or radioiodine therapy. The initial mean nodule volume, 18.5 ± 30.1 mL, demonstrated a significant change, 11.8 ± 26.9 mL at 1 month, and 4.5 ± 9.8 mL in the last month. At the last follow-up, considerable improvement of thyroid-stimulating hormone (TSH), free thyroxine (fT4), and triiodothyronine (T3) levels was observed. On [99mTc] pertechnetate scintigraphy, 35 hot nodules became cold and 9 showed decreased uptake, although they remained as hot nodules.

In a prospective monocentric open parallel-group trial, nodule size was reported as a predictive factor of efficacy in RFA treatment of AFTN.[56] Twenty-nine patients with AFTN were divided into two groups based on thyroid nodule volume: 15 patients with small nodules (<12 mL) in group A and 14 patients with medium nodules (>12 mL) in group B. All patients underwent a single session of RFA; clinical, biochemical, and morphologic changes were evaluated at baseline and at 1, 6, 12, and 24 months after treatment. At 24 months, the rate of responders was greater in group A than in group B (86% versus 45%). A single session of RFA proved to be more effective in restoring euthyroid status in patients with small AFTNs.

Thus RFA has been shown to be a safe and effective alternative treatment of AFTN when radioactive iodine therapy is contraindicated. However, its application needs to be tailored carefully as is most optimal for single, small AFTN.

Recurrent Cancer

Surgery resection followed by radioactive iodine and thyroid hormone therapy is a standard treatment for recurrent thyroid cancers. KSThR has proposed RFA as an alternative to surgery, but it should be limited to patients at high risk for surgery and patients who refuse to undergo repeated surgeries.[4] Several investigators have reported a mean volume reduction of 56 to 93%, an improvement of tumor-related symptoms in 64% of patients,[55] and a decrease in the serum thyroglobulin (Tg) concentration in the majority of patients.[34,57-59] However, long-term follow-up data have not been published. The efficacy of RFA is similar or somewhat superior to that of EA, requiring fewer treatment sessions (mean: 1.2 sessions; range, 1 to 6)[34,58,59] than EA (mean: 2.0 to 2.1 sessions; range: 1 to 6).[60-63] Lewis et al.[64] also suggested that RFA is more favorable in terms of the number of treatment sessions required to treat recurrent thyroid cancers in comparison with EA.

To evaluate the efficacy of treatment, US and computed tomography (CT) are recommended; however, a clear follow-up timeline has not yet been established.

Complications

Please see the Expert Consult website for Figure 16.9.

A variety of complications from RFA have been reported. Understanding the relevant anatomy (specifically the adjacent nerves) and appropriate techniques are important for safe ablation. In a recent multicenter study of 1459 patients, organized by KSThR, the overall complication rate after RF ablation was 3.3% with a major complication rate of 1.4% (see Figure 16.9, available on expertconsult.com).[30] Pain at the ablated site, which sometimes radiated to the head, ear, shoulder, chest, or teeth, was the most common complication.[23,53] It was alleviated when the RF power was reduced or if RF was turned off. Voice change by thermal injury to the vagus or recurrent laryngeal nerve is a serious complication of RFA. It can be reduced by using the moving shot technique or undertreating the thyroid tissue adjacent to the nerves.[6] Hydro-dissection can also be used to protect the nerves.[38] Operators should be familiar with thyroid US and perithyroidal anatomy, including anatomic variations of the nerves.[65-67]

Hemorrhage by vessel injury is usually controlled by a manual compression. A serious perithyroidal hemorrhage can be prevented by examining the perithyroidal vessels with color Doppler before inserting the probe and using small diameter electrodes.[30] Most hematomas usually resolve between 1 and 2 weeks. Skin burn at the electrode puncture site, typically first-degree, can occur, especially with a large nodule bulging into the skin. Skin color changes without any sequelae[30] usually resolve within 1 week after the procedure. Nodular rupture after RFA is very rare with only six cases in a retrospective review of 1491 patients.[30,68] Such cases presented with sudden neck bulging and pain during the follow-up period due to volume expansion by a delayed hemorrhage or tumor wall tear.[30,68] It can often be managed conservatively without any sequelae, but surgery may be necessary in cases of secondary abscess formation or massive hematoma with a mass effect.

Recently, a single center study with a large population achieved a lower complication rate for RFA compared with the previous studies; however, several new complications (e.g., Horner's syndrome, spinal accessory nerve injury and lidocaine-related complications) were reported.[69]

LASER ABLATION

LASER is the acronym for *light amplification by stimulated emission of radiation*. LA refers to ablation with light energy applied via fibers directly inserted into the tissue.[70-78]

Mechanism of Action

Please see the Expert Consult website for Figure 16.10.

Laser light penetrates only a few millimeters as a result of backward and forward scattering and reflection (see Figure 16.10, available on expertconsult.com). Scattering results in a relatively uniform distribution of absorbed energy, which is transmitted to the tissue as heat. Farther from the point of application, the tissue is heated by conduction.[71,73,74] Tissue is destroyed primarily through absorption (about 80%), which is a function of the attenuation coefficient (determined by tissue structure and wavelength), fiber tip shape, and delivered energy (determined by exposure time and output power). High power destroys tissue by means of vaporization, charring around the fiber tip surrounded by a coagulation zone, as seen on US images (Figure 16.11). Heat deposition is greatest near the thermal source, with a rapid energy decay.[79,80] Cell death may continue up to 72 hours after the procedure because of the coagulation of microvessels and ischemic injury.[81] Microscopically, the coagulation zone is surrounded by a rim of reversible damage that separates necrotic from viable tissue.[80,82] Figure 16.12 shows microscopic changes occurring in thyroid nodules resected 1 month and 2 years after LA, respectively. Charring results in decreased energy transmission, which then limits the coagulation zone. In addition, coagulation necrosis itself reduces optical penetration by about 20% in both normal and tumor tissue.[77,82] Using a bare tip, almost spherical lesions with a maximum diameter of 12 to 16 mm can be produced.[83] Lesion size can be increased by using beam splitters for simultaneous use of multiple fibers in an array within the tumor.[76,84] This avoids the difficulty of repositioning a single fiber in

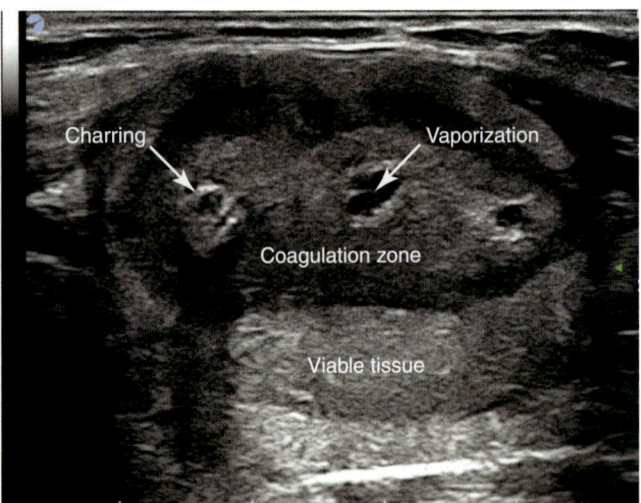

Fig. 16.11 Ultrasound Image of a Three-Fiber Thyroid Nodule Laser Ablation in a Transverse Scan. Laser marks are seen as anechoic spots surrounded by hyperechoic rims. These are cavitation due to tissue vaporization and charring, respectively. The coagulation zone is hypoechoic parenchyma that is clearly cleaved from viable tissue.

the setting of treatment-induced imaging artifact. An important practical advantage over other thermal sources is that the thin and flexible laser fibers make it possible to reach tumors with greater ease and safety.[85]

Procedure and Techniques

Please see the Expert Consult website for Figures 16.13 and 16.14.

LA is performed as an outpatient procedure. Patients are instructed to fast overnight in preparation for the procedure. The flat tip technique, proposed and developed by Pacella et al.,[86] is based on the insertion of a 300-μm plane-cut optic fiber through the sheath of a 21-G Chiba needle. This exposes the bare fiber in direct contact with thyroid tissue for a length of 5 to 7 mm, based on the size of the lesion (see Figure 16.13, available on expertconsult.com). In the thyroid gland, multiple fibers are inserted parallel to each other to obtain an ellipsoid ablation that matches the ellipsoid shape of most thyroid nodules (see Figure 16.14, available on expert consult.com).[87]

The goal of this procedure is to achieve the maximum ablation volume in a single LA outpatient session. The patient is placed on an operating table in the supine position with a hyperextended neck. Light conscious sedation is obtained with intravenous midazolam. Local anesthesia with 2% lidocaine subcutaneous and subcapsular infiltration (2 to 5 mL) is performed under US assistance with a thin (29-G to 30-G) needle. Then, 21-G Chiba needles (1 to 4) are placed manually along the longitudinal, craniocaudal, major nodule axis at a distance of 10 mm from each other, matching the anatomy of the nodule as closely as possible (Figure 16.15). The assistant/sonographer performs multiplanar US images on axial and longitudinal scans throughout laser illumination, which allows for real-time visual control of each source (Figure 16.16). An initial energy of 1200 to 1800 Joules (J) per fiber with an output power of 2 to 4 watts (W) is delivered starting 1 cm from the bottom of the nodule. Highly echogenic areas resulting from tissue heating and vaporization gradually increase over time until coalescing between the fibers (Figure 16.17).

Although nodules as small as 5 mm may be ablated using a single optic fiber, nodules up to 40 to 50 mm in width, 30 to 35 mm in thickness, and 50 to 70 mm in length (i.e., up to 30 to 60 mL) may be treated in a single LA session by combining multiple fiber placement, multiple needle advancements, and high energies. The number of fibers, number of advancements, and total energy delivered are tailored to nodule volume. The duration of laser illumination ranges from 6 to 30 minutes, depending on nodule size.[87] Light irradiation is continuous; it is suspended for fiber repositioning only in the event of severe pain, cough, or other side effects.

Clinical Results

Benign Cold Nodules

According to a literature review on the effects of LA on cold benign thyroid nodule volume, nodule shrinkage ranged from 36% to 82% of initial

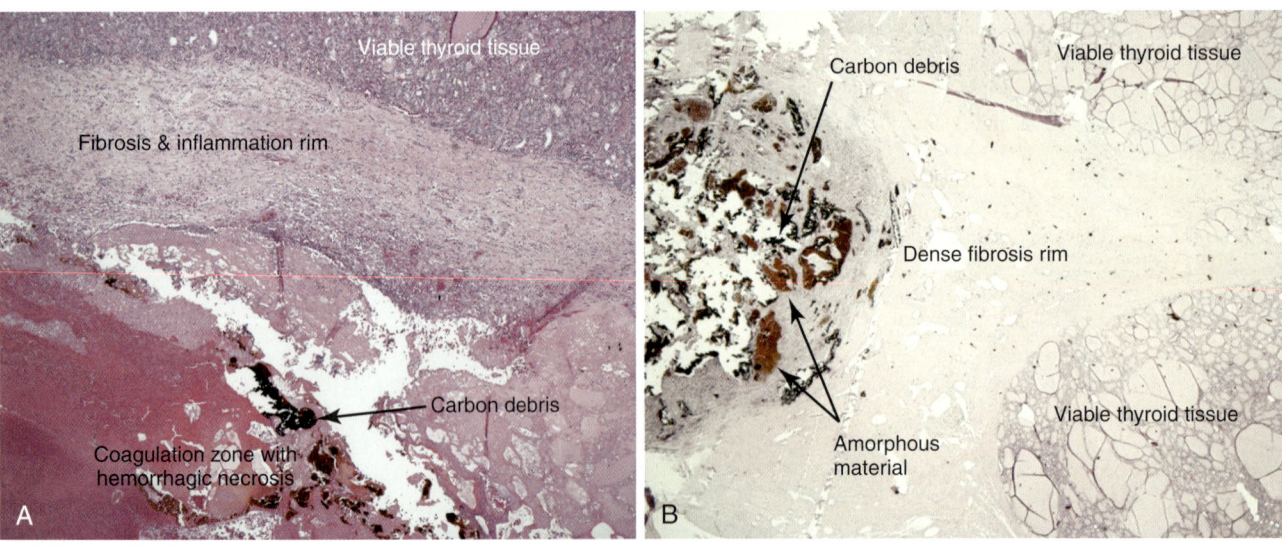

Fig. 16.12 Microscopic Changes Occurring in Benign Thyroid Nodules Resected After Laser Ablation (LA). **A,** One month after LA, nodule section shows the coagulation zone with hemorrhagic necrosis and tissue carbonization. Necrotic and hemorrhagic ablated area with carbonized debris is surrounded by a peripheral rim of fibrous tissue with a strong inflammatory reaction. **B,** Two years after the LA procedure, the ablation zone was reduced, and it has a dense fibrotic rim. The destroyed area is represented by amorphous material, carbon debris, macrophages, or multinucleated giant cells and lymphocytes with no thyroid cells.

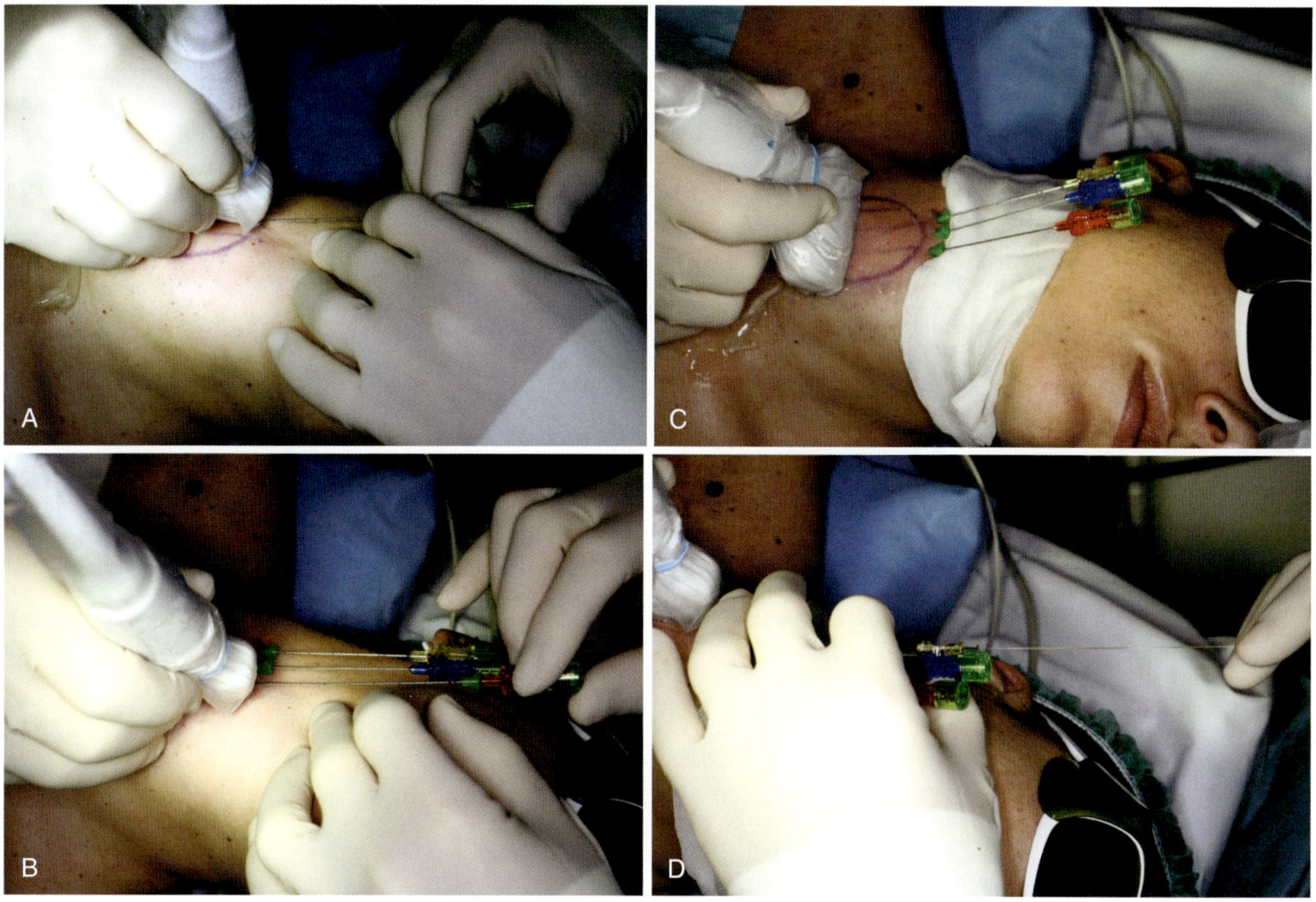

CHAPTER 16 Radiofrequency and Laser Ablation of Thyroid Nodules and Parathyroid Adenoma

Fig. 16.15 Laser Ablation Procedure With Three Fibers. 21-G Chiba needles are placed manually along the longitudinal, craniocaudal, major nodule axis, at a distance of 10 mm from each other. **A,** Placement of the first needle. **B,** Placement of the third needle. **C,** Needles positioned at a taget nodule. **D,** Optic fiber insertion.

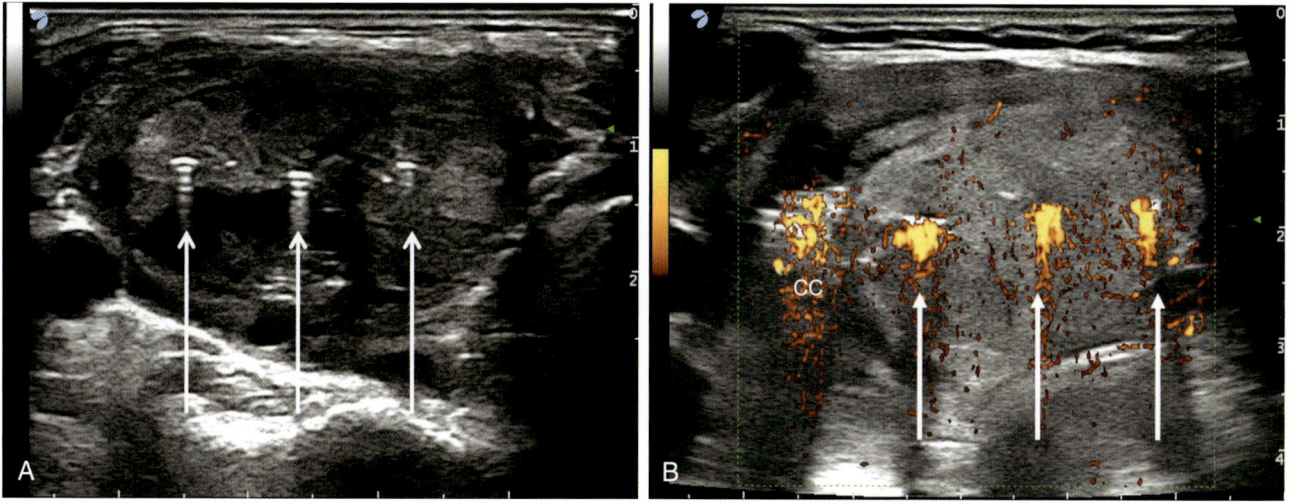

Fig. 16.16 Axial ultrasound images of three needles *(arrows)* fit within a right thyroid nodule. **A,** B mode images. **B,** Color Doppler images during laser illumination.

volume. A 3-year follow-up study of LA of benign nonfunctioning thyroid nodules was reported.[54] One hundred twenty-two patients (95 females, 27 males, ages 52.2 ± 12.3 years) with benign cold thyroid solitary nodules or a dominant nodule within a nontoxic multinodular goiter (volume range: 2.6 to 86.4 mL) underwent thermal neodymium yttrium aluminum garnet (Nd:YAG) LA. The mean energy delivered was 8522 ± 5365 J with an output power of 3.1 ± 0.5 W. Three years after LA, nodule volume had decreased from 23.1 ± 21.3 mL to 12.5 ± 18.8 mL ($-47.8 \pm 33.1\%$ of initial volume, $p \leq 0.001$). After 3 years, symptoms had improved in 89 patients (73%), symptoms were

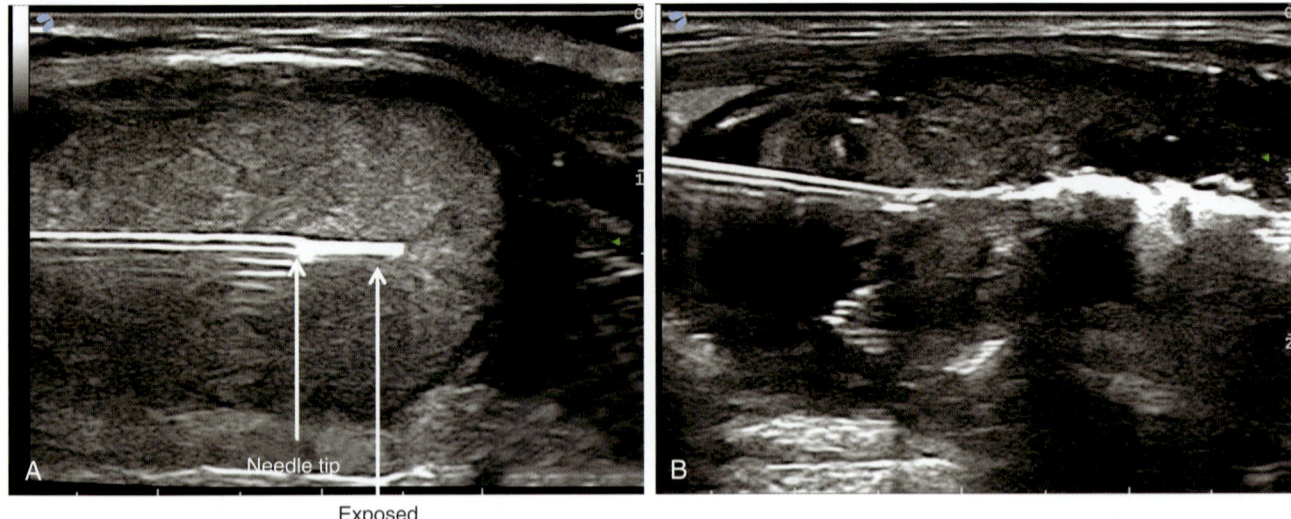

Fig. 16.17 Sagittal Ultrasound Images of a Needle Typically Placed Within a Thyroid Nodule. **A,** The left side of the images is cranial. The needle is parallel to the longitudinal nodule axis. The fiber is exposed about 5 mm out of the tip of the needle. **B,** A highly echogenic area because of the heating, and vaporization is observed during the laser firing.

unchanged in 28 patients (22.9%), and symptoms had worsened in 5 patients (4.1%). Cosmetic signs had improved in 87 patients (71.3%), symptoms were unchanged in 29 patients (23.8%), and symptoms had worsened in 6 patients (4.9%). In 11 patients (9%), nodules regrew above baseline.[54]

A prospective multicenter randomized trial was conducted to compare the 3-year effects of a single LA procedure (Group 1: 101 cases) versus follow-up in a consecutive series of euthyroid patients with benign solid thyroid nodules (Group 2: 99 cases).[88] Volume decrease was 49 ± 22%, 59 ± 22%, 60 ± 24%, and 57 ± 25% at 6, 12, 24, and 36 months, respectively. The reslults showed a nodule reduction of >50% in 67.3% of cases. Local symptoms decreased from 38% to 8% of cases, and cosmetic signs decreased from 72% to 16% of cases. The procedure was well tolerated in most (92%) cases. No changes in thyroid function or autoimmunity were observed. The results of the control group showed the natural course of the untreated euthyroid patients: mean nodule volume increased at the 3-year checkup (25 ± 42%); local symptoms worsened in 20 (20.4%) cases; and after 2 years of follow-up, 8 patients (8.1%) had requested a surgical consultation because of concern about the progression in nodule growth or local symptoms.

 Please see the Expert Consult website for more discussion on this topic.

AUTONOMOUSLY FUNCTIONING THYROID NODULES

The use of thermal ablation techniques for AFTN, either toxic or pretoxic, was initially proposed as a way to avoid surgery and radioiodine therapy. Thermal ablation in AFTN is thus regarded as a palliative rather than a curative treatment. The beneficial effects of repeat LA in a large AFTN have been reported anecdotally.[90] In 16 patients with AFTN, a total of 57 nodule LA treatments (range, 1 to 9 treatments) were performed during 43 sessions (range, 1 to 6 sessions; median 1.5; mean 2.7 ± 2 sessions).[91] The energy used per nodule was 1800 to 14,900 J (median 4200 J), with a total energy deposition of 816 J/mL of nodule volume, which was about twice the mean energy used for cold nodules.[87,91]

Complications

Few complications and side effects of LA have been reported in the published data.[9,54,87,90-100] In a clinical study of 122 patients followed up for 3 years after LA, no patient required emergency care or emergency surgery.[54] Pain during the procedure is usually absent or minimal, but should it occur, the laser should be turned off and fibers should be repositioned to a more central area of the nodule. Persistent pain may occur in 8% to 40% of patients, and it may require additional medication.[9,54,87,91,92,97-99] Intranodular bleeding during needle placement is controlled by rapid fiber insertion and laser illumination; it should not prevent the regular ablation procedure from being completed. In the 3-year follow-up series, thyroid pericapsular bleeding, seen on US as an asymptomatic hypoechoic layer surrounding the thyroid lobe, occurred in 2.3% of patients and disappeared in 3 to 4 weeks.[54] Vagal symptoms with bradycardia occurred in 2% of patients during needle placement, and 2% of patients complained of a cough during laser irradiation; in these latter cases, the fiber closest to the trachea was pulled back and the LA procedure was completed. Furthermore, no patient has ever had intra/perioperative dysphonia, although 2.3% of patients have complained of voice change 12 to 24 hours after the LA procedure; indirect laryngoscopy revealed reduced vocal cord motility in these patients. An additional course of corticosteroids was administered, with complete recovery of dysphonia within 1 to 2 months. A pseudocyst transformation occurred in 4.9% of patients as rapid painful neck swelling 2 to 4 weeks after the LA procedure; these patients received drainage through a 16-G to 18-G Chiba needle. In 2.5% of the 122 cases, some of the fluid leaked into the neck muscle fascia. Subfascial effusion disappeared in 3 to 4 months, with no permanent consequences. In this series, surgical drainage was not required in any patient. Rare (0.3%) side effects were cutaneous burn (0.3%) and transient stridor (0.3%). In the first 6 months after LA, 3.2% of patients developed thyroid dysfunction, either hyper- (1.3%) or hypothyroidism (1.3%). It is not clear whether this was the natural course of the disease or whether it was laser-induced. It should be noted that the list of side effects refers to the series of patients treated with the Nd:YAG laser, including those patients who were treated during the early stages of implementing this technology.[54]

Please see the Expert Consult website for more discussion on this topic.

ALTERNATIVE THERAPIES

Microwave Ablation

MWA generates heat by creating a homogeneous electromagnetic field that interacts with water dipoles and creates a homogeneous ablation zone. MWA permeates can even permeate tissues that are desiccated or evaporated. This differs from comparable thermal procedures, such as RFA, which is dependent on local resistance. An advantage of MWA can be its consistently higher and homogenous intratumoral temperature, which allows for the ablation of nodules of large volume, faster ablation times, and an improved convection profile. However, MWA increases the chance of damaging adjacent structures. Although clinical efficacy and safety have been reported for MWA of thyroid nodules, study limitations include experimental design, small sample sizes, variations in technique, and short follow-up time.[104,105]

High-Intensity Focused Ultrasound

HIFU has been used to treat patients with uterine fibroids or tumors of the prostate, breast, pancreas, and liver. Animal studies on the application of HIFU to the thyroid revealed destruction of particular regions of the gland, but skin burn was also observed.[106,107] In the human, successful HIFU ablation of a single 0.9 cm-diameter AFTN was reported, resulting in the normalization of serum concentrations of TSH and a normal thyroid scan.[108] All complications related to HIFU were transient and included mild subcutaneous edema in three patients and voice change in one.[109] More recent studies show an overall mean volume reduction of 48% to 78% at the 6-month follow-up.[110,111] HIFU appears to be a promising thermal ablation technique considering its noninvasive nature and safety. However, additional studies are required to provide evidence of its long-term follow-up.

PARATHYROID TUMORS

In hyperparathyroidism (HPT), medical therapy alone does not provide a sustained, long normocalcemic period. When parathyroid tumors are refractory to medical therapy, surgery is the treatment of choice with a highly successful cure rate.[112] In the hands of a skilled endocrine surgeon, total or subtotal parathyroidectomy with or without auto-transplantation is safe and efficient. However, nonsurgical options have been developed and used in patient populations who are unsuitable for surgery.[113]

Parathyroid cysts (PCs) are categorized as functioning or nonfunctioning. For functioning PCs with HPT, surgery is the standard treatment. Most of the nonfunctioning PCs are asymptomatic with no need for treatment, but they can cause symptoms such as neck bulging, dysphasia, tracheal compression, recurrent laryngeal nerve palsy, and pain.[114-119] In nonfunctioning PCs, simple aspiration is a first-line procedure for diagnosis and treatment. By simple aspiration only, the therapeutic success rate ranges from 33% to 92%; this broad range in the success rate might reflect the inhomogeneity of the studies in their definitions of success, duration of follow-up, and the incidental inclusion of other lesions.[114,117,118,120,121] In recurrent nonfunctioning PCs, surgery is curative. However, considering the benign nature of nonfunctioning PCs and the surgical risks involved in their removal, nonsurgical methods, such as sclerotherapy with tetracycline or EA, can be applied.[113,122]

The goal of treatment in symptomatic primary HPT commonly caused by adenoma or hyperplasia is a restoration of normocalcemia instead of the complete destruction of all parathyroid tissue, which will result in permanent hypoparathyroidism. For severe secondary HPT with a prevalence in renal disease, parathyroidectomy remains a valid treatment option, especially when medical parathyroid hormone-lowering therapies fail.[123] In lieu of surgery, EA, LA, RFA, MWA, and HIFU have been attempted to control the adenomas or hyperplastic glands with preservation of normal functioning tissue of the glands.[110,124-130] However, due to the anatomic proximity of the parathyroid glands to the critical structures in the danger triangle (see Figure 16.5), the risk of the nerve injury is high, although a few studies reported a transient hoarseness only without any other major complications.[124-126,131] The hydrodissection technique should be used to protect the recurrent laryngeal nerve from irreversible thermal injury. Several studies with the various ablation modalities have achieved some clinical efficacy and safety in the treatment of HPT and secondary HPT with complete or partial remission of parathyroid hormone, calcium, phosphorus, and serum calcitonin.[124-126] However, the number of studies is small with no evidence of long-term efficacy. At present, it seems prudent to apply these nonsurgical ablation modalities in the parathyroid tumors only when the benefits far overweight the surgical risks or when surgery is not feasible.

FUTURE PERSPECTIVES

Please see the Expert Consult website for discussion of this topic.

CONCLUSION

Nonsurgical treatment methods, such as thermal ablations or sclerotherapy, are effective and safe in patients with benign thyroid nodules, recurrent thyroid cancers, and parathyroid lesions. These nonsurgical treatment methods may be as effective as surgery if performed by experienced physicians in optimally selected patients. Therefore the operators performing these procedures should understand neck anatomy, basic ablative techniques, and experience with image-guided interventions.

REFERENCES

For a complete list of references, go to expertconsult.com.

Thyroid Neoplasia

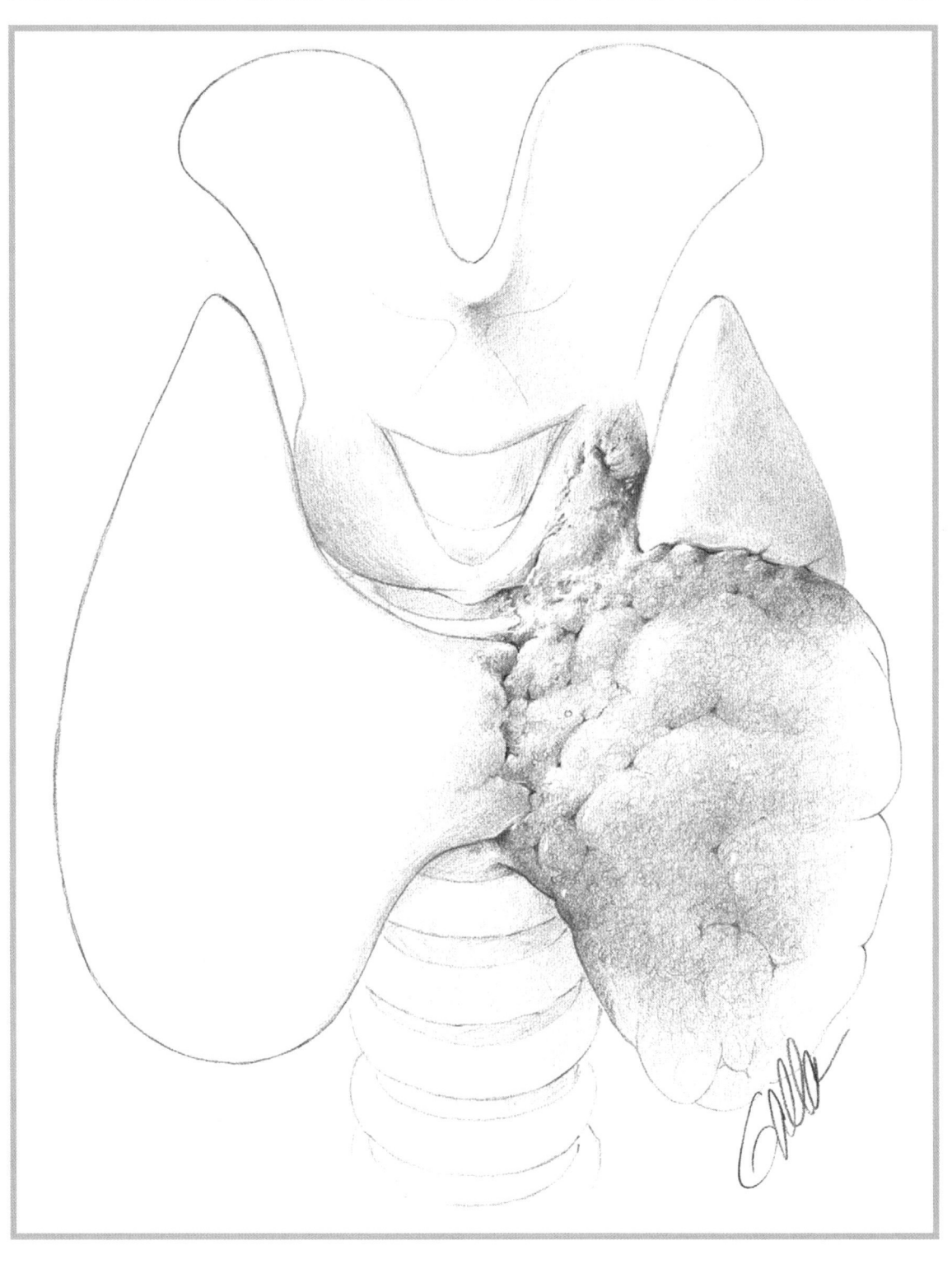

17

Differentiated Thyroid Cancer Incidence

Quinn Dunlap, Louise Davies

> Please go to expertconsult.com to view the related video:
> **Video 17.1** Introduction to Chapter 17, Differentiated Thyroid Cancer Incidence.

INCIDENCE OF DIFFERENTIATED THYROID CANCER

Introduction

Differentiated thyroid carcinoma (DTC) is the umbrella term that encompasses all malignancies arising from thyroid epithelial follicular cells and is the major form of thyroid carcinoma, comprising >90% of total thyroid malignancies. This major category is subdivided into three types: papillary thyroid carcinoma (PTC), which comprises 80% to 85% of all thyroid malignancies, and follicular thyroid carcinoma (FTC), which accounts for 10% to 15% of all thyroid malignancies, and hurthle cell carcinoma, which accounts for 3–4% of all thyroid malignancies. The proportions of each vary by country, and rates are affected by diagnostic practices and iodine sufficiency. Overall, papillary thyroid cancer has a good to excellent prognosis and a generally high rate of 10-year survival (90% to 99%); corresponding survival for follicular thyroid cancer is lower, ranging from 55% to 70% and the corresponding rate for hurtle cell carcinoma is about 75%.[1,2]

PTC has several significant histologic variants: classic, follicular (encapsulated and nonencapsulated), diffuse sclerosing, tall cell/columnar cell, solid, trabecular, and oncocytic, and each varies in aggression and prognosis. PTC has the capability for extrathyroidal extension (ETE) and can involve the adjacent viscera (recurrent laryngeal nerve, larynx, esophagus). It metastasizes through the lymphatics to the regional cervical lymph nodes (central and lateral neck). Follicular thyroid cancer, with a wide range of invasiveness, is less diverse, (3% of all thyroid carcinoma). It spreads hematogenously and exhibits an increased frequency of distant metastasis and decreased incidence of cervical metastasis compared with PTC. In addition, due to its capsular nature, FTC can only be definitively diagnosed via excisional biopsy (in contrast to fine needle aspiration for PTC).[1,3] Hurthle cell was previously thought to be a variant, but recent genotyping research suggests it is a separate entity.[4]

Thyroid cancer is the most common type of endocrine malignancy, accounting for approximately 2.1% of all cancer diagnoses worldwide.[5] It accounted for 3.8% of new cancers diagnosed in the United States (U.S.) in 2014, making it the ninth most common malignancy in incidence overall.[6] The incidence of DTC has tripled between the 1990's and 2010's in the U.S., with similar trends being seen internationally.[6-9] Next, we will describe the magnitude of the increase, the potential causal mechanisms, and the strategies that have been taken to address it.

OVERVIEW OF CURRENT INCIDENCE RATES

In the U.S. there were approximately 57,000 new cases of thyroid cancer in 2017, and thyroid cancer accounted for approximately 3.5% of all new cancer diagnoses in 2015,[10,11] the most recent year for which data are available. As of the mid-2010s, thyroid carcinoma was on pace to rise to the fourth most common malignancy in the U.S. by the year 2030 if trends continue.[12]

Incidence rates of thyroid cancer vary dramatically by country; the highest is South Korea (111.3/100,000).[13] There is no predictable pattern to incidence rates; thyroid cancer rates are high in some countries but low in their nearby neighbors, for instance. Incidence rates are also shifting, with countries such as Brazil and China showing recent increases.[8,10,12,14] See Figure 17.1 for details.

In the U.S., the female incidence of DTC (22.3/100,000) is approximately triple that of males (7.7/100,000). International comparisons mirror this proportionality, showing a worldwide age-standardized incidence rate of 6.1/100,000 for women and 1.90/100,000 for men.[12] The median age at diagnosis is younger for thyroid cancer in comparison with most other major types of cancer and is currently 49 years old for females and 54 years old for males.[15]

In the U.S., non-Hispanic white individuals have the highest incidence of DTC, followed by Asian individuals, Hispanic individuals, and non-Hispanic African American individuals.[16] A family history of a first-degree relative with DTC conveys an increased risk of thyroid cancer (odds ratio [OR] 4.1, confidence interval [CI] 1.7 to 9.9 in one study),[17] but the genetic basis of this observation is not well established. True familial nonmedullary thyroid cancer is rare and generally requires that three first degree relatives be affected (see Chapter 30, Familial Nonmedullary Thyroid Cancer).[18]

RECENT TRENDS IN THE INCIDENCE OF DIFFERENTIATED THYROID CANCER

United States

DTC within the U.S. was relatively stable before the 1990s at a rate of approximately 5/100,000 overall. Over the ensuing decades, the incidence progressively increased—quite rapidly at first, but slowing in recent years—to an overall age-adjusted annual rate of 15/100,000 in 2015 (Figure 17.2).[11] This increased incidence is almost entirely accounted for by changes in the incidence of PTC (>90%), which increased from 3.4 to 12.5/100,000 from 1975 to 2009.[13] Of note, although there has been a slight increase in the incidence of FTC,[19] this increase is not significant, and there has also been no significant increase in the incidence of nondifferentiated thyroid cancers (medullary, anaplastic).[6,20]

CHAPTER 17 Differentiated Thyroid Cancer Incidence

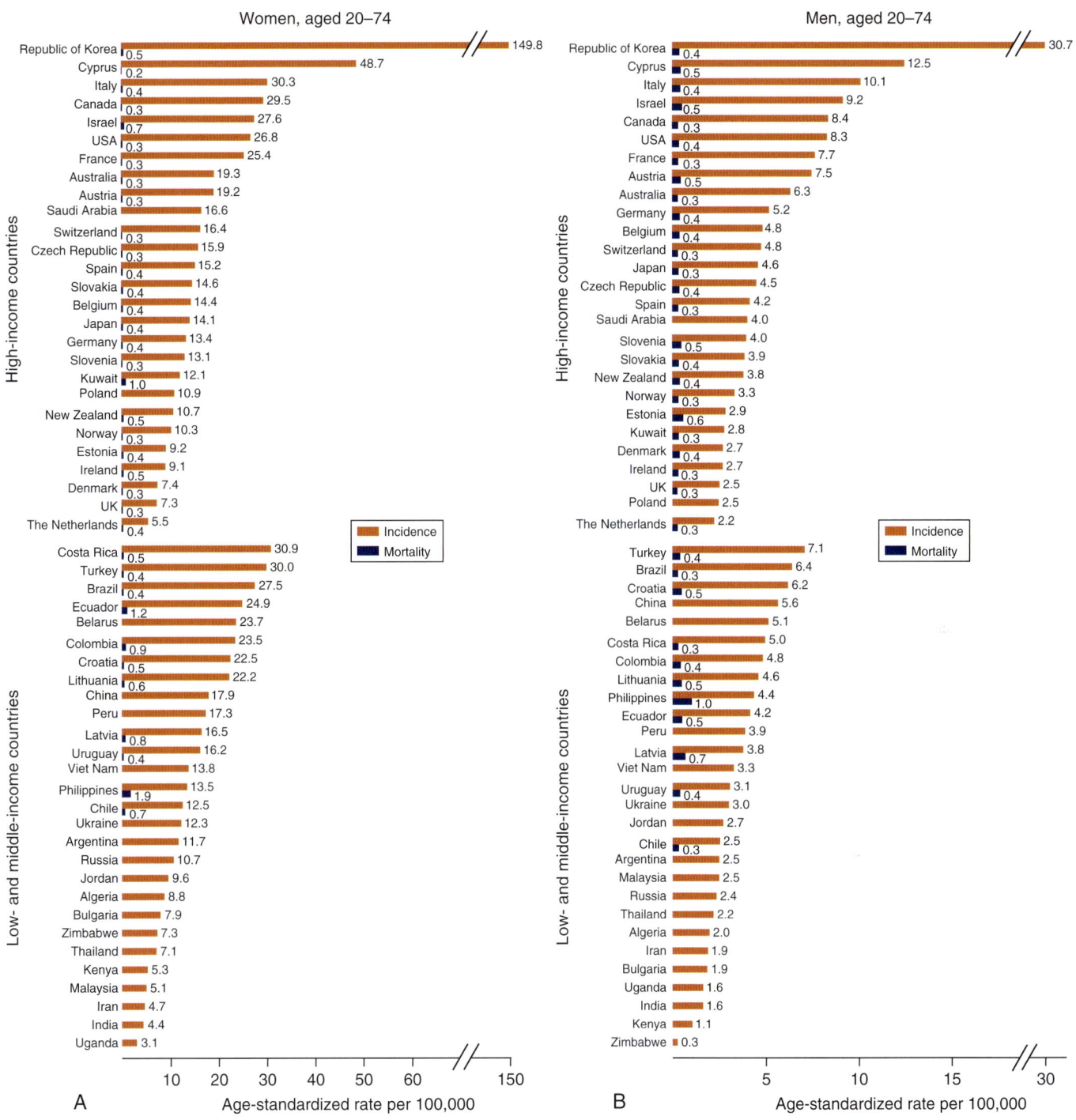

Fig. 17.1 Age-standardized incidence and mortality rates of thyroid cancer per 100,000, ages 20 to 74 years, for 2008 to 2012, in women (**A**) and in men (**B**). The incidence data presented originate from 27 national, 8 regional, and 20 combined regional registries. The data period was 2008 to 2012, except in Slovakia (2008–2010); Costa Rica and Iran, Golestan (2008-2011); Vietnam, Ho Chi Minh City (2009–2012); Latvia; Peru, Lima; and Zimbabwe, Harare (2010–2012). (Reproduced with permission from Bray F, Colombet M, Mery L, Piñeros M, Znaor A, Zanetti R and Ferlay J, editors. *Cancer Incidence in Five Continents*. Vol. XI (electronic version). Lyon: International Agency for Research on Cancer. Available at http://ci5.iarc.fr. Accessed 2019.)

Although the number of thyroid cancer cases has clearly escalated, the disease severity of the average diagnosed case has declined. For example, since 1983, the percentage of patients presenting without cervical lymph node metastatic disease metastases (N0) has increased from 66% to 73%, and the percentage of patients found to have pathologic lymphadenopathy (N1) at the time of surgery has decreased from 30% to 23%. Furthermore, the proportion of patients presenting with distant metastatic disease (M1) has decreased from 3.7% to 3.1%. During the same time period, the 10-year relative survival has improved from 95.4% to 98.6%; interestingly, no changes in 10-year relative survival were observed across this time period when stratified by tumor size and stage.[13]

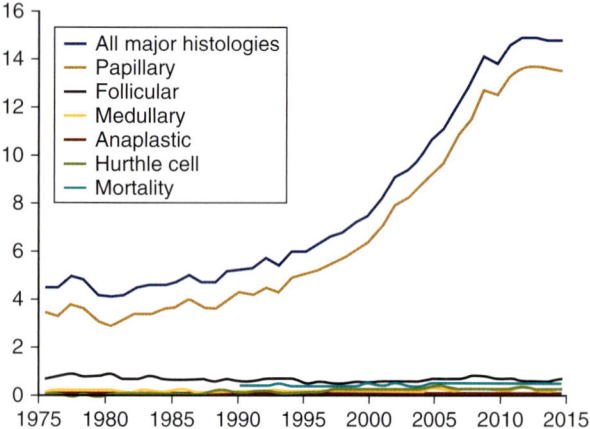

Fig. 17.2 U.S. trends in thyroid cancer incidence by major histologic type, and overall mortality of thyroid cancer, 1975 to 2015. (Data from National Cancer Institute. *Surveillance, Epidemiology, and End Results [SEER] Program*. SEER 9 Registries [1973–2015]. Available at www.seer.cancer.gov; 2018.)

Size

Thyroid cancers of all sizes exhibited an increase over the previous 30 years; the greatest contribution to the overall increase in incidence in both relative and absolute terms was due to malignant tumors <2 cm in size, which were observed to more than quadruple in incidence from 2 to 9.6/100,000.[6] Within this category, the proportion of papillary thyroid microcarcinoma (PMC) (<1 cm) increased from 23% to 36%, with tumors 5 mm or less in size increasing from 15% to 22%.[13] Malignant tumors measuring 2.1 to 5 cm also doubled in incidence, from 1.4 to 3.7/100,000, and cancers measuring >5 cm, although very rare, tripled from 0.2 to 0.7/100,000.

Age Distribution

The incidence rate per 100,000 cases of thyroid cancer has risen dramatically in all age groups since 1975, including among adolescents. Rates grew the most in people over age 65, although this is a small segment of the population, so the largest numbers of cases are still in people younger than age 65.[6]

International Trends

Rates of thyroid cancer differ dramatically across countries, often by degree of human development, although there are notable exceptions. The two largest factors affecting rate differences are iodine availability and access to health care.[9,21,22] Where detailed comparisons can be made, developed countries around the world have experienced increases in thyroid cancer incidence similar to the U.S., including Canada, some countries in Europe and Asia, Australia, and parts of South America.[8,23,24] The most extreme example is South Korea, where the incidence rate of DTC increased 15-fold between 1993 and 2011, almost entirely due to an increase in PTC, with the incidence rate peaking in women ages 50 to 59 years at around 120/100,000.[8,10] This increase began after the introduction of a national cancer screening program in 1999, during which thyroid cancer screening, although not recommended or provided, was offered for a small additional fee when patients were attending other screening programs.[8] An estimated 90% of the cancers detected in this time period were asymptomatic. Less dramatic but similar trends have developed in other countries, such as Italy, France, and Australia, where 70% to 80% of detected lesions are estimated to be small and asymptomatic and likely would have been otherwise undetected, and Japan, where this is the case for an estimated 50% of cancers.[10]

In countries with lower resources or levels of human development, there has in general been a much less dramatic increase, and in these countries there is also a greater FTC to PTC ratio as well as more advanced stages at presentation.[9,21,22,25] Multiple studies have demonstrated that iodine deficiency in developing countries leads to an increase in the relative percentage of FTC and a decrease in PTC, with some studies reporting an FTC to PTC ratio that approaches 1:1.[9,21,26] The higher proportion of FTC likely contributes to the more advanced stages seen at presentation in these countries. Incidence rates of DTC within more developed countries or countries with higher incomes are more than double in comparison with countries without these characteristics.[9]

MORTALITY TRENDS OF DIFFERENTIATED THYROID CANCER

Papillary thyroid cancer, the most common type of DTC, is one of the least deadly human cancers with a 10-year disease-specific survival of >90%.[13] Follicular cancer, as noted earlier, has a significantly worse prognosis with survival rates in the range of 55% to 70%. Although the incidence of papillary cancer has been steadily increasing in the U.S. and developing countries everywhere, the mortality rate has increased only slightly.[27] It is not yet clear whether this shift in mortality is significant.[28]

Follicular cancer mortality has not changed. Since the 1970s, mortality rates in almost all other major countries have either remained stable or decreased, with an average mortality rate from 0.20 to 0.40/100,000 and 0.20 to 0.60/100,000 for women and men, respectively, across all countries.[12]

Interpreting the Incidence and Mortality Trends in Papillary Thyroid Cancer

The qualities of the increasing incidence of thyroid cancer are important. The entire increase in incidence has been due to papillary thyroid cancer, and the majority of the increase has been due to small tumors (<1 cm). This rise of small thyroid cancer incidence coupled without a proportional change in mortality suggests that the majority of the rise in incidence is not a true increase but rather the discovery of a subclinical reservoir.[10,13] Because there has been some increase in larger thyroid cancers as well, there is concern for an underlying true increase in incidence co-occurring with overdiagnosis, although it is possible that the large tumors are also being uncovered as a subclinical reservoir.[8,27,29,30]

There are two hypotheses for the steady and significant increase in the incidence of DTC observed worldwide: (1) advances in medical technology and increased access to health care have led to the detection of a previously undetectable subclinical reservoir: overdiagnosis (2) a true increase in the incidence in DTC exists due to known or new environmental risk factors. It is also possible that both hypotheses are true.

The Overdiagnosis Hypothesis

An increasing incidence without proportional changes in mortality suggests overdiagnosis, but to fully meet the criteria, two other things must be present, a subclinical reservoir of cancer and a way to uncover it.[31] The existence of a subclinical reservoir for thyroid cancer is well known. The earliest studies date back at least to 1947, in which it was shown that people who had died of other causes never knowing they had thyroid cancer nevertheless had one or more foci at the time of their death. The autopsy prevalence is ~10% and varies by method of thyroid examination and whether the whole or half of a gland is examined.[32] The autopsy prevalence has also been stable over time, suggesting that the underlying prevalence of thyroid cancer has not changed.

Methods by which the underlying subclinical reservoir can be uncovered have been identified at the health care system level by showing that increased access to care results in a rising incidence of DTC.[33,34] A more detailed examination reveals the ways in which how we provide health care contributes to the detection of thyroid cancer and provides strong support for the overdiagnosis hypothesis as the main driver of the increasing incidence.

Increased Use of Imaging Studies

As medical technology continues to rapidly progress, the availability of advanced diagnostic imaging studies has become widespread, with a corresponding increase in the number of imaging studies performed. A recent study of a large health care system discovered that patients within the system underwent an average of 1.18 imaging studies/year, of which 35% consisted of either computed tomography (CT), magnetic resonance imaging (MRI), nuclear medicine imaging, or ultrasound. The study, conducted over 15 years, also demonstrated an annual percent change (APC) of 8%, 10%, 3.9% and 57% for CT, MRI, ultrasound, and positron emission topography (PET), respectively (PET data only for 2004 to 2010).[35] Due to the increased resolution and use of these imaging techniques, many patients are referred for evaluation of a thyroid finding, sometimes called an "incidentaloma" because identifying the finding was not the goal of the imaging study.

Diagnostic Cascade

Another path by which patients can end up with a small cancer identified is through inappropriate use of testing, revealing a thyroid finding, but the finding does not explain the person's complaint. An example is ordering a thyroid ultrasound to work up weight gain or hair loss rather than a TSH alone as a first step.[36] The thyroid finding is explored, and a small, asymptomatic cancer is found. As with the incidence of DTC, this trend of broad test ordering has not only been observed in the U.S. but also internationally.[37]

Threshold for Evaluation

Fine-needle aspiration (FNA) biopsy and ultrasound-guided biopsy rates showed a 7-fold and 5-fold increase between 2000 and 2012 in a study of the Veterans Affairs Healthcare System.[38] Another study of the U.S. health care system as a whole that was performed over a 5-year period found a doubling in the rate of FNAs during this time period with an annual growth of 16%.[39] In France, a similar increase in the use of FNA from 1980 to 2000 was seen, showing that shifts in the threshold for evaluation are not limited to the U.S.[37] As more needle biopsies are done, more cancers or nodules of uncertain significance are found, which prompts more surgery.

Management of Thyroid Specimens

In addition to the increased number of specimens sent for analysis, the scrutiny with which specimens are analyzed has also been shown to have significantly increased. Not only are pathologists examining more blocks of tissue per specimen, but the standard pathology report for a thyroid surgical specimen has evolved from 5 to 14 descriptive areas since the 1980s,[6,40,41] highlighting the scrutiny with which each specimen is now analyzed. This means that more cancer is found simply because thyroid glands are examined more closely.

The New or Increased Risk Factors Hypothesis

Although overdiagnosis of subclinical disease is now accepted to be the major contributor to the increasing incidence of DTC, it is also possible that there is an underlying true increase in the incidence of DTC because larger tumors have also increased in incidence, and there has been an increase in mortality of some stages of thyroid cancer.

Exposure to Ionizing Radiation

Ionizing radiation is the most extensively studied and clearly defined environmental risk factor for the development of thyroid cancer, with a somatic mutation signature of a higher frequency of RET (rearranged during transfection) chromosomal rearrangements in comparison with sporadic cases. The risk of thyroid cancer after exposure to radiation decreases with increasing age: the most significant risk is for those exposed under the age of 5, and people age 20 or older have no greater than background risk.[6,8,42]

Ionizing radiation exposure to the general population has doubled in the past 30 years in the U.S.; the majority of this increased exposure is due to increased use of medical imaging studies.[6,8] Nuclear tests have not been performed in the U.S. since the early 1960s, radiotherapy of benign conditions of the head and neck has not been routine since the 1950s, and only a small fraction of the increased use of medical imaging has occurred in those young enough to experience an increased risk from these studies.[6,8,33] Thus, although radiation is a strong risk factor for thyroid cancer, the increased exposure to ionizing radiation in the U.S. has contributed very minimally to the increased incidence of DTC, if at all.[6,33]

Contribution of Iodine Deficiency and Excess

As briefly discussed earlier, iodine deficiency is known to decrease the ratio of PTC to FTC, thus increasing the rate of FTC, as well as producing an increased rate of goiter and anaplastic thyroid carcinoma.[9,21,26,43] The proposed mechanism for this observed trend consists of chronic thyroid-stimulating hormone (TSH) stimulation induced by iodine deficiency.[43] Several studies have been conducted investigating a possible role of iodine excess as a risk factor for the development of DTC, specifically PTC.[44-46] However, no clear biologic mechanism of iodine excess for the development of PTC has been identified. Furthermore, the studies performed thus far demonstrate only minor associations, lack statistical significance, and/or have inconsistencies in subgroup analysis.[6,44,45] Given that the increased incidence of DTC has been primarily attributed to an increase in PTC and that these trends have been most prominent in high income, iodine-sufficient countries, iodine deficiency, although it leads to altered proportions of thyroid cancer, is not responsible for the increased incidence of DTC during the past 30 years.

Obesity and Diabetes

The obesity epidemic has paralleled the rising incidence of DTC in the last 30 years, with the prevalence of obese adults and children increasing by 27.5% and 47.1%, respectively, worldwide.[8] In addition, the prevalence of obesity and incidence of DTC has been noted to increase within the same geographic areas, and obesity has consistently been associated with an increased risk of thyroid cancer in epidemiologic studies,[47-49] particularly in middle-aged adults.[8,50,51] Furthermore, additional studies have concluded that the presence of obesity is associated with more aggressive pathologic features, such as ETE, tumor multiplicity, and cervical metastasis.[52,53] The underlying biologic mechanisms proposed for these observed associations are complex and numerous, including synergistic effects of increased body mass index (BMI), body surface area (BSA), abdominal/central adiposity, chronic TSH elevation, insulin resistance (and thus diabetes), insulin-like growth factor 1 (IGF-1), adipokines, inflammation, oxidative stress, and immune suppression.[6,49,50,54,55] However, associations of contributing obesity-related factors to increased risk of thyroid cancer (such as diabetes and metabolic syndrome) remain weak,[8,55] and associations between obesity and increased prevalence and aggressiveness of DTC remain controversial.[29,52,53,56] A causal relationship between obesity and thyroid cancer has thus not been definitively proven. Some authors have postulated that the associations observed between obesity and thyroid cancer might be due to increased use of health care and diagnostic services due to their associated medical comorbidities.[6,8,50]

Estrogen

Estrogen has historically been proposed as a causal mechanism of thyroid cancer, with the basis of this argument residing in the fact that thyroid cancer is far more prevalent in the female population. Much of the research being performed currently consists of cell line studies, some of which have demonstrated the enhancement of thyroid cancer proliferation by estrogen through various mechanisms, including induction of matrix metalloproteinase activity, leading to increased metastatic phenotype[57,58] and promotion of thyroid cancer cell migration, invasion, and angiogenesis via vascular endothelial growth factor (VEGF).[59] In vitro and animal studies have investigated the role and interplay of estrogen and estrogen receptors (ERs) on thyroid cell proliferation. Thus far these studies have demonstrated that ERs do play a role in the growth of thyroid cancer, but considerable discrepancies with regard to the specific expression patterns seen in thyroid cancer tissues exist.[6,60,61] The complexities of these biologic pathways are not clearly delineated at this point and are also outside of the scope of this chapter.

Clinical and epidemiologic studies with regard to the role of estrogen in the development of thyroid cancer have largely focused on female reproductive factors, including age of menarche, age of menopause, progression of disease during pregnancy, oral contraceptive use, hormone replacement therapy, and parity.[60,62] Although the studies investigating these factors are numerous, they have failed to demonstrate fail to demonstrate strong associations between any of these factors and the development of thyroid cancer, so at this point concrete evidence does not yet exist proving estrogen a risk factor for thyroid cancer development.[6,60,62]

Dietary Nitrates

Nitrates are known to be a natural component of plants, found in high concentrations in leafy vegetables, such as spinach, lettuce, and many root vegetables, such as beets, carrots, green beans, and celery.[63] They are also a contaminant of natural drinking water, making it a possible major source of nitrate intake when levels are above the maximum contaminant level of 25 to 45 mg/L (5 to 10 mg/L of nitrate/nitrogen).[64,65] The proposed mechanism of nitrate-induced development of thyroid carcinoma occurs secondary to competitive inhibition of iodide uptake by the thyroid via nitrates binding to the sodium-iodide symporter, thus hindering production and secretion of triiodothyronine (T3) and thyroxine (T4) and thereby leading to chronically increased production of TSH, proliferative changes in follicular cells, and thyroid gland hyperplasia/neoplasia.[6,64] Other mechanisms, such as formation of N-nitroso compounds (NOCs), which have been shown to be potent carcinogens in animal studies, have also been suggested.[64] In accord, several epidemiologic studies have been conducted to assess the role of dietary nitrate intake in the development of thyroid cancer, and several of these studies have successfully found positive associations between nitrate intake and DTC.[64,65] However, not all studies agree that a true association exists,[66] and ultimately there still exists doubt as to a causal relationship between dietary nitrates and thyroid cancer. To clearly delineate this relationship, larger scale epidemiologic studies with attention to possible confounding factors are both needed and warranted.

Autoimmune Thyroid Disease

Hashimoto's thyroiditis (HT) is the most common autoimmune disease in humans, frequently leading to hypothyroidism.[67] Several recent studies performed on patients undergoing thyroidectomy with coexisting HT report an increased prevalence of PTC in these specimens, leading some to believe that HT may serve as a risk factor for the development of PTC.[67-69] In addition, both disease processes demonstrate some shared risk factors (greater incidence in women, more prevale in iodine-insufficient areas, and history of neck radiotherapy).[68] The predominant hypothesized mechanism for this association consists of hypothyroidism secondary to HT, leading to chronically elevated TSH and thus follicular epithelial cell proliferation and possible neoplasia.[68,70] However, a number of population-based FNA studies find no correlation between HT and PTC,[69,71] and many argue that the positive correlation generally seen in thyroidectomy studies is subject to confounding by indication (patients with abnormal biopsy results are more likely to undergo surgery).[6,71] More prospective studies with longer follow-up are needed to clarify this relationship.

THE EFFECT OF THE INCREASED INCIDENCE OF THYROID CANCER

As the incidence of DTC has dramatically increased in the previous decades, so has the rate of treatment for these newly diagnosed cases. From the mid 2000's until the release of the 2015 American Thyroid Association (ATA) guidelines, total thyroidectomy with or without radioactive iodine (RAI) ablation was the indicated treatment for diagnosed papillary thyroid cancer >1 cm, with lobectomy versus total thyroidectomy for PMC, resulting in a total of 15,888 total thyroidectomies performed on Medicare beneficiaries in the U.S. for a national average rate of 60/100,000 beneficiaries in 2014.[72,73] Black and Welch described the cycle of escalating intervention that has a propensity to occur after advances in diagnostic practices (development of CT, MRI, ultrasound-guided FNA, nuclear medicine imaging), leading to diagnosis of asymptomatic and subclinical disease.[74] The treatment of this disease in accordance with previously established guidelines often results in excellent outcomes (due to the mild nature of disease, as well as lead-time and length biases) and produces the appearance of improving outcomes, thereby reinforcing both diagnostic and therapeutic practices. This phenomenon can ultimately lead to a spurious increase in survival and continued unnecessary treatment of disease as has been seen previously with the epidemic of overdiagnosis that occurred with prostate cancer.[13,74]

Associated Cost Burden

Based on historic incidence trends, the cost of care related to thyroid cancer is projected to reach $18 to $21 billion by the year 2019,[75] with an estimated societal cost of $1.6 billion in 2013 for DTC-associated care for all U.S. patients diagnosed after 1985.[76] Unlike most other cancers, the majority of cost is incurred in the initial and continuing phases of care, with the largest proportion of these costs due to diagnosis, surgery, and adjuvant therapy for newly diagnosed patients (41%), followed by surveillance of survivors (37%), and nonoperative death costs attributable to thyroid cancer care (22%).[76] Although the national health care system may be able to somewhat absorb these costs, the individual patient may not. The Washington State cancer study found that patients with a thyroid cancer diagnosis were more likely to go bankrupt than those without, particularly if they were young female patients (<35 years),[77] less likely to have access to high-quality health insurance, ineligible for Medicaid or Medicare, and more financially vulnerable. As previously discussed, this criterion encompasses a significant number of newly diagnosed DTCs. Even in the absence of a cancer diagnosis, thyroid cancer testing with benign findings leads to significantly increased costs for the system and the individual, with one study demonstrating the FNA biopsy of benign nodules in 1685 individuals led to follow-up imaging in 800 of these patients (47.5%) and a total estimated cost of $879,347 or $1099 per individual.[78] During an average follow-up period of 7.3 years in the same study, 19 (2.4%) of these 1685 were eventually diagnosed with thyroid cancer at a cost of $46,281 per diagnosis.[78]

Treatment Side Effects

The diagnostic cascade was described in detail earlier in this chapter; it may begin with a chance trigger event from an "incidentaloma" on imaging studies or inappropriately ordered tests, and potentially ends with a total thyroidectomy and need for postoperative lifelong thyroid hormone supplementation. Although such a serendipitous finding may enable the early detection and treatment of malignant disease and thus prolonged survival, for a large number of patients with low-risk DTC, particularly those with PMC, the advantages of early detection, diagnosis, and treatment might not outweigh the financial costs, improvement in quality of life, and health implications of treatment.

First, no form of surgical intervention comes without associated risk, and this certainly holds true for surgery within the central neck with the largest volume study to date citing an approximate 20% and 11% complication rate associated with total and hemithyroidectomy, respectively.[79] Complications and associated rates with total and hemithyroidectomy, respectively, from the same study include hypocalcemia (16.1% and 7.1%), hematoma (1.54% and 1.24%), vocal cord paralysis (1.33% and 0.59%), respiratory complications (1.34% and 0.84%), and tracheostomy (0.024% and 0.004%); in addition, a total of 35 postoperative deaths (.00056%) were recorded during the study.[79] Furthermore, even in the instance of total thyroidectomy performed without any complication, lifelong postoperative thyroid hormone supplementation, and thus TSH monitoring, is mandatory.

Second, outside of the possible complications and necessary postoperative care associated with surgical intervention, carrying a thyroid cancer diagnosis alone has been shown to exert a significant negative effect on patient quality of life.[8] One study that performed survivorship studies in colon, glioma, breast, gynecologic, and thyroid cancer found that patients carrying a diagnosis of thyroid cancer reported a similar overall quality of life score (5.56/10) as those with colon (5.20/10), glioma (5.96/10), and gynecologic (5.59/10) cancer; breast cancer patients reported a significantly better quality of life score (6.51/10, p < 0.01).[80] This decrease in quality of life is postulated to be due to the psychological burden of living with a cancer diagnosis, even if indolent in nature, as well as having to repeatedly undergo biochemical and imaging surveillance for progression or recurrence.[8,80]

MANAGING THE INCREASING INCIDENCE OF THYROID CANCER

Given that most or all of the increase in thyroid cancer incidence may be due to overdiagnosis, concerted efforts have been made to understand and change health care system contributors to mitigate overtreatment and provide relief for patients from the effects on health care costs and patient quality of life (Table 17.1).

Guideline Changes

The ATA released an updated, comprehensive set of recommendations in 2009 and then again in 2015, with several refinements made sequentially in direct relation to the overdiagnosis and overtreatment of DTC.[81] Before publication of the 2015 ATA guidelines, PTC of any size was an indication for total thyroidectomy,[6,72] resulting in some thyroid surgeons offering total thyroidectomy for an FNA with atypia or follicular lesion of undetermined significance (AUS/FUS, Bethesda Class III). These recommendations likely contributed to an increased rate of thyroidectomy and thus the number of thyroid specimens for analysis.[6,41] In 2015, the guidelines were also updated to recommend that nodules be 1 cm for biopsy instead of 5 mm in most cases. In addition, other governing bodies as well as the media took action to address the epidemic of overdiagnosis. Clinical data collected since 2010 indicates that these changes have likely been efficacious, with observed stabilization in the incidence of thyroid cancer between 2010 and 2012, notably including stabilization of the incidence of subcentimeter cancers, which was previously rising at >9% APC.[7,11]

TABLE 17.1 Efforts to Address the Overdiagnosis and Overtreatment of DTC

Change	Summary
Do not biopsy thyroid nodules <1 cm	2015 ATA guidelines recommend risk-stratified approach in which nodules <1 cm in size generally should not be biopsied, unless high-risk features are present.
Recommend hemithyroidectomy for PTC <1 cm; option for hemithyroidectomy with PTC >1 cm and <4 cm	2015 ATA guidelines recommend hemithyroidectomy for PTC <1 cm, as well as option for hemi- versus total thyroidectomy for PTC >1 cm and <4 cm in size (previously recommended total for PTC of any size).
Active surveillance acknowledged	2015 ATA guidelines acknowledge active surveillance as a potential management strategy for small PTCs, patients who are poor surgical candidates due to comorbidities, patients with an expected short lifespan, and patients with medical issues more pressing than their thyroid cancer.
Reclassification of some thyroid cancers to NIFTP	Previously termed encapsulated follicular variant of papillary thyroid carcinoma (EFVPTC), a group of international pathologists, endocrinologists, and surgeons recommended a name change in 2016 to noninvasive follicular thyroid neoplasm with papillary-like nuclear features (NIFTP) to better characterize this lesion's indolent nature.
Molecular testing as adjunct to US-guided FNA	The development of molecular testing has enabled closer analysis of biopsy specimens in determination of malignant potential, which is particularly important in Bethesda Class III and IV specimens, potentially saving patients from unnecessary surgery.
Guideline emphasis on patient preference and patient-centered decision making	The 2015 ATA guidelines persistently place an emphasis on ensuring thorough discussion of risks and benefits of surgery (hemi- versus total thyroidectomy), medical management, and observation, encouraging the making of joint decisions between patients and physicians regarding their treatment.
USPSTF recommends against thyroid cancer screening	2017 U.S. Preventative Services Task Force (USPSTF) gave thyroid cancer screening in asymptomatic individuals a grade of "D," renewing their recommendation against screening for healthy asymptomatic people.

DTC, differentiated thyroid cancer, ATA, American Thyroid Association, PTC, papillary thyroid carcinoma, US, ultrasound, FNA, fine-needle aspiration.

Renaming a Papillary Thyroid Cancer Variant—NIFTP

As part of the increased incidence of thyroid cancer, there has been an increase in the identification of a type of papillary cancer called the follicular variant, of which there are two subtypes—encapsulated follicular variant of papillary thyroid cancer (EFVPTC) and a nonencapsulated type. The non encapsulated type is estimated to make up 10% to 20% of all thyroid cancers diagnosed in Europe and North America.[82] Follicular variant papillary thyroid cancer, particularly the encapsulated type, exhibits behavior that is markedly more indolent and genetically distinct from other PTCs.[83-85] In an effort to mitigate the overdiagnosis and overtreatment of these indolent lesions, a combined group of pathologists, endocrinologists, and surgeons collaborated to address this issue by renaming this particular subtype. They showed through their international retrospective study, including 109 patients diagnosed with noninvasive EFVPTC who were followed for at least a decade, that patients with EFVPTC had 100% survival without metastatic disease over this time period.[82] As a result, the group recommended adoption of the new term noninvasive follicular thyroid neoplasm with papillary-like nuclear features (NIFTP) in place of noninvasive EFVPTC, thereby removing the word "cancer" from the diagnosis. The goal is to reduce the psychological and clinical consequences associated with a cancer diagnosis for this large patient population.

CONCLUSIONS AND NEXT STEPS

In summary, the dramatic increase seen in the incidence of thyroid cancer since the early 1990's has mainly been due to the detection of a subclinical reservoir (overdiagnosis). Although investigation into potential new causes or changes in risk factors is warranted to examine the changes in rates of larger cancers and in mortality, tremendous efforts have been put forth to rein in the identification of small thyroid cancers unnecessarily. Recent data shows that there is wide variation in how thyroid nodules and cancer are identified and managed. Among U.S. Medicare beneficiaries in 2014, although 15,888 thyroidectomies were performed, there was a 6.2-fold difference in rates across communities, and these rates did not align with health care availability, regional socioeconomic status, or surgeons per capita, suggesting widely divergent beliefs and practice patterns surrounding the management of thyroid nodules and associated thyroid cancer.[73] To support efforts to further mitigate overdiagnosis and also research efforts to identify potential new causes, decreasing unnecessary variations in thyroid care practices will be a crucial next step.

REFERENCES

For a complete list of references, go to expertconsult.com.

Molecular Pathogenesis of Thyroid Neoplasia

Matthew D. Ringel, Thomas J. Giordano

INTRODUCTION

Over the past decade, there has been an enormous expansion of knowledge regarding the molecular pathogenesis of thyroid tumors and major advances in clinically applying this knowledge to enhance diagnostic approaches to thyroid nodules and informing clinical trials and treatments for patients with progressive disease.[1] This includes not only somatic genomics (i.e., genetic changes only found in tumor cells) but also germline predisposing genomics (i.e., inherited genetic alterations in all cells).[2] In this chapter, we will focus on genomic changes that are currently being used in clinical practice and/or clinical trials to improve preoperative diagnoses, to predict the biological behavior of cancers, and/or to determine treatment options or clinical trial enrollments for patients with established thyroid cancer.

THYROID CANCER EPIDEMIOLOGY

Thyroid carcinoma rates are increasing worldwide (see Chapter 17, Differentiated Thyroid Cancer Incidence).[3] At present in the United States, thyroid cancer is the fifth most common cancer in women and the 11th most common cancer in men. It accounts for ~95% of malignancies of classical endocrine organs.[4-6] It is of considerable interest that among all cancer of nonreproductive organs, the 3:1 ratio of female:male cancer incidence is the highest.[6] It is without question that the marked increased in rise in thyroid cancer that began in the early 2000s reflects increased medical surveillance, the use of thyroid ultrasound, and the development of ultrasound-guided fine-needle aspiration (FNA) technologies.[7-10] The evidence for this includes the much more rapid rise in the diagnosis of small papillary thyroid cancers in the United States[8] and the data from South Korea, where the incidence of diagnosed papillary thyroid carcinoma (PTC) became similar to that of autopsy studies as a result of more universal coverage of thyroid ultrasound in cancer screening.[11] Interestingly, with this emerging data, evidence that many patients with small PTCs can be actively surveilled safely for decades,[12-14] and a consequent increased emphasis on identifying larger PTCs in clinical guidelines,[15] the incidence of diagnosed thyroid cancer has "flattened," or even decreased, in the past few years.[4] It is important to note, however, that whereas the *percentage* of individuals diagnosed with larger thyroid cancers or have died from thyroid cancer has been stable or has decreased, the *absolute number* of individuals with larger cancer or have died from the disease is increasing.[16] The reasons for this are unclear. It still may be in part due to the increase in detection but also may reflect an increase due to other factors such as environmental exposures[17] or genetic drift in the population. Together, these data highlight the need for additional biomarkers to better identify patients destined to have indolent thyroid cancer versus those likely to harbor more aggressive disease to avoid overtreatment and also to minimize the effects of undertreatment.

PATHOLOGY

From a clinical perspective, the thyroid gland is composed of two populations of hormone-producing cells: (1) follicular cells that produce thyroid hormones from the backbone of thyroglobulin and (2) parafollicular cells (C-cells) that represent a minority population of neuroendocrine cells that produce calcitonin and carcinoembryonic antigen (CEA) (see Chapter 2, Applied Embryology of the Thyroid and Parathyroid Glands). These two cell populations likely derive from the same endoderm progenitor cells, a feature of thyroid development only recently discovered.[18] Although rare mixed tumors can produce both thyroglobulin and calcitonin,[19] the vast majority of thyroid cancer derives distinctly from either cell type (called follicular cell-derived thyroid cancers) or medullary thyroid cancers. The cancers that derive from the follicular cells account for ~95% of thyroid cancer cases and can further be divided into subgroups based on histopathological characteristics. The majority of these cancers are well-differentiated and are either PTC or follicular thyroid cancer (FTC) and together are termed as differentiated thyroid cancer (DTC) (see Chapter 19, Papillary Thyroid Cancer; Chapter 20, Papillary Thyroid Microcarcinoma; Chapter 21, Papillary Carcinoma Observation; and Chapter 22, Follicular Thyroid Cancer).[20] The cancer cells in these tumors typically maintain expression of the thyroid-stimulating hormone (TSH) receptor, the sodium-iodide (Na/I) symporter, and thyroglobulin, features that have important treatment and monitoring implications. Classical forms of PTC develop de novo within the normal thyroid without a clear "premalignant" pathology, with tumors less than 1 cm defined as papillary microcarcinoma. By contrast, FTCs are thought to develop in part from benign follicular adenomas[21,22] thereby presenting a multistep premalignant-to-malignant model similar to other cancers,[23] including colon carcinoma.[24] Finally, it is important to recognize that the majority of thyroid nodules detected clinically are not neoplastic but are hyperplastic nodules, colloid nodules, or other benign pathologies that are not known to have malignant potential.[25] Autonomous thyroid nodules ("hot" nodules on radioiodine scanning) rarely develop into malignancy and are characterized by specific mutations that activate protein kinase A signaling, thereby increasing thyroid hormone production (*TSHR* and *GNAS1* mutations).[26,27]

Hürthle (oncocytic) cell thyroid cancers had been classified as a variant of FTC; however, the most recent World Health Organization (WHO) classification considers Hürthle cell tumors a distinct type (see Chapter 25, Hürthle Cell Tumors of the Thyroid). This classification is consistent with recent genomic data that establish Hürthle cells as a distinct form of DTC.[28,29] Cancers composed of these cells typically do not concentrate radioiodine well but express TSH receptor and thyroglobulin. Hürthle cells are eosinophilic polygonal cells characterized by the presence of large and a greater number of mitochondria with atypical features.[30] These cells can be seen not only in cancers but also in benign adenomas and in association with benign thyroid disorders such as Hashimoto's thyroiditis.[31,32]

A highly specific type of thyroid tumor recently classified is termed as *noninvasive follicular tumor with papillary-like nuclear features (NIFTP)* (see Chapter 23, Noninvasive Follicular Thyroid Neoplasm with Papillary-like Nuclear Features [NIFTP]).[33] This tumor type previously was termed under one of several names, including encapsulated follicular variant of PTC, follicular adenoma with cellular atypia, and follicular tumor of uncertain malignant potential.[34] These tumors are intrathyroidal; encapsulated; do not display vascular, capsular, or lymphatic invasion; and exhibit nuclear features of PTC. They appear typically to have a benign clinical course and are often characterized by mutations in the *RAS* genes.[35,36] Although preoperative diagnosis is elusive due to the requirement for thorough assessment of the tumor capsule for invasion, postoperatively, NIFTPs are thought to be largely cured by surgery alone.[37,38]

Follicular cell-derived and parafollicular cell-derived thyroid cancers can become poorly differentiated based on histomorphologic and immunohistochemical features. In the case of follicular cell-derived thyroid cancer, these poorly differentiated thyroid carcinomas (PDTCs) sort into two main groups. According to the Turin classification,[39] PDTC includes so-called insular and trabecular variants that are classically FTC-derived.[40,41] Alternatively, other PDTC are derived from high-grade papillary carcinomas that are enriched for tall and columnar cell variants PTC.[42-44] Anaplastic thyroid cancer (ATC) appears to develop mostly from well or poorly differentiated PTC[45,46] or FTC,[47] although in some cases it may occur de novo[48] and often contains higher numbers of cancer stem cells[49,50] and is characterized by very robust immune cell infiltrates shown to facilitate its progression.[51-53] These tumors typically do not express TSH receptor, Na/I symporter, or thyroglobulin; are remarkably aggressive; and unless diagnosed and fully removed surgically, are uniformly fatal.[54]

THYROID CANCER PROGNOSIS

Individuals with DTCs typically have an outstanding prognosis, and cure is common when diagnosed early. Because these tumors are slow-growing and typically indolent in most cases, there are multiple studies demonstrating the safety of active surveillance rather than surgery for individuals with very small PTCs that have no evidence of metastasis.[13,14,55-57] However, it is important to recognize that some patients with DTCs have local metastasis and others may have or develop distant metastasis that can be life threatening. As outlined in detail in other chapters of this text, current treatment strategies rely on risk stratification of patients based on imaging characteristics, tumors, and demographics as well as response to initial therapies (see Chapter 24, Dynamic Risk Group Analysis and Staging for Differentiated Thyroid Cancer). This wide variety in clinical behavior for DTC tumors highlights the important potential role of molecular markers to optimize and individualize therapy.

Patients with ATC have a poor prognosis as a group with the only chance of cure being early and complete surgical resection disease eradication before metastasis (see Chapter 28, Anaplastic Thyroid Cancer and Primary Thyroid Lymphoma). Because of the poor prognosis, most patients with potentially curable localized ATC are treated aggressively, often with surgery and chemoradiation, unless there are major comorbidities. Less aggressive local approaches are often recommended if the cancer cannot be surgically resected and/or it is metastatic to regional or distant sites. Recent data demonstrate that targeting $BRAF^{V600E}$ may have noncurative treatment benefits or neoadjuvant treatment benefits for patients with ATC,[58-60] as discussed in the treatment section later in this chapter. Thus evaluation of somatic genomics of ATC may influence treatment approaches.

Individuals with medullary thyroid carcinoma (MTC) fall into two categories, those with sporadic MTC (~75%) and those with inherited MTC (~25%) due to an inherited germline mutation in *RET*[61] (see Chapter 26, Sporadic Medullary Thyroid Carcinoma, and Chapter 27, Syndromic Medullary Thyroid Carcinoma: MEN 2A and MEN 2B). For all patients with MTC, primary surgery, including central neck node dissection, can be curative. Such an approach is most effective for patients diagnosed early due to the high frequency of regional nodal spread. Because individuals identified with genetic screening in a family can be diagnosed earlier, even before the cancer develops, they have the best prognosis as a group, whereas individuals with either sporadic MTC or the probands (first in the family) of a family with inherited MTC are typically diagnosed with larger and later stage tumors.[62]

For patients with larger or more aggressive PTCs or PDTCs with incomplete responses after surgery or with known residual metastases, additional treatment with TSH-suppressive doses of thyroid hormone; radioactive iodine; and in selected cases, kinase inhibitors, clinical trials, or external radiation therapy are used. These treatments and their indications are highlighted in the appropriate chapters of this text.

GERMLINE GENETICS OF THYROID CANCER

MTC is the form of thyroid cancer most associated with germline predisposition, a feature that influences clinical management. As described earlier approximately 25% of MTC cases are inherited due to germline mutations in *RET* that cause multiple endocrine neoplasia type 2 syndromes.[63-65] MTC development is nearly universal in individuals who inherit this mutation, which can vary based on the specific mutation and the specific family. Recommendations for "prophylactic" thyroidectomy based on these data are available and reviewed separately but are universally recommended for individuals with germline inheritance of the more aggressive mutations with the highest penetrance of clinically important MTC.[66,67] Interestingly, ~50% of MTC in patients with sporadic disease harbor a somatic *RET* mutation at codon 918, which is associated with more aggressive disease.[68] This same mutation, when it occurs in germline, causes MEN2B. Somatic mutations in *RAS* are also common but not overlapping with *RET*.[69] Recently, loss of expression of cell cycle regulators RB and p18 have recently been associated with a more aggressive course for MTC.[70,71]

In contrast to the high frequency of familial disease in MTC, the vast majority of patients with follicular cell-derived forms of thyroid cancer have clinically sporadic disease. Nonetheless, when considering the entire PTC population (about 80% of all DTCs), PTC has among the highest degree of "familiality"[72-75] (see Chapter 30, Familial Nonmedullary Thyroid Cancer). In addition, both PTC and FTC can occur as part of rarely diagnosed cancer syndromes such as Cowden's syndrome[76] (*PTEN* mutations), Carney Complex[77] (*PRKAR1A* mutations), DICER syndrome[78] (*DICER1* mutations), familial adenomatous polyposis[79] (*APC* mutations), Werner syndrome[80] (progeria), and others.[81] In all of these syndromes, benign thyroid nodules can also develop, thus not all nodules in such patients represent thyroid cancer.

For individuals with nonsyndromic forms of PTC, large genome-wide associate studies (GWAS) have been performed by international consortia that have identified a number of single nucleotide polymorphisms (SNPs) that are associated with PTC diagnosis.[82-85] Several of these have been functionally characterized, and it is possible that they will lead to new approaches to determining who is at risk of having PTC, thereby allowing for population screening recommendations.[86,87]

SOMATIC GENOMICS OF THYROID CANCER

Several large population-based and broad genomic studies have led to the molecular characterization of several forms of thyroid cancer. These data have modified our understanding of the disease, will likely lead to revised pathologic classifications, and have been used to develop molecular diagnostics for thyroid cancer diagnoses and new options for treating some patients with aggressive disease. Several of these studies are highlighted later, and the data are summarized for the most common mutations in Table 18.1.

PTC

The Cancer Genome Atlas (TCGA) was a broad effort funded by the NIH to establish the genomic landscapes of the most common types of cancer in the United States population.[88] PTC was one of the analyzed tumor types.[89] In this study, 496 PTCs and germline blood samples (and in some cases, adjacent normal tissues) from adult patients were analyzed after the careful selection of tumors that would ensure high quality and tumor cell predominate samples (PTC). Whole exome DNA sequencing, global RNA sequencing, and microRNA (miR) sequencing; methylation profiling; and reverse phase protein arrays were performed on all samples. A wealth of data came from this study, but several features of PTC were identified as of key importance to the field:

1. Well-differentiated PTC has a "quiet" genome with not much evidence of global genomic instability, low mutation rates, low growth rates, and fewer genetic and epigenetic changes than most forms of cancer;
2. PTC is largely driven by two oncogenes, *BRAF* and *RAS*, both of which activated MAP kinase pathway signaling; the mutations are mutually exclusive and each is associated with unique RNA expression profiles, miR expression profiles, DNA methylation patterns, and protein expression and phosphorylation patterns that are separable;
3. *BRAF* mutations are associated with classical forms of PTC, whereas *RAS* mutations are most associated with follicular variant of PTC; and
4. A variety of rare mutations and/or rearrangements involving *RET* (RET/PTC rearrangements), *NTRK 1,2* and *3; ROS1, ALK, THADA*; and others were identified, and their signaling was distinct from *BRAF*-mutated tumors. Some of these uncommon genetic changes have important treatment implications (see later).

It is important to note that the TCGA PTC study, which is best described as defining the genomic landscape of well-differentiated PTC, was limited largely to T1 or T2 tumors that were relatively early stage as only 11 cases had distant metastases. Thus it creates a solid baseline of the genomic landscape of the most common PTCs.[90]

It is important to recognize that pediatric PTCs[91-95] and radiation-induced PTCs[40,96-98] appear to have different genomic drivers in comparison to the majority of adult PTC. In both situations, *BRAF* mutations are less common and *RET/PTC* and other gene rearrangements are particularly common (see Chapter 29, Pediatric Thyroid Cancer). The reasons for this distinction in children are not yet clear, but in the case of radiation-related tumors, such as those that developed after the Chernobyl nuclear disaster in 1985, there is evidence that ionizing radiation causes DNA breaks to occur at specific genomic loci,[99] resulting in expression of these fusion proteins, with a particular predilection for *RET/PTC3* (*NCOA4(RFG)-RET* fusion).[96,100,101]

As noted earlier, PTCs have been associated with profiles in miRs both in the TCGA cohort[89] and individual studies.[102-105] These have included consistently increased expression of a panel of miRs, including miR 221, 222, 146b, and 181b.[105,106] These miRs, along with the DNA mutations and rearrangements, have been used to develop molecular diagnostic and potentially prognostic approaches that are described later and in other areas of this text (see Chapter 12, Fine-Needle Aspiration and Molecular Analysis).

From a prognostic perspective, several large retrospective case control studies have reported that PTCs with an activating mutation in *BRAF* are more likely to occur in older patients,[107] and have tumors that demonstrate extrathyroidal invasion,[108] recurrence or residual disease,[109] and in some studies, distant metastasis.[109-114] $BRAF^{V600E}$ expression results in the loss of thyroid-differentiated function, including reductions in expression of the Na-I symporter and TSH receptor, which would predict

TABLE 18.1 Common Genetic Lesions Associated with Thyroid Cancer Types

Genetic Alteration	NIFTP	PTC	FTC	HCC	PDTC	ATC	MTC
BRAF		X			X*	X*	
RAS[†]	X	X[‡]	X		X[†]	X	X
RET rearrangements		X[§]					
PPARγ/PAX8 rearrangements[†]			X				
RET mutations							X
PIK3CA mutations			X		X	X	
PTEN mutations/loss[†]			X		X	X	
TERT Promoter mutations		X	X		X	X	
TP53 mutations					X	X	
TRK mutations/rearrangement		X					
ALK mutations/rearrangement		X				X	
ROS rearrangement		X					
Mitochondrial DNA mutations				X			
ATM mutations				X	X	X	
SWI/SNF mutations					X	X	
ERCC4/5 mutations					X	X	

*Implies derivation from PTC such as tall cell variant or ATC.
[†]Also identified in follicular adenoma.
[‡]Implies derivation from follicular variant of PTC (FVPTC).
[§]Most common in radiation-related and pediatric PTC.

less response to treatment.[115-117] However, it is not clear that $BRAF^{V600E}$ is an independent prognostic predictor, and the power of its predictive capability alone seems unlikely due to the high frequency of this mutation in PTC microcarcinomas (20% to 40%) that are associated with an outstanding prognosis,[118,119] although some studies have identified an increased risk of recurrence.[120] More recently, the co-occurrence of $BRAF^{V600E}$ and TERT promoter mutations has been more strongly associated with poor prognosis,[46,121-125] and they have been mechanistically linked.[126] Similarly PTC and FTCs with both RAS and TERT promoter mutations appear to be more aggressive,[127-129] thus it is possible that this combination of mutations will define a group of patients with thyroid cancers that warrant more aggressive treatment.[130]

FTC

As noted earlier, classical FTCs were excluded from the TCGA of PTC to enable statistical power and diagnostic consistency to the data set. Several groups have performed smaller, single site genomic studies of primary FTCs, albeit in a less "global" manner than TCGA.[21,131,132] These studies have identified mutations in RAS genes as a common event in FTC and premalignant follicular adenomas. Gene rearrangements involving PPARγ and PAX8 have been described in both follicular adenomas and FTC and can induce thyroid pathology in mice thereby constituting a bona fide thyroid oncogene.[133-138] In addition, somatic loss of expression and/or mutations of PTEN and/or mutations in PIK3CA or AKT genes have been identified and observed activating the phosphoinositide 3 (OH) kinase (PI3K) pathway.[139-142] However, similar to RAS and PPARγ/PAX8 genetic alterations, these mutations also occur in benign follicular adenomas, making them not as useful for preoperative diagnosis.[141] As noted earlier, the combination of a driver mutation with a concomitant TERT promoter mutation may prove to have prognostic significance, but further studies in FTC are required. miR profiles have been performed in FTC and several predictors have been reported, including some that are used as part of clinically available profiles, although the FTC data are relatively sparse in comparison to PTC.[143,144]

Hürthle Cell Thyroid Carcinoma

Over the past several years, several studies have been performed in which large panels of cancer-related genes have been assessed for mutations and/or rearrangements in populations with Hürthle cell thyroid carcinoma.[28,29,145-148] This has included several resected distant metastases. In these studies there is evidence that, genomically, these tumors are distinct from other forms of DTC. Mutations in mitochondrial DNA genes, in genes in the mTOR metabolic pathway, and generalized chromosomal loss or gains that are uncommon in other forms of thyroid cancer have been identified.[28,29] The typical mutations in PTC and FTC are rare, and the underlying cause of these more global changes is not certain and requires further study. Nonetheless, the identified changes were not found in normal thyroid tissue, thus it is likely these changes will be incorporated into new molecular panels in the future to enhance diagnosis (see Hurthle Cell Carcinoma, Chapter 25).

PDTC and ATC

As follicular cell-derived forms of thyroid cancer become dedifferentiated, they become genomically more complex and have been reviewed elsewhere.[90] Several groups have applied large genomic panels with targeted sequencing of cancer-related genes to these tumors.[148,149] Several features are common:

1. Combinations of mutations or changes in gene expression are identified that include not only MAPK activation (e.g., BRAF or RAS mutations) but also secondary mutations that cause activation of the PI3K and mTOR pathways
2. Mutations in the promoter to the human telomerase gene (TERT) that cause overexpression are common
3. In ATC, mutations in TP53 become common
4. Mutations in genes that regulate epigenetic marks in cells, such as the SWI/SNF complex, are common
5. Mutations predicted to alter pathways for DNA repair, thereby leading to genomic instability, are common (e.g., ATM and ERCC4 and 5)[46,121,142,148-155]

MTC

As noted earlier, patients with sporadic MTC frequently have somatic mutations in RET at codon 918 or activating mutations in RAS in the primary tumors.[61,63,69,156] Interestingly, in multiple mouse models MTC develops with generalized activation of cell cycle through loss of retinoblastoma (Rb) expression, loss of P18 or P16 expression, or loss of p27.[70,71,157,158] Indeed several recent studies have demonstrated that loss of RB or P16 expression is independently associated with poor prognosis in MTC, together suggesting a unique role for these cell cycle regulators in MTC development and biology.[70]

CLINICAL IMPLICATIONS OF THE SOMATIC GENOMIC DATA

Molecular Diagnostics

Molecular diagnostic tests for thyroid cancer diagnosis have been developed to improve the precision of preoperative diagnosis of clinical and radiographic nodule features and FNA cytology[95,159-178] (see Chapter 12, Fine-Needle Aspiration and Molecular Analysis). FNA is highly accurate for benign and malignant diagnoses; however, ~30% of cases are either indeterminate or insufficient. For the indeterminate group, molecular diagnostic tests have been developed to improve the negative predictive value to a similar rate as a benign FNA and/or to improve the positive predictive value similar to a malignant FNA.[168] These are based on mRNA expression profiling,[159] miRNA profiles,[179,180] and DNA mutations and/or gene rearrangements.[172,174,175] This field is continually evolving and methods are continuing to improve, and applications have been advancing. In general, the appropriate patients for this test are those with indeterminate FNA results and have an indeterminate clinical and radiographic risk of cancer. Patients with indeterminate FNA with very low risk radiographic or clinical features likely can be monitored safely whereas those with high clinical or radiographic risk may benefit from surgical resection rather than molecular testing and monitoring. Thus molecular testing of indeterminate FNA samples should be applied as adjunctive tests only for patients in whom the results will influence clinical management.

Predictive Biomarkers

The role of molecular testing results as predictive biomarkers has been more elusive in terms of clinical management. In MTC there are well-established recommendations for prophylactic thyroidectomy based on the particular germline mutation. For example, individuals with germline MEN2b mutations should undergo prophylactic thyroidectomy and bilateral central neck dissection at a young age, whereas patients with less virulent germline mutations (e.g., V804M) might be able to be closely monitored for years without surgery in early childhood.[181,182]

In follicular cell-derived thyroid cancer there is growing evidence that tumors with a combination of BRAF or RAS mutations with a TERT promoter[125] or TP53 mutation[183] are associated with poor prognosis.[130] TERT promoter and TP53 mutations are uncommon outside of patients with larger primary tumors with high risk features and preoperative features often dictate extent of surgery. Thus additional information for the molecular results are most applicable for the subgroup of patients with indeterminate clinical situations and indeterminate thyroid nodule FNA results. Although not studied yet in a clinical trial for outcome improvement, it may be prudent to plan for a total thyroidectomy in patients with primary thyroid cancers in whom these mutations are known before surgery, even if radiographic or clinical features predict early-stage disease (i.e., if molecular diagnostics are performed).

By contrast the association of $BRAF^{V600E}$ with outcomes is less strong and probably not sufficient alone to drive clinical decision-making for individual patients beyond clinical and radiographic staging.[184,185] Rare mutations, such as ALK mutations and translocations, are uncommon in thyroid cancer, but when present they are associated with more aggressive disease.[93,186-188] It is notable that clinical decision making may be modified in the rare situations when multiple driver mutations or combinations of driver and TERT promoter or TP53 mutations are identified.

Treatment-Related Biomarkers

Over the past decade, there has been a major emphasis on developing "targeted" therapies for cancer, including thyroid cancer. As our understanding of molecular biology and structural biochemistry continues to evolve, target-based therapies rather than organ-based therapies are being developed and approved by the FDA. Some of these therapies are being studied in patients with thyroid cancer, or are approved for thyroid or other types of cancer. Specific examples of target-based therapies include the approvals of "checkpoint" immunotherapy in thyroid cancers and other tumors with high mutational burden, microsatellite instability, or overexpression of PD1 and PDL-1.[189] These biomarkers are rare in thyroid cancer, and although inactive in most patients with thyroid cancer as monotherapy, they are currently being evaluated as part of combinatorial strategies in thyroid cancer.[190] In addition, the FDA-approval of BRAF and MEK inhibitors, specifically for anaplastic thyroid cancers with $BRAF^{V600E}$ mutations,[191] and FDA-approvals for tumors with TRRK1 or ROS1 rearrangements and ALK mutations and rearrangements all suggest that in selected cases,

molecular testing may influence treatment choices and potentially clinical outcomes and have been reviewed elsewhere.[192] In addition to these FDA-approved treatments, current clinical trials using second generation RET inhibitors have led to remarkable responses in RET-mutated MTC and RET-rearranged PTC.[192] Thus, many clinical trials now require some element of genomic testing to determine study eligibility. Finally, the combination of MEK or BRAF inhibitors with I-131 in mutated tumors has been studied in several clinical trials from which final data are emerging.[193] These data have led to new recommendations for molecular testing of ATCs or PDTCs.

Recent data also suggest a role for "liquid biopsy," circulating free DNA in patients undergoing targeted therapy to detect the development of so-called resistance gatekeeper mutations, particularly in MTC.[194] As current clinical trials are completed, recommendations for genomic markers that predict a response or resistance to specific therapies may become recommended for all thyroid cancers as the data evolve.

CONCLUSIONS

The role of molecular diagnostics and predictive molecular testing has evolved in thyroid cancer over the past decade as technologies have evolved and knowledge and available therapies have expanded. Molecular diagnostics are beneficial as an adjunct for selected patients with cytologically and clinically indeterminate thyroid nodules. Predictive molecular testing is possible, but the implications beyond clinical and radiographic testing is less clear. The use of molecular testing to predict sensitivity to specific compounds has become the recommended approach for patients with the most aggressive forms of thyroid cancer, and with more specific compounds being developed, this will likely evolve over time.

REFERENCES

For a complete list of references, go to expertconsult.com.

19

Papillary Thyroid Cancer

Jennifer A. Sipos, Bryan R. Haugen

INTRODUCTION

Classic papillary thyroid cancer (PTC) tends to have an indolent clinical course with low morbidity and mortality. Nonetheless, this disease has a wide spectrum of biologic and clinical behavior that can result in tumor recurrence and death, depending on patient and tumor features and the initial approach to management. The incidence of thyroid cancer is on the rise and though the reasons for this trend remain elusive, it is clear that the majority of the new diagnoses are low-risk tumors. This chapter summarizes the epidemiology and the potential etiologic factors that may be responsible for this trend. Although most tumors have a low-risk profile, it is incumbent upon the clinician to remain cognizant of the potential for a more aggressive cancer (see Chapter 17, Differentiated Thyroid Cancer Incidence). Accordingly, this chapter also explores the various prognostic factors that may shape the risk for recurrent disease and disease-specific mortality. In addition, the initial treatment strategy of PTC, with an emphasis on the effects of therapy on long-term outcomes, is explored. Finally, this chapter will discuss the long-term surveillance to identify recurrent or residual disease.

EPIDEMIOLOGY

Changing Thyroid Cancer Incidence

The incidence of thyroid cancer in the United States has tripled over the past three decades, the majority of which is due to small papillary thyroid carcinomas.[1] This trend has also been noted in many other countries across Europe, Asia, Oceania, and South America.[2,3] The incidence is rising in both genders[4] and across all age groups,[5] including children and adolescents.[6] Fortunately, in the United States, the incidence rates may be stabilizing, though it remains to be seen if the plateau will persist[7] (Figure 19.1).

Although the incidence of thyroid cancer has risen in recent times, PTC remains a relatively rare tumor, representing only 3.1% of all new cancer cases. It is estimated that 56,870 new cases were diagnosed in 2017, and 2010 deaths were attributed to thyroid cancer during this period.[8] In spite of the recent upward trend in thyroid cancer incidence, mortality rates remain stable, suggesting a significant proportion of new cases represent overdiagnosis.[1] Indeed, there is a large reservoir of undiagnosed disease with thyroid cancer identified in up to 36% of cases of autopsy studies, a prevalence that is more than 1000-fold higher than the rates of disease that are clinically diagnosed in the general population (Figure 19.2).[9] Further support of the role of increased diagnostic scrutiny in the uptrend is revealed by the numbers of small cancers detected: 87% of newly diagnosed cancers are 2 cm or smaller and 49% are <1 cm.[10] However, it should be noted that several studies have determined that thyroid cancers of all sizes are on the rise,[11,12] suggesting that overdiagnosis is not solely to blame for increased incidence (see Chapter 17, Differentiated Thyroid Cancer Incidence).

FACTORS THAT MAY CONTRIBUTE TO THYROID CANCER RISK

Exposure to Radiation

Exposure to ionizing radiation during childhood has been the most extensively studied causative factor in the development of thyroid cancer. Factors that increase the risk for developing PTC after radiation exposure include female gender, radiation for childhood cancer (rather than benign conditions), and a family history of thyroid cancer.[13,14] In one study, younger age at exposure and dose of radiation administered significantly influenced the risk of development of cancer.[15]

Polybrominated Diphenyl Ethers

Some have proposed a potential role of polybrominated diphenyl ethers (PBDEs) in the development of thyroid cancer.[16] These ubiquitous flame retardants may be found in plastics, electrical appliances, televisions, computers, building supplies, foams, carpets, and upholstery.[17] PBDEs and their metabolites may accumulate in human tissues and bear a striking structural similarity to thyroxine.[16] These compounds have been shown to be potent endocrine disrupters, with thyroid and estrogen effects being the most common.[17] Although there has been no direct link between an increased risk of thyroid cancer and PBDEs, their increased oncogenic potential in other tissues[18,19] has made them an attractive candidate for further study in thyroid cancer.[16]

Obesity

Obesity and overweight were linked to nearly 18% of all cancer cases and 16% of cancer deaths in 2014.[20] Several studies have identified a significantly higher risk of thyroid cancer in overweight and obese patients.[21-23] The inflection point in the incidence of thyroid cancer occurred in the mid-1970s; there was a similar change in the trend for obesity rates in the United States just a few years prior.[24] Over time the slopes of these two conditions have remained nearly parallel.[24] Consequently, some have posited a potential causal relationship,[25] although the mechanism is elusive.

Obesity affects the secretion of adipokines by adipose tissue, including increased leptin and decreased adiponectin.[26] Through complex molecular signaling, these adipokines interact with key factors in carcinogenesis, including cell proliferation, angiogenesis, and antiinflammatory cytokines.[27,28] Further studies are necessary to delineate the role of obesity in the development of thyroid cancer, particularly as the incidence of obesity continues to climb throughout Europe, North America, and Asia.

CHAPTER 19 Papillary Thyroid Cancer

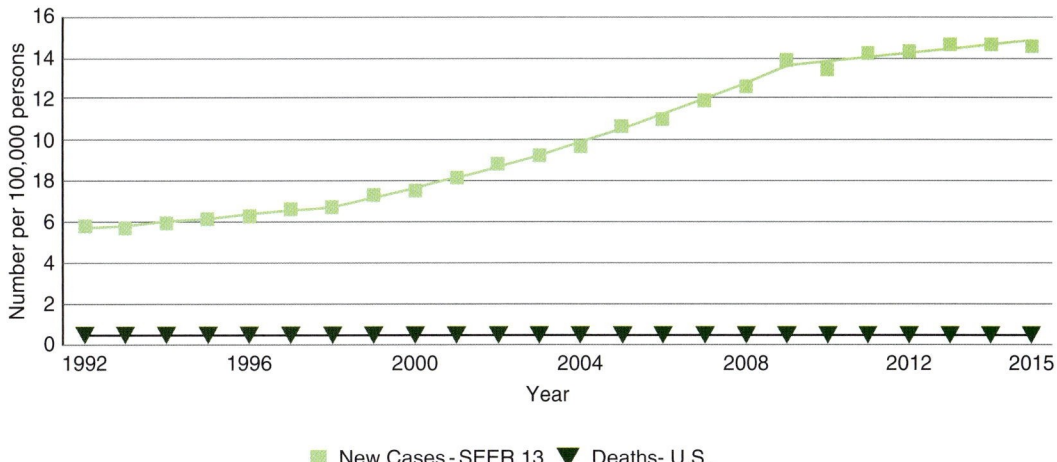

Fig. 19.1 Rising incidence of new thyroid cancer diagnosis in the United States from 1992 to 2015 (light green line). The number of deaths over this same time frame (dark green line). (From National Cancer Institute; Surveillance, Epidemiology, and End Results Program. Cancer stat facts: thyroid cancer. Available at Seer.cancer.gov/statfacts/html/thyro.html. Accessed January 24, 2019.)

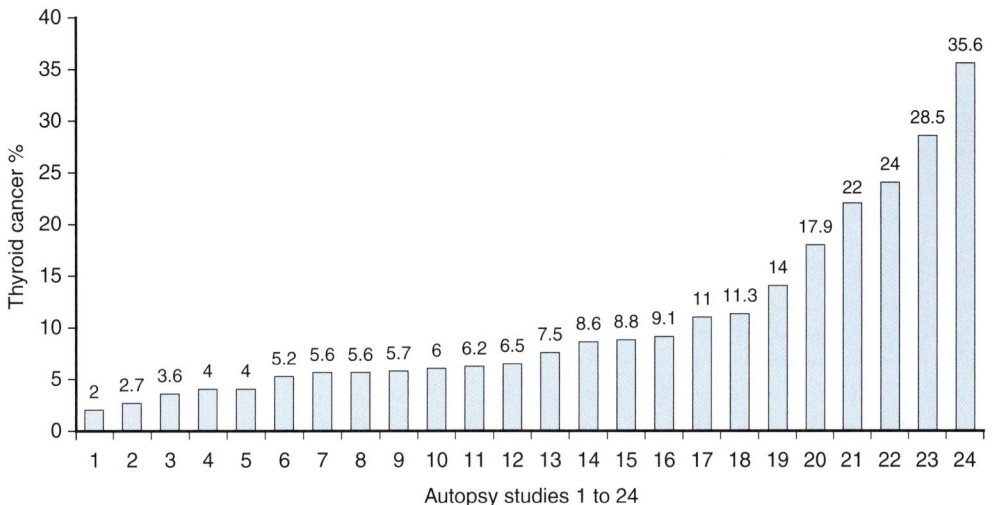

Fig. 19.2 The prevalence of occult incidental thyroid cancer in 24 different autopsy cases. (Data from Pazaitou-Panayiotou K, Capezzone M, Pacini F. Clinical features and therapeutic implication of papillary thyroid microcarcinoma. *Thyroid.* 2007;17[11]:1085–1092.)

Hereditary Syndromes

The majority of thyroid cancers are sporadic; however, approximately 5% of nonmedullary thyroid cancers are hereditary.[29] These hereditary cases have been divided into two groups: those tumors associated with a familial cancer syndrome, such as familial adenomatous polyposis, Gardner syndrome, Cowden disease, Carney complex type 1, or Werner syndrome; and those with thyroid tumors as the primary feature, such as familial nonmedullary thyroid cancer (see Chapter 30, Familial Nonmedullary Thyroid Cancer).

FACTORS INFLUENCING PROGNOSIS

Tumor Histology

Numerous histologic variants of PTC have been described based on architectural or cellular features. Acknowledgement of the tumor subtype is important, as it can contribute to the risk stratification of individual tumors.[30] The classic variant of PTC and the follicular variant of PTC (FVPTC) are associated with very favorable outcomes.[31-33] More concerning histologic subtypes include tall cell,[34,35] hobnail variants,[36] and, perhaps to a lesser extent, columnar cell;[37] these tumors tend to present at an older age and with more advanced disease than is seen in classic PTC (see Chapter 41, Surgical Pathology of the Thyroid Gland). These more aggressive histologic variants also are associated with worse recurrence-free and disease-specific survival rates.[37-39]

Tumor Size

Primary tumor size is closely associated with the outcome of PTC, including both 10-year recurrence and cancer-specific mortality rates.[40] Cancer-specific mortality rates increase incrementally from 2% for tumors <1 cm to 19% for tumors >8 cm.[40,41] Furthermore, larger tumors are associated with a higher rate of locoregional and distant metastases.[41]

Multifocality

Patients with PTC have a 32% to 45% chance of cancer elsewhere in the ipsilateral or contralateral lobe.[42,43] Tumor multifocality is also found frequently in papillary thyroid microcarcinomas (PMCs).[44] Multifocal disease increases the risk of recurrence, particularly in patients who have had a lobectomy.[43-45] With the current trend to performing lobectomy for the majority of low-risk cancers, some have raised concerns about the potential for increased recurrence rates.[46] Indeed, some patients may develop recurrence in the remaining contralateral lobe, necessitating completion thyroidectomy at a later date. Fortunately, it is the minority (7% at 10 years of follow-up) of patients who will require such an intervention.[47] A large, long-term follow-up study of patients undergoing lobectomy for PTC, 14.6% of whom had multifocal disease, demonstrated a recurrence-free 20-year survival rate of 95% in the opposite lobe, 91% for lymph node (LN) recurrence, and a disease-specific survival rate of 97.8%.[48] Predictors of recurrence or worse disease-specific survival were age, primary tumor >4 cm, and clinically apparent LNs, suggesting that properly selected patients will have an excellent prognosis after lobectomy of PTC.

The implications of tumor multifocality on survival are controversial. Some studies have determined that multifocal disease does not increase the risk of disease-specific mortality.[43,49] However, when distinguishing unilateral multifocal from bilateral disease, other studies have demonstrated that survival was lower for bilateral tumors.[50,51]

Extrathyroidal Extension

Extrathyroidal extension (ETE) of tumor beyond the thyroid capsule into the perithyroidal soft tissues and adjacent structures may be seen in up to 40% of surgical specimens and is an important prognostic factor in PTC.[52] The specific extent of ETE should be described on the surgical pathology report. Minimal ETE is defined as microscopic visualization of tumor into the immediate perithyroidal soft tissues. In contrast, extensive ETE is described as gross tumor extension into subcutaneous soft tissues, larynx, trachea, esophagus, or the recurrent laryngeal nerve (RLN).[30] The prognostic implications of ETE in differentiated thyroid cancer is controversial, which may stem largely from a failure to distinguish between these distinct degrees of tumor spread.[53] It is generally accepted that tumor extension into the surrounding tissues, which is visible intraoperatively or on preoperative imaging, is associated with a worse prognosis.[52-54] The implications of minimal ETE on outcomes, however, is less clear. Some retrospective studies have demonstrated that minimal ETE is associated with higher rates of LN metastases[55-58]; other studies found recurrence rates in those with minimal ETE were dependent on primary tumor size.[59] In contrast others have found that minimal ETE is not associated with increased recurrence or decreased survival.[60,61] A recent systematic review and meta-analysis of the effects of minimal ETE on survival and recurrence demonstrated no influence of minimal ETE on disease-related mortality but did indicate an increased risk of recurrence in patients with minimal ETE.[62] The absolute recurrence risk increase for patients with lymph node negative disease was from 2.2% to 3.5% and for patients with lymph node positive disease the increase was from 6.2% to 7%, suggesting that the effects of minimal ETE on absolute risk for disease recurrence was small. Indeed, the 8th edition of The American Joint Committee on Cancer/The Tumor, Node, and Metastases (AJCC/TNM) cancer staging system removed the minimal ETE definition and its influence on overall tumor stage.[63,64] This omission is an acknowledgment of the negligible effects of minimal ETE on tumor-associated mortality.[64]

Lymph Node Metastases

The incidence rates of cervical LN metastases identified at the time of initial surgery in patients with PTC varies widely, depending on the mode of nodal detection. Prophylactic LN dissections yield high rates of LN micrometastases (up to 65%),[65,66] whereas gross nodal involvement detected by preoperative US or during surgery occurs in a smaller, but still substantial, percentage (~20%) of patients.[67] The manner of discovery is important as it is related to the prognostic significance of nodal involvement. Those nodes incidentally identified on surgical pathology with microscopic tumor deposits do not significantly alter risk of recurrence.[68] Prophylactic nodal dissection, therefore, is not recommended as it does not lower recurrence-free survival and risks upstaging patients, resulting in unnecessary additional treatment.[30] In contrast, grossly abnormal nodes are associated with a worse recurrence-free survival[69]; removal of these nodes is thus considered therapeutic.[30]

The number of involved nodes is also related to the recurrence risk. Even with microscopic nodal deposits, more than five involved nodes carries a higher risk of recurrence compared with lower numbers of diseased nodes, 7% to 21%[56,70,71] and 3% to 8%,[56,71] respectively.

The effects of LN metastases on survival is less clear; there are conflicting reports regarding cancer-specific mortality in the presence of nodal involvement.[72,73] An analysis of the Surveillance, Epidemiology, and End Results (SEER) database determined that nodal metastases were associated with increased mortality only in those patients over the age of 45 years.[74] However, a more recent study of patients from the SEER database and the National Cancer Database (NCDB) of patients under the age of 45 years found that increasing numbers of nodal metastases were associated with decreasing overall survival up to six nodes, after which more metastatic nodes conferred no additional mortality risk.[75]

Distant Metastases

Although distant metastases are uncommon in PTC, they are present in approximately 5% of patients at the time of initial diagnosis, and another 2.5% to 5% will develop distant metastases after initial therapy.[76] The most common sites of involvement are lung (50%) and bone (25%), followed by both lung and bone (20%) and other tumor sites (5%).[76,77] One study found a 50% survival rate of 3.5 years.[78] However, subsets of patients have better survival rates, especially postpubertal children, those with microscopic metastases, and patients with iodine-avid tumors.[77,78] Additional prognostic information about distant metastases may be gained by performing 2-[^{18}F]fluoro-2-deoxy-D-glucose-positron emission tomography (^{18}FDG-PET)/computed tomography (CT) scanning. One study found an inverse relationship between survival and degree of ^{18}FDG-PET avidity of the most active lesion as well as the number of (^{18}FDG-PET)–avid lesions. Patients with a positive ^{18}FDG-PET scan had a 7.28-fold increased risk of dying from thyroid cancer compared with patients who had a negative scan.[79]

Oncogenes

The MAPK (mitogen-activated protein kinase) pathway is an intracellular signaling cascade that results in cell growth, proliferation, and apoptosis. A mutation in one of these signaling components in the MAPK pathway is responsible for the majority of PTCs. These mutations are almost always mutually exclusive, suggesting that a single molecular alteration is sufficient to drive oncogenesis.[80] Detection of these mutations may be used to identify malignancy on fine-needle aspiration (FNA), to prognosticate for patients with thyroid cancer, or to guide the systemic agent used in radioiodine-refractory disease.

BRAF

BRAF is a serine/threonine kinase in the MAPK signaling pathway that regulates cellular differentiation, proliferation, and survival. The *BRAF V600E* pathogenic variant is the most common oncogene in sporadic PTC, with an incidence of 36% to 69%.[81] The presence of *BRAF V600E* is associated with higher risk clinic-pathologic features, including LN metastases, ETE, recurrence, and age-associated mortality.[82,83]

The independent prognostic utility of a *BRAF* mutation remains in question, however. With such a high prevalence of this pathogenic variant and the excellent outcomes in the majority of thyroid cancer patients, the specificity of *BRAF* for prognostication is limited. Further, because *BRAF* is often associated with high-risk clinical features, it is difficult to discern what component of the poor outcomes seen with this pathogenic variant are due to the mutation itself, independent of the pathologic elements.[30] Indeed several studies attempting to determine whether *BRAF* serves as an independent predictor of recurrence have produced mixed results.[82,84-87] The identification of a *BRAF* mutation instead may provide direction for the management of radioiodine refractory tumors. A recent clinical trial aimed at redifferentiating noniodine-avid tumors used a BRAF-inhibitor, dabrafenib; 60% of patients exhibited new iodine uptake on diagnostic whole-body scans. After treatment with 5GBq of ^{88}I at 3 months of follow-up, two patients had partial responses and four had stable disease.[89] An ongoing trial is examining the effect of dabrafenib alone or in combination with a MEK inhibitor, trametinib, in progressive, iodine-refractory, BRAF-mutated tumors (clinicaltrials.gov, NCT01723202).

TERT

Newly described in thyroid cancers,[90,91] telomerase reverse transcriptase (*TERT*) promoter mutations are found in low frequency in lower risk PTC (9%), with increasing frequency in more advanced PTC (51%), PDTC (40%), and ATC (54% to 73%).[92-94] Telomerase is responsible for adding tandem repeats of the TTAAGGG sequence to the end of chromosomes to maintain genome stability.[95] Whereas these enzymes are highly expressed in germline and stem cells, expression is reduced or even repressed in somatic cells. The loss of telomeres during somatic cell division results in cells entering senescence.[96] Reactivation of telomerase leads to immortalization by way of unrestricted proliferation and inactivation of replicative senescence.[97]

Although there are conflicting reports[98-101] regarding the effect of a *TERT* mutation on prognosis in PTC, a recent meta-analysis demonstrated that the presence of coexisting *BRAF* and *TERT* mutations was associated with a more aggressive clinical course[102] and another study demonstrated higher mortality rates.[103] Further study is needed to determine the feasibility of pharmacologic therapy targeting *TERT* mutations (see Chapter 18, Molecular Pathogenesis of Thyroid Neoplasia).

Age at Diagnosis

Age at the time of tumor diagnosis is one of the most important contributing factors to prognosis;[41] there is a trend of worsening cause-specific survival for each decade starting at age 60 compared with younger patients (<20 years old).[104] An analysis of the NCDB revealed an incremental increase in 10-year mortality by 30% to 50% per 5 year increment beginning at age 35 years.[105] A recent study determined that the age-associated increasing risk of mortality was associated with BRAF mutational status. This multiinstitutional study found that age is a strong, continuous, and independent mortality risk factor in patients with a *BRAF V600E* mutation but not in those with wild-type BRAF.[83] Older patients are also more likely to harbor more aggressive histologic variants.[106] In patients with distant metastases, those over the age of 40 years are less likely to demonstrate iodine avidity in their lung metastases.[107]

Children and adolescents are more likely to have a more advanced tumor stage at the time of diagnosis; up to 80% harbor nodal involvement and 15% to 20% develop pulmonary metastases rates that are nearly double those seen in adults.[108] Despite the extent of disease at the time of diagnosis, children generally have excellent outcomes. In one systematic review of pediatric patients with pulmonary metastases, a complete response to radioactive iodine (RAI) therapy was seen in up to 50% and disease-specific mortality was 2.7%.[109]

INITIAL TREATMENT OF PAPILLARY THYROID CANCER

Preoperative Imaging

Before removal of thyroid cancer, it is critical to perform a thorough evaluation to determine the extent of disease. Preoperative imaging should include a comprehensive ultrasound (US) of the neck to examine the contralateral lobe of the thyroid, the central neck compartments, and the lateral neck LNs.[30] Such imaging may change the surgical approach in up to 40% of cases.[110,111]

The anterior neck is divided into seven contiguous compartments in which thyroid cancer metastatic LN spread occurs (Figure 19.3). The central neck compartment (level VI) contains the thyroid and poses the greatest challenge to clinicians when deciding the optimal surgery. It is bordered laterally by the carotid arteries, inferiorly by the clavicles, and superiorly by the hyoid bone. Level VI is the compartment that is most frequently involved with LN metastases, but sonographic identification of diseased nodes is hampered by poor preoperative sensitivity. The intact thyroid gland obscures visualization of the majority of nodal metastases.[112]

The lateral neck is further subdivided into four compartments lateral to the carotid. Level IV is bordered laterally by the sternocleidomastoid (SCM), inferiorly by the clavicle, and superiorly by the cricoid cartilage. Level III, located immediately cephalad to level IV, extends superiorly to the carotid bifurcation. Level II is located below the mandible and extends to the hyoid bone. Level V nodes are located in the posterior triangle, lateral to the lateral edge of the SCM.

The presence of malignancy in sonographically suspicious nodes can be confirmed with FNA for cytologic analysis and measurement of thyroglobulin (Tg) in the needle washout.[113,114] If advanced, bulky nodal disease is identified on US, or the patient has clinical signs or symptoms of advanced disease (hoarseness, hemoptysis, a nonmobile thyroid mass), CT or magnetic resonance imaging (MRI) of the neck

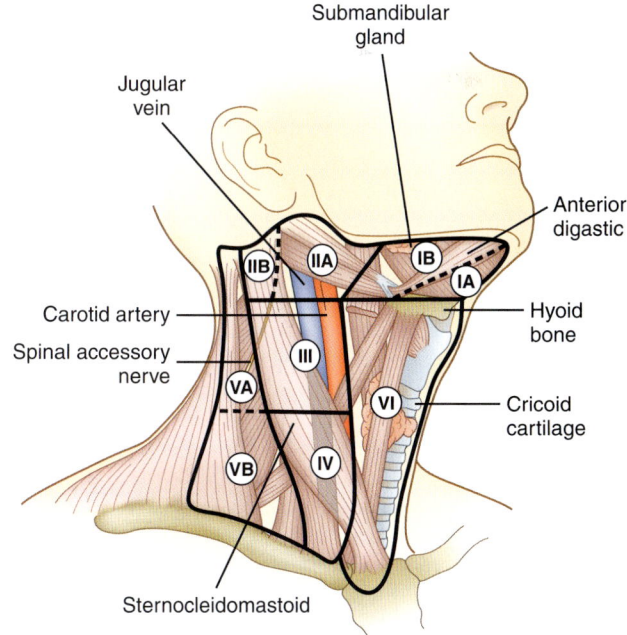

Fig. 19.3 Lymph node compartments separated into levels and sublevels. (From Smith PW, Hanks LR, Salomone LJ, Hanks JB. Thyroid. In: Townsend CM, Beauchamp RD, Evers BM, Mattox KL, eds. *Sabiston Textbook of Surgery: The Biological Basis of Modern Surgical Practice*. 20th ed. Philadelphia: Elsevier; 2017:880–922.)

may be considered to search for additional metastases in areas that cannot be visualized sonographically, including within the mediastinum, at the skull base, and posterior to the trachea.[30]

Initial Thyroid Surgery

Surgery is the initial treatment for most thyroid cancers and is often curative for those with low-risk disease. Historically, the majority of cancers measuring >1 cm were recommended for total thyroidectomy to facilitate surveillance, allow for radioiodine therapy, and reduce the likelihood of recurrence.[115] Newer data, however, has cast doubt on the necessity of removal of the entire gland. The recent trend to the use of less radioiodine therapy has obviated the need to perform total thyroidectomy in many patients with low-risk thyroid cancer.[30] Further strengthening the argument for less extensive surgery is the recognition that the risk of complications with total thyroidectomy is double that seen in lobectomy, regardless of the surgeon's experience level.[116] Most importantly, multiple retrospective studies have revealed that outcomes are equivalent in patients with low-risk disease treated with lobectomy compared with total thyroidectomy when controlled for tumor size and extent of disease.[117-120]

Those tumors measuring <1 cm and lacking metastatic disease or ETE may be treated with lobectomy alone.[30] If there are concerns for cancer in the contralateral lobe, a history of head and neck radiation exposure or a strong family history of thyroid cancer, total thyroidectomy may be appropriate management.[30] Tumors measuring 1 to 4 cm and lacking ETE and metastatic LNs may be treated with lobectomy or total thyroidectomy. The decision to pursue more extensive surgery should include consideration of tumor histology, the potential for contralateral lobe malignancy, presence of abnormal nodes, desire for postoperative radioiodine therapy, and patient preference. Those tumors measuring >4 cm or with preoperative evidence of nodal involvement or ETE, regardless of size, should proceed with total thyroidectomy.[30]

Completion Thyroidectomy

Removal of the contralateral lobe of the thyroid may be necessary after lobectomy, particularly if total thyroidectomy would have been recommended had the diagnosis been known preoperatively.[30] With lobectomy being sufficient therapy for the majority of low-risk cancers, the need for completion thyroidectomy is diminishing.[121] However, in the hands of an experienced surgeon, the complication rates for completion thyroidectomy are comparable to those of total/near total thyroidectomy.[122] The use of RAI therapy to ablate the remaining tissue after lobectomy is not recommended routinely but may be considered in select cases when additional surgery is not feasible.[30]

Lymph Node Dissection

PTC has a high predilection for spread to locoregional LNs, occurring in up to 40% to 90% of cases when prophylactic nodal dissection is performed.[68,123] Though such high rates of metastatic disease may prove enticing to recommend routine prophylactic node dissection, recurrence-free survival is not effected by the removal of sonographically normal, microscopically diseased nodes.[68,124] Instead, prophylactic central neck dissection may be individually considered for those patients with T3 or T4 tumors, or in the presence of lateral neck metastases.[30] Clinically suspicious or biopsy-proven nodal disease warrants a "therapeutic" dissection of the involved compartments. "Berry picking," or selective removal of suspicious LN metastases, is not recommended, as it is associated with significantly higher recurrence rates and does not lower the rate of postoperative complications compared with systematic compartmental dissections.[30,125]

The risk of surgical complications with nodal dissection should be weighed against the benefit of LN removal. Central neck dissections may result in temporary or permanent injury to the RLN and hypoparathyroidism.[126,127] Surgeon case volume predicts patient outcomes; those performing less than 10 cases compared with those performing more than 100 cases per year had complications in 24% and 14.5% of cases, respectively.[116,128] Although dissection of the lateral neck is less often associated with adverse events, injury to the spinal accessory nerve may occur with dissection of level II or V.[129] Similarly, chyle leaks may be seen after removal of nodes in level IV, particularly on the left side (see Chapter 42, Pathophysiology of Recurrent Laryngeal Nerve Injury; Chapter 43, Management of Recurrent Laryngeal Nerve Paralysis; and Chapter 44, Non-Neural Complications of Thyroid and Parathyroid Surgery).[130,131]

Indications for Radioactive Iodine Therapy

There are three main indications for postoperative iodine-131 (131I) use: to treat any known (or unknown) residual disease, to reduce the risk of recurrence, and to destroy remaining noncancerous thyroid cells. This last indication, called *remnant ablation*, improves the sensitivity of serum Tg and may also be used as a staging tool to identify previously undiagnosed tumors (see Chapter 48, Postoperative Radioactive Iodine Ablation and Treatment of Differentiated Thyroid Cancer).

The use of RAI therapy is a contentious issue with conflicting findings regarding recurrence and survival benefit, largely stemming from the lack of prospective, randomized, and controlled trials. The patients for whom RAI may be beneficial can be clarified based on the initial risk stratification of the individual tumor (Table 19.1) and the postoperative disease status.[30] Studies have consistently shown that patients with American Thyroid Association (ATA) low-risk tumors measuring ≤1 cm lacking nodal and distant metastases do not benefit from RAI therapy, and its use is not recommended.[30] Additionally, low-risk tumors measuring 1 to 4 cm lacking local or distant metastases with complete tumor resection and no tumor invasion into the locoregional tissues or structures do not derive mortality benefit from adjuvant RAI therapy.[88,132,133] As such, RAI therapy should not be routinely used in this group unless there is an aggressive histology or evidence of vascular invasion.[30] In contrast, RAI does appear to be beneficial in terms of mortality and disease-free survival for those patients with a high-risk tumor[132,134,135]; its use is routinely recommended in the postoperative management of these patients.[30] For the remaining patients, including those with intermediate risk for recurrence, there is conflicting data regarding the benefits of therapy. Use of RAI in this cohort of patients should be considered on a case-by-case basis[30] (see Chapter 48, Postoperative Radioactive Iodine Ablation and Treatment of Differentiated Thyroid Cancer).

RESPONSE TO THERAPY

Excellent Response

Patients with no biochemical (unstimulated serum thyroglobulin (Tg) < 0.2 or stimulated Tg < 1.0 ng/mL) or radiographic evidence of disease are classified as having an excellent response to therapy[30] (see Table 19.2 and Chapter 24, Dynamic Risk Group Analysis and Staging for Differentiated Thyroid Cancer). Patients with an initial low to intermediate risk of recurrence who meet these criteria are recommended to have serum Tg monitored every 12 to 24 months. Patients with initially high-risk disease should continue to have a serum Tg measurement at least every 6 to 12 months.[30]

Biochemical Incomplete Response

Patients who have undergone total thyroidectomy and remnant ablation and have an unstimulated serum Tg > 1 ng/mL or a stimulated

TABLE 19.1 Indications for RAI Therapy

ATA Risk Stage (TNM)	Description	RAI Improves Disease-Specific Survival?	RAI Improves Disease-Free Survival?	Postoperative RAI Indicated?
ATA low risk, T1a N0, Nx M0, Mx	Tumor ≤1 cm	No	No	No
ATA low risk, T1b, T2, N0, Nx, M0, Mx	Tumor 1-4 cm	No	Conflicting	Not routine—may be considered if aggressive histology or vascular invasion
ATA low to intermediate risk T3, N0, Nx, M0, Mx	Tumor >4 cm	Conflicting	Conflicting	Consider in the presence of other adverse features, including advancing age
ATA low to intermediate risk T3, N0, Nx, M0, Mx	Microscopic ETE, any size tumor	No	Conflicting	Consider based on risk of recurrent disease. Smaller tumors with ETE may not require RAI
ATA low to intermediate risk T1-3, N1a, M0, Mx	Central compartment node metastases	No except patients ≥45 years old	Conflicting	Generally favored due to slightly higher risk of persistent disease especially with increasing number of large nodes or ENE. Advanced age may also favor RAI use.
ATA low to intermediate risk T1-3, N1b, M0, Mx	Lateral or mediastinal node metastases	No except patients ≥45 years old	Conflicting	Generally favored due to higher risk of persistent disease especially with increasing number of clinically evident nodes or ENE. Advanced age may also favor RAI use.
ATA high risk T4, any N, any M	Any size, gross ETE	Yes	Yes	Yes
ATA high risk any T, any N, M1	Distant metastases	Yes	Yes	Yes

RAI, radioactive iodine, ATA, American Thyroid Association, TNM, The Tumor, Node, and Metastases scoring system, ETE, extrathyroidal extension, ENE, extranodal extension.
Modified from Haugen BR, Alexander EK, Bible KC, et al. 2015 American Thyroid Association management guidelines for adult patients with thyroid nodules and differentiated thyroid cancer: the American Thyroid Association Guidelines Task Force on Thyroid Nodules and Differentiated Thyroid Cancer. *Thyroid.* 2016;26(1):1–133.

TABLE 19.2 Response to Therapy Classification

Category	Clinical Description
Excellent response	No clinical, biochemical, or structural evidence of disease
Biochemical incomplete response	Abnormal Tg or rising TgAb levels in the absence of localizable disease
Structural incomplete response	Persistent or newly identified locoregional or distant metastases
Indeterminate response	Nonspecific biochemical or structural findings which cannot be confidently classified as either benign or malignant. This includes patients with stable or declining TgAb levels with definitive structural evidence of disease

Tg, thyroglobulin, TgAb, thyroglobulin antibody.
Modified from Haugen BR, Alexander EK, Bible KC, et al. 2015 American Thyroid Association management guidelines for adult patients with thyroid nodules and differentiated thyroid cancer: the American Thyroid Association Guidelines Task Force on Thyroid Nodules and Differentiated Thyroid Cancer. *Thyroid.* 2016;26(1):1–133.

Tg > 10 ng/mL or a rising thyroglobulin antibody (TgAb) titer with negative imaging are classified as having a biochemical incomplete response to therapy. Such patients should undergo imaging with sonography of the neck, and if the disease is unable to be located, cross-sectional imaging of the neck and chest should be performed. Serum Tg should be followed at least every 6 to 12 months.

Structural Incomplete Response

Those patients with structurally or functionally (on diagnostic whole-body scan [DxWBS] or ^{18}(FDG-PET) evident disease are classified as having a structural incomplete response to therapy.[30] Unfortunately, the majority of patients in this category will have persistent disease in spite of additional treatments.[136] Disease-specific death rates are high in this group, 11% with locoregional metastases, and 50% with distant metastases.[137,138]

Indeterminate Response

Patients with biochemical or structural findings that cannot be confidently classified as either excellent response or persistent disease are deemed as having an indeterminate response to therapy. Such patients may be carefully followed with biochemical testing and serial imaging to better delineate which category is ultimately appropriate. It is estimated that up to 20% of these patients will eventually develop conclusive evidence of disease requiring additional therapy.[30]

LONG-TERM MANAGEMENT AND SURVEILLANCE

Thyroid-Stimulating Hormone Suppression Therapy

Historically, almost all patients were given thyroid hormone to fully suppress serum thyroid-stimulating hormone (TSH). The rationale for this approach was based on the theory that TSH is a stimulant for thyroid cell proliferation and suppression of thyrotropin will inhibit tumor growth.[41] Indeed, early studies supported the role of TSH suppression in reducing the likelihood of disease progression and improving survival, particularly in those with high-risk disease.[41,132] More recent analyses, however, have failed to demonstrate a benefit of such suppressive therapy in those with low-risk tumors.[139-141] In fact, such

TABLE 19.3 Target TSH Ranges Based on Response to Therapy and Individual Risk for Comorbidity

Increasing Risk of TSH Suppression	Excellent	Indeterminate	Biochemical Incomplete	Structural Incomplete
No known risk	0.5–2 mU/L	0.1–0.5 mU/L	<0.1 mU/L	<0.1 mU/L
Menopause	0.5–2 mU/L	0.1–0.5 mU/L	0.1–0.5 mU/L	<0.1 mU/L
Tachycardia	0.5–2 mU/L	0.1–0.5 mU/L	0.1–0.5 mU/L	<0.1 mU/L
Osteopenia	0.5–2 mU/L	0.1–0.5 mU/L	0.1–0.5 mU/L	<0.1 mU/L
Age >60	0.5–2 mU/L	0.5–2 mU/L	0.1–0.5 mU/L	<0.1 mU/L
Osteoporosis	0.5–2 mU/L	0.5–2 mU/L	0.1–0.5 mU/L	<0.1 mU/L
Atrial fibrillation	0.5–2 mU/L	0.5–2 mU/L	0.5–2 mU/L	0.1–0.5 mU/L

TSH, thyroid-stimulating hormone.
Data from Haugen BR, Alexander EK, Bible KC, et al. 2015 American Thyroid Association management guidelines for adult patients with thyroid nodules and differentiated thyroid cancer: the American Thyroid Association Guidelines Task Force on Thyroid Nodules and Differentiated Thyroid Cancer. *Thyroid*. 2016;26(1):1–133.

treatment may prove harmful. A long-term observational study showed a three-fold increased risk of cardiovascular death for each ten-fold reduction in mean TSH level.[142] Patients with subclinical thyrotoxicosis are also at increased risk of atrial fibrillation, ventricular hypertrophy, diastolic dysfunction, and impaired cardiac reserve.[143-145] Additionally, bone turnover may be adversely affected by suppressive doses of levothyroxine.[146] Higher rates of osteoporosis may be seen in thyroid cancer patients[147]; there is an increased risk of fracture when suppressive doses of levothyroxine are used.[144,148,149]

As a consequence of the myriad negative effects of excess levothyroxine, the target TSH range should be determined on an individual basis. It is also worthy of note that lowering TSH to undetectable levels probably does not confer additional benefit beyond that seen with less aggressive suppression below 0.1 mU/L.[140] The optimal TSH range should consider the initial risk for recurrence, the response to therapy, and the risk for thyrotoxicosis-related morbidities in the individual patient (Table 19.3). Furthermore, this target TSH for the individual patient may evolve over time, depending on the response to therapy.[30]

Serum Thyroglobulin

Serum thyroglobulin, a thyroid-specific protein, is measured at routine intervals to detect recurrence of thyroid carcinoma. A rising Tg suggests disease progression, whereas declining values generally provides reassurance of a favorable response to therapy.[150] If detectable, Tg should be measured at the same laboratory each time to analyze the trend in values accurately; there may be as much as a two-fold difference in concentration between assays.[151,152] Furthermore, TgAb levels also should be measured concomitantly as the presence of these antibodies may falsely lower the Tg.[150] A serum TSH also should be measured at the same time of the Tg; there is a direct relationship between serum TSH and Tg levels.

The appropriate intervals for measurement of serum Tg and TgAb during follow-up of thyroid cancer should be based on the initial risk for recurrence and response to therapy.[30] The doubling time of the Tg may also affect the frequency of measurement.[153-155]

As the trend to a less aggressive initial surgery continues to develop, the issue of using serum Tg as a tumor marker moves to the forefront. The optimal Tg value for those patients who have had a less than total thyroidectomy or total thyroidectomy without RAI has not been clearly defined and ascertainment of freedom from disease may be challenging. Recent studies suggest, however, that an unstimulated Tg <0.2 ng/mL or stimulated <2 ng/mL is evidence of an excellent response to therapy for those who have undergone total thyroidectomy without ablation.[156,157] After lobectomy alone, the unstimulated Tg may be significantly higher and is much less sensitive and specific for detection of recurrence, though a value less than 30 ng/mL has been proposed as a threshold for evidence of freedom from disease.[156] Others have questioned the utility of Tg as a tumor marker after lobectomy. Serum concentrations may rise by as much as 10% per year in the absence of disease; when comparing the change in Tg levels over time in those patients with and without recurrence, there was no significant difference.[158] Further study is needed to clarify the optimal management approach for this growing segment of the thyroid cancer population.

An additional challenge in the use of serum Tg is the dedifferentiation of tumors and the subsequent decline in Tg production. In these patients, Tg concentration does not correlate with disease burden. Periodic imaging thus assumes the central role for identification of disease progression.

TgAbs may be present in up to 20% to 25% of thyroid cancer patients,[150] significantly higher than the 10% incidence seen in the general population.[159] TgAbs are more commonly seen in those with lymphocytic thyroiditis.[160] There is significant discordance between assays and the detection of TgAbs, largely stemming from differences in detected epitopes between assays.[161] Because TgAbs can falsely lower serum Tg, undetectable levels of Tg in an antibody-positive patient pose a significant challenge. Serial measurement of the TgAb titer can provide insight into the disease status however. A rising TgAb titer is suggestive of disease progression or recurrence, whereas a declining value may be indicative of reduced tumor burden or absence of disease.[162]

Stimulation Testing

Tg increases with a rise in TSH. This relationship may be used to provide a highly sensitive means of detecting recurrent/residual disease. Once a patient has undetectable Tg and TgAb levels while on levothyroxine therapy, some clinicians opt to perform stimulation testing by raising the serum TSH and subsequently measuring the serum Tg. Stimulation may be achieved either by stopping levothyroxine therapy for 4 to 6 weeks or by injection of recombinant human TSH (rhTSH). A stimulated Tg value of <1 ng/mL in the absence of radiographic evidence of disease has a 98% to 99.5% likelihood of identifying patients completely free of disease.[30,163,164] A highly sensitive Tg assay with a functional sensitivity of 0.1 to 0.2 ng/mL essentially obviates the need for stimulation testing in low- and intermediate-risk patients as the likelihood of identifying clinically significant disease is very low.[165] It should be noted that there is a risk of a false-positive result with stimulation tests, leading to additional unnecessary testing and potentially, treatment.[166]

Imaging

Ultrasound

Postoperative US of the neck is a critical component of the long-term surveillance of thyroid cancer patients, as it is a highly sensitive modality for the detection of recurrent or persistent disease in the thyroid bed and cervical LNs. A comprehensive neck US is typically performed 6 to 12 months after surgery and periodically thereafter, depending on the patient's response to therapy and risk for recurrent disease.[30] A detailed description of sonographically suspicious nodes can be found in Chapter 14, Preoperative Radiographic Mapping of Nodal Disease for Papillary Thyroid Carcinoma.

A suspicious LN identified by US may be followed with serial examinations if it is small (<8 mm in smallest dimension in the central neck and <10 mm in the lateral neck) and located in an area that poses minimal threat of harm if there is enlargement.[30] Larger nodes or those that are smaller yet pose a threat to a vital structure can be considered for aspiration and measurement of Tg in the needle washout.[30] Continued surveillance of small, suspicious nodes and indeterminate US findings is critical; the majority of small metastatic deposits in the neck demonstrate minimal growth or progression when followed for a median of 3.5 years.[167] The delay in removal of those lesions demonstrating progression does not appear to increase the likelihood of local complications or disease-related mortality.[167] There is a balance that must be weighed with performing enough US examinations to identify recurrent disease with performing too many that poses the risk of false-positive findings. One recent study found that there were false-positive US findings in up to 67% of patients with low-risk thyroid cancer when followed for up to 8 years. Of the two patients that demonstrated structural recurrence, one was correctly identified by serial Tg measurement. The authors concluded that in patients with low-risk thyroid cancer, US screening is substantially more likely to identify false-positive results than clinically significant structural disease recurrence.[168] Consequently, the clinician must determine, on an individual basis, the proper intervals for surveillance US examinations during the follow-up of papillary thyroid carcinoma, using the initial risk of recurrence and the trend and concentration of serum Tg.

Diagnostic Whole-Body Scan

Historically, the DxWBS was a cornerstone of the surveillance for recurrent/persistent disease in papillary thyroid carcinoma. Recent data demonstrates, however, that this imaging has a very low sensitivity for detection of disease. It is likewise plagued with false-positive findings.[169] Consequently, DxWBSs are typically not necessary in low-risk patients with an undetectable Tg and negative TgAb on thyroid hormone therapy and a negative cervical US.[30,170,171] In contrast, the patients for whom DxWBSs may prove beneficial include those with abnormal uptake outside the thyroid bed on posttherapy whole-body scan (WBS), those with TgAb, or those with large remnants and high uptake on the posttherapy WBS that may have hindered the visualization of uptake in metastatic nodal deposits.[30] When a DxWBS is deemed necessary, the use of single-photon emission computed tomography (SPECT)/CT radioiodine imaging improves the diagnostic accuracy compared with planar imaging alone.[172]

REFERENCES

For a complete list of references, go to expertconsult.com.

20

Papillary Thyroid Microcarcinoma

Douglas S. Ross

> Please go to expertconsult.com to view related video:
> **Video 20.1** Introduction to Chapter 20, Papillary Thyroid Microcarcinoma.

The World Health Organization (WHO) defines papillary thyroid cancers that are 10 mm or less in maximal diameter as *papillary microcarcinomas*.[1] These are frequently incidentally discovered lesions.[1] Previously, these lesions were called *occult papillary cancers* because they were primarily incidental findings at autopsy or after thyroidectomy. However, they are typically easily identified on high-resolution ultrasonography, which makes the occult terminology obsolete. As a result, the detection of micropapillary cancers has reached epidemic proportions, accounting for over 40% of the thyroid cancers excised in some centers.[2,3] Management of these small papillary cancers generally follows the same principles used to manage American Thyroid Association (ATA) low-risk papillary thyroid cancers.[4,5] Because of the increasing detection and high prevalence of papillary microcarcinomas, this chapter will focus on their natural history and response to therapy, and avoidance of overtreatment (see Chapter 19, Papillary Thyroid Cancer, and Chapter 24, Dynamic Risk Group Analysis and Staging for Differentiated Thyroid Cancer).

PREVALENCE: AUTOPSY SERIES AND INCIDENTAL FINDING AT THE TIME OF THYROID SURGERY

The high prevalence of papillary microcarcinoma has been appreciated from autopsy studies done before the emergence of high-resolution ultrasonography. In the United States, these studies have shown up to a 13% prevalence of micropapillary cancer,[6] whereas in other parts of the world, substantially higher prevalence rates have been noted. For example, in Finland the prevalence in one study was 36%, leading the authors of that study to conclude that the "smallest forms of occult papillary carcinoma of the thyroid are so common in Finland that they can be regarded as a normal finding."[7] The prevalence of micropapillary carcinoma in pathologic specimens is also highly dependent on how carefully one looks for it. In one Spanish study, the initial prevalence based on grossly visible lesions was 5.3%, but when each thyroid was cut into blocks and carefully examined histologically, the prevalence increased to 22%.[8] The prevalence of micropapillary carcinoma in some series was independent of age. For example, in Sweden the prevalence was approximately 7% for patients under age 50 or over age 80,[9] and in Wisconsin, in the United States, the prevalence was 3% in an autopsy study of young adults.[10] Micropapillary carcinoma is frequently an incidental finding at the time of thyroid surgery and has been reported in 2% to 50% of surgical specimens.[11,12]

CLINICAL INCIDENCE AND PREVALENCE

The Surveillance, Epidemiology, and End Results (SEER) database of the National Cancer Institute in the United States provides data that help define the present and predict the future prevalence of papillary microcarcinoma.[13] In 2018, the estimated incidence of new thyroid cancers was 53,990 per year and the measured prevalence of thyroid cancer (all thyroid cancers, not just papillary microcarcinoma) in 2015 was 765,547. Yet if we apply a conservative estimated figure of 6% for the prevalence of papillary carcinoma based on autopsy studies in the United States, the prevalence should be in excess of 18 million individuals. The annual incidence of thyroid cancer in the United States has been increasing, with the 2015 incidence from the SEER database of 15.03 per 100,000, compared with only 4.85 per 100,000 in 1975. In contrast, mortality from thyroid cancer has remained constant: 0.5 and 0.5 per 100,000 in 1975 and 2015, respectively. Although there is controversy as to whether the true incidence of thyroid cancer is increasing in the United States,[14] it is widely accepted that a major component of the increased thyroid cancer incidence is due to ascertainment bias from improved imaging, allowing us to more readily detect both papillary microcarcinomas as well as larger thyroid cancers. This is illustrated by the data from South Korea, where women were offered inexpensive ultrasonographic screening of their thyroid glands coincident with their annual mammograms, resulting in a 14-fold increase in the incidence of thyroid cancer over several years.[15] If indeed there are 18 million individuals with papillary cancer in the United States, we presently have detected about 4.3% of these cancers. With continued improvement in imaging and aggressive use of ultrasound-guided fine-needle aspiration (FNA) biopsy, it should not be a surprise that the annual incidence of thyroid cancer detection has increased by more than threefold since 1975. However, presumably due to guidelines which have recently focused on avoiding overdiagnosis and overtreatment, the annual increase in the rate of thyroid cancer detection peaked at 6.9% in the decade ending in 2009 and has recently fallen to 2.2% per year.[16]

Pathologic data from hospitals also demonstrate that a substantial portion of the increasing incidence of thyroid cancer is due to the detection of papillary microcarcinoma. At the Queen Elizabeth Hospital in Hong Kong, the percentage of papillary microcarcinomas in operative pathology specimens increased from 5.1% in the period from 1960 to 1980 to 21.7% in the period from 1991 to 2000.[17] Publications in 2006 from the University of Wisconsin in the United States and at the University of Ferrara in Italy reported that papillary microcarcinoma represented 43% and surgically excised thyroid cancers represented 40%, respectively.[2,3]

Therefore when reviewing data on the natural history of papillary microcarcinoma, it is important to understand that published series are reporting only on the 4.3% of cancers that have come to clinical attention for one reason or another, and that more recent publications are including higher percentages of incidental cancers that would have gone undetected previously.

CLINICAL SERIES OF PATIENTS WITH MICROPAPILLARY CANCER

There have been many published series of patients with papillary microcarcinoma from single institutions. The Mayo Clinic updated its series in 2008, which includes 900 patients with an average follow-up of 17.2 years (range of 6 to 89 years).[18] Twenty-three percent of the tumors were multifocal, 17% bilateral, 2% extrathyroidal, 30% had nodal involvement, and 0.3% had distant metastatic disease. Less than 25% were under 5 mm and more than a third were 9 to 10 mm. The 40-year cause-specific mortality was 0.7%—all three patients who died presented with lymphadenopathy, one had massive lymphadenopathy, and one had pulmonary metastases upon presentation. Recurrences occurred in 8% of patients, most in cervical nodes, but 1.5% occurred in the thyroid bed. Nodal recurrences occurred in 16% of patients with positive nodes at presentation and only 0.8% of patients without nodes at presentation. Recurrences occurred in 11% of patients with multifocal disease and 4% of patients with unifocal disease.

The Noguchi Thyroid Clinic in Japan also updated its series in 2008, which included 2070 patients with an average follow-up of 15 years.[19] Recurrences occurred in 3.5% of patients at a mean of 10.3 years. Distant metastases occurred in only 0.2% of patients. Recurrence was more likely in patients with larger tumors (greater than 5 mm), more nodes, and invasion (e.g., into the recurrent laryngeal nerve or esophagus), and less likely in patients with coexistent thyroid autoimmunity.

The series of 203 patients from the Queen Elizabeth Hospital in Hong Kong reports a 4.9% rate of nodal recurrence and a 1% rate of local recurrences.[20] Two patients developed pulmonary metastases (1%), and two patients died. The risk of nodal recurrence was increased 6.2-fold when nodes were present at presentation and 5.6-fold when the tumor was multifocal. The researchers did not find higher recurrence rates in tumors greater than 5 mm, but the larger papillary microcarcinomas were more likely to have extrathyroidal extension. Comparing papillary microcarcinomas with larger papillary cancers, there were similar rates of multifocality, but the larger papillary cancers were associated with higher rates of nodal metastases and nodal, local, and distant recurrences.

Recurrence occurred in 4.8% of 293 patients reported from South Korea after a median follow-up of 65 months; cervical nodes at presentation were associated with an increased risk of recurrence.[21] Recurrence occurred in 3.1% of 287 patients from Rome, Italy, and included two patients (0.7%) with distant metastases; multifocal disease, extrathyroidal extension, and a higher number of cervical nodes at presentation were risk factors for recurrence.[22]

Data from several series[3,18-27] demonstrate multifocality in 20% to 40% of patients, bilateral disease in 10% to 19% of patients, extrathyroidal invasion in 2% to 38% of patients, cervical nodal involvement in 17% to 43% of patients, and distant metastases in 0% to 3% of patients (Table 20.1). In one series of 671 patients from Seoul, Korea, 24% had central nodal involvement and 3.7% had lateral nodal involvement.[27]

In a meta-analysis of 17 studies that included 854 patients with incidentally discovered papillary microcarcinoma with 2669 nonincidental cases, the recurrence rates were 0.5% and 6.5%, respectively.[28]

OBSERVATIONAL DATA AND ACTIVE SURVEILLANCE

Important information regarding the natural history of micropapillary carcinoma has been obtained by the ongoing observational trials from Japan (see Chapter 21, Papillary Carcinoma Observation).[29] After excluding those patients with tumors adjacent to the trachea, posterior tumors that might be adjacent to the recurrent laryngeal nerve, tumors associated with lymph nodes, and those with high-grade histology, 1235 patients with biopsy-proven papillary microcarcinomas agreed to observation instead of surgical excision. In patients who were followed for a mean of 75 months (range of 18 to 227 months), 8.0% exhibited tumor growth of more than 3 mm after 10 years of observation (4.9% after 5 years of observation) and 3.8% developed lymphadenopathy (1.7% after 5 years). Ultimately, 191 patients opted for surgery (120 patients because of progression). Of the patients who had surgery after a period of observation, multifocality was present in 69%, 27% had central and 59% had lateral lymph nodes, 1% had minor extrathyroidal extension, and 1 patient had a subsequent recurrence in a thyroid remnant; no patient developed distant disease. Progression was more common in younger patients who were under age 40 years: 5.9% experienced growth and 5.3% lymphadenopathy, compared with 2.2% and 0.4%, respectively, in patients over age 60.

Because of these and similar data from Japan, active surveillance has become an acceptable alternative to immediate surgery for patients with papillary microcarcinoma. Early observational data from New York on 291 patients followed for a mean of 25 months (range of 6 to 166 months) reported that 3.8% of the tumors grew by 3 mm (12.1% after 5 years), but none developed lymphadenopathy.[30] Growth was more likely in younger patients.

Based on the data from Japan, the lifetime risk of progression (to age 85) was estimated to be 60% at age 20; 37% and 27% at ages 30 and 40, respectively; and 15%, 10%, and 3.5% at ages 50, 60, and 70, respectively.[31] The risk of growth during pregnancy was 8%.[32] Serum thyroid-stimulating hormone (TSH) levels greater than 2.5 mU/L are associated with progression during active surveillance, arguing that those patients with higher TSH values should be treated with thyroid hormone to reduce TSH into the lower portion of the normal range.[33]

A "clinical framework" for active surveillance has been suggested in a joint publication from several of these investigators from Japan and the United States.[34] Tumors that should *not* be enrolled in an active surveillance program include those that have subcapsular locations adjacent to the recurrent laryngeal nerve; extrathyroidal extension; lymph node, tracheal or distant spread; or aggressive cytology. The ideal tumor has well-defined margins surrounded by 2 mm or more of normal appearing thyroid tissue. Patients enrolled in an active surveillance program must be compliant with follow-up. Ideal patients are older. Active surveillance requires a center with expertise in neck ultrasonography and thyroid cancer.

Based on observational data of papillary microcarcinomas, the 2015 ATA guidelines do not recommend FNA biopsy of subcentimetric thyroid nodules, even when they have suspicious characteristics.[4] One can argue that the same criteria that excludes a known papillary microcarcinoma from active surveillance should be indications for FNA of a subcentimetric nodule. However, the evaluation of the majority of subcentimetric thyroid nodules by FNA is unnecessary, and implementation

TABLE 20.1 Presenting Characteristics of Micropapillary Thyroid Carcinoma[3,18-27]

Multifocal	20%–40%
Bilateral	10%–19%
Cervical nodes	17%–43%*
Extracapsular invasion	2%–38%
Distant metastases	0%–3%

*In one study, 24% had central nodes and 3.7% had lateral nodes.[27]

of the ATA guidelines appears to have reduced the rate of increase in the incidence of papillary microcarcinoma in the United States.[16] If such a policy is widely accepted, perhaps the increasing annual incidence of micropapillary thyroid cancer could be further reduced.

IMPACT OF INITIAL SURGERY

Unfortunately, there are no randomized prospective trials for the treatment of papillary cancer, and available retrospective data are severely limited by selection bias—patients with apparently worse disease are more likely to have more aggressive therapy. The National Thyroid Cancer Treatment Cooperative Study Group (NTCTCSG) comprises 12 centers in North America that prospectively enrolled patients into a registry and analyzed its database for outcome analysis.[26] Among 710 patients with papillary microcarcinoma, after excluding those with extrathyroidal extension and distant metastases, there were 611 who were disease-free after initial therapy (surgery with or without radioiodine). The median follow-up was 4 years with a range of 0 to 18 years. Recurrences were detected in 6.2% of patients after a mean follow-up of 2.8 ± 2.4 years. In patients who had a near-total or total thyroidectomy, the recurrence rate was identical in patients with multifocal or unifocal disease (6%). However, in patients who had less than a near-total thyroidectomy, recurrence was higher among those with multifocal disease (18%) than those with unifocal disease (4%; $p < 0.01$). Among those with multifocal disease, the difference in recurrence rate after a near-total or total thyroidectomy (6%) was lower than those who had less than a near-total thyroidectomy (18%), but this difference did not quite reach statistical significance ($p = 0.058$). Because 38% of the patients in this cohort had multifocal disease, consistent with the rate of multifocality noted previously in other series, these data could be used to argue that a near-total or total thyroidectomy is the optimal surgical procedure for patients with a preoperative diagnosis of papillary cancer, regardless of size, as long as surgical expertise is available to perform such an operation with minimal morbidity. On the other hand, given the excellent long-term prognosis for papillary microcarcinoma, and the higher complication rate of a total thyroidectomy even among high-volume thyroid surgeons, the ATA guidelines recommend a lobectomy for apparent intrathyroidal disease confined to one lobe.[4]

The Mayo Clinic,[18] the Gustave-Roussy Institute,[35] and the Samsung Medical Center[36] have also reported higher recurrence rates for patients with micropapillary cancer who only had a lobectomy. In contrast, an analysis of the National Cancer Data Base (1985 to 1998) demonstrated a lower rate of recurrence and death after total thyroidectomy for papillary cancers 10 mm or larger but not for tumors smaller than 10 mm.[37] Additionally, an analysis of the SEER Database (1988 to 2005) demonstrated a 99.9% 15-year disease-specific survival rate for patients with micropapillary carcinoma whether the patients had a total or near-total thyroidectomy or lobectomy[38] (see Chapter 31, Principles in Thyroid Surgery).

COMPLETION THYROIDECTOMY

Based on current guidelines,[4] it is unlikely that a patient who had a lobectomy for a papillary microcarcinoma would require an immediate completion thyroidectomy. In the study from the Samsung Medical Center,[36] 3289 patients had a lobectomy and were compared with 5387 patients who had a total thyroidectomy for a papillary microcarcinoma. The recurrence rate *in the contralateral thyroid bed* was lower after a total thyroidectomy (hazard ratio [HR] 0.398, $p < 0.001$), but there was no difference in ipsilateral or nodal recurrence. The authors argued that a lobectomy was therefore reasonable initial surgery, and a completion thyroidectomy could be performed only if there was a contralateral recurrence. Rarely, one would consider a completion thyroidectomy in a patient with a papillary microcarcinoma for whom radioiodine was potentially indicated. This could include a cancer with high-grade histology, a cancer with gross extrathyroidal extension, nodal involvement (more than 5 nodes, more than 2 mm in size), or distant metastases.[4]

NODE DISSECTION

No prospective randomized trials exist to help make decisions regarding the extent of node dissection that is appropriate for patients with micropapillary cancer. Preoperative ultrasonography is important for all patients undergoing thyroid cancer surgery, and there is little argument that in the presence of suspicious nodes there should be a therapeutic node dissection. The SEER data demonstrated a 23% increase in the use of central node dissections for T1 tumors between 2004 and 2008.[39] Whether one should do a prophylactic central node dissection in papillary microcarcinoma requires carefully designed studies that assess both the benefits and risks of central node dissections (see Chapter 27, Syndromic Medullary Thyroid Carcinoma: MEN 2A and MEN 2B; Chapter 38, Central Neck Dissection: Indications and Technique; and Chapter 39, Lateral Neck Dissection: Indications, and Technique).

In one study of 414 patients undergoing thyroid surgery, 24 had a therapeutic node dissection, 235 had a prophylactic node dissection, and 155 who had incidentally discovered papillary cancers had no node dissection.[40] Although there were recurrences in 21% of those who had a therapeutic node dissection, the recurrence rate was 0.4% in those undergoing a prophylactic node dissection and 0.7% in those who had no node dissection. Sixty-one percent of the patients who had a prophylactic node dissection had positive central nodes. However, 79% of those who had no node dissection and 22% of those who had a prophylactic node dissection had tumors that were smaller than 5 mm, so the groups were not comparable. Nonetheless, these data have been used to argue against a prophylactic node dissection.

If patients can be identified preoperatively as being at high risk for positive central nodes, the benefit of a prophylactic node dissection might outweigh the risks. For example, in one study patients whose nodules were positive preoperatively on 2-[^{18}F]fluoro-2-deoxy-D-glucose-positron emission tomography/computed tomography (FDG-PET/CT) scans had more than a twofold increased risk of pathologically involved central nodes compared with those with negative FDG-PET/CT scans.[41] In another study of 2329 patients, 34% had central nodes, but only 4% had greater than 5 nodes; male sex and age <40 years were independent risk factors for large-volume central node metastases.[42]

However, in a meta-analysis of 19 reports and 8345 patients, male sex, age below 45 years, size over 5 mm, multifocality and extrathyroidal extension correlated with positive central nodes, but the presence of positive central nodes did not correlate with recurrence.[43]

Ito and colleagues have argued that central node dissection should be used to avoid the need for radioiodine, although the 2015 ATA guidelines no longer recommend radioiodine for low-risk patients with less than 5 nodes and less than 2 mm in size.[4] They operated on 2638 patients with papillary tumors 20 mm or smaller and reported a recurrence rate of only 2% after a mean follow-up of 91 months (range of 6 to 240 months); 96% of their patients had a central node dissection, and 57% had positive nodes, but only 3 patients received radioiodine.[44] Thus for T1 patients (of whom only 39% were micropapillary cancers), they show a lower recurrence rate with central node dissection and no radioiodine compared with the recurrence rates of approximately 6% reported in the series of patients with papillary microcarcinoma noted previously.

However, in one study, the risk of hypoparathyroidism was threefold higher in patients who had a central node dissection, although the recurrence rate was 1.7% in those patients versus 3.5% in those who did not have a central node dissection.[45]

As noted earlier, the prevalence of positive central nodes in the two studies reviewed were 57% and 61%, yet the recurrence rates in series where prophylactic central node dissection was not routine are 6% or less. Thus the majority of malignant deposits in central nodes appear to have minimal biologic significance.

Because recurrences in papillary microcarcinoma are rarely life threatening, even if one believes that a central node dissection may reduce recurrences (despite the results of the meta-analysis noted earlier), a better strategy might be to avoid initial prophylactic central node dissections and refer the few patients who have a recurrence in the central compartment to a high-volume thyroid surgeon. One group of academic thyroid surgeons reports no difference in long-term complications among patients who required redo central compartment surgery.[46]

RADIOIODINE

The NTCTCSG study of papillary microcarcinoma recurrence also addressed the efficacy of radioiodine.[26] In that study the risk of recurrence was higher in multifocal papillary microcarcinoma (7%) compared with unifocal micropapillary cancer (2%) if the patient did not receive radioiodine. However, in multifocal papillary cancer there was no difference in the risk of recurrence, whether or not adjunctive radioiodine was administered. Similarly, although the risk of recurrence was higher in patients with positive nodes, adjunctive radioiodine did not reduce the recurrence rate in patients with papillary microcarcinoma and positive nodes.

Data from the Mayo Clinic show a higher recurrence rate in node-positive patients with micropapillary cancer who received radioiodine, likely reflecting a selection bias of giving radioiodine to patients with more concerning clinical characteristics. In node-negative patients, the recurrence rate was no different in those who received radioiodine (0%) or those who did not (0.6%).[18] A meta-analysis showed no benefit of adjunctive radioiodine in patients with papillary microcarcinoma.[47]

An analysis of the SEER Database (1988 to 2005) demonstrated a 99.9% 15-year disease-specific survival for patients with papillary microcarcinoma whether patients did or did not receive radioiodine.[38] Several other retrospective studies have failed to show a benefit of radioiodine for stage 1 papillary cancer, including the analysis of the entire NTCTCSG cohort[48] and the stage 1 patients reported by Mazzaferri and Jhiang.[49] In accordance with the ATA guidelines,[4] radioiodine would be indicated in patients with gross extrathyroidal invasion, extensive nodal metastases (more than 5 nodes greater than 2 mm in size), distant metastatic disease, and possible high-grade histology (see Chapter 48, Postoperative Radioactive Iodine Ablation and Treatment of Differentiated Thyroid Cancer).

BRAF

Approximately 45% to 60% of papillary cancer has the BRAF V600E mutation.[50-52] BRAF V600E correlates with advanced stages and mortality[50-52]; however, in some[50] but not all[51] multivariate analyses, BRAF V600E was not an independent risk factor for adverse outcomes. In one study where 39% of 435 patients with papillary microcarcinoma had BRAF V600E mutations, the overall mortality was 0.9%, which is consistent with published series that preceded the widespread use of BRAF analysis.[50] In a meta-analysis of 2247 patients with papillary microcarcinoma, the recurrence rate was increased twofold among patients with mutated BRAF V600E (odds ratio [OR] 2.09, confidence interval [CI] 1.31 to 3.33).[52] In the absence of traditional high-risk features, BRAF V600E should not be considered an indication for aggressive treatment.

POSTOPERATIVE SURVEILLANCE

Surveillance of patients with papillary microcarcinoma follows the same principle as surveillance for all patients with papillary cancer. However, unless there is an indication for radioiodine, whole-body radioiodine scanning is not done. Most patients will be followed primarily with ultrasonography. There are no data that address the appropriate frequency of sonography. A baseline study 4 months after surgery, and follow-up imaging annually for 2 more years (in the NTCTCSG study, more than half of the recurrences occurred in the first 3 years after surgery[26]), then at increasing intervals, should be sufficient to detect nodal and local recurrences. Thyroglobulin measurements are less useful in patients who have had a lobectomy. In patients who have had a total thyroidectomy, baseline thyroglobulin should be obtained while patients are taking thyroid hormone; a subsequent unexpected increase suggests the need for further evaluation. Measurement of thyroglobulin after rhTSH or thyroid hormone withdrawal should be restricted to patients at high risk for recurrence. A financial analysis argues for less intensive surveillance in low-risk patients: at one hospital, the cost of detecting a recurrence in a low-risk patient was $147,819 versus $22,434 in an intermediate-risk patient.[53] Because thyroid hormone suppressive therapy is associated with atrial fibrillation and reduced bone density, the ATA guidelines recommend a target TSH of 0.5 to 2.0 mU/L in ATA low-risk patients with an excellent response to initial treatment.[4]

SUMMARY AND RECOMMENDATIONS

Despite the presence of multifocality and nodal disease in up to 40% to 60% of patients, the overall prognosis for the overwhelming majority of patients with papillary microcarcinoma is excellent, and mortality is well under 1%. Local and cervical node recurrences are almost never life threatening but occur in up to 6% of patients (Table 20.2). Most distant metastases are either present initially or occur in patients who present with bulky cervical adenopathy. The rare deaths from micropapillary cancer occur in this very small subgroup. The risk of death in the majority of patients who do not present with distant metastases or bulky nodal disease is 0.1% to 0.2%.

Recurrences are less common in patients who have had at least a near-total thyroidectomy because most recurrences occur in the contralateral lobe. A lobectomy is recommended for apparent unifocal intrathyroidal tumors. A completion thyroidectomy can be done later if the patient has a contralateral recurrence. The routine use of central node dissection is to be discouraged, because associated complications may result in more morbidity than that associated with a possibly slightly higher recurrence rate among those patients who do not have a prophylactic central node dissection. When central nodal recurrences

TABLE 20.2 Recurrence in Micropapillary Thyroid Cancer

Nodal recurrence	2.5%–5%
Local recurrence	1%–4%
Death	0%–1%

occur, redo surgery should ideally be performed by a high-volume thyroid surgeon. Radioiodine has not been shown to reduce recurrences in ATA low-risk patients, including patients with papillary microcarcinoma and positive nodes. Radioiodine should be used only in select patients with gross extrathyroidal invasion, extensive nodal disease, high-grade histology, or distant metastases. Postoperative monitoring should include annual ultrasounds for at least 3 years, then at less frequent intervals, and annual serum measurement of thyroglobulin (see Chapter 47, Postoperative Management of Differentiated Thyroid Cancer).

REFERENCES

For a complete list of references, go to expertconsult.com.

Papillary Carcinoma Observation

Akira Miyauchi, R. Michael Tuttle

> Please go to expertconsult.com to view related video:
> **Video 21.1** Introduction to Chapter 21, Papillary Carcinoma Observation.

INTRODUCTION

Recognizing that the incidence of papillary microcarcinoma (PMC) detected on autopsy and clinical screening studies far exceeded the prevalence of clinically apparent thyroid cancer more than 20 years ago, Miyauchi from the Kuma Hospital in Kobe, Japan, hypothesized that most PMCs would remain small and never develop into clinically significant disease.[1-8] Furthermore, he posited that immediate surgery for all PMCs may be associated with more harm than good, as it was very likely that the few low-risk papillary thyroid cancers destined to become clinically significant disease would progress slowly and be very effectively treated at the time of documented disease progression. These hypotheses provided the scientific rationale for an observational clinical trial of PMCs that began at the Kuma Hospital in 1993 and then subsequently at the Cancer Institute Hospital in Tokyo in 1995.[9]

Multiple publications from Japan since that time have demonstrated the safety and effectiveness of an observational management approach (also known as active surveillance) in PMCs.[1-6,9-16] As Miyauchi posited, the incidence of having adverse events such as temporary and permanent vocal cord paralysis, temporary and permanent hyperparathyroidism, and the need for levothyroxine administration were all significantly higher in patients that underwent immediate surgery than in patients followed with active surveillance even though the surgeries were performed by well-experienced endocrine surgeons at Kuma Hospital, a center for thyroid care.[17] Furthermore, active surveillance was also demonstrated to be a cost-effective alternative to immediate surgery.[18,19] The calculated total cost of immediate surgery with postoperative management for 10 years, including the cost for reoperative surgery for recurrent disease, was 4.1 times the total cost of active surveillance for 10 years, including the cost for conversion surgery.[20]

More recently, studies from the United States and Korea have reproduced and validated the Kuma Hospital observations.[21,22] In 2011, the Japanese Association of Endocrine Surgeons and the Japanese Society of Thyroid Surgery guidelines endorsed active surveillance as a reasonable management option.[23] Based largely on Japanese experience and an improved understanding of the natural history of low-risk papillary thyroid carcinoma, the American Thyroid Association (ATA) guidelines now endorse active surveillance as an acceptable management option for biopsy-proven, very low-risk thyroid cancer.[24] Furthermore, the ATA guidelines also endorse an observational management approach without cytologic confirmation in subcentimeter thyroid nodules that demonstrate ultrasonographic characteristics that are highly suspicious for thyroid cancer.[24] It is important to note that the active surveillance terminology can be applied to patients with either cytologically confirmed low-risk thyroid cancers or with thyroid nodules classified as having a high risk of being malignant without cytologic confirmation.

Consistent with the practice at the time, Kuma Hospital had previously recommended that thyroid nodules ≥5 mm with suspicious features on ultrasonography be evaluated with ultrasound-guided fine-needle aspiration (FNA). Today, at Memorial Sloan Kettering Cancer Center (MSKCC), patients with highly suspicious thyroid nodules who are deemed to be appropriate for active surveillance are given the option of a cytologic confirmation of malignancy before observational management or active surveillance without cytologic confirmation consistent with the ATA guidelines.[24]

Thus an observational initial management approach is now considered to be a very viable alternative to immediate surgery. It is therefore incumbent on clinicians to understand (1) the low likelihood and pattern of disease progression in low-risk papillary thyroid cancer during active surveillance, (2) the approach to proper patient selection, (3) the characteristics of a successful observational management program, and (4) the criteria used to determine when transition from observation to surgical intervention is warranted.

DISEASE PROGRESSION DURING ACTIVE SURVEILLANCE OF LOW-RISK PAPILLARY THYROID CANCER

In properly selected patients the vast majority of patients demonstrate tumor sizes that are stable or decreasing, whereas only 2% to 8% demonstrate an increase of ≥3 mm in maximal diameter (approximately 100% increase in tumor volume) and 12% to 14% demonstrate an increase in tumor volume more than 50%[11,13,21,22] (Table 21.1). An increase of ≥3 mm in maximal diameter is the minimum change in size that can reliably be measured on serial ultrasonography and has traditionally and effectively been used to be the primary determinate of whether or not a low-risk thyroid cancer has changed significantly. More recently, tumor growth has been described in terms of changes in volume, with a 50% increase or decrease in tumor volume being the smallest change that can be reliably detected.[22] When analyzed based on tumor volume, 12% to 14% of tumors increase in size during the first 2 to 3 years of follow-up. Interestingly, the kinetics of tumor growth demonstrated classic log-linear exponential growth patterns, with rates of change that varied between tumors but were remarkably constant for an individual PMC.[22] As described in subsequent sections (see indications to move from active surveillance to surgical intervention), although tumor volume measurements can reliably determine which small thyroid cancers are slowly growing,

TABLE 21.1 Clinical Outcomes in Active Surveillance Observation Cohorts

First Author	n (Tumor Size)	Median Follow-Up	Maximum Diameter ± 3 mm Increase	Stable	Decrease	Tumor Volume ± 50% Increase	Stable	Decrease	Lymph Node Metastasis
Ito[11]	1235 (<1 cm)	5 yrs	5% (5 yrs)	95% (5 yrs)	—	—	—	—	2% (5 yrs)
			8% (10 yrs)	92% (10 yrs)	—				4% (10 yrs)
Sugitani[13]	415 (<1 cm)	6.5 yrs	6%	91%	3%	—	—	—	1%
Tuttle[22]	291 (<1.5 cm)	2 yrs	4%	92%	4%	12%	79%	7%	0%
Kwon[21]	192 (<1 cm)	2.5 yrs	2%	95%	3%	14%	69%	17%	0.5%

we do not consider a 50% increase in tumor volume as an indication for immediate surgery. Instead, we use tumor volume changes to help guide the frequency of subsequent ultrasound follow-up and view them as just one component in the description of disease progression that needs to be integrated into a decision about whether or not continued observation or immediate surgery is needed.

Interestingly, during active surveillance a decrease in tumor size of more than 3 mm is seen in 3% to 4% of the patients, and a decrease in tumor volume of more than 50% can be seen in 7% to 17% of the patients (see Table 21.1).[21,22] The first report about active surveillance from Kuma Hospital also described a decrease in tumor size of more than 2 mm in 12% of the 58 patients who were surveyed for 5 years or more.[6] The precise reasons for decreasing tumor size over time during active surveillance are unknown but could be associated with either damage to the tumor related to the FNA biopsy procedure, the natural history of these small nodules, or an immune response from the patient.

Identification of novel lymph node metastases during follow-up ranges from 2% to 4% over 5 to 10 years of follow-up.[11,13,21,22] In properly selected patients, it is unusual to identify new lymph node metastases during the first 2 years of follow-up. But as these lymph node metastases usually grow quite slowly, consistent with the primary tumor, they can be identified with high quality ultrasonography during long-term follow-up. Distant metastases have not been identified in any of the patients being followed with observation.[11]

Possible Predictors of Disease Progression

Many published studies have looked for possible predictors of disease progression during active surveillance.[11,13,21,22] They uniformly find that age is a significant predictor of disease progression such that patients <40 years old at the time of a PMC diagnosis have about a 6% risk of having an increase greater than 3 mm, whereas patients ≥60 years old only had a 2.2% risk (p = 0.0014). Similarly the likelihood of identifying lymph node metastases was higher in the younger patients than the older patients (5.3% versus 0.4%, p <0.001).[11] Interestingly, most of the tumors that showed disease progression had either tumor enlargement or the appearance of lymph node metastasis.[25] The risk of disease progression (increase in tumor size greater than or equal to 3 mm or novel lymph node metastasis) was significantly lower in older patients than in younger patients. After 10 years of active surveillance, patients get 10 years older. Miyauchi et al. calculated disease progression rates at 10 years of active surveillance for patients in each age decade. The lifetime disease progression rates estimated with these values were 48.6%, 25.3%, 20.9%, 10.3%, 8.2%, and 3.5% in patients diagnosed in their 20s, 30s, 40s, 50s, 60s, and 70s, respectively.[26] The estimate indicates that more than a half of the patients in their 20s, about 75% of the patients in their 30s, and the vast majority of the older patients will not require thyroid surgery in their lifetime.

Although there is uniform agreement that excess thyroid-stimulating hormone (TSH) stimulation (TSH levels above the normal reference range) should be avoided during active surveillance, it is less certain whether mild TSH suppression would be beneficial. Although Sugitani did not find a correlation between TSH levels and PMC disease progression,[13] a study from Korea did demonstrate that sustained TSH elevations more than 2.5 mIU/mL were associated with PMC disease progression.[27] In the Kuma Hospital series, none of the 50 patients that were treated with levothyroxine to achieve a low normal TSH demonstrated disease progression.[11] Further research on this topic is needed; in the meantime it is certainly reasonable to maintain TSH levels in the low normal reference range during active surveillance.

Pregnancy is known to be a mild growth stimulant to papillary thyroid carcinoma.[28] Although the initial small case series suggested that papillary thyroid microcarcinoma enlargement during pregnancy was common, a follow-up study of 51 pregnancies demonstrated that only 8% of the patients had enlargement of the papillary thyroid carcinoma during pregnancy. After delivery, two patients underwent surgery, and two other patients had disease stabilization again after pregnancy and continue to follow with observation.[12] It is also important to remember that PMCs are more likely to grow in the younger age group, so an increase in the size of a PMC during pregnancy may be due to the underlying growth kinetics of the tumor rather than to the influence of pregnancy (Figure 21.1). Thus we consider women with childbearing potential to be appropriate patients for active surveillance, provided the patient understands the potential for pregnancy to increase the tumor size.

Currently, molecular profiling of PMCs cannot accurately identify the few tumors that are destined to progress and therefore is not used in the selection of patients for active surveillance. Although present in more than 50% of PMCs,[29] *BRAF* V600E mutation was not predictive of tumor progression or identification of nodal metastases and *TERT* promoter mutations were not found in any of these tumors in a small series that went to surgery after a period of observation.[30]

MSKCC is exploring the role of both functional and anatomic characteristics of neck magnetic resonance imaging (MRI) as a noninvasive biomarker to predict disease progression. In small pilot studies, lower apparent diffusion coefficient, diffusion coefficient, and higher perfusion fraction were associated with histologic features of tumor aggressiveness in small thyroid cancers.[31,32]

A histopathological study of PMCs that were resected due to tumor enlargement, appearance of nodal metastases, and other nonprogression-related causes revealed high Ki-67 labeling index being associated with tumor enlargement.[25] Although this was evaluated after surgery, these findings indicate the potential for analyzing aspirates of the tumors to predict tumor progression.

Other factors such as multifocality, family history of differentiated thyroid cancer, gender, and tumor size were not significantly associated with disease progression.[11,13,21,22]

CHAPTER 21 Papillary Carcinoma Observation

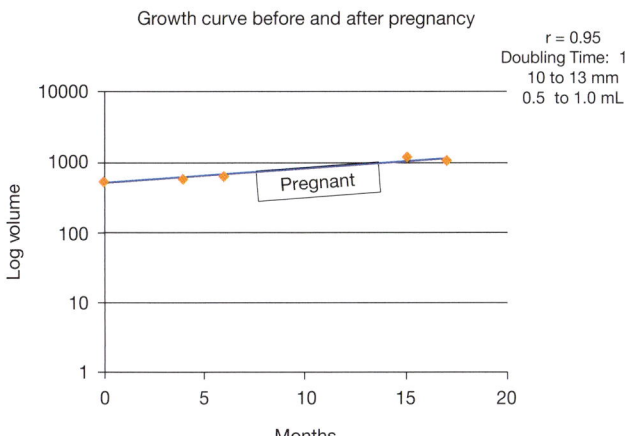

Fig. 21.1 Log-linear growth curve demonstrating a consistent doubling time of 1 year, r = 0.95, as the tumor increased from 10 to 13 mm in maximum diameter and 0.5 to 1.0 mL in tumor volume. Pregnancy had no effect on the growth curve as the tumor sizes after pregnancy had increased to what would have been predicted based on the passage of time alone regardless of pregnancy.

CLINICAL FRAMEWORK FOR AN ACTIVE SURVEILLANCE MANAGEMENT STRATEGY

To facilitate implementation of an active surveillance management strategy in routine clinical practice, colleagues from Kuma Hospital and MSKCC published a clinical framework that incorporated three interrelated domains (tumor/ultrasound characteristics, medical team characteristics, and patient characteristics) to classify patients as either ideal, appropriate, or inappropriate for active surveillance (Figure 21.2).[33,34] Clinicians can use this clinical framework to ensure that appropriate criteria are being considered when evaluating low-risk papillary thyroid cancer patients for a possible active surveillance management approach.

Patients classified as ideal for active surveillance are older patients with PMCs presenting as solitary nodules within an otherwise normal

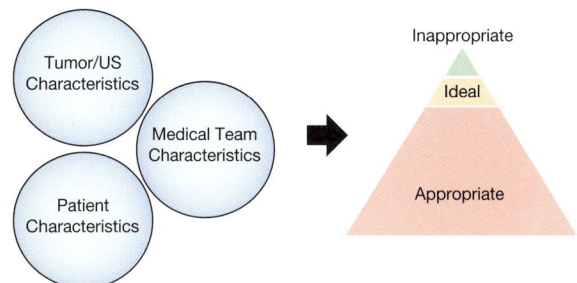

Fig. 21.2 Clinical framework showing the clinical domains used to classify patients as either ideal, appropriate, or inappropriate for an active surveillance management program.[33,34]

thyroid gland (Figure 21.3, A). Furthermore, these patients are motivated to avoid immediate surgery for a variety of reasons and have supportive family members and referring physicians. The ideal patient is also followed by an experienced multidisciplinary team using high-quality neck ultrasonography, prospective data collection, and a tracking/reminder program to ensure proper follow-up.

Conversely, patients classified as inappropriate for active surveillance have evidence of locally invasive or metastatic thyroid cancer at the time of initial presentation. This includes patients with lymph node metastases detected by ultrasonography, distant metastases detected by any modality, vocal cord paralysis due to invasion of the recurrent laryngeal nerve (RLN), or evidence of tracheal invasion. Likewise, patients with tumors (≥7 mm in maximum diameter) immediately adjacent to the RLN that do not demonstrate a rim of normal thyroid tissue between the tumor and the thyroid capsule are also inappropriate for observation because of the risk of invasion to the nerve (see Figure 21.3, A).[3] Tumors ≥7 mm in maximum diameter attaching the trachea with obtuse or nearly right angle carry the risk of tracheal invasion, rendering them to the inappropriate category, while none of

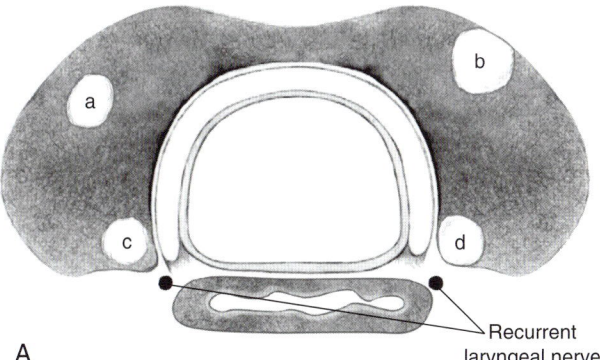
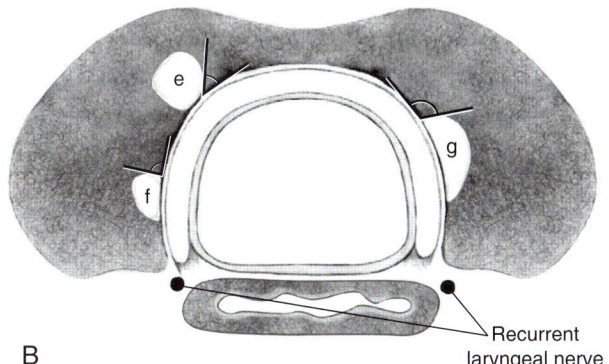

Fig. 21.3 Clinical framework category according to the location of a tumor. **A,** A tumor located within a lobe (A) is ideal for active surveillance. A tumor attaching the anterior or lateral thyroid capsule (B) is regarded appropriate. The presence (tumor C) or absence (tumor D) of a normal thyroid tissue rim in the direction of the RLN is related to the risk of invasion to the nerve. Tumor C is appropriate and tumor D is inappropriate. **B,** The angle formed between the tumor and the trachea is related to the risk of tracheal invasion. Tumor E with an acute angle is appropriate, and tumor F with a near-right angle and tumor G with an obtuse angle are not appropriate. RLNs cannot be demonstrated with ultrasound RLN, recurrent laryngeal nerve.

the tumors attaching the trachea with acute angle had tracheal invasion, rendering them to the appropriate category (see Figure 21.3, *B*).[3] Interestingly, none of the PMCs that were less than 7 mm in maximal diameter demonstrated invasion into a RLN or trachea regardless of their location within the thyroid.[3]

Although very uncommon, a high-grade malignancy on cytology would also be considered a contraindication to active surveillance. Patients who are not willing to accept an observational management approach and patients unlikely to be compliant with follow-up plans are also considered inappropriate for active surveillance. Although the initial studies excluded patients with tumors larger than 1 cm from observation, MSKCC included patients with tumors up to 1.5 cm and demonstrated very similar excellent outcomes compared with the PMCs.[22] Therefore the thyroid cancer disease management team at MSKCC routinely offers active surveillance to properly selected patients with tumors up to 1.5 cm. Less commonly, active surveillance is offered to patients with tumors up to 2 cm if there are concurrent major medical comorbidities that either make the surgery very high risk or are likely to be associated with poor short-term survival.

Interestingly, the majority of patients followed with active surveillance fall into what we defined as appropriate for active surveillance.[22] They are generally classified as appropriate based on either nonspecific, presumably benign findings throughout the rest of the thyroid gland, ill-defined tumor margins which make serial measurements more difficult, FDG-avid PMCs, multifocal PMCs, or primary tumor sizes between 1 to 1.5 cm. As described earlier, women with childbearing potential are also classified as appropriate. Similarly, patients with a strong family history of thyroid cancer who are motivated to follow with observation are also considered appropriate for active surveillance.

Although involvement of the thyroid capsule is considered a contraindication for active surveillance in areas adjacent to the likely path of the RLNs or the trachea, involvement of the capsule and even minor extrathyroidal extension on the lateral and anterior aspects of the thyroid are not considered an absolute contraindication to observation but are rather classified as appropriate for observation (see Figure 21.3, *A*). This is because minor extrathyroidal extension is not associated with adverse outcomes when present in the anterior and lateral thyroid locations, and if it progresses it can be easily treated surgically at the time of disease progression.[35,36]

Patient education and information is a key component to proper patient selection and to the success of an active surveillance management approach.[37] At Kuma Hospital this is accomplished with a short brochure explaining active surveillance before a FNA is performed on suspicious thyroid nodules that are ideal or appropriate for observation. Alternatively, Brito et al. developed a clinical decision aid which facilitated conversation and increased acceptance of active surveillance in a Korean population.[38]

INDICATIONS TO MOVE FROM ACTIVE SURVEILLANCE TO SURGICAL INTERVENTION

As noted earlier, the vast majority of PMC patients followed with active surveillance will demonstrate stable or decreasing tumor sizes. However, some patients will demonstrate clinical disease progression manifest by either an increase in tumor size, identification of lymph node metastases, or direct invasion outside the thyroid. Thus a successful active surveillance management programs requires the development of clinical criteria that should be used to guide the transition from active surveillance to surgical intervention (Box 21.1).

The most common reason to transition to surgical intervention is an increase in tumor size of the primary tumor. The indication for surgical intervention was set as an increase in maximal diameter of ≥3 mm in the Kuma Hospital studies.[7,8] This would correlate to an increase in tumor volume of approximately 100%.[22] This 3 mm cutoff reflects the minimal reproducible measurement difference on serial ultrasonographic examinations, is easily determined, and has been the gold standard that was used to demonstrate the safety of active surveillance.[17] Thus we continue to use an increase of 3 mm in diameter or 100% increase in tumor volume as the primary indication for surgical intervention.

However, surgical intervention can be considered with a confirmed 50% increase in tumor volume (the minimal reproducible measurement difference for tumor volume), based on factors such as (1) proximity of the tumor to the RLN or trachea, (2) patient preference, or (3) primary tumor size >1 cm. Conversely, even with a documented increase in the size of the primary tumor by diameter or volume, surgery may be deferred in patients without other indications for intervention if they have (1) a maximum tumor diameter of <13 mm (at Kuma Hospital) or <15 mm (at MSKCC), and/or (2) a tumor volume doubling time >2 years.

Other indications for surgical intervention include identification of metastatic disease outside the thyroid or evidence of direct invasion into major structures surrounding the thyroid, such as RLN, trachea, or strap muscles. Enlargement of associated thyroid nodules, appearance of primary hyperparathyroidism, and surgical management of associated Graves' disease were also indications for conversion surgery in some of the patients observed at Kuma Hospital.

Although uncommon, patients can choose to abandon an active surveillance management program in favor of surgical intervention even in the absence of structural disease progression. In the MSKCC experience, the decision to move to surgery in the absence of structural disease progression is usually prompted by changes in insurance plans or other socioeconomic factors that make it difficult or impossible for patients to continue observational management at our center.

Treatment Alternatives to Standard Surgical Intervention

Several groups are exploring treatment alternatives to standard surgical intervention (thyroid lobectomy or total thyroidectomy) to destroy these small, low-risk papillary thyroid cancers.[39-41] Although still experimental, options such as alcohol ablation, radiofrequency ablation, and laser therapies may have a role in the future if the goal of therapy is only to destroy the primary lesion. Of course, destruction of the

---

BOX 21.1 Indications for Transition from Active Surveillance to Surgical Intervention

1. Increase in size of the primary tumor*
    a. ≥3 mm increase in tumor diameter and/or,
    b. ≥100% increase in tumor volume
2. Identification of metastatic disease
3. Direct invasion into surrounding structures such as:
    a. Recurrent laryngeal nerve
    b. Trachea
    c. Strap muscles
4. Patient preference

*Surgical intervention can be considered with a confirmed 50% increase in tumor volume based on factors such as (1) proximity of the tumor to the thyroid capsule, (2) patient preference, or (3) primary tumor size >1 cm. Conversely, even with a documented increase in the size of the primary tumor by diameter or volume, surgery may be deferred in patients without other indications for intervention if they have (1) a maximum tumor diameter of <13 mm (at Kuma Hospital) or <15 mm (at MSKCC), and/or (2) a tumor volume doubling time >2 years.

primary lesion would remove one of the key indicators for thyroidectomy during follow-up (increase in size of primary tumor over time). However, these procedures might result in losing only the primary tumor that functions as a marker of the disease progression while leaving possible lymph node metastases.

ACTIVE SURVEILLANCE: PRACTICAL APPLICATION

All patients with primary tumors <1 to 1.5 cm are considered potential candidates for an active surveillance management option (with or without cytologic confirmation). The clinical framework is then used to determine whether a patient is ideal, appropriate, or inappropriate for an active surveillance management approach.[33,34] This requires a careful reevaluation of tumor characteristics on the ultrasound (tumor location, evaluation of cervical lymph nodes, presence of other nodules/thyroiditis) to make sure a patient is appropriately classified as either ideal or appropriate before a decision is made. Thyroid function tests are performed to ensure the patient is not exposed to unwanted excessive TSH stimulation. Importantly, education and information are provided to ensure the patient and any involved family decision makers understand the risks and benefits of observation either with or without cytologic confirmation. Furthermore, information should be shared with other clinicians involved in the care of the patient.

Although patients are provided with a discussion of the risks and benefits of both management approaches, ideal patients are encouraged to consider active surveillance rather than immediate surgery. Similarly, patients classified as inappropriate for active surveillance are given recommendations to proceed with surgical intervention. For patients classified as appropriate for observation, our recommendations may encourage either surgery or active surveillance or potentially either option equally, depending on the specifics of a particular case at MSCKK, whereas active surveillance is recommended as the first line of management at Kuma Hospital. Obviously, the final decision regarding immediate surgery or observation is made by patients and their families, and we strive to achieve a fully informed shared decision.

Ideal or appropriate patients who agree to an active surveillance management approach have neck ultrasonography done at 6- to 12-month intervals for 2 years, then less frequently over time, depending on tumor location, growth rate, and the presence of other nonspecific findings. Thyroid function tests are done yearly. Thyroid hormone replacement is used if needed to maintain the serum TSH to ≤3 mIU/mL. In the absence of disease progression or development of other abnormalities on follow-up ultrasonography, additional FNAs are not routinely planned during observational management.

Patients with tumors that are stable or decreasing continue long-term observation. Patients demonstrating clinical disease progression usually have a confirmatory ultrasound 3 to 4 months later, and if the increase in size is confirmed, they then proceed to surgical intervention based on the criteria described earlier.

RESEARCH NEEDS

Although active surveillance has been established as an acceptable, viable, and safe alternative to immediate surgery in properly selected low-risk papillary thyroid cancer patients, there are certainly areas that require additional research. These include topics such as the following:
1. Defining tumor growth criteria that mandate surgical intervention
2. Optimal TSH level during observation
3. The role of molecular testing in predicting disease progression
4. Psychological effects of observational management
5. Effects of pregnancy on low-risk thyroid cancer
6. Role of alternative interventions, such as alcohol ablation, laser therapy, or radiofrequency ablation

CONCLUSION

Active surveillance is a safe and effective alternative to immediate surgery in properly selected patients with low-risk papillary thyroid cancer. The past 5 years have seen a growing acceptance of active surveillance outside of the original initiating centers in Japan. The continued increase in the incidence of low-risk thyroid cancers makes it more important than ever that clinicians understand and embrace an active surveillance management option for low-risk papillary thyroid cancer.

REFERENCES

For a complete list of references, go to expertconsult.com.

22

Follicular Thyroid Cancer

Cosimo Durante, Sebastiano Filetti

INTRODUCTION

Follicular thyroid cancer (FTC) is a subset of follicular cell–derived thyroid cancer. It falls within the broad category of differentiated thyroid cancer (DTC) and is the second most common histologic subtype behind papillary thyroid cancer (PTC). Unlike PTC, the rate of FTC diagnosis is declining over time due to changes in the diagnostic criteria and maybe due to environmental factors such as iodine sufficiency. Compared with PTC its more common counterpart, FTC carries a more severe prognosis due to more frequent distant metastatic spread. Given the rarity of FTC and the changes of the diagnostic criteria over time, compelling evidence regarding FTC management is lacking, and guideline recommendations nearly reflect that of PTC.

EPIDEMIOLOGY

The frequency of FTC has been estimated between 9% and 40% depending on the population studied, iodine intake, and the pathologic criteria used for the diagnosis.[1,2] In general, FTC represents approximately 10% to 15% of all thyroid cancers, with a majority of these being minimally invasive FTC. The incidence of thyroid cancer in general has nearly tripled since the mid-1970s,[3] but that of FTC has remained stable[3-5] or decreased,[6] suggesting that current thyroid cancer incidence rates are largely the result of increases in PTC diagnoses.

Caucasians account for the majority of new thyroid cancer diagnoses (>90%) in the United States. However, the greatest annual percentage increase for both genders was among blacks (4.6% to 5.8%).[7] In another U.S. cohort,[8] the percentage of FTC relative to all thyroid cancer was estimated to be 14.2% between 1985 and 1990 and 11.4% from 1991 to 1995, and approximately 40% of all new FTC diagnoses involved individuals in their third to fifth decades of life. A more recent U.S. analysis revealed that the incidence of FTC remained stable at 1/100,000 between 1973 to 2002, whereas the rate of new PTC diagnoses more than doubled (from 3/100,000 to over 7/100,000).[1] In a large Italian cohort of 4187 patients with DTCs, the prevalence of FTC in patients diagnosed after 1990 was 9%—roughly half that observed (19.5%) among patients diagnosed between 1969 and 1990.[9] One potential factor in the decline in FTC prevalence is the use of iodine prophylaxis in more recent years, as shown in a world trend analysis.[10] An analysis of French thyroid cancer registries showed a decline in the incidence of FTC cases from 1983 to 2000 but the decrease was not as substantial as that observed in Italy, with absolute decreases of 2.2% and 0.5% annually in men and women, respectively.[11]

Some epidemiologic data suggest that increased iodine intake (secondary to supplementation programs or movement from an iodine-deficient region to an iodine-sufficient one) can alter rates of FTC.[12-14] Like all epidemiologic data correlating iodine status with FTC or DTC, the significance of these data is limited by the lack of a control group and failure to analyze other relevant and potentially confounding variables.

Changes in the pathologic diagnosis of PTCs and FTCs have also influenced the incidence of these tumors. The 1977 description of a follicular-variant PTC by Chen and Rosai[15] stressed the fact that the major criterion for diagnosing a thyroid carcinoma as PTC consists in the presence of altered nuclear morphology rather than the predominance of a papillary rather than follicular pattern, as previously believed (Figure 22.1). This was a paradigm shift that resulted in many cancers previously diagnosed as FTCs (up to 45% according to a study by Verkooijen et al.[16]) being reported as PTCs, reversing the ratio of FTCs to PTCs among DTC diagnoses. This reclassification has strengthened the correlation between thyroid cancer histology and recurrence-free and cancer-specific survival rates: diagnosis of FTC is clearly associated with worse outcomes than those seen with follicular variants of PTC.[17] It is worth noting that with the 2017 edition of the World Health Organization (WHO) classification, Hürthle cell carcinoma is no longer considered a variant of FTC and is now considered a separate entity.[18]

In summary, epidemiologic data suggest that the incidence and prevalence of FTC are declining as a result of changes made in the criteria for pathologic diagnoses of these tumors and of the increasing use of iodine supplementation throughout the world.

ETIOLOGY

The classic clinically evaluable risk factors for DTC include exposure to ionizing radiation (especially in youth) and family history of thyroid cancer. The nuclear reactor accident in Chernobyl, Russia, in 1986, illustrated the effects of radiation exposure on thyroid cancer risk. Most cases of DTC associated with the Chernobyl accident were PTCs with RET/PTC rearrangements, and a few FTC were noted as well.[19] Ionizing radiation appears to be a risk factor for PTC to a greater extent than FTC. FTC can be found in the context of genetic syndromes such as Cowden disease with well-recognized genetic determinants[20] and in familial nonmedullary thyroid cancer (FNMTC) conditions for which no gene signature or gene cluster has yet been identified to predict risk (see Chapter 30, Familial Nonmedullary Thyroid Cancer). In a case control study of a Swedish population of DTC patients, there was no statistically significant increase in parental thyroid cancer for those subjects with FTC, though there was a greater than fourfold increased risk of thyroid cancer if the parent had PTC.[21] As for other environmental and lifestyle factors, there is limited evidence for the role of diet and body mass index (BMI) as a risk factor, although consumption of iodized salt in a cohort study in Sweden did suggest protection against FTC.[22-25]

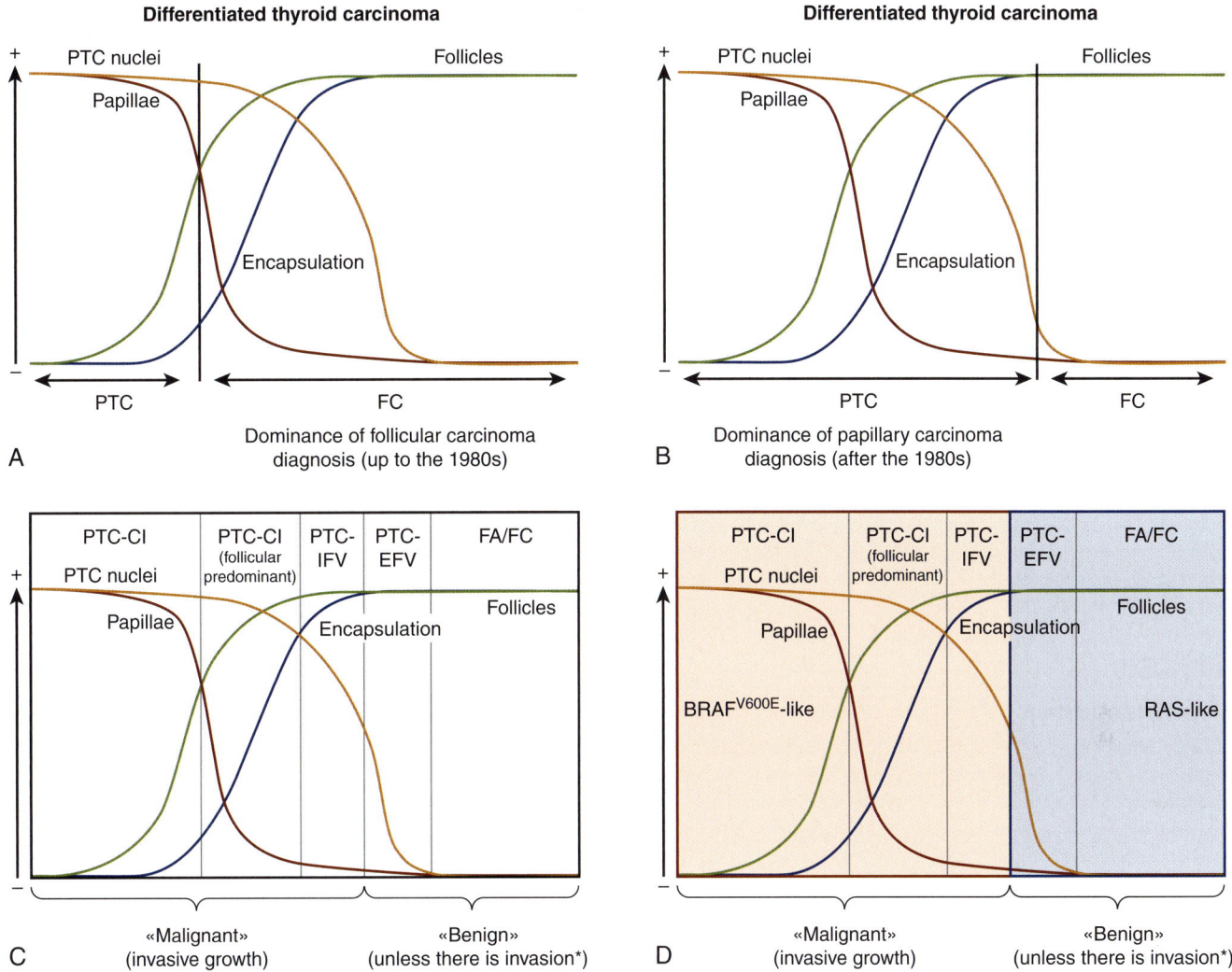

Fig. 22.1 Basic histopathologic concepts for the diagnosis and classification of thyroid carcinoma. Four basic morphologic features are used to diagnose tumors of follicular cell derivation: (1) papillary growth pattern; (2) follicular growth pattern; (3) presence of a tumor capsule and of its invasion, in the form of capsular or vascular invasion; (4) alterations of nuclear morphology typical of papillary carcinoma. The black vertical bar in panels **A** and **B** represents the "histologic border" between the cases diagnosed as papillary carcinoma (on the left) and follicular carcinoma (on the right). These four basic morphologic features correlate with the thyroid carcinoma diagnostic subtypes (**C**) and molecular signatures (**D**). PTC, papillary thyroid carcinoma; FC, follicular carcinoma; PTC-CI, classic papillary thyroid carcinoma; PTC-IFV, infiltrative follicular variant of papillary thyroid carcinoma (infiltrative tumor with partial or absent tumor capsule); FA/FC, follicular thyroid adenoma/follicular carcinoma. *Invasion of the tumor capsule or of vascular spaces. (Redrawn from Tallini G, Tuttle RM, Ghossein RA. The history of the follicular variant of papillary thyroid carcinoma. *J Clin Endocrinol Metab.* 2017;102[1]:15–22.)

The recent era of molecular medicine has identified mutations important in FTC development (see Figure 22.1; see Chapter 18, Molecular Pathogenesis of Thyroid Neoplasia).[26] Kroll et al. described the *PAX8-PPARγ* fusion oncogene that acts as a dominant negative transcription factor and is present in a subset of follicular carcinomas.[27] In a study of 15 patients with histologically proved FTC, 8/15 (53%) had the *PAX8-PPARγ* rearrangement, and of the 3 patients with a history of radiation exposure, 100% had this mutation.[28] A recent review of 17 studies shows that the *PAX8-PPARγ* rearrangement was identified in 36% (112/310) of FTC, 16% (13/83) of FVPTC, and 11% (27/247) of follicular thyroid adenomas (FTAs), suggesting a significant role of this oncogene in the development of follicular tumors.[29] Giordano and colleagues used global gene expression profiling to compare FTA and FTC with and without the *PAX8-PPARγ* rearrangement.[30] They identified a 68-gene signature set that provided insight into potential molecular mechanisms governing *PAX8-PPARγ* dependent FTC. These included genes on chromosome 3p as well as genes involved in fatty acid and carbohydrate metabolism. Another common and distinct mutation associated with FTC is one that activates *RAS* (*N-RAS*, *H-RAS*, or *K-RAS*) through point mutations and thus constitutively activates the mitogen-activated protein kinase (MAPK) oncogenic signaling pathway.[31] *RAS* mutations were identified in 49% of FTC. RAS mutations or the *PAX-PPARγ* rearrangement was present in 88% of this sample of FTC.[32] Additionally, recent studies of FTC tissue show a higher percentage of tumors with activated Akt (pAkt) than activated MAPK (pERK), suggesting that FTC is more dependent on the PI3K-Akt pathway than the MAPK pathway, which is important in PTC.[33] Beyond providing evidence for the underlying genetic defects that

TABLE 22.1 Molecular Markers of Follicular and Hürthle Cell Carcinoma

Tumor Type	Molecular Markers
Follicular carcinoma	RAS, PAX8/PPARγ, PTEN, PIK3CA, TSHR, TERT promoter, CNA
Hürthle cell carcinoma	RAS, EIF1AX, PTEN, TP53, CNA, mtDNA

amp, amplifications; CNA, copy number alterations; del, deletions; fus, fusions; MI, minimally invasive; WHO, World Health Organization; WI, widely invasive.

Data from Landa I, Ibrahimpasic T, Boucai L et al. Genomic and transcriptomic hallmarks of poorly differentiated and anaplastic thyroid cancers. *J Clin Invest.* 2016;126:1052–1066; Pozdeyev N, Gay LM, Sokol ES, et al. Genetic analysis of 779 advanced differentiated and anaplastic thyroid cancers. *Clin Cancer Res.* 2018;24:3059–3068.

may lead to FTC, these genetic signatures have proved to be useful for diagnostic purposes, as will be discussed. Table 22.1 summarizes the principal molecular markers of FTCs identified with next generation sequencing techniques.

DIAGNOSIS

Clinical Presentation

Similar to other forms of DTC, FTC most commonly presents as an asymptomatic mass.[34] The generally accepted risk of thyroid cancer in a nodule is 10% to 15%, including nodules that are discovered by the patient, by clinical neck examination, or incidentally on other imaging procedures (chest computed tomography [CT] scan, carotid ultrasound, etc.) (see Chapter 10, The Evaluation and Management of Thyroid Nodules).[35] Concerning clinical features of thyroid nodules include rapid growth, firm or hard texture with fixation, and occurrence in patients with either a family history of thyroid cancer or a personal history of external radiation to the head or neck, especially in childhood.[36] Distant metastases can be present at initial diagnosis in 15% to 27% of patients.[34] Regardless of the method of initial detection, a complete thyroid and neck ultrasound (US) is recommended to define thyroid nodule characteristics, identify additional nodules, and detect characteristic lymph node metastases,[37] as described elsewhere in this book (see Chapter 13, Ultrasound of the Thyroid and Parathyroid Glands).

To improve the identification of nodules likely to be malignant, US scoring and classification systems have recently been developed and/or endorsed by several scientific bodies, including the American Thyroid Association (ATA),[37] the AACE/ACE/AME Guidelines,[38] the Korean Society of Thyroid Radiology,[39] and the American College of Radiology.[40] These systems are based largely on ratings of nodule features identified as suspicious in studies of PTCs (e.g., marked hypoechogenicity, spiculated margins, lymph-node metastases). The sonographic features of FTCs are substantially different from those of PTCs, and recent findings have demonstrated that the system advocated by the ATA tends to overestimate the risk of malignancy in tumors presenting with high-suspicion US pattern and to underestimate that of lesions with patterns considered low-risk in PTCs.[41] Distinguishing between follicular thyroid adenomas (FTA) and follicular carcinomas is difficult, as they both have a solitary, well-defined, solid, homogeneous nodule; an iso- or hypoechoic with a peripheral halo.[42] The Korean Thyroid Imaging Reporting and Data System[39] also appears to be of little value in distinguishing FTAs from FTC.[43]

As for lymph node metastasis, FTCs are more often subject to hematogenous spread, and this is probably the reason they carry a higher risk of distant metastases.[44,45] However, lymph node metastases are a rare but possible finding in FTC, and surgical planning should be based on a formal preoperative US to evaluate for lymph node metastases.[37,45,46]

Cytopathology and Molecular Diagnostics

No other portion of the diagnostic workup for thyroid nodules causes as much consternation as the interpretation and differentiation of a benign follicular lesion versus a follicular carcinoma on cytology from a thyroid nodule fine-needle aspiration (FNA) biopsy (see Chapter 11, Fine-Needle Aspiration of the Thyroid Gland). Cytopathology expertise and communication between the clinician and cytopathologist are critical to appropriately categorize the risk of malignancy in follicular lesions. In 2007, the National Cancer Institute convened a state of the science meeting to attempt to consolidate and provide guidance regarding thyroid cytopathology terminology. The result was the Bethesda system for reporting thyroid cytopathology,[47] which includes six distinct categories of thyroid FNA cytology findings: benign, atypia of undetermined significance/follicular lesion of undetermined significance, follicular neoplasm/Hürthle cell neoplasm, suspicious for malignancy, PTC, and nondiagnostic. Notably, *FTC* and *suspicious for FTC* are not among these categories (Figure 22.2). In fact, FTCs are distinguished from FTAs solely by the presence of capsular and/or vascular invasion, neither of which can be assessed in cytology specimens. The term follicular neoplasm refers to all tumors characterized by high cellularity, microfollicular architecture, and scant or absent colloid—that is, features indicative of the proliferation of thyroid follicular cells, benign or malignant. These follicular-patterned lesions include FTA, follicular carcinoma, follicular variant of papillary carcinoma, and the newly defined entity referred to as noninvasive follicular thyroid neoplasm with papillary-like nuclear features (NIFTP).[48] Although the reported risk of malignancy for nodules classified as follicular neoplasms varies, the follicular neoplasm diagnosis identifies a larger proportion of FTC (in one study, 28% of malignancies with follicular neoplasm cytology were FTC compared with only 2% of FTC in all other cytologic groups).[49]

In the absence of a definitive diagnosis of FTC on FNA, a variety of cytologic, clinical, US, biochemical, and molecular features can help the practitioner estimate risk and aid in recommending surgery or conservative follow-up. Cytologic features predicting malignancy include transgressing vessels, anisokaryosis, nuclear pleomorphism, greater percentage of single cells, increased cellularity with crowding, nuclear grooves and atypia, and fewer macrofollicular formations. For nodules classified as indeterminate on FNAC, the ATA guidelines suggest that a thyroid scan (^{123}I or ^{99}Tc) can help stratify malignancy risk in a thyroid nodule.[37,52] Novel genetic approaches have been developed to improve presurgical diagnosis. The three assays now being marketed are mainly "rule-out" tests; that is, they are designed to identify benign nodules, thereby reducing rates of diagnostic surgeries. When the ThyroSeq (v.2) assay was independently tested in a cohort of 192 indeterminate nodules, it demonstrated a sensitivity of 70%, specificity of 77% (instead of the originally reported 90% and 93%),[53] and positive and negative predictive values (NPVs) of 42% and 91%, respectively.[51]

The Afirma gene expression classifier (GEC) classifies nodules as benign or suspicious, based on its analysis of transcript levels for 167 genes in mRNA samples extracted from one or two fine-needle aspirates. Its reported NPVs range from 94% to 95%, and its PPV is decidedly lower (37% to 38%).[54,55] False-positive results appear to be especially frequent in nodules with cytology consistent with Hürthle cell proliferation.[56]

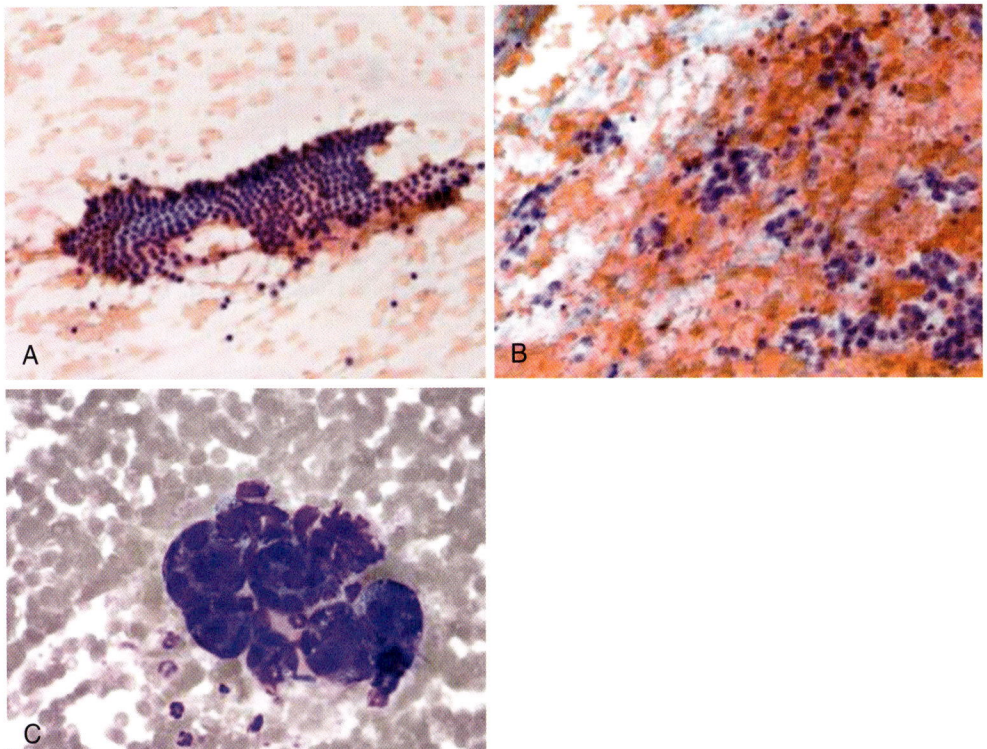

Fig. 22.2 Representative follicular lesion cytology. **A,** Benign colloid nodule (20 ×). The cells are in a broad sheet with no cellular atypia. **B,** FLUS (20 ×). The cells are starting to arrange in microfollicle formations and display some nuclear atypia and crowding. **C,** Follicular neoplasm (40 ×). The cells form microfollicles with nuclear atypia and crowding. **A** and **B** are Papanicolaou stained, and **C** is a Diff-Quick stain. (Images kindly provided by Dr. Sharon Sams.)

The ThyraMIR/ThyGenX assay, which is based on the analysis of microRNA expression levels and a panel of seven gene mutations,[57] has exhibited a sensitivity of 89% and specificity of 85%. The test has been validated in series that include PTC and a smaller proportion of FTC and Hürthle cell carcinoma (HCC). Its performance varies considerably from center to center, and poorer results have been reported in series of indeterminate nodules with high prevalences of FTC and HCC.[58]

Histopathology

Follicular lesions of the thyroid can be separated into distinct clinical entities: FTAs, minimally invasive follicular carcinomas, angioinvasive follicular carcinomas, and widely invasive follicular carcinomas (Figure 22.3). Correct diagnosis requires a thorough evaluation of the entire tumor capsule. Even with a complete appraisal of the tumor capsule, however, the absolute definition of a minimally invasive FTC can be controversial.[37] Minimally invasive FTC is basically defined as tumor penetration or disruption of the tumor capsule in at least one area. Even within this definition, there appears to be a relapse-free survival benefit when there are fewer than four foci of disruption/penetration in the tumor capsule or blood vessels.[59,60] Minimally invasive FTC tends to carry a very low risk of persistent/recurrent disease (estimated at approximately 5%)[37] and generally does not need remnant ablation or adjuvant therapy with radioiodine.[61]

The latest WHO classification[18] distinguishes *encapsulated angioinvasive FTC*—referred to by some as *moderately invasive FTC*[62]—from FTCs with capsular invasion alone because the presence of vascular invasion increases the chances of recurrence and metastases.[18,62] The number of vessels involved (<4 or ≥4 vascular invasion) is also predictive of overall[63] and disease-free survival (DFS).[64-67]

Widely invasive FTCs are characterized by diffuse infiltration of vascular structures and/or adjacent thyroid or extrathyroidal tissues. The capsule is often incomplete, and areas of hemorrhage and necrosis are frequent.

TREATMENT

Surgery

Given the diagnostic challenges discussed earlier, FTCs are almost always identified after a diagnostic thyroid lobectomy (TL), the surgical procedure of choice for solitary, cytologically indeterminate nodules, according to the 2015 ATA guidelines.[37] Total thyroidectomy should be considered if cytologic or ultrasonographic findings are suggestive of an increased risk of malignancy (e.g., lesions exceeding 4 cm in size, those harboring somatic mutations specific for carcinoma, and tumors in patients with a family history of thyroid cancer, a personal history of radiation exposure) or advanced age.

Regardless of the procedure used, it should ideally be performed by a surgeon with high-volume experience (>100 thyroid-related procedures per year), as this has been associated with significantly lower complication rates.[68] Intraoperative frozen sections are sometimes used to guide the extent of surgery (usually determining whether to stop at a hemithyroidectomy versus proceeding with a thyroidectomy). The utility of the frozen section depends on the comfort and expertise of the pathologist. One representative study of 142 patients undergoing

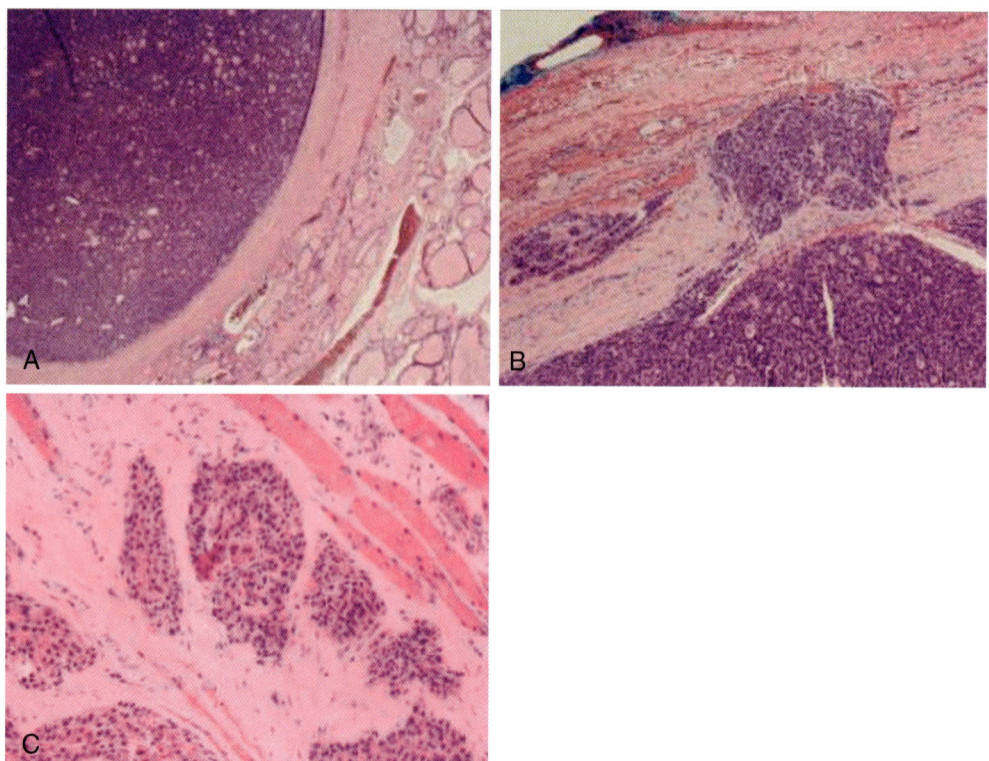

Fig. 22.3 Representative follicular lesion histopathology. **A,** Follicular thyroid adenoma (4×). The tumor capsule is complete and not disrupted in any area. **B,** Minimally invasive FTC (10×). There is an area of penetration into but not through the tumor capsule by FTC. **C,** Widely invasive FTC (20×). FTC has invaded into perithyroidal soft tissue and muscle. (All images are hematoxylin and eosin stained and were kindly provided by Dr. Sherif Said.)

surgery with an indeterminate lesion showed that only 30% of carcinomas were correctly identified by frozen section, suggesting it may not be a cost-effective or reliable procedure.[69] There is not a broad consensus on the utility of frozen section, and the ATA guidelines have no specific recommendation on the use of this procedure.[37,70] In a cost-effectiveness analysis using a Markov decision model, TL alone was superior to both total thyroidectomy (TT) and TL with frozen sections for solitary follicular lesions in terms of both costs and quality-adjusted life years.[71] Approximately 10% of FTCs are multifocal or involve locoregional lymph nodes. Patients with widely invasive FTCs (those with complete penetration of the tumor capsule in multiple areas) on histopathology after hemithyroidectomy should undergo completion thyroidectomy.[72] Minimally invasive FTCs are likely adequately treated with a hemithyroidectomy, especially if the preoperative US shows no lesions on the contralateral thyroid lobe or abnormal lymph nodes. Overall, data analysis from the National Thyroid Cancer Treatment Cooperative Study Group shows improved survival with a total thyroidectomy for moderate to high-risk disease (stages II to IV).[73]

Medical Therapy

FTC generally retains sodium iodide symporter and thyroperoxidase function and can thus be visualized and treated with radioiodine (RAI; see Chapter 47, Postoperative Management of Differentiated Thyroid Cancer, and Chapter 48, Postoperative Radioactive Iodine Ablation and Treatment of Differentiated Thyroid Cancer). Several retrospective observational studies have looked at the effect of RAI in FTC.[74-77] In all these studies, RAI treatment (that given for remnant ablation as well as that administered with therapeutic intent) was compared with no RAI treatment at all. In a cohort of 251 patients with minimally invasive FTCs, cause-specific survival was not significantly different in the treated and nontreated groups.[75,77-79] However, in three other studies[74,78,79] that included FTC patients with higher-risk features (e.g., later-stage disease, widely invasive tumors), survival was significantly improved in those who had received RAI.

RAI remnant ablation does not improve survival or decrease recurrence in most patients with stage I DTC,[73] and its use should be limited to those patients with more aggressive disease (extrathyroidal invasion, extensive lymph node metastases). The National Thyroid Cancer Treatment Cooperative Study Group has shown that RAI improves overall survival for patients with stage II disease.[73] Another large, long-term study of patients with DTC and distant metastases[80] showed that 77% of patients with PTC and 53% of those with poorly differentiated FTC had RAI-concentrating metastatic lesions. In contrast, most well-differentiated FTCs were RAI-avid (92%). Furthermore, patients with positive RAI uptake had a much better prognosis, although only 11.5% of FTC patients achieved complete remission after RAI.

For RAI-refractory FTCs, local treatment, such as surgery or thermal ablation, may be an option if the number of symptomatic or threatening lesions is low. External beam radiotherapy for local or distant disease is reportedly capable of improving relapse-free survival in FTC.[81]

For widespread, progressive, RAI-refractory disease, systemic treatment with tyrosine kinase inhibitors (TKIs) is the best approach.[82] Two large controlled randomized phase 3 studies—the DECISION[83] and

SELECT[84] trials)—showed that these drugs (specifically, sorafenib and lenvatinib) can improve DFS in patients with RAI-refractory DTCs. FTC patients accounted for 25% of those enrolled in the DECISION trial and 19% in the SELECT trial), and 18% of the SELECT population had HCCs.[83,84] A subgroup analysis in the SELECT trial found that, among patients who received lenvatinib, those who had FTCs had longer progression-free survival than those with PTCs (18.8 months; hazard ratio 0.07 [95% confidence interval (CI) 0.03 to 0.21] versus16.4 months; HR 0.30 [95% CI 0.20 to 0.44]).[84] Other novel, systemic treatments are also being tested in clinical trials.[82]

Thyrotropin suppression therapy may be considered in patients with FTC (see Chapter 47, Postoperative Management of Differentiated Thyroid Cancer). This is generally achieved with levothyroxine (T4) at a starting dose of 1.8 to 2 μg/kg/day soon after surgery.[85] There is no evidence of any objective or subjective benefit with combination T4/T3 therapy or desiccated thyroid extract for most patients with DTC.[86] There is evidence of an overall survival benefit in patients with high-risk thyroid cancer with a fully suppressed thyroid-stimulating hormone (TSH) relative to one in the normal range.[73,85,87] The ATA guidelines recommend suppressing TSH with exogenous levothyroxine to a level below 0.1 mU/L for patients at high risk of recurrence or disease-specific mortality and to maintain TSH between 0.1 and 0.5 mU/L for low-risk patients. In patients who are believed to be free of disease, the levothyroxine should be decreased to allow the TSH to rise to the low normal range (0.5 to 2 mU/L).[37,88] TSH-suppression can, in fact, be associated with adverse effects, including increased risks for atrial fibrillation and osteoporosis, notably in elderly patients, and angina in those with ischemic heart disease.[89]

PROGNOSIS

Patient survival for those with DTC (including FTC and PTC) is related to disease stage at initial diagnosis (see Chapter 24, Dynamic Risk Group Analysis and Staging for Differentiated Thyroid Cancer).

Several systems are available for staging thyroid cancers.[90] Some were developed on the basis of studies conducted on PTCs; others are based on data obtained on DTCs in general (i.e., PTC and FTC) or on all histologic types of thyroid carcinoma, including medullary and anaplastic thyroid cancer, and one is based exclusively on data on FTCs.[91]

The AJCC pTNM (tumor, nodes, and metastasis) system is designed to assess the risk of cancer-specific mortality. It has always been the one most widely used, and it has been shown to provide a sufficiently accurate estimate of the prognosis in several studies.[50,90,92] The ATA risk of recurrence classification system was developed to provide an estimate of DFS, and its ability to do so has also been confirmed.[37] Indeed, for this purpose, the ATA risk class is more accurate than the TNM stage (HR 4.67; 95% CI 1.74 to 12.5, p = 0.002 versus HR 1.26; 95% CI 0.98 to 1.62, p = 0.063).[93]

Updated versions of the ATA guidelines and AJCC staging system were published in 2016, and both require independent revalidation. In the new 8th edition of the AJCC/IUCC staging system, the age cut-off for defining stage I disease has been increased from 45 to 55 years, a change made to limit the risk of overtreatment. Moreover, a recent reassessment of the National Thyroid Cancer Treatment Cooperative Study (NTCTCS) thyroid cancer staging systems showed that a new model for FTC, with a threshold at 50 years, outperformed the current system and separate NTCTCS staging systems for PTC and FTC have been proposed.[94]

Metastatic disease at presentation is a major risk factor for mortality, with 67% of patients with this presentation dying of FTC.[78] This risk persisted in a multivariate analysis and predicted a 47-fold increased relative risk for mortality.[78] Extrathyroidal extension of tumor provided a greater than threefold risk of mortality from FTC, and treatment with RAI improved survival.[78] Excluding patients with distant metastases, the local aggressiveness of the primary tumor provides prognostic information. In one study of 132 patients with FTC, the overall mortality was 21%.[95] Patients with gross extrathyroidal extension had 38% recurrence, and 33% died after a mean follow-up of 7.5 years. Similarly, a study of 168 patients with FTC evaluated over a 10-year period revealed a 28% mortality rate.[46] To provide perspective, this study also evaluated 435 patients with PTC, and there was only 9% mortality over 10 years. On a multivariate analysis, the only statistically significant risk factors for FTC mortality were distant metastases (odds ratio [OR] 5.38) and tumor size (OR 2.84). The prognostic importance of tumor size is relevant given that FTC often has a larger tumor size at presentation (75% to 100% larger relative to PTCs).[96,97] FTC tends to have a greater predilection for bone metastases than PTC.[98] Patients with DTC and bone metastases have a 50% mortality rate at 3 years.[99] One large study showed that DTC patients with pulmonary metastases had a much better 10-year survival (63%) than patients with bone metastases who had a grim 25% 10-year survival.[80] In summary, FTC tends to present at a later age, with larger tumors and a greater degree of distant metastases, and thus it has a worse prognosis than PTC. The principal prognostic factors of FTC are summarized in Table 22.2.

TABLE 22.2 Predictors of Recurrence, Survival, or Distant Metastases

Independent Risk Factors	Disease-Free Survival	Survival	Distant Metastases
Older age	In FTC (WI and MI not distinguished): 45 vs. 25 yrs: RR 1.8[1] In MI: ≥45 yrs: OR 14.3 [95% CI 0.02–0.07][2] ≥45 yrs: OR 9.76 [95% CI 2.18–43.78][3]	In FTC (WI and MI not distinguished): (CSS) ≥50 yrs: HR 16.72 [95% CI 2.13–131.37][4] (CSS) >40 yrs (men); ≥50 yrs (women) RR 10.4 [95% CI 1.23–90.9][5] (CSS) >60 yrs at first distant metastases detection: HR 6.71 [95% CI 2.07–31.3][6] (CSS) ≥45 yrs: OR 4.8[7] (CSS) 45 vs. 25 yrs: RR 2.2[1] (OS) ≥45 yrs (risk reduction for patients <45 yrs, RR 0.34 [95% CI 0.24–0.46])[8] (CSS) >40 yrs: OR not available[9] (CSS) continuous variable[10] (OS) ≥45 yrs: HR not available[11]	In FTC (WI and MI not distinguished): ≥45 yrs: OR 19.7[7] >45 yrs: OR not available[14] ≥45 yrs: OR not available[15] Continuous variable, OR not available[16] In FTC and HCC: ≥65 yrs (MI FTC and HCC)[12] >40 ≤ 50 yrs: OR 4.0 [95% CI 1.1–16.1]; >50 ≤ 60 yrs: 5.2 [95% CI 1.3–20.5]; >60 yrs: 17.8 [95% CI 4.8–66.5][17]

Continued

TABLE 22.2 Predictors of Recurrence, Survival, or Distant Metastases—cont'd

Independent Risk Factors	Disease-Free Survival	Survival	Distant Metastases
Tumor size	In FTC (WI and MI not distinguished): >4 cm: OR 6.750 [95% CI 1.01–44.92][18] In MI: ≥4 cm: RR 5.92 [95% CI 0.611–58.824][19] >4 cm: OR 3.509 [95% CI 1.092–11.364][3] In WI: >4 cm: OR 3.83 [95% CI 1.25–11.6][20] In FTC and HCC: per 1 cm increase: HR 1.3 [95% CI 1.1–1.6][17]	In MI: (CSS) ≥45 yrs: OR 11.5 [95% CI 0.03–0.13][2] In FTC and HCC: (CSS) ≥65 yrs: HR 9.11 [95% CI 1.65–50.2][12] (MI FTC and HCC) (CSS) ≥45 yrs: HR 7.2 [95% CI 1.4–131.2][13] In FTC (WI and MI not distinguished): (CSS) ≥4 cm: HR 6.84 [95% CI 1.34–124.9][6] (OS) >4 cm: HR 3.21 [95% CI 1.13–9.16] in patients aged <45 yrs[11] (OS) ≥2 cm (risk reduction for tumors <2 cm, RR 0.72 [95% CI 0.52–0.97])[8] (CSS) for 1 cm increase[21] In MI: (CSS) >4 cm: OR 25.641 [95% CI 1.04–50][3] In WI: (CSS) ≥4 cm, HR not available[22] In FTC and HCC: (CSS) ≥4 cm: HR 13.9 [95% CI 2.9–250][13]	In FTC (WI and MI not distinguished): ≥4 cm: OR 7.9[7] Linear increase[15]
Angioinvasion present		In FTC: (CSS) HR not available[23] (CSS) vascular and lymphatic invasion: RR 40.4 [95% CI 3.3–497.2][24] In MI: (CSS) HR 20.06 [95% CI 1.4–287.06][25]	In FTC: FTC, OR not available[14] In MI: HR 29.06 [95% CI 3.06–209.08][26]
Distant metastasis		In FTC (WI and MI not distinguished): (CSS) M1 at presentation, RR 47.7 [95% CI 17.8–128][27] (CSS) OR 11[7] (CSS) RR 6.4 [95% CI 2.06–20][5] (CSS) RR not available[9] (CSS) HR 5.25 [95% CI 1.90–14.51][4] (CSS) RR 3.2[1] (OS) RR 2.47 [95% CI 1.8–3.31][8] In MI: (CSS) OR 456.9 [95% CI 47.6–1007.5][3] In WI: (CSS) OR 83.3 [95% CI 6.4–100][20] (CSS) >45 yrs, HR not available[22] In FTC and HCC: (CSS) HR 14.77 [95% CI 2.65–82.21][25] (CSS) RR 41.35 [95% CI 3.32–512.99][24] (CSS) HR 14 [95% CI 5.3–37.1][13] (CSS) RR 3.80 [95% CI 2.22–6.520][28]	-
Lymph node metastasis	In FTC and HCC: HR 29.4 [95% CI 8.7–99.4][17]	In FTC (WI and MI not distinguished): (OS) HR 11.23 [95% CI 2.44–61.69] in patients aged <45 yrs; HR 2.86 [1.7–4.78] in patients ≥45 yrs[11] (OS) RR 1.94 [95% CI 1.47–2.5][8] In FTC and HCC: (CSS) RR 50.98 [95% CI 2.78–934.02][24]	FTC, OR not available[14]
Incomplete tumor excision		In FTC (WI and MI not distinguished): (CSS) HR 10.8 [95% CI 3.4–35.1][4] (CSS) RR 5.8 [95% CI 0.99–34.48][5] (CSS) R0, RR 0.06 [95% CI 0.02–0.2][27]	
Extrathyroidal invasion	In FTC (WI and MI not distinguished):	In FTC (WI and MI not distinguished): (CSS) RR 3.8 [95% CI 1.5–10][27]	In FTC and HCC: OR 2.8 [95% CI 1.1–6.9][17]

TABLE 22.2 Predictors of Recurrence, Survival, or Distant Metastases—cont'd

Independent Risk Factors	Disease-Free Survival	Survival	Distant Metastases
Histologic subtype (WI vs. MI)	RR 22.07[29] In FTC and HCC: HR 4.94 [95% CI 1.28–19.06][30] In FTC and HCC: HR 13.12 [95% CI 3.36–51.14][30]	(OS) HR 1.68 [95% CI 1.22–2.32] in patients ≥45 yrs[11] (CSS) HR not available[10] In FTC and HCC: (CSS) HR 9.6 [95% CI 2.8–32.6][12] (mFTC and mHCC) In FTC and HCC: (CSS) WI: HR 3.79 [95% CI 1.03–14.02][25] (OS) HR 2.72 [95% CI 1.33–5.53][31] OS in pts with bone metastases	In FTC and HCC: • WI: OR 7.8[7] • WI: OR 3.0 [95% CI 1.3–6.7][17]

ATA, American Thyroid Association; *CI*, confidence interval; *CSS*, cancer specific survival; *FTC*, follicular thyroid carcinoma; *HCC*, Hürthle cell carcinoma; *HR*, hazard ratio; *MI*, minimally invasive; *OR*, odds ratio; *OS*, overall survival; *RR*, relative risk; *WI*, widely invasive

[1] Mueller-Gaertner HW, Brzac HT, Rehpenning W. Prognostic indices for tumor relapse and tumor mortality in follicular thyroid carcinoma. *Cancer.* 1991;67(7):1903–1911.
[2] Sugino K, Kameyama K, Ito K, et al. Outcomes and prognostic factors of 251 patients with minimally invasive follicular thyroid carcinoma. *Thyroid.* 2012;22(8):798–804.
[3] Ito Y, Hirokawa M, Masuoka H, et al. Prognostic factors of minimally invasive follicular thyroid carcinoma: extensive vascular invasion significantly affects patient prognosis. *Endocr J.* 2013;60(5):637–642.
[4] Lang BH, Lo CY, Chan WF, Lam KY, Wan KY. Prognostic factors in papillary and follicular thyroid carcinoma: their implications for cancer staging. *Ann Surg Oncol.* 2007;14(2):730–738.
[5] Lo CY, Chan WF, Lam KY, Wan KY. Follicular thyroid carcinoma: the role of histology and staging systems in predicting survival. *Ann Surg.* 2005;242(5):708–715.
[6] Sugino K, Kameyama K, Nagahama M, et al. Follicular thyroid carcinoma with distant metastasis: outcome and prognostic factor. *Endocr J.* 2014;61(3):273–279.
[7] Sugino K, Ito K, Nagahama M, et al. Prognosis and prognostic factors for distant metastases and tumor mortality in follicular thyroid carcinoma. *Thyroid.* 2011;21(7):751–757.
[8] Podnos YD, Smith D, Wagman LD, Ellenhorn JD. Radioactive iodine offers survival improvement in patients with follicular carcinoma of the thyroid. *Surgery.* 2005;138(6):1072–1076; discussion 1076–1077.
[9] Gyory F, Balazs G, Nagy EV, et al. Differentiated thyroid cancer and outcome in iodine deficiency. *Eur J Surg Oncol.* 2004;30(3):325–331.
[10] Davis NL, Bugis SP, McGregor GI, Germann E. An evaluation of prognostic scoring systems in patients with follicular thyroid cancer. *Am J Surg.* 1995;170(5):476–480.
[11] Zaydfudim V, Feurer ID, Griffin MR, Phay JE. The impact of lymph node involvement on survival in patients with papillary and follicular thyroid carcinoma. *Surgery.* 2008;144(6):1070–1077; discussion 1077–1078.
[12] Kuo EJ, Roman SA, Sosa JA. Patients with follicular and Hurthle cell microcarcinomas have compromised survival: a population level study of 22,738 patients. *Surgery.* 2013;154(6):1246–1253; discussion 1253–1254.
[13] Sugino K, Kameyama K, Ito K, et al. Does Hürthle cell carcinoma of the thyroid have a poorer prognosis than ordinary follicular thyroid carcinoma? *Ann Surg Oncol.* 2013;20(9):2944–2950.
[14] O'Neill CJ, Vaughan L, Learoyd DL, Sidhu SB, Delbridge LW, Sywak MS. Management of follicular thyroid carcinoma should be individualised based on degree of capsular and vascular invasion. *Eur J Surg Oncol.* 2011;37(2):181–185.
[15] Verburg FA, Mader U, Luster M, Reiners C. Primary tumour diameter as a risk factor for advanced disease features of differentiated thyroid carcinoma. *Clin Endocrinol (Oxf).* 2009;71(2):291–297.
[16] Ban EJ, Andrabi A, Grodski S, Yeung M, McLean C, Serpell J. Follicular thyroid cancer: minimally invasive tumours can give rise to metastases. *ANZ J Surg.* 2012;82(3):136–139.
[17] Kim WG, Kim TY, Kim TH, et al. Follicular and Hurthle cell carcinoma of the thyroid in iodine-sufficient area: retrospective analysis of Korean multicenter data. *Korean J Intern Med.* 2014;29(3):325–333.
[18] Podda M, Saba A, Porru F, Reccia I, Pisanu A. Follicular thyroid carcinoma: differences in clinical relevance between minimally invasive and widely invasive tumors. *World J Surg Oncol.* 2015;13:193.
[19] Ito Y, Hirokawa M, Miyauchi A, et al. Prognostic impact of Ki-67 labeling index in minimally invasive follicular thyroid carcinoma. *Endocr J.* 2016;63(10):913–917.
[20] Ito Y, Hirokawa M, Masuoka H, et al. Distant metastasis at diagnosis and large tumor size are significant prognostic factors of widely invasive follicular thyroid carcinoma. *Endocr J.* 2013;60(6):829–833.
[21] Lin JD, Chao TC, Chen ST, Huang YY, Liou MJ, Hsueh C. Operative strategy for follicular thyroid cancer in risk groups stratified by pTNM staging. *Surg Oncol.* 2007;16(2):107–113.
[22] Asari R, Koperek O, Scheuba C, et al. Follicular thyroid carcinoma in an iodine-replete endemic goiter region: a prospectively collected, retrospectively analyzed clinical trial. *Ann Surg.* 2009;249(6):1023–1031.
[23] D'Avanzo A, Treseler P, Ituarte PH, et al. Follicular thyroid carcinoma: histology and prognosis. *Cancer.* 2004;100(6):1123–1129.
[24] de Melo TG, Zantut-Wittmann DE, Ficher E, da Assumpcao LV. Factors related to mortality in patients with papillary and follicular thyroid cancer in long-term follow-up. *J Endocrinol Invest.* 2014;37(12):1195–1200.
[25] Kim HJ, Sung JY, Oh YL, et al. Association of vascular invasion with increased mortality in patients with minimally invasive follicular thyroid carcinoma but not widely invasive follicular thyroid carcinoma. *Head Neck.* 2014;36(12):1695–1700.
[26] Lee YM, Lee YH, Song DE, et al. Prognostic impact of further treatments on distant metastasis in patients with minimally invasive follicular thyroid carcinoma: verification using inverse probability of treatment weighting. *World J Surg.* 2017;41(4):1144.
[27] Chow SM, Law SC, Mendenhall WM, et al. Follicular thyroid carcinoma: prognostic factors and the role of radioiodine. *Cancer.* 2002;95(3):488–498.

[28] Besic N, Zgajnar J, Hocevar M, Frkovic-Grazio S. Is patient's age a prognostic factor for follicular thyroid carcinoma in the TNM classification system? *Thyroid*. 2005;15(5):439–448.

[29] Yamamoto S, Tomita Y, Uruno T, et al. Increased expression of valosin-containing protein (p97) is correlated with disease recurrence in follicular thyroid cancer. *Ann Surg Oncol*. 2005;12(11):925–934.

[30] Aboelnaga EM, Ahmed RA. Difference between papillary and follicular thyroid carcinoma outcomes: an experience from Egyptian institution. *Cancer Biol Med*. 2015;12(1):53–59.

[31] Mishra A, Kumar C, Chand G, et al. Long-term outcome of follicular thyroid carcinoma in patients undergoing surgical intervention for skeletal metastases. *World J Surg*. 2016;40(3):562–569.

Modified from Grani G, Lamartina L, Durante C, et al. Follicular thyroid cancer and Hürthle cell carcinoma: challenges in diagnosis, treatment, and clinical management. *Lancet Diabetes Endocrinol*. 2018;6(6):500–514.

SUMMARY

FTC is the second most common form of DTC. It tends to present at a more advanced stage and is associated with higher mortality than PTC. A potential reason for the later presentation may be the difficulty in diagnosing FTC by thyroid nodule FNA. Molecular markers may help optimize preoperative diagnosis. Surgical resection remains the best therapy, and patients with higher-risk disease benefit from RAI remnant ablation or adjuvant therapy. For progressive disease that is refractory to systemic RAI therapy, TKIs are currently the best solution, and other systemic approaches are being tested in clinical trials.

REFERENCES

For a complete list of references, go to *expertconsult.com*.

Noninvasive Follicular Thyroid Neoplasm With Papillary-Like Nuclear Features (NIFTP)

Yuri E. Nikiforov, Robert L. Ferris

> Please go to expertconsult.com to view related video:
> **Video 23.1** Introduction to Chapter 23, Noninvasive Follicular Thyroid Neoplasm with Papillary-Like Nuclear Features.

INTRODUCTION

Noninvasive follicular thyroid neoplasm with papillary-like nuclear features (NIFTP) is a recently defined entity[1] that was accepted by the World Health Organization (WHO) in 2017.[2] Before 2016, these tumors were diagnosed as noninvasive encapsulated follicular variants of papillary carcinoma. The nomenclature change was proposed to optimize patient care, eliminate the stigma of malignancy, and optimally de-escalate treatment and follow-up for these patients.

DEFINITION

NIFTP is defined by WHO as a noninvasive neoplasm of thyroid follicular cells with a follicular growth pattern and nuclear features of papillary carcinoma that has a very low malignant potential.[2] It is considered a borderline malignant or premalignant lesion rather than a benign lesion.

The diagnosis of NIFTP is based on the finding of an encapsulated or clearly demarcated nodule with a follicular growth pattern and cells revealing nuclear features of papillary thyroid cancer (PTC) and a complete lack of invasive characteristics, papillary structures, or high-grade microscopic features. A diagnosis of NIFTP can be made only after exclusion of invasion; therefore examination of the entire tumor capsule and tumor interface is required.

EPIDEMIOLOGY

NIFTP is a recently introduced entity, and its exact incidence is currently unknown. Based on retrospective studies estimating the prevalence of noninvasive encapsulated follicular variant papillary carcinoma, it is likely that NIFTP comprises 10% to 20% of the incidence of PTC observed before 2016 in North America and several European countries, as well as in Brazil.[1-4] A significantly lower incidence of the NIFTP diagnosis may be observed in Asia,[2] with NIFTP accounting for 1% to 5% of the papillary carcinomas.[3,5] This may reflect ethnic differences or variation in histopathologic approaches to diagnosing nuclear features of papillary carcinoma by pathologists practicing in different regions. Such an altered higher diagnostic threshold would lead to diagnosing many NIFTP cases as follicular adenomas.

NIFTP is more common in females than males, with a gender ratio of 3:1 to 4:1. The tumor may occur over a wide range of ages, although most patients present during the fourth to sixth decades of life.[1,4,6,7]

ETIOLOGY

The etiologic factors for NIFTP have not been established. For many years these tumors were diagnosed as a variant of papillary carcinoma, and it is likely that NIFTP and papillary thyroid carcinomas share some risk factors, such as exposure to ionizing radiation and preexisting benign thyroid nodules. Similar hormonal factors are probably involved because NIFTP has a female predominance similar to other follicular-cell derived thyroid neoplasms.

Molecular pathogenesis of NIFTP involves gene alterations common in other follicular-patterned thyroid tumors such as follicular adenoma, follicular carcinoma, and follicular variant of papillary carcinoma. NIFTPs are associated with activating mutations of one of the three *RAS* genes (*NRAS* > *HRAS* >> *KRAS*) found in 30% to 60% of cases.[1,8-10] The majority of *RAS* point mutations involve codon 61, although codons 12 and 13 may also be occasionally involved. Other common driver mutations are *PPARG* (most commonly, *PAX8/PPARG*) and *THADA* fusions and occasionally the *BRAF* K601E mutation.[1,9] Mutations in the *PTEN* and *DICER1* genes may also be occasionally seen. *EIF1AX* mutations can be found, typically co-occurring with *RAS* mutations. Before 2016, a large proportion of tumors with these mutations were diagnosed as encapsulated follicular variant of papillary carcinoma,[1,11-15,17] and they met the current diagnostic criteria for NIFTP. Importantly, NIFTP lesions should have no *BRAF* V600E, *RET/PTC*, *NTRK1* or *NTRK3* fusions, or other mutations associated with classical and tall cell variant PTCs.[1,9,10,16-19] Although few studies reported *BRAF* V600E in single cases or in a significant proportion of tumors considered by the authors to be NIFTP,[7,20,21,23] most of those tumors are likely to have at least some well-formed papillae, and using stringent diagnostic criteria should instead be diagnosed as classic papillary carcinoma. NIFTP tumors are early, precancer lesions; therefore they are expected to have no *TERT*, *TP53*, or other mutations common in advanced and dedifferentiated thyroid cancers.[22]

Some studies have shown that NIFTP tumors may have distinct gene expression profiles, with some having the expression profiles resembling those of follicular adenoma and others of infiltrative follicular variant papillary carcinoma.[23] Several specific noncoding miRNAs were reported to have aberrant expression in NIFTP compared with hyperplastic nodules or invasive follicular variant papillary carcinomas.[24]

DIAGNOSIS

Clinical Presentation

NIFTP lesions typically present as a painless, asymptomatic, mobile thyroid nodule that is discovered by palpation or during a neck ultrasound performed for other reasons. Large tumors may cause compression and other local symptoms. Patients are typically euthyroid. On ultrasound, NIFTP is typically present as a solid, well-demarcated, hypoechoic or isoechoic nodule (Figure 23.1).[25-27] No microcalcifications are found. Overall, clinical and ultrasound features of NIFTP are similar to those of follicular adenoma and minimally invasive follicular carcinoma.

Some reports have proposed that ultrasound findings coupled with fine-needle aspiration (FNA) cytology features can be used to triage the intermediate FNA categories.[25,28] In a multicenter study, Hahn et al. demonstrated that NIFTP cases lacked malignant ultrasound features and were better triaged using core biopsy than FNA to facilitate the surgical management.[28] Yang et al. found the ultrasound findings for NIFTP and minimally invasive encapsulated follicular variant of papillary carcinomas were similar and could not be distinguished from each other; these typically exhibited a circumscribed oval or round nodule with a hypoechoic rim and a hypervascular lesion found on Doppler.[25] In contrast, ultrasound findings for overtly invasive encapsulated follicular variant of PTC typically showed a round and oval nodule with irregular margins and a hypervascular Doppler.

Cytology

The FNA of NIFTP usually yields cellular smears with three-dimensional groups of follicular cells and microfollicles and variably expressed nuclear features of papillary carcinoma.[29-31] Colloid can be seen, although it is not abundant. Chromatin clearing, nuclear elongation, and some irregularity of the nuclear contours with scattered groves are typically seen but rarely prominent. Nuclear pseudoinclusions are rare.

The reclassification of the noninvasive follicular variant papillary carcinoma as NIFTP has significant implications for the practice of thyroid cytopathology.[32] The most significant expected change involves a decrease in the implied risk of malignancy, particularly for cases classified into three indeterminate diagnostic categories of The Bethesda System for Reporting Thyroid Cytopathology (TBSRTC):

- TBSRTC Class III. Atypia of undetermined significance/follicular lesion of undetermined significance (AUS/FLUS)
- TBSRTC Class IV. Follicular neoplasm/suspicious for a follicular neoplasm (FN/SFN)
- TBSRTC Class V. Suspicious for malignancy (SFM)[33-35]

Recent studies suggest that the decrease in malignancy risk will be most significant, up to 50%, for thyroid FNA specimens classified as SFM.[33,34] In one analysis of 6943 thyroid FNA specimens from multiple institutions, 173 (2.5%) samples could be diagnosed as NIFTP in the surgically resected nodules. The preoperative FNA cytologic diagnoses for these cases included nondiagnostic in 1%, benign in 9%, AUS/FLUS in 31%, FN/SFN in 27%, SFM in 24%, and malignant in 9%.[34]

NIFTP cannot be reliably distinguished by cytology from invasive follicular variant papillary carcinoma as both lesions typically demonstrate a microfollicular growth pattern and nuclear features of papillary carcinoma, including nuclear enlargement, pallor, crowding, and grooves.[36,37] It may also be difficult to differentiate NIFTP from follicular adenomas with some nuclear atypia. However, cytology can frequently be used to suspect low-risk follicular pattern thyroid lesions and exclude a diagnosis of NIFTP in favor of a classical papillary carcinoma, as NIFTP usually lacks pseudoinclusions and papillary structures.[19,32,33,38,39]

Histopathology

Histopathologic diagnosis of NIFTP rests on identifying four main criteria (Box 23.1).[1,40] These criteria include the following:

1. Encapsulation or clear demarcation of the tumor from adjacent thyroid tissue;
2. Follicular growth pattern;
3. Nuclear features of papillary carcinoma; and
4. Lack of all of the following exclusion criteria: (a) invasion, (b) well-formed papillae or psammoma bodies, (c) >30% solid/trabecular/insular growth pattern, (d) tumor necrosis or high mitotic activity; (e) microscopic features of specific variants of papillary carcinoma.

Additional, secondary diagnostic features may help with the diagnosis but are not required.[40,41]

BOX 23.1 Diagnostic Histopathologic Criteria of NIFTP

Primary Diagnostic Criteria
1. Encapsulation or clear demarcation*
2. Follicular growth pattern
3. Nuclear features of papillary carcinoma
4. Lack of all of the following exclusion criteria:
   a. Vascular or capsular invasion†
   b. Any well-formed papillae or psammoma bodies
   c. >30% solid/trabecular/insular growth pattern
   d. Tumor necrosis or high mitotic activity‡
   e. Microscopic features of other specific variants of papillary carcinoma

Secondary Diagnostic Criteria§
- Lack of *BRAF* V600E mutation detected by molecular assays or immunohistochemistry
- Lack of *RET/PTC*, *NTRK1/3*, *ALK* fusions or high-risk mutations (*TERT*, *TP53*)

*Thick, thin, or partial capsule or well-circumscribed with a clear demarcation from adjacent thyroid parenchyma.
†Requires microscopic examination of the entire tumor capsule interface.
‡High mitotic activity defined as ≥3 mitoses per 10 high power fields (400×).
§Secondary criteria are helpful but not required for NIFTP diagnosis
NIFTP, noninvasive follicular thyroid neoplasm with papillary-like nuclear features.

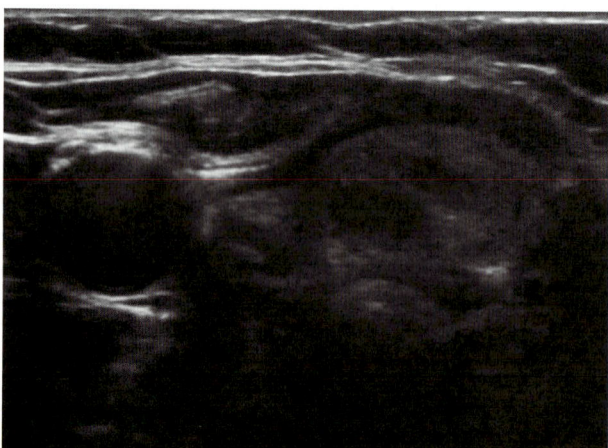

Fig. 23.1 Ultrasound image of noninvasive follicular thyroid neoplasm with papillary-like nuclear features (NIFTP) showing a low American Thyroid Association (ATA) suspicion nodule which is well-circumscribed, with regular margin, mostly isoechoic with hypoechoic areas and no microcalcifications.

CHAPTER 23 Noninvasive Follicular Thyroid Neoplasm With Papillary-Like Nuclear Features (NIFTP)

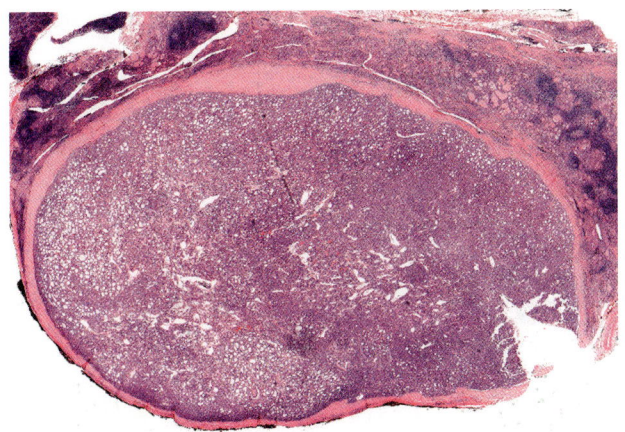

Fig. 23.2 Low-power microscopic image of noninvasive follicular thyroid neoplasm with papillary-like nuclear features (NIFTP) showing complete, moderately thick tumor capsule.

Most NIFTP nodules have a complete capsule (Figure 23.2). Some tumors show no definitive capsule but have a smooth border and are demarcated by a very thin layer of fibrous tissue. Before reclassification, such tumors were called partially encapsulated/well-circumscribed follicular variant papillary carcinomas.[42] NIFTP shows a predominantly or exclusively follicular growth pattern. More often, they are composed of small follicles or show variation in the size of follicles from small to large (Figure 23.3, A). The only other architectural pattern allowed is the solid/trabecular/insular pattern, which should comprise no more than 30% of the tumor. Diagnostic nuclear features of papillary carcinoma should be found. They belong to the three categories: (1) nuclear size and shape (nuclear enlargement/crowding/overlapping and elongation); (2) nuclear membrane irregularities (irregular nuclear contours, grooves, pseudoinclusions); and (3) chromatin characteristics (chromatin clearing with margination, glassy nuclei). To meet the diagnostic criteria for NIFTP, nuclear features from at least two of the three categories should be present (Figure 23.3, B). The working group for reevaluated of the encapsulated follicular variant of papillary carcinoma and proposed a 3-point nuclear score in which each category of nuclear features of papillary carcinoma is assigned a value of 0 (absent) or 1 (present), yielding a summation nuclear score ranging from 0 to 3.[1] A nuclear score of 2 or 3 is required for the diagnosis of NIFTP. The proposed nuclear score has a moderate degree of reproducibility among pathologists[43] and may help standardize the approach to diagnosing nuclear features of papillary carcinoma.[42] Nuclear features of papillary carcinoma may be seen diffusely, affecting all epithelial cells within the nodule, or have patchy, multifocal distribution.

Importantly, none of the exclusion criteria for NIFTP should be found. NIFTP is a noninvasive tumor; therefore no invasion of the tumor capsule or vascular invasion should be present. Invasion is the only histopathological feature that distinguishes NIFTP from invasive encapsulate follicular variant papillary carcinoma, a thyroid tumor with a substantial rate of distant metastasis.[1] To rule out invasion, the entire capsule of the nodule should be examined microscopically. In those samples where the lesion capsule was not fully sampled, the diagnosis of NIFTP cannot be established with certainty.

Another important exclusion criterion is the presence of papillae. The initially proposed diagnostic criteria for NIFTP was "<1% papillae," allowing some papillary structures to be present.[1] The intention was to accept single rudimentary, hyperplastic-type papillae and not true papillae seen in classic papillary carcinoma. However, subsequent studies showed that accepting any well-formed papillae can lead to misdiagnosing classic papillary carcinomas as NIFTP.[7,20] Thus a more stringent criterion permitting no well-formed papillae should be used.[40] As a result the presence of even single papillary structures, particularly when they are lined by cells with prominent nuclear features of papillary carcinoma, should exclude the diagnosis of NIFTP (Figure 23.4, A). However, single simple, hyperplastic-type papillary infoldings are allowed, particularly when they are lined by cells showing no well-developed nuclear features of papillary carcinoma (Figure 23.4, B). Psammoma bodies should not be found, as those provide evidence for preexisting papillary structures characteristic of classic papillary carcinoma.

NIFTP may have a small component of solid/trabecular/insular architecture, which should not exceed 30% of the tumor volume. This criterion was introduced to exclude the solid variant of papillary carcinoma and poorly differentiated carcinoma. Similarly, no increased mitotic activity (defined as 3 or more mitoses per 10 consecutive high power (400×) fields or tumor necrosis should be seen. These are features of poorly differentiated thyroid carcinoma or high-risk papillary carcinoma.

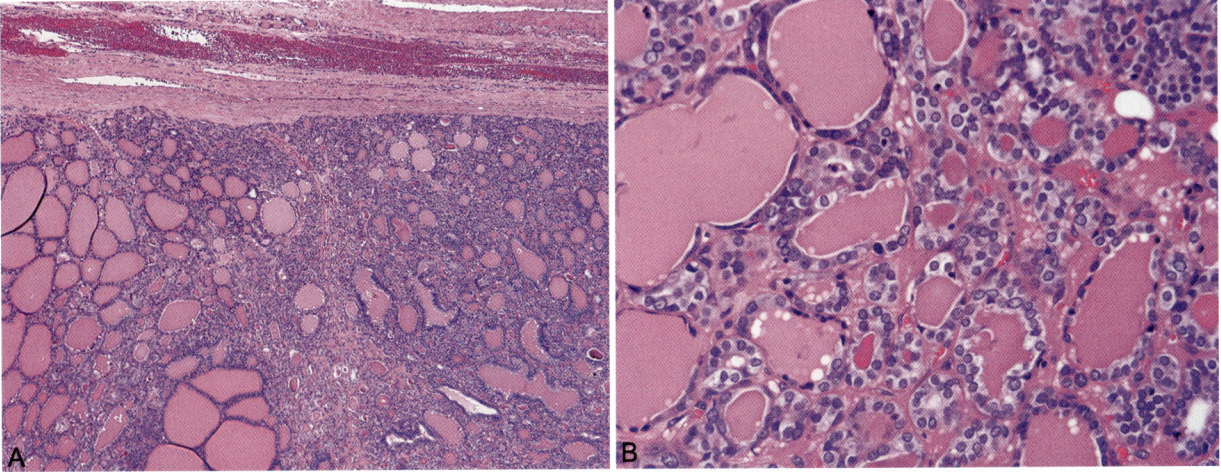

Fig. 23.3 Microscopic features of noninvasive follicular thyroid neoplasm with papillary-like nuclear features (NIFTP). **A,** The tumor shows a thick capsule and is composed of neoplastic follicles that show great variation in size and shape. **B,** High-power image showing follicular cells with enlarged, overlapping nuclei and chromatin clearing. Although no significant nuclear membrane irregularity is noted, the nuclear score of 2 is sufficient for the diagnosis of NIFTP.

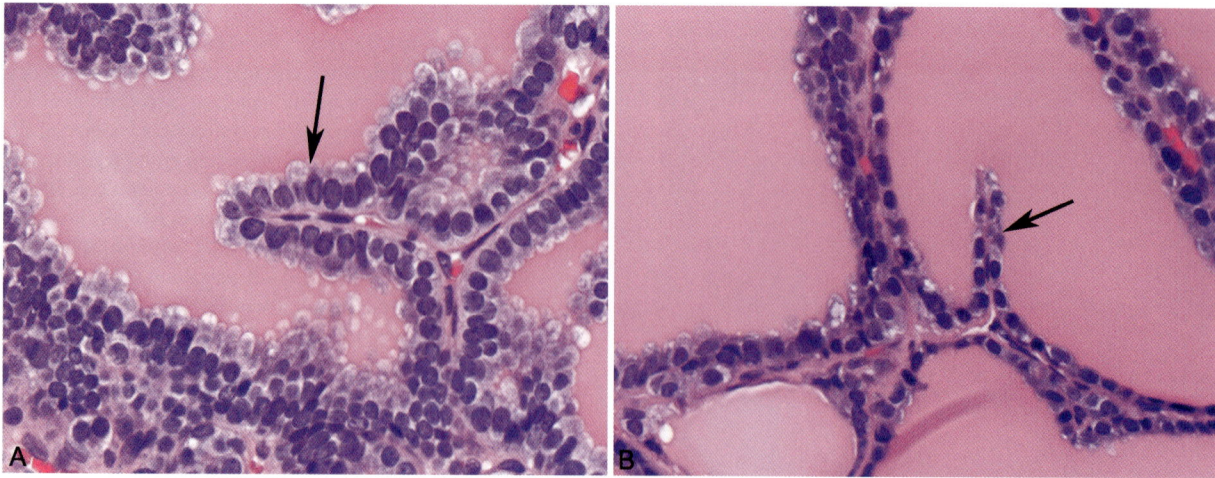

Fig. 23.4 A, A well-formed papilla covered by epithelial cells showing nuclear features of papillary carcinoma is an exclusion criterion for noninvasive follicular thyroid neoplasm with papillary-like nuclear features (NIFTP). **B,** This small simple papillary structure that lacks fibrovascular core, resembling hyperplastic-type papillae, and coved by follicular cells showing no well-developed nuclear features of papillary carcinoma is compatible with the diagnosis of NIFTP.

In addition, no histopathologic features diagnostic of other distinct variants of papillary carcinoma should be present. For example, the presence of tall cells, characteristic of the tall cell variant or cribriform-morular variant of papillary carcinoma, would exclude NIFTP, even if the tumor is encapsulated and shows no papillary structures. The presence of lymph nodes or distant metastases excludes the diagnosis of NIFTP because the presence of such metastases offers evidence for lymphovascular tumor invasion and malignant behavior.[44]

Molecular Diagnostics

None of the molecular markers are diagnostic of NIFTP, as it shares molecular alterations with other follicular-patterned thyroid tumors. Indeed, *RAS* gene point mutations and fusions involving either *PPARG* or *THADA* genes, commonly found in NIFTP, as well as more rarely seen *BRAF* K601E, *PTEN*, and *DICER1* mutations are also found in follicular variant papillary carcinomas, follicular carcinomas, and follicular adenomas. Finding any of these alterations in an FNA sample or resected thyroid nodule indicates that the lesion is a clonal tumor and not a hyperplastic nodule. Furthermore, if found preoperatively in a FNA sample, these alterations would raise the possibility of NIFTP, indicating that surgical excision should be considered in these patients. Importantly, *BRAF* V600E mutations and other *BRAF* V600E-like mutations, such as *RET/PTC* or *NTRK1/3* fusions, are characteristic of classic or tall cell variant of papillary carcinoma, and they should not be found in NIFTP.[1,9,10,17,18] Similarly, high-risk somatic mutations (*TERT*, *TP53*) should not be detected in NIFTP. Overall, molecular profiling of thyroid nodules does not allow a definitive NIFTP diagnosis preoperatively, although it is helpful to preoperatively differentiate a group of follicular-patterned thyroid neoplasms (which includes NIFTP) from classic papillary/tall cell papillary carcinomas and from nonclonal hyperplastic nodules.

Molecular analysis of surgically removed tumors is not required for the diagnosis of NIFTP. However, molecular testing may be helpful in some situations, particularly when histopathologic features are equivocal. In tumors where occasional papillary structures are seen that may not appear microscopically as true papillae, a finding of the *BRAF* V600E mutation or *RET/PTC*, *NTRK1/3*, or *ALK* fusion would strongly support the diagnosis of classic papillary carcinoma. In such cases, not only the entire capsule but also the entire tumor parenchyma should be examined to exclude the presence of papillary structures characteristic of classic papillary carcinoma.[40,41] In those cases where tumor capsule invasion is suspected but not unequivocally evident or the question of whether the capsule is entirely sampled for examination exists, the finding of the *TERT* or *TP53* mutation would provide strong evidence against the diagnosis of NIFTP.

TREATMENT

Surgery

NIFTP is a borderline premalignant tumor which likely serves as a precursor for invasive encapsulated follicular variant of papillary carcinoma. Moreover, due to a significant overlap in clinical presentation and cytologic and molecular features between NIFTP and low-risk follicular-patterned thyroid cancers (minimally invasive follicular carcinoma, follicular variant papillary carcinoma), surgical treatment and a subsequent histopathological examination are required to establish this diagnosis with certainty.[45] However, one of the intended consequences of NIFTP reclassification is to limit surgical management to lobectomy in many appropriately selected patients (Box 23.2). Nevertheless, given our imperfect ability to preoperatively diagnose NIFTP and other factors that may lead to a specific clinical circumstance toward more extensive surgery, total thyroidectomy remains a valid, acceptable, and in some circumstances, a preferable option, even when the ultimate pathology report reveals NIFTP.

Admitting that this is a new entity and long-term prospective follow-up is missing, current practice guidelines consider lobectomy an acceptable treatment for patients with NIFTP, with no completion of thyroidectomy or radioactive iodine treatment required as long as this diagnosis is established after stringent histopathologic criteria.[45-47]

Follow-Up

Based on the absence or very small risk of tumor recurrence in most retrospectively analyzed NIFTP series,[1,48,49] patients with resected solitary NIFTP tumors should require less active follow-up than that recommended for low risk for recurrence differentiated thyroid cancer in patients in the 2015 American Thyroid Association guidelines.[50] Thus maintenance of thyroid-stimulating hormone (TSH) in the normal range should be sufficient and if significant thyroid tissue remains in the neck, as documented by a 6-week postoperative serum thyroglobulin concentration in excess of five, a neck ultrasound examination should be considered every 1 to 2 years for the first decade after surgery to evaluate residual thyroid tissue and lymph node architecture and size. Measurement of yearly quantitative thyroglobulin in NIFTP patients is

> **BOX 23.2 Preoperative Features That May Indicate NIFTP Diagnosis and Are Permissive of Offering Hemithyroidectomy**
>
> I. Physical examination
>   1. No lymph node metastasis
>   2. No fixation
>   3. No voice abnormalities
>   4. No vocal cord paralysis
> II. Ultrasound
>   1. Low and intermediate nodule findings: iso- or hypoechoic, oval to round, sharp regular margin, hypoechoic rim
>   2. Not taller than wide
>   3. No microcalcifications
>   4. No contralateral lobe nodules
>   5. No extrathyroidal extension
>   6. No posterior abutment
>   7. No lymph node metastasis
>   8. No fixation
>   9. No vocal cord paralysis
> III. Cytology
>   Bethesda III, IV, or V with:
>   + Follicular pattern
>   + Microfollicular architecture
>   + Sheet-like architecture
>   - No papillae
>   - No psammoma bodies
>   - No prominent nuclear pseudoinclusions
>   - No prominent nuclear grooves
>   - No necrosis or mitoses
> IV. Molecular Profile
>   1. *RAS* mutation, *THADA* or *PPARG* fusion
>   2. No *BRAF* V600E, *RET/PTC* fusion, *TERT* promoter mutation
> V. Patient/Endocrine Characteristics
>   1. Willing to have second surgery if needed
>   2. Medically fit for possible second anesthesia
>   3. Endocrinologist in agreement with initial lobectomy surgery

NIFTP, noninvasive follicular thyroid neoplasm with papillary-like nuclear features.

appropriate, with expected values 6 weeks after surgery less than 5 ng/mL for total thyroidectomy patients and levels less than 30 ng/mL for lobectomy patients, in the absence of thyroglobulin antibodies.[51] Single thyroglobulin measurements are of less value than mapping the thyroglobulin trend over three or more data points. The intensity of follow-up may be decreased in the future when abundant prospective data for patients diagnosed with NIFTP are accumulated.

The intensity of follow-up may be increased in some situations when the confidence in the diagnosis of NIFTP is low due to either an incomplete histopathologic examination of the tumor capsule or the lack of significant experience of the pathologist in establishing such diagnosis. These scenarios are expected to account for the majority of cases of either classic papillary carcinoma or invasive follicular variant papillary carcinomas being misdiagnosed as NIFTP, and those patients are expected to have a slightly higher risk of regional lymph node or distant metastases, respectively. In some patients, NIFTP tumors may be found in multinodular thyroids coexisting with papillary microcarcinomas or larger cancers.[52] When there is tumor multifocality associated with a NIFTP lesion, follow-up frequency and intensity should be based on the highest risk coexisting malignant lesion as assessed by pathologic evaluation of all excised tissue.

PROGNOSIS

NIFTP is a tumor with very low malignant potential. A less than 1% risk of recurrence for NIFTP has been established based on a retrospective analysis of 109 tumor cases with 13 years median follow-up in the initial reclassification study and 352 cases reported in 2016 in the literature.[1] Incomplete excision of the tumor may lead to local recurrence.[42] Metastatic spread to cervical lymph nodes signifies that that the tumor represents a classic papillary carcinoma misdiagnosed as NIFTP unless the thyroid gland contains another possibly smaller cancer responsible for the lymph node metastasis. These metastatic tumors frequently have the *BRAF* V600E mutation. If vascular or capsule invasion is missed, the tumor (which should have been correctly diagnosed as invasive encapsulated follicular variant papillary carcinoma) is prone to hematogenous spread, more often to the bones and lungs.[1] Such tumors are frequently positive for *RAS* and *TERT* mutations and belong to the spectrum of *RAS*-like follicular-patterned thyroid tumors that progress beyond the noninvasive NIFTP stage.

Since the initial 2016 report, five more recent retrospective studies reported outcome information on large series of NIFTP tumors.[4,6,7,20,49] Among them, three studies found no tumor-related adverse events in 285 patients after a mean follow-up ranging from 5.7 to 11.2 years.[4,6,49] Many patients in these series had multifocal and bilateral tumors and tumors of large-size (>4 cm). However, the other two studies reported that 4% to 6% of patients with nodules meeting the diagnostic criteria for NIFTP had metastasis at the time of surgery.[7,20] Many of these tumors had at least some papillary structures identified, revealed the *BRAF* V600E mutation, and showed lymph node metastasis, which are all features of classic papillary thyroid carcinoma. With thorough histopathologic examination and more stringent criteria that include the exclusion of any well-formed papillae and examination of the entire tumor capsule,[1] it is expected that NIFTP tumors will have a very low probability of tumor recurrence or tumor-related mortality.[1]

SUMMARY

NIFTP is a new entity introduced after the 2016 reclassification of the tumor previously known as noninvasive encapsulated follicular variant of papillary carcinoma. This tumor cannot be definitively diagnosed preoperatively but can be suspected based on a castellation of ultrasonographic, cytologic, and molecular findings. Based on the available data from retrospective studies it should be expected that, when diagnosed based on stringent histopathologic criteria, NIFTP should have a very low (<1%) probability of recurrence. However, the indolent nature of this disease should be further confirmed in additional, preferably prospective series of patients, which should also evaluate the reproducibility and robustness of diagnostic criteria for NIFTP. NIFTP is currently considered a surgical condition, with thyroid lobectomy expected to be adequate for many patients and no immediate completion of thyroidectomy or radio-iodine therapy recommended. Future studies should determine whether if an accurate preoperative diagnosis of NIFTP is possible using cytology and other ancillary techniques, such as molecular testing, and in what situations more conservative management can be safely offered to these patients.

REFERENCES

For a complete list of references, go to expertconsult.com.

24

Dynamic Risk Group Analysis and Staging for Differentiated Thyroid Cancer

Laura Boucai, R. Michael Tuttle

INTRODUCTION

A defined set of clinical factors and pathologic characteristics have been used in different staging systems (e.g., Tumor, Node, and Metastases [TNM] with American Joint Committee on Cancer [AJCC]; metastasis, age, completeness of resection, invasion, and size [MACIS]; age, metastasis, extent, and size [AMES]; and age, gender, extent, and size [AGES]) to predict the risk of death in differentiated thyroid cancer.[1,2] The most important of these include age of the patient at diagnosis, histology, size of the tumor, completeness of resection, and the presence of metastases at presentation. However, in clinical practice a comprehensive initial risk stratification requires review of all available data that is obtained up to 4 months after initial diagnosis and treatment (Table 24.1).[1] Integration of all of these factors allows for an initial estimation of both the risk of death and importantly also the risk of recurrence.

Although each of the major staging systems use risk stratification with respect to disease-specific mortality, they are much less effective at predicting risk of recurrence.[3] For this reason the American Thyroid Association (ATA) endorses a three-tiered system that better predicts risk of recurrence and that can be combined with other staging systems to provide a more comprehensive initial estimate of the risk of death and recurrence for each patient. Unfortunately, these staging systems fail to adequately incorporate the effect of initial therapy (other than completeness of resection).[4] Because the effect of initial therapies is likely to have a major impact on the final outcome of patients, failure to incorporate the effect of initial therapy may result in an inappropriately low estimate of risk in the few "low-risk" patients who do not respond to initial therapy or an inappropriately high estimate of risk in the few "high-risk" patients who have an excellent response to initial therapy.

But more importantly, the current staging systems which classify patients at the time of initial presentation are static and do not change over time.[5,6] In clinical care our risk estimates clearly change over time depending on the response to therapy and biological behavior of each tumor for individual patients, and this risk stratification process should be dynamic. For example a "low-risk" patient who develops a rapidly rising thyroglobulin (Tg) level or new pulmonary nodules would forever be classified as "low risk" based on initial staging when, in reality, the patient is now at increasing risk of developing structurally identifiable progressive disease and may be at increased risk of death from thyroid cancer by virtue of these new clinical findings. It is both the failure to account for the effect of initial therapy and the static nature of our current staging systems that result in the relative inability of these staging systems to guide long-term follow-up recommendations.

The importance of accurate, ongoing risk stratification cannot be overemphasized. The most important clinical aspects of patient care are based on an assessment of individualized risk; therefore implementation of the ATA guidelines into clinical practice requires a thorough understanding of the risk of death as well as of the risk of recurrence for each individual patient we evaluate and treat. This chapter provides an updated guideline on how to practically apply and integrate an initial staging system with the ATA Risk Stratification system, a separate postoperative clinicopathologic system that better predicts recurrence, and the ATA Response to Therapy system, an ongoing reassessment of the patient that incorporates clinical information as it becomes available.

INITIAL RISK STRATIFICATION

Although initial risk stratification using the current staging systems has some limitations, it provides a starting point for initial management recommendations and forms the basis of ongoing risk stratification. The updated ATA guidelines on the management of thyroid cancer and thyroid nodules recommend using both (1) the AJCC TNM system to estimate the risk of death from thyroid cancer and (2) the ATA Risk Stratification system, a separate postoperative clinicopathologic staging system to improve the ability to predict recurrence and to plan follow-up for patients with differentiated thyroid cancer (Box 24.1).[7]

The AJCC recently published the 8th edition of the AJCC/TNM staging system, which is optimized to predict survival.[1] Compared with the 7th edition, (1) the age cutoff has been raised from 45 years of age at diagnosis to 55 years of age; (2) microscopic extrathyroidal extension were removed from the definition of T3 disease; the 8th edition reemphasizes the critical importance of gross extrathyroidal extension as an unfavorable prognostic factor, but it minimizes the significance of minor extension beyond the thyroid capsule that can only be detected on histologic examination; and (3) deemphasizes the importance of locoregional nodal disease such that nodal positivity in itself no longer upgrades the patient to Stage 3 or 4. The net effect of most changes in the 8th edition was to downstage a significant number of patients into lower stages that more accurately reflect their low risk of dying from thyroid cancer.[8-13]

In terms of predicting risk of recurrence, the AJCC TNM system does not adequately implement risk stratification with respect to the risk of recurrence or the risk of biochemical or structural persistent disease (Figure 24.1). Consistent with previous reports,[14-16] Shteinshnaider et al.[17] recently showed that the 8th edition of AJCC adequately predicted disease-specific mortality 0.5% for stage I, 7.5% for stage II patient, 20% for stage III patients and 67% for stage IV patients, but it failed to predict risk of persistent or recurrent disease. In this series the risk of persistent disease at 1 year was comparable between stages II, III, and IV (see Figure 24.1). So although AJCC staging is useful for predicting risk of death, it does not provide adequate predictions regarding the risk of recurrence or persistent disease, which is required to plan follow-up studies.

The three-tiered system endorsed by the ATA and validated internationally performed much better at predicting the risk of recurrence. In our cohort, 23% of the patients were classified as low risk, 50% as intermediate risk, and 27% as high risk for recurrence based on the ATA system.[14] As can be concluded from Figure 24.2, patients classified as low risk had between a 14% and 22% risk of having persistent or recurrent disease, whereas intermediate-risk patients had a much higher likelihood (37% to 48%) of having persistent or recurrent disease. The high-risk group had a 69% to 86% risk of having persistent or recurrent disease.[14,18,19] Interestingly, the persistent/recurrent disease in low-risk patients was a biochemical diagnosis (Tg) without a structural correlate in ~80% of the cases (see Figure 24.2). However, the persistent/recurrent disease was associated with a structural correlate in 30% to 50% of the intermediate-risk group and 60% to 72% of the high-risk group. Therefore the ATA risk stratification system identifies both the risk of having persistent/recurrent disease and the likelihood that the persistent/recurrent disease will be either a biochemical or structurally evident recurrence.

RESPONSE TO THERAPY ASSESSMENT

Although these initial risk assessments provide the basis for ongoing risk stratification, it is clear that new data obtained during follow-up could significantly alter these initial risk estimates.[6] Box 24.2 provides an example of the types of data that are used to modify our initial risk estimates.[20-28] Regardless of the initial AJCC TNM stage or ATA risk group classification, rising values of serum Tg or Tg antibodies would be expected to increase the risk of developing progressive or newly identifiable structural disease. Conversely, declining Tg values, undetectable stimulated Tg values, negative neck ultrasonography, and other cross-sectional imaging would all tend to decrease the risk of disease recurrence and death.

The proposed ATA Response to Therapy system classifies patients as having an "excellent," "biochemical incomplete," "structural incomplete," or "indeterminate response" to initial therapy (Table 24.2).[7] In this system, the response to therapy for each patient is determined on the basis of the standard follow-up testing that is usually done in differentiated thyroid cancer. Patients with an "excellent response" to therapy have no evidence of disease (NED) with negative cross-sectional imaging and undetectable suppressed or stimulated Tg values. Less than 1% of patients in this category die of the disease and the rate of recurrence is 1% to 4%.[14,18,26] "Biochemical incomplete response" represents a group of patients with negative imaging studies and persistent thyroglobulinemia (suppressed Tg ≥1 ng/mL, stimulated

TABLE 24.1 Important Factors to Be Used in Initial Risk Stratification

Preoperative findings	Physical examination
	Vocal cord function
	Cross-sectional imaging
Intraoperative findings	Presence of gross extrathyroidal extension
	Involvement of major structures in the neck
	Completeness of tumor resection
	Lymph node metastases
Pathology findings	Specific histology
	Vascular invasion
	Macroscopic extrathyroidal extension
	Molecular characterization
Laboratory findings	Postoperative serum thyroglobulin
Functional and structural imaging findings	RAI scans
	FDG-PET scans
	Neck US
	CT scans

RAI, radioactive iodine, FDG-PET, [18F]fluoro-2-deoxy-D-glucose-positron emission tomography, US, ultrasound, CT, computed tomography.

BOX 24.1 ATA Risk of Recurrence Group 2015

Low-Risk Patients
Papillary thyroid cancer (with all of the following):
- No local or distant metastases
- All macroscopic tumor has been resected
- No tumor invasion of locoregional tissues or structures
- The tumor does not have aggressive histology (e.g., tall cell, hobnail variant, columnar cell carcinoma)
- If 131I is given, there are no RAI-avid metastatic foci outside the thyroid bed on the first posttreatment whole-body RAI scan
- No vascular invasion
- Clinical N0 or <5 pathologic N1 micrometastases (<0.2 cm in largest dimension)
- Intrathyroidal, encapsulated follicular variant of papillary thyroid cancer
- Intrathyroidal, well-differentiated follicular thyroid cancer with capsular invasion and
- no or minimal (<4 foci) vascular invasion
- Intrathyroidal, papillary microcarcinoma, unifocal or multifocal, including BRAFV600E mutated (if known)

Intermediate-Risk Patients
- Microscopic invasion of tumor into the perithyroidal soft tissues
- RAI-avid metastatic foci in the neck on the first posttreatment whole-body RAI scan
- Aggressive histology (e.g., tall cell, hobnail variant, columnar cell carcinoma)
- Papillary thyroid cancer with vascular invasion
- Clinical N1 or >5 pathologic N1 with all involved lymph nodes <3 cm in largest dimension Multifocal papillary microcarcinoma with ETE and BRAFV600E mutated (if known)

High-Risk Patients
- Macroscopic invasion of tumor into the perithyroidal soft tissues (gross ETE)
- Incomplete tumor resection
- Distant metastases
- Postoperative serum thyroglobulin suggestive of distant metastases
- Pathologic N1 with any metastatic lymph node >3 cm in largest dimension
- Follicular thyroid cancer with extensive vascular invasion (>4 foci of vascular invasion)

ATA, American Thyroid Association, 131I, iodine-131, RAI, radioactive iodine, N0, no regional lymph node metastasis, N1, regional lymph node metastasis, ETE, extrathyroidal extension.

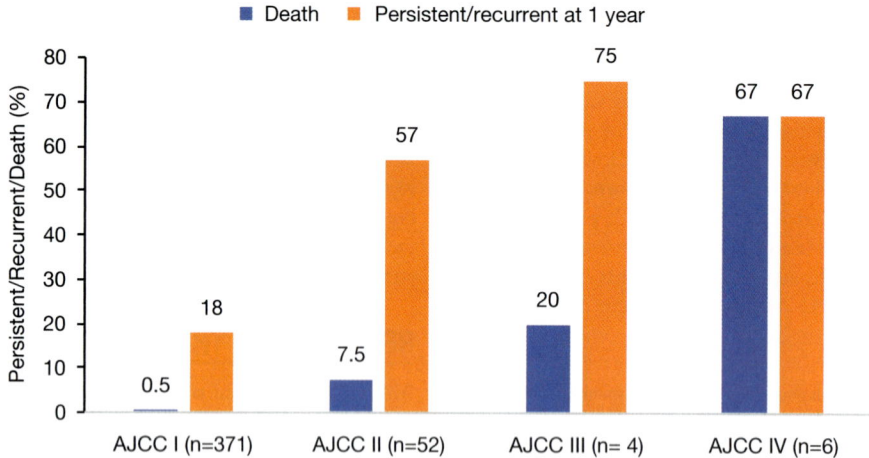

Fig. 24.1 Risk Stratification Based on American Joint Committee on Cancer (AJCC) Staging 8th Edition. Although AJCC staging risk stratifies with regard to the risk of disease-specific mortality, the rates of persistent/recurrent disease are remarkably similar between stages II, III, and IV. Persistent/recurrent: persistent or recurrent disease.

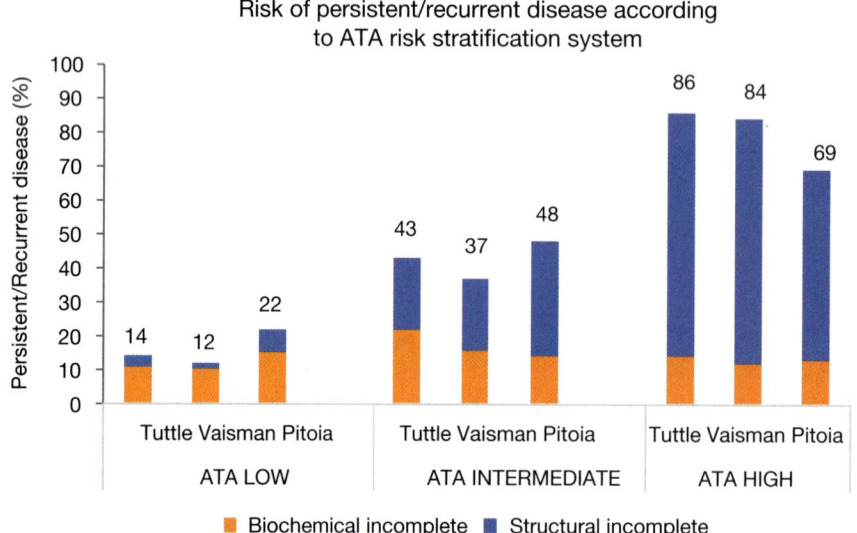

Fig. 24.2 Risk Stratification Based on The American Thyroid Association (ATA) Thyroid Cancer Guidelines Risk of Recurrence Classification System. The ATA risk stratification system provides estimates of recurrent/persistent disease that significantly differs between risk groups. Furthermore, ~80% of the recurrent disease in the low-risk group is biochemical recurrence without a structural correlate (biochemical) compared with 55% of the intermediate-risk and 22% of the high-risk patients. Biochemical: measurable thyroglobulin or rising thyroglobulin antibodies is biochemical evidence of recurrence without structural disease correlate; structural, structurally identifiable disease on functional or cross-sectional imaging.

BOX 24.2 Response to Therapy Variables
Change in serum thyroglobulin levels over time
Change in serum Tg antibodies over time
Results of stimulated thyroglobulin determinations
Results of follow-up neck ultrasound
Results of RAI scanning
Other cross-sectional imaging
Results of FDG-PET imaging
Physical examination

Tg, thyroglobulin, RAI, radioactive iodine, FDG-PET, [18F]fluoro-2-deoxy-D-glucose-positron emission tomography.

Tg ≥10 ng/L, or rising antithyroglobulin antibodies). At least 30% of these patients spontaneously evolve to NED,[29-31] about 20% achieve NED after additional therapy, and 20% develop structurally identifiable disease. Less than 1% of patients in this category die of thyroid cancer.[14,18] Patients with a "structural incomplete response" have structural or functional evidence of disease with any Tg level with or without antithyroglobulin antibodies. Fifty percent to 85% of patients in this category continue to have persistent disease despite additional therapy, and most deaths due to thyroid cancer arise from this category: up to 11% of patients with locoregional disease and up to 50% of patients with distant metastases die of the disease.[14,18] Finally, "indeterminate response" defines a group of patients with nonspecific imaging

TABLE 24.2 Categories of Response to Therapy

Category	Definitions	Clinical Outcomes	Management Implications
Excellent response	Negative imaging **and either** suppressed Tg <0.2 ng/mLa or TSH-stimulated Tg <1 ng/mLa	1%-4% recurrence <1% disease specific death	An excellent response to therapy should lead to an early decrease in the intensity and frequency of follow-up and the degree of TSH suppression
Biochemical incomplete response	Negative imaging **and** suppressed Tg ≥1 ng/mLa or stimulated Tg ≥10 ng/mLa or rising anti-Tg antibody levels	At least 30% spontaneously evolve to NED 20% achieve NED after additional therapy 20% develop structural disease <1% disease specific death	If associated with stable or declining serum Tg values, a biochemical incomplete response should lead to continued observation with ongoing TSH suppression in most patients Rising Tg or anti-Tg antibody values should prompt additional investigations and potentially additional therapies
Structural incomplete response	Structural or functional evidence of disease with any Tg level with or without anti-Tg antibodies	50%-85% continue to have persistent disease despite additional therapy Disease specific death rates as high as 11% with locoregional metastases and 50% with structural distant metastases	A structural incomplete response may lead to additional treatments or ongoing observation depending on multiple clinicopathologic factors including the size, location, rate of growth, RAI avidity, [18]FDG avidity, and specific pathology of the structural lesions
Indeterminate response	Nonspecific findings on imaging studies Faint uptake in thyroid bed on RAI scanning Nonstimulated Tg detectable, but <1 ng/mL Stimulated Tg detectable, but <10 ng/mL or Anti-Tg antibodies stable or declining in the absence of structural or functional disease	15%-20% will have structural disease identified during follow-up[a] In the remainder, the nonspecific changes are either stable or resolve[a] <1% disease specific death	An indeterminate response should lead to continued observation with appropriate serial imaging of the nonspecific lesions and serum Tg monitoring Nonspecific findings that become suspicious over time can be further evaluated with additional imaging or biopsy

NED denotes a patient as having no evidence of disease at final follow-up.
[a]In the absence of antithyroglobulin antibodies.
Tg, thyroglobulin; TSH, thyroid-stimulating hormone, NED, no evidence of disease, RAI, radioactive iodine, [18]FDG, [^{18}F]fluoro-2-deoxy-D-glucose.

findings, faint uptake in the thyroid bed on radioactive iodine (RAI) scanning, nonstimulated Tg detectable but <1 ng/mL, stimulated Tg detectable but <10 ng/mL, or antithyroglobulin antibodies stable or declining in the absence of structural or functional disease. Fifteen percent to 20% of these patients will have structurally identifiable disease on follow-up, and in the remainder, these nonspecific changes will remain stable or resolve over time. The disease-specific mortality rate for this category is <1%.[14,18] The terminology used in the response to therapy system builds on numerous previous publications demonstrating that the risk of persistent disease or recurrence is altered by changes in serum Tg or antithyroglobulin antibody levels (TgAb) over time,[20-25] the degree of RAI avidity of pulmonary metastases,[26] the presence of an undetectable stimulated Tg especially when coupled with a negative neck ultrasound in low-risk patients,[27] and [^{18}F]fluoro-2-deoxy-D-glucose-positron emission tomography (FDG-PET) scanning results in high-risk patients.[28] Recently, this response to therapy system was reassessed in ATA high-risk patients. Age was a major determinant of response to therapy. The proportion of structural incomplete responders was significantly smaller among younger (<55 years) patients compared with older patients (33% vs. 53%, p = 0.002), and disease-specific survival was also significantly better for younger patients compared to older patients (74% vs. 12%, p<0.001), suggesting that age further stratifies patients with respect to response to therapy, especially within the high-risk population.[32]

INTEGRATING INITIAL RISK ESTIMATES WITH RESPONSE TO THERAPY (DYNAMIC RISK ASSESSMENT)

From a clinical management point of view, in most cases it is the response to therapy that should guide our long-term follow-up management recommendations rather than the initial risk estimates made at the time of initial therapy. Therefore the optimal use of these staging systems is to start with an initial risk assessment based on AJCC TNM staging and the ATA risk of recurrence classification system, and then overlay the individual patient's response to therapy to obtain an updated, dynamic, and realistic risk estimate. This response to therapy assessment captures clinical variables related to the specific response of the patient to the therapy administered as well as the behavior of the tumor. Although initially thought to be useful after the first 2 years of treatment, we now understand that this response to therapy assessment can be used as early as immediately after thyroidectomy as well as after 2 years of treatment to define further diagnostic and therapeutic strategies.

The effects of response to therapy assessment on initial risk stratification are best appreciated in Figure 24.3 where the risk of persistent structural disease or disease recurrence is shown for each ATA risk category. An excellent response to therapy significantly decreases the risk of recurrent/persistent structural disease to 2% in patients who were

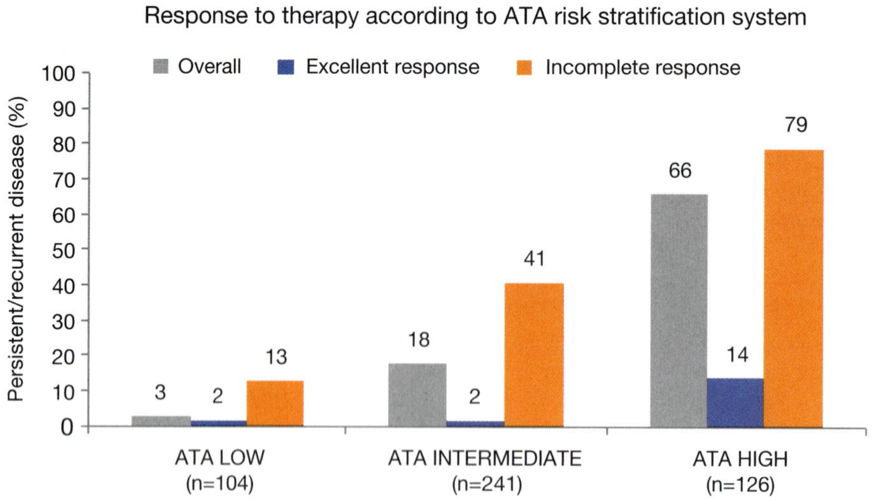

Response to therapy according to ATA risk stratification system

Legend: Overall (gray) | Excellent response (blue) | Incomplete response (orange)

Risk Group	Overall	Excellent response	Incomplete response
ATA LOW (n=104)	3	2	13
ATA INTERMEDIATE (n=241)	18	2	41
ATA HIGH (n=126)	66	14	79

Fig. 24.3 Integrating response to therapy with initial risk stratification based on our cohort of 471 patients on whom we had a stimulated thyroglobulin (Tg) value after 2 years of follow-up. In each group, an excellent response to therapy lowers the risk of recurrent/persistent structural disease. Similarly, an incomplete response to therapy increases the risk of developing recurrent/persistent disease above that predicted by initial staging.

initially classified as low to intermediate risk. Even patients who were initially classified as high risk see a significant improvement in outcomes if they achieve an excellent response to therapy (risk of recurrence/persistent disease decreases from 66% at initial risk stratification to 14% within 2 years of therapy if they had an excellent response to therapy).[14]

Conversely, an incomplete response to therapy in the patient initially classified as low to intermediate risk is associated with a significant increase in the risk of identifying recurrent/persistent structural disease during follow-up. Although low-risk patients are thought to have only a 3% risk of having persistent/recurrent disease, this risk increases to 13% if they have an incomplete response to therapy. Likewise, intermediate-risk patients having an incomplete response to therapy see the initial risk estimate for recurrent/persistent structural disease of 18% rise to 41%.

The impact of these findings is probably most marked in the 50% of our patients who were initially classified as having intermediate risk of developing recurrent or persistent disease. A nearly 20% risk of recurrent/persistent structural disease would demand close, intensive follow-up. However, when these intermediate-risk patients have an excellent response to therapy within the first 2 years of follow-up, the risk of developing recurrent/persistent disease drops dramatically to only 2%. Therefore intermediate-risk patients who have an excellent response to therapy should be followed as "low-risk" patients with the intensity of follow-up tailored to the revised 2% risk estimate and not the initial 18% risk estimate.

REPRESENTATIVE CASE EXAMPLE

Perhaps the best way to illustrate the effect of ongoing risk assessment is to consider an individual case to see how the additional data obtained during follow-up can significantly alter our ongoing risk assessments and our management plans.

Take, for example, a 35-year-old female in whom an asymptomatic palpable thyroid nodule was detected as part of her routine gynecologic yearly follow-up. Ultrasound confirmed a 3-cm thyroid nodule in the right lobe and several abnormal right cervical lymph nodes at levels 3 and 4. Fine-needle aspiration (FNA) confirmed well-differentiated thyroid cancer in the nodule and a representative lymph node. She underwent total thyroidectomy, central neck dissection, and compartment-oriented right neck dissection. The operative report described complete resection of the tumor and lymph nodes with no gross extrathyroidal extension. The final pathology report revealed a 2.5-cm, classic papillary thyroid cancer with minor extrathyroidal extension into perithyroidal fat. Furthermore, 14/24 lymph nodes also contained well-differentiated papillary thyroid cancer. Six weeks postoperatively, she received 100 mCi radioactive iodine (^{131}I), and the posttherapy scan showed uptake in the thyroid bed and perhaps minimal uptake in what were presumed to be right neck lymph nodes with no structural correlate. Her stimulated Tg at the time of ablation was 14 ng/mL, with negative anti-Tg antibodies.

Her initial risk stratification is AJCC stage I (less than 1% risk of death from thyroid cancer), but she has an ATA intermediate risk of recurrence (44% risk of having persistent or recurrent disease according to our cohort). She is followed with suppressed Tg every 6 months for 2 years, neck ultrasonography once a year for 2 years, and also has a stimulated Tg done at 18 months after ablation.

Follow-up Scenario 1

In this scenario, she has an excellent response to therapy. Her suppressed Tg is less than 1 ng/mL (with negative Tg antibodies) every 6 months, and her stimulated Tg is also undetectable at 18 months of follow-up. Her neck ultrasound is completely normal at 1 to 2 years of follow-up. Based on our response to therapy data,[8] her excellent response to therapy allows us to dramatically decrease her likelihood of having persistent/recurrent disease to about 2%.

This restratification essentially allows us to follow her as a "low-risk patient" and not as an "intermediate-risk patient." Consistent with recommendation 63 in the updated ATA thyroid cancer guidelines, she is seen once a year with physical examination and a suppressed Tg value as her primary follow-up. Neck ultrasonography will probably only be obtained if the Tg value changes. Thyroid-stimulating hormone (TSH) will be kept between 0.5 to 2 mIU/L. Additional stimulated Tg values will not be obtained.

Follow-up Scenario 2

In this scenario, she has a structural incomplete response to therapy. Even though she was initially classified as intermediate-risk of recurrence, her serum Tg values remained detectable. In fact they rise from 6 ng/mL at 6 months to 14 ng/mL at 12 months, 36 ng/mL at 18 months, and 77 ng/mL at 24 months of follow-up. Her neck ultrasound did not reveal new disease, but a magnetic resonance imaging (MRI) of the neck reveals a 2 cm high retropharyngeal lymph node that is FDG-avid on PET scanning. Additionally, her chest computed tomography (CT) reveals subcentimeter pulmonary nodules at 6 months that increase to 1 to 2 cm in size over the first year of follow-up and change from FDG-PET negative to PET positive. Post-therapy scanning after an additional therapy of 150 mCi of ^{131}I is negative.

Despite her initial risk stratification as low risk of dying of disease (AJCC stage I) and intermediate risk of having persistent/recurrent disease (44% risk), she has a rapidly progressive, non–RAI-avid metastatic disease and is at significant risk not only of having persistent disease but also of dying from thyroid cancer. Fortunately, this is not the expected outcome for the vast majority of low-risk patients. However, this scenario is very typical for the 1% to 2% of low/intermediate-risk patients who die of thyroid cancer. The lack of response to therapy is usually apparent early in the course, and progressive disease despite numerous therapeutic interventions is the hallmark of low-risk patients who die of thyroid cancer.

In most retrospective publications, she would have been classified as a "low-risk" patient on the basis of MACIS or AJCC staging and then considered to be one of the few "low-risk" patients who unexpectedly died of thyroid cancer. In reality, she would have been considered low risk of death for only the first few months of follow-up with the poor clinical course readily apparent on the basis of chest CT and FDG-PET scanning within 1 year of diagnosis and treatment.

Additionally, the early recognition that she was demonstrating an incomplete response to therapy as early as 6 months after initial therapy and diagnosis led to further evaluations and treatments that would not have been appropriate if she had experienced an excellent response to therapy. Therefore ongoing risk assessment cannot only identify patients who have a lower than anticipated risk of recurrence, but it can also identify those patients whose risk is increasing compared with initial risk stratification, so that additional imaging studies and therapies can be offered in a timely fashion.

PREDICTING CLINICAL OUTCOMES USING RESPONSE TO THERAPY VARIABLES SUPERIMPOSED ON INITIAL ATA RISK STRATIFICATION

Although it is important to identify patients at increased risk of recurrent/persistent disease so that appropriate therapy can be offered in a timely fashion, it is equally important to be able to identify patients at low risk of recurrence who can be followed with a less intense management paradigm. As described earlier, identifying patients at low risk of recurrence over time requires integration of initial risk estimates with response to therapy variables to achieve a dynamic, ongoing risk assessment. But just as is the case with initial risk stratification, a rather small set of variables can be used to determine response to therapy. Chief among these are serum Tg (either suppressed or stimulated), neck ultrasonography, and additional cross-sectional/functional imaging for selected high-risk patients.

To determine the ability of each of these important factors to predict the likelihood of having NED at final follow-up, we analyzed the prognostic importance of each of these key variables, both individually and when combined with cross-sectional imaging in our cohort of 588 patients with differentiated thyroid cancer followed at our center for a median of 7 years after total thyroidectomy and RAI ablation (Figure 24.4).

As would be expected, an undetectable serum Tg value alone (either suppressed or stimulated) was more predictive for having NED at final follow-up in low- and intermediate-risk patients than in high-risk patients. This is not surprising, as the low- and intermediate-risk patients are enriched with well-differentiated thyroid cancer and are usually excellent Tg producers, whereas the high-risk patients will include many patients with poorly differentiated tumors that synthesize and secrete lesser amounts of Tg.

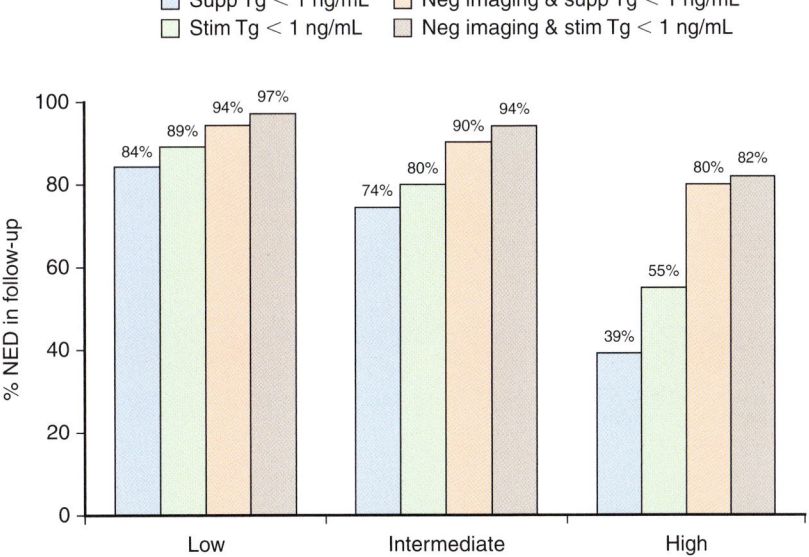

Fig. 24.4 Predictive Ability of Standard Testing With Regard to Final Clinical Outcome. Within each risk group, a combination of negative structural imaging and an undetectable stimulated Tg provided the highest likelihood of being with no evidence of disease at final follow-up. *Supp Tg,* suppressed thyroglobulin; *Stim Tg,* stimulated thyroglobulin; *Neg imaging,* negative cross-sectional and functional imaging, if done.

But optimal negative predictive value for NED at final follow-up is achieved using imaging (usually neck ultrasound) in combination with a stimulated Tg in both low- and intermediate-risk patients.[27] As would be expected, even negative imaging and an undetectable stimulated Tg predict NED at final follow-up in only 82% of high-risk patients.[33] Therefore additional follow-up and imaging studies are often used in these high-risk patients, even after achieving an excellent response to therapy within the first 1 to 2 years of follow-up.

Hence the primary follow-up of low- and intermediate-risk patients can rely heavily, if not almost exclusively, on serum Tg and neck ultrasonography. Additional imaging in patients initially classified as low or intermediate risk is probably only required if the response to therapy is judged to be indeterminate or incomplete. Patients who have a less than excellent response to therapy may benefit from additional imaging and follow-up. These recommendations are consistent with recommendation 63 in the ATA guidelines that notes that "low risk patients who have had remnant ablation, negative cervical ultrasound and undetectable TSH stimulated Tg can be followed primarily with yearly clinical examination and suppressed Tg measurements."[7]

Conversely, additional cross-sectional and functional imaging during follow-up is probably indicated in all of the high-risk patients during early follow-up. Less intense follow-up can be recommended for the few high-risk patients who demonstrate an excellent response to therapy. Obviously, the intensity and type of follow-up should be tailored to the individual risk of recurrence and disease-specific mortality.

SUMMARY

Initial management recommendations should be based on risk estimates obtained from AJCC TNM (or a similar staging system) risk stratification and ATA risk of recurrence estimates. These initial estimates should inform our initial treatment recommendations regarding the extent of initial surgery (extent of thyroidectomy and lymph node dissection), the need for RAI remnant ablation, and the degree of TSH suppression. Data gathered during follow-up (serum Tg, neck ultrasonography, functional/cross-sectional imaging) should be used to judge the individual patient's response to these initial therapies and appropriately modify these initial risk estimates using a dynamic, ongoing risk assessment approach. Long-term follow-up recommendations are then based on the updated, modified risk estimates to better tailor the intensity and type of follow-up to realistic risk estimates.

We view risk-adapted therapy as an ongoing, dynamic process in which all new data are used to either increase or decrease our previous risk estimates. This dynamic approach is a better reflection of the way experienced clinicians manage patients in their own practices and can form the basis of a risk-tailored management approach that maximizes testing and therapy in patients at high risk of recurrence/death while minimizing testing and follow-up in low-risk patients who are very likely to experience full productive lives as thyroid cancer survivors.

REFERENCES

For a complete list of references, go to expertconsult.com.

25

Hürthle Cell Tumors of the Thyroid

Raj K. Gopal, Peter M. Sadow, Ian Ganly

Please go to expertconsult.com to view related video:
Video 25.1 Introduction to Chapter 25, Hürthle Cell Tumors of the Thyroid.
This chapter contains additional online-only content available on expertconsult.com.

INTRODUCTION

Hürthle cell carcinoma (HCC) of the thyroid gland is an uncommon tumor, accounting for 3% to 10% of all thyroid cancers, and therefore few institutions have significant experience with this condition.[1] Because of its rarity, the natural history and optimal management of patients with HCC remain a subject of much debate. The clinical course of these tumors is somewhat unpredictable, and certainly, there are cases initially diagnosed as Hürthle cell adenomas (HCAs) that later behave in a malignant manner and metastasize.[2,3] Furthermore, the often aggressive behavior of HCCs has led many to advocate comprehensive surgical and adjuvant treatments. However, there has been progress over the years, which has led to an updated classification of Hürthle cell tumors (HCTs), based on molecular testing, offering an improved understanding of their biology and the stratification of treatment of these biologically uncertain lesions.

PATHOLOGY

Please see the Expert Consult website for more discussion of this topic.

By definition, Hürthle cell neoplasms are circumscribed lesions composed mainly of Hürthle cells with a predominance greater than 75% of the cell population, although they typically involve 100% of the lesion. Outside of the thyroid, most of these lesions, referred to almost exclusively as *oncocytic lesions*, when mass forming, are referred to as *oncocytomas* or *oncocytic neoplasms*. Lymphocytes are frequently associated with Hürthle cell change, most commonly in chronic lymphocytic (Hashimoto's) thyroiditis, and are an integral component of some oncocytic lesions, such as Warthin tumor of the parotid gland and Warthin tumor-like variant of papillary thyroid carcinoma. Distinguishing a benign neoplasm from cancer based on cytologic analysis of fine-needle aspiration (FNA) biopsy is not possible. Definitive differentiation of HCC from an HCA is based on the presence of vascular or capsular invasion on histologic sections or evidence of extrathyroidal spread and local nodal or distant metastases. The diagnosis of malignancy in HCTs is highly variable, in large part due to subjective interpretation of invasion by pathologists in minimally invasive HCCs, with different tumor submission patterns and diagnostic thresholds.[4] Overall, about 33% demonstrate obvious features of a malignant lesion.[5] This diagnostic variability may be a major factor in the wide-ranging mortality rates reported in different studies, which have caused much of the controversy regarding the natural behavior and history of HCTs.

Please see the Expert Consult website for more discussion of this topic, including Figures 25.1 to 25.5.

PRESENTATION AND NATURAL HISTORY

Most patients with HCC present with a thyroid nodule or mass. The mean age of presentation is between 50 and 60 years of age, approximately 10 years older than the mean age associated with other types of differentiated thyroid cancers.[11,12] Several studies have reported a 3:1 preponderance in females.[12]

Many have traditionally believed that HCCs behave in a more aggressive fashion than other well-differentiated thyroid cancers. However, the reported mortality and survival rates for HCCs are highly variable. Such controversy may be caused by the aforementioned pathologic diagnostic factors as well as small sample sizes, selection biases, and institutional treatment biases. Many earlier studies have reported higher mortality for HCC than for both papillary and follicular thyroid carcinoma, leading many to believe that HCCs are generally aggressive tumors with a worse prognosis than other well-differentiated thyroid cancers.[13-16] In a study of 33 patients treated over 25 years at the University of California at San Francisco, Kushchayeva et al. reported a disease-specific survival (DSS) of 74% and 49% at 5 and 10 years, respectively, and a disease-free survival (DFS) of 65% and 40% at 5 and 10 years.[13] The authors also reported a metastatic rate of 36% with a recurrence rate of 24% in these patients. Lopez-Penabad et al. reported a similarly high mortality rate of 40% associated with HCC in their cohort of 89 patients managed at the MD Anderson Cancer Center over a period of 50 years.[14] These outcomes are in contrast with the 2% overall mortality rate for well-differentiated cancer. Other studies highlight a propensity to regional and distant metastatic behavior of HCCs. In a review of 59 patients with HCC treated over 60 years, Stojadinovic et al. reported a 33% rate of distant metastases and a 21% rate of nodal metastasis.[15] Ruegemer et al. also demonstrated a 34% rate in distant metastases in HCCs compared with only a 7% and 19% rate in papillary thyroid cancer (PTC) and follicular thyroid cancer (FTC), respectively.[16]

However, more recent studies and larger public database surveys have suggested better survival figures for HCCs, comparable to that of other differentiated thyroid cancer types.[12,17,18] A review of 45 HCCs demonstrated a favorable overall outcome (DSS, 96% at 5 years) despite a high incidence of regional cervical metastases (55%).[17] The high incidence of lymphatic spread and the relatively benign clinical course observed in this study is more in keeping with the clinical behavior of well-differentiated PTCs. Bhattacharyya examined the Surveillance,

225

Epidemiology and End Results database (SEER) for the 10-year period between 1988 and 1998 for HCC and identified 555 cases of nonmetastatic HCCs. He reported an overall mean 5-year and 10-year survival rate of 85% and 71%, respectively. Mean survival figures for 411 matched FTCs were comparable. The author reported age and tumor size as the only variables to be predictors of a poorer outcome on multivariate analysis.[12]

GENETICS OF HÜRTHLE CELL TUMORS

Until recently, the genetics of HCTs has been studied using a piecemeal approach and hence has remained poorly understood. Early gene expression analysis suggested that HCTs were derived from the follicular epithelium with some resemblance to FTCs.[19] Their full transcriptional profile, however, hinted that they were molecularly distinct from other differentiated thyroid cancers.[7] Indeed, targeted analysis of genes often altered in papillary and FTCs, such as *BRAF* and *RAS*, showed these genes to be infrequently mutated.[7,20] Hotspot *TERT* promoter mutations were relatively more common but still only detected in a portion of HCC.[21] Furthermore, gene rearrangements, such as the *PAX8/PPARγ* and *RET/PTC* fusions, were also detected subsets of Hürthle tumors.[22] These findings reinforced that HCC harbored a unique molecular foundation, a notion supported by the presence of noncanonical molecular changes in these tumors, including prominent chromosomal losses and mitochondrial DNA (mtDNA) mutations.[23,24]

A more comprehensive understanding of the genetics of HCC has recently emerged from two whole-exome sequencing studies.[8,9] These studies found recurrent nuclear DNA mutations in a diverse set of genes that included *DAXX*, *EIF1AX*, *NRAS*, *KRAS*, *TP53*, *CDKN1A*, *NF1*, *ATM*, and *PTEN*. Furthermore, hotspot *TERT* promoter mutations occurred in ~25% of cases and several novel gene fusions were identified. This heterogeneous catalog of candidate driver events highlights the importance of altered MAPK, PI3K, and DNA damage signaling as well as telomere maintenance in HCC.

The most prevalent alteration found in the nuclear DNA of HCC was widespread chromosomal losses, resulting in loss of heterozygosity (LOH) that, in some cases, spanned the majority of the nuclear genome.[8,9] These striking LOH events resulted in "near-haploid" DNA content that in some cases was accompanied by duplication of the remaining chromosome, resulting in uniparental disomy (i.e., two copies of a chromosome coming from a single parent) or even whole genome duplication. Despite such pervasive LOH events, chromosomes 5, 7, and 12 were rarely lost and instead showed frequent duplication suggesting that important genes were resident on these chromosomes. Although the reason for this marked genomic instability is not yet known, the frequent LOH events appear to contribute to tumor suppressor inactivation.

A concurrent analysis of the mtDNA of HCC identified a number of somatic mtDNA mutations.[8,9] The mtDNA is a small, circular genome with maternal inheritance that is distinct from the nuclear genome and present in multiple copies within each cell.[25] The mtDNA codes for 13 proteins, all of which participate in mitochondrial oxidative phosphorylation (OXPHOS).[26] The mitochondrial genome of HCC was unique in that disruptive mtDNA mutations were frequently observed, which stands in contrast to most other cancers where detrimental mtDNA mutations were not seen.[27] Remarkably, these inactivating mutations nearly always occurred in genes encoding subunits of complex I, the nicotinamide adenine dinucleotide (NADH) dehydrogenase catalyzing the first step in mitochondrial OXPHOS.[26] Although it is not clear how these mtDNA mutations contribute to tumor formation, their high prevalence in HCC suggests that loss of mitochondrial complex I, arguably a version of altered tumor metabolism, is a key genetic feature of this tumor.

STAGING AND PROGNOSTIC FACTORS

Several prognostic scoring (age, gender, extent, and size [AGES]; age, metastasis, extent, and size [AMES]; and metastasis, age, completeness of resection, invasion, and size [MACIS]) and staging systems (Tumor, Node, Metastases; TNM) are used to evaluate well-differentiated thyroid cancers (see Chapter 24, Dynamic Risk Group Analysis and Staging for Differentiated Thyroid Cancer). There is no specific staging system used for HCTs. The validity of the existing prognostic scoring systems has not been extensively evaluated for HCCs. One retrospective study of 40 HCC patients using the AMES risk scoring system showed its utility in predicting recurrence and survival as it found that all 19 low-risk patients remained disease free, whereas 48% of the 21 high-risk patients developed recurrence or died.[28] Furthermore, both recent whole-exome sequencing studies of HCC found a provocative association between LOH and patient prognosis. First, the presence of LOH, or widespread chromosomal losses, was found to be the most frequently encountered event in metastatic HCC.[9] Second, both studies found that the presence of LOH significantly correlated with worse patient outcomes, including progression-free and metastasis-free survival.[8,9] In the future, as the ability to risk stratify thyroid tumors using their molecular features is further refined, this unique DNA copy number change in HCC may help identify tumors with a tendency for more aggressive behavior.

Lymph Node and Distant Metastases

The presence of lymph node metastases associated with HCC at diagnosis, unlike papillary thyroid cancer (PTC), has been consistently shown in many studies to be associated with increased mortality and poorer outcome.[15,29-32] A review of HCC patients treated between 1946 and 2003 by Mills et al. found that independent predictors of DFS were lymph node status, presence of distant metastases, and tumor stage.[31]

Distant Metastases

As seen with other thyroid and nonthyroid cancers, the presence of distant metastases in HCC patients has been shown in numerous studies to be strongly associated with significantly poorer outcomes.[13,15,29,31]

Size

Many studies have demonstrated a correlation between tumor size and risk of malignancy, with HCCs presenting at a larger size compared with HCAs.[12,33] Sippel et al. demonstrated tumor size correlated with malignant potential in HCTs and reported no malignancy in any tumors less than 2 cm and all tumors greater than 6 cm to be malignant with a 50% risk of malignancy in those lesions 4 cm or larger.[32] Similarly, Pisanu et al. showed tumor size greater than 3 to 4 cm to be significantly predictive for malignancy.[34] However, other reports have failed to show a significant association between size and cancer risk.[11,17,29,35] Given the rarity of HCCs, these variable findings may be due to the small study sample numbers and the inherent heterogeneity of the study samples between each study series.

Age

Consistent with other thyroid cancer types, studies have repeatedly shown advanced age in HCC patients (approximately >50 years) to be associated with poorer outcomes.[12,14,29]

Invasiveness

As observed in many human cancers including other thyroid cancer types, the degree of tumor invasion seen on histology has been shown to greatly affect prognosis and outcome in HCCs. Widely invasive HCC has been shown to be an aggressive malignancy with patients at high risk for recurrence and tumor-related death.[15] In a large study of 77 HCCs treated over a 60-year period, the group at Memorial Sloan Kettering found that lesions that were minimally invasive were associated with no relapse or death, whereas those that were widely invasive were associated with a 73% relapse rate and 55% mortality.[15] The same group also found that the presence of vascular invasion was highly associated with disease recurrence, even in the more indolent and well-encapsulated HCCs.[36] Other reports have demonstrated the presence of vascular invasion to be the only risk factor to significantly predict poorer clinical outcome.[17]

Extent of Surgery

Controversy has long existed regarding the extent of surgery necessary for the optimal treatment of HCC. This stems in part from the uncertainty over the natural history and presumed aggressiveness of this tumor type. A recent survey of patients treated at the Marsden Hospital over a 50-year period showed HCCs had a more aggressive disease profile than differentiated thyroid cancers and that extent of surgery was an independent factor affecting DSS, and thus recommended total thyroidectomy.[31] Also, in a review of patients treated with HCC between 1946 and 2003, Mills et al. found that, on multivariate analysis, the extent of surgery was the only independent factor that affected DSS. In contrast, however, many other studies have shown no difference for extent of surgery undertaken and overall outcome.[13-15,17,22]

PREOPERATIVE EVALUATION

Currently, no reliable method exists to differentiate the diagnosis of HCC from HCA and other benign thyroid conditions preoperatively.

Fine Needle Aspiration

Approximately 20% to 30% of patients with an FNA cytology suspicious of Hürthle cell neoplasm will have a malignancy.[32] Several features of Hürthle cells on FNA have been shown to be suggestive of malignant HCCs over benign HCA and benign lesions, including nuclear atypia and crowding, cellular dyshesion, an increased nuclear to cytoplasm ratio, the presence of columnar rather than polygonal cells, and an increased mitotic rate. In neoplastic lesions, the Hürthle cells are poorly cohesive compared with thyroiditis and multinodular thyroid goiters, and colloid is generally absent and lymphocytes are rare compared with abundant colloid and numerous lymphocytes in chronic thyroiditis.[37] However, FNA remains of limited value in definitive diagnosis. Pisanu et al. reported FNA sensitivity of only 23.8% for HCC detection, and these and other authors who have reported similar low predictive rates have thus urged all oxyphil predominate nodules to be referred for surgery.[34]

Ultrasound and Other Imaging Modalities

Please see the Expert Consult website for more discussion of this topic.

SURGERY

In regard to surgical management, presently most advocate initial thyroid lobectomy and completion thyroidectomy if HCC is identified on permanent pathology. However, Kushchayeva et al. showed that extent of surgery had no influence on prognosis.[13] In a large study of 77 HCCs, extent of surgery did not influence outcome in both minimally invasive and widely invasive HCCs.[15] Other authors have similarly observed no benefit from completion thyroidectomy and argue that total thyroidectomy may be overtreatment, in particular for minimally invasive and early-stage HCCs. In contrast a recent survey of patients treated at the Royal Marsden Hospital in London over a 50-year period showed the extent of surgery was an independent factor affecting survival.[26] Other proponents of total thyroidectomy for the diagnosis of HCC argue that completion thyroidectomy also allows the use of thyroglobulin tumor marker surveillance and increases the efficacy of radioactive iodine (RAI) scanning therapy if needed later.

Unlike other well-differentiated thyroid cancers, nodal involvement is associated with poorer outcomes in those with HCC; therefore cervical nodal metastases are generally treated aggressively with a modified neck dissection. Level I cervical involvement is uncommon and does not routinely need to be addressed.

Please see the Expert Consult website for more discussion of this topic.

Intraoperative Frozen Section

Intraoperative frozen section (FS) may be used to guide the need for contralateral thyroidectomy at the initial surgery stage. However, FS examination is limited by many procedural difficulties, including sampling error, variable section thickness, irregularity of the capsule, freezing artifact and distortion such as blood vessel collapse, and the difficulty in distinguishing capsular entrapment from true invasion. The use of FS has been shown to have a variable diagnostic value highly dependent on individual institutional expertise/experience.

In a retrospective review in 2002, Dahl et al. looked at 116 patients diagnosed with a Hürthle cell neoplasm. Forty-nine patients were found to have carcinoma, and 67 patients were found to have benign Hürthle cell neoplasm.[11] FS analysis at the time of the original operation correctly diagnosed only 19% with carcinoma, and for those cases there was 100% correlation with final pathology. However, the majority of FSs (75%) were indeterminate. Similar low-sensitivity figures have been reported for intraoperative FS by others precluding its definitive use to guide the extent of surgery.

HÜRTHLE ADJUVANT THERAPY

Radioactive Iodine

Unfortunately, given the low incidence of these cancers, guidance from definitive large studies is lacking. Compared with other differentiated thyroid cancer types, HCCs are believed to possess lower iodine avidity and thus generally are considered to be poorly responsive to RAI treatment (see Chapter 48, Postoperative Radioactive Iodine Ablation and Treatment of Differentiated Thyroid Cancer). Lopez-Penabad et al. demonstrated in 89 patients with HCCs only a 40% RAI uptake rate in those known to have metastases. Although RAI treatment had no overall benefit on survival, subgroup analysis showed that patients who received RAI for adjuvant ablation therapy had better outcomes compared with those that did not.[14] Another recent study examined the radioiodine uptake rate in recurrent and persistent tumors; it demonstrated an almost 70% (11 of 16 patients) rate of uptake and proposed that RAI treatment may be effective in many of these patients.[38] Ablation of any remaining thyroid tissue would also facilitate the use of serum thyroglobulin as a tumor marker and to allow more sensitive detection of any recurrent or metastatic disease that may take up ^{131}I.

The authors recommend the employment of current guidelines for RAI treatments for well-differentiated thyroid cancers (American Thyroid Association [2015] and British Thyroid Association [2007] guidelines) or treatment paradigms based on metastasis, age, completeness of resection, invasion, and size (MACIS) scoring[34] or postsurgery thyroglobulin level.[39]

Thyroid Hormone Suppression

Patients with HCC generally should have thyroid hormone suppression therapy. Risks of suppression include cardiovascular incidents, including arrhythmias and decreased bone mineral density. General recommendations are to keep thyroid-stimulating hormone (TSH) in the range of 0.01 to 0.1 in patients that have been deemed in the high-risk category and in the range of 0.1 to 0.4 in patients with lower risk to decrease the incidence of side effects.

External beam radiotherapy (EBR) has been shown to be an effective modality of treatment for advanced-stage thyroid cancers at high risk for locoregional tumor recurrence because of associated multiple lymph node metastases, soft-tissue or vascular invasion, and positive surgical margins (see Chapter 49, External Beam Radiotherapy for Thyroid Malignancy). Phlips et al. respectively reviewed 94 patients with well-differentiated thyroid carcinoma treated with adjuvant therapy; 56 patients were treated with RAI alone, and 38 of these patients had an additional course of radiation therapy (55 Gy over 5.5 weeks).[40] They showed no difference in survival despite the fact that the patients who were treated with radiation therapy generally had more advanced disease. Treatment with RAI resulted in a 21% local recurrence, but with the addition of radiation therapy this decreased to 3%. The authors concluded that radiation therapy was very effective for advanced well-differentiated thyroid carcinoma and recommended adjuvant radiation therapy if the patient had macroscopic or microscopic residual disease at the time of the original surgery or if extracapsular extension from cervical lymph node disease was identified.

There is only one study that specifically examined the efficacy of EBR in HCC. Foote et al., in 2003, looked at 18 patients with advanced HCC (including widely invasive disease, presence of positive margins after initial surgery, and unresectable disease) treated with EBR.[41] Their overall 5-year survival in these patients was 66.7%. They observed notable success in the prevention of recurrence in those given EBR as adjuvant treatment for high-risk cancers defined as large tumors (>6.5 cm in diameter), lesions with tracheal invasion, vascular invasion, muscle invasion, metastatic involvement of multiple lymph nodes, metastatic soft-tissue nodules, and positive surgical margins. They concluded that HCC is a radiosensitive tumor and recommended radiation therapy for widely invasive tumors with a high risk of recurrence and incompletely resected or unresectable disease.

Chemotherapy for advanced and metastatic thyroid cancer is generally deemed to be of limited effectiveness. Trials are ongoing for novel targeted therapy with preliminary, yet encouraging, results.[42]

Targeted Therapy

The recent report by Ganly et al. identified the importance of the *RTK/RAS/RAF/MAPK* and *PIK3/AKT/mTOR* pathways in this disease. At least one receptor tyrosine kinase was mutated in 20% of HCC tumors, including *EGFR* (2%), *ERBB2* (11%), *PDGFR* (2%), *TSHR* (4%), *MET* (4%), and *RET* (4%). *PIK3CA* mutations were found in 2% of HCC tumors and were mutually exclusive with *PTEN* mutations (4%). *TSC1/2* mutations occurred in 6% of tumors. *NF1* was deleted or mutated in 9% of tumors. Mutations in *NRAS*, *HRAS*, or *KRAS* occurred in 15% of tumors (*NRAS*, 9%; *HRAS*, 2%; and *KRAS*, 4%). Mutations in *EIF1AX* occurred in 11% of tumors, and mutations in other EIF1, 2, or 3 genes occurred in 9% of tumors. In addition to these mutations, genes which are overexpressed due to whole chromosome duplication of chromosome 7 were found, including *BRAF*, *RHEB*, and *EIF3B*.[8] There is currently a phase II randomized clinical trial of the multiple tyrosine kinase inhibitor sorafenib and the mTOR inhibitor everolimus in patients with widely invasive HCC. The preliminary evidence has shown a significant response rate for these agents, indicating the importance of this pathway in this cancer.

FOLLOW-UP

Please see the Expert Consult website for more discussion of this topic.

SUMMARY

Please see the Expert Consult website for more discussion of this topic.

REFERENCES

For a complete list of references, go to expertconsult.com.

Sporadic Medullary Thyroid Carcinoma

Benjamin R. Roman, Richard J. Wong

 Please go to expertconsult.com to view related video:
Video 26.1 Introduction to Chapter 26, Sporadic Medullary Thyroid Carcinoma.

INTRODUCTION

Medullary thyroid carcinoma (MTC) comprises 1% to 2% of all new cases of thyroid cancer in the United States, a number that is significantly smaller than historically documented, due to the increasing incidence of papillary thyroid cancer.[1] MTC occurs as two distinct clinical entities, hereditary (25%) and sporadic (75%). Although these entities share the same etiology, arising from the neuroendocrine parafollicular or C-cells of the thyroid, sporadic MTCs tend to be more aggressive than hereditary MTC, with more frequent metastasis to cervical lymph nodes. Surgical removal of the thyroid and regional lymph nodes remains the mainstay of therapy for MTC. New advances in targeted therapy with tyrosine kinase inhibitors (TKIs) have recently improved progression-free survival for advanced MTC.

Several organizations have published guidelines on the management of MTC in the last decade. The 2015 guidelines from the American Thyroid Association (ATA) provide the most recent in-depth recommendations on the full spectrum of MTC diagnosis and treatment.[1] This chapter will review pathophysiology; genetics; differences between sporadic and hereditary MTC; clinical presentation; clinical course; diagnostic considerations, including workup and staging; primary surgical treatment decision-making; follow-up and surveillance; surgical management of recurrent disease; radiation therapy; and management of distant metastatic disease, including systemic and targeted therapies.

PATHOPHYSIOLOGY

An understanding of histology and the importance of C-cells, calcitonin, and carcinoembryonic antigen (CEA) form the underpinnings of the appropriate diagnosis and management of MTC. The genetic underpinnings of MTC help distinguish sporadic and hereditary forms of the disease and are important for understanding prognostic and diagnostic considerations when a patient is found to have sporadic MTC.

Histology and C-Cells

During embryogenesis, the ultimobranchial bodies arising from the neural crest migrate to the upper and middle poles of each thyroid lobe. These give rise to C-cells, which make up 1% of thyroid cells. C-cells are neuroectodermal in origin and have neuroendocrine function through the secretion of calcitonin. MTC is only classified as a thyroid cancer because of its location; in truth, it is a neuroendocrine tumor, compared with the more common follicular (thyroid) cell-derived cancers. In noncancer specimens, C-cells normally exist in clusters of six to eight cells at the periphery of thyroid follicles.

MTC was first described in the 1900s as an amyloid tumor and was considered a variant of anaplastic thyroid carcinoma. In 1959, Hazard, Hawk, and Crile first described its unique appearance.[2] Grossly, the tumor is well demarcated, firm, gray-white, and gritty. Microscopically, the cells are uniform round, polygonal, or spindle-shaped cells with finely granular eosinophilic cytoplasm and central nuclei. The cells tend to form sheets or nests with peripheral palisading in a vascular stroma. The presence of amyloid is considered to be a distinctive feature of MTC, although it may not be found in all cases. The amyloid arises from calcitonin or procalcitonin, a different precursor than other amyloid-rich tumors. C-cell hyperplasia is associated with MTC, particularly in the familial form, and is thought to be a precursor in the malignant transformation to MTC.[3,4]

The histologic diagnosis of MTC may be difficult, as it can be confused with papillary or follicular thyroid cancers, as well as paragangliomas, sarcomas, and lymphoma. The diagnosis may be aided by staining for cytokeratins CK7 and CK18, as well as TTF1, and chromogranin A. The most important diagnostic markers, however, are calcitonin chromogranin, CEA, and a lack of thyroglobulin staining. Histologically, MTC can be classified according to dominant patterns. Histologic groups include the classic, amyloid-rich, insular, trabecular, and epithelial variants. Classic variants are most common (48.9%) followed by the amyloid-rich variants (38.3%).[5,6]

Calcitonin and Carcinoembryonic Antigen

C-cells secrete calcitonin and other substances, including CEA, histaminase, neuron-specific enolase, calcitonin gene-related peptide, somatostatin, thyroglobulin, thyrotropin-stimulating hormone, adrenocortical stimulating hormone, gastrin-related peptide, serotonin, chromogranin, and substance P.[7] Calcitonin has been shown to be integral in calcium homeostasis in other vertebrate species, but its role in humans remains unclear.

Calcitonin and CEA are useful tumor markers that can be measured in blood in the basal state. CEA has a longer half-life than calcitonin and is not unique to MTC, making it a less specific marker. Calcitonin levels are almost always elevated in patients with sporadic MTC, and levels are usually correlated with the amount of MTC tumor mass in the body. Measurement of calcitonin is helpful in screening patients at risk for MTC and in the follow-up of patients after treatment. After primary surgery for MTC, persistent or recurrent elevation of calcitonin indicates the presence of local, regional, or distant disease. Imaging may not localize a tumor mass, and some patients in this situation have an indolent course. Historically, calcitonin was often measured after stimulation by administration of the secretagogue pentagastrin. However, this was uncomfortable for patients, causing nausea, diaphoresis, agitation, and urinary urgency. Today, improvements in the accuracy of measuring basal levels of calcitonin have made stimulated testing unnecessary.

GENETICS: SPORADIC VERSUS HEREDITARY

By definition, patients with hereditary MTC have a germline mutation in the *RET* proto-oncogene (see Chapter 27, Syndromic Medullary Thyroid Carcinoma: MEN 2A and MEN 2B). As the name implies, the majority of patients with sporadic MTC do not have germline mutations, although 1% to 7% of patients with no family history of MTC will have germline mutations.[8,9] It is important to refer patients without a family history of MTC for genetic counseling and testing for a germline mutation for several reason. First, if a patient with apparently sporadic MTC is found to have a germline *RET* mutation, other blood relatives harboring the same mutation may be identified by genetic testing, starting with first-degree relatives, and appropriate therapy or preventative surgery can be initiated. Second, if a patient is found to have a germline *RET* mutation, he or she may then be screened for hyperparathyroidism and pheochromocytoma.[10] More studies regarding these issues are needed and future guidelines terminology may change, but it is likely that the specific *RET* mutation will continue to influence the approach to surgical management, risk of recurrence, and need to test for association with other endocrine neoplasms.

Somatic mutations are identified in tumor cells only compared with germline mutations that can be detected in all cells of the body. In the past there has been no routine clinical indication for testing the tumors of patients with apparently sporadic MTC for somatic mutations. However, there is growing evidence that this type of sporadic *RET* mutation may predict responsiveness to systemic therapy with TKIs, suggesting a future clinical role for testing tumors for somatic mutations. Somatic mutations or rearrangements involving *RET* have been identified in 40% to 50% of sporadic MTCs.[11,12] In a tumor with a somatic *RET* mutation, not all cells may harbor the mutation.[13,14] Most of the mutations identified in sporadic MTCs are point mutations involving the same codons associated with the MEN 2 syndromes, including 918, 634, and 883.[11] Of sporadic MTCs with alterations of *RET*, 60% to 80% are found to have the M918T mutation.[11,15-17] Patients with sporadic MTCs bearing a *RET* mutation (particularly M918T) have a more advanced stage at diagnosis, increased rates of recurrent or persistent disease after resection, and poorer long-term survival (10 to 20 years) than those without this *RET* mutation.[11,16,17]

Clinical Presentation and Usual Clinical Course

MTCs occur in two clinical settings, sporadic and hereditary. Hereditary MTC is discussed elsewhere in this book (see Chapter 27, Syndromic Medullary Thyroid Carcinoma: MEN 2A and MEN 2B). Much of the MTC literature combines data on hereditary and sporadic tumors together, making it difficult to compare these entities. Overall, sporadic MTCs behave in a similar fashion to hereditary MTCs with a similar prognosis when adjusted for stage, although hereditary MTCs are more likely to be bilateral or multifocal (>90% compared with 32% in sporadic MTC) and to present at a less advanced stage.

Sporadic MTCs usually present in the fourth to sixth decades of life[18] as a mass in the neck from the thyroid tumor or cervical nodal metastases. In addition to a neck mass, symptoms of dysphagia, shortness of breath, or hoarseness may be present in approximately 15% of cases. Less commonly, they may be discovered after detection of elevated calcitonin or CEA levels in patients with a nodular thyroid.[19] Some patients present with distant metastases or with diarrhea secondary to secretory products from the MTC tumor cells. Rarely, MTC is discovered to be the cause of an elevated CEA level—for example, in a patient being followed after treatment of colon cancer.

MTC frequently metastasizes to regional lymph nodes. Central compartment metastases are present in patients with T1 and T4 tumors 14% and 86% of the time, respectively, whereas lateral compartment metastases are present in patients with T1 an T4 tumors 11% and 93% of the time, respectively.[20] Serum calcitonin levels correlate with nodal disease burden and location.[21] In all, 70% of patients with MTC who present with a palpable thyroid mass also have cervical metastases, and 10% have distant metastases.[20] Hematogenous spread may occur to the lungs, liver, bones, brain, and soft tissues.

Although the clinical course of MTC may be more aggressive than differentiated thyroid cancers such as papillary thyroid carcinoma (PTC), MTC is nonetheless a relatively indolent malignancy, with reported 10-year survival rates from 69% to 89%.[22-24] Multivariate analysis has shown patient age and stage to be significant prognostic factors.[25] Ten-year survival rates for patients with stage I, II, III, or IV are 100%, 93%, 71%, and 21%, respectively.[23] The clinical course is somewhat unpredictable; patients with distant metastases may often live for years.

Patients with normal basal serum calcitonin levels after surgery have better long-term survival rates, with 97.7% survival at 10 years.[23] Studies of survival rates have found close associations with calcitonin doubling times.[26,27] In one study of patients undergoing total thyroidectomy and bilateral cervical lymph node dissection, all patients with calcitonin doubling times >24 months were alive at the end of the study, whereas patients with doubling times <6 months had 5- and 10-year survival rates of 25% and 8%, respectively. Patients with doubling times between 6 and 24 months had 5- and 10-year survival rates of 92% and 37%, respectively.[26]

DIAGNOSTIC CONSIDERATIONS, WORKUP, AND STAGING

ATA guidelines published in 2015 regarding the workup of thyroid nodules recommend a biopsy of nodules greater than 1 cm in size if ultrasonographic features are suspicious for malignancy.[28] ATA guidelines specific to MTC also recommend a biopsy of nodules greater than 1 cm. Fine-needle aspiration (FNA) findings that are inconclusive or suggestive of MTC should undergo further diagnostic workup, including calcitonin measured in the FNA washout fluid, as well as immunohistochemical staining to evaluate for the presence of calcitonin, chromogranin, and CEA, and the absence of thyroglobulin.

Serum calcitonin screening on all patients with a thyroid nodule is not currently recommended due to concerns about cost-effectiveness because MTC is present in only 0.3% to 1.4% of patients with thyroid nodules.[1] Nonetheless, ATA guidelines suggest that physicians decide whether serum calcitonin should be measured for patients with thyroid nodules in their clinic.

Once a histologic confirmation of MTC is made based on FNA, patients should have a physical examination to evaluate for regional lymph node metastases, a serum calcitonin and CEA measurement, and be referred to genetic counseling for *RET* germline testing as discussed earlier. In patients with hereditary MTC, the presence of a pheochromocytoma and hyperparathyroidism should be excluded.

Regarding imaging, ultrasonography of the neck should be performed in all patients with MTC. In addition, a computed tomography

(CT) scan of the neck and chest, cross-sectional evaluation of the liver (three-phase contrast-enhanced multidetector liver CT or contrast-enhanced magnetic resonance imaging [MRI]), and axial MRI or bone scan should be performed in patients with extensive neck disease, signs or symptoms of regional or distant metastases, and in patients with a serum calcitonin level greater than 500 pg/mL. Positron emission tomography (PET)/CT scans are less sensitive in detecting MTC metastases and should not be used during the initial workup.[1]

The American Joint Committee on Cancer (AJCC) 8th edition staging manual defines four stages of disease in MTC (Tables 26.1 and 26.2). As in most solid cancer types, the overall stage groups account for tumor, lymph node, and metastases (TNM). Although there has been some suggestion to incorporate a quantitative assessment of the number of lymph node metastases into staging,[29] the 8th edition staging maintains prior editions' assessments of the presence and location of lymph node metastases. The AJCC 8th edition manual does, however, recommend that the following parameters be recorded for clinical care: number of involved lymph nodes, size of involved lymph nodes and measurement of metastatic focus; completeness of resection; preoperative and postoperative biochemical parameters (calcitonin and CEA); and genetic mutation analysis.[30]

TABLE 26.1 American Joint Committee on Cancer TMN Criteria for Medullary Thyroid Cancer

TMN	Criteria
TX	Primary tumor cannot be assessed
T0	No evidence of primary tumor
T1	Tumor ≤2 cm, limited to the thyroid
	T1a: tumor ≤1 cm
	T1b: tumor >1 cm but ≤2 cm
T2	Tumor >2 to ≤4 cm, limited to the thyroid
T3	Tumor >4 cm, limited to the thyroid or with extrathyroidal extension
T4	T4a: Moderately advanced disease
	Tumor of any size with gross extrathyroidal extension into the nearby tissues of the neck, including subcutaneous soft tissue, larynx, trachea, esophagus, or recurrent laryngeal nerve
	T4b: Very advanced disease
	Tumor of any size with extension toward the spine or into nearby large blood vessels, invading the prevertebral fascia, or encasing the carotid artery or mediastinal vessels
NX	Regional lymph nodes cannot be assessed
N0	No regional lymph node metastasis
	N0a: One or more cytologically or histologically confirmed benign lymph nodes
	N0b: No radiologic or clinical evidence of locoregional lymph node metastasis
N1	Regional lymph node metastasis
	N1a: Metastasis to level VI or VII (pretracheal, paratracheal, prelaryngeal/Delphian, upper mediastinal lymph nodes)
	N1b: Metastasis to unilateral, bilateral, or contralateral cervical or retropharyngeal or superior mediastinal lymph nodes
MX	Distant metastasis cannot be assessed
M0	No distant metastasis
M1	Distant metastasis

From American Joint Committee on Cancer. *AJCC Cancer Staging Handbook*. 8th ed. New York: Springer; 2018.

TABLE 26.2 American Joint Committee on Cancer Staging for Medullary Thyroid Cancer

Stage	T Category	N Category	M Category
I	T1	N0	M0
II	T2 or T3	N0	M0
III	T1 or T2 or T3	N1a	M0
IVA	T4a	N0 or N1a or N1b	M0
	T1 or T2 or T3	N1b	M0
IVB	T4b	Any N	M0
IVC	Any T	Any N	M1

From American Joint Committee on Cancer. *AJCC Cancer Staging Handbook*. 8th ed. New York: Springer; 2018.

PRIMARY SURGICAL TREATMENT

Appropriate surgical extirpation of the primary thyroid lesion and cervical lymph nodes is the most typical approach toward the initial management of MTC. Although there is wide variation regarding the extent of surgery performed, especially for lymph nodes, the principles of surgery and technical aspects related to thyroid surgery remain constant and are covered elsewhere in this book.

The surgical treatment of MTC is influenced by several factors: (1) the clinical course of MTC is usually more aggressive than that of differentiated thyroid cancer, with higher rates of recurrence and mortality, especially in young patients; (2) MTC cells do not take up radioactive iodine; (3) hormone suppression is ineffective; (4) MTC is multifocal and bilateral in >90% of patients with hereditary forms of the disease compared with 32% of patients with the sporadic form; (5) nodal metastases are present in more than 70% of patients with palpable thyroid disease; and (6) the ability to measure postoperative calcitonin levels allows assessment of the adequacy of surgical extirpation.

Extent of Surgery

Total thyroidectomy with central compartment nodal dissection is usually advocated as the initial surgical treatment for the management of MTC. Clinically apparent lateral neck nodes are managed with lateral neck dissection. In cases where the diagnosis of MTC was not known preoperatively and a hemithyroidectomy was performed for a suspicious nodule, current ATA 2015 guidelines recommend completion thyroidectomy for patients with a *RET* germline mutation, an elevated serum calcitonin level postoperatively, or imaging studies showing residual MTC.[1] Completion thyroidectomy should also be considered for patients whose pathology report shows C-cell hyperplasia, multicentric disease, positive surgical margins, or extrathyroidal extension.

Regarding the management of possible occult lateral neck nodal disease, recent guidelines acknowledge two schools of thought. Some surgeons and endocrinologists believe that a high-quality ultrasound examination showing no suspicious lymph nodes negates the need for an elective lateral lymph node dissection. There may be more consensus on this opinion for cases of sporatic MTC microcarcinoma (SmMTC). Conversely, other physicians advocate for elective lateral lymph node dissection based on preoperative calcitonin levels.

Current ATA 2015 guidelines make the following specific recommendations regarding the extent of nodal dissection (in addition to total thyroidectomy): (1) the central compartment lymph nodes should be electively dissected for patients with no evidence of lymph node or distant metastasis on ultrasound; (2) the ipsilateral lateral compartment "may be considered" for elective dissection; (3) in patients with no evidence of lymph node or distant metastasis on ultrasound, lateral compartment dissection may be considered based on serum calcitonin levels; (4) patients with lymph node metastases that are known preoperatively should have central compartment and ipsilateral lateral neck dissection; (5) if preoperative imaging is positive in the ipsilateral lateral neck but negative in the contralateral neck, contralateral lymph node dissection should be performed if the serum calcitonin level is >200 pg/mL.[1]

For the aforementioned case in which a patient has no evidence of lymph node or distant metastasis on ultrasound, the consideration to perform lateral compartment dissection based on serum calcitonin levels did not have consensus among the ATA Guidelines Task Force. Some literature suggests ipsilateral lateral neck dissection for patients with a calcitonin level between 20 and 50 pg/mL and contralateral lateral neck dissection for patients with a calcitonin level >200 pg/mL.[31]

When patients present with advanced MTC, the goals of surgery may change. Specifically, surgery can be considered as a palliative procedure, meant to minimize surgical complications and help avoid the morbidity of locoregional disease progression. In the setting of metastatic disease, unilateral or hemithyroidectomy may be considered to prevent future local invasion, while avoiding the low risks of contralateral recurrent laryngeal nerve injury and hypoparathyroidism. In the setting of locally advanced disease invading the trachea, larynx, esophagus, etc., ATA guidelines recommend considering life expectancy based on extent of disease and other comorbidities, and focusing on preserving speech, swallowing, parathyroid, and shoulder function by considering performing less aggressive central compartment surgery. Other therapies, including external beam radiation, systemic therapy, or other nonsurgical therapies, should be considered in these cases. However, it is the authors' belief that there is still a role for radical extirpative surgery, including laryngectomy, esophagectomy, or laryngopharyngectomy in the presence of locally advanced MTC if there is no evidence of extensive metastatic disease and no reason to suspect a shorter life expectancy based on age or comorbidity.

FOLLOW-UP AND SURVEILLANCE

The follow-up and surveillance of MTC is particularly important when considering the high rates of recurrence after initial surgical management of this disease. The term *biochemical cure* is used to refer to patients with normal calcitonin levels after surgery for MTC. Complete postoperative normalization of calcitonin has been associated with decreased long-term risk of MTC recurrence, though the evidence is less clear for a survival benefit. A persistent or recurrent elevation in calcitonin indicates residual or recurrent MTC and warrants additional investigation. However, patients with borderline elevated but stable calcitonin levels over time often do very well clinically, and follow-up and treatment of these patients should not be overly aggressive.[32-34] Even patients with persistently high levels of calcitonin after surgery may do well for years without radiographic or clinical evidence of disease recurrence; the time it takes for calcitonin levels to double in value is the most reliable marker for disease progression.

Calcitonin, Carcinoembryonic Antigen, and Ultrasound

After surgery for MTC, clinicians should review data that can help predict the outcome and plan long-term follow-up. This includes documented TNM classification from the pathology report, the number of positive lymph nodes removed during surgery, and the postoperative calcitonin level. Although the preoperative calcitonin level serves as a marker of disease burden, the postsurgical reduction of basal levels indicates the success in tumor clearance.

Calcitonin levels drop slowly after surgery.[35,36] Current 2015 ATA guidelines for MTC recommend that serum calcitonin and CEA levels be measured 3 months postoperatively. If undetectable or within the normal range, testing should be repeated every 6 months for 1 year, and then annually thereafter.

For patients with elevated postoperative calcitonin levels less than 150 pg/mL at the 3-month postoperative time point, ATA guidelines recommend a physical examination and ultrasound of the neck. If these studies are negative, the patient should have an ultrasound and physical examination repeated every 6 months (along with ongoing calcitonin and CEA testing every 6 months). If the postoperative serum calcitonin level is higher than 150 pg/mL, patients should have a thyroid ultrasound, chest CT, contrast-enhanced MRI or three-phase contrast-enhanced CT of the liver, and bone scintigraphy and MRI of the pelvis and axial skeleton.

Calcitonin Doubling Time

Most patients with a detectable serum calcitonin postoperatively will have serum values that stay relatively stable over time. Measurement of calcitonin doubling times over months and years of follow-up is recommended, and higher doubling times correlate with more aggressive disease. In one study of patients treated with total thyroidectomy and bilateral lymph node dissection, the 5- and 10-year survival rate for patients with calcitonin doubling times <6 months was 25% and 8%, respectively. In contrast, patients with calcitonin doubling times between 6 to 24 months had 5- and 10-year survival rates of 92% and 37%, respectively. All patients with calcitonin doubling times >24 months were alive at the end of the study (with follow-up ranging up to 29 years).[26] ATA guidelines specifically recommend that in patients with detectable serum levels of calcitonin and CEA after thyroidectomy, the levels of both of these markers should be measured at least every 6 months to determine their doubling times. Reliable estimates usually require at least four data points over a minimum of 2 years. However, doubling times less than 6 months can be reliably estimated within the first 12 months after surgery. The ATA provides a free online calculator for doubling times.[2]

SURGICAL MANAGEMENT OF RECURRENT DISEASE

Patients with findings indicating recurrent disease localized to the neck should undergo reoperation, when possible, with the goal of removing all remaining disease. Reoperation should be considered in patients with elevated calcitonin levels in the setting of an inadequate initial operation, imaging evidence of persisting or recurrent disease, and for expectant palliation of symptoms with continued progression such as local compression, or invasion of critical structures such as the trachea, esophagus, vessels, and nerves. Patients who have systemic symptoms (e.g., pain, flushing, and diarrhea) from metastatic tumor may benefit from a palliative tumor debulking procedure. For patients with a local recurrence in the thyroid bed, a more radical local regional resection may be justified if there is a low burden of distant metastatic disease, helping prevent local tumor recurrence and palliate the neck. Conversely, where there is a high burden of distant disease, the goals of local resection are preservation of swallowing and speech and should be weighed against the potential morbidity of surgery and life expectancy.

Neck recurrence is more common than local recurrence in the thyroid bed. In experienced hands reoperative surgery for regional neck disease can achieve long-term control and biochemical cure in up to one-third of patients. More importantly perhaps, surgery may prevent symptomatic complications of recurrence in the neck.[20,33,37-40] Because of the risks of reoperation, patients with an elevated calcitonin level but no radiographic evidence of disease should not undergo elective exploration. Such procedures may lead to a negative specimens and a minimal chance of biochemical remission. These patients should instead be followed radiographically for any radiographic evidence of recurrent disease.

Before proceeding with neck reoperation, a metastatic workup with imaging is necessary to evaluate the lungs, liver, and bones. This information may alter the decision to approach recurrent disease in the neck with aggressive surgery. Reexploration of the neck to remove metastatic lymph nodes carries a higher risk of complications, including thoracic duct leak, injury to a recurrent laryngeal nerve, and hypoparathyroidism (see Chapter 50, Reoperative Thyroid Surgery). Finding the recurrent laryngeal nerve is always a challenge in revision surgery cases and may be aided by use of an intraoperative neural integrity monitor (IONM) and by finding the nerve in previously undissected regions of the neck. Parathyroid glands may be at risk of removal or being devascularized. Care should be taken to identify parathyroid glands during dissection as well as attached to thyroid specimens after removal. When the blood supply of glands is compromised, they should be reimplanted.

Two recent publications addressing reoperative neck surgery provide guidance on appropriate workup and decision-making before proceeding to the operating room. Although focused on differentiated thyroid cancer, a 2016 American Head and Neck Society (AHNS) consensus statement describes the appropriate use of diagnostic imaging in identifying structural disease recurrence, as well as techniques in reoperative surgery.[41] In addition, recent ATA guidelines focused on MTC weigh in on the extent of surgery in the reoperative setting. In patients with persistent or recurrent locoregional MTC and no distant metastases, neck surgery should include compartmental dissection of image-positive or biopsy-positive disease in the central or lateral neck. The importance of compartment-directed therapy is stressed, with avoidance of limited operative procedures such as resection of only grossly metastatic lymph nodes unless there has been extensive prior surgery in a given compartment.[1]

Outcomes after reoperation for MTC have documented biochemical results and recurrence rates. However, there has been no clinical trial where patients have been staged and randomized to either reoperation or observation alone. In appropriately selected patients, reoperative surgery for locoregional disease can achieve biochemical cure. In about one-third of patients treated by repeat neck operations for persistent or recurrent MTC, the postoperative basal or stimulated serum calcitonin levels are reduced to the "normal range"; however, they are rarely undetectable.[25,33,40,42] Long-term outcomes in patients undergoing repeat neck operations have been fairly good, with excellent prevention of recurrence in the central neck.

RADIATION THERAPY FOR MTC

The role of external beam radiation therapy (EBRT) remains limited in patients with MTC and has not yet shown a survival benefit (see Chapter 49, External Beam Radiotherapy for Thyroid Malignancy). Cohort data indicate that EBRT is sometimes employed after surgical excision. In the patients with sporadic MTC, 13.9% of patients received EBRT.[24] One disadvantage of EBRT is its effects on the tissues (i.e., radiation-induced scarring and fibrosis), which makes any subsequent surgical intervention significantly riskier. Before initiating EBRT, surgeons should be sure that patients are not candidates for reoperation, as the procedure will be more difficult technically and associated with significant complications.

In an analysis of the National Cancer Institute's Surveillance, Epidemiology, and End Results (SEER) data regarding patients with MTC and positive lymph nodes, adjuvant EBRT showed no overall survival benefit.[43] Other cohort studies have demonstrated no difference in local or regional relapse-free survival rates comparing patients with and without adjuvant EBRT.[44] The intent of postoperative EBRT in patients with MTC has been to achieve locoregional control in those at high risk of recurrence, as determined by the operating surgeon and radiation oncologist. Locoregional control is a valid endpoint in patients with MTC, as progression in the cervical region can have a significant effect on quality of life. For this purpose, several cohort studies have demonstrated effectiveness of EBRT. For example, in one study of 34 patients at high risk for recurrence, 5-year locoregional relapse-free survival was 87%, and disease-specific and overall survival rates were 62% and 56%, respectively,[45] an improvement over expected rates without EBRT.

Current ATA guidelines for MTC reflect the aforementioned considerations. The recommendation is that postoperative adjuvant EBRT to the neck and mediastinum should be considered in patients at high risk for local recurrence (microscopic or macroscopic residual MTC, extrathyroidal extension, or extensive lymph node metastases) and those at risk of airway obstruction. The guidelines note that the potential benefits must be weighed against the acute and chronic radiation toxicity.[1] The typical dose is 60 to 66 Gy. Gross residual disease should be treated to 70 Gy or higher. Intensity-modulated radiation therapy (IMRT) should be used to treat MTC adjacent to the spinal cord. EBRT recommendations are undergoing dynamic changes due to multiple new chemotherapeutic agents available for recurrent local and distant disease.

DISTANT METASTATIC DISEASE AND SYSTEMIC THERAPY FOR MTC

The majority of patients with MTC have a relatively indolent course of disease, with either no evidence of distant metastases, or very slow calcitonin doubling time and eventual development of distant disease. However, some patients have a more aggressive clinical course, requiring additional treatment beyond surgery and radiation. This section reviews management of isolated distant metastases, diarrhea, and other complications of metastatic disease, and systemic therapy options including targeted therapy with TKIs. It is important to note that systemic therapy should not be given to patients with increasing serum calcitonin and CEA but no evidence of metastatic disease. Even in the setting of low-volume metastatic disease on imaging, systemic therapy should not be given if the disease is stable, as determined by imaging, and serum calcitonin and CEA doubling times are >2 years (see Chapter 52, Medical Treatment Horizons for Metastatic Differentiated and Medullary Thyroid Cancer).

Management of Isolated Distant Metastases

Patients with distant metastases may exhibit symptoms or have findings on routine imaging leading to the diagnosis. ATA guidelines make the following recommendations for MTC: (1) Patients with neurologic symptoms should have brain imaging performed. (2) Patients with isolated brain metastases are candidates for surgical resection or EBRT, including stereotactic radiosurgery. (3) Whole brain EBRT is also indicated for multiple brain metastasis. (4) Patients with spinal cord compression from MTC metastases should be urgently treated with steroids and surgical decompression. (5) Those who are not surgical candidates may be treated with EBRT. (6) Bony fractures or impending fractures require treatment with surgery, thermoablation (radiofrequency or cryotherapy), EBRT, or cement injection. (7) Patients with solitary lung metastases should be considered for surgical resection. (8) For smaller and peripheral lung metastases, radiofrequency ablation can be considered. However, in the setting of multiple progressive lung metastases, systemic therapy is generally favored. (9) Liver metastases should also be considered for surgical resection. (10) Hemoembolization is an option for patients with multiple small tumors if they involve less than one-third of the liver. (11) Finally, cutaneous metastases should also be considered for surgical resection. Multiple cutaneous metastases are better treated with EBRT or ethanol injection.

Management of Diarrhea and Other Secretory Complications of Advanced MTC

Diarrhea can occur in patients with advanced MTC. The cause is likely a combination of a hypersecretory state due to elevated calcitonin levels made by medullary thyroid carcinoma cells and enhanced gastrointestinal motility. Diarrhea is more often seen in patients with hepatic metastases. Patients with MTC-related diarrhea should avoid alcohol and high-fiber foods. Symptomatic relief may be provided with antimotility agents such as loperamide. Further control may be achieved with treatment or debulking of large tumor deposits. Somatostatin analogue therapy has also been employed. For patients with liver metastases and diarrhea, chemoembolization has been shown to be of benefit.[46,47]

Some patients with metastatic MTC may experience Cushing's syndrome, due to secretion of adrenocorticotropic hormone (ACTH) or Corticotropin releasing hormone (CRH) by their tumors. This is usually a marker of very advanced disease and suggests a poor prognosis. Treatment options include medical therapy or bilateral adrenalectomy for refractory cases.

Systemic Cytotoxic Chemotherapy

Many systemic chemotherapy agents have been studied for the management of metastatic and advanced MTC. Very few have shown any convincing evidence of benefit, and they will not be reviewed in this chapter. Current ATA guidelines recommend the use of cytotoxic therapy with combination doxorubicin and either fluorouracil (5FU) or dacarbazine only in select settings, and not usually as first-line therapy, given the effectiveness of newer targeted therapies. Other potentially promising novel therapies have not been thoroughly studied as of this writing but include treatment with radiolabeled molecules or pretargeted radioimmunotherapy.[48,49]

Tyrosine Kinase Inhibitor Targeted Therapy

The basis for TKI therapy in advanced and metastatic MTC is the implication of the RET, RAS, and endothelial growth factor receptor (EGFR) mechanisms in pathogenesis. Germline RET mutations are present in almost all patients with familial MTC. Somatic RET mutations are present in the tumors of approximately half of patients with sporadic MTC. Many patients without somatic RET mutations have somatic RAS mutations. Additionally, vascular endothelial growth factor (VEGF) receptors are often overexpressed in MTC.[50] TKI therapy has the potential to target these various pathways specifically. Although many TKIs have been studied in MTC, two agents, vandetanib and cabozantinib, have been approved by the U.S. Food and Drug Administration (FDA) after the successful completion of two phase III trials, showing good disease control and durable responses, with significant improvement in progression-free survival (see Chapter 52, Medical Treatment Horizons for Metastatic Differentiated and Medullary Thyroid Cancer).

The phase III trial studying vandetanib enrolled 331 patients with symptomatic or progressive locally advanced or metastatic MTC and compared outcomes in patients treated with the drug versus a placebo. Patients receiving the drug had improvement in progression-free survival from 19.3 months (in the placebo arm) to 30.5 months. The response rate was 45% in patients treated with vandetanib, with a 22-month duration of response. There were also improvements in patient-reported outcomes including quality of life. Responders included patients with and without a RET mutation. Adverse events were relatively rare and low grade.[51]

The phase III trial studying cabozantinib enrolled 330 patients with progressive, metastatic, or locally advanced MTC and compared outcomes in patients treated with the drug versus a placebo. Patients receiving the drug had improvement in progression-free survival from 4.0 months (in the placebo arm) to 11.2 months. The response rate was 28% in patients treated with cabozantinib. Adverse events were significant, including diarrhea, abdominal pain and discomfort, fatigue, hypertension, and more severe complications. In total 16% of patients in the cabozantinib arm had to discontinue treatment due to toxicity, and 79% required a reduction in the dose of the drug.[52] Interestingly, subgroup analysis of patients with a RET M918T mutation demonstrated larger benefits of cabozantinib therapy, with a significant improvement in overall survival.

On the basis of these trials, the FDA and European Medicines Agency (EMA) approved vandetanib and cabozantinib for the treatment of patients with advanced progressive MTC in 2011 to 2012. Current ATA guidelines recommend the use of TKIs in patients with significant tumor burden and symptomatic or progressive metastatic disease according to response criteria in solid tumors (RECIST) criteria.[1]

There are several unresolved issues and questions regarding the use of vandetanib and cabozantinib for advanced MTC. Some issues relate to best practices regarding therapy, including the dose of the drug and optimal strategies for monitoring and managing toxicities. Patients on these drugs are at significant risk for developing hypothyroidism, although the mechanism is poorly understood. In addition, dose reductions and withdrawal of therapy due to toxicity was common, and algorithms for management have not been well established.

Other issues relate to the problem of resistance and the appropriate context for starting therapy with these drugs. Almost all patients will develop resistance over time, making the timing of onset of therapy, which may have benefits of limited durability, an important consideration. Also unresolved is the issue of when treatment with TKIs should be stopped in patients with stable disease or a mixed response. A better understanding of these issues will form the basis for logical combination therapies. Finally, there is limited data on long-term toxicity and overall survival with these drugs. If significant benefits can be demonstrated, there may be a role for first-line therapy with TKIs earlier in the course of disease.

CONCLUSION

Medullary thyroid cancer is a rare malignancy characterized by high rates of regional lymph node metastases and elevated levels of serum calcitonin and CEA. Although germline RET mutations are not common in cases of sporadic MTC, patients without a family history should nonetheless undergo genetic testing for RET mutations. After appropriate diagnostic workup, including evaluation for distant disease in patients with more advanced locoregional disease, surgical removal of the thyroid, the central compartment, and involved lateral neck lymph nodes remains the mainstay of therapy. Postoperatively, calcitonin and CEA levels should be followed, including measurement of doubling times. When regional recurrence in lymph nodes is detected, further surgical therapy is often indicated. There is a limited role for radiation therapy as well as systemic cytotoxic therapies. Recent studies of the TKIs vandetanib and cabozantinib have shown promise for the management of patients with significant tumor burden and symptomatic or progressive disease.

REFERENCES

For a complete list of references, go to expertconsult.com.

Syndromic Medullary Thyroid Cancer: MEN 2A and MEN 2B

Henning Dralle, Andreas Machens

INTRODUCTION

As early as the beginning of the 20th century, medullary thyroid carcinoma (MTC) was noted as a distinct disease entity within the broad spectrum of malignant thyroid tumors.[1-4] By the first half of the century, the peculiar tumor biology of the sporadic type had been described as "small tumors with early lymphatic and hematogenous spread,"[4] whereas multicentric MTC[5] had become the hallmark of familial tumors. Probably the first report of multiple endocrine neoplasia (MEN) 2B regarded a 12-year-old boy presented by Walther Burk in 1901.[1] Yet it was E.D. Williams who clearly defined syndromic MTC as a separate entity in 1965 by publishing the first comprehensive series of hereditary pheochromocytoma (PCC) associated with MTC.[6] The 1993 detection of the susceptibility gene of hereditary MTC by Mulligan et al.[7] and Donis-Keller et al.[8] ushered in the era of genotype-phenotype oriented prophylactic surgery[9-12] (Figure 27.1), completing a 100-year evolutionary saga of clinical, biochemical, and molecular discoveries (see Figure 27.1). Hereditary MTC, unique in many ways among hereditable cancer syndromes, is founded on the following findings:

- The hereditary variant, affecting as many as 25% of MTC patients,[13] is more frequent than many other common hereditary tumors.[14]
- Unlike many other hereditary tumors, hereditary MTC features a strong genotype-phenotype correlation[12,15] that is utilized worldwide for risk assessment.[16-18] This genotype-dependent, age-related tumor progression[12] not only underlies the development of hereditary MTC but also the formation of MEN 2–associated PCC[19,20] and hyperparathyroidism (HPT).[21-24]
- Disease progression from C-cell hyperplasia to MTC, requiring the acquisition of somatic mutations for malignant progression, is a stochastic sequence of events not fully under the control of a gene carrier's genetic makeup.[25] Serum calcitonin, a sensitive diagnostic marker of MTC, better reflects a gene carrier's stage of C-cell disease than his or her underlying germline mutation in the *RET* (*RE*arranged during *T*ransfection) proto-oncogene.[26,27] We may now tailor the timing and extent of surgical intervention in the neck to the gene carrier's stage of disease through consideration of serum calcitonin levels.[17,26,27]
- Lymph node metastases are indicative of progressive disease, portending a worse prognosis for sporadic and hereditary MTC alike.[28] Although multifocal tumor growth is more common in hereditary than in sporadic MTC (65% versus 8%, respectively),[29] no difference in biochemical cure and survival between hereditary and sporadic disease has been found after adjusting for extent of disease.[28,30]
- MEN 2B is a special and virulent variant of MEN type 2 characterized by the presence of MTC in early infancy. More than 90% of MEN 2B *RET* gene carriers harbor de novo germline mutations.[22,31] Such de novo germline mutations are rare in other MTC syndromic settings such as familial MTC (FMTC) and MEN 2A. Therefore indiscriminate DNA-based screening of infants and children for the MEN 2B trait is rarely an option. Intriguingly, there are some early clues in MEN 2B infants, notably "tearless crying" and "pseudo-Hirschsprung's disease." These clinical signs may help identify gene carriers before they develop the more characteristic MEN 2B stigmata, prompting rapid DNA-based screening and immediate surgical intervention.[22,32]

CLINICAL PRESENTATION BY GENOTYPE

Familial Medullary Thyroid Cancer and MEN 2

Activating germline mutations in the *RET* proto-oncogene on chromosome 10q11.2, which cluster in "hot spot" regions, by definition involve all cells of the body (also termed the *first hit* in Knudson's model of oncogenesis).[17,19,24-26,33] These germline mutations do not equally affect all neuroendocrine and nonendocrine tissues, and many tissues may not be affected at all.[25] The appearance of the various syndromic components is largely age-dependent and characterized by a great deal of variability, especially among those gene carriers whose germline mutations have the weakest transforming activity.[15,19] Different tissue-specific susceptibilities are considered the main driver behind FMTC/MEN 2A/MEN 2B phenotypes, all of which share MTC as an integral element.[25]

Familial Medullary Thyroid Cancer (FMTC)

Originally defined as an entity in its own right based on a minimum of four affected kindreds, FMTC is now conceived as an abortive form of MEN 2,[17] which becomes manifest with the subsequent development of PCC or HPT. Such a conversion from an FMTC-only to a MEN 2 phenotype during the patient's lifetime is the rule rather than the exception for *RET* germline mutations in highest ('HST')-risk codon 918 (American Thyroid Association [ATA] category HST) and high ('H')-risk codon 634 (ATA category H), common for mutations in moderate ('MOD')- to high-risk codons 620 and 618, and to a lesser extent for those in codons 611 and 609 (ATA category MOD), and rare for mutations in low- to moderate-risk codons 768, 790, 804, and 891 (ATA category MOD).[15,17-19] Some 6.5% to 9.5% of patients with seemingly sporadic MTC may harbor *RET* germline mutations.[34,35] These gene carriers cannot be recognized unless all relevant exons of the gene have been screened.[17]

Multiple Endocrine Neoplasia Type 2 (MEN 2)

MEN 2 comprises some or all of the following parts: (1) neuroendocrine components: MTC (unifocal or multifocal, unilateral or bilateral),

235

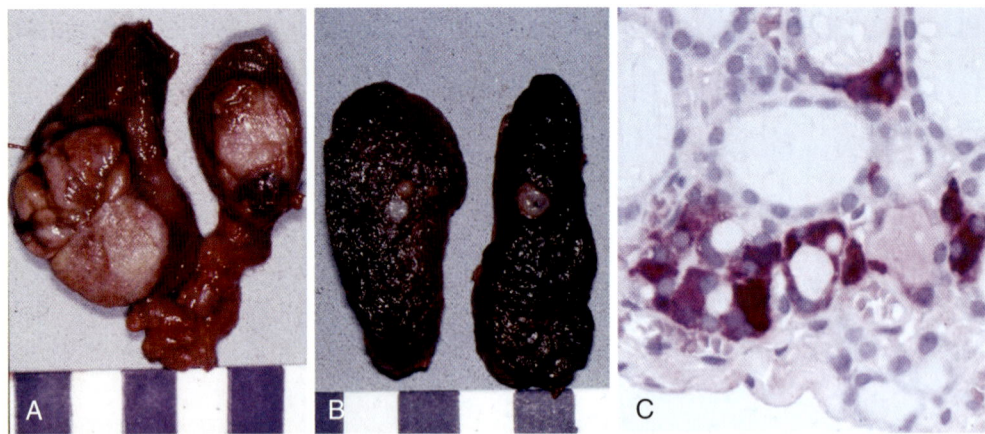

Fig. 27.1 Hereditary C-cell disease in the era of clinical **(A)**, biochemical **(B)**, and molecular **(C)** diagnosis.

PCC (unifocal or multifocal, unilateral or bilateral), or HPT (pseudonodular hyperplasia of one or more parathyroid glands), and (2) nonendocrine components: Hirschsprung's (HSCR) disease and cutaneous lichen amyloidosis (CLA; typically MEN 2A).

The *RET* germline mutations underlying MEN 2A (Figure 27.2) mainly involve high-risk codon 634 (ATA category H) as the classic "MEN 2A codon," infrequently involve moderate- to high-risk codons 620, 618, and to a lesser degree codons 611 and 609 (ATA category MOD), and rarely low- to moderate-risk codons 768, 790, 804, or 891 (ATA category MOD).[15,17]

Neuroendocrine Components in FMTC/MEN 2A
Medullary Thyroid Cancer (MTC)
Representing the usual first component of the MEN 2 syndrome, MTC is the only element common to FMTC, MEN 2A, and MEN 2B phenotypes. *RET* germline mutations are believed to drive C-cell hyperplasia, which can evolve to frank MTC with the acquisition of additional somatic mutations ("second hits") in *RET* or other genes.[12] Annual primary tumor growth is estimated at 0.4 to 0.5 mm in node-negative *RET* carriers, and at 1.2 mm (with low- to moderate-risk mutations) and 2.6 mm (with high-risk mutations) in node-positive carriers.[36] C-cell hyperplasia often is multifocal, involving both thyroid lobes, especially in carriers of the stronger germline mutations in highest-risk codon 918 (ATA category HST) and high-risk codon 634 (ATA category H). Because it takes time to acquire those somatic mutations necessary for malignant transformation, the development of MTC is age-dependent and varies by affected *RET* codon[18,25,26] (see Figure 27.2): highest-risk mutations (ATA category HST) by the time of birth, high-risk mutations (ATA category H) as early as age 1 year, moderate- to high-risk mutations (ATA category MOD) as early as age 5 years, and low- to moderate-risk mutations (ATA category MOD) as early as age 10 years.[15,17]

Pheochromocytoma (PCC)
Owing to the lower susceptibility of adrenal medullary relative to thyroidal C-cells, PCC represents the second most frequent syndromic manifestation.[19,20] Among carriers with PCC, MTC and PCC coexist at the time of diagnosis in 60% with highest-risk mutations in codon 918 (ATA category HST) and in 35% with high-risk mutations in codon 634 mutations (ATA category H). Only rarely is PCC the initial MEN 2 component among carriers with PCC: 0% with highest-risk mutations in codon 918 (ATA category HST), 35% with high-risk mutations in codon 634 (ATA category H), and 4% with moderate- to high-risk mutations (ATA category MOD).[18] Adrenal ganglioneuroma perhaps represents another, though unusual, component of the MEN 2A and 2B syndromes.[37] Because systematic *RET* gene analysis and family screening deplete the pool of unrecognized index patients in the population, PCC is less likely to present before, or together with, MTC in the future.[38]

Activating *RET* germline mutations are also thought to give rise to adrenal medullary hyperplasia from which PCC may develop upon allelic loss at chromosome 1p or deletion of the von Hippel-Lindau gene. This process varies by affected codon[19] (see Figure 27.2): in highest- and high-risk mutations (ATA categories HST and H) as early as ages 8 to 10 years[19,39] and in moderate-risk mutations (ATA category MOD) as early as age 20 years.

Hyperparathyroidism (HPT)
Parathyroid chief cells seem to be less responsive to *RET* activation as parafollicular C-cells of the thyroid or adrenal medullary cells. For unknown reasons, HPT, which is generally mild, is not an integral part of the MEN 2B syndrome. Although HPT is fairly common (19.1% prevalence) among carriers of high-risk mutations in codon 634 (ATA category H),[24] it is infrequent among carriers of moderate-risk mutations in codons 620, 618, 611, 609, and 768, 790, 804, and 891 (ATA category MOD). The development of HPT is age-dependent, due to the need to acquire "second hits" and varies by mutational risk category (see Figure 27.2): for high-risk mutations (ATA category H), the respective mean and minimum manifestation age is 34 years and 10 years, and for moderate-risk mutations age of manifestation ranges from 32 to 41 years (moderate- to high-risk mutations) and from 38 to 54 years (low- to moderate-risk mutations).[19]

Nonendocrine Components in FMTC/MEN 2A
Hirschsprung's Disease
Some 6% to 16% of *RET* families with moderate- to high-risk germline mutations (ATA category MOD) in exon 10 (codons 620 and 618, and more rarely 611 and 609) develop a peculiar phenotype consisting of both a "gain of function" FMTC/MEN 2A phenotype and a "loss of function" HSCR phenotype.[40] These genotypes have been dubbed "Janus genes," referring to the Roman god of doorways facing either way. Frequently, HSCR disease precedes the clinical manifestation of MTC and PCC. The "loss of function" HSCR phenotype is thought to be due to the trapping of precursor RET receptor proteins in the endoplasmatic reticulum, precluding their transport to the cell membrane. Decreased cell surface concentrations of RET receptor proteins are believed to cause the premature arrest of the craniocaudal migration of enteric neurons during the 5th to 12th week of gestation. The absence

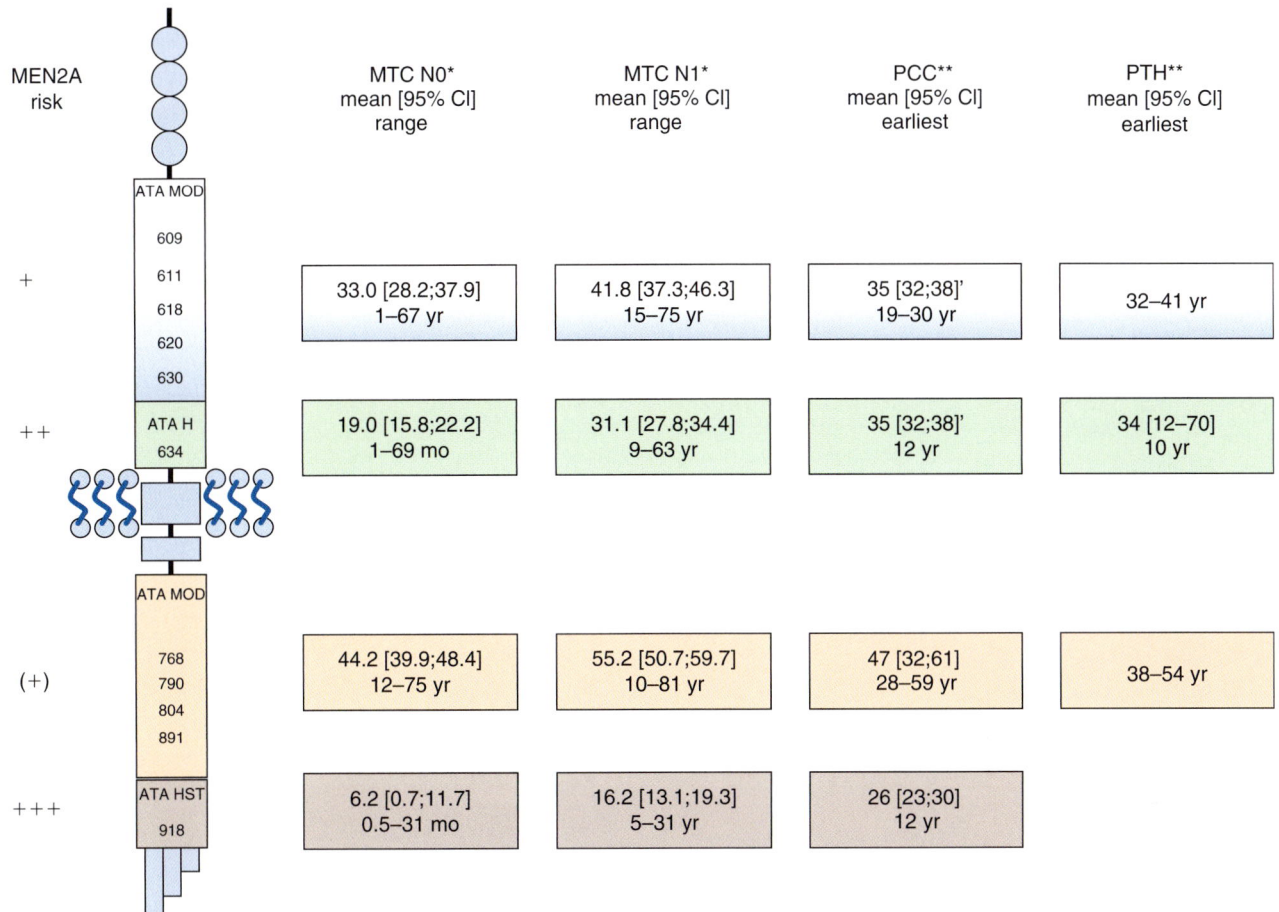

Fig. 27.2 DNA-Based and Age-Related Presentation of MEN 2. ATA, American Thyroid Association, HST, highest, H, high, Mod, moderate, CI, confidence interval, PCC, pheochromocytoma, MTC N0/1, node-negative/positive medullary thyroid cancer, PTH, primary hyperparathyroidism, ', **combined estimate for mutations in *RET* codons 609, 611, 618, 620, 630, and 634. Numbers represent the mean ages (in years) which have been reported (with confidence intervals) followed by the ages of earliest presentation that have been reported. *Data from Machens A, Lorenz K, Weber F, Dralle H. Genotype-specific progression of hereditary medullary thyroid cancer. *Hum Mutat*. 2018;39[6]:860-869; **Data from Machens A, Lorenz K, Dralle H. Peak incidence of pheochromocytoma and primary hyperparathyroidism in multiple endocrine neoplasia 2: need for age-adjusted biochemical screening. *J Clin Endocrinol Metab*. 2013;98[2]:E336–E345.

of autonomic ganglion cells (aganglionosis) within parasympathetic submucosal and myenteric plexuses causes the HSCR symptoms of functional obstruction and megacolon.[40] In stark contrast, gastrointestinal ganglioneuromatosis, also dubbed "pseudo-Hirschsprung's disease," which is a feature of MEN 2B (codon 918), is characterized by the presence of ganglioneuromas in these plexuses.

Cutaneous Lichen Amyloidosis

This condition may occur in as many as 9% of MEN 2A families.[23] It is almost always associated with *RET* germline mutations in codon 634, with one reported kindred each carrying a *RET* germline mutation in codon 804 or codon 891.[41] Itching is usually the first manifestation of CLA. It is typically located in the upper back at either or both interscapular regions in an area of repeated scratching, involving the dermatomes between C4 and T5.[42] The neural crest cells, implicated in the embryonic development of the parafollicular C-cells and adrenal medulla, are also involved in the embryogenesis of the thoracic sensory fibers. These dermatologic symptoms often precede the clinical manifestation of MTC,[41] yet the evolution of CLA is independent of the course of the disease and unrelated to the development of PCC or HPT.[42]

Neuroendocrine Components in MEN 2B

MEN 2B is defined by the combination of MTC and PCC; the absence of HPT; and the presence of ocular, oral, intestinal, and musculoskeletal neuromas, neurofibromas, ganglioneuromas, and unique musculoskeletal disorders.[22] MTC develops so early that it is (1) present in virtually every MEN 2B patient, (2) frequently advanced at the time of diagnosis, and (3) associated with a more adverse prognosis.

Nonendocrine Components in MEN 2B

The nonendocrine components encompass oral, ocular, intestinal, and musculoskeletal stigmata (Table 27.1, Figures 27.3 to 27.5). The oral stigmata include nodules of the anterior tongue, lips, and buccal mucosa,[43,44] as well as dental irregularities.[45] The ocular stigmata comprise conjunctival nodules with recurrent conjunctivitis, thickened corneal nerves (corneal fibers), and infolding of the eyelid margins (i.e., entropium).[43,46-49] The intestinal ganglioneuromatosis usually presents as chronic constipation or bowel obstruction.[50-53] The musculoskeletal

TABLE 27.1 Nonendocrine MEN 2B Stigmata

Stigmata	Clinical Presentation	Pathologic Substrate	Diagnostic Workup
Oral	Nodules on lips, anterior tongue, and buccal mucosa; bumpy lips, prominent labial frenula	Mucosal neuromas and neurofibromas	Clinical examination; tissue biopsy
	Impaired dentition	Unknown	Stomatological examination
Ocular	Conjunctival nodules	Conjunctival neuromas	Ophthalmologic examination; split lamp examination; Schirmer test
	Corneal fibers	Thickened corneal nerves	
	Conjunctivitis sicca	Reduced tear production	
	Entropium	Not known	
Intestinal	"Pseudo-Hirschsprung's" disease with chronic constipation, recurrent abdominal pain, flatulence	Intestinal submucosal and myenteric ganglioneuromatosis	Radiologic examination (contrast-enhanced x-rays); rectal suction biopsy; histologic examination
	Failure to thrive	Combination of intestinal and musculoskeletal symptoms	Physical examination
	Diarrhea	In the event of excessive hypercalcitoninemia, perhaps the action of biogenic amines	Exclusion of the differential diagnosis of lactose intolerance
Musculoskeletal	Marfanoid habitus with hyperflexible joints	Probably caused by a disorder in neurologic development	Neurologic and orthopedic examination; electromyographic studies; special x-ray films
	Muscle weakness		
	Pes cavus; pes excavatus		
	Scoliosis; epiphysiolysis		

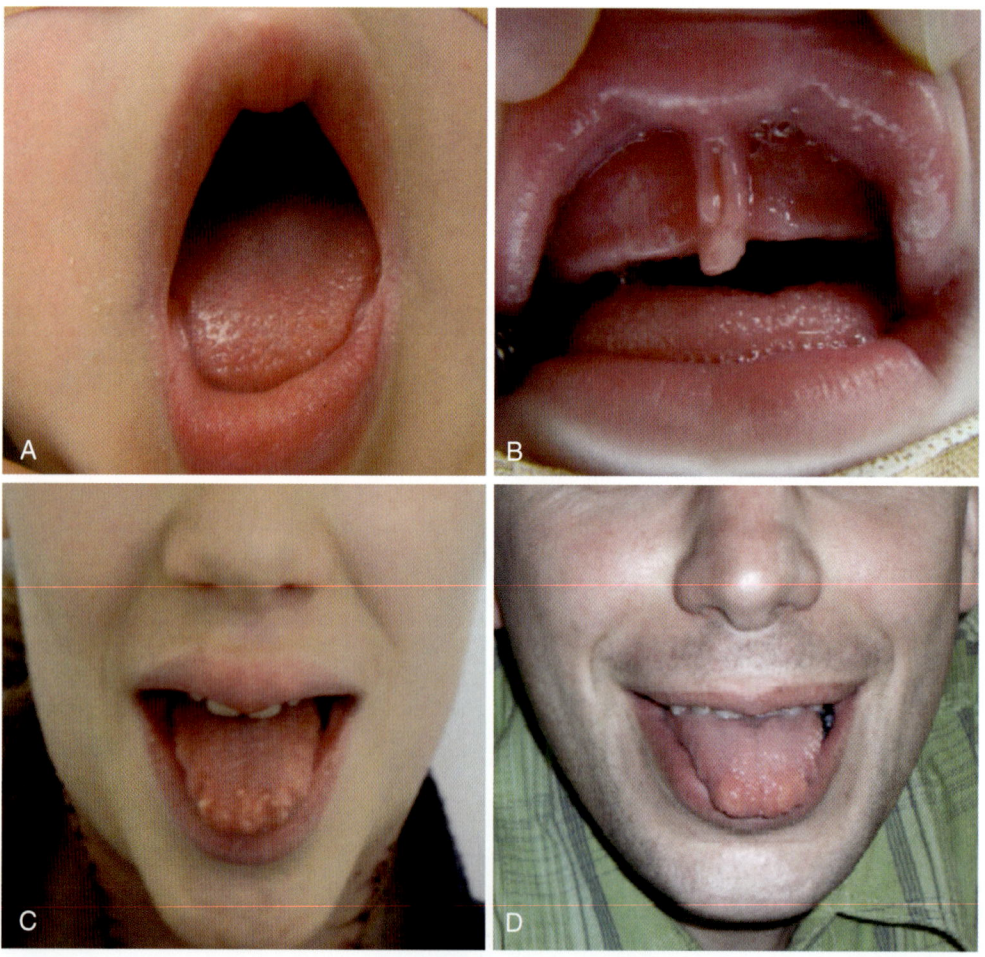

Fig. 27.3 Age-Dependent Presentation of Oral MEN 2B Stigmata (M918T Mutation). **A,** A 6-month-old baby boy. **B,** A 6-month-old baby girl. **C,** A 12-year-old girl with lip and tongue neuromas. **D,** A 30-year-old man with neuromas on his tongue.

CHAPTER 27 Syndromic Medullary Thyroid Cancer: MEN 2A and MEN 2B

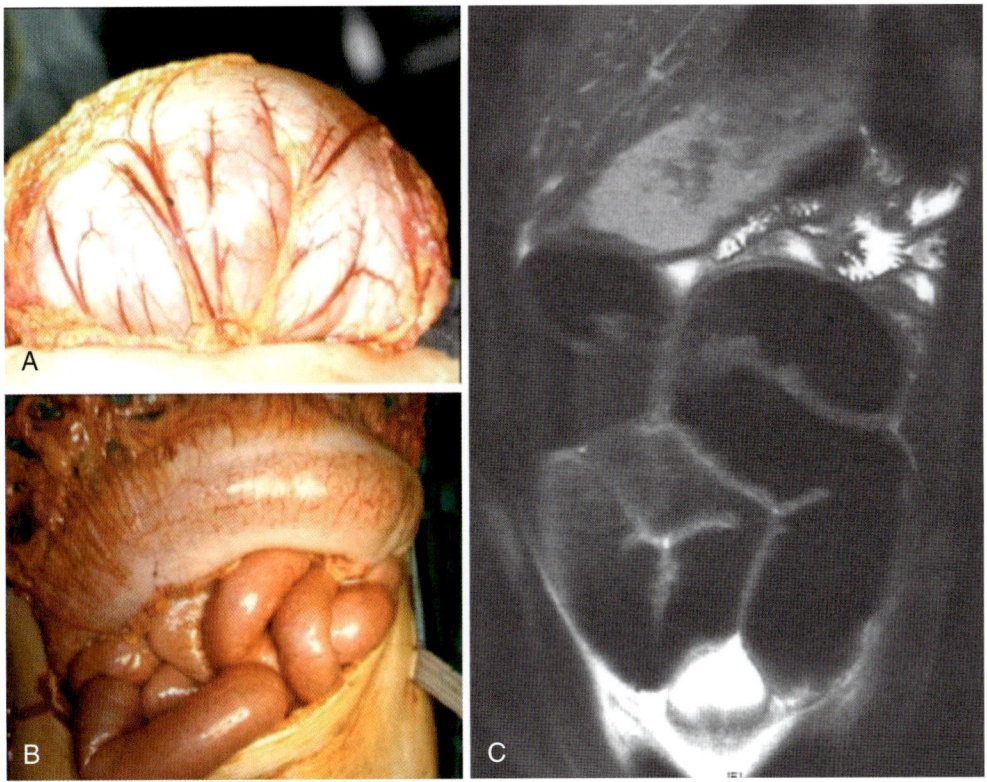

Fig. 27.4 Age-Dependent Presentation of Intestinal MEN 2B Stigmata (M918T Mutation). **A,** Megacolon in a 16-year-old girl with recurrent abdominal pain. **B,** Megacolon in a 15-year-old boy with diarrhea. **C,** Abdominal magnetic resonance imaging (MRI) scan of a 16-year-old boy with recurrent constipation.

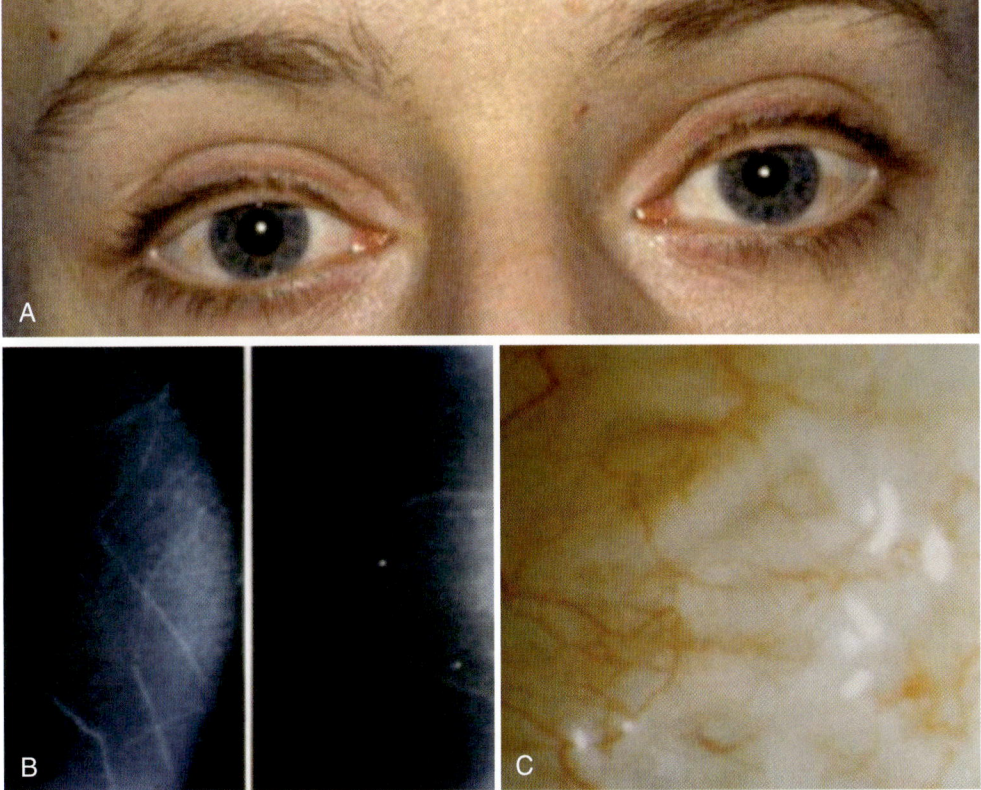

Fig. 27.5 Age-Dependent Presentation of Ocular MEN 2B Stigmata (M918T Mutation). **A,** A 17-year-old boy with entropium and recurrent conjunctivitis. **B,** Split lamp examination revealing prominent corneal fibers in a 30-year-old man. **C,** Close-up ocular view showing thickened corneal fibers in the same 30-year-old man.

stigmata consist of a variety of distinct malformations, such as hyperflexible joints, muscle weakness, mid-face hypergnathism, pectus deformities, scoliosis, slipped capitis femoral epiphysis, and feet abnormalities. The characteristic elongated extremities are reminiscent of a "marfanoid habitus."[54,55]

Although the syndrome was described (at least in parts) much earlier,[1,46,56-59] the term MEN 2B was introduced only in 1975 to signify this "neuroma phenotype" from the classic Sipple's syndrome.[60] Subsequent series disclosed a large variability in the expression of the endocrine and nonendocrine MEN 2B components.[44,61-63]

In fewer than 5% of MEN 2B patients, who may not express the nonendocrine phenotype in full (atypical MEN 2B), other *RET* germline mutations, including double mutations, may be present, including A883F,[64-66] V804M/E805K,[67] V804M/Y806C,[68,69] and V804M/S904C[70] (Table 27.2). These atypical MEN 2B mutations tend to be less aggressive and less penetrant than the classic MEN 2B mutation in codon 918 (ATA category HST), which is consistent with in vitro studies.[71,72]

The endocrine and nonendocrine phenotypes of MEN 2B develop in an age-dependent fashion[32,73] (Table 27.3; also see Figure 27.3). Carriers of the classic MEN 2B mutation in codon 918 frequently harbor MTC in the first months of life[53,74] when surgical cure is still within reach. This window of opportunity closes rapidly within the first years of life so that most MEN 2B patients who are older than 4 years at the time of diagnosis are not curable.[73] PCC as the second part of the endocrine phenotype in MEN 2B is rarely seen before puberty,[19] the youngest MEN 2B patient reported as being 12 years of age.[63]

The majority of carriers of the classic *RET* mutation in codon 918 undergo an uneventful intrauterine development and birth, demonstrating normal body weight and size. No pertinent data are available for the atypical MEN 2B mutations. Some months after birth, failure to thrive due to suckling weakness and chronic constipation may give the first clue of MEN 2B.[32]

Ganglioneuroma and thickened nerve sheaths are probably at the heart of the nonendocrine MEN 2B components, pointing to the *RET* receptor's key role in neural crest development.[75] Prominent corneal nerves, which are visible on split lamp examination, and thickened recurrent laryngeal nerves (Figures 27.5 and 27.6) are common. The neural findings are caused by thickened nerve sheaths, which reduce nerve conduction velocity and action potential amplitudes within the Aa, Ad, and C components of sensory nerves.[54] This pathomorphology is likely the driver not only behind the musculoskeletal stigmata but also behind conjunctivitis and reduced tear production. Ganglioneuromas are expressed ubiquitously but abound in the oral (see Figure 27.3) and intestinal mucosa (see Figure 27.4) and the conjunctiva (see Figure 27.5). In the colon, ganglioneuromatosis interferes with gut motility and digestion, giving rise to pseudo-Hirschsprung's disease[50] (see Figure 27.4).

EVALUATION OF GENE CARRIERS FOR SURGERY

MEN 2A

Medullary thyroid cancer

MTC cells, given their neuroendocrine derivation from the neural crest, synthesize calcitonin. Owing to the presence of nonneoplastic ("reactive") C-cell hyperplasia, biochemical screening occasionally yields false-positive findings, prompting unnecessary thyroidectomies in family members who subsequently are shown not to have inherited the *RET* germline mutation in that family. In very young children, it is important to note that mean serum calcitonin levels are higher in the first (9.81 pg/mL; range 2.0 to 48.9 pg/mL) and second year of life (4.56 pg/mL; range 2.0 to 14.7 pg/mL) than those in adults.[76] Naturally, the risk of harboring occult MTC is the greater the higher these calcitonin levels are. Calcitonin screening, which is superior to neck ultrasonography in predicting MTC,[77] and periodic monitoring of catecholamines and their metabolites greatly diminishes the excess mortality of *RET* gene carriers who used to succumb to metastatic MTC or hypertensive crisis from catecholamine excess from an unrecognized PCC beginning in their late forties.[78]

With the advent of the molecular age, DNA-based screening of the "hot spot" regions in exons 10, 11, 13, 14, 15, and 16 of the *RET* gene has quickly become the diagnostic gold standard.[79] Barring

TABLE 27.2 Genotype-Phenotype Correlations in MEN 2B

Genotype	n	Age at Diagnosis (years)	MTC (%)	Advanced MTC (%)	PCC (%)	Oral Mucosal Neuroma (%)	Intestinal Symptoms (%)	Corneal Fibers (%)	Marfanoid Habitus (%)	Reference
RET Single Mutations										
M918T	32	14	100	68	33	87	95	75	70	32
	22*	13	100	55	48	100	84	69	68	87
	28	11.5	n.i.	n.i.	n.i.	n.i.	93	n.i.	n.i.	52
	18*	13	100	83	33	67	61	71	89	125
A883F	2	19	100	50	50	100	n.i.	n.i.	100	64,66
	2	n.i.	100	n.i.	n.i.	100	n.i.	n.i.	100	65
RET Double Mutations										
V804M/E805K	1	50	100	100	100	100	n.i.	100	100	67
V804M/Y806C	1	23	100	0	100†	100	100	100	n.i.	68
V804M/S904C	4	29	75	0	0	25	0	0	0	70

For inclusion, more than 10 carriers of the M918T RET mutation per study were required.
*M918T confirmed in the majority of patients.
†Adrenomedullary hyperplasia.
MTC, medullary thyroid carcinoma, PCC, pheochromocytoma, n.i., not indicated.

CHAPTER 27 Syndromic Medullary Thyroid Cancer: MEN 2A and MEN 2B

TABLE 27.3 Age-Dependent Development of Extrathyroidal MEN 2B Stigmata and Symptoms (M918T Mutation) Relative to Healthy Controls Within the First Year of Life

	Controls ≤Age 1 year	MEN 2B ≤Age 1 year	MEN 2B Follow-Up
Dry eyes (%)	0	86	91
Chronic congestion (%)	0	61	71
Pes cavus (%)	0	30	75
Conjunctivitis (%)	2	24	55
Hyperflexible joints (%)	0	19	52
Bumpy lips (%)	0	17	96
Oral neuromas (%)	0	17	92
Skeletal disorders (%)	0	0	38
Pheochromocytoma (%)	0	0	28
Conjunctival neuromas (%)	0	0	11

Modified from Brauckhoff M, Machens A, Hess S, et al. Premonitory symptoms preceding metastatic medullary thyroid cancer in MEN 2B: an exploratory analysis. *Surgery*. 2008;144(6):1044–1051.

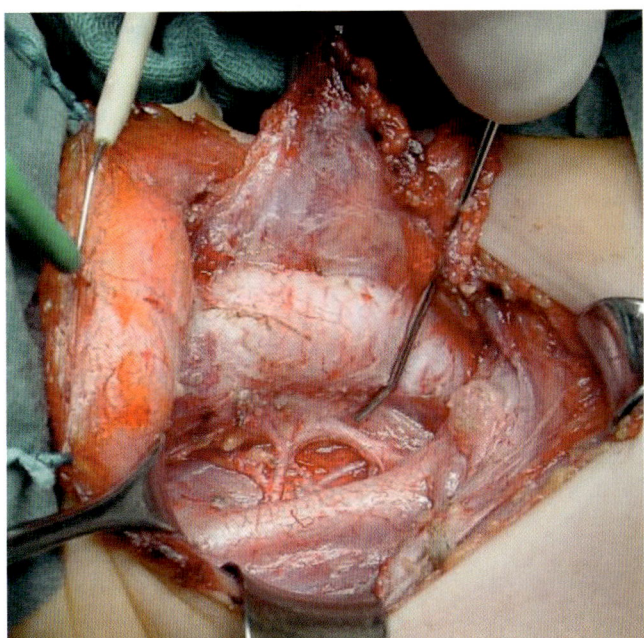

Fig. 27.6 Total thyroidectomy with central compartment dissection in a 19-month-old MEN 2B infant with medullary thyroid cancer.

sample/laboratory error, there are no false-positive findings with DNA-based screening, which has largely replaced calcitonin screening for early diagnosis of gene carriers.[17]

Pheochromocytoma

MEN 2–associated PCC, displaying impairment in terminal differentiation, produces epinephrine more frequently than norepinephrine.[81] This is why more *RET* gene carriers with PCC sustain paroxysmal hypertension than sustained hypertension. When a delay in diagnosis allows PCC to progress, minor triggers can provoke excessive catecholamine secretion, igniting an often lethal hypertensive crisis, typically around the fourth to fifth decade. In the past, this used to be the most common cause of death among *RET* gene carriers. However, with the routine use of sensitive screening tests for catecholamines and their metabolites as noted earlier, PCC is increasingly diagnosed at an asymptomatic stage.[82] These adrenal medullary tumors are usually large enough to visualize on adrenal ultrasonography, computed tomography, and magnetic resonance imaging. To circumvent the risk of sparking a hypertensive crisis, no manipulation of these tumors should be undertaken before an effective alpha-receptor blockade has been put in place.[83]

Hyperparathyroidism

In many *RET* gene carriers, there may be histopathologic evidence of pseudonodular parathyroid hyperplasia, even though the patient's serum calcium and intact parathyroid hormone levels are within normal limits. A diagnosis of HPT should not be based solely on an elevated intact parathyroid hormone level in the absence of hypercalcemia. Enlarged parathyroids frequently visualize on high-resolution ultrasonography so that more sophisticated imaging modalities are needed only for reoperations.

Hirschsprung's Disease

Young *RET* gene carriers from MEN 2A families who present with severe constipation or bowel obstruction secondary to HSCR disease may also harbor C-cell disease in the thyroid gland. The workup for HSCR disease includes a barium enema to show the size contrast between the proximal dilated ganglionic and the distal constricted aganglionic segment. Suction biopsy of the aganglionic segment, supported by histochemical staining of cholinesterase in the ganglion-cell/nerve complex, establishes the diagnosis of HSCR disease, enabling the exclusion of gastrointestinal ganglioneuromatosis, or pseudo-Hirschsprung's disease, associated with the MEN 2B phenotype.

Cutaneous Lichen Amyloidosis

The diagnosis of CLA is made clinically and, if needed, can be histologically confirmed with a punch biopsy from involved skin.

MEN 2B

Challenges of early diagnosis

For MEN 2B carriers, truly "prophylactic" surgery of MTC is exceptional because of the very early onset of the disease. Owing to the typical de novo presentation of MEN 2B, the disease is rarely caught early in the course without targeted screening.[32,33,53,74] Exceptionally, a 6-month-old infant harboring the classic M918T *RET* mutation was found to be free of neoplastic C-cell disease in the thyroid.[84] Another MEN 2B patient with unspecified *RET* mutation revealed C-cell hyperplasia at the age of 14 months.[85,86]

More than 90% of MEN 2B germline mutations arise de novo in the germline.[22,31,32,87] Although familial *RET* germline mutations transmitted to subsequent generations can easily be confirmed in the offspring, most MEN 2B patients will not have children. In the absence of a pertinent family history, identifying a RET germline mutation in an asymptomatic patient can pose a tremendous challenge, the mastery of which hinges on the timely recognition of the MEN 2B-associated nonendocrine stigmata as they emerge. The appearance of these stigmata usually precedes the clinical manifestation of MTC.[22,32] Sadly, even though the classic stigmata are obvious, many patients are not recognized as having MEN 2B in a timely manner.[87]

Intestinal Ganglioneuromatosis

Some 90% of MEN 2B patients develop intestinal symptoms. With a prevalence of 40% to 85%, excessive bloating or flatulence, abdominal distention, constipation, and recurrent abdominal tenderness are frequent MEN 2B symptoms.[52] These clinical complaints often correlate well with the radiologic diagnosis of megacolon. Because intestinal ganglioneuromatosis is an exception outside the setting of MEN 2B,[88,89] current ATA guidelines[17] recommend a *RET* gene analysis on intestinal tissue in these patients. Histologic evidence of ganglioneuromatosis should be based on counts of myenteric ganglion cells using a structured approach.[90] Because many MEN 2B patients develop intestinal symptoms during the first year of life,[32] a *RET* gene analysis may be the patient's only chance of detecting MTC while it is still curable. More than 70% of our patients ages 6 years or younger at the time of diagnosis had prior evidence of intestinal ganglioneuromatosis.

Oral Stigmata

Although oral stigmata (nodular lips, mucosal neuromas, abnormal dentition) are suggestive of MEN 2B, none of these features seems to precede the clinical manifestation of MTC.[32] If present, these stigmata (in particular oral mucosal neuromas) should prompt RET screening, despite the fact that multiple mucosal neuroma are not linked exclusively to MEN 2B.[91]

Thickened Corneal Nerves and Tearless Crying

Thickened corneal nerves, which have been found in a MEN 2B girl as young as 3 months of age,[85] may also be present in MEN 2A.[92-95] Diagnosis is straightforward on split lamp examination. Because they are not usually apparent, thickened corneal nerves are typically an incidental finding of unknown clinical significance. Reduced tear production with subsequent conjunctivitis sicca, rarely appreciated in ophthalmology reports, is a well-known component of ocular MEN 2B.[43,48] A Schirmer test confirms the diagnosis. Nearly all parents spot the low tear production in their babies early on, as they appear to be "crying without tears."[32] The differential diagnosis of this symptom includes a number of rare conditions including Sjögren's syndrome, triple-A syndrome, as well as several environmental and nutritional factors.[96] However, because of the importance of an early diagnosis of MEN 2B, *RET* screening of "tearless crying" children should be considered.

SURGERY

Surgery for Clinically Apparent Hereditary MTC

Synchronous MTC and PCC

According to the underlying *RET* germline mutation, PCC may develop in as many as 30% to 50% of carriers.[19,20] PCC is diagnosed synchronously with MTC in 60% of patients harboring highest-risk (codon 918) and in 35% of patients with the high-risk germline mutations (codon 634), respectively.[18] There are two surgical options in this scenario: subtotal "tissue-sparing" adrenalectomy, minimizing the risk of steroid dependency while leaving the possibility of developing a second PCC in the adrenal remnant,[97] or total adrenalectomy for tumors occupying most or all of the adrenal gland, followed by total thyroidectomy, either (1) in one session for more limited neck disease, or (2) as a two-staged procedure for more advanced neck disease[98,99] (Figure 27.7). At any rate, an effective alpha-receptor blockade should be in place before adrenalectomy.[83,98]

Synchronous MTC and HPT

In MEN 2A patients, most of whom harbor high-risk mutations in codon 634 (ATA category H), the prevalence of HPT is about 20% to 30%.[100] Because often no more than one or two parathyroid glands are involved, the clinical course of HPT in MEN 2A is usually mild. Accordingly, the surgical strategy consists in the removal of grossly enlarged parathyroid glands instead of embarking on subtotal or total parathyroidectomy with parathyroid autografting. Total parathyroidectomy with autografting of parathyroid slivers has been abandoned because it carries a 6% risk of permanent hypoparathyroidism.[101] Wherever feasible, normal parathyroids should be preserved in situ, as is standard practice in neck surgery for hereditary MTC.[102] Only in the event of complete devascularization should normal parathyroids be autografted to minimize the rate of postoperative hypoparathyroidism.[103]

Extent of Thyroidectomy

Because every single parafollicular C-cell has the potential for malignant progression, total thyroidectomy alone can reliably eliminate the risk of hereditary MTC. Moreover, C-cells do not express the sodium/iodine symporter and therefore do not concentrate radioiodine, rendering radioiodine ablation futile for the treatment of MTC.

Extent of Lymph Node Dissection

Patients with MTC and no evidence of neck lymph node metastases on ultrasonography and no evidence of distant metastases should have a total thyroidectomy and dissection of the lymph nodes in the central compartment (level VI).[17] In patients with MTC and no evidence of neck metastases on ultrasonography and no distant metastases, dissection of lymph nodes in the lateral compartments (levels II to V) may be considered based on serum calcitonin levels.[17,80] Patients with MTC confined to the neck and cervical lymph nodes should have a total thyroidectomy, dissection of the central lymph node compartment (level VI), and dissection of the involved lateral neck compartments (levels II to V).[17] When preoperative imaging is positive in the ipsilateral lateral neck compartment but negative in the contralateral neck compartment, contralateral neck dissection should be considered if the basal serum calcitonin level is greater than 200 pg/mL (see Figure 27.7).[17,80] Above that threshold, bilateral lymph node metastases are increasingly present as are mediastinal and distant metastases.[104-106]

Most patients with clinically apparent MTC harbor bilateral lymph node metastases, which require a compartment-oriented microdissection on either side of the central and lateral neck.[98,107-110] By removing tumor deposits from the vicinity of vital neck structures,[111,112] compartment-oriented surgery can aid in preventing tumor-related complications and supporting systemic targeted therapies.[113]

Persistent or recurrent neck disease derives from a less-than-total thyroidectomy, an inadequate lymph node dissection, or both. When tumor recurrence/persistence is amenable to neck reoperation, these foci should be cleared. Systematic lymph node dissection for persistent MTC can be curative in experienced hands after removal of no more than five lymph node metastases at the initial operation and when serum calcitonin levels before reoperation are no higher than 1000 pg/mL.[114] Above these thresholds, biochemical cure is not possible, and the surgical treatment strategy shifts to locoregional tumor control and prevention of tumor-related complications. In the absence of radiographically apparent disease, the decision to reoperate is much less straightforward. Decision making will then have to factor in the extent and meticulousness of the initial operation (as revealed in operating notes and pathology reports) and the excess surgical morbidity attendant to reoperations in the neck. In carriers with gross recurrent disease, it may be prudent to eradicate locally progressive disease as the "pacemaker of disease" from the neck, mediastinum, or distant site, if this is reasonably feasible (Figures 27.8 and 27.9). For detection of recurrent metastatic MTC, an 18-fluoro-dihydroxyphenylalanine (^{18}F-DOPA) or fluorodeoxyglucose (FDG) positron emission tomography/computed tomography (PET/CT) scan is better than conventional imaging.[115,116]

CHAPTER 27 Syndromic Medullary Thyroid Cancer: MEN 2A and MEN 2B 243

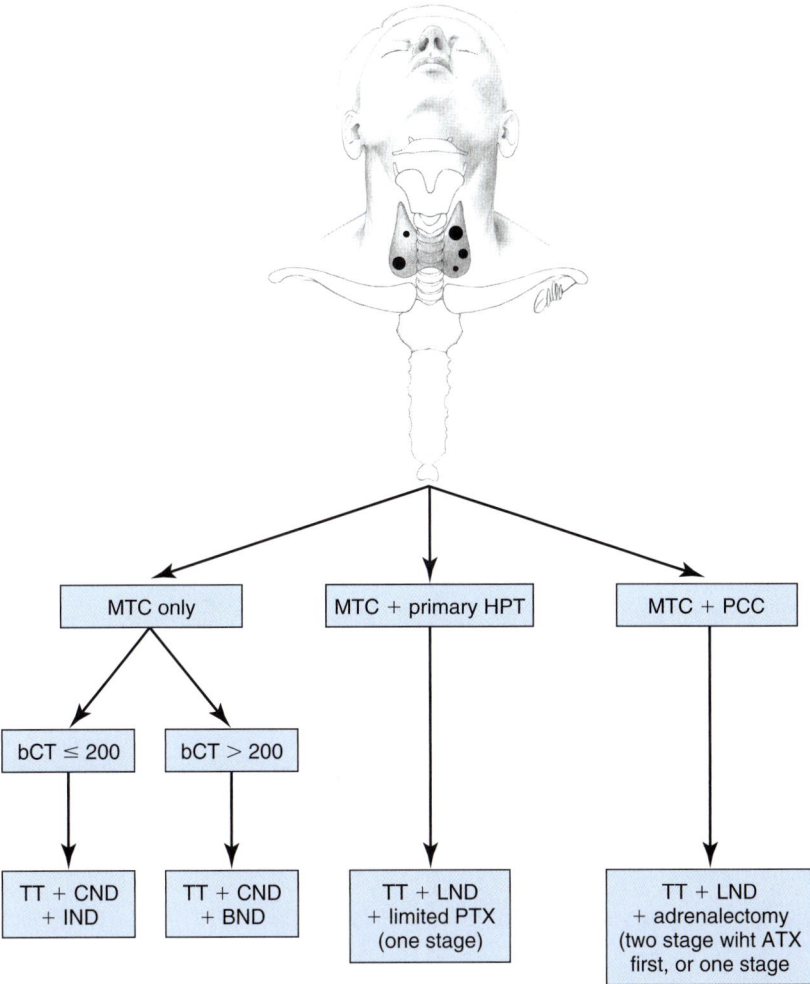

Fig. 27.7 Initial Surgery for Clinically Apparent Hereditary Medullary Thyroid Cancer. ATX, adrenalectomy: preferably subtotal "tissue-sparing" adrenalectomy, bCT, basal calcitonin (reference <10 pg/mL), BND, bilateral lateral node dissection, CND, central node dissection, IND, ipsilateral lateral node dissection, LND, lymph node dissection, PTX, parathyroidectomy, limited parathyroidectomy denotes removal of enlarged parathyroid glands only, as opposed to subtotal or total parathyroidectomy with parathyroid autografting, TT, total thyroidectomy.

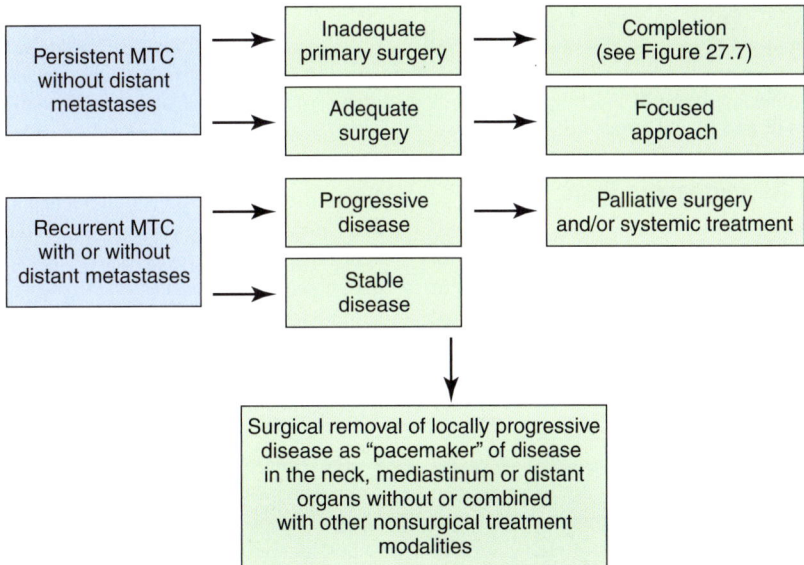

Fig. 27.8 Reoperation for Clinically Apparent Hereditary Medullary Thyroid Cancer.

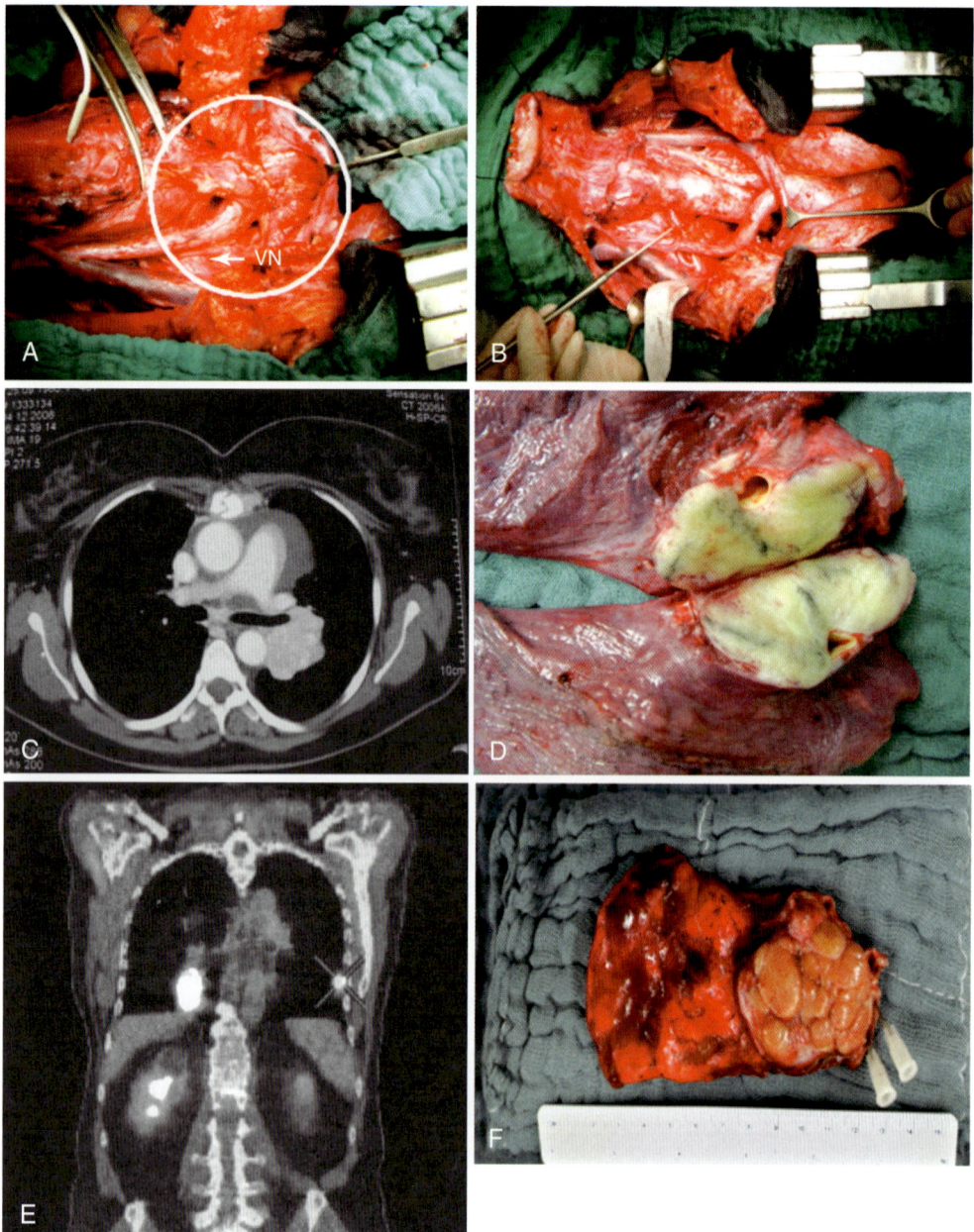

Fig. 27.9 Tackling locally progressive disease as the "pacemaker" of recurrent medullary thyroid cancer in the upper mediastinum **(A and B)**, lung hilum with tumor obstruction of the left main bronchus **(C and D)**, and lung parenchyma **(E and F)**. VN, vagus nerve.

Prophylactic Surgery for Asymptomatic Gene Carriers

There is recent evidence to suggest that an integrated DNA-based/biochemical concept[26,27] (Figure 27.10) may indicate the extent of C-cell disease more effectively than an age-related risk assessment alone.[15,16,18] In an institutional series of 308 RET gene carriers operated on for hereditary MTC, lymph node metastases were found only with increased basal calcitonin levels[26] typically exceeding 30 pg/mL.[17,117] As a corollary, carriers with normal basal calcitonin levels may safely forego lymph node dissection, sparing them the excess surgical morbidity inherent in the procedure (hypoparathyroidism, recurrent laryngeal nerve palsy). If needed, prophylactic thyroidectomy can be postponed beyond the age recommendation for the respective mutation (ATA risk category)[18] until stimulated calcitonin levels start to rise and while basal calcitonin levels are still within normal limits (see Figure 27.10). Such a delay may be relevant to young children who have smaller and more delicate anatomic structures with less space for surgical maneuvering than older children and adults. Smaller children are also less compliant with their thyroxine substitution regimens. For these reasons, the combined DNA-biochemical strategy may offer more leeway than the purely ATA category-based age concept, with less potential for undertreatment or overtreatment.[26]

Most MEN 2B patients have increased basal calcitonin serum levels at the time of diagnosis, necessitating total thyroidectomy and compartment-oriented lymph node dissection without delay.[73] Compartment-oriented surgery should be performed as early in life as possible but may also improve survival in late-onset patients.

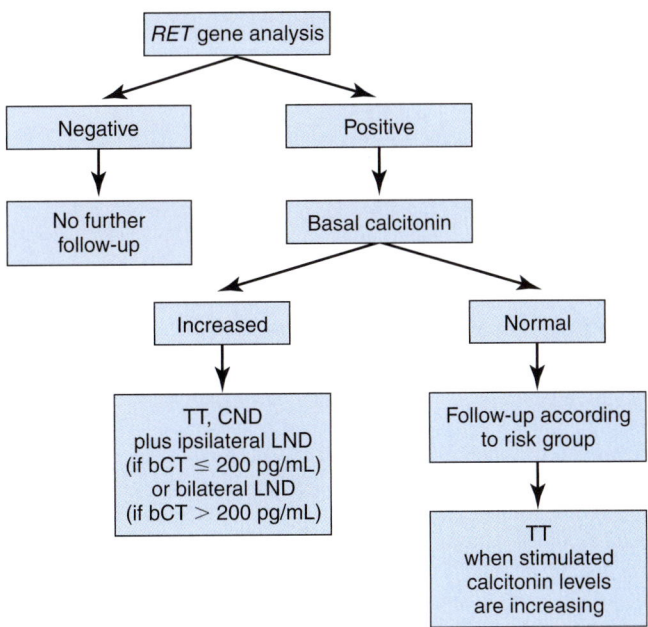

Fig. 27.10 The integrated DNA-based/biochemical concept: Algorithm for genetic diagnosis and surgical management of RET gene carriers at risk of developing hereditary medullary thyroid cancer. TT, total thyroidectomy, CND, central node dissection, ND, node dissection, bCT, basal calcitonin (reference <10 pg/mL), LND, lateral node dissection.

Complications and Outcomes After Surgery for Hereditary MTC

Prophylactic Surgery for Asymptomatic Gene Carriers

In a large study of 167 children,[118] early prophylactic thyroidectomy was a viable surgical concept in experienced hands, sparing older children the postoperative morbidity that may be associated with delayed neck surgery. Postoperative transient hypoparathyroidism was more frequent in older children (32% in the oldest age group versus 3% in the youngest) whether or not central node dissection was carried out. Three children developed transient recurrent laryngeal nerve palsy, all of whom had undergone central node dissection. All complications resolved within 6 months. Postoperative normalization of calcitonin serum levels was achieved in 114 (99.1%) of 115 children with raised preoperative values. No residual structural disease or recurrence was observed.[118]

In children undergoing *prophylactic thyroidectomy without central node dissection*, the transient and permanent hypoparathyroidism rates respectively were 4% and 0% for children ages 3 years or less,[118] compared with 44% and 22% for children ages less than 3 years from another series.[119] The corresponding overall rates were 17.4% and 0% for children ages 18 years or less in the large series,[118] and 27% and 20% in children less than 18 years old in the other series.[119]

In children who had *prophylactic thyroidectomy with central node dissection*, permanent postoperative hypoparathyroidism was 0% (based on 149 children with a mean age of 6 years at thyroidectomy) in the large recent series and 6% (3 of 50 children with a mean age of 10 years at thyroidectomy) in an earlier series.[103]

These data emphasize the need to (1) refrain from central node dissection in gene carriers as long as they have normal basal calcitonin serum levels[26] and (2) to use in situ preservation of normal parathyroid glands[102] to keep postoperative hypoparathyroidism rates to a minimum. After prophylactic surgery, children and adolescents need a careful follow-up, not only for recurrence but also for sufficient thyroxine substitution[120] and psychosocial care.[121]

Surgery for Carriers With Clinically Apparent Hereditary MTC

Compartment-oriented surgery may be beneficial even in the presence of lymph node and distant metastases, both of which signify a worse prognosis.[26,30,117-119,122-124] Bilateral compartment-oriented neck surgery can achieve biochemical cure in at least half the patients with pretherapeutic basal calcitonin serum levels of 1000 pg/mL or less but not in patients with levels greater than 10,000 pg/mL (normal range <10 pg/mL).[80]

CONCLUSION

Early detection of hereditary disease is key to success. Widespread use of systematic *RET* gene analysis in all patients with a personal or family history of MEN 2 or MTC is pivotal in gaining control of hereditary disease at the population level, resulting in (1) depletion of the reservoir of symptomatic gene carriers from previously unrecognized *RET* families (index patients); (2) eradication of MTC, notably node-positive MTC, among all gene carriers from known *RET* families (nonindex patients); (3) an increase of biochemical cure among nonindex patients; and (4) a fall in patient age at thyroidectomy among nonindex patients.[38]

REFERENCES

For a complete list of references, go to expertconsult.com.

28

Anaplastic Thyroid Cancer and Primary Thyroid Lymphoma

Ashish V. Chintakuntlawar, Mabel Ryder, Keith C. Bible

INTRODUCTION

Thyroid cancer incidence is rising rapidly, mostly due to increasing rates of incidentally detected papillary microcarcinoma.[1] Anaplastic thyroid cancer (ATC), however, is a rare form of undifferentiated thyroid carcinoma. Even though the incidence for differentiated thyroid cancer (DTC) is increasing, the incidence for ATC has largely been similar over the years. Overall mortality from DTC is low at ~3%, but ATC disproportionately accounts for ~20% to 50% of all thyroid cancer deaths,[1,2] as ATC is highly lethal with median survival reported at 3 to 6 months.[3,4] On the contrary, primary thyroid lymphoma (PTL) tends to be highly responsive to treatment and thus may have a much better prognosis.[5,6] This chapter reviews the clinical management of aggressive thyroid tumors, specifically ATC and PTL, which present similarly.

EVALUATION OF A PATIENT WITH RAPIDLY ENLARGING NECK MASS

Most patients with aggressive thyroid cancers present with a rapidly enlarging neck mass (Figure 28.1, A). This is often associated with hoarseness, pain or discomfort in the neck, and occasionally erythema of the overlying skin. Other symptoms such as stridor, dysphagia, shortness of breath, or occasional bleeding also occur.[7,8] In occasional cases, aggressive thyroid cancers are alternatively diagnosed incidentally after thyroidectomy for biopsy-proven DTC.[9,10]

It is critical to evaluate patients with aggressive thyroid malignancy rapidly. This is best accomplished by a multidisciplinary team at a tertiary cancer center. Initial evaluation should include a careful history, including autoimmune thyroid disease such as Hashimoto's and DTC, family history, and full physical examination to assess the clinical status of the patient. Airway/vocal cord/upper aerodigestive status should also be assessed by endoscopic examination by an experienced clinician. Although patients may have a large mass causing tracheal deviation or compression of other critical structures such as neck vessels, most patients will not require emergent tracheostomy to maintain the airway. As a rule, guidelines from the American Thyroid Association (ATA) do not recommend routine tracheostomy in these patients but instead only in response to an imminent threat.[11] However, there will be some patients who may require this at initial evaluation, due to impending airway compromise.

Radiographic imaging evaluations for these patients should include a contrast enhanced computed tomography (CT) scan of the neck, chest, abdomen, and pelvis, or alternatively, a whole-body fluorodeoxyglucose-positron emission tomography (FDG-PET) CT. Thyroid FDG uptake on the PET scan is usually very intense in high-grade lymphoma and ATC and is associated with necrosis in some patients (see Figure 28.1, B). Unlike DTC, neck sonography alone has a limited role in these patients, due to limited evaluation of disease posterior to and/or invading the trachea. There is also no role for radioactive iodine in ATC except in cases with a dominant DTC tumor metastatic component requiring therapy itself with radioactive iodine. Imaging of the brain to rule out intracranial metastases is recommended in ATC.[11] This comprehensive evaluation should be completed within a few days so that emergent treatment can be started based on the disease pathology, extent, and patient goals of care. Otherwise, these rapidly growing cancers could soon become life threatening to the patient due to delays.

PATHOLOGIC EVALUATION OF A RAPIDLY GROWING NECK MASS

The role of expert pathologic evaluation cannot be overestimated when evaluating tissue from a rapidly growing neck mass. An accurate, and at the same time, expeditious diagnosis is required to facilitate prompt management. Fine-needle aspiration (FNA) can be helpful in establishing diagnosis,[12] but core biopsy is preferred because morphologic analysis on FNA can be inadequate.[13] FNA cellularity can also vary depending on the diagnosis and extent of tumor necrosis. Additionally, FNA might be inadequate if the diagnosis is uncertain and if additional immunohistochemical stains are required.

ATC can sometimes be difficult to distinguish from PTL, sarcoma, medullary thyroid cancer (MTC) or, in extremely rare cases, primary thyroid squamous cell carcinoma. However, morphology and lymphoid markers can initially differentiate lymphomas, including large cell lymphoma, from ATC. Metastatic adenopathy from upper aerodigestive tract malignancies may also present with rapidly enlarging neck masses. Poorly differentiated cancers also tend to lose immunohistochemical staining for nearly all but cytokeratin markers, often making it difficult to distinguish ATC from metastatic cancers from other sites. In this regard, PAX-8 staining is usually positive in ATC and can point to the increased likelihood of thyroid tumor origin, as can association with adjacent DTC.

If distant disease is present at diagnosis, biopsy of that lesion will help to determine accurate staging, as sometimes metastatic DTC and ATC coexist. If the thyroid is involved in a widespread lymphoma, biopsy from a most easily accessible region with prominent FDG activity on PET CT may help optimally target the biopsy. Once the diagnosis is deemed accurate and agreed upon, treatment is directed by specific pathology. Next we discuss ATC and PTL in detail; specific treatments for squamous cell carcinoma, sarcoma, or MTC are not discussed in this chapter.

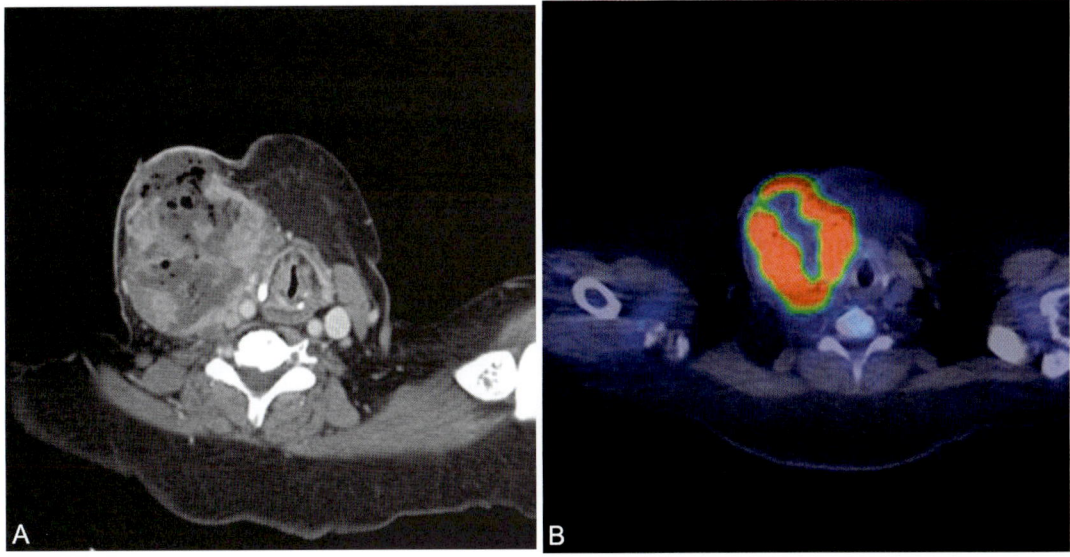

Fig. 28.1 A, Axial view of the computed tomography (CT) scan of the neck, and **B,** fluorodeoxyglucose-positron emission tomography (FDG-PET) for a patient with anaplastic thyroid cancer depicting large mass, with central necrosis, skin invasion, and tracheal deviation.

ANAPLASTIC THYROID CANCER

Staging

The American Joint Committee on Cancer (AJCC) 8th edition has modified ATC staging (see chart) with T designations now being consistent with DTC T designations. The overarching similarity from past AJCC ATC staging, however, should be noted in that all ATC are stage IV:

- Stage IVA represents intrathyroidal
- Stage IVB is associated with gross extrathyroid extension or nodal disease
- Stage IVC implies distant metastasis

ATC AJCC 8th Edition Staging

T	N	M	Stage
T1-T3a	N0/NX	M0	—Stage IVA
T1-T3a	N1	M0	—Stage IVB
T3b	Any N	M0	—Stage IVB
T4	Any N	M0	—Stage IVB
Any T	Any N	M1	—Stage IVC

Epidemiology

ATC comprises only 1% to 2% of all thyroid cancers but is highly lethal and almost universally fatal.[14] The incidence of ATC is largely stable or increasing at a very slight rate.[1] ATC tends to be a disease of the elderly, with a median age of 60 to 65 years and a female preponderance observed in population-based studies.[4,15] Rarely, ATC can present in younger patients in the second or third decades of life. There are no clear regional differences in the incidence of ATC, and there is conflicting evidence about the role of iodine deficiency and supplementation in its pathogenesis.[16,17]

Pathology

FNA in ATC is usually cellular and mixed with acute inflammatory cells. Open biopsy is often not required, but core biopsy is sometimes needed for architectural details and to facilitate additional stains and/or genomic interrogation. Occasionally, ATC is diagnosed incidentally upon evaluation of a surgical pathology sample from a patient in whom DTC was presumed[10] and ATC and DTC commonly coexist. ATC is usually characterized by minimal to no staining for thyroglobulin, calcitonin, and thyroid transcription factor-1 (TTF-1) but may show robust P53 and PAX8 staining. ATC may stain also for cytokeratin and may show focal staining for vimentin, especially in morphologic variants with spindle cells. ATC has different morphologic variants, such as sarcomatoid, squamoid, osteoblastic, paucicellular, rhabdoid, and carcinosarcoma variant, confounding morphologic assessment, and classification is not always possible on FNA analysis. These different morphologic variants do not affect clinical management.

Nearly half of ATCs show coexistent DTC. It is now well known that a large proportion (25% to 41%) of ATCs carry the *BRAFV600E* mutation, suggesting origination from preexisting papillary cancers that commonly carry this alteration.[18–22] Additional genetic alterations occur in ATC, including *P53* (29% to 73% of ATCs) and *TERT* promoter (54% to 73% of ATCs), which have the potential to be associated with incremented mutational burden.[19,23] Other mutated genes in ATC are seen in the PI3-kinase pathway *(PIK3CA, PTEN)*, as cell cycle regulators *(CDKN2A/2B)*, methyltransferases *(KMT2A, 2C, 2D)*, and involved in mismatch repair deficiency *(MSH2, MSH6)*.[19,23] Also, ATCs have been shown to be infiltrated with immune cells, such as tumor-associated macrophages and neutrophils, and have high expression of PD-L1, suggesting a stimulated but restrained immune microenvironment.[24–26]

CLINICAL COURSE AND PROGNOSIS

ATC has a dismal prognosis. In a population-based study from British Columbia, almost all patients not referred for treatment died within 1 month; 1 year overall survival was 19%.[3] In 1961 Woolner et al. reported from the Mayo Clinic that 61% were dead within 6 months, and 77% within 1 year of diagnosis.[27] Almost 50 years later, a study from MD Anderson reported a mean survival of 7 months.[28] Only 8% (20 of 240 patients) from both series survived longer than 1 year. Median survival in a later Mayo Clinic series was only 3 months.[29] Although improvements have been shown in specific publications,[30,31] population-based studies continue to show poor prognosis even today. In a National Cancer Database (NCDB) study from 2017, 1-year survival was still dismal at 11%.[4]

If left untreated, death occurs most commonly from the effects of local tumor invasion, particularly asphyxiation, with over half of patients dead from suffocation from an invasive neck tumor.[32,33] However, in most recent studies, wherein patients were treated with chemoradiation therapy with or without surgery, patients died primarily from distant metastases, suggesting progress in affecting locoregional tumor control.[30,31,34]

In single institutional studies, the presence of a DTC component,[27] younger patient age,[35] and earlier tumor stage at the time of diagnosis[30] have been associated with a better prognosis. In a study of 516 patients from the Surveillance, Epidemiology, and End Results (SEER) database, multivariate analysis showed that only age <60, lesser disease extent, and combined modality therapy with surgical resection and external beam radiotherapy were independent prognostic factors.[36] In the recent NCDB study, age, presence of distant metastasis, administration of chemotherapy, surgical resection, and radiation dose were similarly shown to be independently associated with survival per multivariable analysis.[4] In summary, younger age, limited stage disease (AJCC stage IVA and IVB), and multimodality treatment seem associated with better survival.

Overview of Treatment Planning

Most centers of excellence specifically expedite the care of ATC patients.[37] Effective management mandates focusing on the initially most imminently threatening tumor component, namely the ATC. Treatment of concomitant DTC is put aside until ATC is effectively treated as long as a differentiated tumor does not involve vital structures or is specifically responsible for significant morbidity. In most cases there is no role for radioiodine in the treatment of ATC as ATC is radioactive iodine insensitive. With all due haste, the multidisciplinary treatment team should be assembled (surgery, medical oncology, endocrinology, radiation oncology, and palliative care specialists) to consider treatment options for patients with regard to their disease and clinical status. A meeting with patients and their families should follow, providing full disclosure of the risks and benefits of possible treatment options, including innovative therapy, experimental protocols, and palliative care. Irrespective of available options, every patient's goals of care must guide therapy election. An overview of our approach to a suspected ATC patient is depicted in Figure 28.2.

Initial Assessment for Surgery

Initial assessment of ATC patients should be performed by a multidisciplinary team comprehensively and rapidly. Any unnecessary delay in assessment may permit ATC to progress from potentially resectable to unresectable and imminently threatening. To assess whether a patient is a candidate for surgical resection is complicated due to the inherent complexities of the disease and technical challenges and compromises associated with resection. Box 28.1 enumerates the steps to be considered before a patient is considered for surgical resection.

A few patients may present with stridor and impending airway compromise and may thus require immediate tracheostomy to attain clinical stabilization sufficient to complete the evaluation before a final treatment plan is decided upon. It is critical to evaluate the vocal cords and upper aerodigestive tract tumor invasion, and to determine accurate staging and pathologic diagnosis before surgery is considered. In addition to medical comorbidities, history of previous radiation therapy, extent of the resection required to achieve negative margins, and fitness for anesthesia and surgery should be assessed. It is also important to direct attention to each patient's decision-making capacity and goals of care. The patient and family need thorough and frank discussions of these issues and must participate seminally in the planning process.

As soon as the diagnosis of ATC is made, the treatment team needs to decide if it is confident that it can surgically manage this disease as an initial step. Patient outcomes in thyroid cancer have been closely linked to surgeons experience in thyroid cancer surgery,[38–40] and many studies have shown that surgical resection is a strong predictor of overall survival in ATC.[4,36,41,42] It is no longer appropriate to exhibit uniform therapeutic nihilism for patients with ATC. If needed, expeditious transfer of care to an appropriately skilled surgeon at another center should be accomplished. To do otherwise may allow sufficient tumor progression that can negate all therapeutic intentions, or worse yet, result in an aborted or inappropriate surgery associated with treatment delay, undue patient morbidity, and potentially nonhealing surgical wounds, due to residual tumor involvement.

The distinctly invasive nature of ATC may make effective resection problematic. Attempts at surgical resection are usually made in about half of the presenting patients at large academic centers.[27,35,43] Determination of resectability is achieved by careful assessment of tumor involvement with the visceral compartment, adjacent vascular structures, and the paraspinous structures posteriorly. Radiologic and upper aerodigestive visualization studies provide the best preoperative assessments of adjacent structure involvement. The extent of involvement of the visceral compartment of the neck is the dominant determinant of the morbidity associated with feasibility of surgical resection. Therefore one should preoperatively determine the extent of tracheal, laryngeal, or esophageal involvement by direct review of radiographic studies, choosing when to supplement them with endoscopic evaluation of the hypopharynx, esophagus, larynx, or trachea. It is also critical to rule out distant metastases with systemic staging before surgical resection is planned, as surgical resection in the presence of extensive metastatic ATC may delay systemic therapy and even worsen outcomes. The surgeon also needs to estimate the possible need for thoracic and/or vascular surgical support and should have a skilled team available based on the extent of disease present at the thoracic inlet and upper mediastinum. Control of hemorrhage from thoracic vessels may require emergent sternotomy, and the operating room team should be prepared for that contingency.

Neoadjuvant treatment was generally not considered in ATC. As mentioned above, nearly half of the ATC carry *BRAF V600E* somatic mutation.[18,19,21,22] Personalized therapies are emerging in ATC. Recently, targeted therapy was investigated in *BRAFV600E*-mutated ATC, showing a 69% response rate with the combination of MEK inhibitor, trametinib, and BRAF inhibitor dabrafenib in a small basket study leading to US FDA approval in ATC.[44] This combination therapy was investigated in a pilot study as a neoadjuvant therapy for surgical resection of ATC that was initially deemed unresectable.[45] In this report which included 11 patients, neoadjuvant therapy with dabrafenib and trametinib was feasible in six (55%). Complete resection of local disease was achieved in all six with four of six demonstrating R0 resection. The post-surgical pathology showed <5% tumor viability in four of six patients. Wound infection, temporary unilateral vocal cord palsy and pulmonary embolism were some of the postoperative complications observed in one patient each. This study demonstrates the feasibility of this exciting novel neoadjuvant approach that could be applied at other institutions as rapid testing for somatic mutations becomes available.

Endocrine, hepatic, renal, immunologic, neurologic, and nutritional issues alone may not contraindicate surgery; however, they must be considered when considering radical resection. The rapid growth of ATC mandates rapid initiation of adjuvant therapy after surgery;

CHAPTER 28 Anaplastic Thyroid Cancer and Primary Thyroid Lymphoma

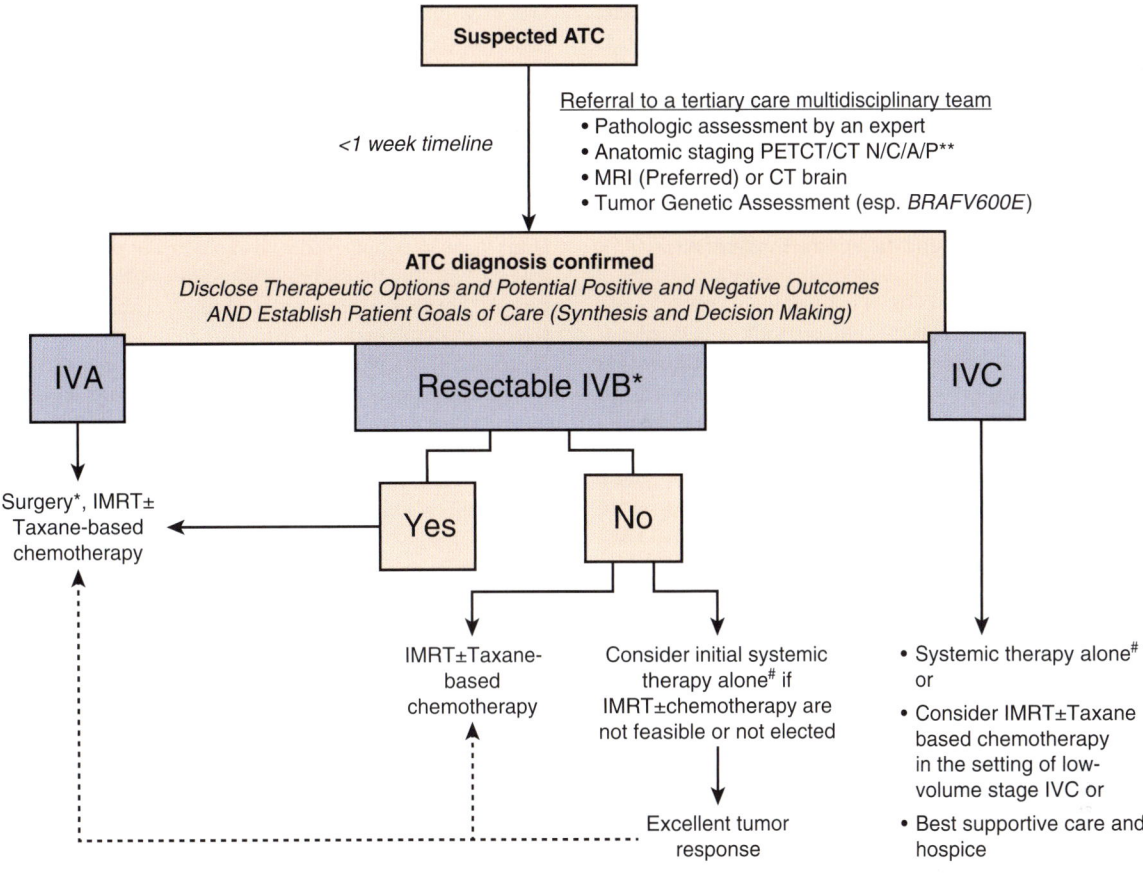

*Goal is R0/R1 resection; refer to detailed pre-surgical checklist in Box 28.1
** CT N/C/A/P - neck, chest, abdominal, pelvic CT
#Dabrafenib/trametinib ± immuno-therapy if *BRAFV600E* mutated (FDA-approved), clinical trial or cytotoxic chemotherapy

Fig. 28.2 Algorithm suggesting evaluation and management of suspected anaplastic thyroid cancer.

BOX 28.1 Surgical Checklist for Anaplastic Thyroid Cancer

	Yes	No
Immediate airway evaluation		
Stridor—Immediate tracheostomy *required*?	☐	☐

Prerequisites/Inclusion Criteria for Surgery
Detailed surgical airway evaluation
- Fiberoptic evaluation including vocal cord status: laryngeal, subglottic and upper tracheal regions ☐ ☐
- Contrast-enhanced axial scanning of neck and upper mediastinum (CT or MR preferred over US) ☐ ☐
- *Consider:* Endoscopic visualization of esophagus to assess invasion ☐ ☐
- *Consider:* Bronchoscopic visualization to assess invasion ☐ ☐

Is R0/R1 resection expected technically realistic?
- Can R0/R1 resection be anticipated to be undertaken without prohibitive collateral damage (no laryngectomy, arterial/tracheal resection; no permanent tracheostomy)? ☐ ☐
- Is assembled/available surgical team optimal for tasks at hand? ☐ ☐

Undertake systemic multidisciplinary evaluation (surgery, endocrinology, radiation oncology, medical oncology, pathology, and possibly palliative care)
- Assured correct pathologic diagnosis—core biopsy, negative calcitonin, expert pathology review ☐ ☐
- Complete radiographic evaluation/clinical staging ☐ ☐
  - Neck and chest axial imaging with contrast ☐ ☐
  - Global staging to assess disease extent (FDG-PET-CT or ☐ ☐
  - CT chest/abdomen/pelvis) to define clinical stage ☐ ☐
  - Brain imaging (MR preferred or contrast-enhanced CT) ☐ ☐
- Assess patient comorbidities and fitness for surgery—acceptable to proceed based upon global patient condition? ☐ ☐
- Is patient competent in terms of capacity and understanding to make decisions? ☐ ☐
  (Recommend involvement of surrogate decision makers as needed)
- Establish patient goals of care and preferences ☐ ☐
- Consensus achieved with patient and team on initial therapeutic plan ☐ ☐

Exclusionary Conditions Before or at Time of Surgery
Anticipated prohibitive morbidity from required surgical procedure?
- Laryngectomy expected/required to achieve R0/R1 resection? ☐ ☐
- Bone, arterial, tracheal resections expected/required to achieve R0/R1 resection? ☐ ☐
- Anticipated time of postoperative recovery prohibitive in the context of anticipated adjuvant treatment (e.g., chemoradiotherapy)? ☐ ☐
- Unacceptably high risk of bilateral vocal cord paralysis from surgery? ☐ ☐
- Apparent distant metastatic ATC stage IVC disease? ☐ ☐
- Patient condition, goals of care, or decision-making capacity unsuitable for surgery? ☐ ☐

prolonged convalescence from surgery may compromise clinical outcomes and should be avoided. Therefore any procedure that is anticipated to include laryngectomy, major arterial or tracheal resection, or permanent tracheostomy may not be advisable.

ATC will typically have potentially profound effects on the initial clinical status consequent to dyspnea, dysphagia, and vocal cord paralysis, and sometimes thoracic outlet obstruction.[43,46] This may require intervention before attempted primary resection and must be dealt with in parallel with other diagnostic and therapeutic interventions.

Airway Management

Maintenance of airway patency in ATC is critical and can be challenging, but tracheostomy should only be undertaken in response to critical airway compromise and not be undertaken electively. Typically there is tracheal deviation, as well as extrinsic compression, and sometimes there is frank invasion of the laryngotracheal airway and potential compromise of one or both recurrent laryngeal nerves. Preoperative assessment for these problems will aid surgical decision making. ATA guidelines do not recommend tracheostomy in patients who have a stable airway, as it neither improves survival outcomes nor quality of life in ATC patients.[47] However, some patients may require tracheostomy, and a thoughtful approach is required.[48,49] We advise tracheostomy for those patients with unresectable tumors in whom imminent suffocation is likely and whose dyspnea does not respond to high-dose corticosteroids. A patient undergoing chemoradiotherapy and not undergoing primary surgical resection with significant and progressing airway compromise may require tracheostomy—a complicated scenario wherein a patient should also be presented with the option of palliative management of dyspnea without tracheostomy.

An overlying tumor often makes a tracheostomy difficult and is better performed under general anesthesia with the patient intubated and not emergently under less-controlled conditions. An experienced anesthesiologist, present for assistance with airway management during induction, is critical. Intubation can be performed with direct laryngoscopy, intubation over a flexible bronchoscope, or by use of a fiberoptic camera mounted on a glide-type laryngoscope. Typically palpated landmarks may be obscured by the tumor, requiring preoperative analysis of imaging studies. With the airway secured, the surgical procedure is started with an incision over the discerned tracheal location. This is rarely midline, and often a portion of the tumor must be resected to expose the trachea, making hemostasis challenging and making the probability of tumor invasion into the surgical wound very great. Extended-length tracheostomy tubes are frequently required, as the distance from the trachea to the surface of the skin is increased due to the tumor. In some cases tracheal stents may provide airway stabilization and symptomatic relief as a last resort, but the placement of such high stems is often very problematic.[50]

Maintenance of Enteral Access

Dysphagia is common at presentation, occasionally with the consequences of malnutrition, weight loss, and dehydration. Typically, this is due to extrinsic compression of the esophagus, but laryngopharyngeal dysfunction may compound this problem, increasing risk of aspiration. Gastrostomy placement should permit critical fluid and nutritional support, particularly when chemoradiotherapy is planned; about three-quarters of patients undergoing chemoradiotherapy will eventually need temporary feeding tube placement.[30] Percutaneous gastrostomy may require variation in technique because of narrowing of the esophagus and compromise of the airway at the thoracic inlet. The endoscopist must therefore be forewarned about deranged anatomy and of any potential airway compromise with sedation, and the endoscopy suite should be prepared for a difficult airway situation.

One may find pediatric or neonatal flexible endoscopes easier to pass, and push techniques may be needed if the esophagus is significantly involved.

Surgical Approach

This section is limited to delineating surgical issues more specific to ATC surgery; descriptions of thyroidectomy, extrathyroidal resections, and nodal resections are well described in other chapters of this text. It is our first choice to perform a complete gross total surgical resection if feasible, realizing that R0 resection may not be achievable. Debulking surgery, however, leaving gross residual disease, is unacceptable and should not be undertaken except under rare circumstances. Because expeditious initiation of adjuvant chemoradiotherapy is intended in the wake of surgery, if possible, 1 to 4 weeks after surgery, significant postoperative complications will delay this and could imperil the overall success of multimodal therapy. It is therefore unclear whether procedures with expected significant delayed convalescence from surgery (as in total esophagectomy or sternal resection) can be justified. Sternotomy or a limited manubrial split may allow resection beyond the upper mediastinum, but should the unhealed sternotomy be within the radiation field, there is risk of additional morbidity. Although extensive resections, such as laryngopharyngectomy and tracheal resections, have been successfully employed for ATC,[51] we do not recommend such radical surgery, as it is seldom reasonable to impose such significant surgical morbidity given the overall poor prognosis in ATC, especially given the alternative availability of chemoradiotherapy, which has a high potential otherwise control locoregional disease. In short, laryngectomy is rarely appropriate in ATC, as its outcomes are often more negative than positive.

Contrary to the current trend toward minimally invasive surgery in thyroid cancer, traditional tenets of surgical oncology are more appropriate for ATC surgery. We prefer an adequately wide incision permitting thorough dissection of uninvolved tissue planes and providing sufficient exposure for optimal surgery. Resection of strap musculature, especially the ipsilateral sternothyroid muscle, or division of the sternocleidomastoid may be done to improve exposure. The surgeon must be prepared for tedious and extensive dissections. For example, although a central approach usually enables locating the recurrent nerve, if this becomes difficult, switching to a lateral approach, from carotid sheath toward the tracheoesophageal groove, may be more successful.

It is usually best to first approach the areas presenting the greatest resection challenge before dealing with areas that are more straightforward. For example, it might be unclear if a left-sided invasive primary tumor can be dissected off the esophagus. One approach is to begin the left-sided dissection before tackling the right thyroidectomy. Placing a bougie dilator or endotracheal tube within the esophageal lumen before surgery will make the esophagus easier to identify within the neck and assist in avoiding violation of its lumen. As another example, initial exploration of the right neck might reveal the right cricoid cartilage to be invaded in a patient unwilling to undergo a laryngectomy, permitting early termination of a procedure before putting the contralateral recurrent laryngeal nerve at risk.

Metastatic cervical lymphadenopathy occurs in approximately 75% of ATC patients, necessitating nodal dissections in these cases.[52] Neck dissection for ATC may require resection of the sternocleidomastoid muscle and jugular vein but is rarely needed for typical thyroid malignancy. Nodal metastases are frequently extracapsular; therefore, unlike other thyroid malignancies, blood vessel wall adventitia is frequently involved. One may peel a layer of adventitia of an artery, but venous wall involvement frequently will require resection of the entire vessel. Often the lower neck nodes and those immediately posterior to the carotid artery are involved with the tumor. These neck dissections will require more extensive dissection lower into the level IV region of the neck than performed with typical thyroid cancer surgical neck dissections. The thoracic duct is frequently encountered in the left neck, and chylous fistulae must be repaired or ligated. Greater care must be taken to avoid injury to the phrenic nerve and the sympathetic ganglia in the neck due to the common posterior invasion seen with ATC.

Management of Surgical Complications

Obviously, the best surgical strategy is to avoid complications by thorough preoperative planning and careful attention to surgical technique. Early recognition of postoperative complications may expedite their resolution so that adjuvant treatment progresses without delay, which is especially critical as adjuvant therapy should begin as soon as possible in ATC. Hemorrhage, wound infection, chylous fistulae, vocal cord paralysis, dysphagia, hypoparathyroidism, and salivary fistulae are the possible complications of an ATC resection. Management of these problems is covered in detail elsewhere in this text (see Chapter 36, Surgical Anatomy and Monitoring of the Recurrent Laryngeal Nerve Chapter 43, Management of Recurrent Laryngeal Nerve Paralysis, and Chapter 44, Non-Neural Complications of Thyroid and Parathyroid Surgery). Thyroplasty and arytenoid adduction procedures should be delayed until the airway stabilizes, adjuvant therapy is completed, and the primary disease is controlled.

RADIOTHERAPY

Radiotherapy, in particular, intensity modulated radiation therapy (IMRT), has become a cornerstone of locoregional treatment in ATC. Effective local control can be achieved by combined modality treatment partnering radiation and chemotherapy with or without surgery. Based on the population and single institutional based studies, about 20% of patients with ATC survive 2 years or beyond after multimodality therapy.[4,7,30,31,53] Alternative fractionation of radiotherapy also has been investigated, but toxicity is high, with benefits uncertain.[31,35,54–56] With IMRT now widely available in the U.S. and Europe, it is feasible to include combination chemotherapy with radiation therapy, and is utilized in our Mayo Clinic protocol.[30,57] The utility of IMRT perhaps points to the fact that total dose, rather than a fractionation approach, may be of greater importance. Indeed, a total radiation dosage >40 to 50 Gy has been consistently associated with improved survival.[4,7,35,56] At our institution we routinely aim to achieve a dose of 66 to 70 Gy in 33 to 35 fractions over 6.5 to 7 weeks with IMRT, especially in IVA and IVB patients (R1, R2 resection or unresectable disease) wherein we are treating unresectable disease with curative intention.[58] Sixty-six Gy in 30 fractions can be considered for small-volume disease or as an adjuvant dose in R0 resection. Similar dosages with IMRT for stage IVC disease may be of greater toxicity and limited benefit. This has the potential to attain locoregional control, but it does not seem to improve survival.[7,31,58] Therefore this decision requires thoughtful consideration by a multidisciplinary team and an individualized approach discussed with each patient.

Concurrent Chemoradiotherapy

There is no consensus regarding the selection of chemotherapeutic(s) to be given concurrently with radiotherapy. Selection of drugs is often based upon side effects, fitness of the patients, and institutional preferences. Doxorubicin, platinum agents, and taxanes remain the most commonly used agents, administered either alone or in combination. Our own practice in general is to offer docetaxel and doxorubicin (15–20 mg/m^2 each, weekly) or paclitaxel and carboplatin (50 mg/m^2 and AUC 2, respectively, weekly) concurrently with radiotherapy.

Studies from multiple institutions describe the apparent benefit from multimodality therapy in ATC, but most are retrospective and subject to potential biases. Major studies are noted in Table 28.1. In 1983 a regimen of combining weekly doxorubicin (10 mg/m^2) and hyperfractionated radiation (160 cGy twice daily, 3 days/week) was reported for ATC,[59,60] delivering 5760 cGy over 40 days. The protocol was well tolerated with little morbidity. Median survival was 1 year, but most patients ultimately developed distant metastases and died.

Multiple studies by Swedish groups[54,61,62] used hyperfractionated radiotherapy, chemotherapy (bleomycin, cyclophosphamide and 5-fluorouracil [BCF]), or most recently, with 20 mg/week doxorubicin, and debulking surgery. Radiotherapy was administered preoperatively at 30 Gy for 3 weeks and postoperatively with an additional 16 Gy, or the same cumulative radiation dose given preoperatively. Death was attributed to local failure in eight patients (24%), but median survival was only 2 to 3 months.

In 1991, a French group reported results in 20 ATC patients treated; depending on the patient's age, two types of chemotherapy were used every 4 weeks: those <65 years received doxorubicin (60 mg/m^2) and cisplatin (90 mg/m^2); those >65 received mitoxantrone (14 mg/m^2) alone.[34] Radiotherapy (17.5 Gy) was given in seven fractions to the neck

TABLE 28.1 Major Studies About Multimodal Therapy for Anaplastic Thyroid Cancer

Study	Years	N	Median Age (Yrs)	Surgery (%)	RT Dose (Gy)	Chemotherapy Regimen	Median OS* (months)	Local Control (%)	Distant Control (%)
Werner	1975–80	19	68–72	63	30–40	Bleomycin, cyclophosphamide, and 5-FU	7–12	NR†	16
Kim	1979–87	19	60	53	56	Doxorubicin	12	68	21
Schlumberger	1981–90	20	NR	60	52	Mitoxantrone or doxorubicin, and cisplatin	2–6	75	35
Tennvall	1984–99	55	76	73	46	Doxorubicin	2–4.5	60	22
Crevoisier	1999–2000	30	59	24	40	Doxorubicin and cisplatin	10	47	37
Sherman	1984–07	37	63	51	58	Doxorubicin	6	50	NR
Prasongsook	2003–15	30	60	90	66	Doxorubicin and docetaxel	21	93	22

*OS – overall survival.
†NR – not recorded.

and superior mediastinum intercurrently. Three patients (15%) survived longer than 20 months. All developed pharyngoesophagitis and tracheitis after the first or second cycle of radiotherapy. The same group published another prospective study in 2004 involving 30 ATC patients. Two cycles of doxorubicin (60 mg/m^2) and cisplatin (120 mg/m^2) were delivered before radiotherapy and four cycles after radiotherapy. Radiotherapy consisted of two daily fractions of 1.25 Gy, 5 days per week, to a total dose of 40 Gy. Surgical resection was possible in 24 patients (80%). Median survival with this protocol was 10 months, and only 5% succumbed to locoregional disease.[31]

In the newer studies from the Mayo Clinic, chemoradiotherapy (doxorubicin and docetaxel at 20 mg/m^2/week each or at 60 mg/m^2 every 3 weeks each, and combined with IMRT to 60 to 66 Gy) has been combined with surgery as feasible. A pilot study published in 2011 demonstrated promise,[57] prompting an expanded cohort of 48 patients confirming these results; median overall survival was 21 months in the patients with multimodal therapy compared with 4 months in patients treated with palliative therapy or best supportive care. Locoregional relapse was seen in only 2 of 27 evaluable patients treated with multimodal therapy.[58] Similar results were seen from a Memorial Sloan Kettering study where patients (N7) treated with doxorubicin 10 mg/m^2/week and radiotherapy of >60 Gy had a median survival of 17 months.[35]

Palliative Systemic Therapies

Cytotoxics have had low efficacy in metastatic ATC, with no U.S. Food and Drug Administration (FDA)-approved cytotoxic agents other than doxorubicin. Doxorubicin, however, has low efficacy and a response rate of 16% in a phase 2 trial.[63] In the same study, the combination of cisplatin and doxorubicin demonstrated a numerically higher response rate of 26%. Paclitaxel has been shown to have a 50% response rate in ATC;[64] however, in another multiinstitution study, paclitaxel demonstrated a lower response rate of 21% and median overall survival of 6.7 months.[65] Based on these studies, taxanes and anthracyclines can be considered for palliative treatment, but modest benefit is anticipated.

Fortunately, personalized therapies are increasingly being used in ATC. Recently a phase-2 study demonstrated efficacy of targeted therapy in *BRAFV600E*-mutated ATC, showing a 69% response rate with the combination of MEK inhibitor, trametinib, and the BRAF inhibitor dabrafenib.[44] These studies led to FDA approval of this combination in locally advanced or metastatic *BRAFV600E*-positive ATC. There are also reports of *BRAF* inhibitors used as a single agent in ATC, but most responses are brief.[66,67] Multikinase inhibitors (MKIs) also have emerged as effective agents in DTC,[68–70] but MKI treatment of ATC has been disappointing.[71–74] Extremely rare cases of thyroid cancer, including ATC, demonstrate ALK fusions that respond exquisitely to ALK inhibitors.[75,78]

With better radiation techniques, an improved understanding of the ATC genetic landscape and the pathogenesis and molecular drivers of ATC, and emerging knowledge of outcomes from molecularly targeted personalized therapies in ATC, further innovative treatment strategies are being planned and studied. The first fully accrued randomized study involving ATC patients, RTOG 0912, examining the potential benefit from adding the MKI pazopanib (or not) to initial chemoradiation therapy in ATC, completed accrual in 2016, with results pending. Multiple other clinical studies incorporating immunotherapy and targeted agents such as BRAF inhibitors and the PPAR-gamma agonist efatutazone are currently underway. In addition, immunotherapy is also being studied in ATC (e.g., NCT02688608, NCT03211117, NCT03181100). Lessons learned from these and other studies have fostered new interest in systemic therapies in ATC for the first time in several decades, hopefully leading to an emerging renaissance in ATC therapeutic innovation.

Failure Patterns and Follow-Up

Despite grim prognosis, treatment with multimodal approaches results in long-term survivors in stage IVA and sometimes in stage IVB ATC. Local recurrence rates have gone down but still could occur in response to multimodal therapy. Inherently, ATC is a systemic disease at diagnosis, and the majority, if not all patients, will eventually develop distant metastases. Both locoregional and distant recurrences can be rapid and fatal. Therefore after completion of primary treatment or during ongoing palliative treatment, ATC patients should be followed closely at a much shorter schedule than other cancers employing regular physical examinations and imaging studies such as FDG-PET or CT scans.

PRIMARY THYROID LYMPHOMA

PTL, along with ATC, should be considered prominently in the differential diagnosis of any rapidly expanding thyroid mass. PTL is a rare, but potentially life-threatening, malignancy that often poses diagnostic challenges based on paucicellular FNA samples alone, making core biopsy critical. PTL typically arises in the setting of chronic thyroiditis, sometimes in patients with long-standing hypothyroidism.[77] Treatments and prognoses differ vastly between ATC and PTL, making expeditious diagnosis (distinguishing it from ATC and other differential considerations) and therapy critical, as PTL prognosis is generally excellent.[5,6,78]

Epidemiology

The annual incidence of PTL is 0.5 to 2 per million, accounting for only 1% to 2% of all extranodal lymphomas.[6,79] The thyroid gland is alternatively sometimes secondarily involved by widespread lymphoma; in such cases, origin is difficult to determine. Therefore we limit our discussion to stage IE and IIE, and not IIIE or IVE PTL. Although many PTLs were incorrectly diagnosed in the past as anaplastic small-cell thyroid carcinoma, adequate pathologic materials and appropriate immunohistochemistry (IHC) interrogation allows differentiation. Pathologists also have become more adept at distinguishing lymphoma from advanced Hashimoto's thyroiditis, which is absolutely critical because PTL typically develops in the setting of coexisting lymphocytic thyroiditis.

Contrary to other lymphomas, females predominate in PTL, probably because PTL originates from activated and transformed lymphoid cells in chronic lymphocytic thyroiditis, which occurs more often in women. Median age is 60 to 70, but a wide age range has been reported.[5,6]

In one study, the relative risk of PTL among people in Sweden with Hashimoto's thyroiditis was 67-fold greater than expected in the absence of thyroiditis (mean follow-up 8.5 years).[77] Another study from Japan found an 80-fold increased frequency of PTL among 5592 women ages 25 years or older with chronic thyroiditis.[80] The average interval between the diagnosis of chronic thyroiditis and PTL was 9.2 years. It is important to remember that Hashimoto's is a common autoimmune disorder, and yet PTL is still extremely rare.

Histopathology

Virtually all PTLs are B-cell non-Hodgkin's lymphomas, which can be identified and elegantly characterized using monoclonal antibodies.[5,81] Most PTLs are diffuse large B-cell lymphomas (DLBCLs), with mucosa-associated lymphoid tissue (MALT) lymphoma less common, pointing to the embryonal origin of the thyroid from the endodermal epithelium in the primitive pharynx. Rarely, DLBCL and MALT lymphoma coexist, likely resulting from transformation associated with poor prognosis.[5,82] Less common PTLs include indolent B-cell lymphomas and others such as T cells and Hodgkin's lymphoma.

The histologic features of Hashimoto's disease and PTL are often difficult, yet critical, to differentiate. PTL demonstrates normal thyroid tissue that is extensively infiltrated with abnormal and invasive lymphoid cells that often penetrate the thyroid capsule, extending into adjacent soft tissues. It is usually composed of monotonous small cells, distinct from autoimmune thyroiditis.

The interface between lymphocytic thyroiditis and PTL may be sharply defined, or there may be a transitional zone in which elements of both are intermixed. Lymphoma cells tend to displace, distort, and replace the thyroid epithelium. Antibodies against molecules, such as CD5, CD10, CD20, CD23, CD43, CD30, BCL-2, c-myc, and cyclin-D1, can be used for subclassification of PTL.[83]

Clinical Diagnosis and Imaging

Diagnostic possibilities in a rapidly enlarging thyroid mass are PTL and ATC; MTC, multinodular goiter, and colloid nodule with acute hemorrhage; and inflammatory disorders, including acute, subacute, and Hashimoto's thyroiditis. Much like ATC, most PTLs present with compressive symptoms caused by a rapidly expanding thyroid mass over the course of days or a few weeks.[82,84] Common symptoms include dysphagia, dyspnea, stridor, neck pressure and neck pain—potential indicators of extrathyroidal tumor extension that should alert clinicians to possible malignant goiter. Stridor and hoarseness often occur together, and when they do, laryngeal nerve paralysis is of concern. The disease may present focally, with only one thyroid lobe or a discrete nodule involved, or there may be diffuse thyromegaly. By palpation the gland is nearly always firm or hard, usually nontender, and often fixed, a sign of invasion. Other signs of extrathyroidal spread include ill-defined thyroid borders with extension laterally or retrosternally on imaging. Nodal involvement is often present but B-symptoms are uncommon.[81] Almost all patients with PTL have clinical or histologic evidence of lymphocytic thyroiditis at the time of diagnosis.[6]

Although laboratory evidence of autoimmune thyroiditis is common, most patients are euthyroid or only mildly hypothyroid, showing minimal elevation in serum thyroid-stimulating hormone (TSH) and otherwise normal thyroid function tests.[6,13,78] Thyrotoxicosis is extremely uncommon but can occur in PTL.[5] Routine serum chemistries and hematologic studies are usually normal. Lactate dehydrogenase may be elevated. Thyroid function testing may disclose subclinical or overt hypothyroidism, and serum antimicrosomal and antithyroglobulin antibodies are often positive.

In general, when ATC or PTL are of consideration, it is best to obtain a core biopsy rather than an FNA.[13] Immunophenotyping with IHC markers is crucial in classifying lymphoma for accurate diagnosis and treatment. Occasionally, an open (surgical) biopsy is necessary to obtain sufficient architectural detail to allow for an accurate histologic subtype.[85]

Once PTL is diagnosed, imaging is required to define disease extent. CT scan, magnetic resonance imaging (MRI), and ultrasonography can be used, but FDG-PET is best used to determine disease extent (Figure 28.3, A).[86–89] Radioactive iodine diagnostic thyroid imaging is typically not appropriate or helpful. On CT scans, PTL usually manifests as one or more areas of low thyroid density, either as areas of isoattenuation or low attenuation on contrast-enhanced CT scan of the neck as solitary nodules and multiple nodules, or sometimes as diffuse goiter.[90] On MRI, PTLs contain homogeneous iso- or high-intensity areas performed weighted images compared with uninvolved thyroid tissue, which appears homogeneously high-intensity on T2-weighted images. MRI and CT scans are comparable in identifying extrathyroidal extension and cervical lymphadenopathy and in staging of lymphoma.[90] Hashimoto's thyroiditis often shows homogeneous signal intensities on MRI that are indistinguishable from those of lymphoma.

Ultrasound is often performed as an initial test, and PTL may appear as a markedly hypoechoic solid mass with significant posterior acoustic enhancement (see Figure 28.3, B) intermingled with coexisting Hashimoto's thyroiditis in the remainder of the gland. Calcifications are usually lacking in PTL. Ultrasonography may disclose contiguous

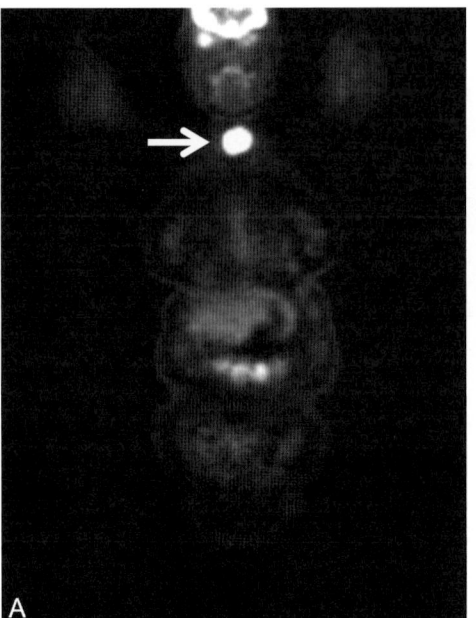 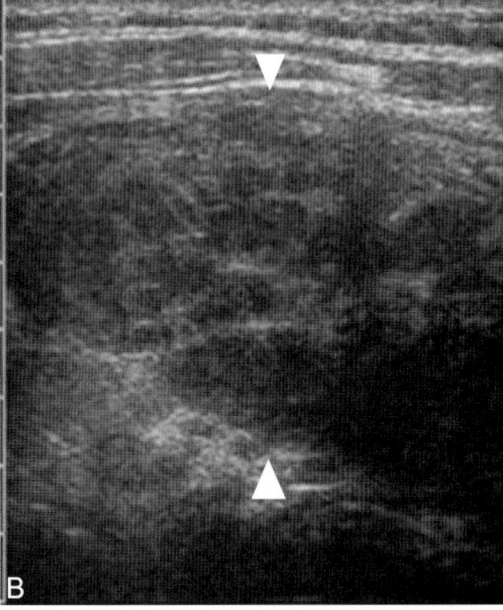

Fig. 28.3 **A,** Skull to thigh fluorodeoxyglucose-positron emission tomography (FDG-PET) imaging of a patient demonstrating uptake in thyroid *(white arrow).* Biopsy demonstrated the mass to be a diffuse large B-cell lymphoma. **B,** Ultrasound image of the left thyroid gland of a patient with enlarged thyroid gland demonstrates largely hypoechoic, heterogeneous appearance *(white arrowheads).* No discrete thyroid nodule is seen. Initially Hashimoto's disease was suspected but biopsy demonstrated diffuse large B-cell lymphoma.

TABLE 28.2 Ann Arbor Classification System for Non-Hodgkin's Lymphoma

Ann Arbor Non-Hodgkin's Lymphoma Stage	Features
I	Single nodal or visceral site of lymphoma only (thyroid)
II	Two or more nodal sites of disease, both on same side of the diaphragm
III	Nodal involvement on both sides of the diaphragm
IV	Involvement of additional distant visceral sites (beyond E)

A, no symptoms; B, fever, drenching sweats and/or >10% loss of body weight in 6 months; E, a single, extra nodal site (thyroid in this instance) contiguous or proximal to known nodal site

tumor spread into both thyroid lobes, is sensitive in detecting abnormal cervical lymph nodes, and represents an important adjunct to a physical examination.[91,92]

Staging for PTL is according to the Ann Arbor classification system (Table 28.2).[93,94] PTL is macroscopically confined to the thyroid gland (stage IE) in almost 60% of patients, with spread to regional lymph nodes (stage IIE) in the other 40% of patients.[5]

Treatment

Large, randomized, multicenter trials for PTL have not yet been performed; thus therapy in PTL is generally defined based upon analogy to similar histologic lymphoma types otherwise occurring at other locations. As in other lymphomas, chemotherapy—and sometimes external beam radiation therapy—have emerged as preferred therapies, especially for high grade PTLs.[5] Overall survival for stage I disease approaches 90%, and for stage II, 60% to 80%, depending on the lymphoma subtype and the therapeutic modality.[81,95]

Airway Protection

Patients commonly present with a rapidly enlarging thyroid mass. Occasionally, tracheal compression with respiratory distress may necessitate emergency surgery or tracheostomy, but this is rare in PTL. Most often, however, rapid institution of therapy using corticosteroids can induce brisk responses in PTL to avert the need for tracheostomy. However, procurement of robust biopsy materials must be undertaken before corticosteroid initiation, as PTL diagnosis can be obscured if corticosteroids are initiated before core biopsy.

Surgery

Surgery is now infrequently undertaken in PTL, due to improved efficacies of systemic therapies. Earlier reports,[96] however, suggested that patients undergoing total macroscopic tumor removal fared considerably better than those with persistent tumor after surgery; 5-year survival rates in the two groups were approximately 65% and 22%, respectively. Similar results were reported from the Mayo Clinic,[97] where 5-year survival rates were 75% in patients with complete resection and 49% in patients with residual disease. Perhaps the least controversial reasons for surgery are for diagnosis and tumor staging and to relieve airway obstruction. In the largest population-based analysis, 68% patients underwent resection with statistically better disease-specific survival reported.[81] However, surgery as monotherapy is of consideration only in stage I disease, mostly low-grade lymphomas such as follicular and MALT lymphomas.[98] Should surgery be considered, RLN resection should not be performed as RLN paralysis from lymphomatous involvement can improve with non surgical treatment.

Radiotherapy

Radiation therapy is employed in the setting of lymphoma subtypes with a lesser risk of systemic dissemination, especially for patients with stage IE or IIE PTL. Control of disease in the neck is related both to radiation dosage and selection of radiation fields and may also be dependent on the degree of surgical debulking (if performed) before radiotherapy. The thyroid, bilateral neck, and mediastinum are treated with at least 40 Gy (4000 rad) given in divided doses over 4 to 5 weeks. An earlier Mayo Clinic study achieved a 59% disease-free survival with about 40 (24 to 60) Gy in 38 patients, most of whom had intermediate-grade histology and stage IE or IIE disease.[97] None experienced substantial side effects. Results are best for patients with stage IE and IIE disease. Another study reported 5-year survival rates of 91% in patients with stage IE disease who were treated with 40 Gy.[99]

Chemotherapy

Historically, chemotherapy was administered to almost half of the patients with PTL based upon recent reviews.[5,100] The most commonly used regimens were R-CHOP (rituximab, cyclophosphamide, doxorubicin, vincristine and prednisone) or CHOP previously. These regimens are well tolerated even in elderly patients with PTL and can be curative even in disseminated PTL.[78] A review of the published literature suggested that the addition of chemotherapy to radiation therapy significantly lowered distant and overall recurrence.[101] More recent studies indicate a 5-year overall survival rate of 74% to 87%.[5,78,95] Older age, advanced stage, aggressive histologic subtype, and lack of combined modality treatment were associated with worse survival.[81]

Failure Patterns and Follow-Up

Recurrence rates vary dramatically; most recurrences (75%) are detected within the first 2 years after therapy, and recurrences were detected by both physical examination and imaging studies.[97,102,103] Routine use of PET CT for surveillance is increasingly discouraged in low-grade lymphomas[104] but may have a greater role in the situation of high-grade PTLs. Indolent lymphomas such as follicular or MALT lymphomas may need longer clinical follow-up.

Both locoregional and distant recurrences can occur.[5] One study of 245 patients found that the gastrointestinal tract was infrequently involved.[102] An autopsy study, however, found the most common sites of involvement to be the gastrointestinal tract (100%), lung and kidney (each 63%), and liver and pancreas (each 50%).[105]

REFERENCES

For a complete list of references, go to expertconsult.com.

29

Pediatric Thyroid Cancer

Gillian Diercks, Andrew J. Bauer, Jeff Rastatter, Ken Kazahaya, Sanjay Parikh

Please go to expertconsult.com to view related video:
Video 29.1 Introduction to Chapter 29, Pediatric Thyroid Cancer.

INTRODUCTION

Much like many childhood diseases, there are major differences in the diagnosis and management of pediatric patients with thyroid cancers compared with adults. This chapter highlights some of those differences and reviews the current approach to the etiology, diagnosis, and treatment of pediatric thyroid cancer. Thyroid cancer accounts for approximately 1% to 3% of all childhood malignancies and 7% of all pediatric head and neck tumors.[1,2] Although thyroid malignancy in children is less common than thyroid cancer in adult patients, a similar annual increase in the number of thyroid cancer diagnoses has been reported in children, with an increase between 2% to 3.8% per year per the Surveillance, Epidemiology, and End Results (SEER) database.[3] The largest increase is found in female patients between 15 to 19 years of age where thyroid cancer accounts for 8% of all cancers.[3] Over 85% of childhood thyroid carcinomas are papillary thyroid cancer (PTC) with the remainder divided between follicular thyroid cancer (FTC) and medullary thyroid cancer (MTC), with the majority of MTC associated with multiple endocrine neoplasia type 2 (MEN 2).[4]

ETIOLOGY

For the majority of children and adolescents diagnosed with thyroid cancer or thyroid nodules, there is no identifiable risk factor. A cohort of pediatric patients is at higher risk of developing thyroid cancer—those with a history of exposure to ionizing radiation and those with a genetic predisposition. Genetic predisposition may present as a family history of isolated differentiated thyroid cancer (DTC; familial nonmedullary thyroid cancer) or with de novo or inherited mutations in oncogenes that increase the risk of developing thyroid malignancy.

The association between thyroid cancer and prior radiation exposure is well established and has been documented for decades. Initial observations about this relationship were made in patients receiving radiation for the treatment of benign diseases, such as tonsillar hypertrophy, thymic hyperplasia, acne, and tinea capitis.[5,6] The development and use of nuclear weapons resulted in further understanding of the relationship between radiation exposure and the development of thyroid cancer after observations that residents exposed to nuclear fallout after atomic bomb testing and survivors of nuclear attacks in Hiroshima and Nagasaki, Japan, had an increased incidence of thyroid cancer.[7,8] By 1954, nuclear power plants for commercial production of energy were in operation. By 2017, there were more than 450 nuclear power plants in operation across the world, and, fortunately, only three significant accidents (meltdowns) have occurred as of 2018: Three Mile Island, United States (1979), Chernobyl, Ukraine (1986), and Fukushima Daiichi, Japan (2011). Each accident has provided valuable lessons, but Chernobyl stands out as providing the most informative data on the risks of inhaled and ingested ^{131}I in the development of thyroid cancer in pediatric patients as the incidence of thyroid cancer increased by a factor of more than 60 in the populations of both Belarus and Ukraine.[9] The initial cohort of pediatric patients who developed PTC after Chernobyl presented within 5 years of the accident and presented with clinically advanced disease, with regional lymph node (LN) metastases and pulmonary metastases in 60% and 24% of patients, respectively, and 50% of tumors exhibiting extrathyroidal extension.[10]

Medical exposure to ionizing radiation is also associated with an increased risk of thyroid cancer and may occur during diagnostic, radiologic imaging, as well as part of treatment regimens for nonthyroid malignancy. Across the various imaging modalities, the increased use of computed tomography (CT) scans is believed to account for up to 47% of the collective effective dose of radiation exposure from diagnostic imaging across the world.[11] Although radiation exposure resulting from a single CT scan is low, and this exposure is further reduced by using pediatric-specific protocols, cumulative exposure from serial CT imaging may contribute to an increased risk of thyroid nodules and thyroid cancer, especially in pediatric patients due to increased proliferative cellular activity observed during childhood.[12,13]

In childhood cancer survivors who received therapeutic radiation therapy (RT), thyroid nodules develop at a rate of about 2% annually, reaching a peak incidence 15 to 25 years after treatment. Approximately 20% of long-term pediatric cancer survivors will have a >1 cm nodule detected by ultrasound (US) that is not clinically apparent on physical examination alone.[14,15] This risk is greatest after RT at a young age (<10 years) and with doses up to 20 to 29 Gy.[16-18] Overall, the standard incidence ratio for radiation-induced DTC ranges from 5- to 70-fold, with younger age and dose of exposure correlating with the highest risk.[19]

The second most common identifiable risk factor for the development of thyroid cancer is genetic predisposition, which may be divided into two broad categories: nonsyndromic and syndromic (thyroid cancer associated with other tumors). Familial nonmedullary thyroid cancer (FNMTC) is an inherited predisposition to DTC without an increased risk for the development of additional tumors (see Chapter 30, Familial Nonmedullary Thyroid Cancer). In families with two or more first-degree relatives with DTC, there is an 8- to 10-fold increased risk of developing either PTC or FTC.[20] Similar to sporadic DTC, 85% of FNMTC is composed of patients with PTC. The

TABLE 29.1 Inherited Tumor Syndromes Associated With Differentiated Thyroid Cancer

Tumor Syndrome	Thyroid Pathology	Risk of Developing Thyroid Cancer	Other Cancers	Gene
PTEN Hamartoma Syndrome	Papillary thyroid cancer or follicular thyroid cancer	35% (>75% develop multinodular goiter)	Women—breast cancer and endometrial cancer (Cowden syndrome) Men and women—intestinal polyps, colorectal cancer, renal cell carcinoma, cutaneous melanoma	PTEN
Familial adenomatous polyposis (FAP, also known as Gardner's syndrome)	Papillary thyroid cancer (cribriform-morular variant)	12%	Intestinal polyps, colorectal carcinoma, small bowel cancer, hepatoblastoma, osteomas, dental and cutaneous abnormalities (cysts and dermoid tumors), hypertrophy of the retinal pigment epithelium (CHRPE)	APC
DICER1 syndrome	Papillary thyroid cancer or follicular thyroid cancer	16% (>50% develop multinodular goiter)	Pleuropulmonary blastoma (birth to age 5 years), Sertoli-Leydig cell tumors, cystic nephroma, Wilms tumor, eye and nose tumors, botryoid embryonal rhabdomyosarcoma, pituitary blastoma	DICER1
Carney complex	Papillary thyroid cancer or follicular thyroid cancer	<5% (>50% develop follicular adenomas)	Lentigines, nerve sheath tumors (schwannomas), myxomas, primary, pigmented nodular adrenocortical disease, growth hormone-secreting pituitary adenomas, large-cell calcifying Sertoli-cell tumors (males)	PRKAR1A
Multiple endocrine neoplasia, type 2	Medullary thyroid cancer	>98%	Parathyroid adenoma, pheochromocytoma	RET proto-oncogene

transmission pattern is most consistent with an autosomal dominant mode of inheritance; however, to date, a single germline locus has not been identified.[20,21] Compared with sporadic DTC, FNMTC appears to present at a younger age and exhibits clinical anticipation between generations, whereas subsequent generation family members present with earlier and more invasive disease.[20] In families with three or more affected individuals, US screening of other at-risk family members has been shown to detect disease at an earlier stage, allowing for less aggressive treatment.[21]

Syndromic forms of thyroid cancer in which there is a familial genetic tumor predisposition to the development of thyroid malignancy and other tumors include PTEN hamartoma tumor syndrome (PHTS),[22] familial adenomatous polyposis (FAP),[23] DICER1 syndrome,[24-26] Carney complex,[27] and MEN 2[28] (Table 29.1).

Additional risk factors for the development of thyroid nodules and thyroid cancer include iodine intake and a personal history of autoimmune thyroiditis. The roles of iodine deficiency and iodine excess in thyroid cancer tumorigenesis have both been examined. Current data suggest that iodine deficiency is a weak initiator but a strong promoter of DTC, in particular for FTC, likely secondary to chronic thyroid-stimulating hormone (TSH) stimulation.[29] Autoimmune thyroiditis, both hypothyroidism (Hashimoto's thyroiditis) and hyperthyroidism (Graves' disease), have also been associated with increased risk.

PATHOLOGY

PTC and its variants are the most common histologic subtype of childhood thyroid cancer (>85%; see Chapter 41, Surgical Pathology of the Thyroid Gland). PTC subtypes include classic PTC (CPTC), follicular variant PTC (FVPTC), and, additionally, more invasive forms of PTC, including diffuse sclerosing variant PTC (DSVPTC), widely invasive (diffuse) follicular variant PTC, solid-trabecular PTC (SPTC), and tall-cell variant PTC (TCVPTC).[30-32] In radiation-induced tumors, a solid-trabecular growth pattern is more common than a dominant papillary growth pattern.[33] The remainder of thyroid cancers diagnosed in children and adolescents are FTC, MTC, and, very rarely, poorly DTC.

Within each variant, the histologic appearance of thyroid cancer in children is similar to adults. Childhood PTC has a high predilection to invade lymphatics, giving rise to multifocal disease through intraglandular spread in 30% to 80% of patients, a high incidence of regional LN metastases in up to 70% to 90% of patients (Figures 29.1 and 29.2), and an increased rate of distant metastasis, primarily to the lungs, in 8% to

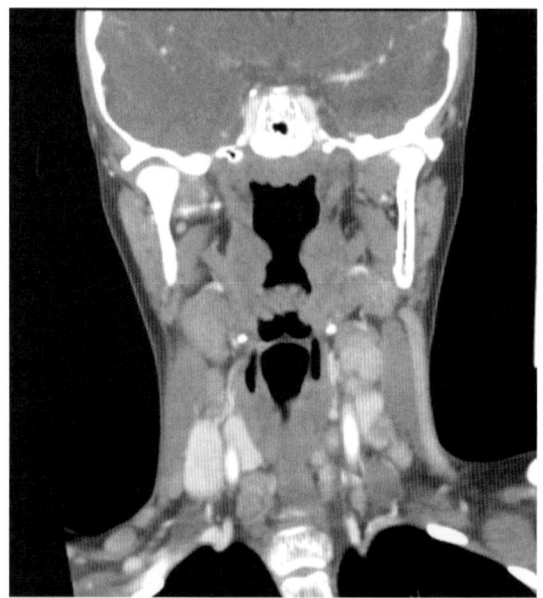

Fig. 29.1 Coronal computed tomography (CT) with contrast demonstrating bilateral, lateral, and central compartment lymph node metastases in an 11-year-old patient with diffuse sclerosing variant papillary thyroid cancer (DSVPTC).

CHAPTER 29 Pediatric Thyroid Cancer 257

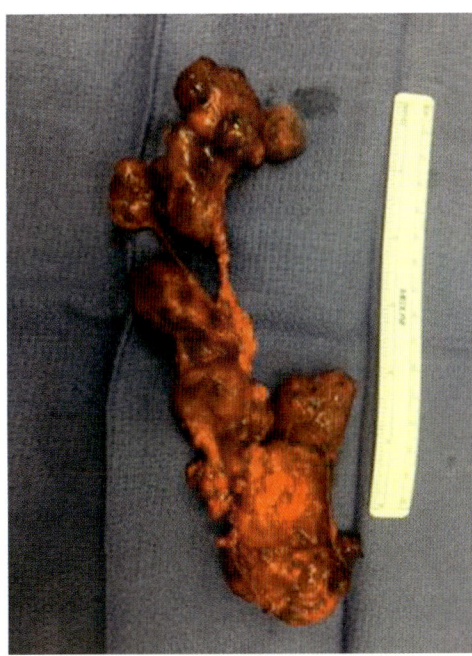

Fig. 29.2 Right lateral compartment neck dissection specimen of an 18-year-old with diffuse sclerosing variant papillary thyroid cancer (DSVPTC).

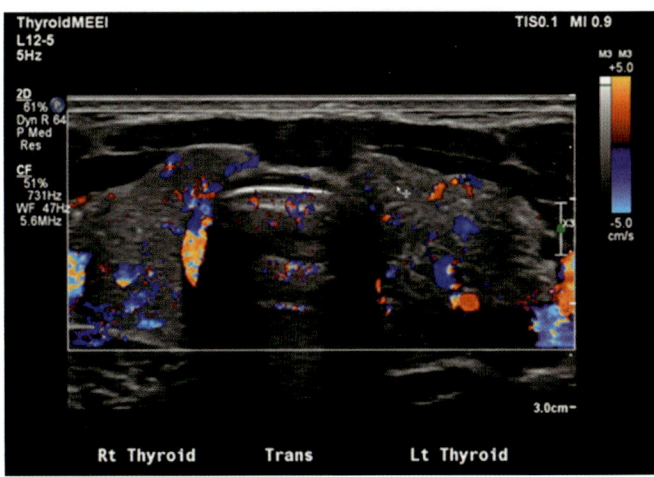

Fig. 29.3 Thyroid ultrasound (US) showing diffuse vascularity and microcalcifications in an 11-year-old girl with diffuse sclerosing variant papillary thyroid cancer (DSVPTC).

20% of patients at the time of diagnosis.[3,30] Additionally, PTC can directly invade local structures, such as the esophagus, trachea, recurrent laryngeal nerve (RLN), and blood vessels, creating significant local morbidity.

DTC usually presents as a firm, partially encapsulated or nonencapsulated, infiltrative mass. Encapsulated CPTC appears to have a similar risk for regional LN metastasis compared with partially or unencapsulated CPTC; however, under strict criteria for diagnosis, encapsulated FVPTC (EFVPTC) has a lower risk for intrathyroidal or LN metastasis.[34,35] The most indolent form of EFVPTC is referred to as a *noninvasive follicular thyroid neoplasm with papillary-like nuclear features (NIFTP)*—a recent change in nomenclature to designate the benign behavior of this neoplasm subtype.[36] Although most data suggest that NIFTPs are indolent, there are reports that associated LN metastasis may arise, emphasizing the need to ensure the diagnosis is used following strict criteria and that surveillance may still be appropriate to ensure noninvasive behavior.[37]

Invasive or aggressive forms of PTC, including DSVPTC, widely invasive (diffuse) follicular variant PTC, SPTC, and TCVPTC, are associated with an increased risk of regional and distant metastasis. DSVPTC typically does not present as a distinct thyroid nodule; rather, it displays diffuse infiltrative invasion of part or all of the thyroid with innumerable microcalcifications (the "snow-storm" appearance on US; Figure 29.3) (see section dedicated to DSVPTC at the end of this chapter).[38] Other forms of invasive PTC may display similar behavior, including aggressive local invasion with extrathyroidal and extranodal extension and an increased risk of pulmonary metastasis. On occasion, a mixed histology will be present. In these cases, one should direct treatment and surveillance based on the most invasive variant.

FTC, like PTC, is a well-differentiated cancer that produces thyroglobulin (Tg) and has the capacity to transport iodine across the cell membrane via the sodium-iodine symporter (NIS). FTC is less common than PTC but shows an increased incidence in iodine deficient regions of the world as well as in certain thyroid tumor predisposition syndromes, in particular PHTS.[39,40] In contrast to PTC, FTC metastasizes hematogeneously.[41,42] The risk of local and distant metastasis is determined by the extent of capsular invasion as well as the extent of metastasis into blood vessels in the tumor capsule and pericapsular space. Within pediatrics, minimally invasive FTC defined as microscopic invasion into the capsule with <4 capsular or pericapsular blood vessels showing evidence of invasion is more common than widely invasive FTC. Angioinvasive FTC is associated with an increased risk of distant metastasis with higher rates of recurrence and poorer outcomes in tumors with metastasis into >4 blood vessels.[43,44] Due to the rarity of FTC in pediatrics, it is unclear if the size criteria established in adults, FTC >4 cm, increases the risk of invasive behavior. Widely invasive FTC and Hürthle cell carcinoma are uncommon in pediatrics but are associated with an increased risk of regional and distant metastasis (lungs and bone).

Medullary thyroid cancer (MTC), unlike thyroid cancers of follicular cell origin, originate from the parafollicular C cells. These cells are derived from neural crest derivatives and do not express the TSH-receptor, Tg, or NIS. Thus MTC does not respond to TSH suppressive therapy, and ^{131}I therapy is ineffective in the treatment of MTC. In addition, calcitonin, along with carcinoembryonic antigen (CEA) rather than Tg, is secreted and used as a marker of tumor progression. With uncommon exception, MTC in pediatrics is associated with MEN 2 with only case reports of sporadic MTC. MTC tumorigenesis follows the same pattern of development in pediatrics as in adults, starting with C-cell hypertrophy (CCH) with progression to MTC. The CT level is predictive of MTC development, progression, and metastasis[45] (see Chapter 26, Sporadic Medullary Thyroid Carcinoma, and Chapter 27, Syndromic Medullary Thyroid Cancer: MEN 2A and MEN 2B). Surgical management of MTC in children is similar to its management in adult patients, with early total thyroidectomy recommended for patients with American Thyroid Association (ATA) "high" and "highest" risk *RET* proto-oncogene mutations.[46]

GENETICS

Alterations in the oncogenes (mutations and fusions) that drive tumorigenesis in DTC and MTC are similar between pediatric and adult patients.[47] However, differences in clinical behavior of these tumors, most importantly, maintenance of cellular differentiation, suggest that there are likely differences in gene expression and downstream signaling pathways between pediatric and adult DTC. The consequences of these differences are reflected by increased disease-specific mortality in adult patients with regional and distant metastasis compared with pediatric patients with similar disease burden.[44,48]

In DTC, thyroid tumorigenesis and progression are associated with somatic point mutations of *BRAF*, *DICER1*, and the *RAS* genes, as well as fusions involving the rearranged during transfection (*RET*), neurotrophic tyrosine receptor (*NTRK*), and anaplastic lymphoma (*ALK*) kinases, with resultant constitutive activation of the mitogen-activated protein kinase (MAPK) and phosphoinositide 3-kinase (PI3K) signaling pathways (see Chapter 18, Molecular Pathogenesis of Thyroid Neoplasia). With uncommon exceptions, these oncogene mutations are mutually exclusive events, and there is a fairly predictable relationship between oncogenic genotype and histopathologic phenotype, with RET-PTC *(RET/PTC)* rearrangements and B-rapidly accelerated fibrosarcoma *(BRAF)* point mutations common in PTC, paired-box gene 8 *(PAX8)*-peroxisome proliferator-activated receptor gamma *(PPARγ)* common in FTC, and *RAS*, *DICER1*, and *PTEN* mutations found across the spectrum of thyroid tumors, from benign follicular adenomas to FVPTC, FTC, and poorly differentiated thyroid carcinoma.[47] Additional point mutations and fusions have been reported and more recent data in adults suggest that second or third mutations, in particular telomerase reverse transcriptase *(TERT)* + *BRAF* or *RAS* and *EIF1AX* + *RAS*, are associated with tumor progression and dedifferentiation.[51] In pediatrics, *RET/PTC* and *NTRK*-fusion genes are associated with an increased risk of invasive disease, although there are no data to suggest that these alterations are associated with increased disease-specific mortality.[47] In children, *BRAF* mutations may not increase the risk of invasive or refractory disease.[47] A summary of the most common oncogenes and their association with DTC and clinical behavior is provided in Table 29.2.

Overall, MTC in adults may either develop secondary to sporadic, somatic mutations (75%) or be associated with germline *RET* mutations (25%). Sporadic MTC is uncommon in pediatrics and is most commonly associated with somatic mutations in the *RET* proto-oncogene and *RAS*, as well as several additional genes, including fusion genes involving anaplastic lymphoma kinase (*ALK*).[52] Familial MTC is one of several tumors syndromes that define MEN 2. MEN 2 is caused by activating mutations in the *RET* proto-oncogene that are transmitted via the germline in an autosomal dominant pattern of inheritance.

The expression and penetrance of the tumors associated with MEN 2, including MTC, parathyroid adenomas, and pheochromocytoma, correlate with the specific *RET* proto-oncogene codon mutation (i.e., there is a correlation between genotype and phenotype; see Chapter 27, Syndromic Medullary Thyroid Carcinoma: MEN 2A and MEN 2BMTC). Mutations in codon M918T are associated with the most aggressive form of MTC and designated as "highest" risk under the ATA guidelines with a risk of MTC developing before 1 year of age.[46] MEN 2B is also associated with early signs and symptoms, including alacrima (the inability or decreased ability to make tears), constipation (associated with ganglioneuromatosis), and hypotonia, (feeding difficulties with failure to thrive, club feet, hip dislocation). The more classically defining symptoms, including oral and lip mucosal neuromas and elongated, marfanoid facies, are not clinically evident until school age, around 5 years of age.[53,54] Because in MEN 2B germline mutations in codon 918 are more often de novo, recognition of the early clinical signs and symptoms is critically important to diagnose the syndrome before MTC metastasis, which often occurs before 4 years of age.[55] Fifty percent of patients will develop a pheochromocytoma; however, unlike patients with MEN 2A, there does not appear to be an increased risk for developing hyperparathyroidism.[46]

There are multiple codon mutations associated with MEN 2A, with the highest risk of developing MTC associated with mutations in C634 and A883F. The remaining mutations carry an increased risk of developing MTC, although for individual patients, the course from CCH to MTC may be quite indolent with MTC not developing until the third, fourth, or later decades of life. There is a 10% to 50% risk of developing hyperparathyroidism and/or pheochromocytoma, defined by the individual codon mutation. Two additional features associated with MEN 2A are cutaneous lichen amyloidosis, a pruritic, plaque-like rash typically on the upper back associated with mutations in C634 and V804M, and Hirschsprung's disease, associated with mutations in C609, C611, C618, and C620.[46]

PRESENTATION AND PREOPERATIVE EVALUATION

Clinical Presentation

The clinical presentation of pediatric DTC can be variable. Small thyroid masses may be incidentally noted on imaging studies obtained for another indication. Larger lesions can present as a neck lump notable on physical examination. Owing to the attachment of the thyroid gland to the airway, associated tumors classically elevate along with the laryngo-tracheal complex as the patient swallows. In the context of thyroid cancer, masses located more laterally in the neck raise concern for disease metastatic to the lateral neck nodes. Involvement of cervical LNs in the central neck may be less easily distinguishable from the primary lesion or thyroid gland by physical examination alone. Imaging studies, including cervical US and, in select cases, cross-sectional imaging, can further demonstrate the relationship between the thyroid gland, associated intrathyroidal masses, and worrisome cervical lymphadenopathy. Clinical suspicion for thyroid cancer is higher in patients with a history of neck radiation, autoimmune thyroiditis, select cancer predisposition syndromes, or a family history of thyroid cancer.[56,57] Along with obtaining a comprehensive patient and family history, the initial clinical evaluation should include a complete head and neck examination, including confirmation of the status of vocal fold mobility through fiberoptic laryngoscopy preoperatively.

Flexible Fiberoptic Laryngoscopy

Office-based flexible fiberoptic laryngoscopy (FFL) is well established as a safe and effective procedure for evaluating laryngeal dynamics in conscious patients of all ages from infants to adults.[58-60] FFL is useful

TABLE 29.2 Molecular Genetics of Pediatric Thyroid Cancer

Oncogene	Increased Risk of Differentiated Thyroid Cancer	Increased Risk of Invasive Disease
BRAF	Yes	Adults (yes) Pediatrics (no)
RET-PTC fusion	Yes	Yes
NTRK-fusion	Yes	Yes (limited data)
BRAF-fusion	Yes	Yes (very limited data)
DICER1	Yes, but also found in benign disease (NIFTP and FA)	No
RAS		May be associated with dedifferentiated disease (uncommon in pediatrics)
PAX8-PPARγ	Yes (FTC)	No
TSHR, THADA, GNAS	No	Not applicable

FA, follicular adenoma, FTC, follicular thyroid cancer, NIFTP, noninvasive follicular thyroid neoplasm with papillary-like nuclear features.
Data from Bauer AJ. Molecular genetics of thyroid cancer in children and adolescents. *Endocrinol Metab Clin North Am*. 2017;46(2):389–403.

for establishing the functional status of the vocal cords both pre- and postoperatively for thyroid surgery. Pre- and postoperative confirmation of vocal cord function should be performed in all pediatric patients undergoing thyroid surgery. Confirming function of the vocal folds is particularly important if the patient's symptoms (e.g., hoarse voice, stridor, aspiration) suggest paresis of one or both vocal folds secondary to RLN compromise either from invasive thyroid disease or iatrogenic injury. Preoperative vocal fold assessment is important as paresis or paralysis may suggest more advanced disease and influences the discussion regarding the risks of surgery. Preoperative vocal cord assessment also has implications for intraoperative laryngeal neuromonitoring.[61,62] Postoperative vocal cord assessment is useful to confirm preservation of vocal cord function or assist in directing further management in the case of paresis.

Ultrasound Vocal Cord Visualization

Transcutaneous laryngeal US is a safe and effective alternative to FFL for evaluation of vocal cord function.[63-66] It can be particularly useful in patients who are unable or unwilling to tolerate FFL. The laryngeal cartilages in children are not yet ossified and will allow sonographic visualization of vocal cord mobility. The cricothyroid membrane may also act as a window to evaluate the vocal cords if the thyroid cartilage has become too ossified. Vocal cord mobility can be assessed during normal respiration with the active abduction that occurs with inspiration, and vocalization will cause the vocal cords to adduct. It should be noted, however, that the larynx also elevates during vocalization so the US probe will need to be moved in conjunction with the larynx to maintain visualization of the vocal cords during phonation. Providers may prefer sonographic evaluation if they have access to an US machine but not FFL.[64] Laryngeal US should be considered a preliminary and somewhat veiled laryngeal examination—any abnormality or questionable findings should be followed up with fiberoptic laryngoscopy.

Preoperative Imaging

Cervical US is the most common imaging modality employed while evaluating thyroid disease in both pediatric and adult patients.[67] Modern US machines can provide a wealth of detailed information regarding the overall size and vascularity of the thyroid gland as well as the size, location, and features of associated thyroid masses.[68-70] US is well suited to evaluate the neck for associated central and lateral neck lymphadenopathy and is commonly used to provide visualization for fine-needle aspiration (FNA) biopsy of both thyroid nodules and abnormal LNs. In many patients US alone provides sufficient imaging information. In select situations, such as in patients with bulky thyroid lesions or metastatic lymphadenopathy, cross sectional imaging by CT or magnetic resonance imaging (MRI) can provide useful information beyond that obtained by US.[67,71] Cross-sectional imaging is often required to adequately examine for the presence of suspicious lymphadenopathy in the superior mediastinum, retropharynx, parapharynx, and subclavicular regions—regions that are typically inadequately visualized using US.[48] Cross-sectional imaging is particularly beneficial for preoperative planning in the setting of advanced disease, including concern for any aerodigestive invasion, bulky lymphadenopathy, or with a preoperative vocal cord paresis. Chest imaging, with either x-ray or CT, may be considered preoperatively for children with significant lymphadenopathy to assess for the presence of pulmonary metastases.[48]

The decision to obtain a preoperative CT or MRI may be based on traditional factors such as whether more bone or soft tissue detail is desired, but often the decision is based upon provider preference. With pediatric patients specifically, the choice of an MRI or CT should involve consideration for radiation exposure and the potential need for sedation or anesthesia. The potential health consequences of radiation exposure from CT imaging has influenced many pediatric providers to use this modality less frequently.[72-75] Additionally, with very young patients, both CT and MRI may require sedation or general anesthesia. Recent studies have also raised concern for the potential negative effects of general anesthesia on cognitive development in young children.[76,77] Iodinated contrast agents may be used; however, there is concern that radioactive iodine (RAI) treatment may need to be delayed.[48] However, given the time from when a preoperative CT with contrast is performed, through surgery and the postoperative period, typically enough time will pass for the iodine load to be metabolized before diagnostic and/or therapeutic RAI administration.

Fine-Needle Aspiration

FNA in pediatrics has been shown to have the same accuracy, and positive and negative predictive values as in adults; similar to adults, these findings are institution-dependent. In a meta-analysis of 12 studies, the pooled estimated sensitivity and specificity were 94% and 81%, respectively, and assuming a 20% risk of malignancy, the accuracy, positive and negative predictive values were 84%, 55%, and 98%, respectively.[78] The 2015 ATA Guidelines for pediatric patients advocate for the use of US for FNA in pediatric patients to improve diagnostic yield.[48] Conscious sedation or local anesthesia with distraction techniques should be used to reduce the anxiety for the procedure. Real-time slide review during the procedure can assure that the sample is adequate in regard to cell number (6 groups of at least 10 well-preserved thyroid cells is an adequate specimen). When evaluating lateral neck nodes for thyroid malignancy, the FNA samples should be sent not only for cytology but also for Tg rinsing, which can improve diagnostic yield.

Controversy, however, remains in the management of "inadequate" or "nondiagnostic" FNA as well as nodules with indeterminate cytology. High-risk lesions can be, in part, defined by US characteristics, positive family history, or exposure to ionizing radiation. Otherwise, either repeat FNA or surgical removal remains a reasonable option. If, however, the FNA is inconclusive again, surgical removal is advised. For pediatric patients with indeterminate cytology, diagnostic lobectomy should be considered based on an increased likelihood of malignant histology compared with adults (28% to 50% for The Bethesda System for Reporting Thyroid Cytology (TBSRTC) category III and 50% for category IV).[79,80]

Genetic Testing

Similar to adults, FNA in children with TBSRTC-indeterminate cytology occurs in up to 35% of biopsies. The risk of malignancy in pediatric indeterminate specimens is higher than in adult patients.[47] Preoperative genetic panels, including oncogene testing, gene expression classifiers and microRNA (miRNA), are used in clinical practice of adults with indeterminate pathology. Children have a higher risk of malignancy and a higher pretest probability; however, access to utilization of molecular testing has been limited by a decreased likelihood of obtaining prior authorization from health insurance companies. In patients <21 years of age, somatic oncogene panels are the only genetic tests that should be used as gene expression or sequencing classifiers, and miRNA panels have not been validated in the pediatric age group.

Within the list of known oncogene drivers, there are several with high specificity for thyroid malignancy and several that may be found across the spectrum of pathology. Oncogenes that may be associated across the spectrum of thyroid neoplasia include *RAS, DICER1,* and *PAX8/PPARγ*. Oncogenes that have a high specificity for thyroid malignancy include *BRAF, RET/PTC,* and *NTRK*-fusions. Diagnostic lobectomy, at least, should be considered for unilateral nodules with indeterminate cytology (Bethesda categories III, IV, and V) and lower risk oncogenes (*RAS,*

DICER1, PTEN, and *PAX8/PPARγ*) whilie nodules with oncogenes associated with a higher specificity for malignant pathology and invasive behavior should undergo total thyroidectomy with central LN dissection (*BRAF, RET/PTC,* and *NTRK*-fusions).[47] Lateral neck dissection should only be performed for patients with suspicious lateral nodes on US and confirmed by FNA (see Table 29.2).[47]

Germline testing should be considered based on family history of a known tumor predisposition syndrome or a family pedigree that is consistent with a known inheritable syndrome, including PTEN hamartoma syndrome, DICER1 pleuropulmonary blastoma syndrome, FAP, Carney complex, and MEN 2. Routine serum calcitonin measurements for patients being evaluated for nodules are not typically performed in the United States, although this is a common practice in other countries. Serum calcitonin or calcitonin immunohistochemistry should be considered if there are physical examination features consistent with MEN 2B or cytology that raises suspicion for MTC.

TREATMENT

Surgical Management of PTC

As previously mentioned, thyroid cancer is less common in children and adolescents, and treatment recommendations are based on retrospective data and expert opinion only. Therefore analysis from data gathered over decades from different practices challenge us to draw definitive conclusions. This, combined with the fact that childhood PTC is an indolent, typically nonfatal disease, makes randomized prospective trials nearly impossible. Most recommendations come from small cohorts, multicenter retrospective reviews, and extrapolations from adult studies and guidelines. In 2015, the ATA published guidelines for the management of pediatric thyroid nodules and nonmedullary DTC in recognition of these challenges. These guidelines attempted to stratify those populations at risk, guide appropriate levels of treatment, and reduce the risk of long-term morbidity in pediatric patients undergoing treatment.[48]

The ATA recommends that most children with PTC undergo total or near-total thyroidectomy due to the increased risk of bilateral and multifocal disease in children. Compared with lobectomy, total or near-total thyroidectomy is associated with a significantly reduced risk of recurrence in children over a 40-year period (6% versus 30%).[81] Total thyroidectomy also allows for use of Tg levels postoperatively to monitor for persistent and recurrent disease.[48] More recent data suggest that lobectomy may be considered for pediatric patients with low-invasive PTC, including encapsulated FVPTC.[30] On US, these nodules are typically mostly solid with smooth margins and no evidence of microcalcifications or lymphadenopathy.

Prophylactic central neck LN dissection should be considered in pediatric patients undergoing surgery for nodules suspicious for, or consistent with PTC (Bethesda category V and VI) secondary to a high risk of central neck (level VI) metastasis. Up to 36% of pediatric patients with tumors <4 cm have cervical metastases,[82] and cervical nodes have been reported in children with small tumors <1 cm in size.[48] In adult patients there is concern that pursuing this approach upstages the patient without any benefit on reducing disease-specific mortality and exposes the patient to a potentially increased risk of surgical complications as well as an increased likelihood that RAI will be administered. In pediatrics this approach should be considered secondary to the high rate of central neck metastasis. Neck dissection is associated with decreased risk of persistent or recurrent locoregional disease, leading to long-term disease-free survival in children.[48] When children are treated with total thyroidectomy with prophylactic central neck dissection, 5- and 10-year disease-free survival approaches 95%, and the risk of reoperation may be reduced.[48] If the patient is found to have <5 LN with metastatic disease, then there is a high likelihood of surgical remission affording an opportunity to avoid RAI therapy as well.[48,83] Although there is concern for an increased risk of surgical complications associated with central neck dissection, the rate may be significantly reduced by referral to a high-volume thyroid surgeon.[84]

Therapeutic central neck dissection should be performed in all children found to have central and/or lateral neck LN metastases. Lateral neck dissections should only be performed in the presence of FNA-proven metastatic lateral neck disease. Tg-washout may be useful in the detection of metastasis. Prophylactic lateral neck dissection is not recommended.[48]

When nodal dissection is performed, a complete dissection of the affected compartment should be performed, rather than "berry picking." For children undergoing prophylactic central neck dissection, frozen section or intraoperative findings, the size of the primary tumor, as well as the experience of the operating surgeon may guide the aggressiveness of nodal dissection, including whether or not to pursue contralateral dissection.[482]

SURGICAL MANAGEMENT OF FTC

Unlike PTC, FTC is often unifocal and does not have a propensity toward LN invasion but may exhibit early hematogenous spread even in patients without evidence of LN metastases. Minimally invasive FTC is defined as FTC with microscopic or no capsular invasion and/or limited vascular invasion (<4 vessels in or adjacent to the tumor capsule). Widely invasive FTC is defined as FTC with widespread capsular invasion, widespread vascular invasion, or extension into surrounding thyroid tissue. Invasion of four or more vessels is associated with more aggressive disease, an increased risk of distant metastases, and a poorer prognosis.[48]

Similar to adult patients, children ultimately diagnosed with FTC will have indeterminate FNA cytology. Thus the majority will undergo initial ipsilateral thyroid lobectomy and isthmusectomy, with consideration of total thyroidectomy for patients with underlying thyroid disease, bilateral nodules, or a known diagnosis of a thyroid tumor predisposition syndrome. Frozen section may rule out the presence of PTC; however, many institutes do not use frozen section as the process distorts the nucleus, obscuring the ability to accurately confirm a diagnosis. Frozen section cannot be used to rule out FTC as the diagnosis is based on complete histologic evaluation of the nodule to assess for invasive behavior. For minimally invasive FTC <4 cm, lobectomy with or without isthmusectomy is considered to be sufficient. For widely invasive FTC or tumors >4 cm, completion thyroidectomy should be performed along with postoperative RAI based on ^{131}I diagnostic whole-body scanning and TSH stimulated Tg levels.[48]

SURGICAL MANAGEMENT OF MTC

Historically, all patients with a germline *RET* proto-oncogene mutation were referred for surgical intervention, regardless of calcitonin levels, as the goal of surgery was to remove the thyroid before the onset of invasive MTC (see Chapter 27, Syndromic Medullary Thyroid Cancer: MEN 2A and MEN 2B). More recent recommendations suggest that the timing for thyroidectomy should be based on the specific codon mutation.[46,85] For patients with "highest" MTC risk mutations, such as codon 918, thyroidectomy should be performed at the time of diagnosis. Patients with MEN 2B have been found to have MTC within the first year of life. If thyroidectomy is completed after age 4 years, there is a reduced likelihood for surgical remission.[46] Patients with "high" risk codon mutations, codon 634 and 883, should have thyroidectomy by 5 years of age. All other codons are considered "moderate" risk with the timing for thyroidectomy based on family and patient preference or based on an upward trend in calcitonin levels based on serial measurement as well as ultrasonographic evaluation.[46] LN dissection is determined based on calcitonin level and preoperative imaging with a risk of extrathyroidal metastasis increasing in patients with a calcitonin >40 pg/mL, thereby minimizing operative morbidity in the setting of a prophylactic operation.[46,86]

Before any operation, patients with MTC should be screened for pheochromocytoma.[87] A confirmed pheochromocytoma must be treated with pharmacologic blockade and adrenalectomy before proceeding with any thyroidectomy.

Postoperative Management and Complications

In recent years, multiple studies have established that complication rates after pediatric thyroidectomy are increased compared with similar surgery in adult patients. Because pediatric patients generally have an excellent life expectancy, even in the setting of advanced disease, they are at risk for enduring the long-term effects of these complications, particularly those involving calcium metabolism and airway compromise. This highlights the importance of technical skill in the surgical management of children with thyroid disease as well as proper judgment regarding the extent of surgery, particularly in the central neck compartment.

The risk of vocal fold paralysis from RLN injury ranges from 0% to 8.1% in the literature, with the risk of permanent injury reported between 0% to 78%.[82,88-91] Bilateral nerve injury presents a particular challenge, due to respiratory distress and the potential need for a tracheotomy, and occurs in 0% to 2.3% of cases.[82,89-91] The risk of injury is highest in children under 1 year of age undergoing prophylactic total thyroidectomy, approaching 14.3%, and decreases with increasing age.[92] Infants are also at significantly higher risk for requiring a tracheotomy.[92] Risk of nerve injury is significantly associated with advanced tumor stage, complete thyroidectomy, and dissection of both the lateral and central neck compartments as well.[90]

Due to the significant morbidity associate with bilateral RLN paresis in a child, ipsilateral RLN function should be assessed during a total thyroidectomy after completing the dissection of the first thyroid lobe. RLN function can be monitored actively with neuromonitoring and manually by palpating the posterior aspect of the larynx while stimulating the RLN as well as the ipsilateral vagus nerve. If the RLN is intact but not responsive to stimulation, aborting the procedure should be considered before addressing the second side, especially in the setting of benign or unilateral disease. Staging the procedure until the RLN function has a chance to recover may help avoid bilateral vocal cord paresis and the need for a surgical airway.

For children undergoing total or completion thyroidectomy procedures with or without central neck dissections, the risk of transient (<6 months) or permanent (>6 months) hypoparathyroidism is also a concern, with transient hypoparathyroidism occurring in 5.7% to 51.6%[89,93] and permanent hypoparathyroidism occurring in 1.1% to 12.3%[82,93] of cases. The risk of postoperative hypoparathyroidism, similar to the risk of RLN injury, increases with younger age,[92,94] history of parathyroid reimplantation,[92] tumor stage, and nodal dissection.[82]

Thyroid surgery in children is significantly associated with an increased risk of endocrine complications compared with adult patients (p <0.01).[91] Statistically, the majority (52.2%) of children undergoing thyroidectomy have surgery with a low-volume endocrine surgeon (<30 endocrine cases annually) who does not specialize in pediatrics; on average these providers perform one pediatric endocrine case per year.[95] Only 20.8% of pediatric patients are cared for by high-volume endocrine surgeons, but these surgeons perform only an average of two pediatric cases per year.[95] Despite this low pediatric volume, compared with low-volume endocrine surgeons, high-volume endocrine surgeons have a statistically lower cost and length of stay (p <0.05).[91] Facilities caring for a high volume of pediatric thyroid and parathyroid patients have a statistically lower complication rate than low-volume facilities (p < 0.01)[91] as well as statistically lower rates of short-term complications and readmission after surgery (p = 0.01).[96] Volume is a better predictor of postoperative outcome than surgical specialty (general surgeon versus otolaryngologist).[95]

These differences in outcomes underscore the need for careful and appropriate surgical planning, meticulous dissection, and appropriate postoperative monitoring and interventions. Whenever possible, children with thyroid disease should be cared for by high-volume providers and facilities. Additionally, standardized vitamin D screening and supplementation; measurement of intraoperative and/or postoperative intact parathyroid hormone levels; and postoperative calcium management, monitoring, and treatment protocols have not been established for pediatric patients and represent an important area for future research.

The 2015 ATA Guidelines also recommend that children with DTC be cared for by a team experienced in the management of DTC in children. In addition to high-volume surgeons, the team should include experts in pediatric medical and oncology services, such as endocrinology, oncology, radiology, nuclear medicine, cytology, and pathology. A team experienced in the management of thyroid cancer in children will help with interdisciplinary decisions to provide optimal therapy and reduce the potential for either overly aggressive or inadequate treatment.

RADIOACTIVE IODINE THERAPY FOR CHILDREN WITH THYROID CANCER

The benefits of RAI include destruction of thyroid cancer cells as well as any postsurgical remnant thyroid tissue, thereby increasing the future sensitivity of surveillance Tg. RAI is a highly effective, targeted medical therapy to treat persistent postsurgical disease; however, there are concerns regarding future secondary cancers over decades of life expectancy after RAI therapy. Although there is a paucity of long-term prospective data to define the lifetime risk of RAI-induced nonthyroid malignancies, given the potential risk of secondary malignancy, careful consideration should be given to the benefits and potential short- and long-term harms of RAI therapy for medical treatment of well-differentiated thyroid cancer in children.

The risk of secondary malignancy after RAI for DTCs in children has been investigated but only through retrospective analysis. In a report of 215 children and adolescents with PTC treated from 1940 to 2008, with a median duration of follow-up of nearly 30 years, cause-specific mortality at 40 years was only 1%.[84] However, the number of deaths (all causes) was significantly higher than predicted, with 15 of 22 deaths (68%) from a second, nonthyroid primary malignancy (SPM).[84] The authors concluded that survival from childhood PTC should be expected, but they speculated that later death from nonthyroid malignancy may be related to postoperative therapeutic radiation.[84] In review of this data set, it is important to remember that of the 15 patients that died from nonthyroid malignancy, only 4 received RAI along with the remaining 7 receiving radium seed or external beam radiation. In a population-based analysis of 3850 children and young adults in the SEER registry, 26 SPMs were observed compared with 18 SPMs expected. The relative risk of SPM was higher for patients who received RAI compared with those who did not, 1.42 versus 1.01, respectively. Most notably there was a 34-fold increase in the standardized incidence ratio for post-RAI exposure salivary gland cancer.[97] Although the increase in salivary gland cancer was only attributable to three patients, this is a rare tumor and very likely

TABLE 29.3 Risk Stratification for Pediatric Differentiated Thyroid Cancer

Low risk	Disease grossly confined to the thyroid with N0/Nx disease or patients with incidental N1a disease (microscopic metastasis to a small number of central neck lymph nodes)
Intermediate risk	Extensive N1a or minimal N1b disease
High risk	Regional extensive disease (extensive N1b) or locally invasive disease (T4 tumors), with or without distant metastasis

developed secondary to RAI exposure. Overall, despite a 16-fold increased use of RAI over the study time frame, between 1973 and 2008, there was no improvement in overall disease-specific mortality which was >98%.

Based on this data, the 2015 ATA management guidelines for children with thyroid nodules and DTC recommended stratifying pediatric patients with DTC into three risk categories—low risk, intermediate risk, and high risk—based on the extent of the primary tumor and LN and distant metastases to promote the use of RAI ablation in patients with more advanced disease, rather than all patients, in an attempt to reduce long-term morbidity from therapy that in many patients may be unnecessary[48] (Table 29.3).

Postoperative staging should be performed within 6 to 12 weeks after surgery to help identify patients who may benefit from further interventions, including additional surgery or RAI therapy. ATA pediatric low-risk patients may be initially assessed and followed with TSH-suppressed Tg alone. A TSH-stimulated Tg and diagnostic whole-body scan (DxWBS) should be performed in ATA pediatric intermediate and high-risk patients to evaluate for persistent disease. ^{123}I should be used for DxWBS whenever possible. If RAI uptake is identified, further imaging, including US or single-photon emission computed tomography/computed tomography (SPECT/CT), may be used to further evaluate and define regions of uptake.

Therapeutic RAI is recommended for the treatment of iodine-avid persistent locoregional and nodal disease that cannot be readily resected as well as when avid distal metastases are present. RAI uptake is improved with a TSH level above 30 mIU/L; this can be achieved for most children by withdrawing LT3 or LT4 for 2 weeks. Children with functional thyroid cancer, thyroid cancer that produces T3 and T4, or with reduced pituitary function (ie. survivors of a non-thyroid primary malignancy with pituitary dysfunction) may require recombinant human TSH (rhTSH) to achieve a TSH > 30 mIU/L.[49,50] In children, data are lacking regarding whether outcomes are different using empiric RAI dosing or dosimetry. Dosimetry may be particularly useful for children <10 years of age, in children who exhibit distant metastases that are likely to require additional RAI treatments, or children with limited bone marrow reserve. A posttreatment DxWBS should be performed for all children 4 to 7 days after completing RAI therapy to identify additional regions of uptake that may not have been visualized on the DxWBS. The addition of SPECT/CT may help better define anatomic locations of focal uptake.

When children exhibit persistent disease after initial RAI ablation therapy, the decision to pursue additional RAI therapy or other therapies is individualized and should be based on available clinical data (Tg trend and change in size and/or number of lesions being followed with serial radiologic imaging), weighing the risks and benefits of further RAI.

The recent ATA guidelines have helped with risk stratification and decision making regarding the use of RAI after thyroid surgery in children with well-differentiated thyroid cancers. It may be appropriate not to offer RAI in select low-risk children to avoid unnecessary toxicity and secondary malignancy where there is no clear benefit from the exposure. Families should be educated regarding the benefits and risks of RAI, both short- and long-term, and included in the decision about whether to proceed with RAI therapy.

Follow-Up

The treatment goal is to achieve negative radiologic imaging (whole-body scan or negative neck US) and a Tg level below the level of detection. Once this has been accomplished, yearly follow-up with a physical examination, cervical neck US, Tg and anti-Tg level on LT4 therapy (when antibody-negative on thyroid hormone suppressive therapy), and serum TSH should be performed.[48] Differing approaches to surveillance should be used based on the initial degree of invasiveness and surveillance data. For patients with disease limited to the thyroid and central neck, a basal Tg and neck US may be adequate to define remission. In contrast, for patients with pulmonary metastasis, a TSH-stimulated Tg and DxWBS should be considered to define remission. Based on historic data showing an increased risk of long-term recurrence, lifelong surveillance with intermittent ultrasonography and TSH and Tg levels should be pursued.[81]

Currently, we remain somewhat limited in our knowledge of how to treat children with detectable serum Tg but negative imaging studies.[98] One can hope that genetic and molecular markers such as BRAF, RET/PTC, and RAS, among others, may better help us stratify risk among children in the future (see Chapter 18, Molecular Pathogenesis of Thyroid Neoplasia). Lifelong follow-up with special attention to secondary malignancies in children who have been treated with RAI is essential.

Diffuse Sclerosing Variant PTC

DSVPTC was first described by Vickery and colleagues in 1985[99] and represents only about 0.7% to 6.6% of papillary thyroid cases overall.[100] However, DSVPTC represents a larger proportion of thyroid cancer cases in children and adolescents, approaching up to 41% of cases in some series.[38] DSVPTC is more invasive than CPTC and is associated with increased risk of LN metastases (see Figures 29.1 and 29.2), diffuse or multifocal involvement of the thyroid gland (see Figure 29.3), lymphovascular invasion, extrathyroidal extension, nerve invasion, and increased risk of locoregional recurrence after initial treatment.[100-102]

Because of diffuse gland involvement, DSVPTC may present as enlargement of the gland without a discrete mass, highlighting the importance of US imaging in children presenting with thyroid enlargement and goiter. US characteristics concerning DSVPTC include solid composition, poorly defined margins, heterogeneous echotexture, and scattered microcalcifications[101] (see Figure 29.3). Microscopically, in addition to showing nuclear features of PTC, DSVPTC also demonstrates squamous metaplasia, numerous psammoma bodies, fibrosis, and lymphocytic infiltration.[100] Lymphocytic thyroiditis and Hashimoto's thyroiditis are associated with DSVPTC, with up to 85% of patients demonstrating positive antithyroglobulin antibodies.[101,103] Compared with CPTC, DSVPTC shows higher rates of RET/PTC rearrangement[100,104] and less frequent BRAF and rare RAS mutations.[104] RET/PTC3 mutations are associated with a higher risk of advanced disease at presentation and persistent disease, whereas RET/PTC1 mutations are associated with improved remission rates after RAI therapy.[104]

Up to 80% of patients with DSVPTC have clinical evidence of LN metastases at diagnosis,[101,102] and up to 40% to 50.4%[102,105] have extrathyroidal extension. Younger patients with DSVPTC are more likely to have LN metastases and distant metastases than older patients with this variant.[106] Rates of distant metastases range from 5% to 14.9%[100-102,107]; metastatic disease most commonly affects the lungs.

Overall, the risk of recurrence approaches 14% to 22%[101,102] and disease specific mortality is approximately 3%.[100] The presence of lateral LN metastases is significantly associated with a risk of recurrence.[101] Tumor size and extrathyroidal extension have been associated with a shorter time to recurrence.[38] Some series have suggested a poorer prognosis compared with low-risk, classical type PTC,[108] whereas other studies have suggested no difference in overall or disease-free survival, despite these more aggressive features, with proper surgical management followed by RAI therapy.[106,107] Compared with classical-type PTC, Malandrino et al. noted an up to three times higher risk of recurrence in patients with DSVPTC; however, when the study was restricted to patients who received postoperative RAI, the risk of recurrence was no longer significantly elevated.[106]

Providers caring for children with thyroid cancer must be aware of DSVPTC and recognize when this variant may be present at the time of presentation, allowing for proper preoperative imaging to identify LN and distant metastases. This allows for appropriate surgical planning and management as well as proper postoperative care to minimize the risk of recurrent disease. Given the high rate of recurrence in this population, long-term follow-up is recommended.

SUMMARY

Thyroid cancer in children and adolescents is less common than in adult patients. Providers caring for children with thyroid disease must be knowledgeable about the unique pathology and behavior of pediatric thyroid cancers, including DSVPTC, as well as the ATA guidelines (https://www.thyroid.org/professionals/ata-professional-guidelines/) for the treatment of pediatric DTC and MTC. Treatment of most childhood PTCs should entail total or near-total thyroidectomy and appropriate nodal resection (not "berry picking"). Every effort should be made to preserve parathyroid and RLN function, and neural monitoring is recommended. Surgery should be performed by a high-volume surgeon and all care provided by an experienced multidisciplinary team composed of endocrinology, radiology, pathology, and behavioral health specialists familiar the unique aspects involved in caring for pediatric patients. These efforts are targeted to minimize surgical and adjuvant treatment morbidity while maintaining low recurrence and low disease-specific mortality. RAI benefits children in intermediate and high ATA risk categories, including those with more aggressive tumor variants and invasive behavior. More work is needed to better understand pediatric tumor genetics and outcomes to further individualize treatment plans and optimize long-term outcomes.

REFERENCES

For a complete list of references, go to expertconsult.com.

Familial Nonmedullary Thyroid Cancer

Wilson Alobuia, Aarti Mathur, Electron Kebebew

INTRODUCTION

In 1955, Robinson and Orr published the first report of isolated familial papillary thyroid cancer affecting 24-year-old identical twins.[1] Twenty years later, Němec and colleagues described differentiated thyroid cancer without environmental exposures in a mother and son.[2] Since that time, numerous reports have been published describing families with thyroid cancer of follicular cell origin without other familial syndromes. Population-based studies have established that individuals with a close relative with thyroid cancer have a five- to nine-fold increased risk of developing thyroid cancer. The familial clustering of thyroid cancers of follicular cell origin is now recognized as a discrete entity called *familial nonmedullary thyroid cancer (FNMTC)*, which is characterized by distinct clinicopathologic characteristics. This chapter reviews the epidemiology, classification, clinical features, genetics, treatment, prognosis, and outcomes of FNMTC.

EPIDEMIOLOGY

A familial occurrence and association with multiple endocrine neoplasia (MEN) types 2A and 2B have been well described for medullary thyroid cancer.[3] FNMTCs are nonmedullary cancers that arise from thyroid follicular cells with four predominant histologic subtypes: papillary (85%), follicular (11%), Hürthle (3%), and anaplastic (1%).[4,5] Although the majority of cases are sporadic, numerous reports have described familial clustering, now known as FNMTC, which accounts for 3.2% to 9.6% of all thyroid cancer cases.[6-10]

CLASSIFICATION OF FAMILIAL DISEASE

Currently, FNMTC is defined by the presence of well-differentiated thyroid cancer of follicular cell origin in two or more first-degree relatives in the absence of other predisposing hereditary or environmental causes. However, statistical estimates by Charkes suggest that 62% to 69% of cases with only two affected family members may, in fact, be sporadic. The likelihood of sporadic disease falls to less than 6% in families with three or more affected members.[11] Furthermore, patients with FNMTC from families with ≥3 affected members (compared with those with 2 affected family members) have been shown to have a statistically significant higher risk of bilateral/multifocal thyroid disease, extrathyroidal extension, lateral lymph node metastasis, and an overall worse prognosis compared with patients with sporadic disease.

FNMTC encompasses a heterogeneous group of nonsporadic diseases in isolation but also occurs as part of a syndromic complex. Familial syndromes with a known FNMTC association include familial adenomatous polyposis (FAP), Gardner syndrome, Cowden disease, Carney complex type 1, Werner syndrome, and papillary renal neoplasia, or may occur in isolation (i.e., without other syndromic association).[12-24] McCune-Albright syndrome, Peutz-Jeghers syndrome, and ataxia-telangiectasia (Louis-Bar syndrome) may also be associated with the development of FNMTC, but there are more limited data linking these syndromes with FNMTC.[25-27] Known clinical characteristics and genetic causes of some of these syndromes are shown in Table 30.1.

Evidence that FNMTC is a distinct entity caused by an inherited genetic predisposition comes in large part from epidemiologic and kindred studies that demonstrate an increase in familial clustering of nonmedullary thyroid cancers (FNMTC) affecting multiple generations.

Several epidemiologic studies have documented a 5- to 10-fold increased risk of thyroid cancer in the first-degree relatives of subjects with FNMTC.[24,28,29] In a population-based case-control interview study of 159 cases of thyroid cancer with 285 age- and sex-matched controls in Connecticut, the odds ratio of a first-degree relative developing thyroid cancer was 5.2 times that of the general population.[28] A Utah population database study demonstrated an increased relative risk (8.6, 95% confidence interval [CI], 4.7 to 13.7) of thyroid cancer in first-degree relatives of thyroid cancer subjects.[29] Similarly, a Canadian analysis of 339 patient pedigrees compared with 319 unaffected ethnically matched controls found that 5% of patients with NMTC reported at least one first-degree relative with thyroid cancer.[24] A population-based study of the Swedish cancer registry demonstrated that the risk of developing thyroid cancer in a given individual is higher when the affected family member is a sibling and is even higher when the sibling is an affected sister.[30] The relative risk of developing papillary thyroid cancer (PTC) was 3.21 when a parent was diagnosed with thyroid cancer and 6.24 when a sibling was diagnosed with thyroid cancer. The relative risk was the highest when the two affected siblings were sisters (relative risk, 11.9). From an affected mother, the risk was equally high for sons and daughters; however, when either parent was diagnosed with thyroid cancer, the risk for sons was 4.98 (95% CI, 2.13 to 9.86) and for daughters 3.44 (95% CI, 1.96 to 5.60).

A major drawback of population-based studies is that they cannot control for a selection bias or for confounding factors such as environmental exposures (e.g., radiation exposure, or iodine deficiency or excess) that might contribute to a higher risk of thyroid cancer. However, FNMTC has also been reported in large multigenerational kindreds with up to 16 family members affected and where environmental factors were not uniform.

These studies of affected familial groups also demonstrate characteristics that appear to be unique compared with sporadic disease, further supporting the fact that FNMTC is a distinct entity. These

TABLE 30.1 Syndromes Associated With FNMTC: Clinical Characteristics and Genetic Causes of Syndromes

Name	Responsible Gene/Mutation	Histologic Subtype of Thyroid Cancer	Extrathyroidal Clinical Characteristics
Familial adenomatous polyposis (FAP)	Inactivating mutations of APC	PTC with cribriform pattern	Multiple adenomatous polyps with malignant potential lining mucosa of GI tract, particularly colon
Gardner syndrome	Inactivating mutations of APC	PTC with cribriform pattern	Variant of FAP with extracolonic manifestations (supernumerary teeth, fibrous dysplasia, fibromas, desmoid tumors, epithelial cysts, hypertrophic retinal pigment epithelium, upper GI tract hamartomas, hepatoblastomas)
Cowden disease	PTEN	FTC	Hamartomas of the breast, colon, endometrium, and brain
Werner syndrome	WRN	PTC, FTC, ATC	Premature aging, scleroderma-like skin changes, cataracts, subcutaneous calcifications, muscular atrophy, and diabetes
McCune-Albright syndrome	GNAS1	PTC, clear cell	Café-au-lait skin pigmentation, polyostotic fibrous dysplasia, and hyperfunctioning endocrinopathies (precocious puberty, hyperthyroidism, growth hormone excess, and Cushing's syndrome)
Carney complex	PRKAR1α	PTC, FTC	Myxomas of soft tissues; skin and mucosal pigmentation (blue nevi); schwannomas, tumors of the adrenal, pituitary, and testicle

APC, PTC, papillary thyroid cancer, GI, FTC, follicular thyroid cancer, ATC, anaplastic thyroid cancer.

include association with second site malignancy, younger age at presentation (30 ± 11), and a higher rate of affected males than in sporadic cases. For example, a metareview of 15 case reports described a median age of 39 years and a male-to-female ratio of 1:2.2.[31] FNMTC, unlike sporadic cancers, has been associated with nonthyroid adenocarcinomas. Pal and colleagues found that the incidence of any type of cancer was 38% higher in relatives of patients with thyroid cancer.[24] The Utah population database revealed a highly significant association between thyroid tumors with familial clustering and leukemia, and breast, prostate, and soft tissue tumors.[29] Similarly, other studies have demonstrated an association with breast, kidney, colon, and bladder cancers, and melanoma and lymphoma.[32,33] When comparing 47 cases of first- and second-generation FNMTC patients, Capezzone and colleagues found that offspring show an earlier age at disease onset and have more aggressive disease compared with their parents, a feature known as *genetic anticipation*.[34] This phenomenon is defined as the occurrence of a genetic disorder at progressively earlier ages and with increased severity in successive generations and is characteristic of inherited neoplasia. In a prospective screening of at-risk family members, thyroid cancer was detected in 4.6% of kindreds with two affected family members compared with 22.7% in kindreds with three or more first-degree relatives.[35] These data taken together suggest that FNMTC is a true familial disease rather than a chance occurrence of sporadic disease, especially in families with three or more first-degree relatives affected.

CLINICAL FEATURES

Most studies suggest that FNMTC is more aggressive than sporadic thyroid cancer of follicular cell origin with higher rates of extrathyroidal invasion, multicentric tumors, lymph node metastasis, and recurrence rates.[36] It is also often associated with concomitant benign thyroid pathologies. Uchino and colleagues identified 258 patients from 154 families and found that compared with patients with sporadic disease, the FNMTC group had significantly higher rates of coexistent benign thyroid tumors, multicentric tumors, and lymph node metastasis.[37] The 30-year rate of recurrence in local lymph nodes was about 40% for FNMTC compared with 20% in the sporadic cases. There was also a higher recurrence rate and worse disease-free survival in this group. There was no difference in age at diagnosis, primary tumor size, rate of extrathyroidal invasion, distant metastasis, or overall survival between the two groups. However, this study diagnosed patients with FNMTC when at least one first-degree relative was affected by thyroid cancer, thereby possibly including cases of sporadic disease as FNMTC.

A retrospective review of 14 patients with FNMTC found a 93% rate of multicentricity and a 43% rate of bilateral disease.[32] Patients with FNMTC had higher rates of extrathyroidal invasion in 57% compared with 5% to 14% in sporadic cases in addition to an increased recurrence rate of 50%.[32] Another large cohort study with a multicenter case-matched design found a higher recurrence rate of 44% compared with 17% in its control group.[38] The researchers also found that the median disease-free survival rate was significantly shorter for patients with FNMTC compared with their matched controls. The number of family members affected with thyroid cancer and distant metastasis is a known significant predictor of disease severity and disease-free survival in familial cases.[35] Perhaps the most compelling study to demonstrate the aggressive nature of FNMTC is the descriptive study by Lupoli and colleagues of 119 patients with papillary thyroid microcarcinoma, of which seven had FNMTC.[39] The rates of tumor multicentricity, bilobar disease, lymph node metastasis, vascular invasion, and recurrence rates are all significantly higher compared with sporadic cases. Despite the multiple studies suggesting an aggressive nature of FNMTC, not all investigators have found this to be the case. Ito and associates found no difference in disease-free survival after comparing 273 patients with FNMTC to sporadic cases of PTC.[40] The patients with familial PTC had a higher rate of multicentricity but no difference in overall prognosis compared with sporadic cases. The authors also found six families with presumptive familial follicular thyroid cancer (FTC), a prevalence of 1.9%.[41] Aggressive features such as extrathyroidal invasion, tumor size, and lymph node and distant metastases, as well as overall prognosis, did not differ from those with sporadic FTC. A metareview conducted by Loh also did not demonstrate a more aggressive biology when evaluating rates of multicentricity, local invasion, lymph node and distant metastases, and recurrence rates.[31]

TUMOR HISTOLOGY

Familial PTC is the most common type of FNMTC, followed by Hürthle cell carcinoma, then FTC. Familial PTC is characterized by multicentric tumors without any distinguishing pathologic features and multiple adenomatous nodules with or without oxyphilia.[42-45]

Familial Adenomatous Polyposis

Thyroid cancer associated with FAP is usually bilateral and multifocal with a prognosis similar to sporadic PTC.[46,47] The histologic features are different from sporadic tumors with the characteristic cribriform pattern having solid areas and a spindle-cell component most often associated with marked fibrosis. The cribriform-morular variant is a rare subtype of PTC in this patient population accounting for approximately 0.1% to 0.2% of cases.[16]

Cowden Disease

Multiple adenomatous nodules are a characteristic finding in Cowden disease.[48] Gross examination reveals firm yellow-tan, well-circumscribed nodules diffusely involving the thyroid gland. Microscopically, they appear as well-circumscribed, nonencapsulated solid cellular nodules sharing features similar to follicular adenomas. Some nodules may have a discontinuous rim of fibrous tissue simulating a capsule. Multiple follicular adenomas are common in Cowden disease. Follicular carcinomas may also arise from a preexisting follicular adenoma. PTC has rarely been associated with this disease.[48]

Werner Syndrome

Patients with this syndrome have an increased risk of a variety of neoplasias, including benign thyroid lesions and an increased rate of PTC (only type of thyroid cancer present in Caucasian patients), followed by FTC (14%), and anaplastic thyroid cancer (ATC) (2%).[21,44,49,50]

Carney Complex

The thyroid gland is usually multinodular with multiple adenomatous nodules, follicular adenomas, and both PTC and FTC are present in about 15% of patients with Carney complex.[22]

GENETICS OF FNMTC

Syndromic

FNMTC encompasses thyroid cancer cases associated with other hereditary cancer syndromes (syndromic) for which many of the susceptibility genes are known (see Table 30.1).

Familial Adenomatous Polyposis

FAP is caused by germline mutations in the adenomatous polyposis coli (*APC*) gene on chromosome 5q21.[15] It is characterized by the development of multiple adenomatous polyps with malignant potential lining the mucosa of the gastrointestinal tract, particularly the colon, with an early age of onset and a nearly 100% lifetime risk of colorectal cancer.[51] Extracolonic manifestations in FAP include osteomas, epidermal cysts, desmoid tumors, upper gastrointestinal tract hamartomatous polyps, congenital hypertrophy of the retinal pigmented epithelium (CHRPE), hepatoblastomas, and thyroid tumors. Thyroid nodules can be found in 38% of patients with FAP,[52] with a diagnosis of thyroid cancer preceding a diagnosis of FAP in one-third of patients.[46] In patients with FAP, thyroid cancer occurs at about 10 times greater frequency than that expected for sporadic cases.[42] Among these patients, PTC occurs with a frequency of about 0.7% to 12%.[47,52,53] Isolated FTC and concomitant PTC and FTC are the most commonly seen thyroid cancers in FAP, although one case of medullary thyroid cancer has also been reported in a patient with FAP.[46] Young women with FAP have a 160 times higher risk for PTC than other individuals.

The majority of *APC* mutations are either frame-shift or nonsense mutations leading to a truncated protein.[54] However, most female patients with FAP and PTC also have a *RET/PTC* somatic mutation in addition to the *APC* germline mutation.[14,51]

There are three subtypes of FAP: (1) Gardner syndrome, caused by mutations in the *APC* tumor suppressor gene; (2) Turcot syndrome type 1, a rare autosomal recessive disorder caused by a mutation in two DNA mismatch repair genes, *MLH1* and *PMS 2*; and (3) Turcot syndrome type 2 (Crail's syndrome), an autosomal-dominant syndrome secondary to the mutations in the *APC* gene. The MLH1 and PMS2 proteins form a complex that coordinates with other proteins to repair mistakes that arise during DNA replication.

The overall prognosis of FAP-related NMTC is excellent. NMTC in patients with FAP is usually multifocal and bilateral, with rare metastases and a prognosis similar to sporadic cases.[42,47] Only one case of distant metastasis to the spine was observed among 36 patients (2.7%) with FAP-associated NMTC.[46] In another study, thyroid cancer was described as a cause of death in 1 of 45 patients with FAP.[55] The recommended treatment for FAP-associated NMTC is a total or near-total thyroidectomy.

Gardner Syndrome

This is a variant of FAP, polyposis of the large bowel, associated with extracolonic manifestations of supernumerary teeth, fibrous dysplasia of the skull, osteomas of the mandible, fibromas, desmoid tumors, epithelial cysts, hypertrophic retinal pigment epithelium, upper gastrointestinal hamartomas, hepatoblastomas, and thyroid tumors. Thyroid neoplasms occur at a younger age and mostly in females. The overall risk of developing thyroid cancer is about 2%.[17-19]

Cowden Disease

This autosomal dominant disorder is associated with a mutation in the *PTEN* tumor suppressor gene on chromosome 10q22-23.[56] It is characterized by hamartomas and other tumors of the thyroid, breast, colon, endometrium, and brain. The most frequent extracutaneous manifestations of this disease are thyroid neoplasms, both benign as well as FTCs, occurring in approximately two-thirds of the subjects.[20,56]

Werner Syndrome (Adult Progeria)

This autosomal recessive disease, also known as *adult progeria*, has been linked to mutations of the *WRN* gene on chromosome 8p11-p12. The *WRN* gene is critical in the replication and repair of DNA, mutations of which lead to truncated, nonfunctional WRN proteins and thus slower, decreased cell division. It is characterized by premature aging, scleroderma-like skin changes, cataracts, subcutaneous calcifications, muscular atrophy, diabetes, and a high incidence of malignant neoplasms. A systematic review of published Werner syndrome cases showed the frequency of thyroid neoplasms to be 16.1% among all patients diagnosed.[57] The relative risk of developing FNMTC was estimated to be 8.9% for Japanese residents with Werner syndrome.[57] Among patients with Werner syndrome, thyroid cancer occurs at a young age and is predominantly follicular, although papillary and ATCs may also occur.[21]

Carney Complex

This autosomal dominant disease is caused by germline mutations of the *PRKAR1A* gene located on chromosome 17q24.2 (type 1) or chromosome 2p16 (type 2). The *PRKAR1A* gene codes for a regulatory alpha subunit of protein kinase A, an enzyme that promotes cell growth. It is characterized by myxomas of the soft tissues, skin, and mucosal pigmentation (blue nevi); schwannomas; and tumors of the adrenal gland, pituitary, and testicle. Major diagnostic criteria for Carney complex include the presence of thyroid cancer at any age or multiple hypoechogenic nodules on thyroid ultrasound in a prepubertal child.[58] Thyroid gland disease occurs in approximately 11% of patients and includes adenomatous hyperplasia, cysts, and PTC or FTC.[22] Up to 60% of all individuals with Carney complex may have thyroid nodules detected by ultrasound, and two-thirds of them occur in children and adolescents.[59,60] Thyroid nodules appear during the first 10 years of life.[61] In general, the life span is decreased in patients with Carney complex, with the major cause of death (57%) being cardiovascular complications from the disease. Fourteen percent of patients reportedly die of cancer progression, but thyroid cancer as a cause of death has not been reported.[58]

Pendred Syndrome

Described as a disease of "deaf-mutism and goiter," Pendred syndrome was first described by Pendred in 1896. The syndrome is inherited in an autosomal recessive fashion and is primarily caused by germline mutations in three genes: *SLC26A4, FOXI1,* and *KCNJ10*. Thyroid involvement ranges from minimal enlargement to large multinodular goiters and thyroid cancer.[62] The prevalence of thyroid cancer in Pendred syndrome is estimated to be 1%, with FTC being the most common histologic subtype,[63] although a follicular variant of PTC, metastatic FTC, and anaplastic transformation from FTC have all been reported.[64-67]

Nonsyndromic FNMTC

Review of the different kindreds and the genetic studies suggests that nonsyndromic FNMTC inheritance is autosomal-dominant with incomplete penetrance and variable expressivity. However, the causative genes predisposing to FNMTC have not yet been identified.

Linkage analyses have identified five different chromosomal regions that may harbor putative susceptibility genes for the development of nonsyndromic FNMTC (Table 30.2). The first study by the French NMTC Consortium identified the thyroid cancer with oxyphilia (TCO1) locus on chromosome 19p13.2 in a French family with oxyphilic thyroid tumors.[68] An Australian group identified NMTC1 on 2q21 in a Tasmanian kindred with follicular variants of PTC.[69] The PRN1 locus on chromosome 1q21 was identified in an American kindred with PTC, nodular thyroid disease, and papillary renal neoplasia.[70] Attempts to validate these results have been met with varying success. In particular, the TCO1 and NMTC1 loci have been confirmed in a few independent families, and there is some evidence to suggest that the two loci may, in fact, interact with one another, further increasing the risk of thyroid cancer.[69,71] Novel variants of *TIMM44*, a gene that maps to the TCO locus, appear to cosegregate with the TCO phenotype, although in vitro functional experiments suggest that they do not lead to loss of function.[72] When evaluated in tumor specimens from patients with FNTMC, the loss of heterozygosity at the TCO and NMTC1 loci was demonstrated in some but not all specimens.[73]

These findings suggest that alterations at TCO and NMTC1 are important only in a fraction of cases with FNMTC, which is not surprising as most cases are PTC, rather than TCO (Hürthle cell) or a follicular variant of PTC. Prazeres and colleagues reported the finding of loss of heterozygosity at the 19p13.2 and 2q21 loci in tumors from familial clusters of NMTC, providing evidence that the inactivation of putative tumor suppressor genes in these regions may be involved in the development of FNMTC.[74] In contrast, the de novo linkage analysis studies on FNMTC family cohorts have shown little to no linkage to suggest the presence of chromosomal susceptibility loci. These conflicting results underscore the main limitations of the positive studies mentioned earlier. They were characterized in one or a few affected families, and all but one examined rare variants of FNMTC. Linkage analyses have excluded *MNG1, TCO,* and *RET* as major genes of susceptibility to FNMTC and have demonstrated that this trait is characterized by genetic heterogeneity.[75]

Another approach used to understand the genetics of FNMTC is to identify and characterize common somatic mutations associated with thyroid cancer of follicular cell origin and determine whether they occur as germline mutations in FNMTC. Such studies have excluded the presence of germline mutations of genes associated with sporadic thyroid cancers, including *BRAF, RET, RET/PTC, MET, MEK1, MEK2, RAS,* and *NTRK*.[73,76] Although no germline mutations were found, Cavaco and colleagues observed a similar prevalence and distribution in the common somatic mutations (*RAS* and *BRAF*).[73] The investigators suggest that these somatic mutations may be involved in tumor progression in FNMTC.

A Portuguese group, using a single-nucleotide polymorphism (SNP) array platform, recently identified a locus on 8p23.1-p22 in a Portuguese FNMTC family.[77] A susceptibility locus on 8q24 was also identified in a large family with PTC, and melanoma and was subsequently validated in 25 additional families without a history of melanoma.[78] Another group also performed an SNP array-based linkage analysis of 38 families and found linkage on 1q21 and 6q22.[79] A large genome-wide association study in Iceland compared SNP array profiles of 192 patients with PTC or FTC to healthy controls and identified strong association signals at markers on 9q22.33 and 14q13.3.[80] A genome-wide linkage analysis in a family pedigree including 13 affected members with PTC or ATC across three different generations identified a locus on 4q32.[81]

It is currently unclear whether such population-based study results can be extrapolated to the narrower cohort of families with FNMTC.

An alternative approach is to study the telomere-telomerase complex based on previous reports of high telomerase activity and short

TABLE 30.2 Susceptibility Loci for Nonsyndromic FNMTC

Tumor Type	Chromosome Location	Candidate Gene	Ref.
Familial papillary thyroid cancer with papillary renal cell neoplasia (fPTC/PRN)	1q21	Unknown	70
Familial papillary thyroid cancer	2q21	Unknown	69
FNMTC	6q22	Unknown	79
Familial papillary thyroid cancer	8q24	Unknown	78
Familial papillary thyroid cancer with oxyphilia (TCO)	19p13.2	TIMM44	68

FNMTC, familial nonmedullary thyroid cancer.

telomere length in the development of other types of cancers. Capezzone and colleagues evaluated the telomere-telomerase complex in the peripheral blood of patients with FNMTC and found that relative telomere length was significantly shorter, whereas hTERT mRNA expression and telomerase activity were significantly higher in patients with FNMTC.[82] The relative telomere length of patients of the second generation was similar to that of the parents and was significantly shorter, compared with unaffected siblings. This demonstrates that an imbalance of the telomere-telomerase complex may have a role to play in FNTMC.

SCREENING AND SURVEILLANCE

Syndromic FNMTC

Among patients with syndromic FNMTC, there are no clear recommendations regarding screening. All young patients with thyroid cancer should be examined clinically for other manifestations of syndromic disease, and a meticulous family history should be taken to rule out other possible syndromes.

In patients with FAP, annual surveillance with a physical examination or thyroid ultrasound has been recommended. The American College of Gastroenterology recommends an annual thyroid ultrasound in individuals with FAP, *MUTYH*-associated polyposis, and attenuated polyposis (conditional recommendation, low quality of evidence.)[83] When thyroid nodules are detected, total thyroidectomy is recommended, as hemithyroidectomy carries a risk of recurrent thyroid cancer.

In patients with Carney complex, a thyroid ultrasound is recommended as a baseline examination and is a satisfactory, cost-effective method for determining thyroid involvement in pediatric and young adult patients.[59,60] Thyroid ultrasound may be repeated in regular intervals as needed.

Given the high prevalence of NMTC in Werner syndrome and the high rate of more aggressive histologic subtypes, screening and surveillance for thyroid nodules and NMTC by thyroid ultrasound is justified.[84]

Thyroid ultrasound evaluation and routine thyroid examination in patients with hypothyroidism and Pendred syndrome may be recommended for early identification of NMTC. There is no role for routine prophylactic thyroidectomy in patients with Pendred syndrome, but thyroidectomy should be considered in hypothyroid patients with thyroid nodules.

Nonsyndromic FNMTC

Screening programs in patients at risk of cancer are usually recommended when the risk of cancer (penetrance) is high, and when the results of the screening will direct subsequent treatment and improve the outcome, mortality, or quality of life of patients as a result of early detection. It is important, however, to realize that active screening can be expensive and may be associated with the risk of overtreatment.

Currently, there are no definite screening and/or surveillance recommendations for FNMTC. A prospective cohort study of 25 kindreds (12 families with 2 members affected, and 13 with 3 or more members affected) was recently performed to determine the utility of screening using yearly neck ultrasound and fine-needle aspiration (FNA) biopsy of thyroid nodules in at-risk individuals whose relatives were diagnosed with FNMTC.[35] In this population of patients, screening led to an earlier detection of low-risk disease (smaller tumor size, low rate of central neck lymph node metastases) and was associated with a less aggressive initial treatment (lower rates of total thyroidectomy, use of radioactive iodine ablation). Based on these findings we recommend the following:

1. Screening with thyroid ultrasound should be considered in kindreds with three or more first-degree relatives affected by FNMTC.
2. Screening should begin 10 years before the peak incidence or before the earliest age of the diagnosis in the family, whichever occurs first.
3. Screening should be performed in all generations of kindreds affected by FNMTC at regular intervals (every 2 to 3 years).

The findings of this study provide a framework for the development of screening guidelines for patients with FNMTC.

TREATMENT

A total or near-total thyroidectomy with a prophylactic central neck lymph node dissection is the best surgical treatment for patients with FNMTC because these patients, theoretically at least, have the remaining "normal" follicular cells predisposed to tumor formation, and they also have a high rate of multicentric disease. They may, based on the majority of clinical studies, have more aggressive disease with extrathyroidal invasion, lymph node metastasis, and higher recurrence rates. A therapeutic lateral lymph node neck dissection should be performed only if lymph node involvement is observed by preoperative imaging or by physical examination. We also recommend high-dose radioiodine ablation I-131 after a thyroidectomy because of the higher risk of recurrence associated with FNMTC in most studies. Although there are no data to compare treatment approaches in this patient population, the advantage of such an aggressive approach is similar to that observed for patients with sporadic disease in that it renders basal or stimulated serum thyroglobulin levels more sensitive for postoperative surveillance for persistent/recurrent disease and may be associated with a lower recurrence rate.

PROGNOSIS/OUTCOME

Despite the aggressive treatment approach used in most cases of FNMTC, up to 12% of patients will have persistent disease after an operation, and 44% will develop recurrent disease requiring multiple operations.[5,38] Several studies have tried to examine the effects of FNMTC on disease-free and overall survival (Table 30.3). These studies are limited by the fact that the overall mortality rate for all differentiated thyroid cancer is low and would require a large patient population and extended follow-up time to show any difference between groups. However, a retrospective study of 139 affected patients compared with 757 unaffected family members found that the survival of patients with FNMTC who had been treated was similar to that of their unaffected family members.[85] Survival was, however, significantly shorter for patients with three or more affected family members and for patients diagnosed before the familial setting was recognized. This would suggest that earlier treatment among patients with FNMTC may improve survival. Uchino et al. also examined survival in their large case series and found that disease-free survival was significantly shorter for patients with FNMTC than for patients with sporadic disease. However, there was no difference in overall survival.[37]

CHAPTER 30 Familial Nonmedullary Thyroid Cancer

TABLE 30.3 Summary of Outcome Studies in Patients With FNMTC

Author	Sample Size	Study Type	Type of Thyroid Cancer	Extent of Disease Difference in Patients With FNMTC Versus Sporadic	Difference in Recurrence Rate in FNMTC Versus Sporadic	Overall Survival
Uchino, et al.[37]	258	Retrospective	Papillary or follicular carcinoma	Increased intraglandular dissemination versus sporadic (40.7% versus 28.5%) Additional multiple benign nodules versus sporadic cases (41.5% versus 29.8%)	Recurrence rate 16.3% (versus 9.6% sporadic)	No difference
Grossman, et al.[32]	14	Retrospective	Papillary (13) and Hürthle cell (1) carcinoma	Presented with larger primary tumor (2.7 cm versus 2 to 2.2 cm) Multifocal (93%) Invasion beyond thyroid capsule (57%) Metastasis to regional lymph nodes (57%)	Recurrence rate 50%	Not assessed
Alsanea, et al.[38]	48	Retrospective matched-case control	Papillary (45) and Hürthle cell (3)	Younger age at presentation (39 ± 11 versus 46 ± 15)	Recurrence rate 44% (versus 17%)	No difference
Lupoli, et al.[39]	119 (7 with FNMTC)	Retrospective	Papillary microcarcinoma	Increased multicentricity (72%) Lymph node metastases (43%) Local and vascular invasion (43%)	Recurrence rate 43%	Difference not assessed
Triponez, et al.[85]	139	Retrospective	Papillary follicular Hürthle cell anaplastic	Not assessed	Not assessed	Shorter survival for patients with three or more affected family members diagnosed before familial setting recognized

FNMTC, familial nonmedullary thyroid cancer.

SUMMARY

Familial NMTC accounts for approximately 5% of all thyroid cancers. It is defined by the presence of thyroid cancer of follicular origin in two or more first-degree relatives. FNMTC is associated with an early age at onset, an increased incidence of multifocality, and aggressive tumor biology compared with sporadic tumors. Patients typically have a worse prognosis than those with sporadic tumors. Therefore aggressive treatment is warranted and should consist of at least a total or near-total thyroidectomy with central lymph node dissection and a therapeutic lateral neck dissection, only for clinically-positive lymph nodes. It is important to identify the causative genes to allow for better risk stratification, early detection, and management of FNMTC.

REFERENCES

For a complete list of references, go to expertconsult.com.

Thyroid and Neck Surgery

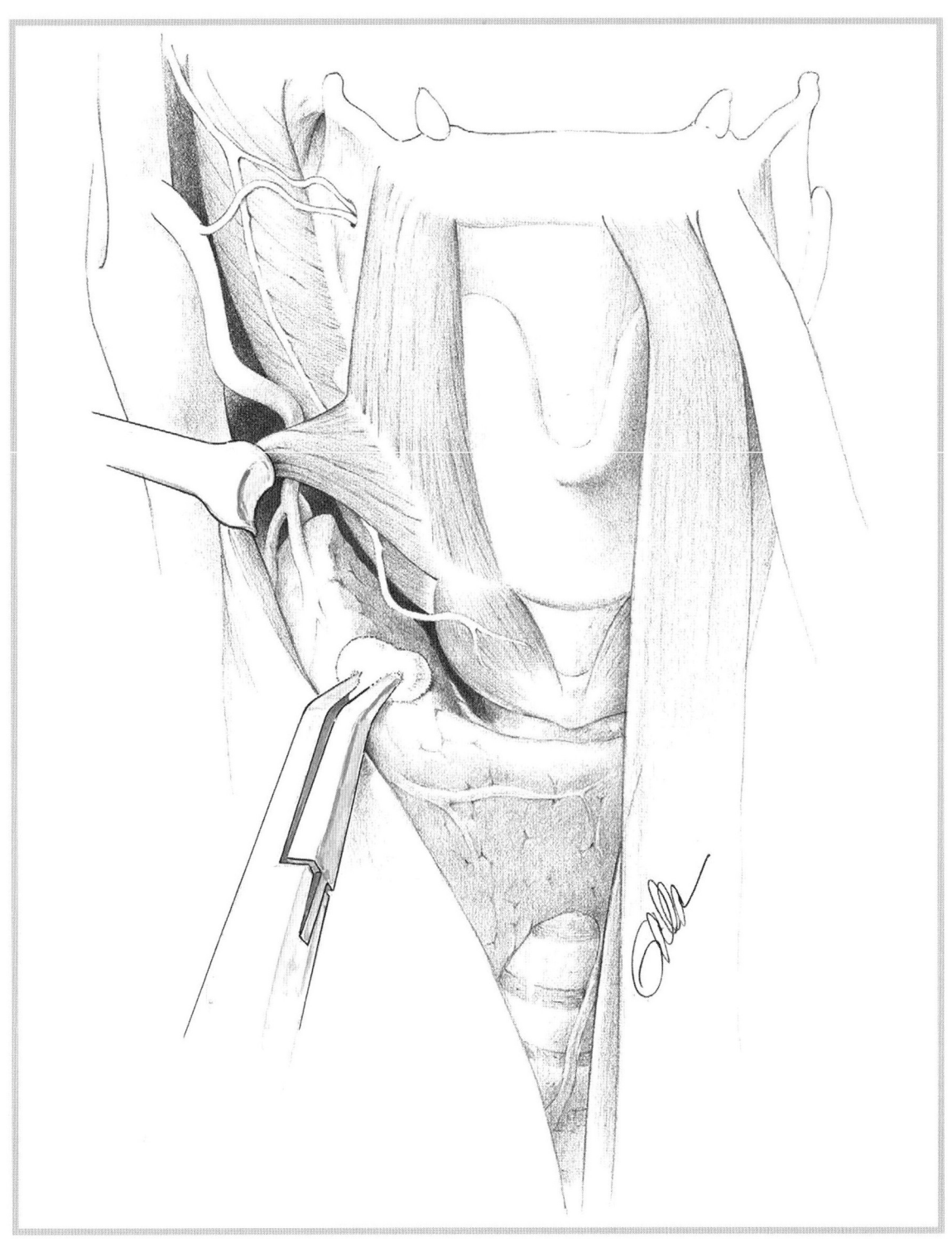

31

Principles in Thyroid Surgery

Whitney Liddy, Juliana Bonilla-Velez, Frédéric Triponez, Dipti Kamani, Gregory Randolph

> Please go to expertconsult.com to view related video:
> **Video 31.1** Basic Thyroid Surgical Maneuvers.
> **Video 31.2** Advanced Thyroid Cancer Surgery.
> **Video 31.3** Total Thyroidectomy: Autofluorescence and Parathyroid Angiography.

INTRODUCTION

There are a number of chapters in this text devoted to specific thyroid surgical approaches, ranging from minimally invasive to extracervical, robotic, and transoral approaches (see Chapter 32, Robotic and Extra Cervical Approaches to the Thyroid and Parathyroid Glands, Chapter 33, Transoral thyroidectomy, and Chapter 34, Minimally Invasive Video-Assisted Thyroidectomy). In this chapter, we review when to perform thyroid surgery, the extent of surgery recommended, as well as the basic technical principles in standard thyroid surgery; these principles are, to some degree, applicable to all forms of thyroid surgery. Standard open thyroid surgery may be considered the basic starting point for all thyroid surgeons; familiarity with these surgical anatomic principles is an essential first step for other less routine surgical approaches.

EXTENT OF THYROIDECTOMY

Although fine-needle aspiration (FNA) is the procedure of choice for the evaluation of clinically indicated thyroid nodules, Chapter 11, Fine-Needle Aspiration of the Thyroid Gland: The 2017 Bethesda System and Chapter 12, Fine-Needle Aspiration and Molecular Analysis there are clinical parameters other than cytology that can affect the decision to operate and the extent of a thyroidectomy (see Chapter 11, Fine-Needle Aspiration of the Thyroid Gland—The 2017 Bethesda System); these include age (higher malignancy risk <20 and >60 years of age), sex of the patient (males have increased risk of malignancy), family history of thyroid malignancy syndromes such as familial papillary carcinoma, Cowden syndrome, multiple endocrine neoplasia (MEN) type 2A or 2B (see Chapter 27, Syndromic Medullary Thyroid Carcinoma: MEN 2A and MEN 2B and Chapter 30, Familial Nonmedullary Thyroid Cancer), personal history of exposure to ionizing radiation (especially as a child), and a history of a rapidly growing thyroid mass (see Chapter 10, The Evaluation and Management of Thyroid Nodules).[1] On physical examination, size, firmness, and fixation of the nodule are important to note as well as hoarseness. Especially important and predictive of malignancy are the findings of vocal cord paralysis (VCP) and lymphadenopathy (see Chapter 15, Pre- and Postoperative Laryngeal Examination in Thyroid and Parathyroid Surgery and Chapter 14, Preoperative Radiographic Mapping of Nodal Disease for Papillary Thyroid Carcinoma). Thyroid-stimulating hormone (TSH) elevation has been associated with higher risk of malignancy in a thyroid nodule as well as with more advanced cancer stage.[2,3] Certain ultrasonographic findings also increase the risk of malignancy, such as solid hypoechogenicity, irregular margins, microcalcification, rim calcifications (especially if interrupted with extrusion of soft tissue), central blood flow, taller than wide morphology, extrathyroidal extension (ETE), and increased elastography measures of firmness and density (see Chapter 13, Ultrasound of the Thyroid and Parathyroid Glands).[4] Focal 18 fluorodeoxyglucose-positron emission tomography (^{18}FDG-PET) positivity of a thyroid nodule is also found to increase malignancy risk.[5] Molecular assessment of FNA cytology has emerged as a useful tool to reduce the diagnostic uncertainty of the indeterminate cytologic categories and to aid in preoperative malignancy risk assessment. The most commonly used tests today include microarray analysis of messenger RNA (mRNA) expression of certain genes implicated in thyroid cancer and next-generation sequencing analysis of panels of common genetic alterations (e.g., *BRAF, RET/PTC1, RET/PTC2, RAS, HRAS, NRAS, PAX8/PPAR gamma, PIK3CA*) (see Chapter 10, The Evaluation and Management of Thyroid Nodules; Chapter 12, FNA and Molecular Analysis; and Chapter 18, Molecular Pathogenesis of Thyroid Neoplasia).[6] However, given the continued need for long-term outcome data on the use of molecular testing in therapeutic decision making, patients should be counseled on the potential benefits and limitations of molecular testing. Just as cytopathologic analysis is of central importance in the decision to operate and in discussions of extent of thyroidectomy, equally important is the interpretation of these data not in isolation but in the context of other key clinical parameters already described.

EXTENT OF SURGERY BASED ON FNA RESULT

In 2007, the National Cancer Institute convened a state of the science meeting to consolidate and provide guidance regarding thyroid cytopathology terminology.[7] This meeting resulted in the Bethesda System for Reporting Thyroid Cytopathology, which recognizes six distinct categories of thyroid FNA cytopathology: nondiagnostic, benign, atypia of undetermined significance or follicular lesion of undetermined significance (AUS/FLUS), follicular/Hürthle cell neoplasm (or suspicious for follicular or Hürthle cell neoplasm), suspicious for malignancy, and malignant. The Bethesda System was revised in 2017 to incorporate new data into malignancy risk stratification, such as the reclassification of some thyroid neoplasms as noninvasive follicular thyroid neoplasm with papillary-like nuclear features (NIFTP); however, the names of the categories did not change (see Chapter 11, Fine-Needle Aspiration of the Thyroid Gland—The 2017 Bethesda System).[8] Each of these categories confers an estimated risk of malignancy, which in turn influences the surgeon's management recommendations. However, as noted earlier, the overall clinical scenario (history, physical examination parameters, specific FNA data, etc.) must factor into the surgeon's decision making. For example, certain unfavorable clinical parameters may appropriately lead the surgeon to recommend surgery in the setting of an FNA reported as benign. Typical surgical management recommendations for each of these cytopathologic categories is presented below. These recommendations are summarized in the 2015 American Thyroid Association Management Guidelines for Adult Patients with Thyroid Nodules and Differentiated Thyroid Cancer.[4]

Nondiagnostic

The nodule reported as nondiagnostic should undergo repeat aspiration with ultrasound guidance; 50% of such repeated aspirates yield diagnostic information.[9] Diagnostic lobectomy can be considered for the nodule with multiple nondiagnostic results; core needle biopsy may also be considered. Approximately 10% of such nodules are malignant. Nodules that are highly suspicious on ultrasound or demonstrate significant growth on ultrasound surveillance should be considered for surgery. Clinical risk factors for malignancy should also be considered in surgical decision making.

Benign

When the needle biopsy returns with adequate cellularity and is clearly benign, surgery is deferred generally in lieu of serial ultrasonographic surveillance (see Chapter 10, The Evaluation and Management of Thyroid Nodules). Occasionally, because of size of the nodule especially over 3 to 4 cm, compressive symptoms, or the need for absolute assurance by the patient, surgery can be considered. The extent of surgery will depend on the clinical scenario but is most often unilateral.

Indeterminate

Atypia of Undetermined Significance or Follicular Lesion of Undetermined Significance

When cytology is read as AUS/FLUS, the mean risk of malignancy is estimated around 15% to 20%; however, notable challenges have been discussed in the literature regarding this estimate.[8] In this setting, repeat ultrasound-guided FNA and molecular testing may be offered to aid in malignancy risk assessment. If surgery is decided upon without these further investigations, the surgery is typically a lobectomy. In the setting of repeat FNA with AUS/FLUS or suspicious molecular testing results, surgery is considered. Either a lobectomy or total thyroidectomy may be recommended as the initial treatment of choice based on clinical risk factors, specific molecular testing results, sonographic pattern, and patient preference. Rarely in this category, frozen section can confirm malignancy intraoperatively (such as with classic papillary thyroid carcinoma) and allow for conversion to total thyroidectomy if indicated. However, given the limited utility of frozen section with other diagnoses (such as follicular variant papillary thyroid cancer [PTC] and follicular thyroid carcinoma), many surgeons choose to forego frozen section intraoperatively. In any case, if lobectomy is decided upon as the initial management strategy, the patient must be counseled regarding the possible need for completion thyroidectomy.

Follicular or Hürthle Cell Neoplasm

When the needle biopsy result reveals follicular or Hürthle cell neoplasm (or suspicious for follicular or Hürthle cell neoplasm), a lobectomy without frozen section is generally offered for complete capsular histologic evaluation. The patient is counseled about the potential need for completion thyroidectomy, which occurs in approximately 20% to 30% of cases. Alternatively, molecular testing may be offered for further malignancy risk assessment. Total thyroidectomy may be considered when the lesion is more likely to be malignant, based on molecular testing results or clinical factors such as male sex or larger size of the lesion (generally >4 cm).[10] Initial total thyroidectomy may also be considered in patients who, based on their age, have a less favorable prognosis should a cancer be diagnosed or if there is substantial unbiopsied contralateral lobe nodularity.

Suspicious for Malignancy

Needle aspirates that read as suspicious for malignancy are most often suspicious for papillary carcinoma; the risk of papillary cancer up to 70%.[8] These have traditionally been best treated with lobectomy with frozen section and intraoperative touch cytologic prep (see Chapter 11, Fine-Needle Aspiration of the Thyroid Gland—The 2017 Bethesda System). If a diagnosis of papillary carcinoma can be made intraoperatively, total thyroidectomy can be offered. Biopsy of suspicious lymph nodes may be helpful for diagnosing papillary carcinoma. Alternatively, molecular testing may be considered before surgery if a positive result would lead to an altered surgical plan, such as proceeding straight to total thyroidectomy.[4] Total thyroidectomy may be considered for nodules that have known mutations, nodules that are larger than 4 cm, or nodules in patients with a strong history of radiation exposure or familial thyroid carcinoma.[4]

Consideration for Total Thyroidectomy in Patients With Indeterminate Nodules

In general, a completion thyroidectomy would be recommended for patients if the diagnostic lobectomy resulted in a malignant diagnosis. Consideration can be given to proceed with a total thyroidectomy at initial surgery in patients with bilateral nodular disease, significant medical comorbidities, coexisting hyperthyroid disease, or in patients who prefer to undergo bilateral surgery to avoid the risk of a second surgery.[4]

Malignant

Diagnostic for Medullary Carcinoma, Anaplastic Carcinoma, or Lymphoma

An initial biopsy that is read as diagnostic for medullary carcinoma of the thyroid requires a workup to exclude pheochromocytoma, hyperparathyroidism, and radiographic evaluation for nodal disease; consideration must be made for total thyroidectomy, central neck dissection, and often unilateral or bilateral lateral neck dissection (see Chapter 26, Sporadic Medullary Thyroid Carcinoma and Chapter 27, Syndromic Medullary Thyroid Carcinoma: MEN 2A and MEN 2B). Blood testing for calcitonin, carcinoembryonic antigen (CEA), calcium, parathyroid hormone (PTH) and pheochromocytoma laboratory testing should be performed. Germline RET mutational analysis informs whether the patient has an inherited or a sporadic disease. With no evidence of nodal disease, total thyroidectomy with central neck dissection is considered often, with some surgeons considering lateral neck dissection depending on calcitonin levels.[11]

With a diagnosis of anaplastic thyroid carcinoma, surgery is offered in the relatively uncommon circumstance where all gross disease can be resected; surgery is sometimes offered for palliative purposes.[12] Given the significance of the diagnosis of anaplastic thyroid cancer, open biopsy confirmation rather than FNA alone can be considered. A common surgical procedure appropriate for anaplastic carcinoma is isthmusectomy; it can confirm tissue diagnosis and is often combined with tracheotomy if the airway is deteriorating.

Aspirates read as diagnostic for lymphoma often need to be subtyped; this frequently requires core biopsy or sometimes open biopsy/isthmusectomy (see Chapter 28, Anaplastic Thyroid Cancer and Thyroid Lymphoma). Recommended management for thyroid lymphoma, as is the case for other lymphomas, typically involves chemotherapy and radiation rather than surgery.

Diagnostic for Papillary Carcinoma of the Thyroid

The extent of thyroidectomy for patients with well-differentiated thyroid carcinoma, specifically PTC, has been actively debated within head and neck and surgical oncologic circles for decades. In the past, total thyroidectomy was performed for PTCs >1 cm.[13-15] However, according to current guidelines (2015 American Thyroid Association Management Guidelines for Adult Patients with Thyroid Nodules and Differentiated Thyroid Cancer), thyroid lobectomy is now acknowledged as an acceptable treatment option in certain cases of PTC <4 cm.[4] In most cases, PTC is associated with prolonged survival.[16] The controversy as to the relationship between thyroidectomy and the prolonged, long-term survival enjoyed by the majority of patients with papillary thyroid carcinoma, has made randomized prospective studies impractical. The best surgical plan for a patient with a preoperative FNA read as diagnostic of papillary carcinoma of the thyroid has been controversial, in part, because of the unique features of PTC (see Chapter 19, Papillary Thyroid Cancer and Chapter 20, Papillary Thyroid Microcarcinoma).

Unique Features of Papillary Carcinoma
The Prevalence and Favorable Prognosis of Small PTC Lesions

The first of these unique features of papillary cancers is the entity of occult or microscopic carcinoma. Such lesions are typically defined as less than 1 cm and typically as intrathyroidal.[17,18] Such lesions are highly prevalent in humans and are often found incidentally during thyroidectomy performed for other lesions. The lesions occur, on average, in 8.5% of surgical specimens.[19,20] When comparing data from the Surveillance, Epidemiology, and End Results Program (SEER) clinical prevalence rates to known autopsy rates of PTC, which range from 5% to 36% depending on the country, it is estimated that only 2% of existing PTC lesions in humans ever present with clinical disease.[21,22] Although small occult carcinomas may metastasize to regional nodal beds in the neck, they are rarely associated with clinically significant metastatic disease or death.[23,24] The favorable prognosis of small PTC lesions has been well studied. In 1960 Woolner described six patients with occult PTC diagnosed through an excisional biopsy of cervical lymph node(s) who were followed clinically (i.e. without any thyroid surgery) and found to have no progression of disease over many years.[17] In Japan, a large prospective study of observation alone for patients with biopsy-proven papillary microcarcinomas (PMC) was performed. Among 162 patients observed, 72.3% demonstrated no local disease progression (PTC size was stable or smaller) on surveillance ultrasounds during long-term follow-up (at least 5 years) (See Chapter 21, Papillary carcinoma observation).[25]

Cervical Lymph Node Metastases in PTC: Micrometastatic versus Macrometastatic (Clinically Apparent) Disease

The second unusual feature of papillary carcinoma is that cervical lymph node metastasis at presentation, although highly prevalent in microscopic form in regional nodal beds, seems for many patients to have little prognostic implication.[16,26] Some evidence suggests that the presence of cervical lymph node metastasis may increase recurrence rate and have a greater prognostic significance in elderly patients.[27,28] Data from the SEER database suggests that nodal disease, when in macroscopic form, is an important determinant of tumor-related survival, especially when present in patients over 45 years of age, or patients with other high-risk features (large tumor size or distant metastasis). Macroscopic nodal disease was found to be an independent risk factor for decreased survival in patients with papillary cancer over age >45 years of age, or in patients with follicular cancer.[29-32] For patients <45 years of age, Adam et al. analyzed data from SEER and the National Cancer Database (NCD) and showed that the overall presence of lymph node metastasis (without differentiating between macroscopic and microscopic disease) was associated with a small but increased risk of death (hazard ratio of approximately 1.3, $p < 0.05$).[33] Therefore, the overall effect of PTC regional metastases on survival is thought to be small.[4]

Papillary carcinoma frequently spreads to both central and lateral regional nodal beds. Thirty percent of patients have clinically positive (i.e., macroscopically positive) nodes at presentation when based upon physical or ultrasound examination; however, histologic studies show microscopic spread to regional neck nodes in a wide range of patients (up to 90%); up to 80% of patients experienced spread to the contralateral thyroid lobe.[34-42] This high prevalence of microscopic disease in the neck stands in stark contrast to the low rate of development of clinical disease in the untreated N0 neck.[29,43] Presumably, in the majority of cases, microscopic disease in the neck is inherently inactive. The discordance between the presence of microscopic disease in the neck and its lack of clinical significance has led to the abandonment of past recommendations for elective lateral neck dissection in the N0 setting.[40,42] Controversy still exists as to the applicability of this argument in the ipsilateral central neck.[46]

PTC's Robust Prognostic Risk Grouping Segregation

Several groups have proposed risk stratification strategies that use key demographic and oncologic characteristics to categorize patients with well-differentiated thyroid cancer (WDTC) into risk categories with distinct patterns of recurrence and survival (see Chapter 24, Dynamic Risk Group Analysis for Differentiated Thyroid Cancer).[47-49] The most frequently used schemes are listed in Table 31.1. Risk-group stratification appropriately allows aggressive treatment in the high-risk group and avoidance of excessive treatment and its complications in low-risk groups (Table 31.2). Brierley reviewed 382 patients with 10 different commonly used prognostic scoring systems; he found the following systems to be comparable in predicting prognosis: age, grade, extent, size (AGES); tumor, node, metastases (TNM); European Organization for Research and Treatment of Cancer (EORTC); metastases, age, completeness of resection, invasion, size (MACIS); and age, metastases,

TABLE 31.1 Key Factors in Various Prognostic Schemes

MEMORIAL SLOAN KETTERING	MAYO CLINIC		LAHEY CLINIC	KAROLINSKA INSTITUTE
Games	Ages	Macis	Ames	Dames
Grade	Age	Metastases	Age	DNA
Age	Grade	Age		Age
Metastases	Extension	Completeness of resection	Metastases	Metastases
Extension		Invasion	Extension	Extension
Size	Size	Size	Size	Size

TABLE 31.2 Effect of Risk Groups on Survival

Institution	Risk Group	Number	Percent Distribution	Death Rate (%)
Memorial Sloan Kettering	Low	264	40	1
	Intermediate	357	38	15
	High	210	22	54
Mayo Clinic	Low	737	86	2
	High	121	14	46
Lahey Clinic	Low	277	89	1.8
	High	33	11	46

extent, size (AMES).[50] Key elements of existing prognostic schemes for papillary carcinoma include the following:

1. Age over 45 years
2. Degree of invasiveness or ETE (increased invasiveness increases risk of local, regional, and distant recurrence and decreases survival)
3. Metastasis (presence of distant metastasis decreases survival)
4. Sex (males generally have a poorer prognosis than females)
5. Lesion size (lesions >4 cm have a poorer prognosis and lesions <2 cm have better prognosis)
6. Bulky lymph node metastasis, especially with extracapsular extension
7. Poorly differentiated histology

Other factors that affect prognosis for well-differentiated thyroid carcinoma have been studied. If gross disease is left at the completion of initial surgery, prognosis worsens.[51] Postoperative treatment with radioactive iodine (RAI) and thyroxine (T4) suppression generally improves prognosis, although a minority of thyroid cancer experts do not accept this.[52,53] Some have used histologic grading in prognostic schema.[54]

The most widely used system for prediction of disease-specific survival in risk stratification strategies is the American Joint Committee on Cancer's Tumor-Node-Metastasis staging system in its 8th edition (AJCC/TNM, www.cancerstaging.org).[55,56] The American Thyroid Association (ATA) recommends the AJCC/International Union Against Cancer (UICC) TNM staging system be employed for all patients with differentiated thyroid cancer (DTC).[14] Although this widely used AJCC/UICC TNM staging system for DTC provides a convenient and familiar method of assessing the extent of the tumor, it does not take into account several independent prognostic variables; it was developed to predict primarily the risk of death, not recurrence. Current risk stratification schemes also do not account for certain aggressive histologic subtypes of cancer and other pathologic findings, such as frequent mitosis, tumor necrosis, microscopic degrees of ETE capsular invasion, or molecular characterization of the primary tumor. TNM data are based primarily on clinical and pathologic data available after thyroidectomy and therefore do not change over time; however, risk of recurrence or death may change depending on the patient's response to treatment (see Chapter 24, Dynamic Risk Group Analysis for Differentiated Thyroid Cancer). To improve the estimation of risk of recurrence, the ATA has offered a risk of recurrence stratification system that segregates patients into low-risk, intermediate risk, and high-risk of recurrence.[14] The ATA low risk of recurrence group includes patients without distant metastasis, with all macroscopic tumor resected, without tumor invasion of local structures, without aggressive histology or vascular invasion, and without uptake outside of the thyroid bed after initial whole-body scanning (WBS). The ATA intermediate risk of recurrence group includes patients with microscopic local invasion, cervical nodal disease, uptake outside of the thyroid bed at the first WBS after ablation, and patients with aggressive histology or vascular invasion. The ATA high risk of recurrence group includes patients with macroscopic tumor invasion, patients with incomplete tumor resection, and patients with distant metastasis or with thyroglobulin out of proportion to findings on initial WBS.[14] The risk of recurrence for the low, intermediate and high ATA risk groups are 14%, 44%, and 86%, respectively (see Chapter 24, Dynamic Risk Group Analysis for Differentiated Thyroid Cancer).

Treatment for PTC <1 cm or Papillary Microcarcinoma (PMC)

Subcentimeter papillary thyroid carcinomas (i.e., papillary microcarcinoma [PMC]) i.e. often take an indolent course. With the 2015 update to the ATA guidelines for DTC, FNA of thyroid nodules <1 cm is no longer routinely recommended for sonographically suspicious nodules, unless ETE or suspicious lymph nodes are observed.[4] Furthermore, there is compelling evidence from observational studies in Japan, which shows active surveillance for PMCs as a safe and effective alternative to surgery (see Chapter 21, Papillary Carcinoma Observation).[57,58] However, additional studies are needed to define (1) specific risk factors that may differentiate the poorer-behaving cancers that may lead to favoring surgery over observation, (2) management issues related to long-term surveillance especially as it relates to different age groups, and (3) acceptability of the active surveillance approach in other regions outside Japan.[4] When surgery is planned for PMC, there is a variety of work supporting the notion that lobectomy is equivalent to total thyroidectomy (as described previously).[13,59] Bilimoria's recent work revealed no difference in survival or recurrence rates between lobectomy and total thyroidectomy for lesions less than 1 cm.[13] Given the status of current evidence, the ATA recommends that patients with PMC and without other risk factors (multifocality, ETE, regional or distant metastasis, history of head and neck radiation, or familial thyroid carcinoma) who are not undergoing active surveillance undergo a lobectomy, unless there are surgical indications to remove the contralateral lobe[4] (see Chapter 20, Papillary Thyroid Microcarcinoma).

Extent of Thyroidectomy for PTC >1 cm and <4 cm

The extent of thyroidectomy for patients with especially low risk PTC has been actively debated for decades, fueled by the prolonged long-term survival of the majority of patients with PTC and the possibility of higher complication rates with more extensive operations. Although well-differentiated thyroid carcinoma certainly can be a lethal disease, it is associated with prolonged survival in a majority of patients. Multiple studies have examined survival outcomes and recurrence to support[16,27,28,52,67] or argue against[24,43,49,54,71,72,76] total thyroidectomy for PTC patients. Bilimoria et al. studied a group of more than 52,000 patients with papillary carcinoma and found—using Cox hazards modeling adjusting for age, race, income, lymph node status, distant metastasis, RAI use, and year of diagnosis—that for lesions ≥1 cm there is significant, yet small, improvement in survival and decreased recurrence at 10 years with total thyroidectomy; this is opposed to patients with less than total thyroidectomy.[13] However, data on certain high-risk parameters, such as ETE, completeness of resection, and other comorbid conditions were not available for analysis and could have had a significant effect on survival.[13] A more recent analysis of data from the 61,775 patients treated between 1998 and 2006 showed that the survival advantage for patients with PTC between 1 and 4 cm from the Bilimoria study disappeared when adjusting for demographic, clinical, and pathologic factors related to complexity and severity of the disease.[59] Additional data from the SEER database on DTC and PTC showed similar results. Barney et al. compared outcomes from lobectomy and total thyroidectomy in 23,603 patients with DTC; the patients were treated between 1983 and 2002 and showed no difference in 10-year overall or cause-specific survival.[60] Mendelsohn et al. examined SEER data specifically addressing PTC and found no difference in overall or disease-specific survival when comparing 16,760 patients who underwent total thyroidectomy to 5964 patients who had a lobectomy.[61] Other studies have also supported the excellent survival outcomes observed with lobectomy in selected patients.[62,63] This evidence led the ATA to modify their recommendations for surgical treatment of PTC in their 2015 guidelines. Recommendation 35 states that in patients with cancers >1 cm but <4 cm without high risk features (ETE, lymph node metastasis), initial surgery may consist of lobectomy or total thyroidectomy based on disease features, need for RAI therapy, or patient preference.[4] The National Comprehensive Cancer Network (NCCN) guidelines also suggest that patients with intrathyroidal disease <4 cm who do not have a history of radiation exposure or regional or distant metastasis can be treated with either lobectomy or total thyroidectomy.[83] The extent of thyroidectomy for a preoperatively identified PTC should be a team decision made by the surgeon, the endocrinologist, and the patient.

Extent of Thyroidectomy for PTC >4 cm

Patients with PTC that is greater than 4 cm in size have more advanced disease and should be treated with a total thyroidectomy. There is a linear relationship between tumor size, recurrence, and cancer-specific mortality for DTC. Furthermore, total thyroidectomy should be performed in cases of tumor size >4 cm, gross ETE, or gross regional or distant metastatic disease to facilitate adjuvant therapy with RAI and oncologic surveillance.[4,52,83] This concept is supported by recommendations from the ATA and NCCN guidelines.[4,83]

Total Thyroidectomy for PTC: Additional Considerations

Radioiodine ablation of thyroid gland remnants after total thyroidectomy can allow for WBS and the sensitive use of thyroglobulin as a postoperative marker.[84] Measurement of serum thyroglobulin as a tumor marker is most reliable when normal thyroid tissue is absent.[85] It should be noted that some practitioners feel that thyroglobulin can also be followed when a lobe or a fraction of a lobe is present. Schlumberger found that thyroglobulin was useful even in patients who had less than total thyroidectomy without ablation.[86] Harvey et al. measured serum thyroglobulin in 84 patients with WDTC after lobectomy and 58 patients after total thyroidectomy. Tumor recurrence was heralded by increased thyroglobulin in both groups. The authors concluded that despite residual thyroid tissue, serum thyroglobulin could exclude the presence of significant metastatic disease in most patients after lobectomy for thyroid cancer.[87]

After a total thyroidectomy, even in expert hands, a significant number of patients have residual thyroid tissue that requires postoperative ablation. Auguste showed that after total thyroidectomy, 13 out of 80 patients required radioiodine ablation.[88] Marchetta also noted average neck uptake of 15% after total thyroidectomy.[89] Surprisingly, Szilagy et al. noted that in their series, 20% of patients having had total thyroidectomy did not require T4 replacement.[90] There is no question, however, that when a complete total thyroidectomy is done, hypothyroidism is achieved sooner than with less than total thyroidectomy and postoperative RAI ablation. The three regions that often contribute to postoperative uptake after total thyroidectomy are discussed later in this chapter.

Total thyroidectomy also treats any potential contralateral lobe papillary carcinoma foci that could be the source of additional recurrence or dedifferentiation; however, dedifferentiation is rare. One must keep in mind that management of PTC varies in different parts of the world with quite different approaches. In Japan, one common approach is a partial thyroidectomy leaving a large remnant in the contralateral lobe but performing ipsilateral or bilateral nodal surgery. Interestingly, this algorithm, which takes on a different perspective for targeting microscopic disease with emphasis on the ipsilateral nodal beds and de-emphasis on the contralateral thyroid lobe, has been met with favorable results.[91]

As a final point, in the surgical literature, appreciation of "risk groups" has appeared since the 1990s. Confusion has been evident, however, between (1) occult carcinomas and microcarcinomas and (2) the AMES and AGES low-risk groups. These two are not synonymous. It is, however, obvious that many more patients are included in the low-risk groups than just patients with papillary lesions ≤1 cm. Most patients in these low risk groups enjoy excellent long-term prognosis.[77]

Extent of Thyroidectomy for PTC Detected on Lobar Specimens: Completion Thyroidectomy

The finding of PMC in lobar specimens is a common problem occurring on average in 8.5% of patients in a number of recent studies (range 1.3–21.6% of patients).[92-102] Recent ATA guidelines recommend completion thyroidectomy be offered to those patients for whom a near-total or total thyroidectomy would have been recommended had the diagnosis been available before the initial surgery. Completion thyroidectomy may be avoided in patients with low-risk unifocal tumors <4 cm, patients without evidence of ETE or clinically apparent nodal or distant metastatic disease, and patients without a history of head and neck radiation or familial thyroid carcinoma.[4] NCCN recommendations for completion thyroidectomy also allow for observation in favorable lesions up to 4 cm (negative margins, no ETE, no macroscopic multifocal disease (>1 cm), no cervical lymphadenopathy, no vascular invasion, nonaggressive pathologic variants, and no contralateral lesions).[15,15a]

When contemplating completion thyroidectomy, practical management issues also need to be considered. Thyroid hormone availability to the patient and an expressed desire by endocrinologists for WBS and postoperative thyroglobulin assessment are important determinants of this decision. Other important considerations for completion thyroidectomy are the postoperative laryngeal examination[103] and the intraoperative and pathologic assessment of parathyroid preservation from the first side. These factors relate to risk of completion surgery. Most important, this should be a team decision made jointly by the patient, the endocrinologist, and the surgeon after thorough discussion.

Surgical Complications

Surgical treatment must blend an aggressive oncologic approach with a commitment to minimize the potential risk of complications. In skilled hands, total thyroidectomy can be offered with low morbidity.[104] Interestingly, a review of the Healthcare Cost and Utilization Project—National Inpatient Sample (1998-2009) identifying 16,954 patients who underwent total thyroidectomy showed a median annual surgeon volume of 7 cases, 51% of surgeons performing only one case per year, and 81% of patients undergoing surgery by low-volume surgeons (≤25 cases/year).[105] Complications have been demonstrated to occur more frequently from surgeries performed by low-volume surgeons.[105,106] The bulk of the literature also clearly shows increased complication rates, mainly recurrent laryngeal nerve (RLN) paralysis and permanent hypoparathyroidism, with bilateral compared with unilateral thyroid surgery.[54,107] (see Chapter 42, Pathophysiology of Recurrent Laryngeal Nerve Injury; Chapter 43, Management of Recurrent Laryngeal Nerve Paralysis; Chapter 44, Non-Neural Complications of Thyroid and Parathyroid Surgery; and Chapter 45, Quality Assessment in Thyroid and Parathyroid Surgery).

RLN paralysis. In general, permanent RLN paralysis rates in expert hands are in the 1% to 3% range.[108a,b,109,110] However, many reports reveal significantly higher rates, in the 6% to 8% range; rates as high as 23% have been reported (see Chapter 36, Surgical Anatomy and Monitoring of the Recurrent Laryngeal Nerve).[72,81,82] In studies by Hockauf, who reviewed more than 1000 patients, and Segal, who reviewed 61 pediatric patients, a 10% incidence of VCP was reported.[111,112] Sinclair, on the other hand, reported a 1.1% incidence of RLN paralysis with routine thyroidectomy and a 17.5% incidence in surgery for retrosternal goiters.[113] Martensson showed that the incidence of RLN paralysis increased with bilateral thyroid surgery, revision thyroid surgery, and surgery for malignancy or in patients brought back for bleeding.[114] The reported prevalence of RLN injuries after thyroid surgery varies widely. A recent analysis of 27 articles reviewing more than 25,000 patients undergoing thyroidectomy found the average immediate postoperative VCP rate was 9.8%. The rate of permanent VCP varied 10-fold, according to the method of examining the larynx; the rate ranged from 0% to 18.6%.[109] With the advent of nationwide surgical outcome databases, we have broad cross-sectional perioperative information, which may give insight into these issues. In 2008, the Scandinavian Quality Register (SQR) for Thyroid and Parathyroid Surgery reported on 40 endocrine surgical units from Sweden and Denmark that specializing in endocrine surgery; SQR noted an immediate VCP rate of 4.3%.[115] In the National Audit by the British Association of Thyroid and Endocrine Surgeons (BAETS), a permanent VCP rate of 1.0% (95% confidence interval 0.7–1.6%) found.[116] One must keep in mind that both Scandinavian and British quality registers derive from surgeon-reported data without routine postoperative laryngeal examination. For the SQR, the rate of VCP doubled when patients were subjected to routine laryngeal examination as opposed to selective performance of postoperative laryngoscopy only in patients with persistent and severe voice changes. The BAETS audit showed increasing rates of nerve paralysis with increasing postoperative laryngoscopy rates. The administrators of these two national databases, therefore, deem the rates of temporary and permanent RLN palsy to be severely underestimated.[115,116] We may then surmise that RLN paralysis rates in the wider literature are also likely to be underestimated because not all patients in these studies undergo postoperative laryngeal examination. Lo found a 6.6% incidence of VCP when all patients had postoperative laryngoscopy. Of these, only 1.1% had nerve damage recognized during thyroidectomy.[117]

Bilateral thyroidectomy is a unique offering within head and neck surgery because both left and right cranial nerves innervate the airway introitus; both are at risk during one surgical procedure. Experienced practitioners who champion total thyroidectomy have reported rates of transient bilateral VCP requiring tracheotomy between 2% and 3% of thyroidectomy patients.[118] Rates of RLN paralysis should be appropriately described as incidence of paralysis per nerve at risk. De Roy Van Zuidewijn found a 3.1% incidence of paralysis per nerve at risk.[119] Thomusch found RLN injury was associated with extent of surgery, surgery for recurrent disease, and with cases where the surgeon failed to visualize the nerve.[120] RLN injury rates are lower when the nerve is clearly identified during surgery.[4,110] There is not enough evidence in the literature to show that overall RLN injury rates are decreased with intraoperative neural monitoring, possibly secondary to the difficulty with sufficiently powering these studies, higher volume and more experienced surgeons are increasingly using nerve monitoring to facilitate RLN management. Such stimulation is safe and allows the surgeon to identify a neuropraxic nerve injury and possibly defer contralateral thyroid surgery (see Chapter 36, Surgical Anatomy and Monitoring of the Recurrent Laryngeal Nerve).[121,122]

Hypoparathyroidism. Hypoparathyroidism is the most common complication seen after total thyroidectomy and revision thyroid surgery.[124-127] Calcium and often vitamin D are required several times a day with careful monitoring. Temporary hypoparathyroidism, as defined in a recent position statement from the American Thyroid Association, is an intact PTH level less than the lower limit of the laboratory standard (usually 12 pg/mL) combined with resultant hypocalcemia for less than 6 months after surgery; however, permanent hypoparathyroidism continues beyond 6 months.[127] Low calcium levels can result in troublesome and sometimes life-threatening symptoms, whereas high calcium levels can result in renal stones. A 2014 meta-analysis of temporary and permanent rates of hypoparathyroidism showed a mean incidence of 19% to 38% and 0% to 3%, respectively.[126] In an American College of Surgeons survey, which reviewed 24,108 thyroid surgeries, Foster noted a permanent hypoparathyroidism rate of 8%.[128] Mazzaferri reported a 13% incidence of permanent hypoparathyroidism after total thyroidectomy in the community setting.[73] Even in selected tertiary care settings, rates of 29% to 48% have been described.[48,129] Thomusch found parathyroid injury was associated with extent of resection, surgery for recurrent disease, advanced age, female sex, and surgery for Graves' disease.[120] The risk of hypoparathyroidism increases with invasive cancers and when lymph node dissection is performed with thyroidectomy. The risk of hypoparathyroidism is also vitally linked to the experience of the surgeon. One experienced surgeon noted hypoparathyroidism in only 3.2% of patients after total thyroidectomy overall, but he described a 25% incidence in his first 25 total thyroidectomy cases.[28] Risk factors for permanent hypoparathyroidism include prior central neck surgery, bilateral surgery, simultaneous thyroidectomy and parathyroidectomy, autoimmune thyroid disease, central neck dissection, substernal goiter, low-volume surgeon, and prior gastric bypass.[127] And although parathyroid autotransplantation has been associated with high rates of temporary hypoparathyroidism, rates of permanent hypoparathyroidism are very low.[130] Recently, different intraoperative techniques that help identify parathyroid glands and/or identify vascularity are being actively studied and reported. They are described in the next section.

Extent of Surgery PTC Summary: Encompass Gross Disease in Thyroid and Nodes at First Surgery

A rational surgical plan for patients with WDTC can be constructed despite the divergent information available in the literature. It is also important to not be overly dogmatic about any one approach, given the retrospective nature of the data.

A clear-cut divergence in prognosis exists in patients with WDTC. A large group of patients enjoy an excellent prognosis, and a small group of patients are associated with a very poor prognosis. Age and presence of distant metastatic disease at presentation are probably the most important prognostic determinants. Most specialists believe that, as Schlumberger has written, the "extent of treatment and follow-up care should be tailored to the level of risk."[131] This philosophy should be kept in mind when one is considering the extent of thyroidectomy for WDTC. The bulk of the data available suggests that the overriding principle in the surgical treatment of WDTC is that the surgeon should, at first surgery, encompass the gross disease in the thyroid and neck nodes; the surgeon must understand that, although present, microscopic disease in the contralateral lobe and the neck nodes has little clinical significance. Tsang wrote, "the goal of surgery should be macroscopic complete resection of tumor. Microscopic residual disease in our series did not differ significantly from its absence in terms of cause specific survival and local control…in these patients."[72] Such microscopic disease is indolent and is not clinically manifest in the majority of cases. Gross disease should be encompassed at the first operation. Enlarged lymph nodes should be excised. Patients with obvious invasion of the trachea should be managed with segmental airway resection.

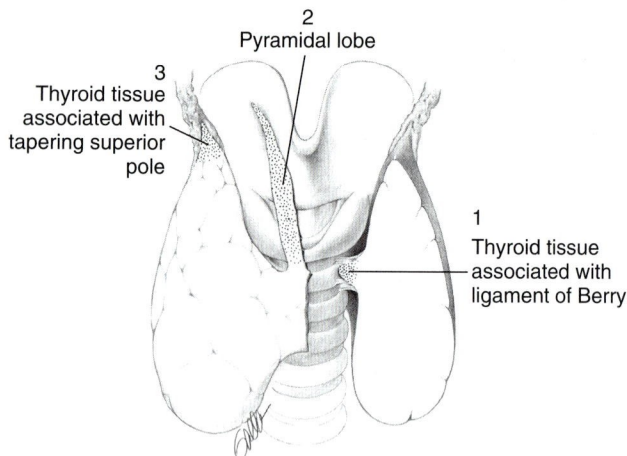

Fig. 31.1 Front view of thyroid and larynx, showing three areas that may contribute to thyroid bed radioactive iodine uptake after total thyroidectomy: *1*, thyroid tissue associated with ligament of Berry; *2*, thyroid tissue associated with unresected pyramidal lobe; *3*, thyroid tissue associated with unrecognized tapering of the superior thyroid pole.

Total thyroidectomy is an excellent procedure in skilled hands and should be considered based on the patient's risk group and tumor characteristics as long as significant postoperative morbidity is not expected. However, the feasibility of total thyroidectomy, even in experienced hands, has been questioned because residual thyroid tissue remains (typically centered at the ligament of Berry, pyramidal lobe, or superior pole) in a small but substantial fraction of patients (Figure 31.1). Aggressive bilateral thyroidectomy, therefore, may not obviate the need for postoperative ablation. Leaving a small contralateral lobe remnant is a reasonable option if it is away from the cancer, if it is anodular, if leaving the lobe is necessary to preserve parathyroid function, or to limit neural dissection. Education is required at the resident level regarding proper technique in the performance of a total thyroidectomy. This involves careful preservation of the parathyroid glands with intact blood supply and untraumatized RLNs.

It is important to emphasize that the extent of thyroidectomy should be tailored not only to the patient's risk group and operative findings but also to the progress of the specific surgery; this is particularly the case if the contralateral lobe is not involved by cancer. If dissection of the first side has revealed two parathyroids of good color with good vascular pedicles and an RLN that has been identified, preserved, and that stimulates well electrically at the end of the dissection, contralateral thyroid surgery can be safely contemplated. If the first side has not gone well, then elective contralateral lobe resection should be deferred, at least on that day. Parathyroid color changes associated with devascularization may not always be reliable. Characteristic blackened color change may be associated with venous disruption and certainly implies parathyroid injury and potential dysfunction. However, arterial interruption may be unassociated with this color change yet result in significant parathyroid dysfunction. Parathyroid autofluorescence and ICG angiography are new avenues in optimal parathyroid management. Proponents of RLN monitoring feel it is helpful in identification and dissection of RLN; they also feel it can be helpful in assessing neural function at the end of surgery (see Chapter 36, Surgical Anatomy and Monitoring of the Recurrent Laryngeal Nerve).[122]

Parathyroid Identification Using Parathyroid Autofluorescence and Preservation of Parathyroid Vascularization by Parathyroid Angiography

Many efforts have been made to reduce the rate of hypoparatyroidism. However, until very recently, visual detection of the parathyroid glands, capsular dissection very close to the thyroid gland, and autotransplantation of nonperfused glands have been the mainstay of parathyroid preservation.

Mahadevan-Jansen et al. discovered a special optical characteristic of the parathyroid glands; when excited in the near infrared light (at about 785 nm), parathyroid tissue reemits at another wavelength (at about 820 nm), which is a much stronger signal when compared with other surrounding tissue (thyroid, fat and muscle, Figure 31.2).[132] The autofluorescence of the parathyroid glands comes from a fluorophore that is resistant to heat, freezing, and formalin fixation,[134-136] but the exact nature of this fluorophore is still unknown.

The main difficulty with autofluorescence of the parathyroid glands is that the difference of the intensity of autofluorescence between parathyroid tissue and surrounding tissues varies and is not always as high as in Figure 31.2. In general, parathyroid tissue is 2 to 10 times more autofluorescent than thyroid tissue, but there are several issues:

1. The intensity of autofluorescence differs from one patient to another.
2. Autofluorescence is slightly weaker in diseased parathyroid glands compared with normal ones (Figures 31.3 and 31.4).
3. Thyroid tissue can be as autofluorescent as the parathyroid tissue in some patients (particularly in patients with thyroiditis).
4. False positives signals may also occur from colloid nodules, brown fat, and metastatic lymph nodes.[135]

Despite these limitations, several studies have shown that near-infrared-based systems are highly accurate for parathyroid identification.[133,134,136] Most of these studies report that the identification of parathyroid glands is more accurate with autofluorescence-based systems than with the naked eye only; autofluorescence-based systems are associated with better postoperative outcomes.[139,148,150]

Currently, two different techniques are available. The first one is a probe-based spectroscopy system. With this device, the surgeon holds a sterile, pen-style probe in their hands and touches the tissue in the neck. The system analyses the optical properties of the tissues next to the probe and gives a distinct audio and visual signal when the probe is touching

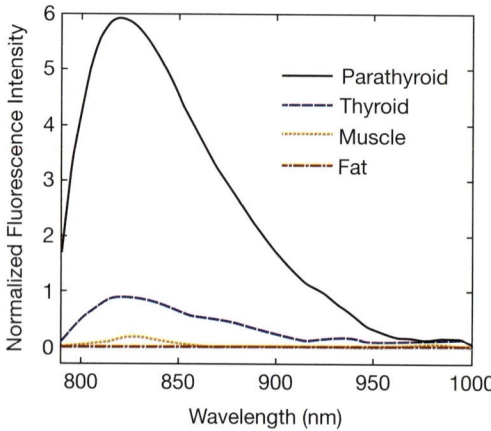

Fig. 31.2 Typical near-infrared fluorescence spectra of parathyroid, thyroid, muscle, and fat in a single patient. (From McWade MA, Sanders ME, Broome JT, Solórzano CC, Mahadevan-Jansen A. Establishing the clinical utility of autofluorescence spectroscopy for parathyroid detection. *Surgery.* 2016;159[1]:193–202.)

CHAPTER 31 Principles in Thyroid Surgery   279

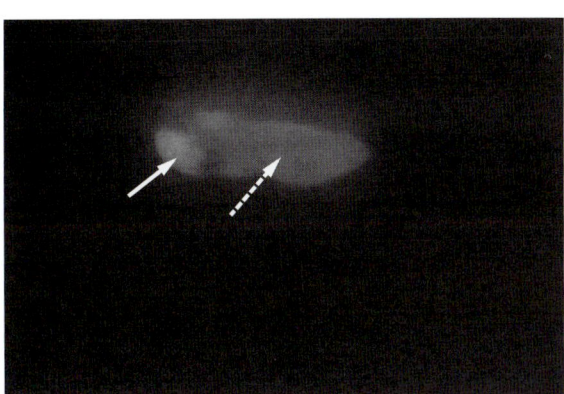

Fig. 31.3 Autofluorescence of a thyroid lobe and a parathyroid adenoma showing that the autofluorescence of the adenoma *(solid arrow)* is only slightly more intense than that of the thyroid *(dashed arrow)*.

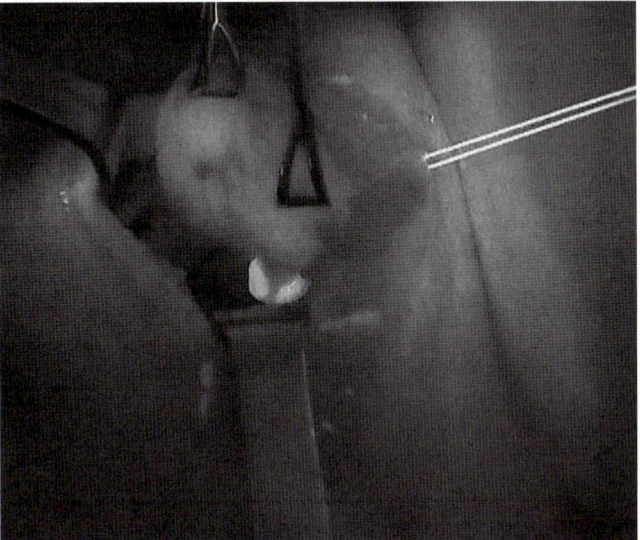

Fig. 31.4 The left thyroid lobe is retracted by Babcock clamps and two autofluorescent spots are clearly apparent. They correspond to both normal left parathyroid glands. Of note is the autofluorescence of Vicryl thread used to retract the skin.

parathyroid tissue. The second technique is an optical system that generates a grayscale visualization of the surgical field with enhancement of autofluorescent tissues. With this system, the surgeon looks at the surgical field with a special camera once the thyroid lobe has been medialized and searches for autofluorescent foci (see Figure 31.3). Both devices have been approved by the U.S. Food and Drug Administration (FDA) to help detect parathyroid tissue in real-time during thyroid and parathyroid surgery (PTEye from AiBiomed, a probe-based system and Fluobeam from Fluoptics, an optical system). Other commercially available optical systems exist and can also be used for parathyroid detection.

As mentioned previously, the autofluorescent properties of the parathyroid glands are maintained even after the parathyroid is removed; therefore autofluorescence does not allow assessment of the function of the parathyroid glands. For this reason, angiography of the parathyroid glands with the fluorescent dye indocyanine green (ICG) has been developed.

In 1907, Halsted described[154] that parathyroid glands are vascularized by tiny, terminal vessels that need to be carefully dissected and preserved to preserve their vascularization and therefore function. Several studies have shown that some of these parathyroid vessels run very close to the thyroid gland and are sometimes difficult to preserve.[155,156] Delattre reported that in 5.5% of the dissected specimen, all four parathyroid glands would have been devascularized by standard capsular dissection.[43] This emphasizes that capsular dissection is not always adequate for preserving parathyroid gland vascularization.

ICG is a water-soluble, albumin-bound fluorescent FDA-approved dye, initially used to test for liver function. For many years, ophthalmologists employed ICG for retinal angiography with safety. Its fluorescent properties are in the near-infrared light wavelengths (peak absorption at 800 nm, peak emission at 830 nm) that penetrate the tissue up to 1 cm in depth. This allows good visualization of vascularization of different tissues, including parathyroid glands in the thyroid surgical field. ICG can be reinjected many times because the half-life is 2 to 3 minutes, and the toxic dose is 5 mg/kg.

The main goal of ICG angiography of the parathyroid gland is to ascertain the vascularization and ultimately the ongoing function of the parathyroid glands after thyroid resection[158-164] (see Figures 31.5 and 31.6). Studies show that ICG angiography is more reliable than visual evaluation alone in defining the vascularization of the parathyroid glands; the technique demonstrates a good correlation between vascularization of the parathyroid glands and parathyroid function and has an almost 100% positive predictive value (no hypoparathyroidism in patients with at least one well-vascularized parathyroid gland).

Presently, the main limitation of this technique is the lack of standardization of vascularization assessment. The currently available devices lack numerical evaluation, making it difficult to compare the evaluations of different groups and of different devices. Some studies suggest that some parathyroid glands evaluated as "well-vascularized" by some authors would have been evaluated as "moderately-well vascularized" by other groups.[164,165] However, in the long term, patients with "moderately-well vascularized" parathyroids recovered good parathyroid function, which suggests "some" perfusion of the parathyroid glands might be enough to avoid long-term hypoparathyroidism.

From a practical point of view, most modern operating rooms are equipped with some kind of ICG fluorescence endoscopic camera; surgeons interested in evaluating parathyroid glands with ICG angiography can use the equipment available in their institution. Initially, a well vascularized parathyroid gland should be evaluated before thyroid resection. According to the device used and its sensitivity to ICG, a standard dose of ICG (between 1.25 and 7.5 mg) is injected intravenously (IV), and the vascularization of the parathyroid gland is seen a few seconds after ICG injection (20 to 60 seconds depending on the length of the IV line and the flushing speed). This gland is used as the local standard for "well vascularized parathyroid gland." After thyroid resection, visualized parathyroid glands are reevaluated with ICG angiography. According to some studies,[158] if at least one parathyroid gland is well-vascularized, the patient may be managed without measuring calcium and PTH postoperatively.

ICG angiography can also be used to identify the parathyroid vessels before thyroid resection. This is a current area of research with few published papers; different authors are developing this method not just to predict parathyroid function post thyroidectomy but also to prevent postsurgical hypoparathyroidism by adapting the thyroid resection according to the vessel mapping indicated by ICG angiography.[148,166]

Thyroidectomy in Pregnancy

The recommended workup of thyroid nodules is generally the same for pregnant versus nonpregnant patients. However, thyroid surgery is often delayed until after pregnancy, if judged clinically prudent, given the significantly higher associated risks. A large study of the Healthcare Cost and Utilization Project—National Inpatient Sample reviewed 201 pregnant patients undergoing thyroidectomy (or parathyroidectomy)

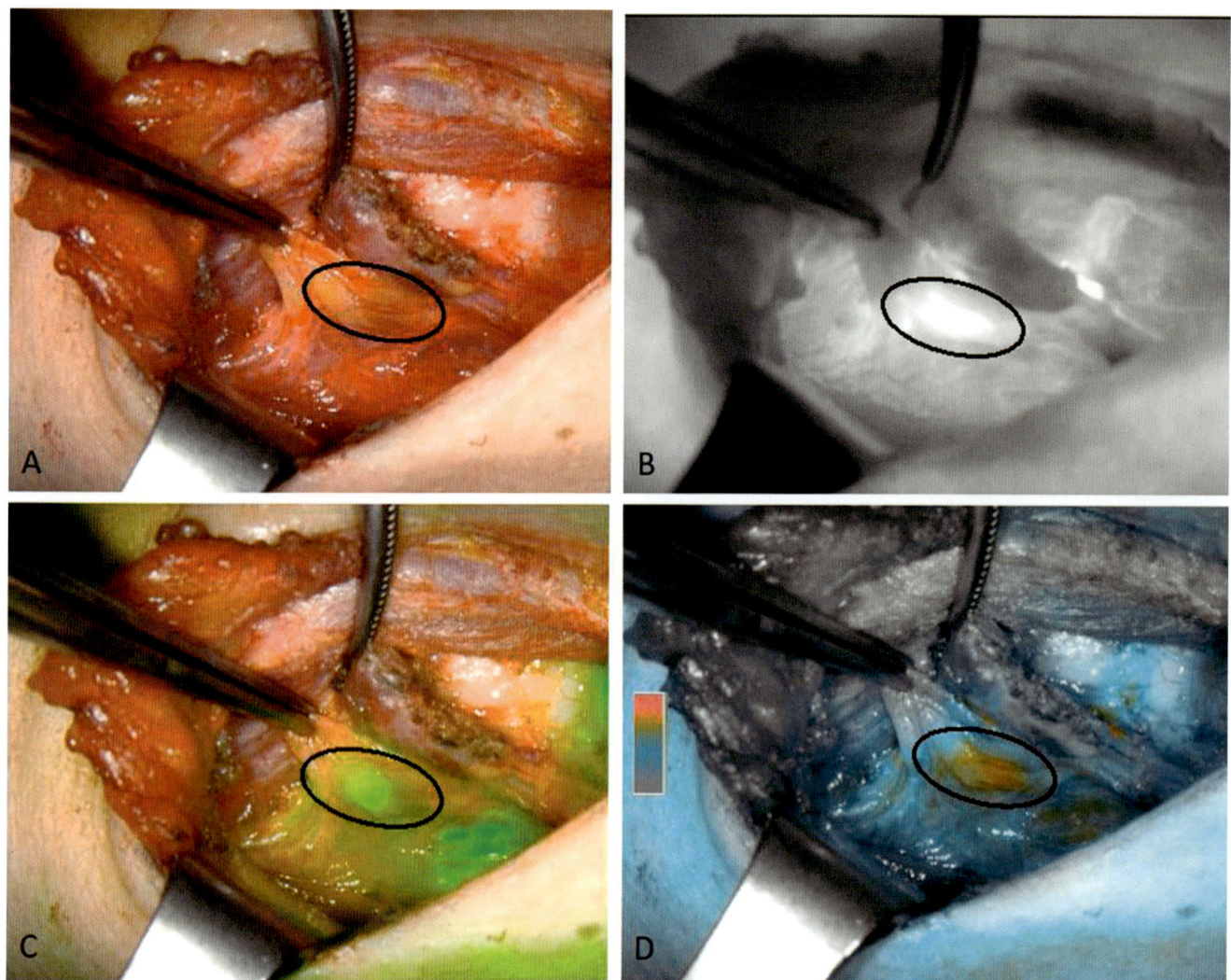

Fig. 31.5 Indocyanine green (ICG) angiography images taken after right thyroid lobectomy; the superior parathyroid gland is well vascularized. **A,** Standard color view; **B,** Near-infrared, black and white view; **C** and **D,** Combined standard + near-infrared view in green scale (**C**) and color-scale (**D**). (See the video for details.)

and showed that the patients had twice the risk of perioperative complications for both benign and malignant conditions than nonpregnant controls, with 5.5% having fetal complications (e.g., fetal distress and abortion) and 4.5% having maternal complications (e.g., cesarean section and hysterectomy).[167] In the setting of WDTC, most studies have shown no difference in prognosis if surgery is delayed until the postpartum period.[168,169] However, in some high-risk cases of thyroid cancer (medullary or anaplastic thyroid cancer, high-risk WDTC), surgery has been advised during pregnancy. The latest ATA guidelines recommend that, when necessary, surgery should be performed in the second trimester, which is typically before 24 to 26 weeks gestation; this represents the time before fetal viability but after organogenesis.[170,171] Clearly, discussion between the patient, obstetrician-gynecologist, endocrinologist, and surgeon should be thorough; surgery, especially for low-risk PTC, should be avoided, if possible, for most pregnant patients until postpartum.[172]

NOMENCLATURE OF THYROIDECTOMY

The name of the procedure performed should reflect, in a straightforward manner, the extent of resection. *Partial lobectomy*, performed in rare cases, implies that a portion of the lobe has been removed. *Lobectomy* implies that an entire lobe has been completely removed with its capsule intact and without isthmus resection. *Hemithyroidectomy* implies that a lobe has been completely removed along with the isthmus and usually with any associated pyramidal lobe. *Subtotal thyroidectomy* implies that a lobe and the isthmus have been completely removed, and that the contralateral lobe has been partially removed; this usually involves its medial and ventral portion and typically leaves a posterior element. *Bilateral subtotal* implies a significant portion of both lobes has been removed. In a *near-total thyroidectomy*, all thyroid tissue is removed except for a 1-gram-or-less remnant on one side, typically left to assist in preserving the adjacent parathyroid tissue or to avoid distal RLN dissection.[173] Such a remnant must be anodular and away from the cancer focus. When thyroid tissue is left during a thyroidectomy, it is important not to just clamp across the remaining parenchyma without identification of the course of the RLN. In a *total thyroidectomy*, the surgeon resects all gross thyroid tissue. *Isthmusectomy* implies complete removal of the isthmus, typically as a biopsy technique for thyroid lymphoma, anaplastic carcinoma, or Riedel's thyroiditis, where it may be combined with tracheotomy. Less frequently, and generally not recommended, isthmusectomy may be performed for

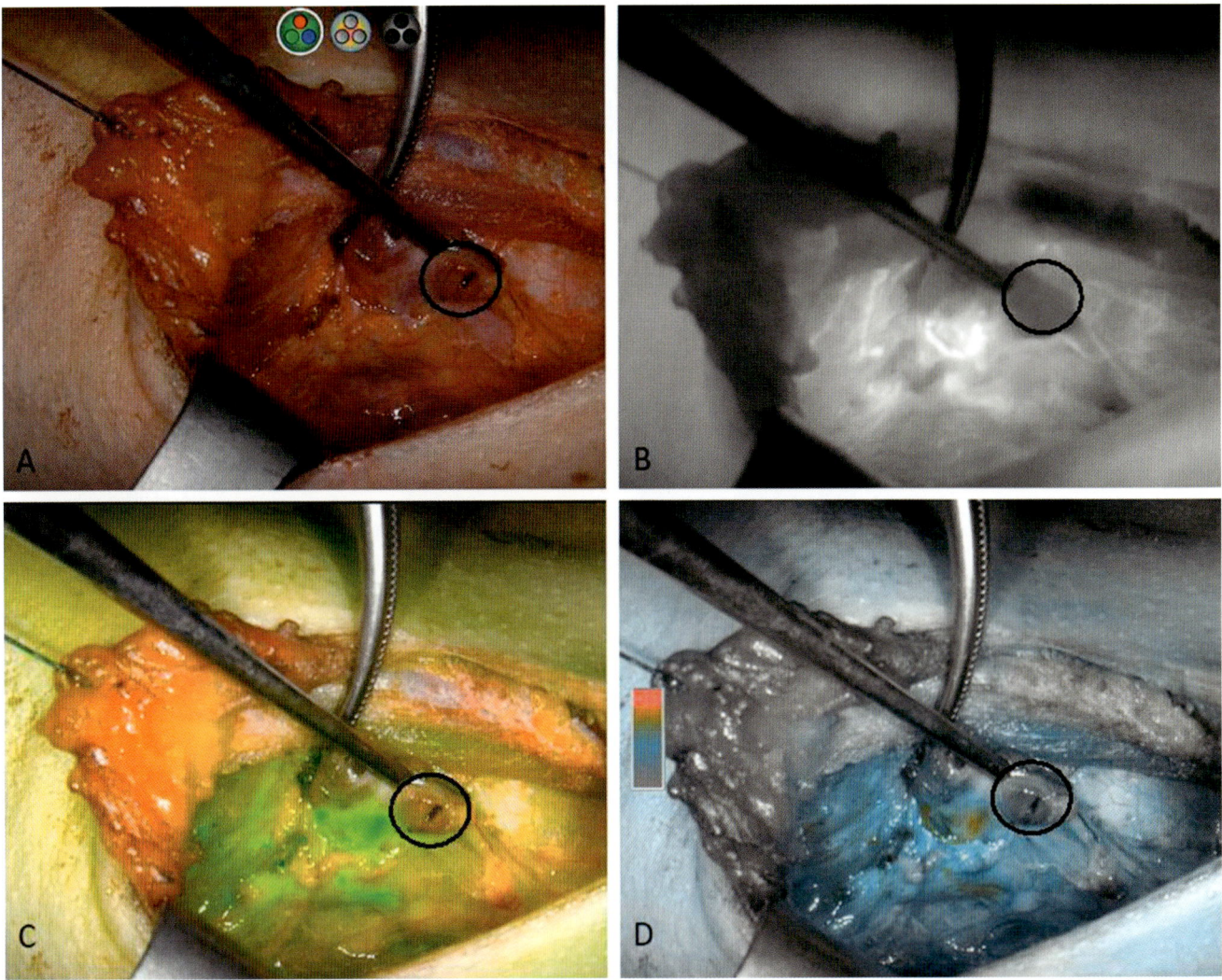

Fig. 31.6 Indocyanine green (ICG) angiography images after right thyroid lobectomy; the inferior parathyroid gland is not vascularized. The pictures are taken after a small incision of the parathyroid gland has been performed. **A,** Standard color view; **B,** Near-infrared, black and white view; **C** and **D,** Combined standard + near-infrared view in green scale (**C**) and color-scale (**D**). (See the video for details.)

benign disease that is confined to the isthmus, such as the isthmus toxic nodule or follicular or Hürthle neoplasia. In this chapter, we describe hemithyroidectomy (total unilateral extracapsular lobectomy and isthmusectomy) as the minimum surgical procedure for unilobar WDTC. Partial lobectomy for thyroid cancer is unacceptable because reoperation in a previously dissected field is technically complex and fraught with risks to the RLN and parathyroid glands.

THYROIDECTOMY SURGICAL STEPS

Overview

Thyroidectomy can be considered an endeavor that proceeds in a logical sequence of steps from ventral (skin of the ventral neck) to dorsal (toward the vertebral column). After skin incision and dissection past the platysma muscle, the surgeon interacts with the strap muscles (which are separated in the midline) and then the ventral surface of the thyroid isthmus. The next most dorsal structure encountered is the middle thyroid vein. This attaches to the lateral thyroid lobe in a ventral position (Figure 31.7). The next most dorsal anatomic structure of importance to be encountered during thyroidectomy is often the inferior parathyroid gland, which is almost always situated anterior/ventral to the RLN. Once this is dissected free from the inferior pole, the next most dorsal important structure is the RLN. After RLN identification, the final and deepest (most dorsal) structure of consequence encountered is the superior parathyroid gland, which is almost always situated at the level of the cricoid cartilage adjacent to the RLN laryngeal entry point. Again, we think it is helpful to consider these sequential structures encountered as one proceeds from ventral to dorsal during thyroidectomy.

Some experts prefer to mobilize the lower portion of the thyroid gland first and identify the inferior parathyroid and RLN, followed by identification of the superior parathyroid gland at the ligament of Berry before mobilizing the superior pole vessels. Others prefer to start with mobilization of the pyramidal lobe and prelaryngeal tissues cephalad to the thyroid isthmus (the site of Delphian lymph nodes) and then mobilize the superior portion of the thyroid lobe. Dissection of the superior lobe cephalad to the cricoid cartilage should be lateral to the inferior constrictor and cricothyroid muscles to help avoid injury to the external branch of the superior laryngeal nerve

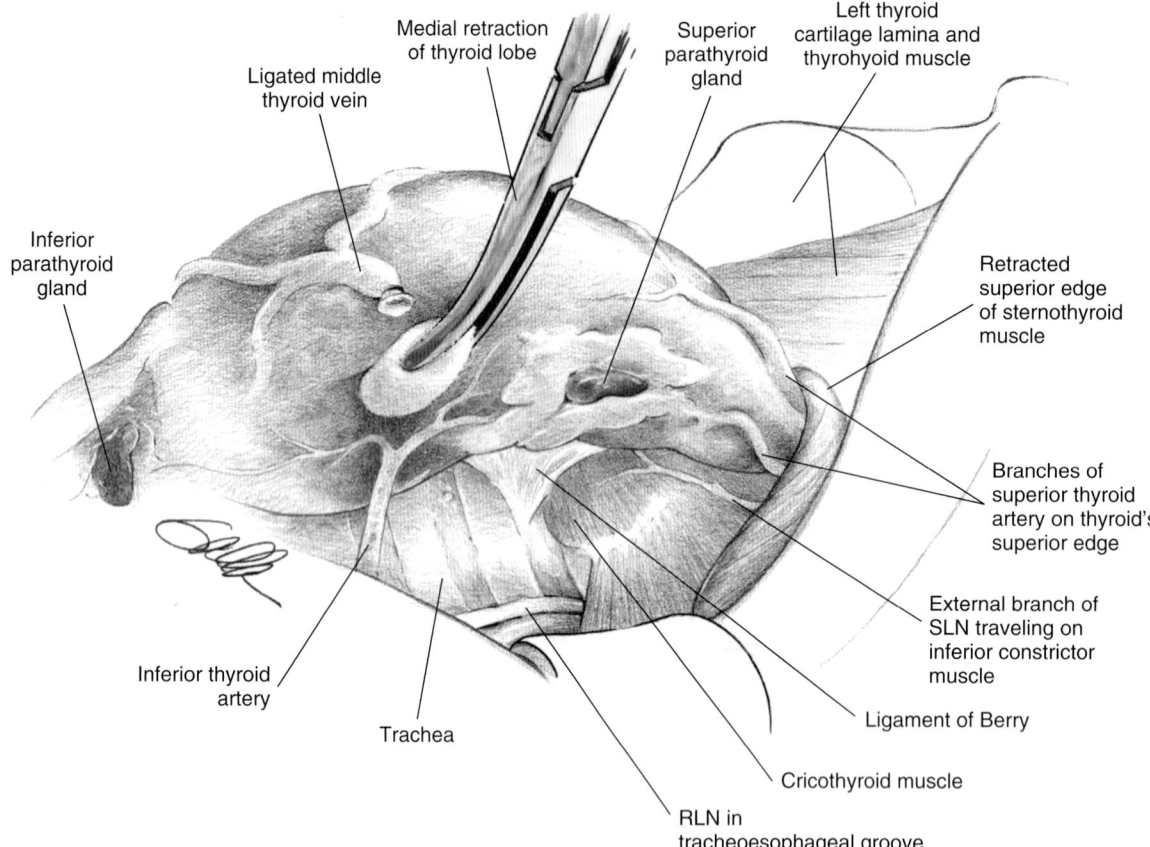

Fig. 31.7 Left lateral view of lateral thyroid region, showing exposure. Exposure of the region is facilitated by ligation of the middle thyroid vein and lateral retraction of strap musculature. Once this is performed, the thyroid lobe is retracted medially. As this is done, deeper anatomy—including the inferior thyroid artery, parathyroid glands, and recurrent laryngeal nerve—becomes apparent.

(EBSLN) (i.e., the "high note" or Amelita Galli-Curci nerve) (see Chapter 35, Surgical Anatomy of the Superior Laryngeal Nerve). Neural monitoring has great application to EBSLN identification and preservation at superior pole dissection. Neural stimulation under the laryngeal head of the sternothyroid muscle provides a positive glottic electromyography (EMG) response and a gross cricothyroid muscle twitch with EBSLN stimulation. The laterally reflected superior pole pedicle is stimulated as negative then progressively dissected and controlled. Dissection of the superior portion of the thyroid can usually be done by reflecting the superior pole laterally and caudally (Figure 31.8). Luckily, the RLN is not at risk cephalic to the cricoid cartilage unless there is a right-sided, nonrecurrent laryngeal nerve. The superior pole vessels should also be individually divided and ligated relatively low on the thyroid gland to avoid injury to the EBSLN (see Figure 31.1). Once the superior pole vessels have been ligated, the superior parathyroid gland, if not already identified, can be observed at the ligament of Berry and tubercle of Zuckerkandl. If bleeding is encountered in this area, it should be controlled with gentle pressure with no vessel clamped until the RLN is positively identified. We also often place a small clip adjacent to the parathyroid glands, both to minimize gland manipulation during dissection from the thyroid and for easier identification of these glands intraoperatively or subsequently, especially in patients with extensive lymphadenopathy. The thyroid lobe is then dissected free from the trachea

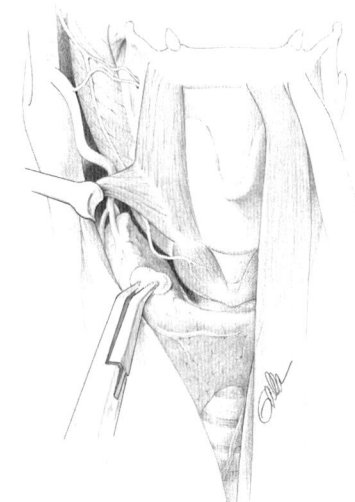

Fig. 31.8 The external branch of the superior laryngeal nerve must be protected during dissection of the superior pole and ligation and division of superior pole vessels. The superior pole vessels are ligated and divided directly on the thyroid capsule of the superior pole to avoid inadvertent injury to the external laryngeal nerve. Note how the sternothyroid laryngeal head insertion runs parallel to the distal course of the EBSLN.

using sharp dissection. For patients undergoing total thyroidectomy, the same operation is repeated on the contralateral side.

Initial Surgical Considerations

Successful thyroid surgery implies meticulous technical skill and attention to detail. Preoperative evaluation must be robust with the establishment of the patient's disease status, preoperative laryngeal examination, and evaluation for any significant comorbidity, including anticoagulation (see Chapter 14, Preoperative Radiographic Mapping of Nodal Disease for Papillary Thyroid Carcinoma and Chapter 15, Pre- and Postoperative Laryngeal Examination in Thyroid and Parathyroid Surgery). Patients being operated on for hyperthyroidism should be rendered euthyroid preoperatively. Presurgical evaluation for medullary thyroid carcinoma must include exclusion of pheochromocytoma before surgery. Close communication with the anesthesiologist is also important, especially if goitrous change or thyroid malignancy is affecting the glottic or tracheal airway. No paralytic agents beyond induction are used when laryngeal nerve monitoring and stimulation are planned. Preoperative history or evidence on preoperative CT of cervical arthritis, cervical degenerative joint disease, atlantoaxial subluxation, or an inability to hyperextend the neck should be discussed. Patients with cervical spine issues should be positioned preoperatively to determine the degree of extension possible, pain, or other symptoms accompanying extension.

Today, most thyroid surgeons recognize that exposure and full identification of the RLNs and parathyroid glands with their blood supplies are essential to reduce the risk of complications and achieve the goal of complete thyroid resection. This requires maintenance of a strictly bloodless field; many thyroid surgeons consider an additional method: the use of magnification during thyroid surgery. In the past, some surgeons believed that, "the dissection at no time should be directed at identification or uncovering of the recurrent laryngeal nerve," and that identification of the parathyroid glands amounted to "an erroneous guess work implying a risk of inducing hypoparathyroidism."[174] Not that long ago, it was written that "the parathyroids and RLN are not routinely sought [during thyroidectomy]; rather the main object is to avoid them."[175] We, on the other hand, share the opinion of Lennquist that "it is always better to see what you are doing."[176] In fact, routine visual identification of the RLN during thyroid surgery is now considered the gold standard for prevention of RLN injury. Early proponents of this method were Lahey and Hoover in 1938.[177]

Patient Positioning

The patient is placed in the supine position, with the neck extended and arms tucked and padded at the patient's side. When padding the arms, one must avoid pressure at the elbow on the radial or ulnar nerves and pressure from the IV line, blood pressure, or pulse oximetry line equipment. Neck extension is achieved by using an inflatable balloon or shoulder roll. The appropriate amount of extension is individually modified for each patient (Figure 31.9). Support is placed from scapula to scapula beneath the shoulders, allowing the neck to extend and the shoulders to fall posteriorly. These maneuvers allow the thyroid to move both anteriorly and superiorly. Careful attention must be paid to the degree of neck extension; the head must be supported with a soft donut pillow. The surgeon should check the adequacy of head support. The anesthetist should independently check the patient to be certain the head is properly supported. Hyperextension can cause serious posterior neck pain postoperatively. Inadequate head support must be avoided. These concerns are magnified in patients with cervical spine disease. Minimal to no neck extension is advisable for such patients (see Figure 31.9).

Venous pressure is reduced when a reverse Trendelenburg (head and back up) position is obtained. Preoperative antibiotics are generally not employed. The eyes are lubricated and taped shut to prevent corneal abrasion. Alcohol or Betadine preps can be used. There is little evidence that the timing of postoperative RAI is so crucial that iodine-containing preps cannot be used. The operative field is draped widely to include the chin, bilateral lateral neck, and the suprasternal notch. These landmarks are important for making a symmetric incision that maximally blends with the form and contour of the neck. The earlobe, jawline, and lower lip may be left in view to permit orientation for neck dissection.

Incision and Flap

Once the patient is fully extended, prepped, and draped, a surgical pen can be used to outline the important landmarks of the anterior neck, such as the midline mentum, the laryngeal notch, cricoid anterior arch, sternal notch, and bilateral clavicles. Generally, an incision placed approximately 1 fingerbreadth below the cricoid anterior arch will be strategic in terms of localizing the region of the isthmus of the thyroid gland. An incision planned *in or parallel* to normal skin creases is ideally camouflaged postoperatively (Figure 31.10). Stretching a silk ligature over the planned incision site facilitates making a balanced and symmetric incision (Figure 31.11). Regardless of the planned laterality of the procedure, the incision is generally to be placed in the midline. The skin should never be crosshatched with a scalpel, but a midline crosshatch may be drawn with the surgical pen. An incision placed too low, especially in women with larger breasts, may descend onto the sternum with the increased tendency for keloid formation. An incision too high will leave a visible scar above normal clothing. The incision should be long enough to perform the operation and should adequately allow for full visualization during a procedure. There has

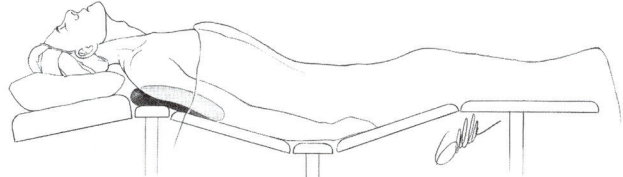

Fig. 31.9 The neck is extended with a shoulder roll but adequately supported with a sponge donut. Twenty degrees of reverse Trendelenburg position are maintained to avoid venous engorgement in the neck.

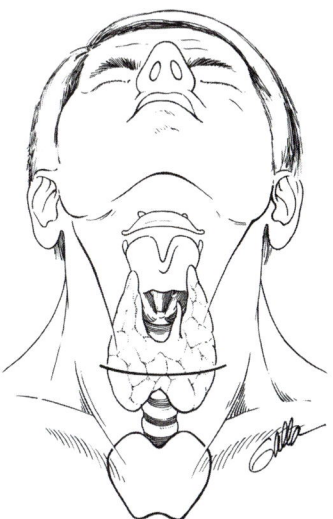

Fig. 31.10 Appropriate position of thyroidectomy incision, approximately one fingerbreadth below the anterior arch of the cricoid cartilage. The incision is ideally placed in a normal cervical skin crease in this region.

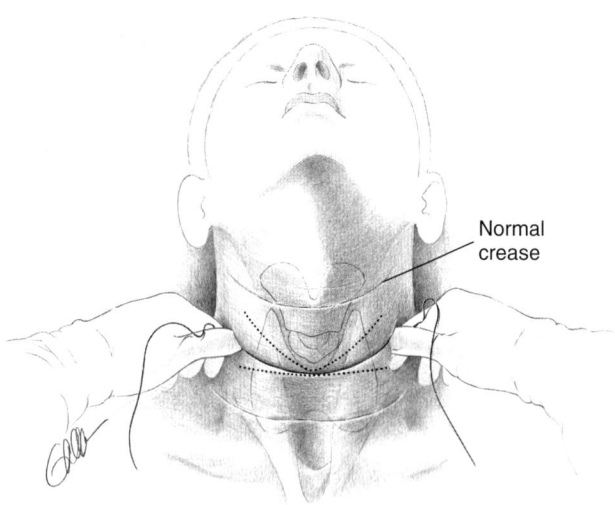

Fig. 31.11 The incision is planned and fashioned symmetrically over the thyroid isthmus in a natural skin crease or parallel to Langer's lines. A 2-0 silk tie pressed against the neck is used to mark the incision site. The incision is fashioned 1 cm below the cricoid cartilage. A sterile marking pen is used to mark the midline, the incision itself, and the lateral borders of incision. The dotted lines above and below the suture show incorrect incision lines.

been a tendency toward greater emphasis on smaller incisions in the 4 to 5 cm range. However, patients with larger lesions, short or heavy necks, or a low-set larynges and thyroids may require larger incisions for optimal exposure (see Figure 31.11) (see Chapter 40, Incisions in Thyroid and Parathyroid Surgery).

The skin incision is carried down through the platysma. Attention is then turned to creating the superior platysma flap. The platysma layer laterally and an analogous plane in the midline are grasped with Alice or Kelly clamps and are superiorly retracted with downward counterretraction provided by the surgeon's finger (Figure 31.12).

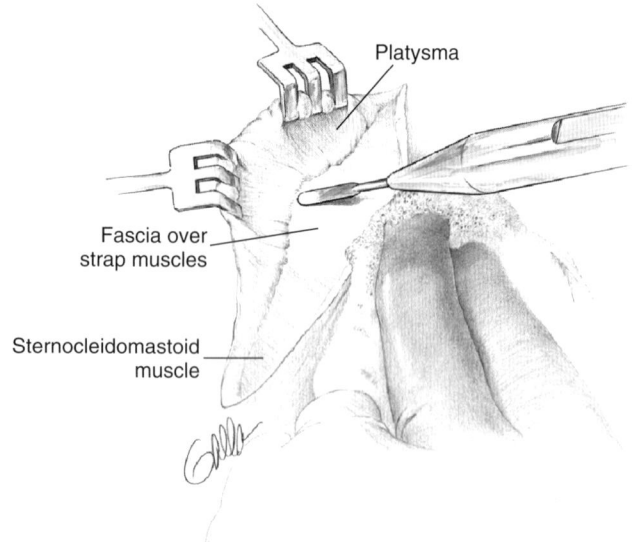

Fig. 31.12 An avascular plane is developed superficial to the anterior jugular veins and deep to the platysma. The plane is developed superiorly up to the thyroid cartilage and inferiorly down to the suprasternal notch and clavicles. A midline incision is fashioned through a superficial layer of deep cervical fascia between the strap muscles to expose the thyroid. The incision is made from the suprasternal notch to the thyroid cartilage.

The anterior jugular veins are kept down as dissection proceeds superiorly in a subplatysmal plane, paying careful attention to avoid buttonholing the skin, which is especially important at the level of the thyroid cartilage notch where skin can be quite thin and adherent to underlying tissue. An inferior flap can also be raised (see Figure 31.12). Some thyroid surgeons feel a platysma flap is unnecessary.[178] The flaps may be sutured or retracted with Mahorner, Gelpi, Goldman spring, or Joll retractors.

Strap Muscles and the Midline Airway

The superficial layer of the deep cervical fascia is dissected in the midline between the strap muscles (midline raphe or linea alba). The outer layer of strap musculature includes the sternohyoid and omohyoid muscles. The more lateral omohyoid muscle is important because nodal disease can track from the central visceral compartment to the lateral neck chain along the omohyoid muscle. In such circumstances, a large node can be found associated with the omohyoid as it extends laterally over the jugular vein to the lateral neck. The inner layer of strap muscles includes the sternothyroid muscle and, more superiorly, the thyrohyoid muscle. Thyroid gland dissection primarily involves the outer sternohyoid and inner sternothyroid muscles, which together ensheathe the ventral aspect of the gland. The sternohyoid muscle is the more robust and thicker strap muscle. Deep to it and recessed laterally is the thinner sternothyroid muscle. Thus the medial edge of the sternohyoid muscle must be lifted to see the underlying sternothyroid muscle. The laryngeal head of the sternothyroid muscle inserts along the oblique line of the thyroid cartilage lamina and to a varying degree "hoods" the superior pole. The division of the laryngeal head of the sternothyroid muscle is occasionally helpful to improve exposure of the superior pole of the thyroid gland (Figure 31.13).

After the platysma flap is raised and the strap muscles are separated at the median raphe, it is helpful to next identify the midline trachea just above and below the thyroid isthmus. While dissecting below the isthmus, the surgeon must watch for the right and left inferior thyroid veins, which can blend in to form an inferior venous plexus, termed the *plexus thyroideus impar,* below the isthmus. The surgeon must also watch for a high-riding innominate artery or a thyroid ima artery. This artery arises as an unpaired inferior vessel from the innominate, carotid, or aortic arch and occurs in 1.5% to 12% of cases. The identification of the trachea at this stage in the case, just above and below the thyroid isthmus, affords constant midline orientation throughout the rest of the case; the midline orientation is especially helpful in subsequent identification of the RLN. This constant midline tracheal reference point can also be helpful if the neck base anatomy is distorted by malignant or benign goitrous disease (see Figure 31.8).

The pyramidal lobe represents the inferior-most portion of the embryologic remnant of the thyroglossal duct tract and is present in 30% to 40% of individuals. Typically, this arises from the midportion of the isthmus but can arise more laterally, even from the right or left upper poles. The relatively dense fascia overlying the cricoid cartilage can obscure the pyramidal lobe. One should check the appearance of any transected tissue in this interval just superior to the isthmus because the cut edge of thyroid tissue representing the transected pyramidal lobe is easily recognized. The pyramidal lobe extends to a varying degree superiorly, often in close association with the midline notch in the superior thyroid cartilage, and occasionally extends to the hyoid bone (see Figure 31.1). Prelaryngeal or Delphian nodes should be looked for as this region is dissected. As this prelaryngeal dissection proceeds, care is taken to avoid damage including cautery to the cricothyroid muscles, which have a negligible fascial covering.

As the strap muscles are then reflected off the ventral surface of the thyroid gland, the loose connective tissue that fills the interval between

CHAPTER 31 Principles in Thyroid Surgery

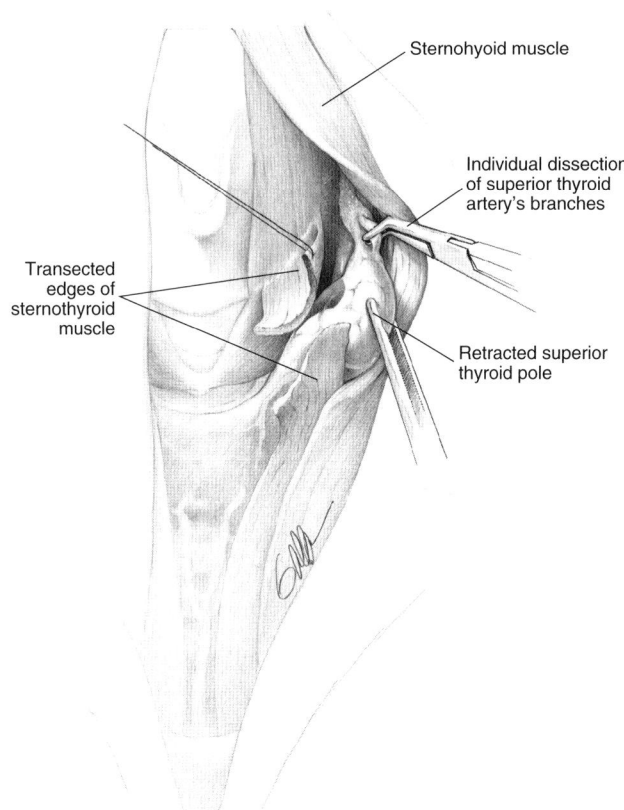

Fig. 31.13 Front view showing left thyroid superior pole dissection. Lateral and inferior retraction on the superior pole after sternothyroid muscle transection can increase exposure of the superior pole region, allowing individual dissection of the superior thyroid artery's branches at the level of thyroid superior pole capsule.

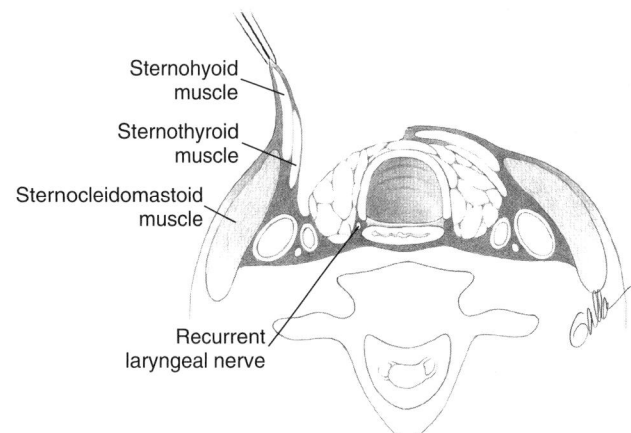

Fig. 31.14 Separation of the sternohyoid muscle and sternothyroid muscle to the level of the ansa hypoglossal nerve and jugular vein laterally facilitates greater exposure for thyroid lobectomy.

the undersurface of the strap muscles and the true thyroid capsule is seen as a cobweb-like network of thin fascia. This interval, referred to as the *perithyroidal sheath* or *false thyroid capsule,* represents a pretracheal portion of the middle or visceral layer of the deep cervical fascia. Occasionally, small bridging vessels extend from the true thyroid capsule to the undersurface of the strap muscles. These vessels are best identified individually and cauterized. They can cause troublesome bleeding if the interval between the strap muscles and the true thyroid capsule is bluntly dissected digitally. The true thyroid capsule is tightly adherent to the thyroid parenchyma and is continuous with fibrous septa that divide the thyroid's parenchyma into lobules. The true thyroid capsule usually has large capsular vessels, which can cause significant bleeding if the thyroid gland is too aggressively handled during retraction.

During reflection of the strap muscles off the ventral surface of the thyroid gland, some fibrotic reaction can occasionally be seen as a result of FNA. If the plane cannot be established with relative ease, malignant infiltration of the strap muscles should be considered. In such circumstances, the sternothyroid muscle should be left on the thyroid. If lateral retraction of the strap muscles does not provide adequate exposure, they should be divided without hesitation. This maneuver can be helpful not only when the thyroid lesion is large but also when the thyroid and larynx are low-set, especially when the trachea drops away dorsally in the neck base; this dorsal drop is often the case with barrel-chested males with chronic obstructive pulmonary disease (COPD). Strap muscle transection results in no loss of function or cosmetic concern.[179] Strap muscle transection should be high on the strap muscles to prevent significant muscle denervation. As mentioned earlier, the superior division of the sternothyroid muscle is a preferred maneuver to expose the superior pole region of the thyroid gland. If the strap muscles are divided, the lateral border of the muscle should be identified relative to the carotid sheath contents, which are directly adjacent (Figure 31.14). During strap muscle mobilization, as in all steps of the thyroidectomy, the field must be kept meticulously bloodless.

Lateral Thyroid Region Exposure—Middle Thyroid Vein

Once the strap muscles are retracted or divided off of the ventral surface of the thyroid, a preliminary dissection lateral to the thyroid is performed to mobilize the lobe preliminarily and to identify the middle thyroid vein. The lateral thyroid region is opened by the division of the middle thyroid vein. The middle thyroid vein or veins run without arterial complement (Figure 31.15). The lateral thyroid region, after division of the middle thyroid vein, is exposed through lateral retraction of the strap muscles and, to some extent, the carotid sheath and sternocleidomastoid muscle. This lateral strap muscle retraction is ideally performed with an army-navy type of retractor towed out and lifted upward, keeping the carotid contents in view. Medial retraction of the thyroid and laryngotracheal complex exposes the parathyroid glands and RLN. Kocher referred to this maneuver as "the medial dislocation of the goiter" (Figure 31.16). With this maneuver, the surgeon's hand engages the thyroid with the gauze (this is critical to prevent slipping on the surface of the thyroid gland) and retracts the thyroid and larynx medially and to some degree rotates the thyroid slightly up and over the trachea. As the thyroid lobe is progressively mobilized, it is also drawn up medially on the laryngotracheal complex. It is best to avoid Lahey or other clamps that can penetrate the thyroid and may result in bleeding or spillage of malignant cells. Gauze overlying the thyroid with digital retraction works best.

Inferior Parathyroid

Proceeding dorsally, the next step after strap muscle retraction and middle thyroid vein division is dissection of the plexus of inferior pole-related veins. It is essential that, as these veins are dissected close to the surface of the thyroid, the inferior parathyroid is identified and swept away and preserved, with dissection being medial to the upper cranial aspect of the inferior parathyroid gland. It is ideal if the inferior parathyroid gland can be identified, marked with a small surgical clip, and reflected inferiorly and laterally before one searches for the RLN.

SECTION 5 Thyroid and Neck Surgery

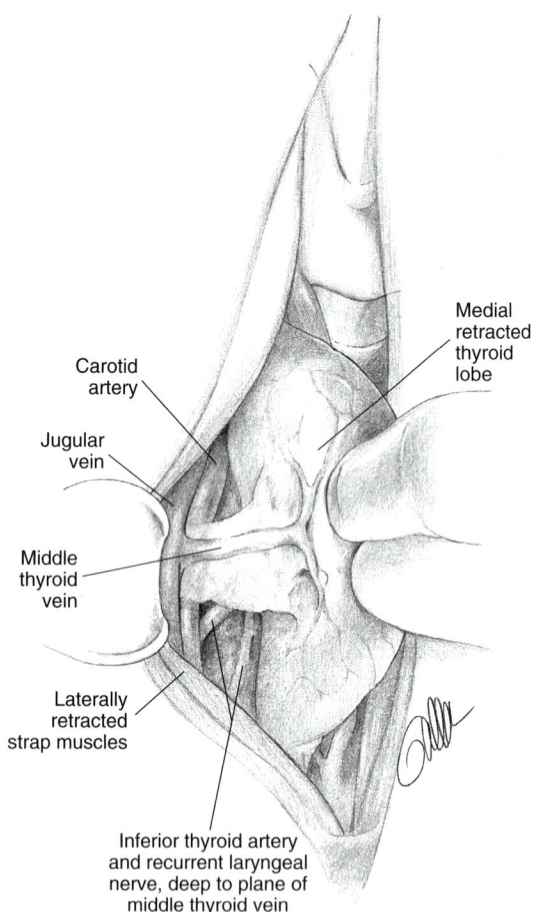

Fig. 31.15 The surgeon's hand retracts the gland anteriorly and medially to expose the posterior surface of thyroid gland. A moistened gauze can be used to grasp the thyroid gland. The middle thyroid vein(s) is (are) subsequently identified, ligated, and divided.

Recurrent Laryngeal Nerve

There are several approaches to finding and carefully preserving the RLN (see Chapter 36, Surgical Anatomy and Monitoring of the Recurrent Laryngeal Nerve). The RLN can be found in the thoracic inlet in the recurrent laryngeal triangle, which has been defined by Lore.[180] The advantage of finding the RLN in the thoracic inlet is that it lies as a single nerve trunk (before branching) in a soft-tissue bed. In revision cases, this is typically "below the last surgeon's scar." Most of the extralaryngeal branches occur more superiorly once the nerve has crossed the inferior thyroid artery (ITA). If found at such an inferior location, it is best to avoid a tendency to trace the RLN superiorly along its entire course. If this is done routinely, inferior parathyroid blood supply extending from lateral to medial may be sacrificed unnecessarily. It is better, once the RLN is found inferiorly, to further identify it superiorly in skip areas, leaving most of its course undissected as it ascends the lateral thyroid region. The presence of a small vessel on the RLN helps in its identification. As the RLN is dissected superiorly, it relates to the ITA. A variety of specific relationships between RLN and ITA have been described; the ITA or its branches intersect with the nerve, which typically is deep to the artery (Figure 31.17). The reliability of the intersection between the RLN and the ITA can be exploited to find the nerve once arterial pulsation of the ITA has been identified. The relationship between artery and nerve may vary from side to side within the same patient. The ITA need not specifically be identified in all cases; however, doing so may help with identification of not only the RLN but also, when medial ITA branches are traced, parathyroid tissue.

The ITA ascends as a branch of the thyrocervical trunk off the subclavian artery and then enters the lateral thyroid region from behind the carotid artery. At this point, it often loops downward and branches to vascularize the inferior and often superior parathyroids in addition to the lateral aspect of the thyroid, which it typically meets at the level of the midpole. The superior parathyroid may be vascularized by an anastomotic loop that arises from the superior and inferior thyroid arteries (see Figure 31.7). The ITA also has a branch that vascularizes the lower edge of the ligament of Berry (Figure 31.18).

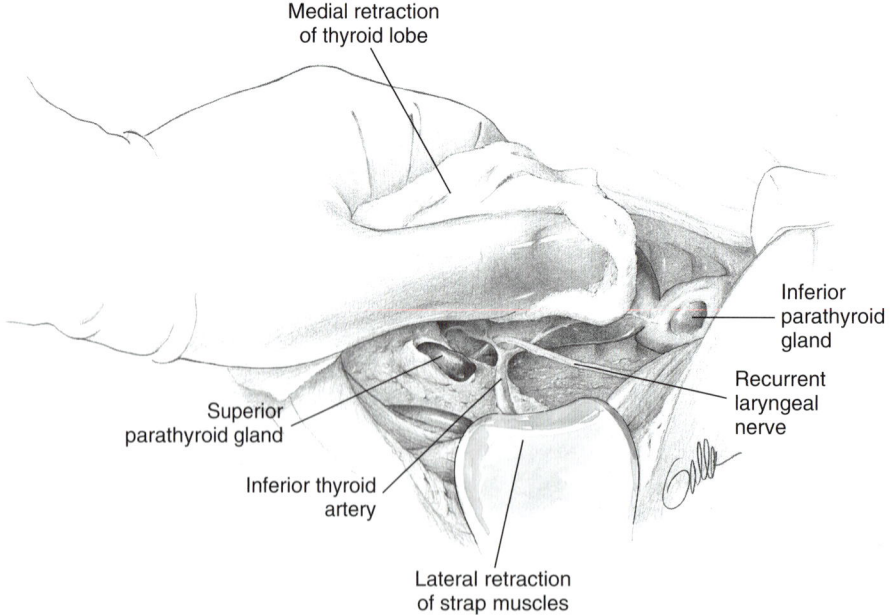

Fig. 31.16 Appropriate traction on the thyroid gland in an anteromedial direction places the inferior thyroid artery under tension and facilitates exposure of the recurrent laryngeal nerve. The inferior parathyroid is usually located anterior to the nerve and approximately 1 cm inferior to the point at which the inferior thyroid artery crosses the nerve. The superior parathyroid gland is usually located superior to the inferior thyroid artery and posterior to the nerve, where it passes deep to the inferior constrictor muscle.

CHAPTER 31 Principles in Thyroid Surgery   287

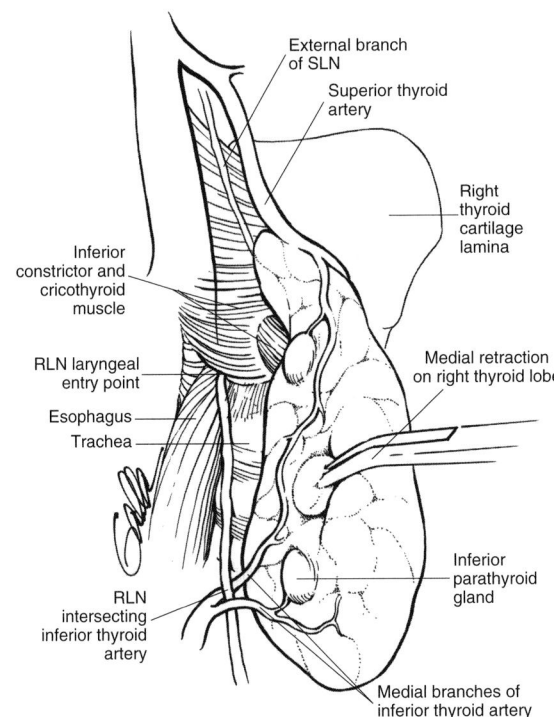

Fig. 31.17 Right lateral view of the lateral thyroid region, showing intersection of the recurrent laryngeal nerve, as it ascends the neck, with the inferior thyroid artery.

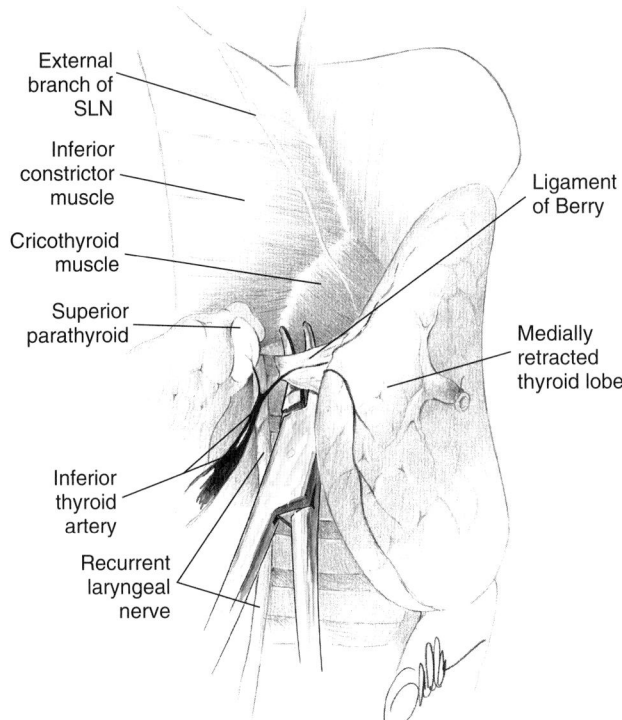

Fig. 31.18 Resection of the thyroid gland and division of the ligament of Berry. The recurrent laryngeal nerve passes through the ligament of Berry and passes deep to the inferior constrictor muscle at the level of the cricoid cartilage. A small crossing vessel or vessels may traverse this posterior suspensory ligament. If bleeding occurs in this area, it should be controlled with pressure or thrombin-soaked Gelfoam while keeping the nerve under direct vision.

While dissecting the RLN superiorly above the ITA, one encounters the ligament of Berry. This ligament, also known as the posterior superior suspensory ligament of the thyroid or as the adherence zone, anchors the thyroid to the lateral aspect of the lower edge of the cricoid and to the first and second tracheal rings. The anchoring effect is responsible for the upward motion of the thyroid because the larynx and trachea elevate during deglutition. This tough and well-vascularized interval has a close and variable relationship with the RLN (see Chapter 36, Surgical Anatomy and Monitoring of the Recurrent Laryngeal Nerve). Typically, the RLN runs deep to the ligament or between a larger anterior and smaller posterior leaflet of the ligament (Figure 31.19). The thyroid capsule in the region of the ligament of Berry becomes relatively dissolute. The ligament of Berry can be considered a condensation of the capsule in this region. As a result, a varying degree of thyroid tissue infiltrates the substance of the ligament of Berry, which brings thyroid tissue directly adjacent to the nerve.[181] The tubercle of Zuckerkandl, a lobule of thyroid tissue that can be present to a variable degree, can extend posteriorly behind the RLN or anteriorly just below the ligament of Berry (see Chapter 2, Applied Embryology of the Thyroid and Parathyroid Glands).[179] This tubercle, when present, also brings thyroid tissue directly adjacent to the RLN. The ligament of Berry is dense, easily bleeds, and has a very close relationship to adjacent thyroid tissue. Within all of this are the RLN, its extralaryngeal branches, and (often) the superior parathyroid. For this reason, this region is the most challenging to dissect during thyroid surgery (see Figure 31.18). Indiscriminate clamping and cautery risk neural injury. Transient compression with gauze or a pledget often controls smaller vessels in this area safely. Pledgets soaked with dilute epinephrine are additionally helpful. Careful transient use of a fine-tipped bipolar cautery is encouraged in this area. The RLN should be dissected and visualized until it disappears from the surgical field by entering under the inferior-most fibers of the inferior constrictor muscle lateral to the cricothyroid muscle at the lower edge of the lateral cricoid cartilage. This is the precise point of the exit of the RLN from the thyroid surgical field and is termed the *laryngeal entry point* (see Chapter 36, Surgical Anatomy and Monitoring of the Recurrent Laryngeal Nerve).

As one is dissecting the RLN, the opposite hand can be used to retract the thyroid and larynx and to provide slight cranial retraction. This impacts on the nerve at its laryngeal entry point and has the effect of straightening the path of the nerve, making it somewhat less redundant and more amenable to careful atraumatic dissection. One must be cautious when a portion of the ligament of Berry is posterior to the RLN; even judicious thyroid lobe retraction may cause upward bowing of the nerve onto the lateral aspect of the trachea or kinking of the nerve. Such retraction-induced positional changes to the nerve could lead to, at the very least, transient neuropraxia; such occurrences likely cause most cases of transient paralysis that surprise surgeons postoperatively. Data from neural monitoring studies show that RLN injury is most often from stretch at the ligament of Berry, so great care and ongoing visual inspection during related maneuvers are extremely important and cannot be overemphasized. In all circumstances, as one retracts the thyroid lobe, one must keep the RLN in constant view to determine the effect of thyroid retraction on the nerve. This is especially true during ligament of Berry dissection.

Another approach to the identification and preservation of the RLN avoids dissection and identification of the nerve at the thoracic inlet altogether; this is termed the *superior approach*. In the approach, the nerve is found initially near its laryngeal entry point. The method requires that the upper pole be dissected and reflected so the laryngeal entry point can be approached (see Figure 31.13). Selective division of the sternothyroid muscle can be helpful in gaining exposure of the

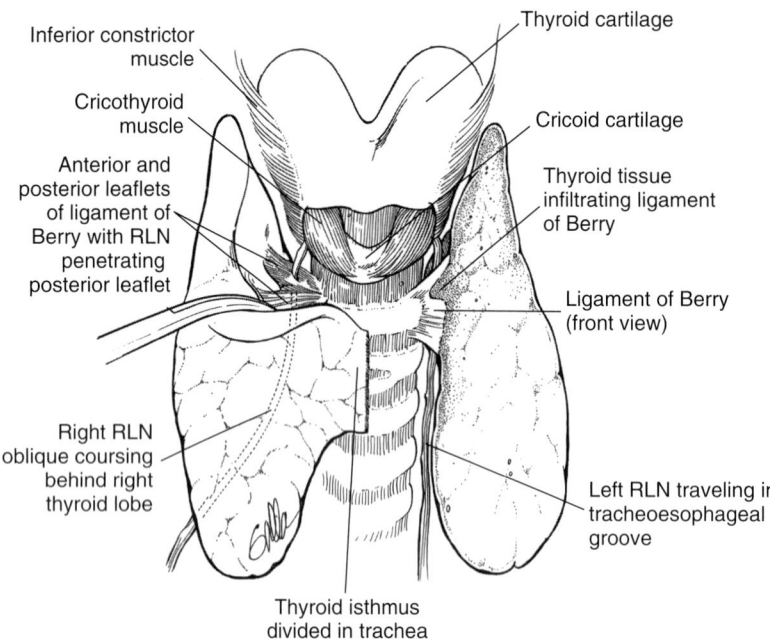

Fig. 31.19 Front view of the thyroid and larynx, showing the course of the recurrent laryngeal nerve through the ligament of Berry. The recurrent laryngeal nerve (RLN) may pass deep to, or through portions of, the ligament of Berry. Thyroid tissue may infiltrate the ligament of Berry, which can bring thyroid tissue in direct apposition to the RLN in this area.

superior pole and may improve visualization of the EBSLN during dissection (see Chapter 35, Surgical Anatomy of the Superior Laryngeal Nerve).

Parathyroid Glands

After the RLN and inferior parathyroid gland are identified, the surgeon begins the search for the superior parathyroid. Parathyroid position relates to embryologic migration paths. Knowing parathyroid embryology (see Chapter 2, Applied Embryology of the Thyroid and Parathyroid Glands) is of extreme importance for successfully identifying these tiny structures, which range in their location from the mandible to the middle mediastinum. A normal parathyroid gland weighs 35 to 40 mg and typically measures 5 × 3 × 1 mm. Parathyroid gland localization requires meticulous dissection to avoid interrupting the lateral to medial orientation of the blood supply of the parathyroid glands. The dissection must also remain bloodless, as blood staining of tissue limits the surgeon's ability to identify subtle cues in parathyroid identification; of key importance is the characteristic of parathyroid color. Magnification is strongly recommended. Parathyroid tissue can be recognized by a variety of characteristics (Table 31.3). First is the gland's unique color, which is typically brown to reddish tan and is often described as a salmon color. Normal fat, in contrast, is bright yellow, whereas brown fat is similar in color to normal parathyroid glands.

Thyroid tissue is firmer and a mottled reddish brown, whereas lymph nodes, often with a notable pitted surface, are a variable gray to tan to red and are generally firmer than parathyroid glands. Importantly, parathyroids—unlike thyroid tissue, lymph nodes, or fat—have, upon detailed inspection, a characteristic distinct hilar vessel (a "vascular strip"). The parathyroid surface is smooth because it represents an encapsulated organ within the neck. The surfaces of lymph nodes and the thyroid are typically more mottled, especially when viewed with loop magnification. Parathyroid shape is also an excellent distinguishing characteristic. Wang has beautifully described common shapes.[182] Parathyroid glands are usually shaped like a kidney bean but may assume other shapes. Lymph nodes are generally less flat and more spherical. Parathyroids, unless truly intrathyroidal or engulfed in surface lobules of the gland, are discrete from the adjacent thyroid surface and can be dissected off the thyroid surface on a laterally based vascular pedicle. Thyroid surface nodules can be mistaken for normal or abnormal parathyroid glands but are usually partially intrathyroidal. Their dissection off the thyroid gland's surface typically results in more hemorrhage than when a true capsular parathyroid is dissected with care.

An important distinguishing feature of parathyroid glands is their unique encapsulated organoid appearance, identified most easily when the adjacent fat, in which they commonly rest, is manipulated. Parathyroid tissue has a discrete edge. Manipulation of the surrounding

TABLE 31.3 Parathyroid Characteristics

Structure	Color	Firmness	Shape	Discrete Sliding Movement	Vascular Hilum
Thyroid	Red	Yes	Varies	No	No
Fat	Bright yellow	No	Amorphous	No	No
Lymph node	White-gray to red	Yes	Spherical to elliptical	+/−	No
Thymus	White-yellow	No	Amorphous	No	No
Parathyroid	Tan, brown, salmon	Soft	Elliptical, flat	Yes	Yes

amorphous fat (thymic fat for the inferior parathyroids and fat lobules on the posterolateral surface of the lateral aspect of the thyroid lobe for the superior parathyroids) results in a discrete gliding motion of the encapsulated abnormal parathyroid within the fat; the motion is likened to a rowboat riding on a wave on the windswept water. This can be described as a *glide sign*. This unique motion results from the encapsulated nature of the parathyroid; the motion, confirmatory color, shape, and vascular strip help to definitively identify parathyroid tissue during thyroidectomy. Parathyroid adenomas are typically darker and firmer than normal parathyroid glands because of less intra- and intercellular fat.

In cases of bilateral thyroidectomy, symmetry in parathyroid conformation and location can be tremendously helpful. Akerström noted positional and shape symmetry of the superior glands in 80% of cases and symmetry to the position and shapes of the inferior parathyroid glands in about 70% of cases (see Chapter 60, Surgical Management of Multiglandular Parathyroid Disease).[183] Gilmore noted that over 90% of normal superior parathyroid glands are situated at the level of the cricoid cartilage.[184] Finding one parathyroid on one side should prompt the surgeon to dissect the corresponding location contralaterally and to expect a similarly shaped parathyroid. It should be noted that although symmetry exists right to left, the inferior parathyroids may not have the same shape as the superior parathyroids. As noted earlier, the relationship of the RLN and the ITA may differ from side to side within the same patient.

Parathyroids have a clear-cut location relative to the plane of the RLN in the neck, which has been described by Pyrtec[185] (Figure 31.20). If the RLN's path through the neck is taken as a coronal plane, the inferior parathyroid is ventral or anterior (i.e., more superficial in the neck) to the plane and the superior parathyroid is dorsal or posterior (i.e., deeper in the neck). This positioning of the parathyroids relative to the RLN is very helpful, especially when one is trying to identify inferior and superior parathyroids during parathyroid exploration.

> BOX 31.1 **Inferior Parathyroid/Parathyroid III**
>
> - Path: Travels with thymus, position more variable than superior parathyroid
> - Location: Within 1 cm inferior or lateral to the inferior thyroid pole
> - Relationship to recurrent laryngeal nerve: Superficial
> - Vessel: Inferior thyroid artery
> - Maneuver to identify: Often seen with gentle manipulation of thyrothymic fat directly underneath the strap muscles, extending from the anterior mediastinum to the inferior surface of the inferior thyroid pole

The normal locations of the superior and inferior parathyroids have been reviewed by Wang, Gilmore, and Akerström.[183-185] The inferior parathyroid glands (parathyroid III arising from the third branchial pouch) enjoy a more variable position in the adult neck than the superior parathyroids (parathyroid IV arising from the fourth branchial pouch) because of variations in their longer embryologic path of migration (Box 31.1). The inferior parathyroid migrates with the thymus and so typically rests within 1 to 2 cm inferiorly or posterolaterally to the inferior pole of the thyroid. It may also rest in the thyrothymic ligament, thymus, or fat lobule adjacent to the thyroid's inferior pole. When this fat is thickened, discrete, and relatively encapsulated, it is called the thyrothymic horn; this is a thymic remnant that has undergone fatty degeneration. Failure of the inferior parathyroid to attain its full migration to the root of the neck base results in a location much higher in the neck, such as at the level of the carotid bifurcation, where it is typically found in close association with a rest of thymic tissue; this is an embryologic testament to its origin and identity as an inferior gland. Such an inferior parathyroid gland has been termed an *undescended parathymus*. Finding the ITA and dissecting along its medial branches can help one to find the inferior parathyroid. However, the distal arterial vessels are diminutive and subject to injury.

The superior parathyroid arises from the fourth branchial pouch and migrates with the lateral thyroid anlage C-cell complex; the superior parathyroid tracks closely with the posterolateral aspect of the bilateral thyroid lobes (Box 31.2). Its location in the neck is most characteristically at the level of the cricothyroid cartilage articulation—that is, laterally at the junction of the upper margin of the cricoid cartilage and the lower margin of the thyroid cartilage lamina. Its location is less reliably described as being approximately 1 cm above the intersection of the RLN and the ITA. These two linear structures in the neck and their intersection point, however, enjoy a reasonably variable relationship and so provide a less reliable clue to superior parathyroid location.

> BOX 31.2 **Superior Parathyroid/Parathyroid IV**
>
> - Path: Travels with lateral anlage/C-cell complex, which forms upper portion of the lateral thyroid lobes
> - Location:
>   - More constant: within 1 cm of cricothyroid articulation
>   - Less constant: 1 cm cranial to the intersection of the inferior thyroid artery and recurrent laryngeal nerve
> - Relationship to recurrent laryngeal nerve: Deep
> - Vessel: Inferior thyroid artery or an anastomotic branch formed between the inferior thyroid artery and the posterior branch of the superior thyroid artery
> - Maneuver to identify: As the thyroid lateral lobe is dissected serially, thin fascial bands are taken down to maintain dissection at the level of the true thyroid capsule; superior parathyroids typically are seen in fat lobules closely adherent to the posterior lateral aspect of the thyroid lobe's superior pole

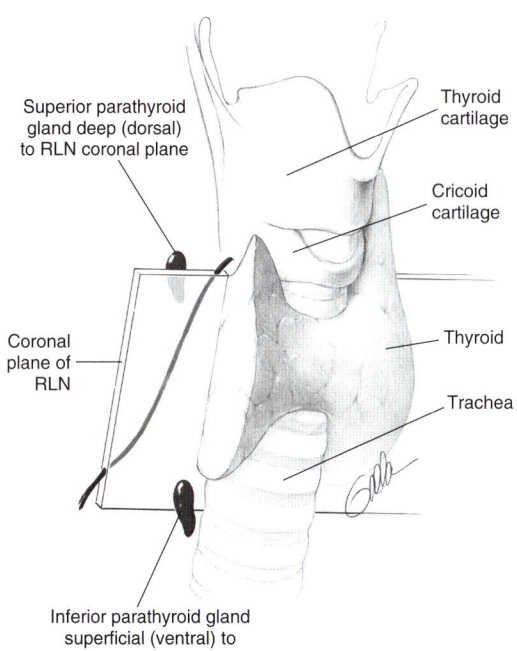

Fig. 31.20 Right anterior oblique view of the thyroid and airway. If the recurrent laryngeal nerve's course in the neck is taken as a coronal plane, the superior parathyroid gland is deep (dorsal) and the inferior parathyroid is superficial (ventral).

The superior parathyroids typically reside in fat lobules closely associated with the posterolateral surface of the thyroid lobe, deep to the plane of the RLN. One identifies the parathyroids and the adjacent fat as one dissects the posterolateral aspect of the thyroid lobe by serially reflecting all the thin layers of fascia overlying the true thyroid capsule in this area. Although both the inferior and superior parathyroid glands are usually supplied by the ITA, Halstead and Evans in 1907, and more recently Nobori et al., have shown that the superior parathyroids can also be vascularized by the superior thyroid artery.[186] As this area is dissected, one should be aware of the possible arterial contribution to the superior parathyroid by the posterior-most branch of the superior thyroid artery. Care should be taken to preserve this branch, if at all possible, as one dissects the superior thyroid pole vascular pedicle (see Box 31.2 and Figure 31.7). During dissection of this region, occasionally the lateral edge of the thyroid blends with adjacent musculature overlying the hypopharynx and esophagus because of the fascial layers that overlie these structures. It is beneath these fascial layers that the superior parathyroid gland resides. When the superior parathyroid gland is ectopic, it tends toward a retrolaryngeal and retroesophageal location that may typically be difficult to visualize sonographically. Because of the deep posterior location of the normal superior parathyroid gland, ectopic superior parathyroid adenomas tend to migrate in the tracheoesophageal groove from these posterior locations into the posterior mediastinum along prevertebral fascial planes; this occurs perhaps secondary to forces of repetitive deglutition and negative intrathoracic pressure.

As mentioned previously, one undertakes dissecting the thyroid lobe on its posterior surface close to its capsule, reflecting away all the fascia, fat, and soft tissues containing the parathyroid glands and the blood vessels. This ensures preservation of not only the parathyroid glands but also their blood supply. The ITA generally runs in a lateral-to-medial direction. The superior thyroid artery's contribution to the superior parathyroid gland often runs directly inferiorly (i.e., caudally) and is visualized as one dissects the superior pole.

Having identified the parathyroid glands, the surgeon reflects them along with their associated fat off the thyroid gland, based on an undissected, laterally oriented soft-tissue pedicle containing their blood supply (Figure 31.21). During this dissection, one identifies and controls the distal branches of the ITA, medial to the parathyroid at the level of the thyroid capsule, as described by Attie[187] (Figure 31.22). Kocher originally performed ligation of the ITA laterally in an effort to prevent blood loss during thyroidectomy. Halstead subsequently modified this maneuver and suggested that the ITA should be controlled at the level of its distal-most medial branches on the gland to preserve the parathyroid blood supply.[188] Lahey, in 1938, resurrected lateral thyroid artery ligation, but he combined this with subtotal thyroid resection and found that this combination resulted in low rates of hypoparathyroidism.[189] Vessels bridging the interval between the medial surface of the parathyroid and the lateral surface of the thyroid gland are generally believed to be insufficient to vascularize the parathyroid gland.[187,190] Curtis, in 1930, suggested that distal parathyroid artery segments may be fed by anastomotic vessels from the trachea and esophagus, which are maintained in the setting of subtotal thyroidectomy.[190] Thus, left undissected on a thyroid remnant, parathyroid glands may receive their blood supply through these tracheal and esophageal anastomotic vessels. However, this practice is not recommended because it leaves portions of thyroid gland behind. It is preferable to excise all thyroid tissue by performing an extracapsular complete thyroidectomy. The blood supply to the parathyroid glands must be safely preserved to maintain their viability by careful and meticulous dissection. When a parathyroid gland cannot be dissected from the thyroid, it should be biopsied and then transplanted into the sternocleidomastoid muscle.

Superior Pole and EBSLN

Some practitioners suggest dissection of the superior pole as an initial step during thyroidectomy, some reserve it as a final maneuver, and others do it in between. We prefer to first dissect the inferior pole, reflect the inferior parathyroid laterally in the lateral thyroid region, find the RLN, and then dissect the superior pole. Leaving the superior pole until this point in the dissection allows greater lobe mobilization, which facilitates retraction from the superior pole downward, and allows greater visualization of the superior pole region and the EBSLN (see Chapter 35, Surgical Anatomy of the Superior Laryngeal Nerve). Keeping the superior pole in this final phase of lobectomy also allows the superior pole management after the superior parathyroid has been reflected on a good vascular pedicle. Given its dorsal location, dissection of the superior parathyroid gland is necessarily kept until a final phase of the surgery. Once this gland is reflected posterolaterally and preserved, the superior pole can be aggressively mobilized and downwardly retracted, at which point the superior pole vessels can be dissected with optimal exposure afforded for the EBSLN. As the superior pole vessels are dissected, downward mobilization of the gland is facilitated by using a Mayo clamp or DeBakey forceps on the superior pole parenchyma (assuming there is no tumor in the superior pole), which facilitates downward retraction. Once the inferior pole has been dissected upward and the superior pole has been fully dissected downward, the ligament of Berry and the final centimeter of RLN can be exposed with greater ease. When the superior pole is significantly enlarged or if the dissection is difficult, two steps can be taken to improve exposure of the superior pole region. The first is sternothyroid muscle transection, as mentioned earlier. The sternothyroid muscle tends to "hood" the superior pole as it extends superiorly to insert on the oblique line of the thyroid cartilage. Lateral retraction of the sternohyoid muscle and medial retraction on the thyroid-laryngotracheal complex allows visualization of this discrete muscle band as it extends medially to its laryngeal insertion. The transected sternothyroid muscle need not be reapproximated. We have found that the insertion of the laryngeal head of the sternothyroid muscle on the oblique line of the thyroid cartilage is a very robust indicator of the position of the EBSLN as it runs down just posteriorly along the inferior constrictor muscle on

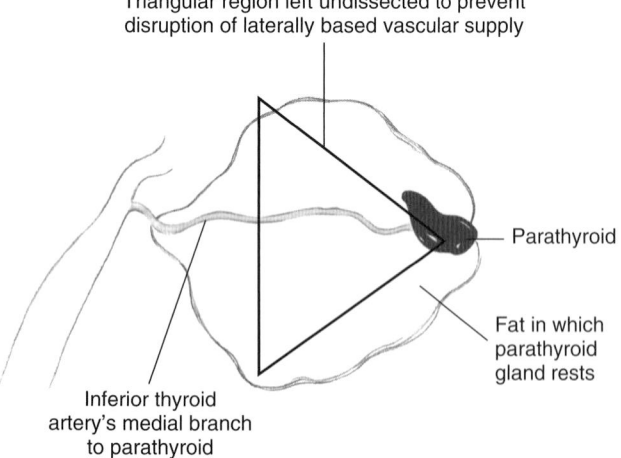

Fig. 31.21 Preserving parathyroid gland vascular supply. Color alone is insufficient to judge parathyroid health after dissection. If the parathyroid has not been dissected from adjacent fat and if a triangular region is left undissected lateral to the parathyroid to prevent disrupting the laterally based vascular supply, then the parathyroid should be judged well vascularized.

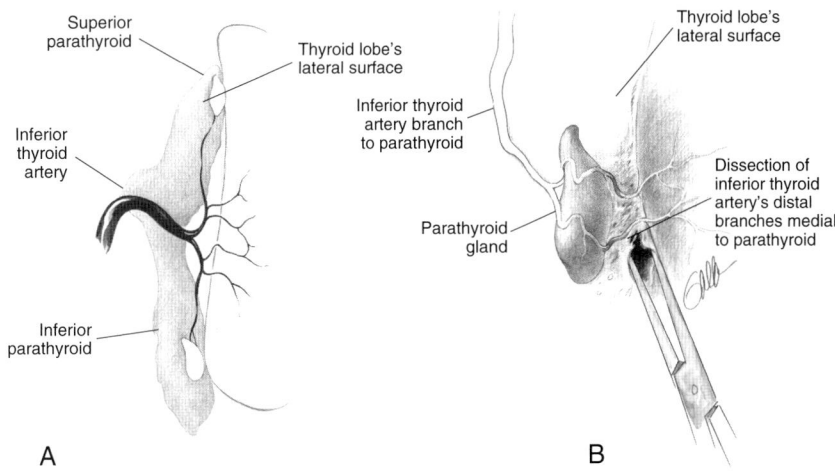

Fig. 31.22 A, Parathyroid glands resting in fat on lateral thyroid lobe's surface. **B,** Dissection on the capsule of thyroid medial to the parathyroid to preserve the laterally based parathyroid blood supply.

the lateral edge of the larynx on its way to the cricothyroid muscle. Patients experience no additional pain, edema, or drainage from this "mini strap division" (see Figure 31.13). The second maneuver for exposure during superior pole dissection involves simply dividing the isthmus and dissecting the ligament of Berry; this allows the thyroid to be pedicled entirely by superior pole attachments. This also allows full mobilization of the lobe and facilitates downward lobe retraction to dissect the superior pole. The superior pole vessels should be taken individually to optimize their control and avoid risk of injury to the EBSLN. Posterior branches of the superior thyroid artery may contribute to the superior parathyroid blood supply and should be reflected posteriorly and maintained if possible.

The superior laryngeal nerve branches from the vagus high in the neck and extends to the larynx, running deep to the external and internal carotid arteries (see Chapter 35, Surgical Anatomy of the Superior Laryngeal Nerve). We have found that the EBSLN can be identified visually in 80% of cases and identified through electrical stimulation in virtually 100% of cases. As it extends to the larynx inferomedially along the lateral surface of the inferior constrictor muscle, it innervates both vertical and oblique portions of the cricothyroid muscle, which is a primary tensor of the vocal cord. Lennquist has shown that in about 20% of cases, the EBSLN follows an intramuscular course in the inferior constrictor muscle.[191] The nerve in this circumstance can still be identified with nerve stimulation through identification of a discrete cricothyroid muscle twitch. Cernea has shown that in 20% of patients, the EBSLN is vulnerable to surgical injury crossing the superior thyroid artery vessels at or below the level of the superior pole of the thyroid[192] (see Chapter 35, Surgical Anatomy of the Superior Laryngeal Nerve). Mooseman and Cernea have beautifully reviewed the anatomy of the superior laryngeal nerve, its external branch, and the relationship of this nerve to the superior pole.[192,193]

To summarize, a 20% to 20% rule can be considered for the EBSLN: 20% of the time it is deep to the fascia of the inferior constrictor as it runs along the lateral larynx traveling to the cricothyroid muscle, and 20% of the time it extends caudally to interact with the superior pole vessels extending below this uppermost limit of the superior pole, placing it at risk as the superior pole vessels are controlled. The path of the EBSLN is reliably along the lateral aspect of the inferior constrictor as it runs caudally to innervate the cricothyroid muscle. It is always just posterior to the laryngeal insertion of the sternothyroid muscle as already noted. This sternothyroid muscle insertion onto the thyroid lamina represents an obliquely oriented line on the thyroid cartilage laminae.

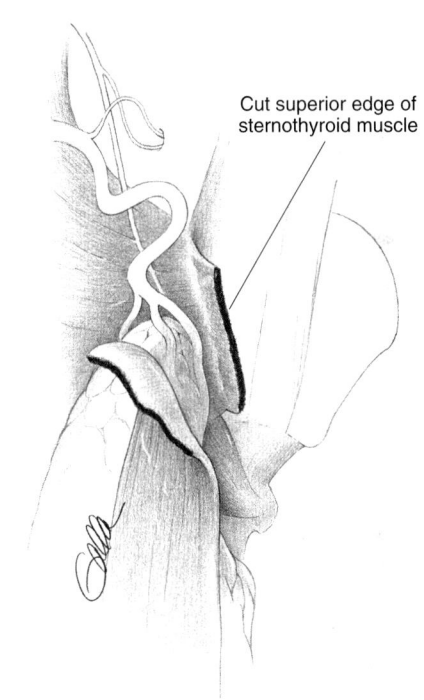

Fig. 31.23 Incision is made in the sternothyroid muscle with cautery, increasing superior pole exposure.

Even when the nerve is traveling deep to the muscular fascia and cannot be visualized (approximately 20% of cases), it can be electrically traced out using this muscle's laryngeal insertion as a landmark (see Figures 31.8 and 31.23).

Isthmus

The thyroid isthmus can be divided easily at any point during thyroidectomy. For this reason, we prefer to perform this as a final step. Generally, the isthmus is divided at the junction with the contralateral lobe opposite to the tumor (taking care to stop dissection before entering the contralateral tracheoesophageal groove and risking injury to the contralateral RLN). It is best to have no remaining thyroid tissue left on the anterior aspect of the upper cervical trachea in the event of a need for reoperation (see Chapter 9, Reoperation for Benign Disease and

Chapter 50, Reoperative Thyroid Surgery). It may also be more cosmetically acceptable because some patients will develop compensatory thyroid hypertrophy status post-lobectomy. The stump of the isthmus can be oversewn with 2-0 chromic or silk suture if not divided and treated with an energy device. The specimen side of the isthmus may be tagged with a silk suture as an isthmus margin. This helps to ensure that the pathologist has properly oriented the specimen. Except in the setting of Hashimoto's thyroiditis, the remaining half of the thyroid is generally sufficient to maintain a euthyroid state without supplementation. However, thyroid function tests should be obtained on all patients approximately 6 weeks postoperatively.

Contralateral Surgery: Safety Checklist

Before the surgeon begins dissection of the contralateral thyroid lobe, he or she should confirm the rationale for total thyroidectomy. Is there malignancy that warrants contralateral surgery? Is there benign nodularity that requires contralateral lobectomy? To avoid the possibility of bilateral VCP and possible need for tracheotomy, it is also extremely important to ensure normal functioning of the ipsilateral RLN before moving to the contralateral side. This is determined not only through confirmation of a visually intact nerve but (if neural monitoring is employed) also through review of the electrophysiologic data with final vagal nerve stimulation at completion of lobectomy[122] (see Chapter 36, Surgical Anatomy and Monitoring of the Recurrent Laryngeal Nerve). A second safety check before moving to the contralateral lobe is an assessment of whether the parathyroid glands on the first side appear to be viable. If they were clearly preserved, have good color, were relatively undissected from the surrounding fat, and have a well-vascularized, laterally based pedicle, their normal function is likely. If, on the other hand, they required autotransplantation, were maintained in situ but became significantly dark, or have a questionable vascular pedicle, one might be more reluctant to remove the opposite lobe. ICG angiography can be used if available.

Thyroid Bed Uptake after Total Lobectomy

Although the bulk of the thyroid lobe is an encapsulated discrete structure that can generally be completely excised, there are three regions where the integrity of the thyroid capsule can degrade: the ligament of Berry, the pyramidal lobe, and the superior pole. Depending on the degree of thyroid gland infiltration in these regions and the diligence of the surgeon, thyroid tissue can, with the best of efforts, be left in situ, resulting in thyroid bed radioiodine uptake after "total lobectomy" (see Figure 31.6). Such tissue can also result in recurrent hyperthyroidism in patients being operated on for Graves' disease (see Chapter 8, The Surgical Management of Hyperthyroidism). Emerick found that 82% of 65 patients with follicular carcinoma who underwent total thyroidectomy had "residual functioning thyroid bed activity and represented ablation candidates."[194] Attie and Auguste found that 15% of patients who underwent total thyroidectomy had postoperative thyroid bed uptake greater than 1.5% and required ablation.[88,195] Marchetta found that mean thyroid bed uptake after total thyroidectomy was 15% (range 4% to 33%).[89] Clark et al. found that 47 of 82 patients undergoing total thyroidectomy had thyroid bed uptake of greater than 1%.[196] The amount of thyroid tissue left after "total thyroidectomy" can be significant.

The most common area in which thyroid tissue remains is at the posterior superior suspensory ligament or ligament of Berry. This ligament, described in detail in Chapter 36, Surgical Anatomy and Monitoring of the Recurrent Laryngeal Nerve, can be thought of as a condensation of the true thyroid capsule. It extends from the undersurface of the thyroid to the corresponding surface of the anterior lateral trachea and lower cricoid. Thyroid tissue can be present in this ligament, bringing it in very close relationship to the RLN, as Berlin and, more recently, Wafae described.[181,197] In addition, the tubercle of Zuckerkandl, which resides to a varying degree inferior to the ligament of Berry and can extend behind the RLN, also can be left during an attempted total thyroidectomy. In both circumstances, unless the distal-most course of the RLN is meticulously dissected, thyroid tissue may remain adjacent to the ligament of Berry region. This is obviously of less importance during dissection for benign disease. If thyroid tissue is left at the ligament of Berry, it can appear as a roundish profile of thyroid tissue approximating the cut edge of the ligament of Berry; it appears on postoperative scanning as two symmetric foci of uptake on either side of the upper trachea in the thyroid bed. Some authors suggest that "a small remnant of thyroid tissue may be retained [at the ligament of Berry] to preserve the integrity of the nerve."[175] We believe that the degree of dissection when the ligament of Berry is infiltrated with thyroid tissue should consider the caliber of the nerve and the degree to which that nerve is lifted off its bed. If a nerve is very thin and lifted off its bed, we feel significant dissection in this area may result in a neuropraxia, typically transient. If the tissue in this area is anodular and away from the cancer, it can be maintained as a very small remnant at the ligament of Berry to decrease the risk of nerve or parathyroid injury. If the nerve is thick and firmly anchored to the dissection bed, then it is our experience that it will be able to tolerate the distal dissection required to resect all gross thyroid tissue (see Chapter 36, Surgical Anatomy and Monitoring of the Recurrent Laryngeal Nerve).

The second area that can result in postoperative thyroid bed uptake is the pyramidal lobe.[198] The pyramidal lobe can be quite flattened and ensheathed in thick precricoid fascia and can exist off the midline to some extent, even arising from the medial aspect of the left or right superior pole. The pyramidal lobe must therefore be sought and dissected superiorly, typically to the level of the thyroid cartilage notch.

The third area that can result in postoperative thyroid bed uptake is the superior pole. The superior pole is usually more tapered than the more bulbous and discretely encapsulated inferior pole. Frequently, it can taper so extremely that the distal-most portions of the superior pole represent small wisps of thyroid tissue that can be present within fascial bands formed as the superior pole vessels are dissected. Clamps placed on the superior pole vessels need to be placed high enough to encompass such thyroid tissue. At the same time, the more superiorly the superior pole dissection extends, the greater the risk to the EBSLN (see Figures 31.6 and 31.7). This is particularly hazardous if a single right-angled clamp is used for "mass ligature" of the upper pole vessels. We recommend that each of the branches of the superior thyroid artery be individually dissected, divided, and ligated (see Figure 31.13).

Closure and Final Steps

If appropriate, the lobectomy specimen is sent for frozen section. This is usually done for nodules that are suspicious but not diagnostic of papillary carcinoma on preoperative FNA. Once the result is back and no further surgery is contemplated, the neck is examined for nodal disease. The ipsilateral paratracheal, pretracheal, and prelaryngeal regions are carefully examined visually and through palpation, as are the adjacent jugular nodal regions 3 and 4.

Every parathyroid gland should be considered the last parathyroid gland. Contralateral surgery may be subsequently necessary, but before the hemithyroidectomy specimen is sent for frozen section, it should be meticulously inspected for parathyroid glands that may have been removed inadvertently with the lobe. Lee found that 11% of 414 thyroidectomy specimens contained parathyroid glands. Nearly 60% of these were extrathyroidal and could have been preserved in situ or autotransplanted.[199] The inferior pole and the posterolateral aspect of the superior pole are key regions to examine carefully. Any presumptive parathyroid should be biopsied for confirmation and then autotransplanted. The bulk of the biopsied parathyroid should be kept in iced saline on the surgical field as one awaits the frozen section result. Parathyroids that have been identified in the surgical field should be inspected before closure. Black parathyroid glands are likely to be ischemic; they should be biopsied for confirmation and then reimplanted. We believe the lack of black color change does not prove that the parathyroid vascular supply is intact. A parathyroid that is blackened has likely undergone venous outflow disruption. A parathyroid gland may have arterial interruption and retain normal color. Also, little color change is typically seen in parathyroids that are resected on thyroidectomy specimens. It is therefore important not to be lulled into a false sense of security by normal parathyroid color. It is important to honestly assess the vascular pedicle supplying the parathyroid. If there is a wide span of tissue extending laterally from the parathyroid that has been undissected, and if the parathyroid itself has not been dissected away from its surrounding fat and is of good color, then it is reasonable to assume that it will function well postoperatively.

Parathyroids that are to be autotransplanted should be maintained in cold saline solution on the surgical field. When frozen section confirmation is obtained, the parathyroid remnant should be divided into 1-mm² pieces and placed into several muscle pockets in the sternocleidomastoid muscle and marked with a nonabsorbable suture or clip.[201-204] If muscular pockets are used, then it is important that no bleeding occurs within these pockets. These pockets should be marked with clips or nonabsorbable suture because primary hyperparathyroidism after parathyroid autotransplantation during thyroidectomy has been reported.[204] Postoperatively, symptoms of hypocalcemia should be treated promptly. The treatment of hypocalcemia likely does not result in a decrease in autotransplant take.[201] Fresh parathyroid grafts begin functioning in 6 to 10 weeks. Liberal autotransplantation schemes at thyroidectomy may be associated with higher transient but generally low permanent rates of hypoparathyroidism.

An assessment for hemostasis should be made in the thyroid bed and on the airway, strap muscles and platysma-skin flap. It is helpful to have the anesthesiologist give positive pressure ventilation through several respiratory cycles to increase venous pressure to detect any occult venous bleeders (i.e., Valsalva maneuver). Scant oozing around the ligament of Berry is best controlled with suture ligation with fine silk (if possible), simple pressure, or with thrombin-soaked gel foam. Careful transient bipolar cautery with fine-tipped forceps can be very useful. Clamping and cautery in this area without identification of the RLN may result in RLN injury.

Drains are infrequently needed after thyroidectomy.[205] This decision must be made on an individual basis. With a large amount of dead space, extensive dissection, and strap muscle transection, drainage may be appropriate. A 15 French Jackson Pratt drain works well in these circumstances; it can be drawn out through the incision and kept loosely in place with a platysma level dissolvable stitch. In the adjacent skin edge, 5-0 nylon can be placed and left long to tie when the drain is removed, typically the next morning. Strap muscles are reapproximated with 3-0 absorbable suture. An effort should be made, as the strap muscles are closed, to cover all exposed strap muscle fibers. Uncovered strap musculature tends to scar to the undersurface of the platysma/skin flap and occasionally leads to unsightly puckering of the superior skin flap with swallowing. The platysma layer can be closed with an absorbable suture. The deepest portion of the dermis can be encompassed with these sutures to ensure that the skin edge comes to evert properly and align. The skin closure we prefer is with a subcuticular running dissolvable suture followed by overlying Steri-Strips, removed at 2 weeks postoperatively (see Chapter 40, Incisions in Thyroid and Parathyroid Surgery).

Dictation and Synoptic Reporting

The findings and conduct of surgery are of great importance and need to be conveyed to the endocrinologist managing the patient postoperatively. This information is important in calculating prognostic parameters such as MACIS scores and has great utility in interpreting postoperative RAI uptake, ultrasound, and thyroglobulin data, which can significantly affect the need for RAI ablation and treatment. Chambers et al. have found that an online synoptic data form required at the completion of surgery yielded significantly improved information flow beyond routine dictated reports; such reports have been the traditional way of communicating surgical information. Chambers recommended that a preoperative laryngeal examination, key anatomic data (as it relates to the parathyroid, RLN, and SLN), and details of invasion, tumor size, and completeness of resection were essential ingredients of such a surgical reporting system.[206]

REFERENCES

For a complete list of references, go to expertconsult.com.

32

Robotic and Extracervical Approaches to the Thyroid and Parathyroid Glands

Emad Kandil, Ehab Alameer, Woong Youn Chung, Hyun Suh, David J. Terris

> Please go to expertconsult.com to view related video:
> **Video 32.1** Transaxillary Robotic Thyroidectomy
> **Video 32.2** Postauricular Robotic Thyroidectomy

INTRODUCTION

Advances in surgical technology have enabled surgeons to develop multiple minimally invasive and remote access approaches to the thyroid gland.

In the early 2000s, Miccoli introduced the minimally invasive endoscopic thyroidectomy (MIVAT) using a small cervical incision, which initially gained significant interest in the United States.[1-4]

Following that, remote-access approaches were attempted using endoscopes through small incisions placed on the anterior chest, breast, or axilla, or combinations of these sites.[5]

It was believed that such extra-cervical, "scar-less in the neck" approaches would be desirable for many patients interested in cosmetic outcomes, specifically young patients and patients with a history of keloid or hypertrophic scars.

However, initial experience proved that endoscopic remote-access thyroidectomy was limited by two-dimensional visualization and rigid instruments.[5]

The surgical robot technology was then introduced to thyroid surgery through the work of Chang and colleagues, who pioneered a gasless transaxillary approach, and the work of Terris and colleagues, who described the facelift (or retroauricular) approach. The robot system provided three-dimensional visualization and multi-articulated endoscopic arms, which proved ideal for the limited workspace of the neck.[6-8]

Development of multiple remote-access thyroid surgery techniques prompted the American Thyroid Association (ATA) to issue a statement on this topic in 2016.[9]

In this statement, the authors acknowledged that remote-access thyroid surgery has a role in selected circumstances when done by surgeons performing high volume thyroid surgery. Adherence to strict selection criteria was recommended to help ensure safe outcomes.

At the time of publication of this ATA statement, the four most commonly utilized remote-access approaches to thyroidectomy in the United States were: the endoscopic breast approach, the endoscopic and robotic bilateral axillo-breast approach (BABA), the endoscopic and robotic transaxillary approach, and the endoscopic and robotic facelift (retroauricular) approach.

In recent years, there has been a trend moving away from the robotic facelift approach in favor of transaxillary and transoral approaches, as was noted in a U.S. multi-institutional study.[10] In that study, robotic facelift approach operative time was significantly longer than the other two remote-access approaches.

The transoral endoscopic thyroidectomy vestibular approach (TOETVA) was introduced to clinical practice by Anuwong,[11] and this technique has been adapted to include modifications such as transoral endoscopic parathyroidectomy vestibular approach (TOEPVA), transoral robotic thyroidectomy vestibular approach (TORTVA), and transoral robotic parathyroidectomy vestibular approach (TORPVA; see Chapter 33, Transoral Thyroidectomy).[12]

Some suggested advantages proposed by the proponents of TOETVA include shorter distance from the incision to the thyroid or parathyroid gland, thus decreasing the amount of dissection needed to create a sufficient working space, and reducing the operative time.[13]

TOETVA also provides a midline, symmetrical view of the anatomic landmarks. It is performed with standard, reusable laparoscopic instruments, which may reduce cost compared with robotic-assisted techniques. The healing of oral mucosa occurs quickly and the incisions are usually not visible within weeks after surgery. However, the procedure continues to evolve. Recently submental incision was described to facilitate the extraction of the thyroid gland.

A recent publication attempted to establish a basic framework necessary for a safe and responsible implementation of transoral techniques that may also be applicable to the evaluation and potential integration of other technologies or techniques.[12] The authors suggested a list of requirements that a surgeon must meet before considering this approach:

- High-volume thyroid practice
- Competence with necessary instrumentation
- For robotic cases, surgeons must be facile and credentialed in robotic surgery

The authors also stressed the importance of institutional support, surgeon and team education, and preparation and outcomes recording.

PATIENT SELECTION, INDICATIONS, AND CONTRAINDICATIONS

For the two most commonly performed robotic thyroidectomy techniques in the United States—the robotic-assisted gasless transaxillary and retroauricular approaches—an "ideal" patient is typically a young female, who have a small or average body mass index (BMI) less than 30 kg/m^2.

However, our group has demonstrated that robotic transaxillary thyroidectomy can be safely done in North American patients with BMI above 40 kg/m^2,[14] and other groups have shown that robotic retroauricular approach can be safely done for patients who are obese, but with a BMI less than 40kg/m^2.[15]

Like other remote-access approaches, these techniques may be considered especially in patients meeting such criteria with a history of keloid or hypertrophic scar formation.

TABLE 32.1 Contraindications for Robotic-assisted Transaxillary and Retroauricular Approach

Thyroid	Parathyroid
Absolute:	
Large substernal or retropharyngeal goiters	Nonlocalized parathyroid adenoma
$\geq$T3 or more thyroid cancer or any suspicious gross invasion	Possibility of multiglandular hyperplasia
Medullary thyroid cancer	Anatomic or pathologic contraindications to the required positioning
Relative:	
Nodules greater than 5 cm	
Large goiters with volumes greater than 40 mL	
Known T2 well-differentiated thyroid cancer	
Graves' disease with substernal extension	
Obesity (body mass index [BMI] >40 kg/m^2)	
History of previous neck surgery or radiation.	
Anatomic or pathologic contraindications to the required positioning (e.g., rotator cuff pathology or cervical spine stenosis)	

TABLE 32.2 Indications and Contraindications for Transoral Endoscopic Approach

Indications	Contraindications
Thyroid diameter no more than 10 cm, and	**Absolute:**
Dominant nodule size no more than 6 cm, when benign or indeterminate (Bethesda II, III, IV), and no more than 2 cm when Bethesda V, suspicious for malignancy or confirmed well-differentiated thyroid cancer.	History of head and neck surgery—including mandibular surgery
	History of head/neck/ upper mediastinum irradiation,
	Preoperative recurrent laryngeal nerve palsy
Multinodular goiter	Lymph node metastasis
In carefully selected patients, a surgeon may also consider Graves' disease, lesions that are cytologically suspicious, and well-differentiated thyroid cancer with the above size caveat.	Extrathyroidal extension such as tracheal or esophageal invasion
	Presence of oral abscesses
	Evidence of substernal thyroidal extension
	Relative:
	Severe chronic lymphocytic (Hashimoto's) thyroiditis
	Elevated body mass index

Data from Razavi CR, Russell JO. Indications and contraindications to transoral thyroidectomy. Ann Thyroid. 2017;2(5).

Moreover, patients selected for the trans-axillary approach should also be free from any anatomic or pathologic contraindications to the required procedural positioning, such as rotator cuff pathology or cervical spine stenosis.

As previously stated, obese patients may undergo these procedures safely by experienced. Due to the learning curve of 25 to 40 cases associated with these procedures, conservative patient selection is recommended for surgeons new to these techniques.

Thyroid tumor characteristics and surgeons operative experience should also weigh in when selecting patients for robotic-assisted approaches. Although we suggest partial thyroidectomy as the procedure for surgeons new to the robotic-assisted techniques, several studies have reported that robotic-assisted total thyroidectomy and neck dissection are equivalent in oncologic outcomes and safety to open technique, when performed by surgeons who are experienced with both thyroid surgery and neck dissection as well as robotic techniques.[16,17] This has allowed for the expansion of clinical pathology successfully treated by robotic-assisted procedures.

For patients with parathyroid pathology, this approach should only be offered to those with a well-localized parathyroid adenoma preoperatively on imaging studies. Patients with higher possibility of multi gland disease should not be offered this approach.

Absolute clinical contraindications to robotic-assisted thyroidectomy (Table 32.1) include large substernal or retropharyngeal goiters, thyroid tumor size $\geq$ 4 cm ($\geq$T3) or any suspicious gross invasion, and medullary thyroid cancer.[18] Relative clinical contraindications have previously included nodules greater than 5 cm, large goiters with volumes greater than 40 ml, known well differentiated thyroid cancer between 2-4 cm (T2), Hashimoto's thyroiditis, and Grave's disease, as well as obesity, a history of previous neck surgery or radiation.[16,17,19-21]

The indications for TOETVA include the following: thyroid diameter no more than 10 cm and dominant nodule size no more than 6 cm, when benign or indeterminate (Bethesda II, III, IV), and no more than 2 cm when Bethesda V, suspicious for malignancy or confirmed well-differentiated thyroid cancer.[22] Contraindications include history of head and neck surgery—including mandibular surgery, history of head/neck/upper mediastinum irradiation, patients unfit for general anesthesia, evidence of acute clinical hyperthyroidism, preoperative recurrent laryngeal nerve (RLN) palsy, lymph node metastasis, extrathyroidal extension, such as tracheal or esophageal invasion, presence of oral abscesses, and evidence of substernal thyroidal extension. Relative contraindications include chronic lymphocytic (Hashimoto's) thyroiditis and an elevated BMI, due to the potential increased friability of the thyroid and greater difficulty with elevating skin flaps, respectively. These cases would warrant more extensive patient and surgeon preparation. Table 32.2 summarizes indications and contraindications for TOETVA.

SURGICAL TECHNIQUE

Robotic-assisted Retroauricular (Facelift) Thyroidectomy

Steps in a standard robotic-assisted retroauricular (facelift) thyroidectomy procedure are as follows:
- Ideally intubation with an electromyographic endotracheal tube for intraoperative RLN monitoring.
- Positioning in supine with arms tucked bilaterally on the operating table. The head is rotated slightly 20 to 30 degrees to the contralateral side of the planned incision. The hair at the base of the occipital hairline is shaved 1 cm posteriorly along the planned incision.
- The inferior end of the incision is marked at the inferior extent of the lobule in the postauricular crease and is carried superiorly and posteriorly into the shaved region of the occipital hairline in a gentle curve (Figure 32.1). The incision is infiltrated with local anesthetic and the neck is prepped and draped in a sterile fashion.

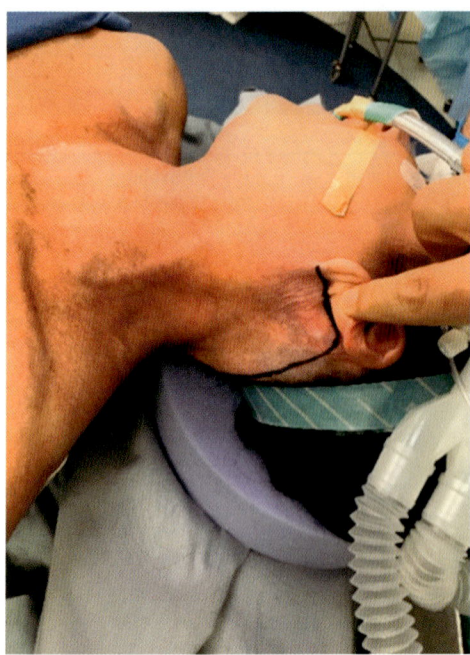

Fig. 32.1 Preoperative view of retroauricular or "facelift" incision.

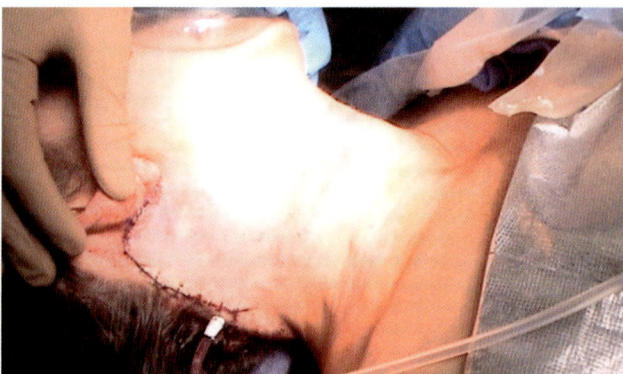

Fig. 32.2 Postoperative view of retroauricular or "facelift" incision.

- The skin is incised with a scalpel, and electrocautery is used to develop a subplatysmal flap, exposing the sternocleidomastoid (SCM) muscle; dissection continues anteriorly and inferiorly along the SCM muscle.
- The great auricular nerve is identified, and dissection superior to this reveals the external jugular vein and the anterior border of the SCM. If necessary for exposure, the external jugular vein can be divided.
- Dissection continues down to the anteromedial border of the SCM to the clavicle and reveals a muscular triangle bordered by the SCM, the omohyoid, and the sternohyoid muscles. The omohyoid, sternohyoid, and sternothyroid muscles are retracted ventrally, exposing the ipsilateral superior pole of the thyroid gland, and the superior thyroid pole pedicle is isolated.
- The self-retaining modified thyroidectomy or Chung retractor is secured on the contralateral side of the operating table and positioned to retract the strap muscles ventrally. A Singer hook (Medtronic, Jacksonville, FL, USA) or army-navy retractor is attached to a Greenberg retractor (Codman & Shurtleff, Inc., Raynham, MA, USA) and secured to the ipsilateral side of the operating table, and it serves to retract the SCM laterally and dorsally. Alternatively, a modified approach creates the plane between the two heads of the SCM.
- The daVinci robot system is positioned in the operative field contralateral to the incision. The endoscopic camera in the "30 degrees down" configuration is introduced first into the incision. One disadvantage of this procedure is the limitation of utilization of only three arms. A vessel sealer device and a Maryland grasper are placed in arms two and three and brought into the operative field under direct visualization. The vessel sealer is usually placed in the surgeon's dominant hand.
- The upper thyroid pole is retracted ventrally and caudally, exposing the superior thyroid vessels, which are dissected and divided near the capsule. The gland is then retracted medially, allowing for identification of the RLN in the tracheoesophageal groove. The nerve monitor is used to confirm integrity of the nerve, which is dissected along its path until the insertion under the inferior constrictor muscle at the laryngeal entry point. The superior and inferior parathyroid glands are identified and preserved.
- The inferior thyroid pole is then dissected, and feeding vessels are divided with the thyroid dissected from the trachea. The isthmus is divided, and the thyroid is removed. Integrity of the RLN monitoring signal and hemostasis is verified.
- If used, a drain is placed posterior to the retroauricular incision. The incision is closed in two layers. Interrupted absorbable subdermal sutures are placed, and the skin is closed with interrupted or running absorbable sutures or nonabsorbable interrupted sutures, which must be removed in clinic (Figure 32.2).
- When appropriate, excision of redundant skin can be performed before closure, allowing for a simultaneous "facelift" procedure.

Robotic-assisted Transaxillary Thyroidectomy

Steps in a standard robotic-assisted transaxillary thyroidectomy procedure are as follows:

- The patient is positioned supine and undergoes general anesthesia and intubation with an electromyogram (EMG) endotracheal tube for intraoperative nerve monitoring. The neck is slightly extended with a shoulder roll, and the arm ipsilateral to the lesion or the larger lobe of the thyroid is placed cephalad and flexed above the head into the modified Ikeda's arm position (Figure 32.3). The contralateral arm is padded and tucked. Somatosensory evoked potentials (SSEP; Biotronic, Ann Arbor, MI, USA) can be used to monitor the median and ulnar nerve signals (Figure 32.4). Intraoperative ultrasound is performed after positioning (Figure 32.5).
- To mark the inferior point of the incision, a transverse line is drawn from the sternal notch, laterally to the axilla. The superior point of the incision is marked with a 60-degree oblique line from the thyrohyoid membrane to the axilla (Figure 32.6).
- These points are connected with a longitudinal mark approximately 2 inches in length running along the border of the pectoralis major muscle. The neck and anterior chest are prepped and draped, and the incision site is infiltrated with local anesthetic, then incised.
- Monopolar electrocautery is used to dissect through the subcutaneous tissues of the incision to expose the lateral border of the pectoralis major muscle and continues cephalad toward the clavicle to create a flap in the subplatysmal plane, superficial to the pectoralis fascia. This may require the extender tip of the electrocautery.
- Lighted breast retractors are used to facilitate flap creation. The clavicle is identified and followed medially to the sternal notch, leading to identification of the ipsilateral SCM muscle. The sternal (medial) and clavicular (lateral) heads of the SCM are identified.
- The avascular plane, which exists between the sternal and clavicular heads of the SCM, can be developed with electrocautery or a vessel

CHAPTER 32 Robotic and Extracervical Approaches to the Thyroid and Parathyroid Glands

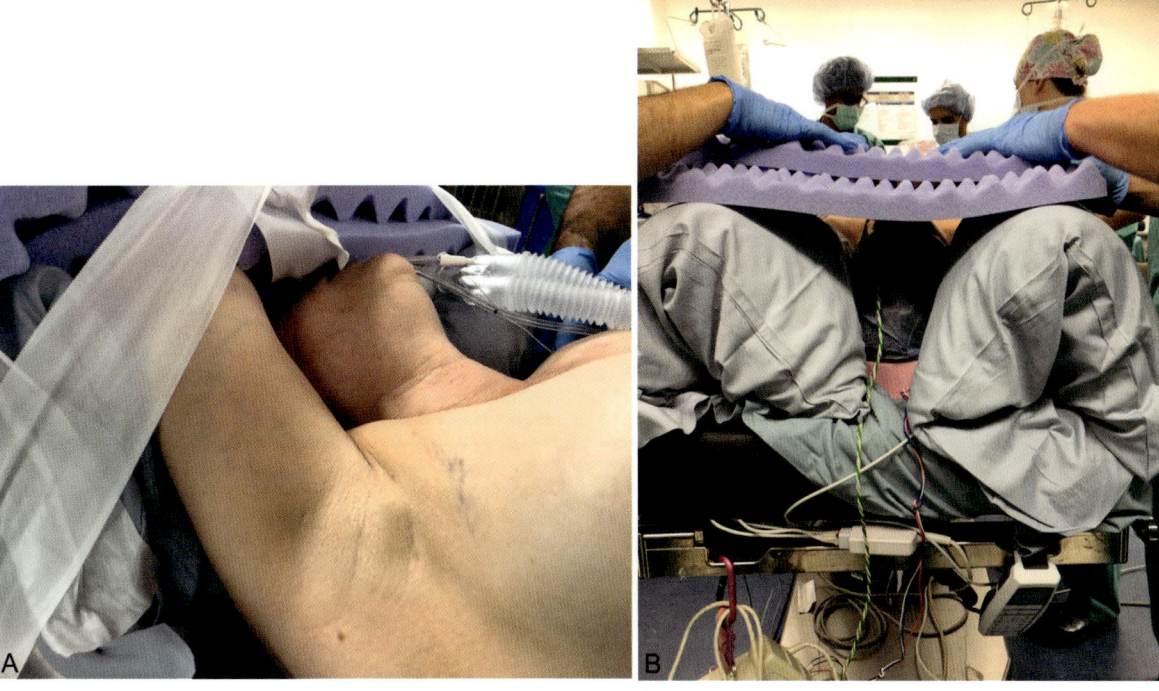

Fig. 32.3 **A** and **B,** Modified Ikeda arm position for transaxillary thyroidectomy.

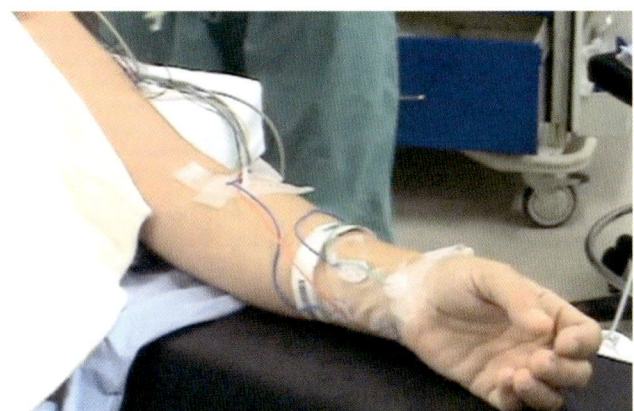

Fig. 32.4 Electrodes for somatosensory evoked potential (SSEP) monitoring in transaxillary surgery.

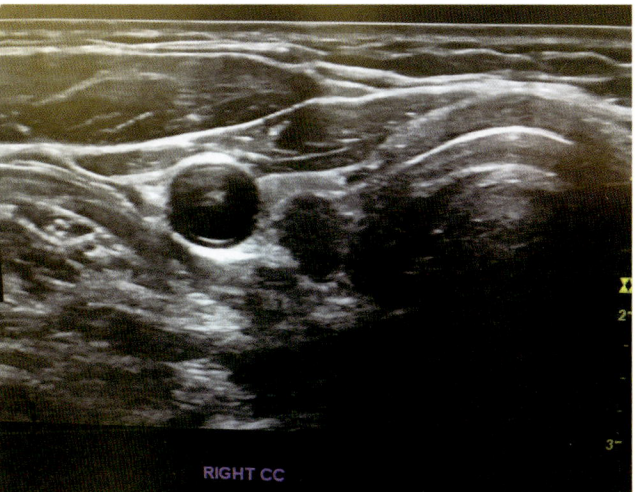

Fig. 32.5 Preoperative ultrasound showing a parathyroid adenoma.

sealer and anterior retraction of the sternal head of the SCM, exposing the omohyoid muscle.
- Dissection of the uppermost fibers of the omohyoid muscle with electrocautery or a vessel sealer will reveal the superior pole of the thyroid gland. The surgeon must avoid damage to the internal jugular vein. Once the superior pole is exposed, a self-retaining Chung retractor or modified thyroidectomy retractor (Marina Medical, Davie, FL, USA) is mounted to the contralateral side of the operating table and used to lift the strap muscles anteriorly (Figure 32.7).
- The daVinci surgical robot (Intuitive, Sunnyvale, CA, USA) is brought into the operative field from the contralateral side (Figure 32.8). The dual-channel camera configured in the "30-degree down" mode is docked first in the central position. A second and third arms are placed with instruments to the right or the left of the central camera arm under direct visualization. The sealing device is placed on the surgeon's dominant side and a Maryland dissector in the contralateral robot arm. The fourth arm is equipped with a Prograsp and is placed on the upper edge of the incision.
- The assisting surgeon inserts a laparoscopic suction/irrigation device through the axillary incision. This serves also to retract the clavicular SCM head or trachea downward during the dissection. The assistant is also responsible for placement of the nerve monitoring device and can troubleshoot robotic arm positioning and maintenance.
- The vagus nerve is stimulated in the carotid sheath. If a bilateral dissection or neck dissection is planned, an electrode may be placed on the vagus nerve for continuous nerve monitoring. The upper pole of the thyroid (Figure 32.9) is retracted medially and inferiorly,

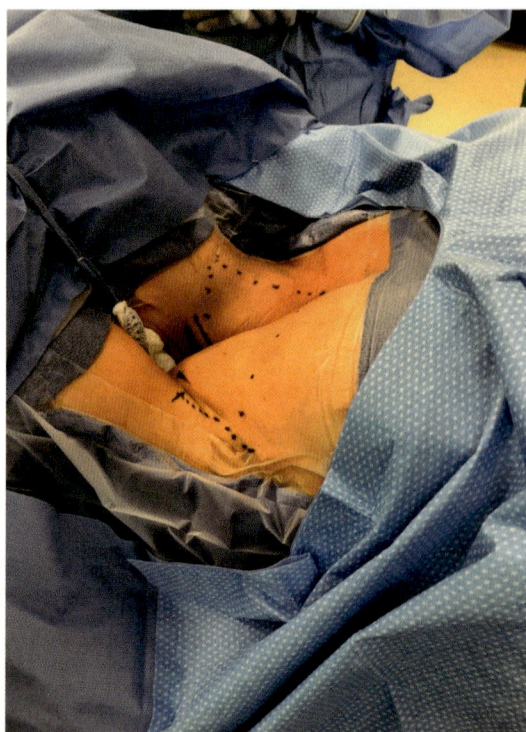

Fig. 32.6 Marking of landmarks for transaxillary incision.

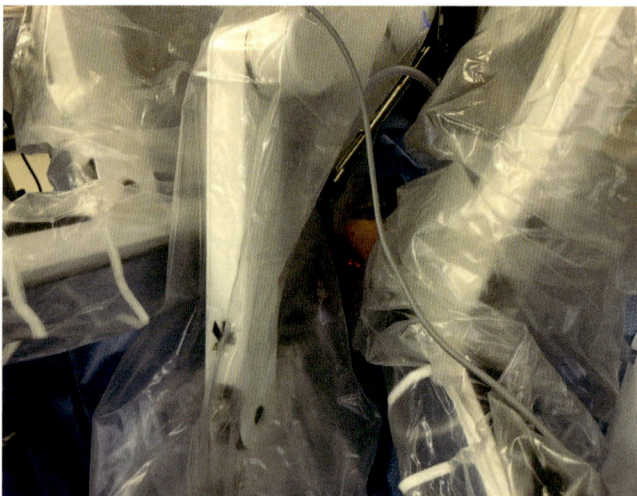

Fig. 32.8 Robot docked for transaxillary procedure.

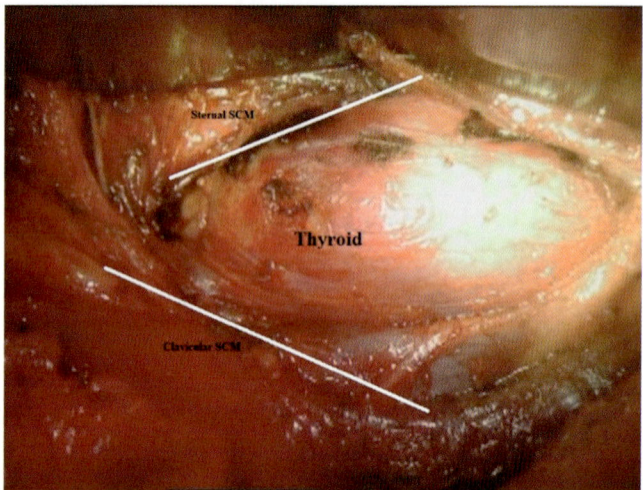

Fig. 32.9 Intraoperative photo of dissection of thyroid lobe.

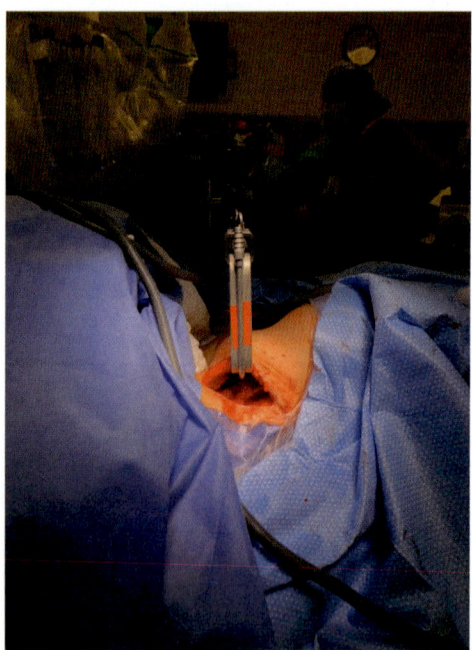

Fig. 32.7 Retraction of skin flap for transaxillary approach before robot docking.

and the superior thyroid vessels are dissected and divided close to the thyroid to avoid injury to the external branch of the superior laryngeal nerve. The superior pole is freed from the cricothyroid muscle, and the superior parathyroid gland is identified and preserved.
- The thyroid is retracted medially, and the middle thyroid vein is dissected and divided. The RLN is identified at the tracheoesophageal groove and is carefully followed until its insertion at the laryngeal entry point. The functional integrity of the RLN, once identified, is confirmed.
- The inferior pedicle is dissected and divided. The inferior parathyroid is identified and preserved. The inferior thyroid is dissected medially to the RLN and is separated from the trachea until reaching the contralateral side. The thyroid lobe and isthmus are divided, and the specimen extracted.
- If a central lymph node dissection is incorporated into the procedure, the central lymph nodes are dissected en-bloc circumferentially from the nerve and removed en-bloc with the thymus and the thyroid.
- For total thyroidectomy, once the ipsilateral lobe has been removed, subcapsular dissection of the contralateral lobe from the trachea is performed. When the contralateral tracheoesophageal groove is reached, the RLN is identified and stimulated. The superior and inferior pedicles are dissected and ligated, the RLN is traced to the laryngeal entry point, and the remaining thyroid is dissected and extracted through the axillary incision.
- If a parathyroidectomy is to be performed, the diseased parathyroid gland is identified, dissected, excised, and removed in an endobag (Figure 32.10).

CHAPTER 32 Robotic and Extracervical Approaches to the Thyroid and Parathyroid Glands   299

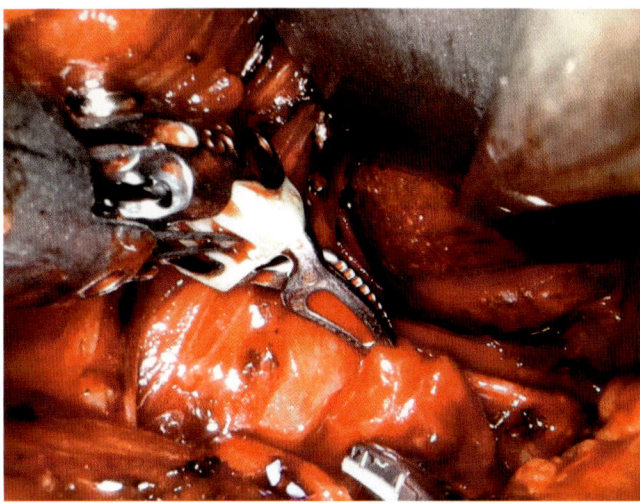

Fig. 32.10 Intraoperative photo of a parathyroid adenoma dissection.

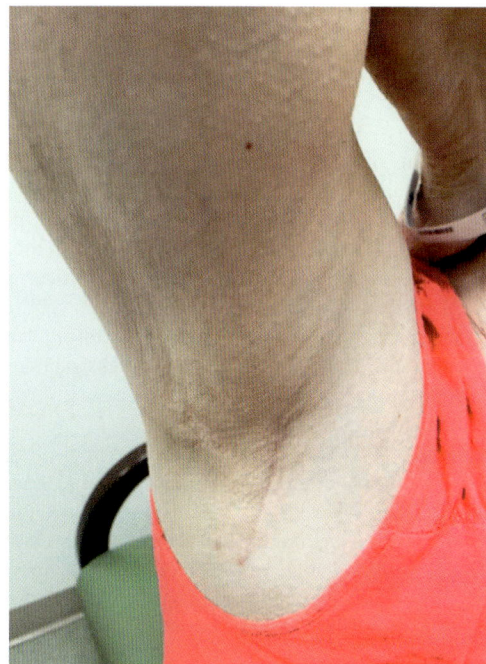

Fig. 32.12 Well-healed postoperative photo of transaxillary incision.

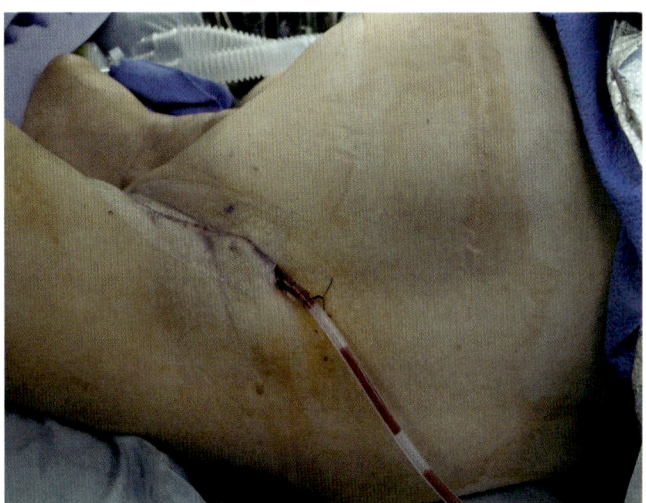

Fig. 32.11 The transaxillary wound is closed in layers and a drain is placed.

- Final stimulation of the RLN and vagus nerve is performed, and hemostasis is ensured. A drain is placed, and the axillary incision is closed in two layers with interrupted subcutaneous and continuous subcuticular closure (Figures 32.11 and 32.12).

Transoral Endoscopic Thyroidectomy Vestibular Approach (TOETVA)

Steps in a TOETVA procedure are as follows:[23-25]
- The TOETVA is performed under general anesthesia with nasotracheal intubation.
- Oral tracheal intubation can be used but may limit the movement of instruments during operation.
- The patient is placed in supine position with a sandbag under the shoulders to slightly extend the neck.
- Preoperative antibiotics are given and the oral cavity is cleaned with normal saline and Betadine (povidone iodine) before incision.
- After identifying the landmarks of the oral vestibular area (the area between the lower lip and lower teeth), three incisions are performed.

- A 10-mm incision is made in the gingivobuccal sulcus above the frenulum.
- This incision and its surrounding tissue are infiltrated with a saline and epinephrine solution (alternatively, local anesthetic can be used) and then bluntly dissected over the midline mandible into the submental subplatysmal plane.
- Two 5-mm incisions are made lateral to each canine in the sulcus near the level of the lip. These incisions and the surrounding tissue are also infiltrated.
- Ports are placed in all three incisions, with the camera in the central port.
- Carbon dioxide insufflation is maintained at 6 mm Hg.
- The working space between the strap muscles and platysma is then dissected using the dilator first, followed by dissection under direct vision using a monopolar hook and an ultrasonic energy device (Harmonic Scalpel).
- Thyroid exposure is approached by opening the deep fascia between strap muscles in the midline. Next, to retract the strap muscle, silk 2-0 suture is passed through the neck skin.
- The following steps are: identifying and cutting the isthmus. The superior thyroid vessels are then ligated using an ultrasonic scalpel. The upper parathyroid, RLN would be revealed, and the lower parathyroid is also preserved.
- Thyroidectomy is completed by Harmonic device. The specimen is put into an endobag and taken out through the 10-mm incision in the oral cavity.
- The deep fascia and the vestibular port locations are closed using 4-0 absorbable sutures.

This approach has been described for both endoscopic and robotic techniques.

POSTOPERATIVE CARE

Postoperative care for both robotic-assisted retroauricular and robotic-assisted transaxillary approaches is as for the open approach. For the TOETVA,[26] no dressing or skin wound care is required. Oral antibiotics and mouthwash three times per day are usually prescribed for 3 to 5 days. Most patients start an oral soft diet the same day of surgery and can be discharged home on the same day or per surgeon's preference.

Complications

Complications of the robotic-assisted thyroidectomy procedures include not only those observed with conventional cervical procedures, such as recurrent laryngeal nerve injury, postoperative pain, neck hematoma, wound infection, and hypocalcemia, but also those unique to the type of access technique, such as brachial plexus neuropraxia for the trans-axillary technique.[8]

Several metanalyses[27-31] have found no significant differences between robotic and open thyroidectomy in terms of transient and permanent recurrent laryngeal nerve injury, permanent hypoparathyroidism, or hematoma formation.

With robotic transaxillary thyroidectomy, brachial plexus neuropraxia is reported in about 0.2–2.2% of cases.[32,28] This complication can be avoided with the use of somatosensory evoked potential (SSEP) monitoring for radial, ulnar and median nerves. A recent study by our group at Tulane Medical Center evaluated a series of 137 robotic transaxillary surgeries performed on 123 patients using SSEP. Seven patients (5.1%) developed significant changes intraoperatively, but immediate arm repositioning resulted in prompt recovery of signals and complete return to baseline parameters with no postoperative positional brachial plexus injuries.[33] Also, rare cases of esophageal and tracheal injuries, as well as mortality, have been reported with this approach's early experience.[14,34]

Complications of the transoral endoscopic approach were reviewed by Shan and Liu in a systemic review.[35] The authors evaluated 10 articles containing 211 cases. In this review, hypoparathyroidism and RLN injury were the most common complications in thyroid surgery. The overall incidence of temporary hypoparathyroidism was 7.1%. The overall incidence of temporary RLN injury was 4.3%. Mental nerve palsy was reported in 2 articles[36,37] published in 2011 and 2014 with an overall incidence of 4.3%. Of note, the mental foramen is most commonly located below and between the mandibular premolar, so care must be taken to identify and avoid this nerve injury while making the lateral incisions. Also, the presence of clean-contaminated wounds in transoral thyroid surgery raises concerns for development of surgical site infection, therefore, prophylactic antibiotics are given for patients who undergo this procedure.

Possible complications specific to the type of access are shown in Table 32.3.

TABLE 32.3 Possible Complications Specific to the Type of Access

Approach	Complication
Transaxillary	Brachial plexus neuropraxia
Retroauricular	Mouth corner deviation from indirect injury to the marginal mandibular nerve
	Ear lobe numbness from indirect injury to the greater auricular nerve
Transoral	Mental nerve injury
	Skin burns
	Temporary chin numbness
	Oral commissure tears

CONCLUSIONS

- Remote-access approaches to the thyroid and parathyroid may be considered for appropriately selected patients, including those with a history of keloids or hypertrophic scars.
- Reports of successful, safe application of remote-access thyroidectomy for multiple pathologies, including thyroid cancer, have been reported with increasing case numbers in the United States.
- Robotic-assisted technology allowed surgeons to overcome limitations of the endoscopic approach to thyroidectomy. Multiple robotic-assisted extra-cervical approaches to thyroidectomy have been developed, taking advantage of the three-dimensional visualization and multiarticulated arms of the robot, which proved ideal for operating in the limited workspace of the neck.
- Transaxillary and transoral thyroidectomy are currently the most commonly performed remote-access procedures in the United States. A recent multi-institutional study showed that the facelift approach is falling out of favor due to longer operative time, lack of access to the contralateral thyroid lobe, and increased complications compared with the other remote-access approaches.
- TOETVA is safe and feasible. It has a shorter learning curve compared with the other remote-access approaches.

REFERENCES

For a complete list of references go to *www.expertconsult.com*.

Transoral Thyroidectomy

Jeremy D. Richmon, Angkoon Anuwong, Zhen Gooi, Jonathon O. Russell

> Please go to expertconsult.com to view related video:
> **Video 33.1** Introduction to Chapter 33, Transoral Thyroidectomy.
> **Video 33.2** Transoral Endoscopic Thyroidectomy Vestibular Approach.

HISTORY OF TRANSORAL THYROIDECTOMY

Since Kocher introduced the modern era of thyroid surgery well over a century ago, the surgical approach has remained virtually unchanged: a lower midneck transverse incision. With improved instrumentation, lighting, and safer operating conditions over the decades, the size of the incision has decreased, but a resultant scar persisted in the anterior neck as a conspicuous hallmark of the surgery. However, there has been recent interest in the development of remote access approaches to the thyroid with the primary goal of avoiding a visible postoperative scar. Although the value of avoiding a visible thyroidectomy scar has been fiercely contested by various experts over the years, there is a growing body of evidence (to be discussed later) that suggests a visible scar may have a significant quality-of-life effect on a patient. This patient-centered perspective, combined with a focus on nonmalignant disease in predominantly a young, female population, has motivated both patients and surgeons to explore alternative approaches to the thyroid (See Chapter 31, Principles in Thyroid Surgery and Chapter 32, Robotic and Extracervical Approaches to the Thyroid and Parathyroid Glands).

Since 1997, there have been approximately 20 different thyroidectomy techniques proposed as minimally invasive alternatives to the conventional transcervical approach.[1] Most of the novel thyroidectomy approaches effectively move the incision to a concealed area of the chest, axilla, or hairline. A minimally invasive procedure should strive to minimize tissue dissection, be safe, respect surgical planes, minimize surgical trauma, and avoid scarring.[2] With these criteria in mind, it is clear that many of these procedures are actually more invasive than the transcervical approach. These alternative approaches have engendered much controversy because they necessitate a compromise between minimal tissue dissection, a visible cervical scar (the status quo), and extensive tissue dissection with a remote, imperceptible scar. The challenge to minimize tissue dissection while still achieving an optimal, scarless cosmetic result has led to the evolution of transoral thyroidectomy.

Natural orifice transluminal endoscopic surgery (NOTES) has garnered increasing enthusiasm in various surgical fields over the past decade.[3,4] By accessing surgical targets deep in the abdomen and pelvis using transoral, transvaginal, or transanal endoluminal approaches, tissue dissection can be minimized; this can result in a favorable risk profile and improved recovery. Within the field of head and neck surgery specifically, there have been advances in transoral surgery for pathologies in the oropharynx and laryngopharynx that have been made possible by technologic innovations in robotic and laser microsurgery. In the context of remote access thyroid surgery, a transoral approach offers several key advantages that make it particularly attractive; the advantages include the following: reduced tissue dissection to reach the central neck; a midline approach, which affords equal exposure to both sides of the neck; and anatomy that is more familiar to the head and neck surgeon (in contrast to the chest and axillary approaches).

In 2007, Witzel et al. published the first report demonstrating the feasibility of a transoral approach to the thyroid in two human cadavers and 10 porcine models through a single, sublingual incision.[5] With the proof of concept established, there were further preclinical experiments establishing the potential of the transoral route.[6-8]

The first clinical use of transoral endoscopic thyroidectomy was reported in 2011 by Wilhelm et al.[9] In this series of eight patients, three patients required conversion to an open approach, and one patient had a permanent recurrent laryngeal nerve (RLN) injury. Nakajo et al. next described their transoral video-assisted approach in eight patients with a premandibular (rather than sublingual) incision and the use of Kirschner wires to elevate the anterior neck skin flap.[10] All patients experienced anterior chin sensory disorders for more than 6 months, which demonstrated one of the risks inherent in this technique. In 2011, Richmon et al. modified the transoral endoscopic approach by introducing the da Vinci robotic system (Intuitive Surgical, Inc., Sunnyvale, CA).[11] Advantages of the robotic over endoscopic technology include the following: a high-resolution, three-dimensional image; wristed and tremor free instrumentation; and precise robotic motion scaling, which allows for superb tissue visualization and handling. The initial approach included a single midline sublingual port for the camera and two lateral vestibular ports for the effector arms. Although feasible, the camera position through the floor of mouth resulted in restricted motion with collisions against the nose and maxilla. The technique was modified by moving the camera port anterior to the mandible such that all three ports were transvestibular; this allowed for unrestricted translation of the camera.[12] The transvestibular approach was subsequently described via a purely endoscopic approach as well.[13] This approach would subsequently become the accepted standard for transoral endoscopic and robotic thyroidectomy. Notable preclinical developments in transoral thyroidectomy can be found in Table 33.1.

Initial experience with transoral robotic thyroidectomy (TORT) was fraught with an unacceptable rate of mental nerve injury.[14] This was due to the placement of the lateral trocars low in the vestibule and close to the mental nerve foramen, which resulted in excessive tension on the nerve with instrument movement. This setback was overcome in

TABLE 33.1 Summary of the Notable Preclinical Developments in Transoral Thyroidectomy

Author	Year	Journal	Subject	Methods
K. Witzel	2008	Surg Endosc	2 cadavers, 10 pigs	Transoral access for endoscopic thyroid resection
T. Wilhelm	2010	Eur Arch Otorhinolaryngol	5 cadavers	Anatomic study
T. Wilhelm	2011	Surg Endosc	5 pigs	Transoral endoscopic thymectomy
T. Wilhelm	2011	World J Surg	8 humans	eMIT: transoral thyroidectomy
E. Karakas	2010	Surg Endosc	10 cadavers, 10 pigs	Transoral thyroid and parathyroid surgery (lateral approach for hemithyroidectomy)
E. Karakas	2011	Surgery	2 patients	Transoral thyroid and parathyroid surgery (lateral approach for hemithyroidectomy)
J.D. Richmon	2011	Head Neck	2 cadavers	Transoral robotic-assisted thyroidectomy
A. Nakajo	2013	Surg Endosc	8 patients	TOVANS (transoral video-assisted thyroidectomy)
J.O. Park	2014	Eur Arch Otorhinolaryngol	6 cadavers	Transoral endoscopic thyroidectomy (trivestibular approach)

eMIT (endoscopic minimally invasive thyroidectomy)

Anuwong's landmark publication of his initial 60 patients of transoral endoscopic thyroidectomy by vestibular approach (TOETVA); the patients had excellent surgical outcomes.[15] There were no mental nerve injuries as the lateral port sites were moved closer to the commissure and away from the mental nerve foramen. Since this publication and the dissemination of this technique through conferences and cadaveric courses, there are currently more than 50 centers, in 13 countries worldwide, that perform transoral thyroidectomy.[34] Enthusiasm for this technique continues to expand, and the rapidly growing body of evidence further supports the safety and feasibility of this procedure.

BETTER COSMETIC RESULTS ARE A NATURAL OUTCOME OF PROCESS IMPROVEMENT

Thyroid surgery has evolved in various facets over the years. Examples of process improvements that have become common include the avoidance of surgical drains, use of intraoperative nerve monitoring (IONM), and outpatient thyroid surgery. Each of these changes has been passionately debated by the experts; however, over time, these and other improvements have become well-accepted among most high-volume thyroid surgeons. The excellent safety profile and low morbidity of thyroid surgery is the product of continuous improvements made over more than a century.

The midline cervical incision represents possibly the final, and likely most contentious, area of potential improvement. Despite myriad approaches developed to either reduce the size of the scar or move the incision away from the middle of the neck, none of these have become widespread in North America or Europe.[16] Almost all Western world surgeons and patients continue with the Kocher incision (popularized more than 100 years ago), even though some patients find it undesirable and even though repeated attempts have been made to improve cosmesis.

REMOTE-ACCESS THYROID SURGERY IS MORE POPULAR IN ASIA THAN IN THE WESTERN WORLD?

Much of the evolution and dissemination of remote access thyroid surgery has occurred in Asia. Patient selection and operative indications likely play a role in the more tempered adoption of remote access approaches in the United States (US).[17] Historically, an elevated body mass index (BMI) was a contraindication for remote access surgery. Many Western patients have a different body habitus; series of remote access patients from the US demonstrate a higher BMI on average than most series from Asia.[18] Authors have suggested that this factor may contribute to the novel complications that were noted with remote access thyroid surgery in the US. Furthermore, the size of thyroid tumors was found to be larger in US series than in those from Asia.[16] Nodules or tumors larger than 3 cm have traditionally been contraindicated for remote access thyroidectomy. Because Western patients have a higher BMI and have larger tumors than their Asian counterparts, they are less likely to be considered as candidates for most remote access approaches.

More nuanced explanations likely exist and may contribute to the discrepancy between the remote access thyroidectomy experience in Asia and the Western world. Some authors have alluded to the fact that there is less interest in avoiding a cervical incision in Western populations.[16] Unfortunately, there is little evidence to support such conclusions as will be discussed later. The cost of robotic remote access approaches has been found to be higher than open controls, but this decreases as operative times decrease.[19] There is also the role of compensation; in societies where robotic remote access approaches reimburse at a higher rate than open thyroidectomy, these approaches are more common. On the other hand, in a fee-for-service system, prevalent in the US, there is a financial disincentive for surgeons to perform cases that take longer; this is especially the case if there is a learning curve associated with proficiency. Perhaps all of these and/or other explanations are valid, but it is clear that remote access thyroid surgery has lagged in adoption in the Western world despite a recognized demand among some patients and despite an excellent safety profile among patients in Asia.

WHY OFFER REMOTE ACCESS THYROID SURGERY AT ALL?

If patients are less likely to be candidates for remote access approaches in the Western world, and if the procedures are costlier and may have additional risks, why should it be offered to patients at all?

There is a growing body of research evaluating the effect of a cervical incision on quality of life demonstrating that a scar may appear to negatively affect some patients in both Asia and North America. Reports from one South Korean series suggest that the characteristics of the scar are not as important as the presence of the scar itself. In other words, no matter how well an incision heals, having a cervical incision is detrimental to the overall quality of life at least during the initial period after surgery.[20] The authors reported that a well-healed cervical incision affected the health care-related quality of life at a level similar to the effect of psoriasis, vitiligo, or severe atopic dermatitis. Another series from the Midwestern US suggests that approximately 20% of patients are self-conscious about a cervical incision more than 1 year after thyroid surgery; however, a majority are satisfied with their scar.[21] The authors noted that more than 10% of patients were considering additional intervention to correct a thyroid scar. This subset of patients affected negatively by a cervical incision was further characterized in a large quality-of-life series focused specifically on thyroid cancer survivors.[22] In their research, Goldfarb and colleagues suggest that young patients especially are more likely to suffer a worse quality of life owing to a cervical incision. The authors hypothesize that this may be related to stigma or a negative body image; this may be seen with some pediatric cancers.

To better understand the demand for improved cosmesis in the US, Coorough and colleagues administered nearly 1000 questionnaires to healthy volunteers in the US; they asked for insight on open thyroidectomy versus transaxillary thyroidectomy.[17] They found that more than 80% of respondents preferred to avoid a cervical incision, and a majority were willing to pay more to avoid an incision. Perhaps most importantly, a majority of patients were willing to accept a hypothetical increase in surgical risk to avoid a cervical incision. Finally, 20% of respondents were more likely to choose avoidance of a cervical incision even if it was less likely to cure their thyroid cancer. Although these responses came from nonpatients, the authors suggest that ethical dilemmas exist regarding autonomy in such situations. When it is clear that a patient may prefer to avoid a cervical incision even with increased risk and expense, should they have the option of selecting such a procedure?

Finally, Nellis and colleagues recently presented data regarding the effect of a cervical incision by asking 193 casual observers to compare patients with a cervical scar to controls without a scar. They found that patients with a cervical scar were perceived negatively in regard to overall attractiveness, attractiveness of the neck, and perceived quality of life. These same casual observers were, on average, willing to pay more than $10,000 to avoid a cervical incision.[23]

There is sufficient evidence to demonstrate that some patients prefer to avoid a cervical incision, even in cases of cancer, even if the surgery is more expensive, and even if the complication rates may be higher. It is clear that, to some patients, a cervical incision is a cause of morbidity. Because most thyroid pathology is indolent, the onus is on the surgeon to minimize all morbidity as much as possible and engage with patients to develop an individualized treatment plan. Thus, minimizing the effect of a cervical incision becomes a priority for every thyroid surgeon.

TRANSORAL THYROID SURGERY (TOTS) VERSUS OTHER REMOTE ACCESS APPROACHES

It is beyond the scope of this chapter to address all the remote approaches to thyroid surgery, and some of these approaches are addressed elsewhere in this text (see Chapters 31, Principles in Thyroid Surgery, and Chapter 32, Robotic and Extra Cervical Approaches to the Thyroid and Parathyroid Glands). The bilateral axillo-breast approach (BABA), robot assisted transaxillary surgery (RATS), and retroauricular facelift approach (RFA) have all found success in some hands but are used in a very limited fashion in North America. Primary limitations that have been cited for each include difficulty visualizing the contralateral lobe (RFA), extensive dissection (BABA, RATS, RFA), unfamiliar angle of dissection (BABA, RATS), and increased operative times (BABA, RATS, RFA). None are truly "minimally invasive," and none avoids a cutaneous incision. Additionally, the learning curve for these procedures is generally felt to be between 35 to 50 cases.[24-26] In addition to the financial disincentive identified previously, it is difficult for practicing surgeons to dedicate 50 cases to mastery of a novel technique. For these and other reasons, none of these approaches have gained a significant following in the Western world.

Compared with each of the previously mentioned approaches, the potential technical advantages of TOTS are obvious. It is the only approach without any cutaneous incision, and therefore provides the best cosmetic outcome. It has the shortest dissection route of any of the other methods, and therefore may be expected to have a shorter operative time and less postoperative pain.[27,28] The midline approach of TOTS allows equal visualization of both the right and left central necks, allowing total thyroidectomy to be completed without the need for repositioning or additional incisions. The superior to inferior angle of dissection is a vantage point that is familiar to most high-volume thyroid surgeons who may regularly find the RLN at the insertion (as for the superior approach to the RLN, see Chapter 36, Surgical Anatomy and Monitoring of the Recurrent Laryngeal Nerve). Same day discharge is more common in the Western world and is more likely for TOTS compared with other remote access approaches.[29]

In addition to the technical advantages of TOTS, there are patient selection advantages as well. The indications for the procedure are broader; body habitus has not affected outcomes in some US series, and patients with larger nodules (up to 6 cm with a thyroid lobe up to 10 cm in maximal dimension) remain potential candidates for the approach.[30] Our own unpublished review of the last 300 cases of thyroid surgery by a single surgeon found that more than 50% of patients were candidates for TOTS. Finally, the learning curve for this approach has been anecdotally described as 7 to 10 cases[28] and more recently has been defined as approximately 11 cases for a laparoscopic naïve surgeon in a North American population.[31] For all of these reasons, TOTS offers distinct patient and surgeon advantages over the other remote access approaches to the thyroid.

Compared with all other remote access approaches, it is apparent that TOTS has broader indications in a Western population,[31] allows for faster discharge,[29] has lower pain scores,[28] bilateral central neck access, and a faster learning curve[30] than other remote access approaches. TOTS also offers the best cosmetic outcome with no cutaneous incisions.

TOTS: Robotic Versus Endoscopic Approaches

Transoral thyroidectomy can be performed safely via a purely endoscopic approach using laparoscopic instruments (i.e., transoral endoscopic thyroidectomy vestibular approach (TOETVA), or with the assistance of robotic technology (TORT). Each camp has its proponents. The advantages and disadvantages of each approach are listed in Box 33.1. The primary difference is that TOETVA can be performed with routine laparoscopic instrumentation that exists in most modern hospitals and is therefore widely accessible. This is in contrast to the additional expense and limited access to robotic technology. The robot's primary advantage is the use of wristed instrumentation and three-dimensional imaging as opposed to straight arm laparoscopic instruments with a two-dimensional screen. The procedures are identical in scope and capability; however, they use different instrumentation to achieve the desired extent of surgery. Nonetheless, TOETVA has garnered significantly more practitioners with currently >50 centers worldwide in contrast to TORT, which is primarily practiced in a few centers in South Korea.

BOX 33.1 Relative Advantages and Disadvantages of Robotic Versus Laparoscopic Technology for Transoral Thyroidectomy

Endoscopic	Robotic
PROS	
• Less expensive, more accessible equipment • Less overall instrumentation • Familiar to general surgeons • Fewer admin/credentialing burdens	• Better optics (3D view) • Ability to control 3-4 instruments precisely • Finer, articulated, tremor-free instruments • Quicker learning curve • Familiar to OTO-HNS
CONS	
• 2D-view • No wristed instrumentation • New skillset for OTO-HNS surgeons	• Still need endoscopic instruments • May need more ports • More expensive • More admin/credentialing burdens

OTO–HNS - Otolaryngology–Head and Neck Surgery

PATIENT SELECTION AND CONTRAINDICATIONS

Given the excellent safety and efficacy of modern conventional transcervical thyroid surgery, it is paramount that patient selection for transoral thyroid surgery is geared toward achieving similar outcomes.[32] Although this approach affords the patient the opportunity to avoid a visible scar, it poses technical challenges. Such challenges include altered surgical view, working space, haptic feedback, and limitations posed by the central vestibular incision in extracting the resected thyroid lobe/gland. In determining ideal patient selection criteria and contraindications for this approach, it is worth examining the experiences of pioneering centers. Anuwong described an initial series of 60 patients in Thailand; the patients were operated on between April 2014 and January 2015 women accounted for 95% of patients with a mean age of 41 years.[15] Patient selection for their series included 57% of patients with a single-thyroid nodule, most of whom received a hemithyroidectomy and isthmusectomy. There were 2 patients who had papillary microcarcinomas. The average nodule size for the entire series was 5.4 cm. The incidence of transient hypoparathyroidism and RLN injury was 5% and 3.3% respectively; however, there were no instances of permanent hypoparathyroidism or RLN injury. This group reported on an expanded cohort of 425 patients that included 45 patients with Graves' disease operated on with similar inclusion criteria until the end of 2016.[28,33] In these expanded cohorts, three patients experienced conversions to open thyroidectomy because of excessive blood loss, two of these patients had a history of Graves' disease, and one patient had a thyroid goiter >12 cm.

Within North America, surgeons from Johns Hopkins University described a case series of 15 patients. The majority of patients had thyroid nodules biopsied as either benign or having atypia of undetermined significance.[34] This cohort of patients had a mean BMI range of 30.3. TORT was used in 6 patients, TOETVA in the rest. The median maximal dimension of the excised thyroid lobes was 6.5 cm. One patient required conversion to open surgery that was attributed to substernal and retroesophageal extension of the thyroid that was not detected on preoperative ultrasound.

Yi et al. have described their experience with using transoral thyroidectomy for the treatment of papillary thyroid cancer in 20 patients.[35] Their inclusion criteria were patients with an intrathyroidal cancer <2 cm with no evidence of central or lateral lymph node metastasis. Twelve patients (60%) received a lobectomy. There was one instance of transient vocal cord paresis. Three patients who received total thyroidectomy had transient hypocalcemia.

Overall, the indications, ideal patient selection criteria, and contraindications for transoral thyroid surgery are evolving, which is reflective of its ongoing development and adoption by new practitioners. A study group convened at the 1st International Transoral Thyroidectomy NOTES (i.e., natural orifice transluminal endoscopic surgery) Conference in Bangkok, Thailand, in February 2016. The group published their recommendations for inclusion criteria for transoral thyroid surgery to encompass thyroid lobe size <10 cm, benign tumors, papillary microcarcinoma and Graves' disease.[36] It is worth noting that reported conversions to open surgical procedures in the literature have been attributed to either substernal goiters or Graves' disease. Razavi and Russell have proposed contraindications for transoral thyroid surgery to include a history of head and neck surgery, head/neck/upper mediastinal irradiation, active clinical hyperthyroidism, preoperative RLN palsy, lymph node metastasis, extrathyroidal extension of tumor, intraoral abscesses, and substernal thyroid extension.[31]

Current Recommendations for Patient Selection

Considerations for patient selection and contraindications to transoral thyroid surgery, together with further considerations for beginning surgeons who are adopting this technique, are as follows:

1. Patient motivation: The ideal patient should be very motivated to avoid a visible neck scar. Furthermore, patients with a history of keloid/ hypertrophic scarring should also be considered candidates for the transoral approach.
2. Patient past medical history: Patients with a prior history of neck surgery and irradiation should be excluded given the high likelihood for intraoperative bed scarring, limiting clear visualization of tissue planes. Hashimoto's thyroiditis (HT) can make the thyroid gland more adherent to surrounding tissue planes; this may lead to increased difficulty with dissection. The hypervascularity associated with Graves' disease also increases the risk of intraoperative bleeding during dissection, which can limit visualization of the operative field.
3. Thyroid factors: Within the published data, there have been variations on inclusion criteria for the maximum size of thyroid lobe and thyroid nodules; however, it is recommended that for beginning surgeons, maximal thyroid dimension should be ≤6 cm in length with a maximal nodule dimension of ≤4 cm. As surgical experience is accumulated, the maximal thyroid dimension size may increase to 10 cm in the absence of malignancy. One additional consideration is thyroid nodule location and side. As the initial mobilization of the thyroid lobe focuses on upper pole dissection, and identification of the RLN typically occurs in a more proximal location close to its insertion point compared with traditional open thyroid surgery, a prominent upper pole nodule can present additional difficulty. A more ideal location for thyroid nodules, for the surgeon learning the procedure, is the mid or lower pole. For increased ease of laparoscopic instrumentation and dissection, a thyroid nodule on the ipsilateral side of the dominant surgeon's hand is ideal for the beginning surgeon as well, (e.g., right thyroid lobectomy is performed by a right-handed surgeon).
4. For oncologic safety, initial surgical cases should not include patients with thyroid nodules having Bethesda classification V or VI. Patients with radiologic and cytologic evidence of central or lateral neck metastasis should be excluded.

5. Oral cavity, neck anatomic features and the thyroid gland: Although there should be no exclusion criteria based on gender, men are not ideal initial patients for surgeons accumulating experience in this surgery; the (typically) more prominent chin and thyroid notch of male patients further limits maneuverability of instruments and retraction of the dissected portions of the thyroid. Anecdotal experience suggests that a more medial placement of the lateral ports may counteract this effect but does not completely negate this fact. The presence of oral cavity braces decreases the space for camera and instrument placement and increases difficulty of specimen extraction. Mandibular prognathism or orthognathism are additional anatomic features that should be considered preoperatively. During extraction of the thyroid specimen, the surgeon must negotiate the curvature of the submental space and bony projection of the mandibular symphysis; these anatomic characteristics depending on the patient specific anatomy may increase technical difficulty.

Informed Consent

As with any alternative procedure, the patient needs to have a full understanding of the risks inherent to the transoral approach as compared with those of traditional thyroidectomy. Risks inherent to the transoral approach include the following: numbness and paresthesia to the lip and chin; sensation over the central neck; bruising to the lip, chin, and central neck; and the potential need to convert to an open approach.

Preoperative counseling and the informed decision-making process should include disclosure on the part of the surgeon regarding their experience with this technique and its longer operative times (should the surgeon be early in their experience).

PREOPERATIVE WORKUP

Preoperative workup should include a thyroid ultrasound as well as fine-needle aspiration (FNA) of thyroid nodules per American Thyroid Association (ATA) criteria.[36] There should be a low threshold toward obtaining cross-sectional imaging for any concern regarding substernal/retroesophageal extension, which is a contraindication for the transoral approach.

TECHNIQUE

The surgical techniques for TOETVA and TORT are very similar as mentioned previously. The procedure will be described for TOETVA later[15,30,37] with key differences for TORT specifically mentioned.

Patient Positioning

The patient is intubated with a nasotracheal or orotracheal tube and placed supine with slightly more neck extension than conventional open thyroidectomy (Figure 33.1). A nerve-integrity monitoring endotracheal tube is recommended to allow IONM. The patient is prepared and draped from the nose to the areolae in case conversion to open thyroidectomy or specimen retrieval (via the axilla) are required. Anesthesia should be on one side of the patient across from the operating nurse. The endoscopic tower is at the foot of the bed and the surgeon stands at the head of the bed with one or two assistant surgeons on each side (Figure 33.2).

Trocar Placement

The lip is marked and infiltrated with lidocaine with epinephrine (Figure 33.3). The procedure is initiated with ~2 cm horizontal midline vestibular incision for the camera port (Figure 33.4). Monopolar cautery is used to control mucosal bleeding. The midline is then divided

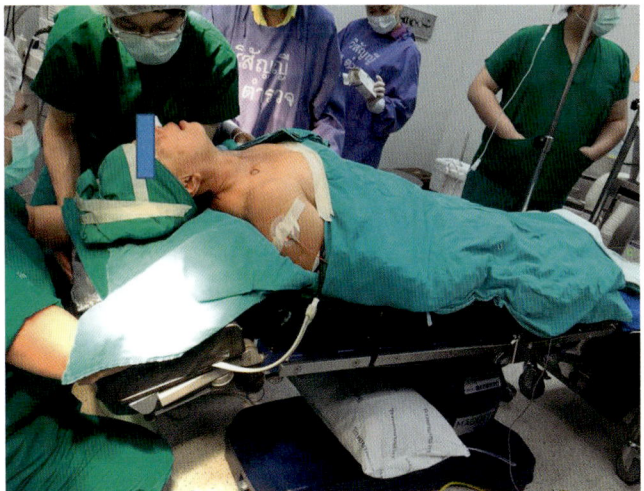

Fig. 33.1 Patient positioning for transoral endoscopic thyroidectomy by vestibular approach (TOETVA).

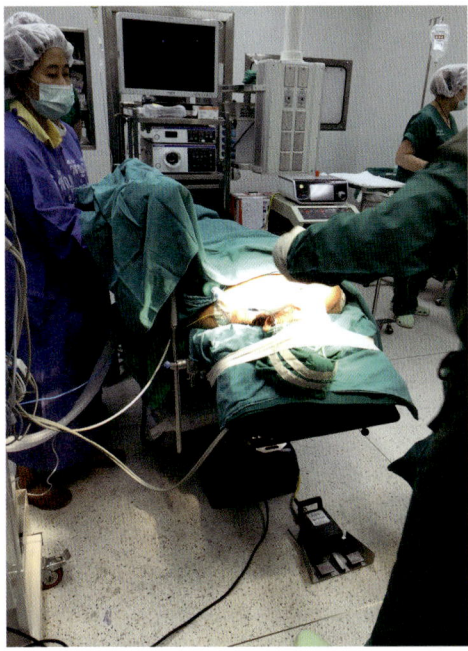

Fig. 33.2 The endoscopic tower is at the foot of the bed with anesthesia positioned on one side. The surgeon stands at the head of the bed with one or two assistant surgeons on each side.

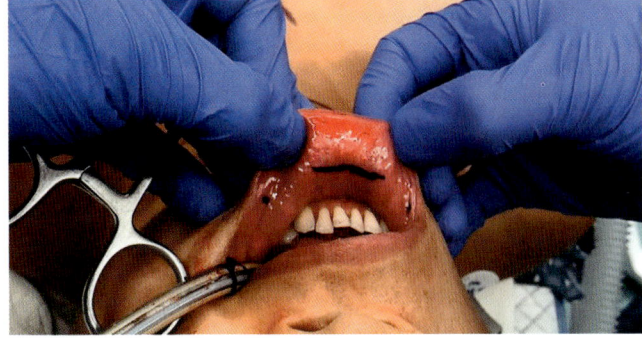

Fig. 33.3 Location of the Incisions for Trocar Placement. Note the two stab incisions close to the lateral commissure. This position avoids mental nerve injury.

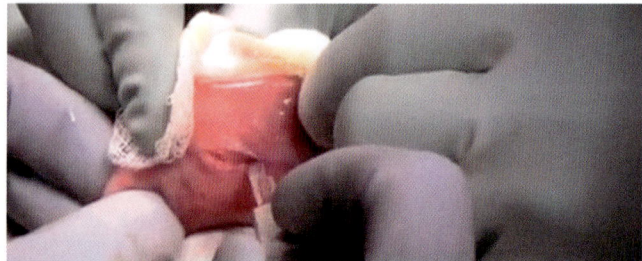

Fig. 33.4 The procedure is initiated with an incision through the lower lip mucosa.

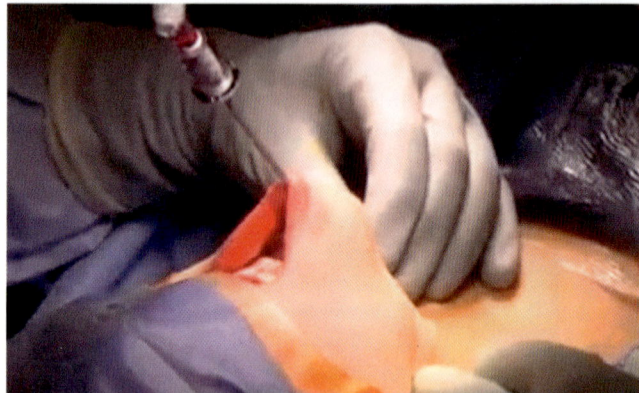

Fig. 33.5 Lidocaine with epinephrine is infiltrated in the subplatysmal plane in a fanning fashion between the sternocleidomastoid muscles.

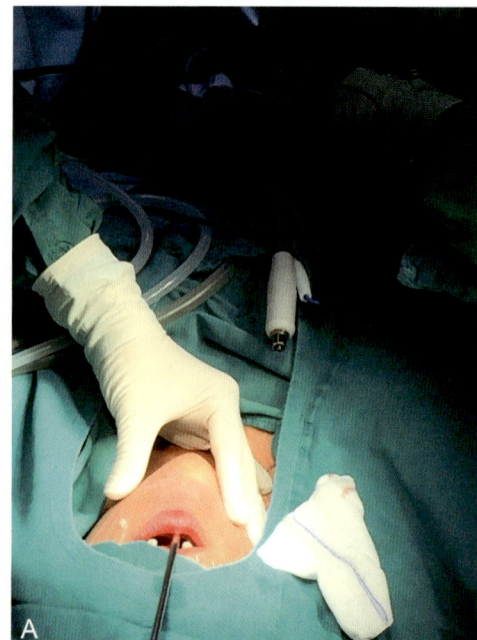

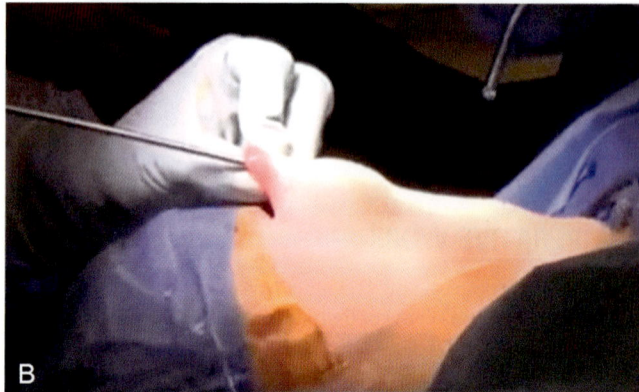

Fig. 33.6 A and B, A blunt tip probe is used to dissect the subplatysmal space.

bluntly, or cautery is used to divide the fascicles of the mentalis muscles that direct toward the anterior arch of the mandible. Care should be directed to avoid penetrating the skin. Once a tunnel to the tip of the chin has been developed, some surgeons advocate hydrodissection with a solution of 500 mL of saline with 1 mg of epinephrine. This is performed with a Veress needle; first, infiltrate is placed at tip of the chin to create a subcutaneous wheel. The skin is then manually elevated as the needle is advanced in the subplatysmal plane to the sternal notch. Infiltrate is advanced in this layer in a fanning fashion between the sternocleidomastoid muscles (Figure 33.5). At this point, a blunt dilator (e.g., Hegar, Pratt) is passed through the central vestibular incision in the subplatysmal plane, in the same fanning fashion, to assist with making the working space (Figure 33.6).

A 10 mm cannula is placed inside and through the central incision with the tip advanced just beyond the mandible into the neck. Continuous CO_2 insufflation is established at 6 mm Hg and flow 15 to 25 L/min. A suspension suture can be placed just beyond the tip of the cannula (through the skin to assist in elevation of the skin flap).

Stab incisions for each lateral port are then created. This is best made at the upper lateral edge of the lower lips (just medial to the commissure) (Figure 33.7), and slightly more medial for men. This location optimizes port mobility while avoiding the mental foramen and resultant mental nerve injury. The Veress needle is used again to hyrodissect a tract to the inferior edge of the mandible. Subsequently, 5 mm cannulas are then advanced through each stab incision with the inner trocars to the same level as the central trocar just below the inferior edge of the mandible (Figure 33.8). Care must be taken so as not to puncture the skin as the trocars are passed over the edge of the mandible.

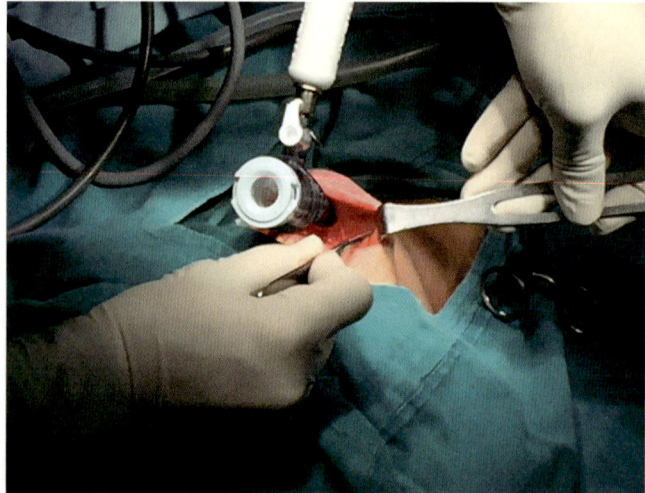

Fig. 33.7 Location of the stab incision for the lateral ports.

CHAPTER 33 Transoral Thyroidectomy

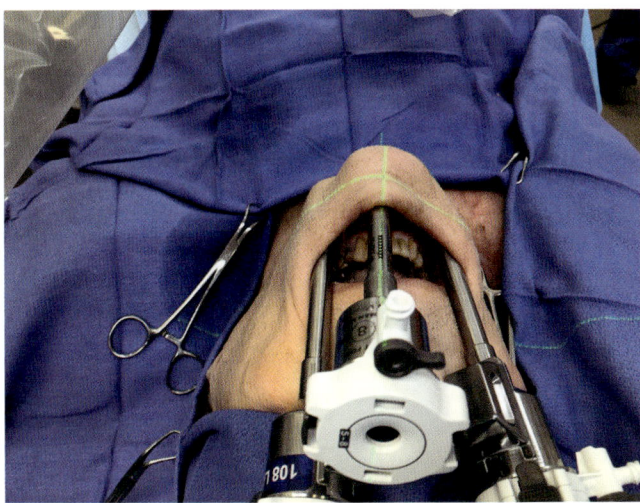

Fig. 33.8 Transvestibular port placement with all ports (robotic in this case) placed anterior to the mandible. The central trocar houses the camera and each lateral port has a surgical instrument for tissue manipulation.

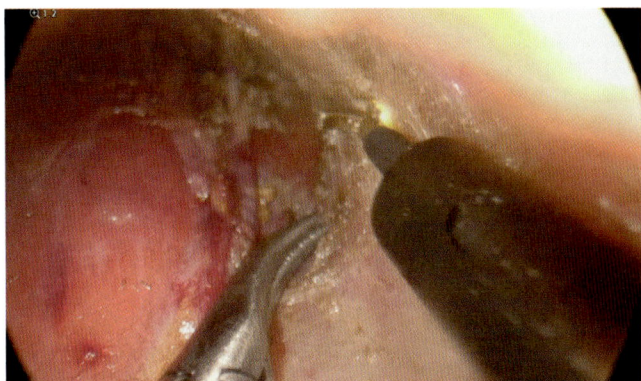

Fig. 33.9 The fibrous attachments remaining after blunt dissection are then taken with hook cautery, and the subplatysmal space is widely opened between the sternocleidomastoid muscles.

Working Space Creation

A 10 mm 30-degree downward telescope is introduced through the central trocar, and it is supported and adjusted by a bedside assist surgeon. A laparoscopic Maryland dissector and monopolar spatula (or hook or other energy device) are placed in the 5 mm ports. The fibrous attachments remaining after blunt dissection are then taken down from the level of the cannulae tips to the sternal notch, which creates a wide subplatysmal working space (Figure 33.9). The boundaries of flap dissection extend down to the clavicle and medial borders of both sides of the sternocleidomastoid muscles. Opening a vent on one or both of the side cannulae can assist with smoke evacuation and fogging of the scope. During TORT, the robot may be docked immediately after cannula placement to perform this step, or after the subplatysmal flaps have been elevated laparoscopically. Furthermore, some TORT surgeons use an additional port through the axilla with the fourth robotic arm entering from below to assist with retraction.

Thyroid Dissection

The following steps may be performed either robotically (TORT) or laparoscopically (TOETVA). The midline raphe of the strap muscles is identified and divided with cautery or an advanced energy device (e.g., Harmonic, Ligasure [Medtronic, Minneapolis, Minnesota]) (Figure 33.10). The strap muscles are elevated off the target lobe (Figure 33.11) until the carotid is visualized. The superior-most attachments at the cricoid may be released to facilitate exposure to the superior pole. A second transcutaneous suture may be passed into the working space and around the strap muscles. The bedside assist can retract this suture to increase the working space around the thyroid lobe.

With a view of the midline, the pyramidal lobe is elevated, the avascular pretracheal fascia is identified, and the isthmus is divided from superior to inferior. Attention is then turned to the cricothyroid space (e.g., Joll's space), as graspers or Kittner dissectors elevate and retract the superior pole to the contralateral side. The external branch of superior laryngeal nerve (EBSL) may predictably be found during this maneuver. The energy device is then used to divide the superior thyroid vessels (Figure 33.12). As the thyroid is retracted to the contralateral side, the superior parathyroid gland can be found (Figure 33.13). Gently dissect and lateralize the parathyroid gland to preserve its blood supply.

The next step is to identify the RLN that lies dorsal to the inferior parathyroid gland and ventral to the superior gland. In the transoral technique, it is usually found at its insertion site and dissected caudally, which may be unfamiliar to some surgeons. Meticulous dissection and hemostasis is mandatory to correctly identify the distal branch or branches. The use of the IONM stimulator is invaluable during this step

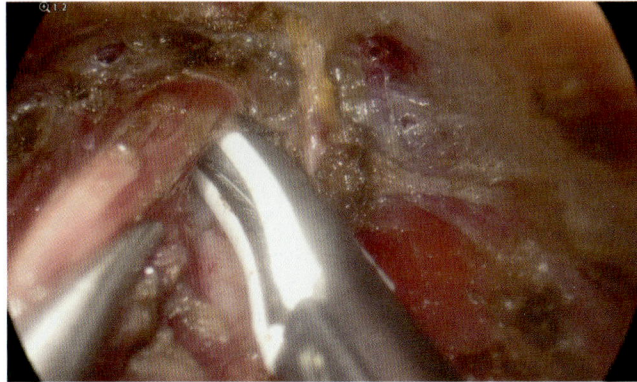

Fig. 33.10 The midline raphe of the strap muscles is identified and divided with cautery or an advanced energy device.

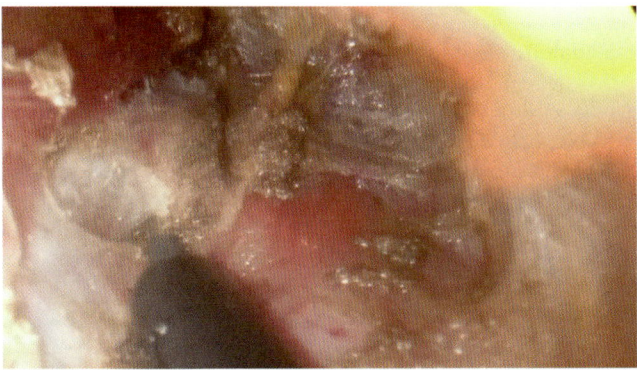

Fig. 33.11 The strap muscles are elevated off the underlying thyroid lobe.

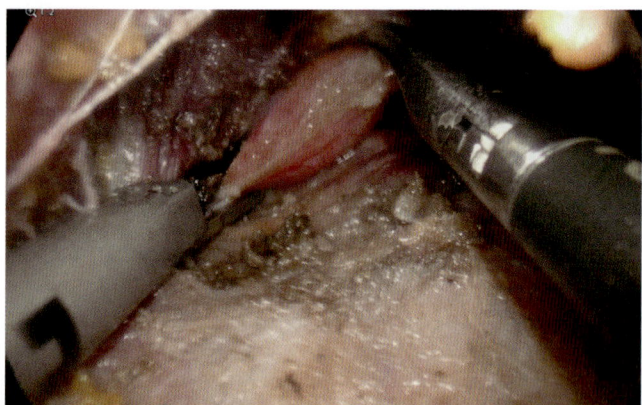

Fig. 33.12 The superior pole is grasped, pulled medially, and the vessels are divided with an advanced energy device.

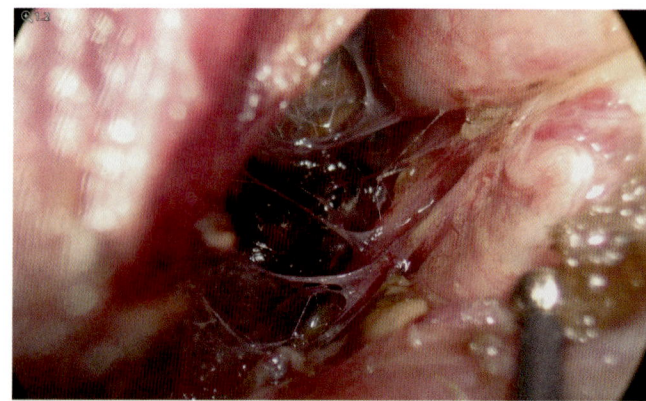

Fig. 33.14 Use of the nerve-stimulating probe to confirm identification of the recurrent laryngeal nerve. Note the location of the inferior parathyroid in relation to the nerve.

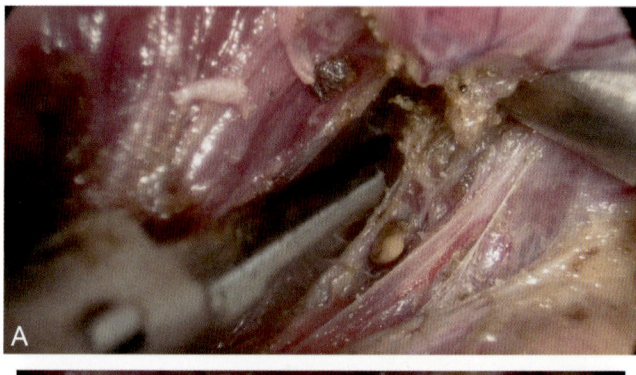

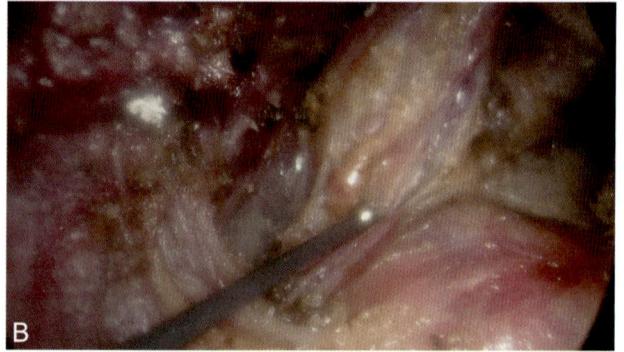

Fig. 33.13 A and B, Identification of the superior parathyroid gland and use of the nerve stimulator to map out the recurrent laryngeal nerve.

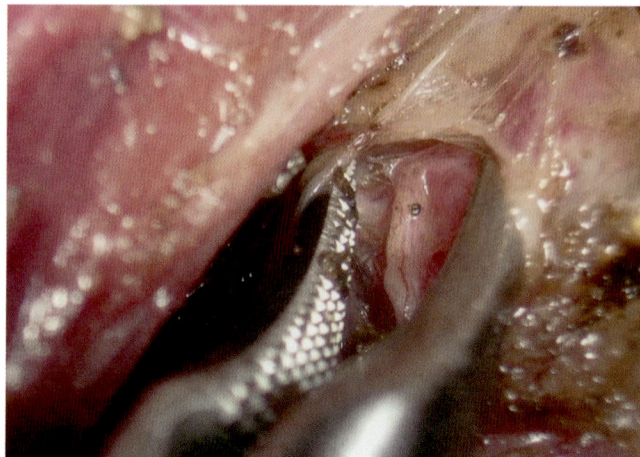

Fig. 33.15 The nerve is gently dissected free as the overlying thyroid is reflected medially.

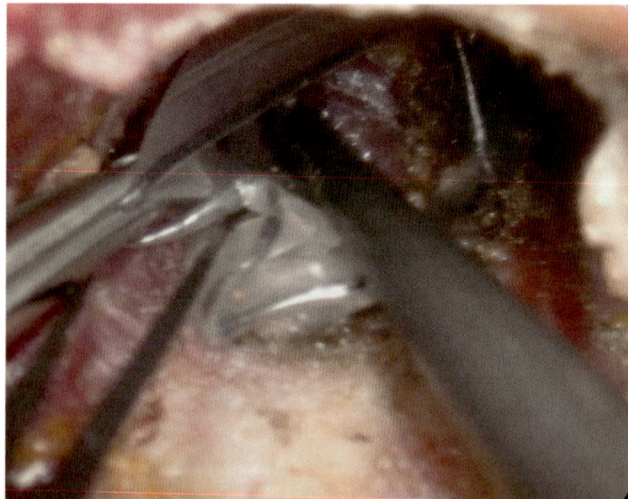

Fig. 33.16 The specimen is placed in an endoscopic retrieval bag before being extracted through the central incision.

(Figure 33.14). Oozing can be controlled with gentle pressure, a pledget, and precise bipolar cauterization. No tissue should be divided without assurance that the nerve is stimulated and protected. The magnified, high-definition view afforded by the telescope can greatly aid in the identification of the terminal nerve branches. Once the nerve is identified, it should be dissected caudally as the thyroid lobe is retracted medially (Figure 33.15). Berry's ligament is then divided, and the inferior vascular pedicle is divided to fully mobilize the lobe. If a total thyroidectomy is being performed, the procedure is repeated on the contralateral side. A central neck dissection can also be performed on one or both sides (if indicated).

With resection complete, attention is turned to specimen extraction. An endoscopic specimen bag is advanced through the central cannula and pushed into the working space by the scope. The specimen is placed into the bag and pulled out through the central vestibular incision (Figure 33.16). Specimens <4 cm can usually be teased through the

CHAPTER 33 Transoral Thyroidectomy   309

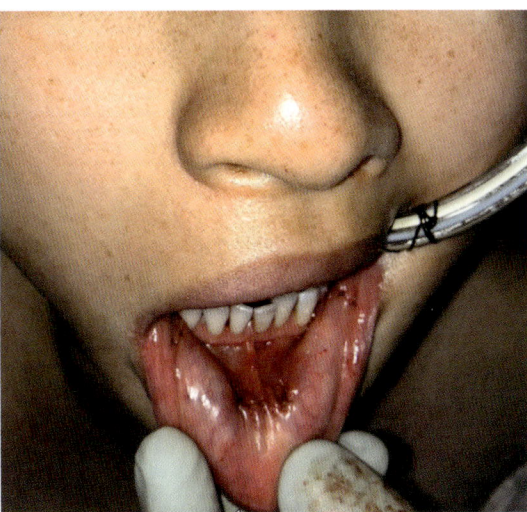

Fig. 33.17 Immediate appearance of the lower lip after closure at the end of the procedure.

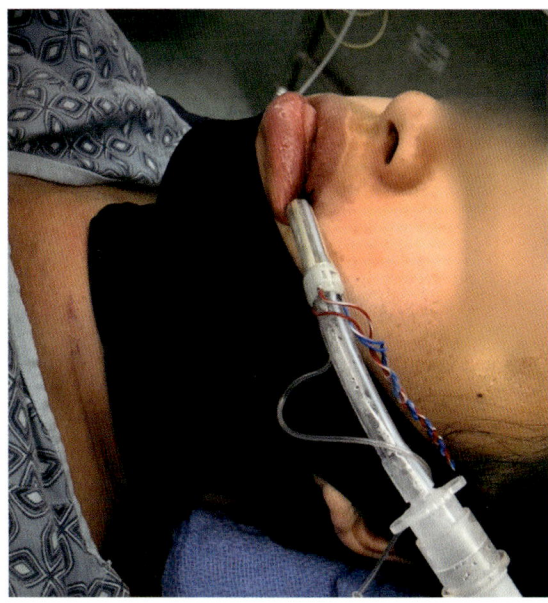

Fig. 33.18 A Jaw Bra or compression dressing is placed to obliterate dead space. Drains are usually avoided.

incision intact. To assist with extraction of larger specimens, some authors have described controlled cuts into the specimen while it is within the bag; however, this is not advised for malignancy. Our personal experience has suggested that using serial dilation of the central incision with the Hegar dilators is usually sufficient to remove all nodules smaller than 6 cm. Once removed, the endoscopic instruments are replaced, the wound is irrigated, and hemostasis is confirmed. Integrity of the RLN should be confirmed again with the IOMN stimulator. Thrombin glue may be used. The midline raphe of the strap muscles may be reapproximated with a barbed suture and the three oral mucosal incisions are closed with a 4.0 absorbable suture material (Figure 33.17).

After surgery, a pressure dressing or Jaw-bra is placed around the chin for 24 hours to obliterate the dead space (Figure 33.18). Drains are not required. Patients may be started on a liquid diet the day of surgery and advanced as tolerated thereafter. Perioperative antibiotics for 24 hours are sufficient. Discharge planning and postoperative care is otherwise similar to that of traditional transcervical thyroidectomy. There is usually minimal postoperative edema or bruising afterward (Figure 33.19), which is essentially imperceptible by 1 month (Figure 33.20).

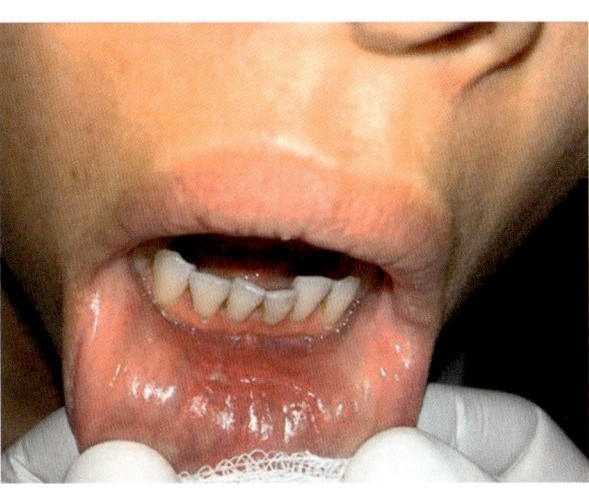

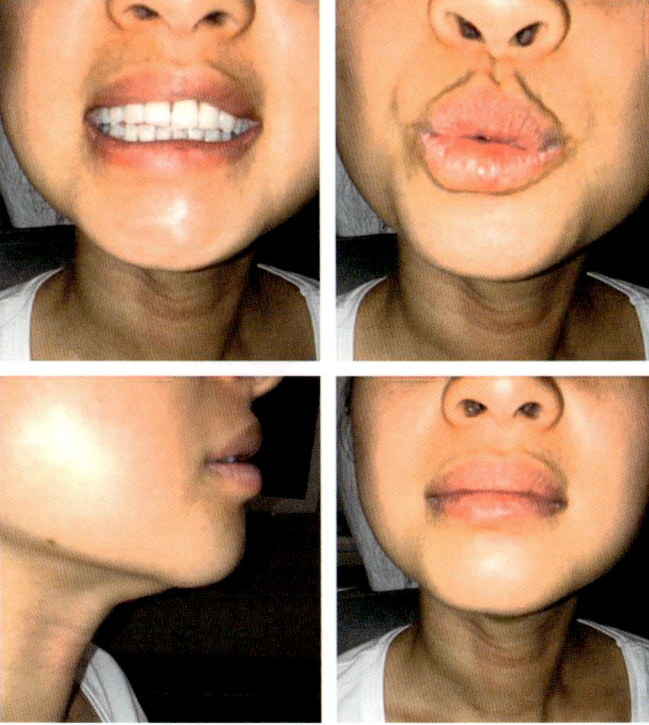

Fig. 33.19 Postoperative appearance at 1 week.

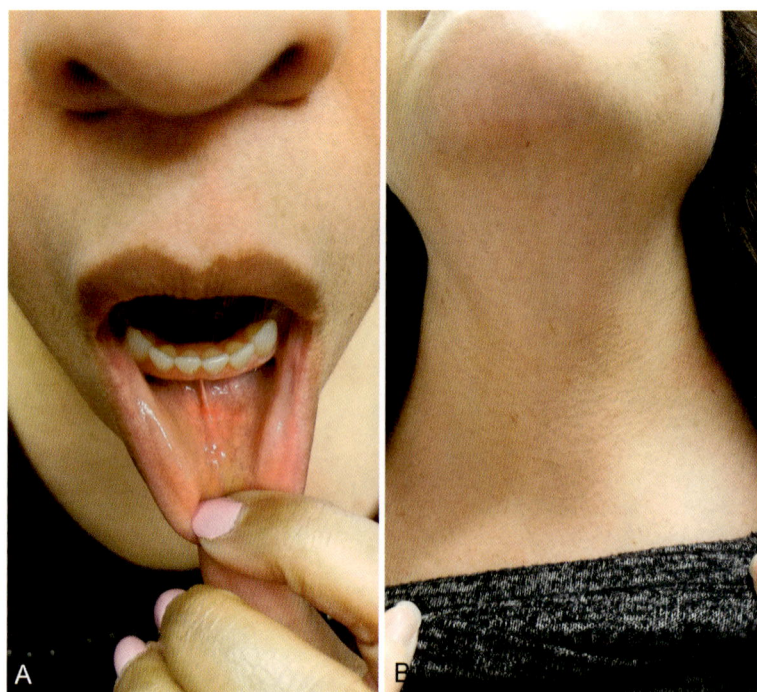

Fig. 33.20 **A** and **B**, Postoperative appearance at 1 month.

OUTCOMES

We are still in the early experience of transoral thyroidectomy. The largest series to date is that of Anuwong and colleagues reviewing their experience with 425 TOETVA patients.[28] There were three conversions to an open procedure due to excessive bleeding. Twenty-five patients (5.9%) had transient RLN palsy and 46 patients (10.9%) had transient hypoparathyroidism. There were no permanent instances of these complications. Only three patients had transient mental nerve injury, which resolved. Hematoma formed in a single patient and seroma in 20 patients. These patients were matched with 216 patients who underwent open thyroidectomy. The operative time for TOETVA was significantly longer than that for open thyroidectomy (hemi was 78.6 minutes versus 64.2 minutes, respectively; and total operative time was 135.1 minutes versus 103.3 minutes, respectively). Using a visual analog scale, patients reported less pain with TOETVA than with open thyroidectomy. There were no significant differences in complications between the groups. These data are very encouraging and bolster the role of the transoral approach to thyroid surgery but should be interpreted with caution and may not be extrapolated to surgeons and centers that have not yet attained proficiency.

FUTURE DIRECTIONS

Transoral thyroid surgery is a relatively new procedure that will likely see considerable evolution as patient awareness and demand increase, and instrumentation continues to advance. Current instrumentation is limited in that it is not designed for this procedure. TOETVA is limited in that it uses standard laparoscopic instrumentation that is not wristed, requires an experienced bedside assistant surgeon to hold the scope, and has a two-dimensional view. Each of these limitations will likely be addressed in the near future. Wristed instrumentation allows for increased range of motion of the distal arm of the instrument and avoids line-of-site issues that occur while looking down the shaft of rigid endoscopic instrumentation. Custom-made scope holders will free up one of the hands of the assistant surgeon and prevent fatigue, drift, and tremor, which can affect the endoscopic view. Three-dimensional endoscopes may one day rival the view afforded by the robot. TORT is hampered by the size and cost of the surgical robot, which has been limited primarily to the da Vinci Si and Xi (Intuitive Surgical, Inc., Sunnyvale, CA) although these are recent reports with the S_p.[38,39] However, surgical device companies are working on smaller and less expensive robots that will likely have applicability in TORT. What is certain is that future technologic evolution will continue to lead to novel innovations in remote access, "scarless" thyroid surgery.

REFERENCES

For a complete list of references go to expertconsult.com.

34

Minimally Invasive Video-Assisted Thyroidectomy

Rocco Bellantone, Francesco Pennestrì, Celestino Pio Lombardi

Please go to expertconsult.com to view related video:
Video 34.1 Minimally Invasive Video-Assisted Thyroidectomy.
This chapter contains additional online-only content, including exclusive video, available on expertconsult.com.

INTRODUCTION

The conventional surgery for neck endocrine diseases is generally performed using traditional Kocher incision, which is characterized by a standard skin incision and results in a visible, large scar on the neck (see Chapter 31, Principles in Thyroid Surgery). For minimally invasive neck endocrine surgery, a variety of techniques are available, some of which require the use of a surgical endoscope;[1-5] however, others do not.[6] The different minimally invasive techniques using an endoscope can be classified in purely endoscopic[2,3,7,8] and video-assisted[5,9,10] procedures. In the totally endoscopic techniques, surgical dissection is completely carried out under endoscopic vision.[11] This requires a continuous carbon dioxide (CO_2) insufflation[1,2,8] or the use of external devices (retractors) to maintain the operative space for dissection and trocar positioning.[11] These totally endoscopic approaches are generally more technically demanding in comparison with the conventional techniques and can be difficult to reproduce in different settings.[11] As a general result, the totally endoscopic procedures have a more limited acceptance.[12] However, minimally invasive video-assisted parathyroidectomy (MIVAP) (see Chapter 58, Minimally Invasive Video-Assisted Parathyroidectomy) and minimally invasive video-assisted thyroidectomy (MIVAT), have gained large, worldwide acceptance, which began shortly after their introduction during the late 1990s.[4,5] This is likely attributable to the advantages related to endoscopic magnification coupled with the fact that these procedures share many features of conventional surgery. MIVAP and MIVAT are completely gasless procedures that reproduce all the steps of the conventional operation. The endoscope represents a tool that allows performance of the same basic operation through a very minimal skin incision thanks to magnification.[5,9,13,14]

MIVAP and MIVAT are associated with a minimal incision and optimal cosmetic result. Moreover, the absence of neck hyperextension and extensive dissections results in less postoperative pain. Several comparative studies have demonstrated MIVAT superiority in terms of reduced postoperative pain, better cosmetic results, and higher patient satisfaction over the conventional thyroidectomy.[15-18] Furthermore, data from multicenter studies on a large series of patients showed that MIVAT is a safe, effective, and reproducible technique.[16,19,20] MIVAT also allows for the option of locoregional anesthesia (cervical block).[21]

In one retrospective study,[22] we demonstrated that thyroid gland manipulation is not substantially different from MIVAT and conventional thyroidectomy; there is no additional risk of thyroid capsule rupture with thyroid cells seeding in patients who undergo MIVAT. Many authors[23-25] have demonstrated the applicability of treating thyroid malignancy with a video-assisted approach. Studies comparing the results of MIVAT and conventional thyroidectomy, in terms of adequacy of surgical resection, showed that MIVAT is safe and effective for the treatment of small papillary thyroid carcinomas (PTCs) and has similar oncological effectiveness when compared with traditional thyroidectomy.[25]

Please see the Expert Consult website for more discussion of this topic.

INDICATIONS

Appropriate patient selection is key to the success of MIVAT. In early experiences with MIVAT, the indications were quite limited; initial contraindications included thyroiditis and prior neck surgery.[11] With increasing experience, selection criteria for MIVAT have become widened. Based on the surgeons' experience, patients with previous contralateral video-assisted neck surgery or thyroiditis can be safely selected for MIVAT. Expanded indications include patients who have undergone video-assisted thyroid lobectomy needing a completion thyroidectomy and for selected patients with Graves' disease, where MIVAT can be performed safely with results comparable with open surgery.[28] In our experience, it has also been possible to perform MIVAT in cases of nodules >35 mm in diameter.[11] We believe that a preoperative diagnosis of PTC with lymph-node involvement represents a contraindication for MIVAT.[11] More recently, some have applied the technique to carry out a prophylactic thyroidectomy and central compartment lymphadenectomy in patients carrying the rearranged during transfection (RET) oncogene mutation for familial medullary thyroid carcinoma (see Chapter 27, Syndromic Medullary Thyroid Carcinoma: MEN 2A and MEN 2B).[29,30]

INSTRUMENTS

For the most part, surgical instruments necessary for MIVAT are typically available in almost all operating rooms. The only instruments not commonly used for a conventional thyroidectomy are small (2 to 3 mm in diameter), dedicated, reusable tools (e.g., spatulas and spatulas-shaped aspiration) necessary for dissection (Figure 34.1). Ultrasound knife system (Ultracision®, Harmonic Focus Plus®) (Figure 34.2) is of great utility in this kind of operation and has been shown to be associated with reduction of operative time.[31]

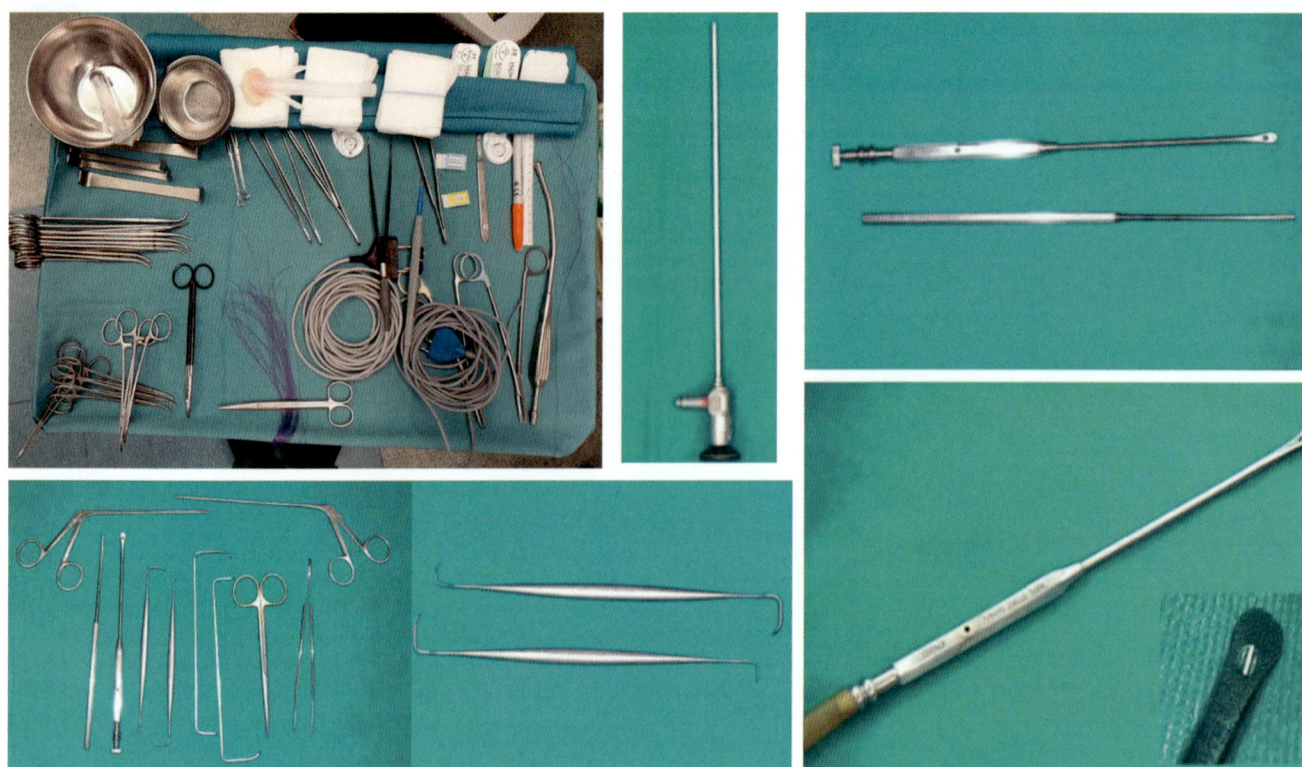

Fig. 34.1 Surgical instruments.

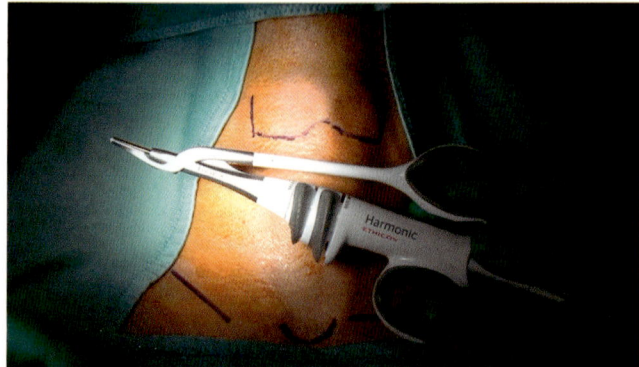

Fig. 34.2 Harmonic Focus Plus® an ultrasound knife system.

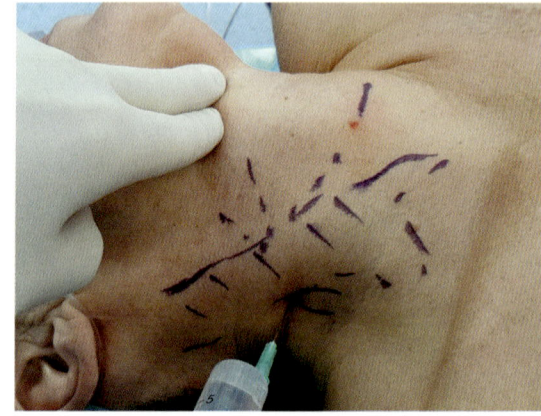

Fig. 34.3 Superficial modified deep cervical block.

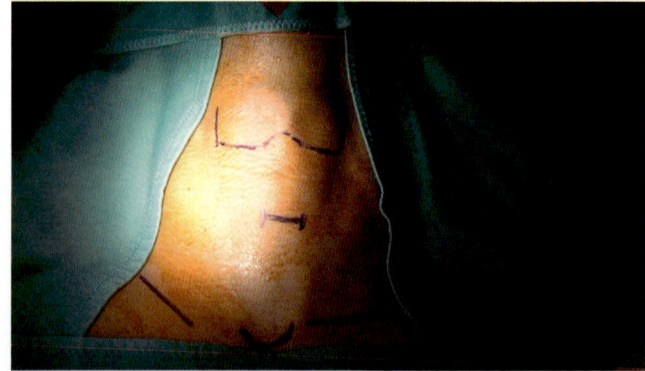

Fig. 34.4 Patient position.

SURGICAL TECHNIQUE

The operative technique has been previously described in detail.[14]

Anesthesia

Traditionally MIVAT was described as requiring general anesthesia with orotracheal intubation. More recently, and with increasing experience, the feasibility of MIVAT under locoregional anesthesia (MIVAT-LA) with superficial modified deep cervical block (Figure 34.3) has been demonstrated.[21] In our experience, MIVAT-LA is most optimal in patients with relative contraindications for general anesthesia, such as pregnant patients with PTC.

Patient Position

The patient under general or locoregional anesthesia is positioned supine with the neck in slight extension (though less than in conventional surgery, Figure 34.4). The lesser extension may contribute to lower postoperative pain as compared with those patients who have undergone conventional thyroidectomy.

Surgical Equipment

The surgical team is composed of the surgeon and two assistants, one of whom handles the endoscope. The need for at least three surgeons involved in the procedure has been considered one of the main limitations of this approach. The monitor is positioned at the head of the patient in front of the surgeon, who is positioned on the right side of the patient. A second monitor is usually positioned in front of the assistants who are on the left side of the patient. The absence of any external support allows modulating and changing the position of the endoscope in relation to the different steps of dissection. This represents an important advantage of the video-assisted procedure over purely endoscopic techniques. The tip of the endoscope is usually oriented toward the head of the patient, but it can be changed to expose and explore the upper mediastinum when, for example, a concomitant central compartment lymphadenectomy is required.

Surgical Steps

A small (1.5 to 2 cm) skin incision is performed between the cricoid cartilage and the sternal notch, in the midline (Figure 34.5). The skin incision is usually higher than in conventional cervicotomy and can also be modified according to the neck conformation and the thyroid position. However, the skin incision is usually performed just below (1 cm) the cricoid cartilage to obtain a good exposure and a safe control of the superior pole vascular peduncle. The skin incision is ideally placed in an existing skin line to optimize the cosmesis. After incising the platysma muscle and preparing the upper and the lower flaps (Figure 34.6 A and B), the cervical *linea alba* is opened as far as possible. At the beginning of our experience, the procedure included a short period of CO_2 insufflation to facilitate dissection of the thyroid lobe from the strap muscles. After this initial experience, the procedure became completely gasless. The thyroid lobe is separated from the strap muscles by means of small conventional retractors (Farabeuf retractors), which are also used to maintain the operative space. The thyroid lobe is medially retracted while the strap muscles are retracted laterally using two Farabeuf retractors. At this point, the endoscope (5 mm – 30°) and the dedicated small surgical instruments (2 mm in diameter) are introduced through the single skin incision (Figure 34.7). The first step of the procedure consists of the complete freeing of the thyroid gland from the strap muscles to have a good exposure of the prevertebral fascia, which represents the posterior aspect of the dissection. The lateral edge of the dissection is represented by the medial aspect of common carotid artery, and the medial edge is represented by the tracheal esophageal groove. The dissection is carried out by a blunt

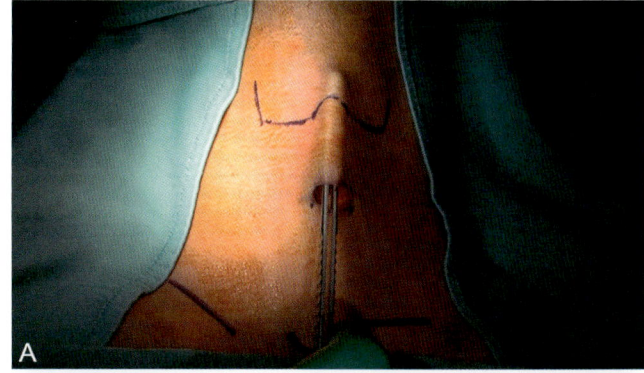
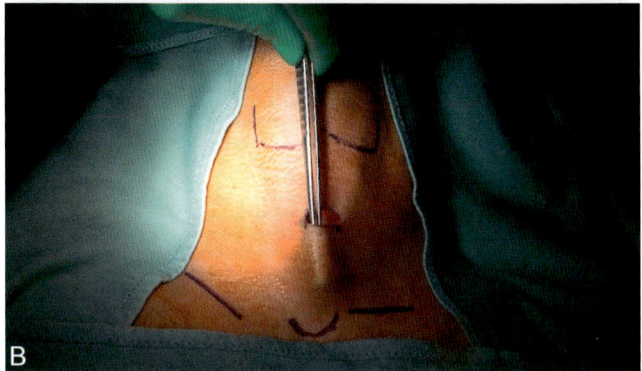

Fig. 34.6 A and B, Preparation of the upper and the lower flaps.

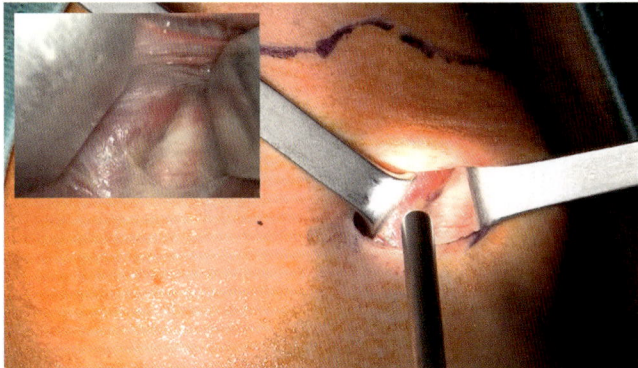

Fig. 34.7 The thyroid lobe is medially retracted while the strap muscles, first on the most affected side, are retracted laterally, using two little Farabeuf retractors. At this point, the endoscope (5 mm – 30°) is introduced through the single skin incision.

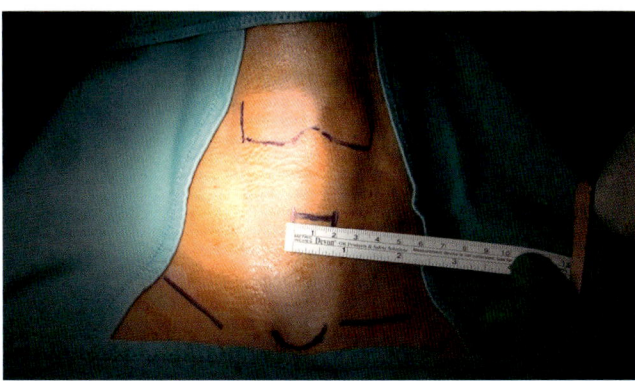

Fig. 34.5 Skin incision.

technique using two dedicated spatula instruments; one of the instruments is connected to an aspiration system. After its complete separation from the muscles, the thyroid lobe is retracted downward to expose the superior peduncle vessels; these are dissected using the spatula and the spatula-shaped aspirator (Figure 34.8) and then selectively clipped and cut, or directly cut using an ultrasound knife system (Figure 34.9). It is very important to accurately control the tip of the instrument to avoid any pharynx or larynx thermal injury. During this phase, it is usually possible, thanks to the magnification of the endoscope, to identify the external branch of the superior laryngeal nerve (Figure 34.10). After controlling the superior thyroid vessels, the thyroid lobe is retracted medially and slightly upwards to identify the recurrent laryngeal nerve and the parathyroid glands (Figure 34.11). The magnification (two- to three-fold) of the endoscope permits straight forward identification

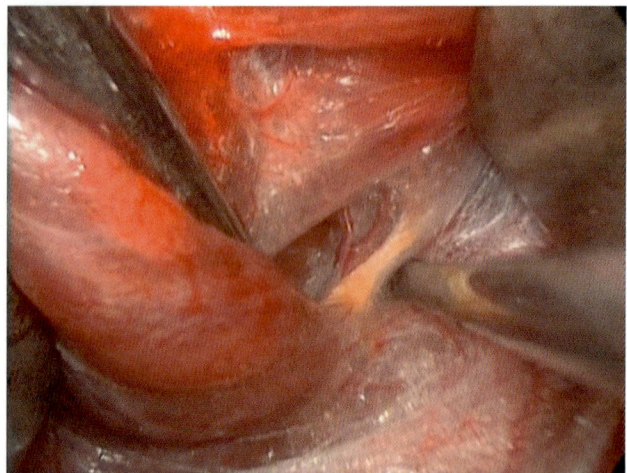

Fig. 34.8 The thyroid lobe is downward retracted to expose the superior peduncle vessels that are dissected using the spatula and the spatula-shaped aspirator.

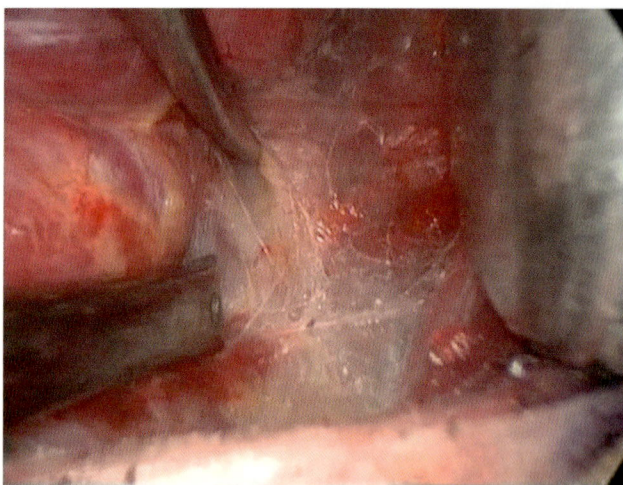

Fig. 34.11 After cutting the superior thyroid vessels, the thyroid lobe is medially and slightly upwards retracted to identify the inferior laryngeal nerve and the parathyroid glands.

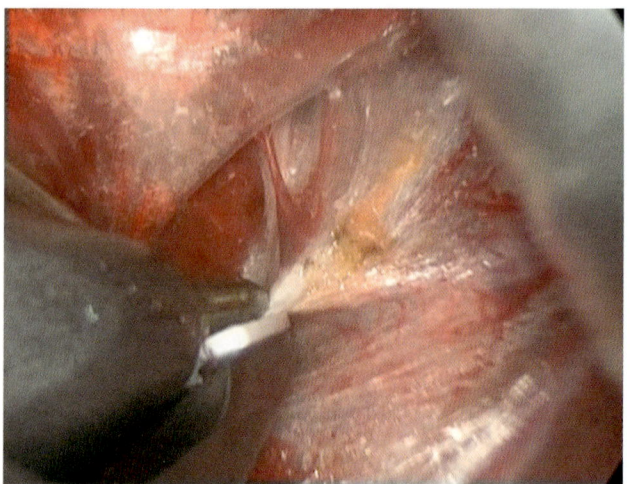

Fig. 34.9 The superior peduncle vessels are cut using Harmonic Focus Plus®.

of these structures as long as the dissection is performed bluntly and bloodlessly. The traction on both the thyroid lobe (medially) and the strap muscles (laterally) provides exposure of the tracheal esophageal groove and the inferior thyroid artery; this allows for exposure of the nerve, typically where it crosses the inferior thyroid artery. Once identified, the recurrent laryngeal nerve is prepared and bluntly dissected under endoscopic vision, inferiorly to its entry point in the larynx (Figure 34.12). The parathyroid glands are usually easy identified and preserved assisted by endoscopic magnification. It is important to carry out a completely bloodless dissection, which is facilitated using the spatula-shaped aspirator. At this point, the thyroid lobe is extracted from the skin incision as the procedure is completed under both endoscopic and direct vision. When performing this maneuver, it is very important not to strongly pull the thyroid lobe ventrally because it is not yet completely freed; an excessive traction may result in traction injury of the nerve at the ligament of Berry. Although the separation of the thyroid from the trachea is usually carried out using an ultrasound knife system (Figure 34.13), dissection close to the nerve and the parathyroid glands is best done by nonthermal vessel division after putting titanium clips or conventional ligature. If a total thyroidectomy is planned, the same steps are performed in the contralateral side. After checking the hemostasis, the strap muscles are sutured along the midline as well as the platysma. The skin is closed by means of a nonreabsorbable subcuticular running suture (Figure 34.14) or by a skin sealant. Typically, no drains are placed.

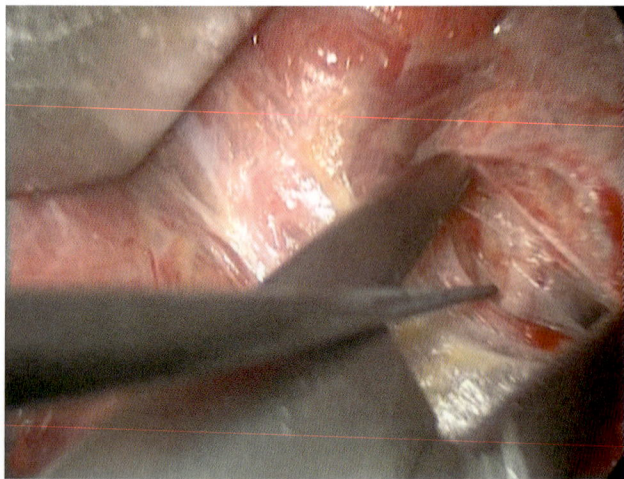

Fig. 34.10 Identification of the external branch of the superior laryngeal nerve.

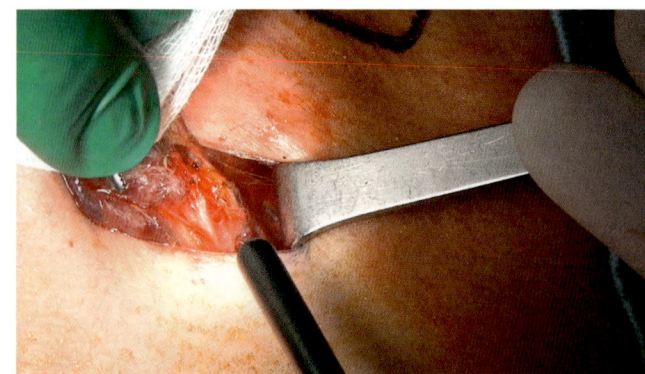

Fig. 34.12 Once identified, the inferior laryngeal nerve is prepared and bluntly dissected, under endoscopic vision, from the thyroid gland until its entrance in the larynx.

CHAPTER 34 Minimally Invasive Video-Assisted Thyroidectomy

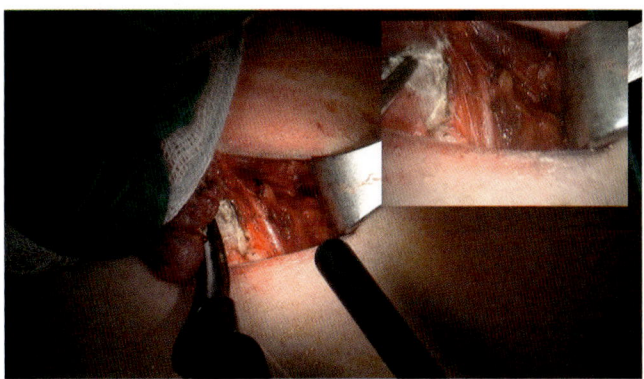

Fig. 34.13 The separation of the thyroid from the trachea is usually carried out using an ultrasound knife system.

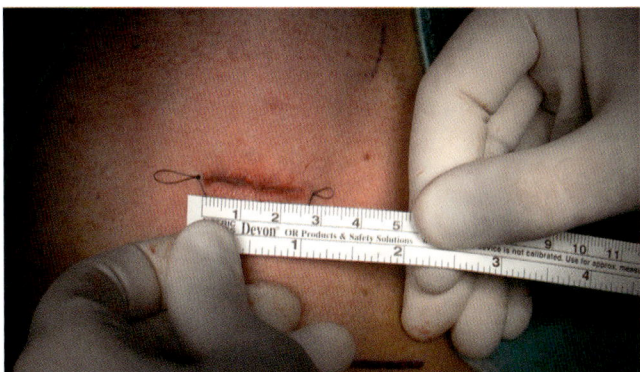

Fig. 34.14 The skin is closed by means of a nonreabsorbable subcuticular running suture.

PERSONAL EXPERIENCE

In 2009, we published a review of our experience[32] in a series of patients selected for MIVAT over a 10-year period with a total of 1363 video-assisted thyroidectomies studied. Conversion to the conventional procedure was necessary in only seven cases. In 126 patients, central neck nodes were removed through the same access. Pathologic results showed the following: benign disease in 986 cases, PTC in 368 cases, C-cell hyperplasia in one case, and medullary microcarcinoma in one patient with RET germline mutation. Postoperative complications included 27 transient and one definitive recurrent laryngeal nerve paralysis, 230 patients with transient hypocalcemia, 10 definitive hypoparathyroidism, four patients with postoperative hematoma, and five wound infections.

MINIMALLY INVASIVE VIDEO-ASSISTED NECK DISSECTION

Central compartment lymph node metastases, often microscopic, are frequent in patients with PTC[23-25] and in RET gene mutation carriers.[29] According to the current international guidelines on prophylactic central compartment, in the case of differentiated thyroid carcinoma, dissection is not mandatory and generally should be performed only in cases of macroscopic/clinically apparent lymph node involvement[33,34] (see Chapter 38, Central Neck Dissection: Indication and Technique). Preoperatively identified macroscopic/clinically apparent lymph node involvement has been always considered an absolute contraindication for a video-assisted approach. However, it is difficult to accurately and preoperatively assess the status of the central compartment, and intraoperative detection of central neck nodes enlargement at MIVAT thyroidectomy occurs. In these circumstances, a video-assisted central compartment dissection (VA-CCD) can be undertaken.

Please see the Expert Consult website for more discussion of this topic.

Supported by the results of video-assisted approach for selected cases of differentiated thyroid carcinoma and encouraged by the results of VA-CCD, we also evaluated the feasibility of a minimally invasive video-assisted approach to the functional lateral neck dissection (VALNED) in patients with PTC. We considered eligible two patients with low-risk PTC and lateral neck nodal metastases <2 cm without evidence of great vessels involvement. One patient underwent bilateral VALNED and one patient underwent unilateral VALNED. The mean number of removed nodes was 25 per side. Both patients experienced transient hypocalcemia. No evidence of residual tissue or recurrent disease was found at follow-up.[27] These results are encouraging, but it should be considered a preliminary experience. For definitive conclusions, larger comparative series studies will be necessary.

Accurate patient selection plays an important role in ensuring the success of any video-assisted procedure, especially at the beginning of a surgeon's experience. At the present time, we feel, given our experience, that ideal candidates for video-assisted approach are the following: patients with small benign or low and intermediate-risk differentiated thyroid carcinoma and patients who are RET gene mutation carriers without preoperative evidence of lymph node metastases. The results of the studies discussed previously have demonstrated that VA-CCD can be carried out if unexpected suspicious or simply enlarged lymph nodes are found during MIVAT; the outcomes are equivalent with the outcomes of a conventional open operation. Of course, surgeons should be well trained in both open endocrine and endoscopic surgery.[19,20,41]

MIVAT: Evidence-Based Recommendations

Immediately after the first described case of minimally invasive thyroidectomy, several smaller single institution reports, two multicenter studies, and several large retrospective studies (consisting primarily of technical description of different video assisted techniques) have been published showing the safety and utility of MIVAT.[2,3,5,8,10,19,32,42-48] Gal et al.[17] and El Labban,[18] in two well-designed randomized controlled trials (evidence level II B), have also confirmed the safety and utility of MIVAT. These studies show the complication rate is comparable between the two approaches. Overall, conventional thyroidectomy involves less operative time, whereas MIVAT offers distinct Hegazy et al.[49] compared MIVAT with minimally invasive open thyroidectomy using the Sofferman technique (strap muscle transection). This prospective randomized study (evidence level II B) demonstrated that MIVAT offers a significantly improved postoperative course and smaller incision. Miccoli et al.[50] recently published a prospective, randomized study that confirmed postoperative pain was less for MIVAT than after conventional open surgery.

In 2008, to stress other advantages of MIVAT over conventional thyroidectomy, we published a prospective, randomized study[51] comparing MIVAT and conventional thyroidectomy. The study demonstrated with a level II B of evidence that the incidence and the severity of early voice and swallowing postthyroidectomy symptoms are significantly reduced in patients who undergo MIVAT compared with patients undergoing conventional surgery. A recent retrospective cost analysis shows that the cost of MIVAT appears to be equal to that of open thyroidectomy.[52]

REFERENCES

For a complete list of references, go to expertconsult.com.

35

Surgical Anatomy and Monitoring of the Superior Laryngeal Nerve

Marcin Barczyński, Claudio R. Cernea, Catherine F. Sinclair

> Please go to expertconsult.com to view related video:
> **Video 35.1** Introduction to Chapter 35, Surgical Anatomy and Monitoring of the Superior Laryngeal Nerve.
> **Video 35.2** Superior Laryngeal Nerve Anatomy and Monitoring.
> **Video 35.3** Stimulation of the Right-Sided External Branch of the Superior Laryngeal Nerve During Thyroidectomy.

The technical aspects of operations on the thyroid gland have changed very little since the original papers by Kocher.[1] Usually, the complication rate of thyroidectomy is very low when an experienced surgeon performs the operation. The most common complications include hypoparathyroidism and injury of the recurrent laryngeal nerve (RLN). However, injury to the external branch of the superior laryngeal nerve (EBSLN) can occur during the dissection and control of the superior thyroid vessels. This injury causes paralysis of the cricothyroid muscle (CTM), impairing the production of high tones, and altering the voice's fundamental frequency; this is especially problematic for individuals requiring vocal projection and professional singers. The effects of EBSLN paralysis are difficult to detect during routine postoperative laryngoscopy, yet functional consequences can be disastrous for those people who depend professionally on their voices. Armed with complete knowledge of the anatomic variations of the superior thyroid pole area, and through meticulous dissection of the superior thyroid pedicle, one may avoid such injury. In addition, this chapter will briefly discuss the use of the internal branch of the superior laryngeal nerve (IBSLN) to continuously monitor vocal fold function via the laryngeal adductor reflex (LAR).

HISTORY

In 1892, Fort reported the anatomic features of the CTM, including its motor supply by the EBSLN.[2] Several publications have studied the anatomy of the EBSLN,[3-9] generally in cadaver series. The largest report, by Moosman and DeWeese, included 200 fresh cadavers.[6]

Little attention was paid initially to the surgical anatomy of the EBSLN during the beginning of the 20th century. In fact, even Kocher[1] did not specifically mention this nerve in his book, which was once considered the cornerstone of thyroid surgery. Kocher's book entitled "Surgical operations teaching manual" in a chapter "Indications and results in goiter operations" documented his personal experience with more than 3000 thyroidectomies. The importance of the preservation of the EBSLN was made clear as a result of a thyroidectomy performed in 1935. At that time, Amelita Galli-Curci was the most famous soprano of the world. She underwent a thyroidectomy for a 170-g goiter. The surgeon used local anesthesia and asked his patient to speak during the surgery to be sure that the RLNs incurred no damage. The surgeon made careful identification and preservation of the RLNs. However, Galli-Curci's vocal registry dramatically lowered postoperatively, and her voice became permanently hoarse. She had to give up singing; the press of the time wrote, "the surprising voice is gone forever; the sad specter of a ghost replaced the velvet softness."[10] Since that time, the EBSLN has been known as "the nerve of Amelita Galli-Curci." Interestingly enough, some authors have recently questioned the veracity of this event.[11]

In 1957, Gregg stated that, despite the large experience of his service (8000 thyroidectomies), he was unsure how to prevent or detect damage to the EBSLN.[12] Subsequently, several authors proposed that the dissection of the superior thyroid pole should be performed with great care to avoid including the nerve in the ligature of the superior thyroid vessels.[13-17]

Some reports in the literature have described methods to identify the EBSLN during a thyroidectomy. Some authors have based their identification only upon the anatomic appearance of the nerve.[8,10] Others have tried some form of electrical stimulation to aid in identification,[18-22] mainly when dealing with markedly enlarged thyroid glands.[23]

ANATOMY

The superior laryngeal nerve (SLN) is one of the first branches of cranial nerve X (i.e., the vagus). It usually separates from the vagus at the nodose ganglion, which is about 4 cm cranially to the carotid artery bifurcation.[24] About 1.5 cm inferiorly, the SLN divides in two branches: the IBSLN and EBSLN.[7] The IBSLN descends within the carotid sheath posterior to the internal carotid artery before passing anteromedially to pierce the thyrohyoid membrane with the superior laryngeal artery. The IBSLN supplies sensation to the supraglottic larynx, piriform fossae, and valleculae. The EBSLN descends from behind the carotid vessels, extends from the vessels medially, and continues medially to the larynx. The nerve is usually about 0.8 mm wide,[25] and its total length varies between 8.0 cm[7] and 8.9 cm[26] (Figure 35.1). In 1968, Moosman and DeWeese defined the sternothyroid-laryngeal triangle (Joll's space). The limits of Joll's space are as follows: medially, the inferior pharyngeal constrictor and the CTM; anteriorly, the sternothyroid muscle; and laterally, the superior thyroid pole[6] (Figure 35.2). According to the anatomic study encompassing 200 cadaver dissections, the EBSLN almost invariably approached the larynx within this triangle.

The surgical importance of this nerve relates to its proximity to the superior thyroid vessels. In most instances, the EBSLN crosses the superior thyroid artery and vein well above the superior border of the superior thyroid pole. At least in theory, the EBSLN is protected against surgical injuries; however, Droulias et al. reproduced the

CHAPTER 35 Surgical Anatomy and Monitoring of the Superior Laryngeal Nerve

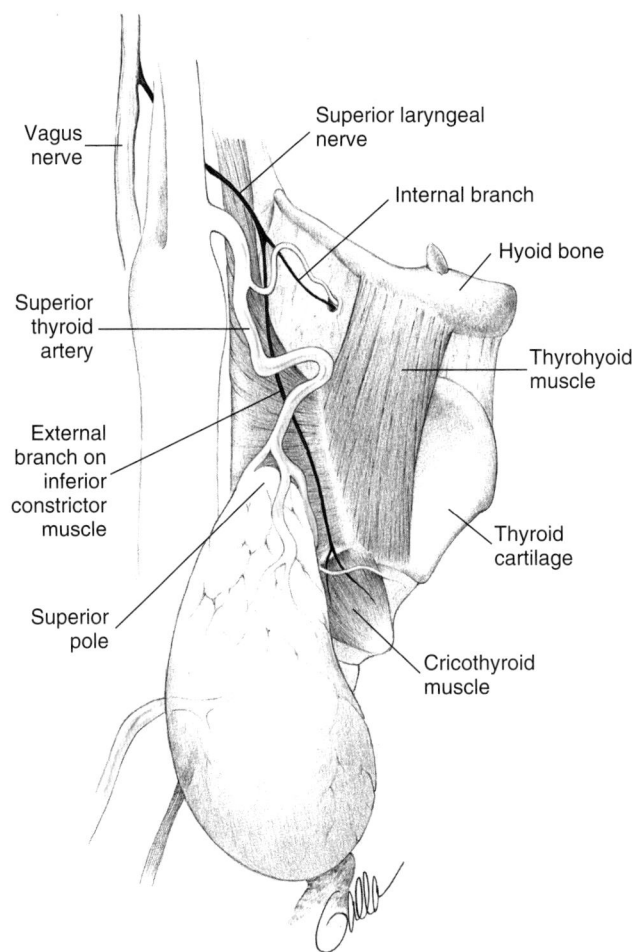

Fig. 35.1 External branch of the superior laryngeal nerve (EBSLN) descends from behind the carotid vessels, then crosses them medially, routing to the larynx.

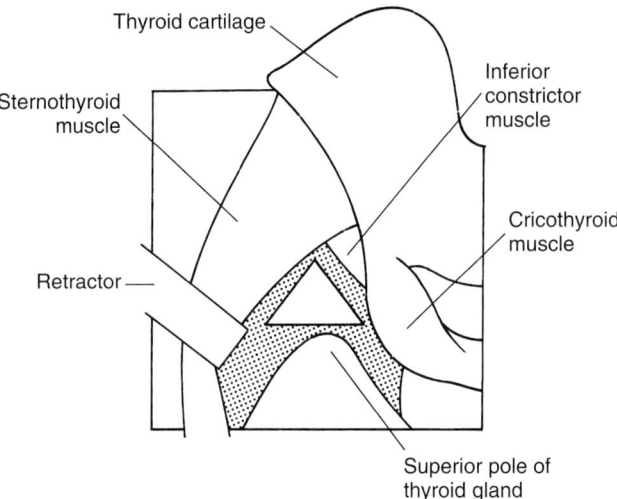

Fig. 35.2 The sternothyroid-laryngeal triangle (Joll's space).

surgical conditions of a thyroidectomy in 24 cadavers. They clamped the superior thyroid pedicle adjacently to the superior thyroid pole and found that the nerve was entrapped in most situations.[26] Clader, Luter, and Daniels dissected 48 cadavers and found that 68% of the EBSLNs were intimately associated with the superior pole vessels and were at risk during thyroidectomy.[27] On the other hand, Espinoza, Hamoir, and Dehm[28] and Lennquist, Cahlin, and Smeds[8] noted lower rates of "at-risk" EBSLNs (15% and 18%, respectively). In addition, Lennquist, Cahlin, and Smeds stated that only 80% of the EBSLN could be identified during a thyroidectomy because, in the remaining 20%, the nerve was located within the fibers of the inferior pharyngeal constrictor muscle.[8]

In a study, Wu et al. processed 27 human hemilarynges with Sihler's stain, a technique that clears soft tissue and counterstains nerve. Of the 27 specimens, 44% had a neural connection that exited the medial surface of the CTM (on the outside of the larynx) and then entered into the larynx. The neural connection then extended through the cricothyroid membrane and ramified the anterior third the ipsilateral thyroarytenoid muscle (also known as the *vocalis muscle* in the endolarynx).[29] Similar observations were made in the canine by Nasri et al. who identified cross-innervation of the thyroarytenoid muscle by the EBSLN in 42.9% of subjects. This was confirmed by electromyography (EMG) recordings from thyroarytenoid muscle that followed the electrical stimulation applied to the EBSLN.[30] Sanudo et al. found that in 68% of 90 human microdissected specimens, the EBSLN (after innervating the CTM) continues on, extending through the cricothyroid membrane to innervate the anterior thyroarytenoid muscle region.[31] Using microdissection technique in 103 human larynges obtained from necropsies, Maranillo et al. studied the existence of a neural connection between the external laryngeal nerve and the RLN. The human communicating nerve was identified in 85% of cases in this study (bilaterally in 44% and unilaterally in 41%).[32] Masuoka et al. investigated the prevalence of functional innervation of the CTM by the RLN during 70 thyroid lobectomies in humans. Responses after stimulation of unilateral vagal and RLN were evaluated in this study by visual observation of the CTM twitch and by EMG through needle electrodes inserted into the CTM. The RLN stimulation resulted in possible CTM contractions and clear electromyographic responses (>300 μV) in 39%, either response in 34%, and neither response in 27% of the CTMs.[33] These findings have been questioned by subsequent electrophysiologic studies; the later studies suggest that although the EBSLN may innervate the vocal cord through the human communicating nerve, the RLN does not innervate the CTM.[34] Thus the human communicating nerve provides documented connection to the to the vocal fold in 41% to 85% of patients.[29-36] The variability of this neural connection, variability in recording the small and early glottic waveform associated with EBSLN stimulation, and variability in endotracheal tube position are all likely responsible for defined waveforms being recordable in fewer than 100% of patients during EBSLN stimulation (using currently available standard monitoring technology).[37,38] However, use of a novel endotracheal tube with additional anterior surface electrodes allows for quantifiable EBSLN electromyographic activity in 100% of cases. Monopolar and bipolar stimulator probes produced similar electromyographic data.[39]

There are few surgical classifications of the EBSLN anatomic variations. However, the most widely recognized surgical classification of the EBSLN was proposed in 1992 by Cernea et al.[9] This classification is based on the potential risk of injury to the nerve during thyroid surgery. It categorizes the nerve in relation to superior thyroid vessels and the upper edge of the superior thyroid pole (Figure 35.3).

Cernea EBSLN Classification Scheme

Type 1. Nerve crosses the superior thyroid vessels more than 1 cm above the upper edge of the thyroid superior pole and occurs in 68% of patients with small goiter and in 23% of patients with large goiter.

Type 2A. Nerve crosses the vessels less than 1 cm above the upper edge of the superior pole and occurs in 18% of patients with small goiter and 15% of patients with large goiter.

Type 2B. Nerve crosses the superior thyroid pedicle below the upper border of the superior thyroid pole and occurs in 14% of patients with small goiters and 54% of patients with large goiters.

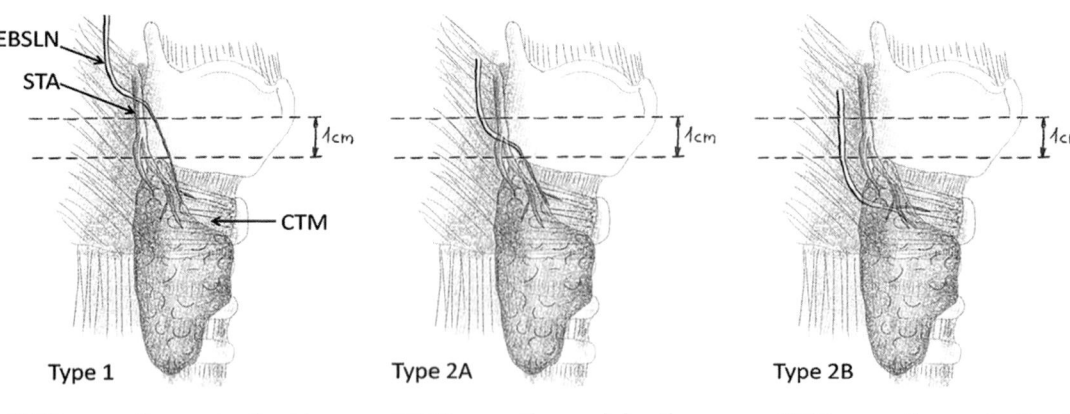

Fig. 35.3 Cernea's external branch of the superior laryngeal nerve (EBSLN) surgical anatomic classification scheme. (From Barczyński M, Randolph GW, Cernea CR, et al. External branch of the superior laryngeal nerve monitoring during thyroid and parathyroid surgery: International Neural Monitoring Study Group standards guideline statement. *Laryngoscope*. 2013;123[suppl 4]:S1–S14.)

Types 2A and 2B are particularly prone to injury during dissection and ligation of the superior thyroid vessels due to their low-lying course.[9,21] It is of interest to note that most studies on the anatomy of EBSLN have been performed in Western countries. Hence studies may have some limitations in their application to other nations, particularly to patients in Asian countries. Hwang et al. investigated 92 EBSLNs during 50 thyroid operations performed on adult Korean patients in Seoul and found that type 1 EBSLN was observed in 15 of the 92 nerves (16.3%), type 2A EBSLN was noted in 52 (56.5%) and type 2B EBSLN was noted in 25 (27.2%). Patients with types 2A and 2B were at higher risk of injuries, and these types were more frequently observed (83.7%) compared with previous Western studies. It was also found that 35.9% of distal insertion sites of EBSLNs were located within 1 cm of the center of the cricoid cartilage.[40]

In 1998, Kierner et al. published a similar classification; however, they added a fourth category in which the EBSLN runs dorsally to the superior thyroid pedicle, making its identification more difficult.[41] They observed this anatomic relationship in 13% of their dissections. They observed fewer type 1 nerves (42%) than in the Cernea series (Figure 35.4).

Kierner EBSLN Classification Scheme

Type 1. Nerve crosses the superior thyroid vessels more than 1 cm above the upper edge of the thyroid superior pole.
Type 2. Nerve crosses the vessels less than 1 cm above the upper edge of the superior pole.
Type 3. Nerve crosses the superior thyroid pedicle below the upper border of the superior thyroid pole.
Type 4. Nerve runs dorsally to the superior thyroid pedicle.

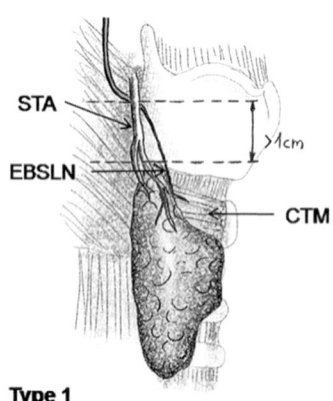 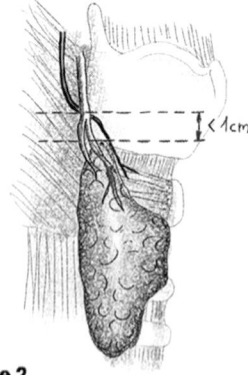 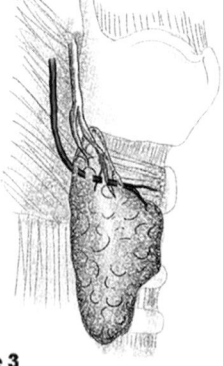 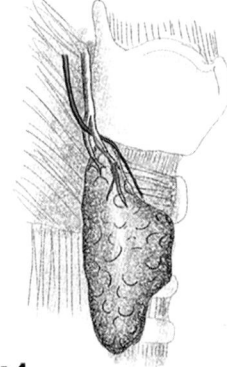

Fig. 35.4 Kierner external branch of the superior laryngeal nerve (EBSLN) surgical anatomic classification scheme. (From Barczyński M, Randolph GW, Cernea CR, et al. External branch of the superior laryngeal nerve monitoring during thyroid and parathyroid surgery: International Neural Monitoring Study Group standards guideline statement. *Laryngoscope*. 2013;123[suppl 4]:S1–S14.)

In 2002, Friedman et al. proposed a different classification for the EBSLN that focuses on the relationship between the nerve and the inferior constrictor at its junction with the CTM. Based on their experience with 1057 nerves exposed in 884 patients, they were able to identify and to classify 900 (85.1%) of the nerves.[42] Friedman's classification system was not intended to replace the classification system proposed by Cernea et al. In contrast, it should be considered as a complementary classification system, useful for intraoperative identification of the nerve. Three variations have been described by Friedman et al. for the main trunk of the EBSLN before its terminal branching (Figure 35.5).

Friedman EBSLN Classification Scheme

Type 1. Nerve runs its whole course (superficially or laterally) to the inferior constrictor and descends with the superior thyroid vessels until it terminates in the CTM.

Type 2. Nerve penetrates the inferior constrictor in the lower portion of the muscle. In this case, it is only partially protected by the inferior constrictor.

Type 3. Nerve dives under the superior fibers of the inferior constrictor and remains covered by this muscle throughout its course to the CTM.

In a 2009 report, Selvan et al. proposed a new clinical typing of the EBSLN based on a prospective, descriptive dissection study of 70 nerves in 35 patients; using EMG, the cricothyroid compound muscle action potential (CMAP) was recorded to identify EBSLNs and classify them according to clinical variation during routine thyroid operations.[43] The system categorizes the nerve in relation to superior thyroid vessels and the cricoid cartilage (Figure 35.6).

Selvan EBSLN Classification Scheme

Type 1a. Nerve that was located within 1 cm of the entry of the vessels into the gland either anterior or between the branches of the superior thyroid vessels and within 3 cm from the cricoid cartilage (9% of patients).

Type 1b. Nerve that was located posterior to the vessels but within 1 cm of the entry of the superior thyroid vessel into the gland. This entry point is close to the anterior insertion line of the CTM onto cricoid cartilage (present in 3% of patients).

Type 2. Nerve that was located within 1 to 3 cm of the entry of the vessels into the gland or within 3 to 5 cm from the cricoid cartilage (present in 68% of patients).

Type 3. Nerve that was located between 3 and 5 cm of the entry of the vessels into the gland or more than 5 cm from the cricoid cartilage (present in 20% of patients).

In many recent papers, the anatomic classification proposed by Cernea et al. has been widely accepted. Some authors have reported similar proportions of the high-risk type 2b EBSLN as in the original Cernea et al. results. Ozlugedik et al.[44] studied 40 necks and observed a 17.5% frequency of type 2b nerves. In a prospective study involving 78 superior thyroid poles in surgical patients, Mishra et al.[45] found an even lower percentage (10.25%) of type 2b nerves. In other publications, the frequency of type 2b nerves was significantly higher than the original findings reported by Cernea et al.[9] Pagedar and Freeman[46] evaluated 178 EBSLNs in 112 consecutive patients; 48.3% were type 2b. Chuang et al.[47] performed an anatomic study of 86 EBSLNs in 43 cadavers; 38.3% were type 2b.

Some authors pointed out that some individual "intrinsic factors" could be related to an increased incidence of type 2b EBSLN.

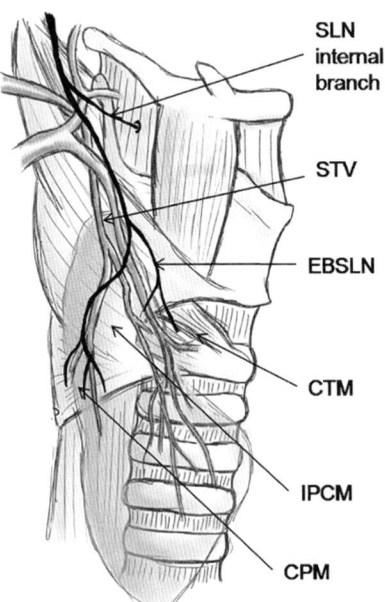
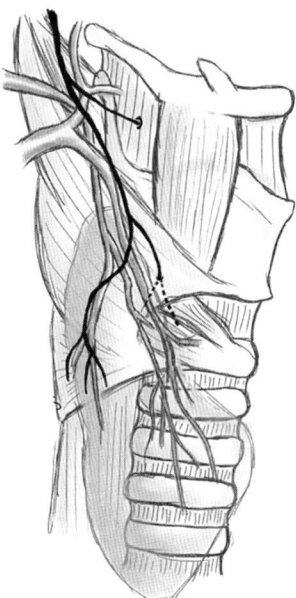
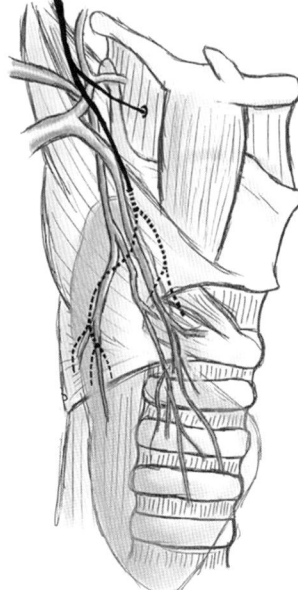

Type 1
EBSLN runs its whole course superficially or laterally to the inferior constrictor, descending with the superior thyroid vessels until it terminates in the cricothyroid muscle

Type 2
EBSLN penetrates the inferior constrictor in the lower portion of the muscle. In this case, it is only partially protected by the inferior constrictor.

Type 3
EBSLN dives under the superior fibers of the inferior constrictor, remaining covered by this muscle throughout its course to the cricothyroid muscle.

Fig. 35.5 Friedman external branch of the superior laryngeal nerve (EBSLN) surgical anatomic classification scheme. CPM cricopharyngeus muscle, IPCM inferior constrictor muscle, STV superior thyroid vien (From Barczyński M, Randolph GW, Cernea CR, et al. External branch of the superior laryngeal nerve monitoring during thyroid and parathyroid surgery: International Neural Monitoring Study Group standards guideline statement. *Laryngoscope.* 2013;123[suppl 4]:S1–S14.)

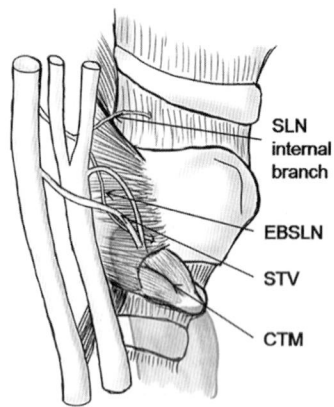 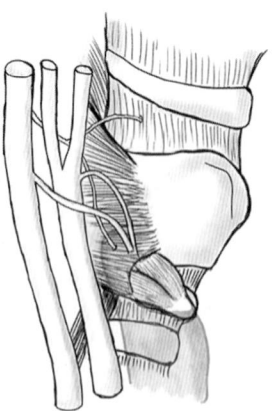 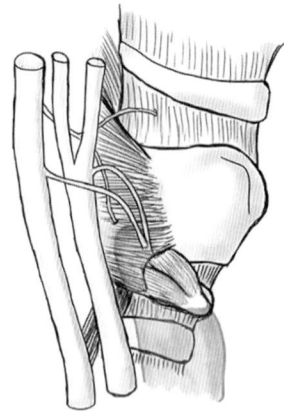 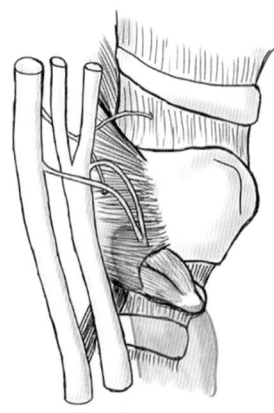

Type 1a
EBSLN is located within 1 cm of the entry of the vessels into the gland either anterior or between the branches of the STV and within 3 cm from the cricoid cartilage

Type 1b
EBSLN is located posterior to the vessels but within 1 cm of the entry of the STV into the gland. This entry point is close to the anterior insertion line of the CTM onto cricoid cartilage

Type 2
EBSLN is located within 1 to 3 cm of the entry of the vessels into the gland or within 3 to 5 cm from the cricoid cartilage

Type 3
EBSLN is located between 3 and 5 cm of the entry of the vessels into the gland or more than 5 cm from the cricoid cartilage

Fig. 35.6 Selvan external branch of the superior laryngeal nerve (EBSLN) surgical anatomic classification scheme. (From Barczyński M, Randolph GW, Cernea CR, et al. External branch of the superior laryngeal nerve monitoring during thyroid and parathyroid surgery: International Neural Monitoring Study Group standards guideline statement. *Laryngoscope.* 2013;123[suppl 4]:S1–S14.)

Furlan et al.[48] conducted an anatomic study on 36 nonpreserved cadavers. Type 2b nerves were statistically more prevalent among individuals with lesser stature ($p = 0.0006$) and with increased glandular volume ($p = 0.0007$).

Morton et al.,[49] in a review article, criticized all existing anatomic classifications of the EBSLN. In their view, all classifications failed to establish a reliable anatomic landmark to safely identify and protect the nerve during a thyroidectomy. However, we strongly believe that the way the surgeon approaches the superior thyroid pole is the most important factor concerning the protection of the nerve during a thyroidectomy, especially when dealing with a large goiter.

PHYSIOLOGY AND PATHOPHYSIOLOGY

The EBSLN is the only motor supply to the CTM. Tschiassny, in 1944,[50] and Arnold, in 1961,[51] demonstrated the influence of the contraction of this muscle on voice production. The CTM has two bellies, the *pars recta* and the *pars obliqua*. The action each of these two subunits is not fully understood, but the combined contraction of these two components is important in adjusting the vocal fold length and tension.[52]

The frequency of vocal fold vibration is influenced by the vocal fold tension, which is controlled, in large part, by a balance between the actions of two muscles: the thyroarytenoid muscle—which tends to shorten the fold length—and the CTM. The CTM muscle promotes elevation of the cricoid cartilage, shortening the distance with the thyroid cartilage. This motion of the cricoid cartilage increases the vocal fold length and tension. Arnold called this CTM-induced vocal cord tension "external tension" of the vocal fold; the classification is distinct from the more refined increase in "internal tension" offered by the action of the thyroarytenoid muscle. The CTM-induced vocal cord tension is thought to be of central importance in the production of high-frequency sounds during phonation. Besides this phonatory function of the EBSLN, some authors have suggested it has a role in respiration, noting respiratory activity, mainly during expiration.[53,54]

The injury of the EBSLN causes a complete paralysis of the CTM that is evidenced by a so-called electrical silence at EMG.[21] Functionally, the fundamental frequency of the voice is lowered, and voice performance is worsened markedly, especially in producing high-frequency sounds (see Chapter 42, Pathophysiology of Recurrent Laryngeal Nerve Injury and Chapter 43, Management of Recurrent Laryngeal Nerve Paralysis).[21]

SURGICAL TECHNIQUE

A surgical approach to the superior thyroid pole is necessary in most operations involving the thyroid gland. Some surgeons prefer to start the thyroidectomy with the superior pole dissection;[14,21] for others, this is the final step.[17] Regardless of the sequence, the dissection of the superior thyroid pole usually starts with initial mobilization of the whole thyroid lobe. Ligation of the middle thyroid vein is advisable to facilitate this initial mobilization. It is highly recommended that the sternothyroid-laryngeal triangle be completely exposed before any superior pole suture is placed (see Figure 35.2). In most instances, when the thyroid lobe is of normal size or only slightly enlarged, there is no need for complete section of the strap muscles. However, if required, a partial incision of the sternothyroid muscle with cautery may improve the access to the superior thyroid pedicle (Figure 35.7) (see Chapter 31, Principles in Thyroid Surgery).

Several techniques have been described to minimize the potential risk of injury to the EBSLN during superior thyroid vessels dissection and ligation:

1. Ligation of the individual branches of the superior thyroid vessels under direct vision on the thyroid capsule without attempts to visually identify the nerve
2. Visual identification of the nerve before ligation of the superior thyroid pole vessels
3. The use of either a nerve stimulator or intraoperative nerve monitoring (IONM) for mapping and confirmation of the EBSLN identification

CHAPTER 35 Surgical Anatomy and Monitoring of the Superior Laryngeal Nerve

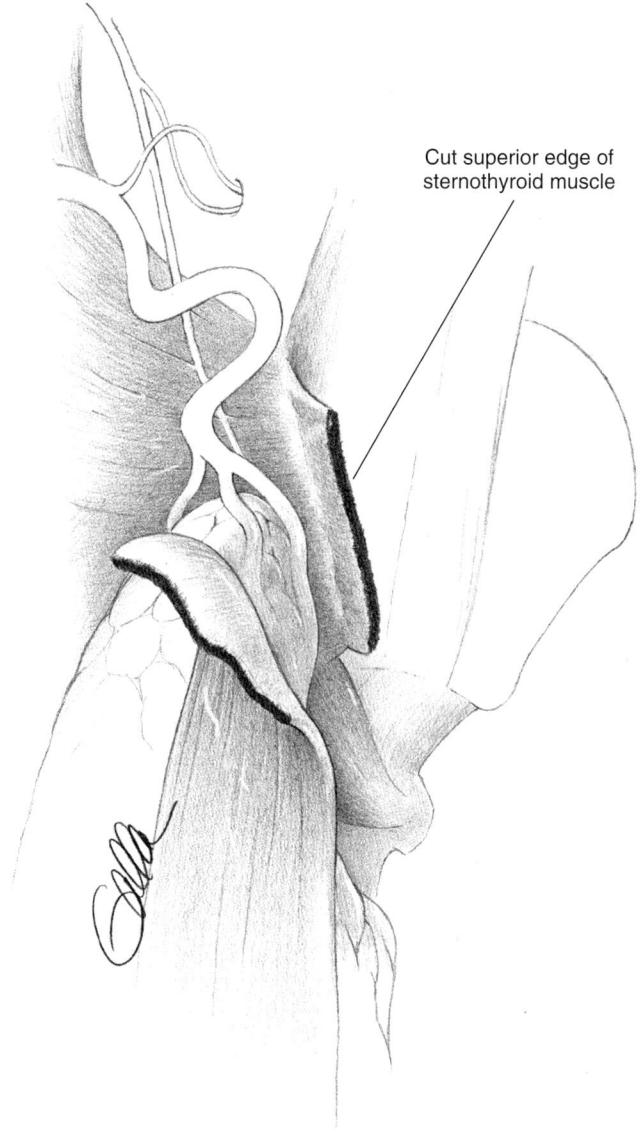

Fig. 35.7 Incision is made in the sternothyroid muscle with cautery, increasing superior pole exposure.

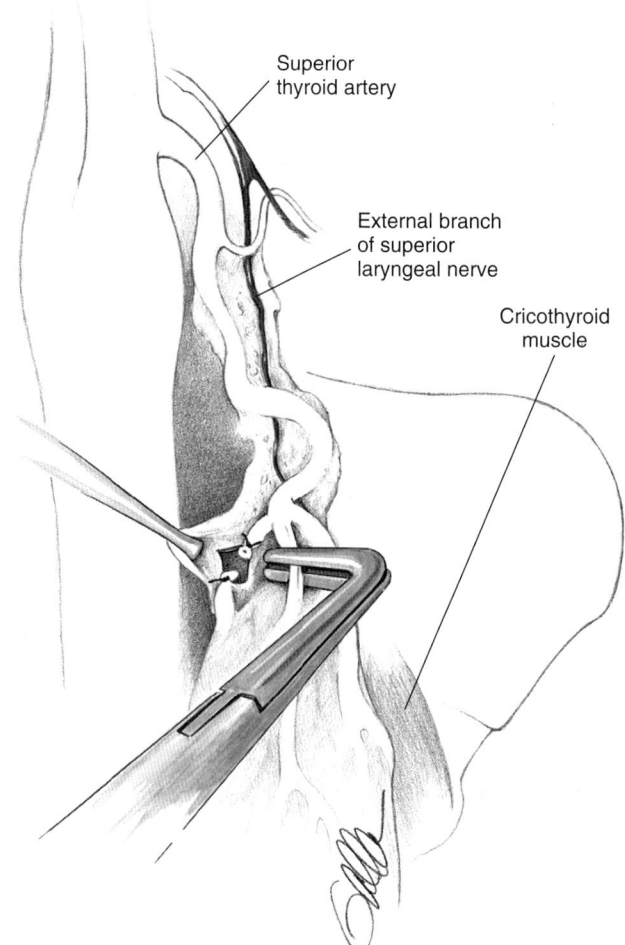

Fig. 35.8 Superior thyroid pole dissection with individual superior thyroid artery branch ligation. Sutures should be placed as far caudally as possible.

The superior thyroid vessels usually divide into three branches that embrace the superior thyroid pole; two are located anteriorly and one runs dorsally to the thyroid superior pole. It is imperative that the surgeon dissect and ligate these branches individually and as caudally as possible (Figure 35.8). Loré et al. emphasized that gentle traction of the thyroid lobe caudally may help preserve the integrity of the EBSLN.[17]

Generally, the EBSLN will be situated cranially to the superior border of the thyroid lobe, and strict adherence to the aforementioned principles will offer reasonable protection. However, in 15% to 20% of cases, the nerve may be type 2B. Thus in all cases, superior pole vessel ligature and dissection in the sternothyroid-laryngeal triangle and along the medial surface of the thyroid's superior pole must be performed meticulously, with wide exposure. The surgeon should have a low threshold for use of a nerve stimulator when dissecting in this area. This is especially useful in those circumstances (approximately 20% of cases) in which the EBSLN is deep to the inferior constrictor muscle fascia.[8] When the nerve is electrically stimulated, a quick but powerful contraction of the CTM is immediately obtained (see this chapter's video on EBSLN). Once the EBSLN is visualized, it must be kept constantly under direct vision during the entire dissection of the superior thyroid pole (Figure 35.9). After completion of superior thyroid pole dissection, the integrity of the nerve may also be documented through electrical stimulation (see also Chapter 36, Surgical Anatomy and Monitoring of the Recurrent Laryngeal Nerve).

Some authors have based their identification and preservation of the EBSLN only on surgical anatomic findings.[8,10] One clear advantage of using nerve stimulation in EBSLN management is the ability to stimulate the nerve superiorly and get a positive signal even if the nerve is subfascial within the fibers of the inferior contrictor. The positive signal results in CTM twitch as well as a typical, small, short-latency response on endotracheal monitoring systems (through the human communicating nerve). The bands of tissue taken as part of superior pole management can then be stimulated as negative before they are divided (see also Chapter 36, Surgical Anatomy and Monitoring of the Recurrent Laryngeal Nerve). Nevertheless, like many others in the international literature,[18-20,22] we prefer a positive electrical identification.[21,23] Barczyński has studied 210 patients in a randomized controlled study of RLN and EBSLN visualization versus visualization and IONM. Barczyński found significant improvement in ability to identify the EBSLN with monitoring (83% with monitoring versus 34% without monitoring) as well as significant improvement in multiple early voice postoperative parameters with monitoring (see also

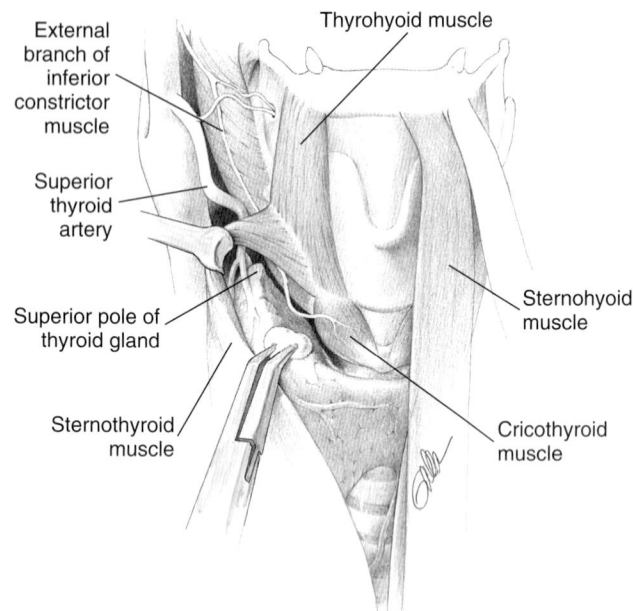

Fig. 35.9 Gentle caudal traction of the thyroid lobe is recommended to preserve the external branch of the superior laryngeal nerve (EBSLN).

Chapter 36, Surgical Anatomy and Monitoring of the Recurrent Laryngeal Nerve).[35]

Dissection of the superior thyroid pole is much more difficult when the surgeon is dealing with a large goiter. In this instance, the upper border of the pole is elevated markedly, putting it in close contact with the EBSLN (Figure 35.10). An additional consideration is enlargement of the superior thyroid vessels, which usually parallel the dimensions of the goiter and demand an even more careful dissection. Sectioning of the strap muscles can improve exposure and facilitate safer dissection. We have demonstrated that the probability of a high-risk 2B nerve in patients with goiter may rise to 54%.[23] Hence attempts to obtain a positive identification of the EBSLN in such goiters are especially important.

Recently, some authors have employed minimally invasive techniques to approach the thyroid gland, including video-assisted thyroidectomy. It is important to emphasize that the anatomic classification that Cernea proposed in 1992 was developed using nonpreserved cadavers after rigor mortis to enable the neck to be hyperextended, which is exactly the same position as in a conventional thyroidectomy.[9] However, no neck hyperextension is applied during a video-assisted thyroidectomy, thus approximating the EBSLN to the superior thyroid pole. In a limited series of 12 cases, Dedivitis and Guimarães were able to clearly identify the nerve in 83.3% of the cases; the authors noted that the nerves ran medially to the branches of the superior thyroid vessels in 80% and laterally in 20% of the cases.[55] They found that the magnification and illumination offered by the scope probably facilitates visualization and preservation of the EBSLN.

A prospective study of 10 patients submitted to minimally invasive thyroidectomy under local anesthesia, with nerve monitoring of the EBSLN.[56] Among the 15 nerves at risk, 8 were identified and successfully preserved, with their normal function assessed during the operation by the IONM and, postoperatively, by video laryngoscopy.

Monitoring of the EBSLN

Contrary to routine dissection of the RLN, most surgeons tend to avoid rather than routinely expose the EBSLN during thyroidectomy.[57] The

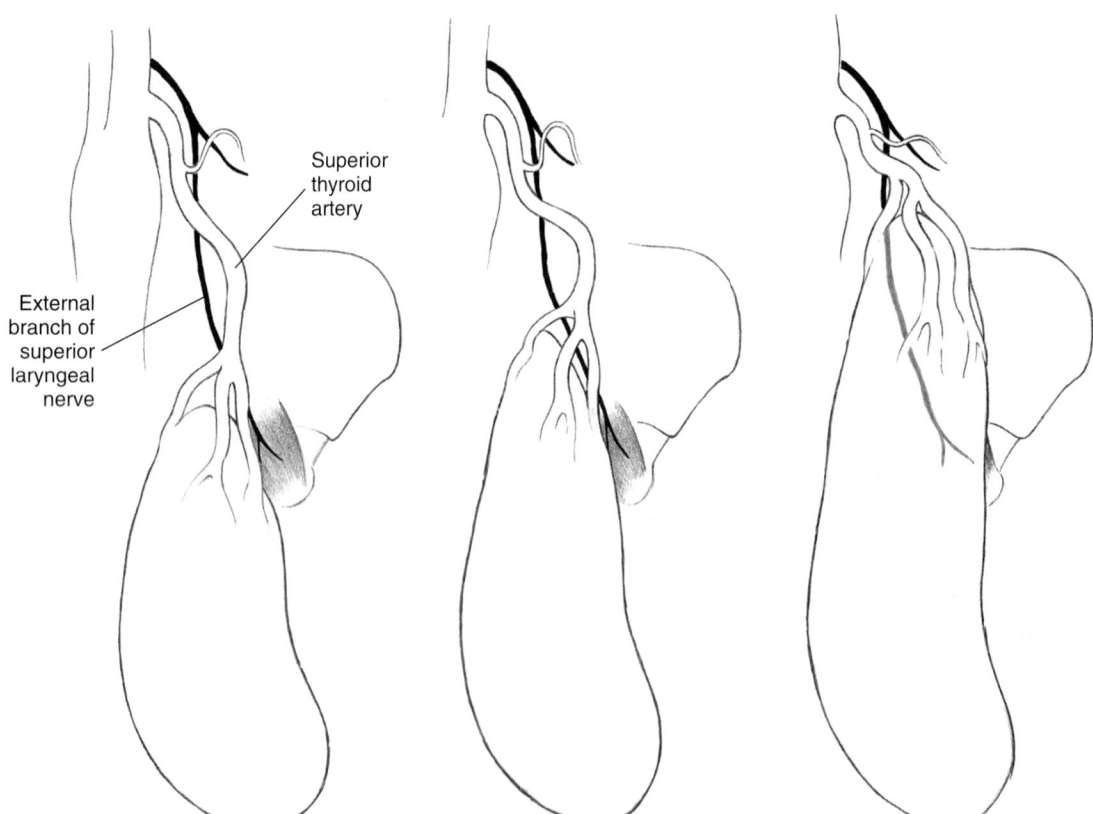

Fig. 35.10 Dissection of the superior thyroid pole is more difficult when the surgeon is faced with a large goiter.

rate of visual EBSLN identification by experienced thyroid surgeons has been reported to exceed 98%. However, in most published studies, visual inspection of the EBSLN was not successful in more than two-thirds of patients.[58] The most recent guideline statement the International Neural Monitoring Study Group highlighted the importance of visually searching for the nerve in all cases. These guidelines recommended that attempts to visually identify the EBSLN should be facilitated by implementation of neural stimulation techniques and evaluation of the CTM twitch response or, preferably, glottic endotracheal EMG monitoring to assure functional preservation of the nerve during thyroidectomy (Figure 35.11).[58] As shown by data from the current international survey on the identification and neural monitoring of the EBSLN during thyroidectomy, IONM was used for recognition of the EBSLN in the majority of patients by 5/19 (26.3%) low-volume versus 39/57 (68.4%) highest-volume surgeons (>200 thyroidectomies per year) based on the CTM twitch assessment ($p = 0.004$), and 3/16 (15.8%) low-volume versus 35/57 (61.4%) highest-volume surgeons based on the evaluation of endotracheal surface EMG ($p < 0.001$). Eight of 19 (42.1%) low-volume surgeons versus 39/57 (68.4%) highest-volume surgeons were aware of the EBSLN Neural Monitoring Guideline Statement ($p = 0.041$).[57]

Barczyński et al. published a study comprising 210 patients who were randomized into two arms (N = 105, each): visual identification of the EBSLN and RLN versus additional EBSLN and RLN monitoring. Use of IONM corresponded to both improved EBSLN identification rates during surgery (34.5% without IONM and 83.8% with IONM), as well as reduced incidence of transient EBSLN damage in latter group (5.0% versus 1.0%, respectively; $p = 0.02$), findings which correlated to a diminished risk of early phonation changes after surgery in the monitored arm.[35] Similar conclusions were drawn by Uludag et al. based on the outcomes of a study of 133 patients undergoing thyroidectomy. The patients were randomized into two groups: (1) patients with 105 nerves at risk and upper thyroid pole dissection without visual identification of the EBSLN, and (2) patients with 106 nerves at risk with IONM used to map out the EBSLN during thyroidectomy. The EBSLN Voice Impairment Index-5 (VII-5) was administered during 6 months of postoperative follow-up to assess for altered postoperative voice performance. EBSLN damage was diagnosed in nine (8.6%) nerves at risk in group 1 and in one (0.9%) nerve at risk in group 2 patients ($p = 0.015$ and $p = 0.010$, respectively). IONM was considered to markedly assist in both visual identification and functional neural preservation among group 2 patients in this study. The VII-5 revealed significantly altered voice in group 1 versus group 2 during the entire 6-month postoperative follow-up period. Authors concluded that IONM plays a major role in functional preservation of the EBSLN that leads to a decreased rate of EBSLN damage during the upper thyroid pole management.[59]

Lee et al. recently reported the outcomes of a prospective study of 490 thyroid operations (299 total thyroidectomies and 191 hemithyroidectomies) wherein IONM was used to facilitate RLN and EBSLN identification and preservation. Outcomes for these patients were compared with outcomes of 500 thyroidectomies performed by the same surgeon without IONM.[60] In this study, demographic characteristics, type of operation, pathology, RLN and EBSLN identification and classification, functional and electrophysiological data, as well as surgical morbidity were analyzed. Interestingly, the added value of IONM defined as improved identification rate of the EBSLN compared with the visual inspection alone was in this study equal to 13.8% ($p < 0.0001$). This value was even higher at 15.8% for type 2b EBSLNs. The usefulness of IONM could not have been predicted by analysis of preoperatively-known factors including indications for surgery. Hence routine use of IONM, even by high-volume thyroid surgeons, may allow for better intraoperative management of the RLN and EBSLN than visual identification technique alone.[60]

CTM twitch and glottic EMG recordings are both methods of IONM that are recommended for thyroid surgeries where there is a risk of jeopardizing the EBSLN. The International Neural Monitoring Study Group recently proposed an optimal management strategy for superior thyroid pole dissection to ensure EBSLN preservation. This strategy involves two maneuvers:[58]

1. The EBSLN should be stimulated with observation of the CTM twitch or endotracheal EMG waveform (if present) cranially and medial to the upper thyroid pole vessels (a true positive stimulation).
2. Stimulation of the tissues neighboring the upper thyroid vessels before their division at the given level should be negative for EBSLN identification, which means that there is no CTM twitch or endotracheal EMG waveform after this stimulation (a true negative stimulation).

Contrary to the RLN monitoring, EBSLN monitoring relies on evaluation of clearly visible CTM twitch (present in all patients after a positive identification of the nerve), and EMG glottic waveform analysis recorded by the surface endotracheal tube electrodes; this is observable in 70% to 80% of patients when using standard EMG tubes or close to 100% of patients when using NIM TriVantage tubes (Medtronic, Minneapolis, MN). NIM TriVantage tubes have additional electrodes located on the anterior and more proximal surfaces of the tube.[39,58] IONM of the EBSLN with EMG assessment provides the potential additional benefits of prognostication, quantification, and documentation of neural function rather than solely stimulating the nerve with CTM twitch assessment.[35-38]

In a group of 105 patients and 210 EBSLNs at risk, Barczyński et al. found that after EBSLN stimulation at 1 mA, 73.9% of patients exhibited evoked potentials recorded by standard surface endotracheal tube EMG electrodes, with a mean amplitude of 249.5 ± 144.3 μV. The mean amplitude after EBSLN stimulation was significantly lower than the mean amplitude of evoked potential observed during stimulation of

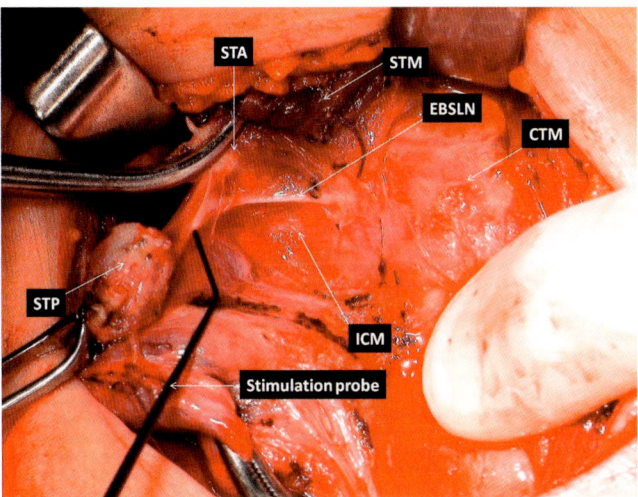

Fig. 35.11 Meticulous dissection and ligation of individual branches of the superior thyroid artery with visual identification and electric stimulation of the EBSLN to assure functional preservation of the nerve. EBSLN, external branch of the superior laryngeal nerve, CTM, cricothyroid muscle, ICM, inferior constrictor muscle, STM, sternothyroid muscle, STA, superior thyroid artery, STP, superior thyroid pole. (From Barczyński M, Randolph GW, Cernea CR, et al. External branch of the superior laryngeal nerve monitoring during thyroid and parathyroid surgery: International Neural Monitoring Study Group standards guideline statement. *Laryngoscope*. 2013;123[suppl 4]:S1–S14.)

the RLN, which was equal to 638.5 ± 568.4 µV ($p<0.001$).[35] Similar observations were made recently by Randolph et al., who reviewed data from 72 consecutive patients undergoing thyroid surgery. Ninety-three RLNs were stimulated and 73 EBSLNs were found and stimulated with either 1 or 2 mA. A clear EMG waveform after EBSLN stimulation was obtained in 57 (78.1%) of the cases. The mean amplitude of response for the EBSLN was 269.9 ± 178.6 µV, approximately one-third that of the mean RLN amplitude (782.2 ± 178.6 µV).[37,39]

Overall, it is advisable to stimulate the EBSLN at the most cranial arc of dissection during the final stage of upper thyroid pole dissection to confirm not only anatomic preservation but, more importantly, functional preservation of the nerve.[58] However, the possible role of measuring waveform amplitude in the prognostication of EBSLN function remains to be determined in future studies.

The mnemotechnic formula of "EBSLN" facilitates memorization of the steps necessary for safe dissection and identification of the EBSLN (Figure 35.12).

DIAGNOSIS OF EBSLN PARALYSIS

EBSLN dysfunction is difficult to confirm based solely on clinical and endoscopic findings (see Chapter 42, Pathophysiology of Recurrent Laryngeal Nerve Injury and Chapter 43, Management of Recurrent Laryngeal Nerve Paralysis). Voice changes are variable and, in male patients, can be subtle. However, in female patients and voice professionals, voice alteration can be significant with symptoms, such as lowering of fundamental frequency, inability to produce high-tone sounds, and vocal fatigue with high vocal loads. If a more elaborate voice evaluation is performed, shortening of the phonic time of the consonant /z/ as well as lowering of high tones and contraction of the vocal range are usually detected.[21] Teitelbaum and Wenig reported that videolaryngostroboscopy may help in the diagnosis of EBSLN paralysis after thyroidectomy.[61] They have suggested that the paralysis results in bowing of the affected vocal fold, posterior glottic rotation toward the side of the paralysis, inferior displacement of the affected vocal fold, and asymmetry of the vocal fold mucosal wave. However, these findings are not uniform in all patients with EMG proven CTM dysfunction; thus clinical diagnosis remains elusive.

The most objective method for detecting an injury of the EBSLN is EMG of the CTM.[21,48] Using the inferior border of the thyroid cartilage and the superior aspect of the cricoid cartilage as external anatomic landmarks, an electrode is placed percutaneously in the muscle, and the patient is asked to produce a high-tone /e/. If the nerve is intact, a marked increase in the electrical activity of the CTM is immediately verified. However, if the EBSLN is injured, no increase in background electrical activity is observed. The contralateral muscle may be used as a control. EMG is an invasive and sometimes painful examination; thus it is not used routinely.

From a practical viewpoint, intraoperative electrophysiologic testing of the EBSLN at the end of the operation can serve to prognosticate postoperative EBSLN function, and it has the potential to become a new standard of care in thyroid surgery. A positive CTM twitch after stimulation of the EBSLN at the end of the operation can be regarded as a sign of good functional preservation of the nerve that denotes an extremely low risk of intraoperative nerve injury.[58]

Incidence of EBSLN Injury

It is difficult to compare the incidence of EBSLN injury among the few available series in international literature because laryngeal examination methods are heterogeneous and examination findings are unreliable. Loré et al. reported 0.9% injury in 111 patients, employing only indirect laryngoscopy.[62] Rossi et al. found only 0.3% injury in 309 patients, but the examination method was not described.[63] Lennquist, Cahlin, and Smeds attempted to actively preserve the nerve and found 2.6% injury in 38 patients studied prospectively.[8] Lekakos et al. noted 11% nerve injury in 27 patients in whom a "high ligation" of the superior thyroid vessels was executed, compared with 0% incidence of injury among 122 patients in whom the branches of the superior thyroid pedicle were separately ligated.[15] In evaluating 20 patients before and after thyroidectomy with EMG and acoustic analysis, Jansson et al. reported a 58% rate of "partially" injured EBSLNs.[64] Teitelbaum and Wenig found 5% incidence among 20 patients.[61] Loré et al., in a more recent paper, reported only 0.1% with laryngoscopic changes consistent with paralysis of the EBSLN among 934 nerves at risk.[17] In our own prospective clinical series, we found from 12% to 28% incidence of injury when the EBSLN was not identified intraoperatively; some of these injuries were permanent, as confirmed by long-term electromyographic evaluation.[21] There is a growing body of evidence, based on more recent reports, that routine visual identification of the EBSLN, together with electrical stimulation or nerve monitoring, may improve outcomes of the superior thyroid pedicle management in terms of diminished risk of neural injury.[35,38,59,65-70] Careful dissection should be continued once the nerve is identified to assure functional nerve preservation. In cases when the nerve is not seen, but mapped out in the operative field, this dissection should involve optimizing the level of superior thyroid artery ligation to ensure intact functional integrity of the EBSLN (provided by electrical nerve testing).[58,70]

Treatment of EBSLN Injury

Unfortunately, once injury of the EBSLN has occurred, no truly effective treatment is available. Intensive phonotherapy is highly recommended. If the paralysis is permanent, the consequences for the career of a voice professional may be significant; this was likely the case with Amelita Galli-Curci, despite the existing controversy in historical literature.[11] Hong et al. suggested, based on their experimental work, that laryngoplasty might be useful in such a situation.[52] However, to the best of our knowledge, outcomes of this procedure have not been validated in any prospective clinical series.

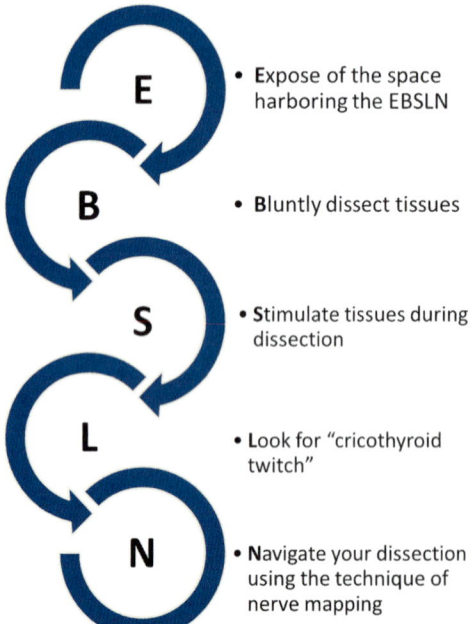

- **E** • Expose of the space harboring the EBSLN
- **B** • Bluntly dissect tissues
- **S** • Stimulate tissues during dissection
- **L** • Look for "cricothyroid twitch"
- **N** • Navigate your dissection using the technique of nerve mapping

Fig. 35.12 The mnemonic "EBSLN" can aid in remembering the steps necessary for safe dissection and identification of the external branch of the superior laryngeal nerve (EBSLN).

IBSLN MONITORING

In contrast to the EBSLN, the IBSLN is a purely sensory nerve that supplies the pharynx and supraglottic larynx. It enters the larynx via the thyrohyoid membrane and runs with the superior laryngeal vessels. Although not directly in the surgical field for neck endocrine procedures, the IBSLN can be injured during excision of high retropharyngeal lymph nodes or during cervical spine approaches for upper cervical vertebral levels. Monitoring of this nerve branch has recently become possible with the discovery that the laryngeal adductor reflex (LAR) is preserved in humans under total intravenous general anesthesia.[71,72] The LAR is a primitive airway protective reflex that prevents inhalation of potentially noxious objects. Its afferent pathway is via the IBSLN and vagus, nerve with efferent fibers running in the RLN to cause bilateral vocal fold adduction. This adduction can be recorded on EMG endotracheal tubes as for regular RLN monitoring; however, the exception is that the latency of response of LAR is longer (at around 22 milliseconds) (Figure 35.13). This technique of continuous IONM requires no equipment other than an EMG endotracheal tube. The tube electrodes are used to both elicit the reflex (via stimulation of laryngeal mucosa) and to continuously record the bilateral contractile response for the duration of a surgical procedure. We have shown that the posterior supraglottis is the optimal site of stimulation because it elicits a robust bilateral response in all patients.[73] We have now continuously monitored more than 200 patients with this technique; we have found the technique to provide real time information about nerve function that is complementary to that obtained by traditional intermittent RLN monitoring techniques. In addition, because it results in bilateral vocal fold adduction, it is possible to separate the afferent and efferent limbs of the reflex and to monitor either the purely sensory IBSLN (by stimulating mucosa on the side ipsilateral to the IBSLN at risk, and then recording vocal fold adduction on the side contralateral to the IBSLN at risk) or to monitor the RLN (by stimulating the IBSLN on the side contralateral to the RLN at risk and recording vocal fold adduction on the side ipsilateral to the RLN at risk). This technique continues to evolve, but it may prove to be a valuable addition to the IONM armamentarium for both the purely sensory IBSLN and for the RLN.

CONCLUSION

The EBSLN is a terminal branch of the SLN and has a close anatomic relationship with the superior thyroid pedicle. In 15% to 20% of cases, the nerve may be a type 2b that crosses the superior thyroid vessels below the upper border of the superior thyroid pole. In these circumstances, it may be at high-risk of injury during a thyroidectomy. Therefore it is advisable to ligate the branches of the superior thyroid artery and vein separately, as far caudally as possible. Intraoperative stimulation of the EBSLN, with or without IONM, can improve the visual identification rate of the nerve, and diminish the prevalence of nerve injury and possible postoperative voice impairment. Monitoring of the EBSLN provides an additional and sufficient reason to use IONM during thyroid surgery, especially when dealing with a grossly enlarged thyroid lobe.

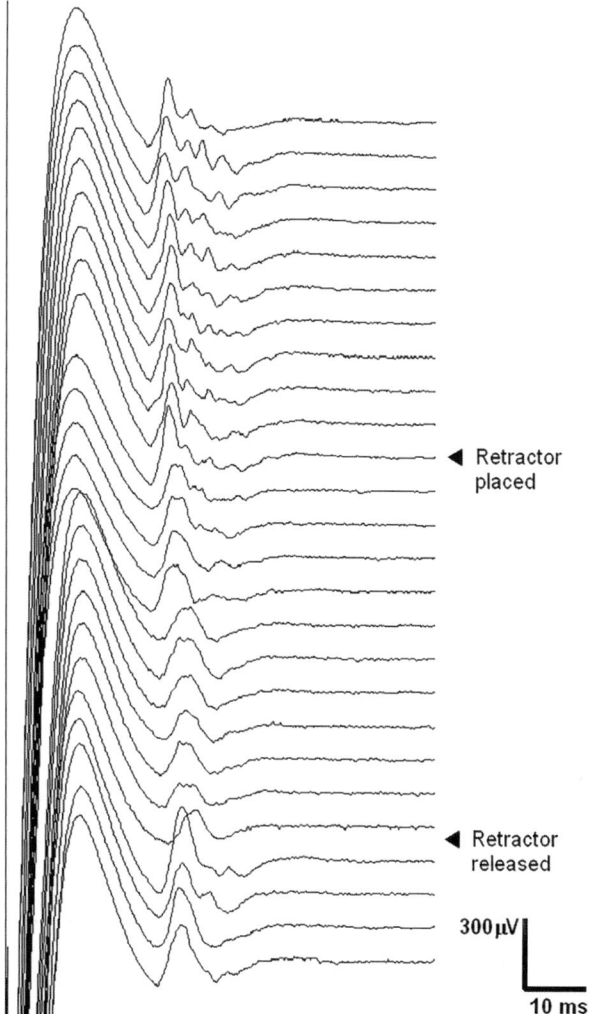

Fig. 35.13 LAR traces from a C3/4 cervical spine approach during retractor placement. Nerve at risk was the left internal branch of the superior laryngeal nerve (IBSLN). Note the decrease in amplitude with placement of deep retractors. Also note the return of activity once the retractors were released and their location adjusted.

REFERENCES

For a complete list of references, go to expertconsult.com.

36

Surgical Anatomy and Monitoring of the Recurrent Laryngeal Nerve

Gregory W. Randolph, Dipti Kamani, Che-Wei Wu, Rick Schneider

"The accident of hemorrhage is a minor evil…Although there are others more terrible and frightening, the cutting of the recurrent nerves is dangerous in the highest degree, [for when] this unfortunately occurs, either the patient dies of it miserably or at least loses for the rest of his life the most beautiful prerogative given to man by God, which is (la favella) speech; but this danger can easily be avoided by that Surgeon who, with the provision of Anatomy, knows the site of these nerves."

Dr. Fulvio Gherli, Doctor of Philosophy and Medicine, Scandiano, Italy, 1724[1]

Please go to expertconsult.com to view related video:
Video 36.1 Introduction to Chapter 36, Surgical Anatomy and Monitoring of the Recurrent Laryngeal Nerve.
Video 36.2 Recurrent Laryngeal Nerve Monitoring.
Video 36.3 Continuous Vagal Nerve Monitoring.
This chapter contains additional online-only content, including exclusive video, available on expertconsult.com.

INTRODUCTION

Please see the Expert Consult website for discussion of this topic.

This chapter reviews the surgical anatomy of the recurrent laryngeal nerve (RLN), related surgical and management maneuvers, and monitoring techniques for the RLN. The superior laryngeal nerve (SLN) is discussed in a limited capacity, only in relation to complement RLN as it relates to thyroidectomy. For in-depth information on SLN, refer to Chapter 35, Surgical Anatomy of the Superior Laryngeal Nerve.

Reported Incidence of RLN Paralysis

RLN paralysis is one of the most feared postoperative morbidities after thyroid surgeries. Unilateral vocal cord paralysis (VCP) can lead to voice changes accompanied by dysphagia and aspiration; bilateral VCP may result in tracheostomy. Given the frequency and significance of RLN paralysis at thyroidectomy, the knowledge of the anatomy, surgical maneuvers, and monitoring techniques for the RLN is important. The reported incidence of RLN paralysis is reviewed in depth in Chapter 15, Pre- and Postoperative Laryngeal Examination in Thyroid and Parathyroid Surgery.

Permanent RLN paralysis rates in expert hands have been reported in the 1% to 2% range.[4] However, the rates of RLN paralysis after thyroidectomy in many studies are likely underestimates for several reasons. First, the thyroid units with unfavorable data are less likely to report findings. Second, most injuries are not detectable intraoperatively by surgeons. Lo found that surgeons had recognized intraoperative injury in only 1% of cases, although surgical injury had actually occurred in nearly 7% of patients.[5] The third reason is the variability in practice of postoperative laryngeal examination in these studies; typically, only patients with significant and persistent symptoms undergo laryngoscopy. Several practitioners have shown the lack of reliability of clinical symptoms in VCP (see Chapter 15, Pre- and Postoperative Laryngeal Examination in Thyroid and Parathyroid Surgery).[6-9] Variability in symptoms results from variation in degree of injury, cord position, contralateral cord compensation, and the evolution over time in position of the paralyzed cord. The Scandinavian Quality Register has found that the rate of RLN paralysis doubles when all patients receive postoperative laryngeal examination.[10] The true rate of RLN injury can only be appreciated if all patients uniformly receive preoperative and postoperative laryngeal examination.

Although the rate of RLN injury with thyroidectomy in expert hands may be low, Djohan recently wrote that "the estimated incidence of RLN injury in standard thyroidectomy is from 2% to 13%."[11] In patients undergoing surgery for thyroid cancer, 15% were found to have VCP when laryngoscopy was performed within 1 week.[8] Foster, in reviewing 24,108 thyroidectomies, described a rate of 2.5% for tracheotomy.[12] Recently, a large systematic review of the literature reviewing 25,000 patients found a postoperative rate of 9.8%.[13]

Bilateral thyroidectomy is unique in head and neck surgery in that both left and right cranial nerves are subject to risk in one surgical procedure. Bilateral cord paralysis occurs frequently enough in patients undergoing bilateral thyroid surgery that indications for tracheotomy in patients undergoing bilateral thyroidectomy have been developed.[14] Several practitioners have shown that rates of RLN paralysis during thyroid surgery are greater in cases associated with (1) lack of intraoperative RLN identification, (2) bilateral surgery, (3) surgery for cancer, (4) significant lymph node resection, (5) surgery for Graves' disease or thyroiditis, (6) revision surgery, (7) surgery associated with substernal goiter, (8) surgery associated with longer operating room times or greater blood loss, and (9) patients brought back to surgery because of bleeding. Also, surgeon experience has been related to RLN paralysis rates with rates of <1% being associated with surgeons performing greater than 45 nerve dissections per year.[4,5,15-18] Kandil et al. specifically reported on post total thyroidectomy complications and found that low-volume surgeons were likely to have higher postoperative complications compared with high-volume surgeons (odds ratio 1.53, 95% confidence interval 1.12, 2.11, $p = 0.0083$).[19] A large German multicenter study yielded the following risk factors, in descending order of their importance (odds ratio), for permanent paresis of RLN: carcinoma recurrence (6.66), goiter recurrence (4.67), carcinoma first operation (2.04) (comparison in each case with benign nodular goiter), hemithyroidectomy versus subtotal resection (1.76), no nerve identification versus nerve identification (1.41), hospital experience (1.34), and surgeon experience (1.23).[18]

Laryngeal Examination in All Patients Preoperatively and Postoperatively

Surgical management of the RLN and RLN monitoring are necessarily wedded with knowledge of pre- and postoperative glottic function (see Chapter 15, Pre- and Postoperative Laryngeal Examination in Thyroid and Parathyroid Surgery).

Preoperative laryngeal examination is necessary for the following reasons:
1. VCP may present preoperatively in the absence of voice complaints.
2. VCP present preoperatively suggests invasive malignancy. Its identification informs preoperative planning and radiographic evaluation.
3. VCP may be present preoperatively even in the setting of benign disease (discussed later).
4. Management of the invaded RLN found at surgery is, in part, affected by the knowledge of preoperative functional status.
5. Responsibility for postoperative VCP can be wrongly attributed if one fails to demonstrate its presence preoperatively.
6. Preoperative laryngeal examination provides a preoperative baseline for postoperative laryngeal assessment.

Postoperative laryngeal examination is necessary for the following reasons:
1. Glottic examination is the only existent accurate postoperative RLN outcome measure. Voice changes may occur without VCP, and VCP may occur without voice changes.
2. Postoperative functional glottic information allows for maximum interpretation of intraoperative electromyography (EMG) data from the neural monitoring.
3. Postoperative VCP has significant implications on swallowing and for the planning of future contralateral surgery. The presence of postoperative unilateral VCP is therefore important whether or not it is associated with symptoms. VCP has been found to have significant adverse effects to work-related outcome measures in up to 40% of patients affected.[20]

Shonka and Terris discuss the latest American Thyroid Association (ATA) guidelines regarding voice assessment and laryngeal examination for patients in selective thyroid surgery; however, they note such a selective approach is insufficient, and preoperative and postoperative laryngeal examination should be performed routinely for all thyroid surgical patients. This is because these examinations provide important information to the surgeon, aid in patient counseling and medical decision making, and are imperative in assessing the quality outcomes of thyroid surgery.[21]

This chapter assumes that all patients undergoing thyroid and parathyroid surgery have pre- and postoperative laryngeal examinations (see Chapter 15, Pre- and Postoperative Laryngeal Examination in Thyroid and Parathyroid Surgery). Without this basic framing information, a discussion of intraoperative RLN management is not rational.

Preoperative Vocal Cord Paralysis

Please see the Expert Consult website for discussion of this topic.

Preoperative Laryngeal Examination and Intraoperative Electrical Stimulability

The relationships among laryngeal examination, electrical stimulability, and nerve invasion are interesting. In our series of monitored patients, we have reviewed the laryngeal function and intraoperative EMG data in several interesting subsets of patients (Figure 36.1, A and B).[9] Out of 22 cases with malignant nerve invasion, 45% of cases had normal preoperative laryngeal examination. RLN was routinely identified above and

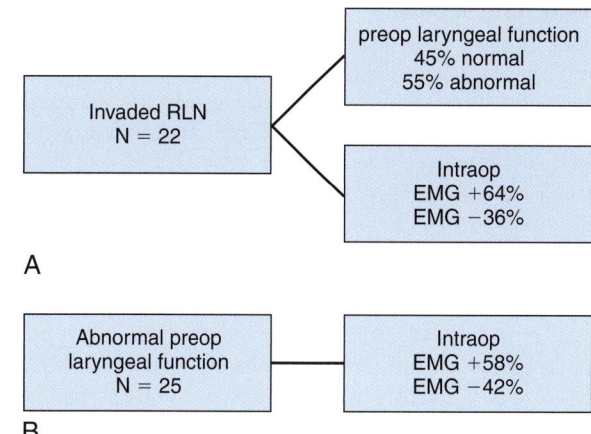

Fig. 36.1 A, Nerves found invaded with carcinoma: preoperative laryngeal function and intraoperative electric stimulability. B, Patients with preoperative laryngeal nerve dysfunction and intraoperative electrophysiologic stimulability. (From Ditpi Kamani and Gregory Randolph, unpublished data, 2011.)

below the area of invasion as well as electrically stimulated, and 63% of invaded nerves were detected to retain electrical stimulability despite the intraoperative finding of nerve invasion. Among the invaded nerves that retained electrical stimulability, the average EMG amplitude in invaded nerves with normal preoperative laryngeal function was 180 µV, whereas in the invaded nerves with known preoperative VCP, it was only 63 µV.[9] Thus invaded nerves are associated approximately one half of the time with preoperative clinical nerve paralysis, yet they retain electrical stimulability in two thirds of cases (with a low level of EMG response) (see Figure 36.1, A). With maintenance of neural activity in the setting of invasion even when preoperative VCP is present, resection of such a nerve is expected to worsen glottic function; this affects the voice as well as swallowing. These patients should receive appropriate preoperative counseling. In fact, Chi et al. have demonstrated when invaded nerves with preoperative VCP and retained intraoperative stimulability are preserved, postoperative vocal cord atrophy and decline of vocal function are prevented.[24]

In the same study, among 25 patients presenting with abnormal preoperative laryngeal function, 58% patients demonstrated intraoperative stimulability. In these patients who retained electrical stimulability, if the laryngeal dysfunction was due to past surgery, the average amplitude was only 93 µV; if laryngeal dysfunction was due to malignant invasion, the average amplitude was only 63 µV. Notably, in patients with abnormal preoperative laryngeal function, the RLN failed to be electrically stimulable in 42% of patients. Chi et al. have presented a small series of such patients who retained some electrical stimulability despite preoperative paralysis.[24] Thus in patients with abnormal preoperative laryngeal function, almost 60% maintain electrical stimulability with low-level EMG (see Figure 36.1, B).

Visualization of Nerve

Please see the Expert Consult website for discussion of this topic.

SURGICAL ANATOMY

"People see what they are prepared to see."
Ralph Waldo Emerson, *Journals*, 1863

A thorough knowledge of vagal, RLN, and SLN anatomy, including branching patterns and anatomic variations, is vital knowledge for any thyroid or parathyroid surgeon.

Vagal Neural Anatomy

The modern vagus nerve anatomy was first described by Willis in the 1600s.[43] The vagus derives its blood supply from a discrete vagal artery, a branch of the inferior thyroid artery (ITA), and it is reinforced by branches from the internal carotid, common carotid, aortic arch, and bronchial and esophageal arteries.[44] The cervical branches of the vagus nerve of concern during thyroid surgery include the SLN, both internal and external branches, and the RLN. The SLN's *internal branch* brings general visceral afferents to the lower pharynx, supraglottic larynx, vocal cords, base of the tongue, and special visceral afferents to the epiglottic taste buds. The SLN's *external branch* (external branch of the superior laryngeal nerve; EBSLN) brings branchial efferents to the cricothyroid muscle and inferior constrictor. As is described later, the internal branch of the SLN may also provide motor contributions to the posterior cricoarytenoid (PCA) muscle and intraarytenoid muscle, and the EBSLN may provide, at least in some patients, limited motor input to the thyroarytenoid muscle. The RLN contains branchial efferents to the inferior constrictor, cricopharyngeus, all laryngeal intrinsics except the cricothyroid muscle, general visceral afferents from the larynx (vocal cords and below), upper esophagus, and trachea.[45] RLN branches also convey sympathetic and parasympathetic branches to the lower pharynx, larynx, trachea, and upper esophagus. Apart from the larynx and pharynx, the vagus nerve provides afferent and parasympathetic innervation to the heart, esophagus, stomach, intestines, liver, spleen, and kidneys.

Cortical areas (including Broca's area, the motor cortex, and the anterior cingulum) that control laryngeal function project to brainstem nuclei bilaterally (primarily from the nucleus ambiguous).[46] The nucleus ambiguous projects to the ipsilateral portion of the larynx.[31,47] Gacek's work in the cat has identified laryngeal motor supply arising in the ipsilateral nucleus ambiguous with adductor function, primarily in the dorsal division of the nucleus and abductor neurons primarily in the ventral division. He identified a second source of laryngeal innervation in the retrofacial nucleus, from which neurons extend to the cricothyroid and PCA muscles with abductor fibers arising centrally and adductor fibers more peripherally.[31,48]

Please see the Expert Consult website for more discussion of this topic, including Figure 36.2.

Dionigi et al. have shown the vagus nerve is located directly posterior to the carotid artery and jugular vein in 73% of cases, lies directly posterior to the carotid artery in 15% of cases, lies directly posterior to the jugular vein in 8% of cases, and lies anterior to the carotid and jugular vein in the carotid sheath in 4% of cases.[50]

RLN Neural Anatomy

As the heart and great vessels descend during embryologic life, the RLN is dragged down by the lowest persisting aortic arch (see Chapter 2, Applied Embryology of the Thyroid and Parathyroid Glands). The right vagus runs from the posterior aspect of the jugular vein in the neck base to cross anterior to the first part of the subclavian artery. The RLN branches and courses up and behind the subclavian artery (fourth branchial arch) running medially along the pleura and cranially behind the common carotid artery into the right thoracic inlet in the base of the neck. The left vagus courses from the carotid sheath in the left neck base anterior to the aortic arch (sixth arch, ligamentum arteriosus). The RLN branch curves up under the aortic arch just lateral to the obliterated ductus arteriosus (Figure 36.3, *A*).

Because of its course around the right subclavian artery, the right RLN enters the neck base at the thoracic inlet more laterally compared with the left RLN[51] (see Figure 36.3, *A*). The right RLN then ascends the neck, enters the thoracic inlet, emerges from under the common carotid artery, tracks laterally to medially as it travels superiorly, and ultimately crosses the ITA. It assumes a paratracheal position in the last centimeter of its course as it approaches the lowest edge of the inferior

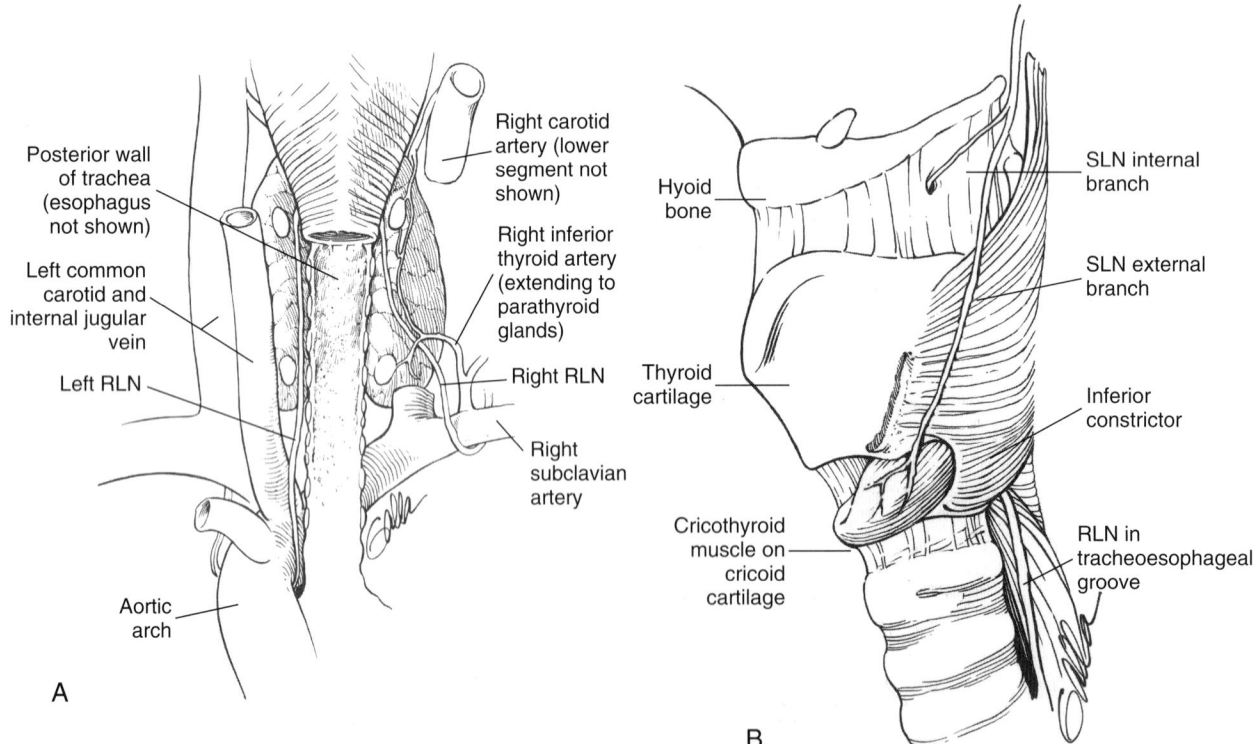

Fig. 36.3 A, Posterior view of recurrent laryngeal nerve course in the neck and upper chest. **B,** Side view of recurrent and superior laryngeal nerve innervation of the larynx.

constrictor. Shindo et al. found in their distal course both right and left RLNs typically form an angle of between 15 and 30 degrees relative to the trachea; they showed the right RLN as having a more oblique course in paratracheal region as compared with the more vertical/strictly tracheoesophageal groove course of the left RLN.[29]

At the lower edge of the cricoid cartilage posterolaterally, the RLN travels under the inferior-most fibers of the inferior constrictor (i.e., the cricopharyngeus muscle), extending deep to the inferior constrictor and up behind the cricothyroid articulation to enter the larynx. In approximately 30% of cases, the RLN actually penetrates the lowest fibers of the inferior constrictor on its way to the larynx[27] (see Figure 36.3, B). Incorrect descriptions of this anatomy exist, in which the RLN is described to pass deep to the cricothyroid, rather than the inferior constrictor muscle.[28,30] In this chapter, the point at which the RLN disappears under the lowest fibers of the inferior constrictor will be termed *the laryngeal entry point*; it marks the distal-most exposure of the RLN in the thyroid surgical field. For the last centimeter or so before laryngeal entry, the RLN travels close to the lateral border of the trachea.

The vagus diameter in its cervical course is approximately 4 mm with the epineurium and 3 mm without. The diameter decreases to approximately 2 mm after the RLN takeoff point.[32] The RLN diameter averages approximately 2 mm and ranges between 1 and 3 mm.[32,33] The average length of the vagus from the second cervical vertebra to the separation of the RLN (based on 30 dissections in 15 adult humans) is 11.5 cm on the right and 13.5 cm on the left. The length of the RLN from vagal takeoff to laryngeal entry point is 8.5 cm on the right and 10 cm on the left.[32] The different lengths result in discretely different latencies in the evoked EMG, and the specific latencies allow recognition of the corresponding nerve when electrically stimulated (discussed later).

Superior Laryngeal Nerve

The SLN arises immediately beneath the nodose ganglion of the upper vagus and descends medial to the carotid sheath. It divides into its internal and external branches about 2 or 3 cm above the superior pole of the thyroid, although this point may vary (see Chapter 35, Surgical Anatomy of the Superior Laryngeal Nerve). The internal branch travels medial to the carotid system and enters the posterior aspect of the thyrohyoid membrane, which provides sensation to the ipsilateral supraglottis and base of the tongue. The EBSLN descends to the region of the superior pole and extends medially along the inferior constrictor fascia to enter the cricothyroid muscle. As the EBSLN slopes downward on the inferior constrictor musculature, it has a close association with the superior thyroid pedicle.[34] Several practitioners have shown that in approximately 20% of cases, the EBSLN is closely associated with the superior thyroid vascular pedicle at the level of the capsule of the superior pole; this places it at risk during ligation of these superior pole vessels.[33-35] In approximately 20% of cases, the EBSLN runs subfascially on the inferior constrictor muscle and may not be directly visualized, yet it can be stimulated electrically.[34,35] Depending on the degree of superior pole development, the sternothyroid muscle may "hood" the superior pole region. Isolated sternothyroid division can help with exposure in this region. With EBSLN injury, there is a loss of vocal cord tensing, which is manifested by increased vocal tiredness and a loss of higher registers. Postoperative examinations after unilateral external branch injury are subtle and controversial, but they are generally believed to include a bowed and somewhat lower cord and a larynx rotated to the affected side. Such an injury ended the operatic career of Amelita Galli-Curci; however, there is intrigue regarding the veracity of this claim (see the "SLN Monitoring" section presented later in the chapter and also Chapter 35, Surgical Anatomy of the Superior Laryngeal Nerve).

Microanatomy of the RLN

Please see the Expert Consult website for discussion of this topic.

At the laryngeal entry point in the RLN, the adductor and abductor fibers lack spatial segregation; they are diffusely distributed throughout the entire nerve.[31,48,54] The RLN contains two to four times as many adductor fibers as abductor fibers.[31,48,56]

VISUAL APPEARANCE

The RLN is white and approximately 2 mm wide. Although it generally follows a linear course, it can have a somewhat curved profile and be similar in appearance to the spinal accessory nerve in surgery of the lateral portion of the neck. Virtually always, the normal RLN has a vessel running on its surface (vasa nervosum), which can be seen as a ventral "red strip." This may be less apparent if the nerve has been attenuated over time, as in massive goiter or if the nerve is placed on stretch. All that visually appears to be the RLN may not be. Electrical confirmation complements the visual impression and avoids visual false-positives. Raffaelli and colleagues noted that sympathetic chain branches to the distal RLN branch can be large enough to mimic a nonrecurrent nerve.[57] They also describe rare, medially directed branches of the sympathetic system that can mimic the normal RLN. They have found at least one such case, in which the nerve that "perfectly mimicked the RLN, when dissected fully, originated from the sympathetic stellate ganglion, not the vagus."[57] Sympathetic nerve branches, when stimulated, should not yield laryngeal EMG activity; thus functional information provided by RLN monitoring aids in distinguishing such nerves. The RLN is amendable to surgical dissection without injury. Chiang et al. have shown that RLNs that require extensive dissection of >5 cm in the setting of goiter did not have higher rates of paralysis than nerves requiring less dissection.[58]

Nonrecurrent RLN

The right nonrecurrent RLN (NRLN) occurs in 0.5% to 1% of cases and is associated with a right subclavian artery takeoff from the distal aortic arch.[59] The right subclavian artery in these cases follows a retroesophageal course to the right or, less commonly, between the esophagus and the trachea.[59] The left NRLN is extremely rare, with only 0.04% cases reported in the literature; it is associated with situs invertus.[59] Henry found that the symptoms of dysphagia secondary to subclavian interaction with the esophagus (dysphagia lusoria) were not consistently present in cases of right NRLN. When dysphagia is present, dysphagia lusoria is difficult to separate from dysphagia referable to a pathologic condition of the thyroid.

Please see the Expert Consult website for more discussion of this topic.

Several preoperative imaging such as barium swallow, ultrasonography, computed tomography (CT), magnetic resonance imaging (MRI), and angiography are employed and shown to provide successful identification of associated vascular anomaly and hence the NRLN.[59,61,62] However, preoperative identification of NRLN may be difficult, especially when limited preoperative imaging is performed before thyroid surgery. NRLN has no functional implications, but it is prone to intraoperative injury due to abnormal anatomy. A study of 31 patients at-risk of NRLN demonstrated a 12.9% paralysis rate.[63] Recently, an intraoperative electrophysiological and anatomic algorithm has been shown to reliably identify NRLN before dissection in the related area[64] (discussed later under RLN monitoring section). The NRLN derives from the vagus as a direct medial branch in the neck and extends generally with a downward looping course from behind the carotid artery to the laryngeal entry point; however, it can follow more horizontal or ascending paths.[57,59,65,66]

Please see the Expert Consult website for more discussion of this topic, including Figures 36.4 and 36.5.

RLN Displacement

RLN position may be significantly abnormal in the setting of goitrous change, especially when substernal or retrotracheal extension exists. RLN position and identification may also be more difficult if significant paratracheal RLN chain nodal disease exists. The nerve in the setting of goitrous change can be displaced in any direction and may even come to lie ventral to the inferior pole. Importantly, goitrous enlargement can be associated with fixation and splaying of the RLN to the undersurface of the enlarged thyroid lobe. In such cases, routine identification of the RLN in the thoracic inlet is prohibited because of the size of the goiter. Recommendations have been made that blunt dissection will allow delivery of the goiter from the wound or the substernal goiter into the neck without RLN identification. In our study of large cervical and substernal goiters, 16% were associated with abnormally positioned RLNs, which were either fixed to the undersurface of the goiter or splayed significantly over the surface of the goiter.[74] Left and right lobes were equally affected. In 184 cases not involving goiter, we did not find any nerves that were fixed or splayed except in the presence of invasive malignancy. We noted that fixation and splaying of the RLN occurred more frequently in larger goiters and goiters with substernal extension, with tracheal compression evident on preoperative CT scan, and in goiters with intubation difficulties. Sinclair reported a 17.5% rate of postoperative RLN paralysis in patients with retrosternal goiter in whom the RLN was not specifically identified during blind digital goiter delivery. Sinclair reported several cases in which the nerve was associated with the thyroid gland and was thus at serious risk when the retrosternal mass was mobilized into the neck (a maneuver usually achieved by dislocating the mass with a finger from below and behind). We believe that this hazard must be recognized by all thyroid surgeons and that every strand of tissue stretched over the retrosternal component of the goiter should be presumed to be nerve until anatomically proven otherwise.[75]

Lahey, in 1938, recommended RLN identification "even in deep intrathoracic goiter extending nearly to the diaphragm."[76] We believe that because of the possibility of nerve fixation and splaying on the undersurface of a goiter, blunt dissection without nerve identification risks stretch injury. Identification of the RLN in such cases is a necessary initial step. The nerve that is fixed to or splayed on the undersurface of the goiter should be dissected off before the gland is delivered. The nerve can be identified through a superior approach (discussed later) and can be dissected retrograde off the goiter before digital delivery of the goiter. After goiter resection, the nerve so dissected can appear to be significantly redundant, but it will stimulate normally and function postoperatively despite the intraoperative appearance of laxity. We have noted that goiters associated with retrotracheal extension as identified by preoperative CT scanning may be associated with RLN displacement to the ventral surface of the goiter. This is a disorienting position and places the nerve at extreme risk, even in experienced hands. Therefore analysis of preoperative CT scanning in patients with retrotracheal goiter may empower the surgeon to have low suspicion for such ventral RLN displacement (see Chapter 6, Surgery of Cervical and Substernal Goiter).

Tubercle of Zuckerkandl

Aside from thyroid tissue that may actually infuse the ligament of Berry (LOB; see the discussion of the LOB presented later in the chapter), surface nodules and lobulation of the thyroid gland near the ligament may make distal RLN dissection more difficult. The tubercle of Zuckerkandl (TOZ) is a lobule of thyroid tissue, which, if present, typically occurs just caudal to the LOB at the posterolateral margin of the thyroid lobe. The tubercle was described by Zuckerkandl in 1904 as the "processus posterior glandulae"[28,77] and by Madelung in 1867 as the "posterior horn of the thyroid"[78] (see Chapter 2, Applied Embryology of the Thyroid and Parathyroid Glands, Figures 2.2 and 2.3, D).

The adult orthotopic thyroid is derived from the fusion of medial and lateral elements (see Chapter 2, Applied Embryology of the Thyroid and Parathyroid Glands).

Please see the Expert Consult website for more discussion of this topic.

When thyroid tissue is present as a posterior lateral projection of the lateral thyroid lobe, it can be termed the TOZ, and it is believed to represent the point of fusion between the lateral anlage and the medial thyroid elements; its association with the RLN and upper parathyroid glands (PIV) are of special surgical importance.

When present in its typical position, the tubercle is caudal to the LOB. The tubercle points to the nerve as the nerve interacts with the LOB and laryngeal entry point. The nerve is typically deep to the tubercle and may be entrapped in a cleft between the tubercle's deep surface and the adjacent deep surface of the thyroid lobe (Chapter 2, Applied Embryology of the Thyroid and Parathyroid Glands, Figures 2.2 and 2.3, D). The nerve is said to be in this deep position relative to the TOZ in 93% of cases, but in the remaining 7% of cases the nerve may ride ventral to the tubercle and thus be in an extremely vulnerable position at surgery.[78] Hisham reported that the RLN was located anterior to the tubercle in 6% of patients and felt this variation was more common in revision patients[26] (see Chapter 2, Applied Embryology of the Thyroid and Parathyroid Glands, Figures 2.2 and 2.3, D). When the tubercle is extending dorsally and the nerve is brought ventrally, the TOZ is felt to be the initial manifestation of what would be in the neck: a retrotracheal goiter and a posterior mediastinal goiter (in the mediastinum); both of these are associated with such high-risk "ventral" RLNs (see Figure 6.7, B in Chapter 6, Surgery of Cervical and Substernal Goiter). Even if the nerve is in its more typical position (deep to the TOZ), it may be relatively entrapped in the cleft between the TOZ and adjacent thyroid; it may be stretched, as the TOZ is serially dissected and retracted to expose the RLN.

Please see the Expert Consult website for more discussion of this topic.

A TOZ grading scheme has been offered: grade 1 (less than 5 mm), grade 2 (between 5 and 10 mm), and grade 3 (greater than 1 cm).[81] Significant TOZ (i.e., grade 3) is felt to be present in 14% to 61% of patients and seems to vary in its prevalence in relation to country of origin. One study has shown that significant TOZ may be more common on the right side than on the left side (69.6% versus 53.2% respectively).[78,82,83] Of course, as thyroid tissue, the TOZ is subject to any benign or malignant process. This variability in existence of the tubercle from patient to patient has hindered this as being a reliable landmark for nerve identification (see Chapter 2, Applied Embryology of the Thyroid and Parathyroid Glands, Figures 2.2 and 2.3, D).[84]

Extralaryngeal RLN Branching

Various surgical and cadaver dissection series show the RLN branches before the laryngeal entry point in from 30% to 78% of cases.[69,70,85-88] These studies do not usually distinguish between the small branches arising from the RLN and extending to the adjacent trachea (sensory), esophagus (sensory and motor), inferior constrictor (sensory and motor), and sympathetic chain, and the typically larger branches arising as a terminal division of the nerve destined to innervate laryngeal musculature. Of course, branches that contain laryngeal intrinsic motor fibers must together enter the larynx at the laryngeal entry point and not extend more ventrally or posteriorly, which implies their sensory or non-laryngeal motor nature. Obviously, only the branches extending to the laryngeal entry point will affect laryngeal motor function. Both the research of Serpell et al. and our own research has noted that 50% to 60% of patients have some small branches of the RLN to the trachea, esophagus, or inferior constrictor; however, only 20% to 30% have true RLN extralaryngeal branches that enter the larynx and with stimulation resulting in laryngeal EMG activity.[89,90] This is in agreement with the older work of Morrison (who noted true extralaryngeal branches in approximately one third of patients on at least one side)[91] as well as more recent studies.[90] Endotracheally based monitoring systems identify only thyroarytenoid depolarization, whereas assessment of laryngeal twitch or posterior laryngeal electrodes will inform regarding PCA depolarization. In our experience, the small RLN branches to the esophagus and inferior constrictor, when stimulated, usually result in local contraction of the associated esophageal or inferior constrictor musculature. With careful dissection, Brok found four or five branches of the RLN to the cricopharyngeus in nine of nine patients.[45]

Any true extralaryngeal RLN branches not recognized during surgery are at risk for injury. The total diameter of the normal RLN in the neck is only approximately 1 to 2 mm, so these branches are often less than 1 mm. Most laryngeal branches of the RLN arise from the distal RLN segment, with 90% of branching occurring above the intersection of the RLN and the ITA.[69] Reed found that only 5.4% of 506 dissected nerves branched at the level of the RLN and ITA crossing.[92] It is known that the distal-most RLN intralaryngeal branches are always given off by the time the RLN is above the cricothyroid joint.[43] Serpell's group has shown that the most common branch point occurred in the distal 2 cm course of the RLN measured from the bottom of the inferior constrictor and averaged approximately 18 mm with a range of 5 to 34.[89,90] True "extralaryngeal RLN branches" (i.e., major branches destined to enter the larynx) can be assumed to be analogous to intralaryngeal branches, except that they are premature and occur more proximally below the lower edge of the inferior constrictor. The lowest segment of the inferior constrictor is termed the *cricopharyngeus*.

Thus extralaryngeal nerve branches, when present, usually exist at the level of the LOB and are usually not present below the ITA. The lack of branches below the ITA is part of the rationale for the inferior approach to the RLN in the thoracic inlet (as described by Lore).[93] We have seen that RLN branching occurrence and pattern vary from side to side within the same patient; this observation is in agreement with the work of Morrison and Katz.[69,91] Katz noted, in a study of 1771 nerves, that if extralaryngeal branches occur on one side, 39% of patients will have branching on the opposite side.[68]

The most important message regarding patients with extra laryngeal branching, because of this increased anatomic complexity and narrow diameter of the branched RLN, is that they are at increased risk for both transient and permanent VCP. Sancho et al. suggested that branched nerves are twice as likely to have transient postoperative VCP (15.8%) than nonbranched nerves (8%).[94] Cassella's work also suggested an increased rate of paralysis in patients with branched RLN: about 7 to 12 times that of patients with unbranched RLNs.[95]

Functional Variability of RLN Branches: Abductor and Adductor Fibers

See Figure 36.6.

Please see the Expert Consult website for discussion of this topic, including discussion of Figure 36.6.

Galen's Anastomosis

See Figure 36.7.

Please see the Expert Consult website for discussion of this topic, including discussion of Figure 36.7.

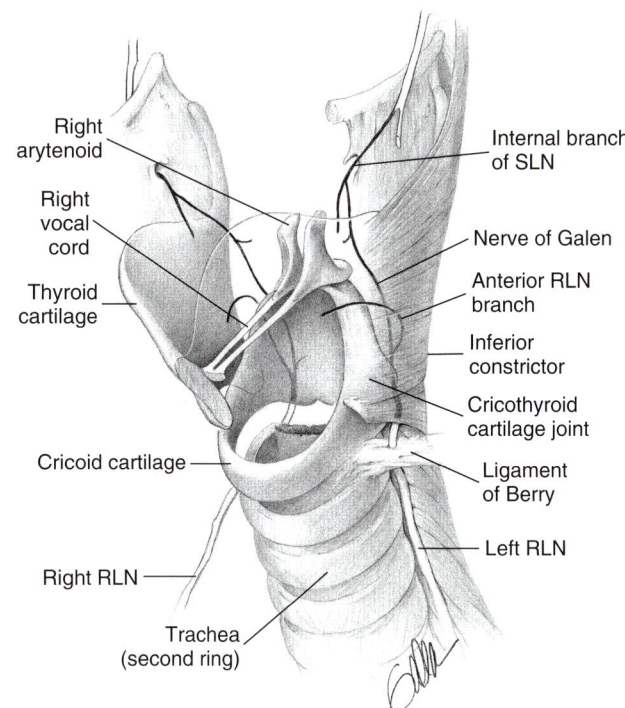

Fig. 36.6 Three-dimensional view of bilateral recurrent laryngeal nerve (RLN) entry into the larynx underneath the lower edge of the inferior constrictor, showing the anterior and posterior RLN branches within the larynx. The left thyroid lamina is not shown.

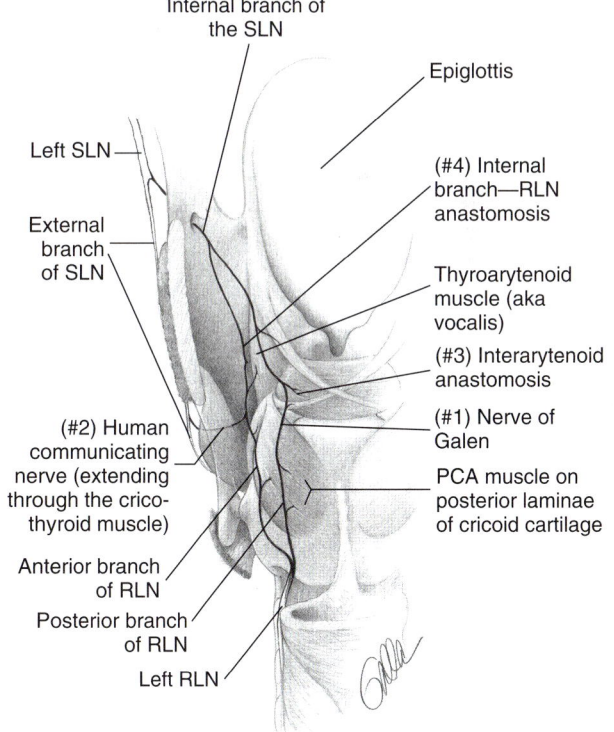

Fig. 36.7 Posterior view of the left hemilarynx, detailing four main anastomotic regions between the superior and recurrent laryngeal nerve (RLN) systems: (1) nerve of Galen, (2) human communicating nerve extending through cricothyroid muscle, (3) interarytenoid region anastomosis, and (4) superior laryngeal nerve (SLN) internal branch-RLN thyroarytenoid (TA) region anastomosis.

Adductor and Abductor Laryngeal Musculature: Stimulation Frequency and Glottic Function

 Please see the Expert Consult website for discussion of this topic.

RLN-SLN Connections: Significance During Thyroid Surgery

To appreciate fully the functional significance of extralaryngeal branching and to interpret intraoperative RLN monitoring information, the thyroid surgeon needs to understand not only the anatomy of the RLN and SLN systems but also their interconnections (see Figure 36.7 available on expertconsult.com). The SLN internal branch chiefly relates to the afferent innervation of the hypopharynx, base of tongue, supraglottis, and vocal cords. The SLN's external branch provides motor innervation to the cricothyroid muscle and sensory innervation to the anterior subglottis. It is believed that the afferent activity, important in regulating laryngeal protective mechanisms, resides primarily in the IBSLN.[121]

Connections between the RLN and SLN systems have been documented in a variety of dissection studies in 15% to 83% of cases.[49,122-124] Sato, in 201 dissections of 113 cadavers, found direct connection between the RLN and the IBSLN in 53.7% of cases.[125] Most have regarded these connections as primarily anastomotic connections between distal sensory branches of SLN and RLN, although some have speculated that these anastomotic links are associated with the possible motor complement within SLN branches. Dilworth noted that anastomotic interconnections between vagal branches innervating a given organ are a pattern seen throughout the body.[126] Galen, and later Martin, believed that return of function (i.e., voice) that sometimes occurs after RLN transection resulted from regrowth from branches of the SLN.[127] More recently, practitioners have again suggested that one method of vocal cord recovery after RLN injury involves reinnervation through supplemental motor branches of the SLN.[127] Functionally important connections between the SLN and RLN systems can be divided into four groups (see Figure 36.7 available on expertconsult.com): I. Galen's anastomosis, II. SLN external branch/distal RLN anastomosis (human communicating nerve), III. interarytenoid anastomosis, and IV. SLN internal branch—RLN TA region anastomosis.

I. Galen's Anastomosis

 Please see the Expert Consult website for discussion of this topic.

II. SLN's External Branch-Distal RLN Anastomosis (the "Human Communicating Nerve")

 Please see the Expert Consult website for discussion of this topic.

III. Interarytenoid Muscle Plexus

 Please see the Expert Consult website for discussion of this topic.

IV. SLN Internal Branch—RLN Thyroarytenoid Region Anastomosis

 Please see the Expert Consult website for discussion of this topic.

RLN and Inferior Thyroid Artery

The ITA derives as an upwardly directed branch of the thyrocervical trunk and extends under the carotid artery into the central neck. It loops downward more medially, extending to the thyroid at the midpolar level (not at the level of the inferior pole, as its name would imply). The RLN and the ITA have a variable relationship. The RLN may be deep, superficial, or may ramify branches of the artery. The basic relationship, however, is that the artery and nerve intersect. Hollingshead found that the RLN is deep to the ITA in about 50% of cases, runs between the branches of ITA in 25% of cases, and runs anterior to the ITA in 25% of cases.[145] Reed found 28 different RLN ITA patterns and noted bilateral symmetry to this pattern in only 17% of patients.[92] Sturniolo et al. noted that of 192 patients, in which 48.8% were undergoing bilateral surgery; the relationship of the RLN and ITA varied from side to side.[146] Sato and Shimada found that 8% of cadaveric RLNs ran parallel to the ITA rather than crossing.[103] Hollingshead noted that the division of the ITA into superior and inferior branches may occur quite laterally, even behind the carotid artery. Hollingshead also stated that the ITA may be absent in 0.2% to 5.9% of cases.[145] The superior thyroid artery or the thyroid ima assumes the vascular distribution of the ITA in these circumstances.[147] The RLN itself is vascularized by a posterior branch of the ITA that travels the distal course of the RLN.[147] We believe that the highly variable patterns of nerve-artery crossing, the varying course of the ITA, and the potential for its absence and parallel course to the RLN make it a poor landmark for routine RLN identification.

Ligament of Berry

The fibrous LOB anchors the thyroid to the laryngotracheal complex (Figure 36.8, A). Also described as the posterior suspensory ligament of the thyroid, the ligament was described by Gruber and also Henle in 1880 as well as James Berry in 1888. The ligament's tethering of the thyroid to the airway is responsible for the elevation of the thyroid with the larynx with deglutition. In 1888, Berry wrote the following:

> I have noticed in operations of this kind, which I have seen performed by others upon the living, and in a number of excisions, which I have myself performed on the dead body, that most of the difficulty in the separation of the tumor has occurred in the region of these ligaments. ... This difficulty, I believe, to be a very frequent source of that accident which so commonly occurs in the removal of goiter, I mean division of the recurrent laryngeal nerve.[148]

Berlin's superb work describing the relationship of the RLN to the LOB, which he described as the "adherent zone," was published in 1935.[123] The LOB can be regarded as a condensation of the thyroid capsule, which arises from: the posterolateral aspect of the cricoid and the first, second, and, occasionally, third tracheal rings; the LOB extends to the corresponding deep surface of the medial aspect of the bilateral thyroid lobes.[123,149] Sasou has measured the ligament as having a length of 11.5 mm (range: 8 to 14 mm) and a width of 4.4 mm (range: 2 to 7 mm).[149] The LOB is separate and distinct from the significantly less robust anterior suspensory ligament, which arises from the midline and paramidline upper cervical trachea to extend to the corresponding deep surface of the thyroid isthmus. The LOB is both dense and well vascularized and derives a branch along its inferior edge from the ITA. This artery is well known to thyroid surgeons and can result in troublesome hemorrhage during the final phase of dissection. The ligament can be very closely associated with adjacent thyroid tissue that, to a varying degree, can infuse the substance of the LOB and, in so doing, approximate the RLN (see Figure 36.8, A and B). Berlin, in 1935, reviewed the relationship between the RLN, the LOB, and adjacent thyroid tissue. He performed 140 cadaver dissections and 72 surgical dissections. Despite the classic description of the RLN's crossing deep to the LOB, Berlin found that in 30% of cases, the RLN coursed through the ligament itself.[150] Lore also has described cases of the RLN's traveling through leaflets of the ligament rather than posterior to the ligament.[93] In cadaveric dissections, Berlin (in 10% of cases) and Armstrong (in 15% of cases) noted that the RLN penetrated the thyroid gland.[88,123] This work is supported by the more recent work of Wafae, who found that the thyroid gland involved the RLN at the LOB in 38% of cadaveric dissections.[27] Anatomically, the LOB is believed to represent a condensation of

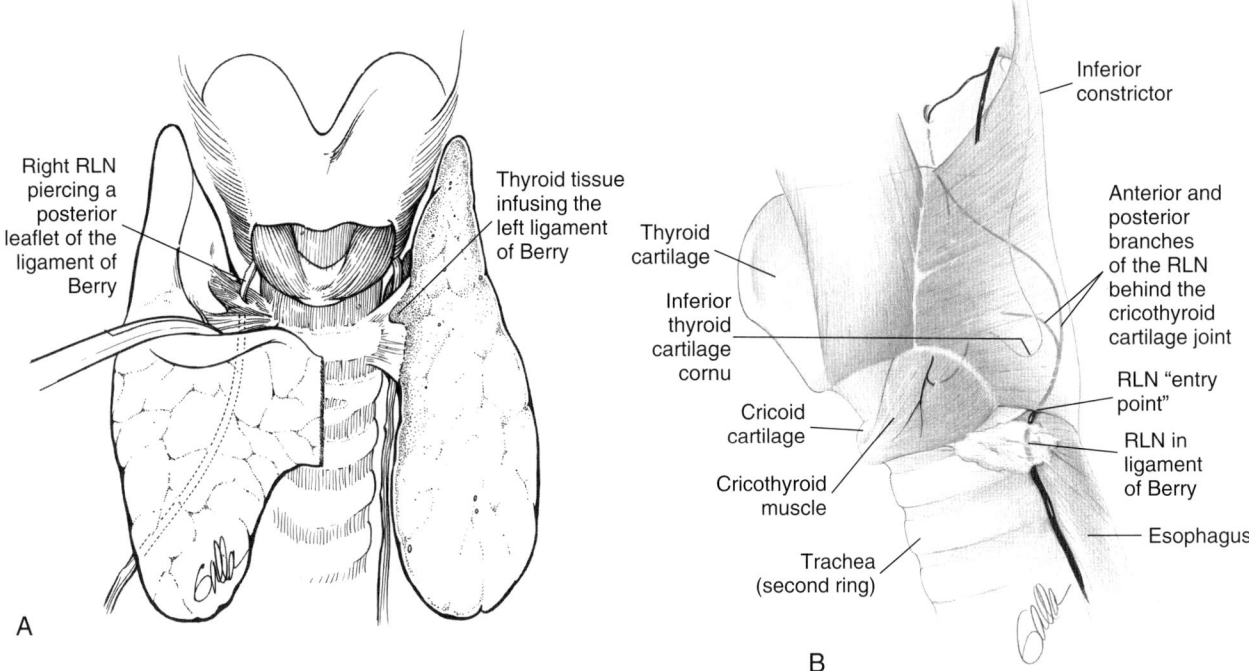

Fig. 36.8 **A,** Anterior view of the thyroid and airway, detailing anterior and posterior leaflets of the ligament of Berry. On patient's right, the nerve is piercing through the posterior leaflet of the ligament of Berry. On the left, there is potential for thyroid tissue infusion within the substance of the ligament, bringing thyroid tissue adjacent to the nerve within the ligament of Berry in some patients. **B,** Side view of the larynx, showing the ligament of Berry and laryngeal entry point relative to palpable landmark of inferior thyroid cartilage cornu.

perithyroid sheath, not true thyroid capsule; the true capsule in this region blends with the adjacent tissue of the LOB. The thyroid tissue that infuses the ligament is the most common site where thyroid tissue is left behind inadvertently after "total thyroidectomy." Occasionally, the tissue is seen in the thyroid bed as a small, round profile of thyroid tissue approximating the transected edge of the LOB and may result in thyroid bed uptake postoperatively.

This set of anatomic concerns prohibits capsular dissection as a method to prevent RLN injury. Despite this anatomic reality, some still think that blind capsular dissection is sufficient to avoid RLN injury.

There is debate in the literature as to the exact relationship of the ligament and the RLN. Certainly, all agree the RLN is generally posterolateral to the ligament, but some argue that the RLN may penetrate the ligament in from 0.6% to 10%,[51,123,151] whereas others feel the nerve virtually never penetrates and is always posterolateral.[26,149]

In its distal course, the RLN can also have a bend or genu just before entering the larynx.[152] Within the LOB, we estimate that this occurs in 1% to 2% of cases and requires extreme vigilance and good exposure as the nerve is dissected through the ligament. The dense and vascular nature of the LOB, the multiple branches of the RLN that can be present at this level, the potential for a bend or genu of the nerve at its laryngeal entry point, and the close relationship of thyroid tissue to the LOB all make this area the most difficult region of nerve dissection during thyroidectomy. Slow, meticulous dissection is required. Minimal oozing is best controlled with several moments of gentle pressure with a neurosurgical pledget. Bipolar cautery with full exposure of the nerve is useful. It is recommended that the course of the nerve should be followed throughout the LOB as one would follow the facial nerve through the parotid gland during parotidectomy, rather than following the thyroid capsule. Indiscriminate clamping and cautery will likely result in nerve injury (Figure 36.9, A and B).

Inferior Thyroid Cartilage Cornu: Landmark for the RLN Laryngeal Entry Point

The laryngeal entry point represents the most constant position of the RLN in the neck. Regardless of goitrous displacement or nonrecurrence of the RLN, it is here where the nerve can be always found. Finding the nerve at the laryngeal entry point can be difficult despite its anatomic constancy because of the adjacent tough, fibrous, and well-vascularized LOB. The nerve may be behind or within the ligament and may have thyroid tissue very closely associated with it in this region. A consistent landmark indicating the laryngeal entry point is the inferior cornu of the thyroid cartilage, as described initially by Berlin (1935) and subsequently by Rustad (1952), Riddell (1970), and Wang (1975).[38,86,150,153] The RLN's laryngeal entry point is approximately 1 cm below caudal to the thyroid cartilage's inferior horn, which can be easily palpated (see Figure 36.8, B).[154]

We suggest that, rather than palpating for what can be a variable tubercle of the thyroid cartilage, the cricoid represents an excellent landmark for RLN identification during thyroid surgery. The anterior arch of the cricoid is a clear landmark available during thyroidectomy and marks the lower edge of the cricoid cartilage. Directly lateral is the RLN laryngeal entry point, reliably.

SURGICAL APPROACHES TO THE RLN

"It is a fundamental surgical principle that to avoid damaging any vital structures at operation, that structure must be clearly identified by the surgeon. The RLN at thyroidectomy is no exception…There should be few, if any, instances in which the RLN cannot be identified."

Wheeler, 1999

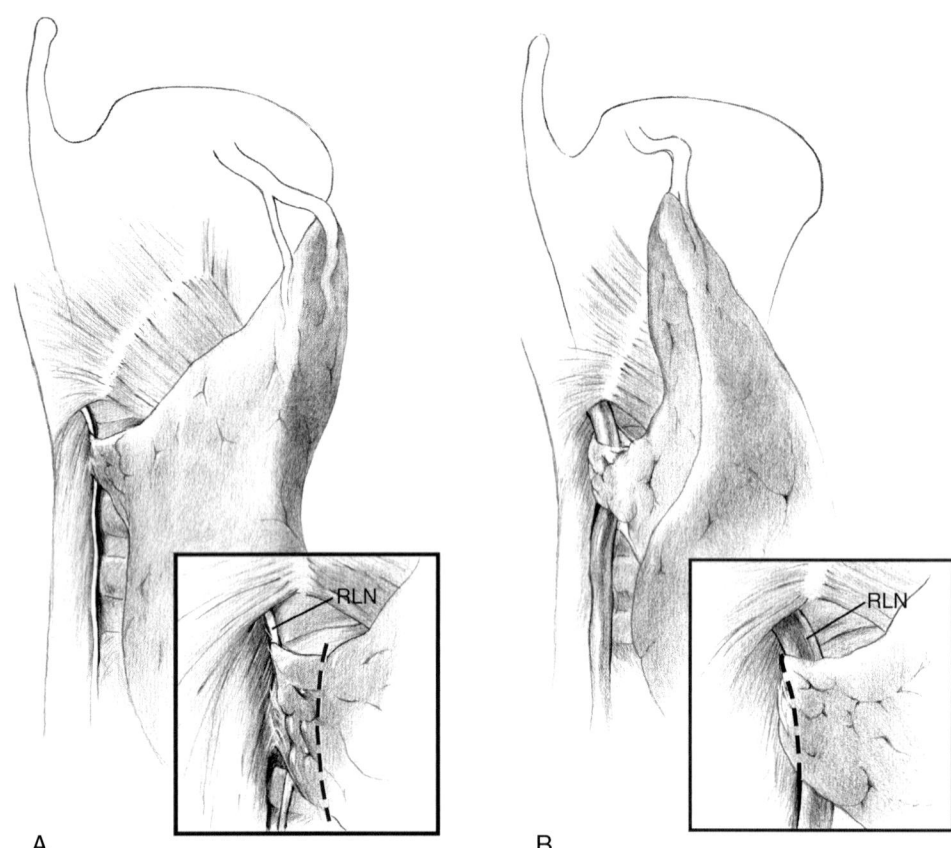

Fig. 36.9 A, If a nerve is identified as of reduced caliber, especially if its dissection has lifted it off its surgical bed, stretch is likely to occur with significant ligament of Berry dissection, so maintaining an anodular small remnant of thyroid tissue here would be suggested. **B,** If a nerve is thick and cordlike, resting stably on its surgical bed, it would likely withstand more aggressive dissection implicit in complete thyroid tissue resection at the level of the ligament of Berry.

"It is an axiom in thyroid surgery that an RLN seen is injured"
Prioleau, 1933

We agree with Dr. Wheeler. Despite the many studies that show a lower rate of injury when the RLN is identified (discussed earlier), some have still recommended blind capsular dissection without RLN exposure.[28, 155] The work of Berlin and Wafae has shown, as discussed previously, the potential for thyroid tissue to partially or completely surround the RLN at the LOB.[27,150] This and the close relationship of the RLN with thyroid surface nodularity make capsular dissection as the sole method of RLN preservation flawed.

Despite intentions of finding the RLN, some surgeons have difficulty. In a report of 192 patients in which a "systematic intraoperative search" was made for the RLN, in nearly 18% of the cases, the RLN could not be found on either side. In the reoperative subgroup, the nerve could not be localized in 42% of cases. These practitioners noted that the RLN was "extremely varying [in] conformation…without… any constant relationship between the nerve and anatomical structures of the ITA, the tracheoesophageal furrow and the thyroid lobes."[146] With this in mind, three approaches can be used routinely for systematic search and identification of the RLN.

General Identification Principles

The most important rule to follow is that no structure is transected until the RLN is identified visually and electrically. If this single rule is strictly adhered to, then RLN injury and transection injury will be rare. To identify the RLN, a bloodless field is essential. The RLN is identified in its characteristic location with a wavelike profile and a characteristic vascular strip. In cases of goitrous enlargement of the gland, the strap muscles can be retracted, but they should be cut without hesitation if additional exposure is needed. As the strap muscles are retracted laterally, the thyroid and laryngotracheal complex should be retracted as one unit medially to open up the lateral thyroid region. Excessive retraction on the thyroid can lead to nerve traction injury, which has been clearly shown to occur through anterior vertebral column neurosurgical procedures.[156]

The distal course of the RLN may extend ventrally and follow a course along the upper cervical trachea obliquely upward out of the tracheoesophageal groove. As the thyroid is dissected and freed from its cervical attachments, it is progressively pulled medially and the airway, to some degree, is displaced upward and rotated through this retraction (Figure 36.10). This distal upward course of the RLN may become accentuated through these maneuvers; it may become vulnerable to injury, especially during subtotal lobectomy, which may not involve visualization of the last centimeter or so of the RLN's course.[51,157] A nerve in this circumstance may be injured through placement of clamps or suturing of the thyroid remnant.

Palpation of the nerve has been recommended as a technique for nerve identification. One method involves upward retraction of the partially mobilized thyroid lobe and palpation or "plucking" of the nerve, thereby allowing identification.[158] Proponents believe that the thyroid retraction stretches the ITA and that this, in turn, brings

CHAPTER 36 Surgical Anatomy and Monitoring of the Recurrent Laryngeal Nerve

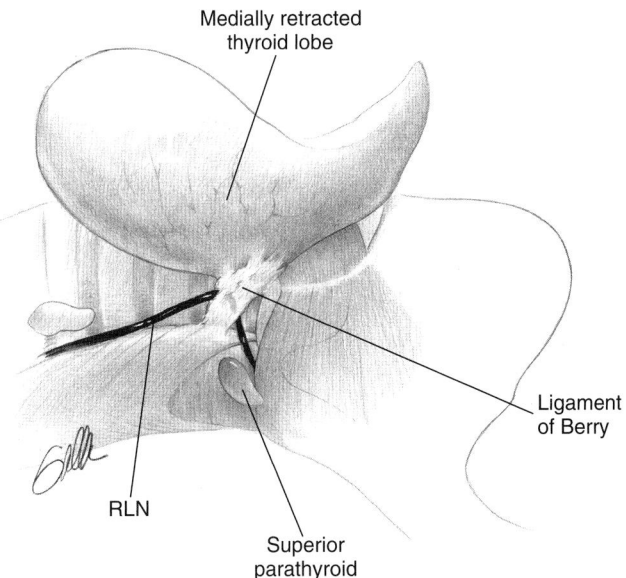

Fig. 36.10 Side view of the thyroid and larynx, demonstrating that thyroid retraction in some circumstances can bring the distal-most course of the recurrent laryngeal nerve quite ventral in the neck, potentially placing it at risk.

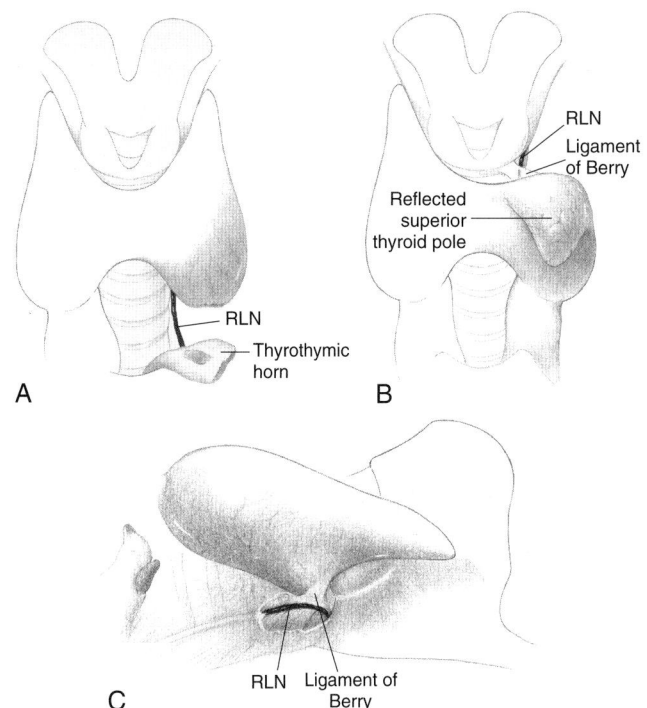

Fig. 36.11 Approaches to the recurrent laryngeal nerve. **A,** Inferior approach. **B,** Superior approach. **C,** Lateral approach.

the RLN upward and into more of a ventral relationship. We believe that this technique may, in some cases, results in traction injury of the nerve; we have not had occasion to use it.

Once total lobectomy is complete, blood often oozes from the LOB area. To control bleeding, patience is recommended, rather than indiscriminate cautery or clamping. Use of a neurosurgical pledget to brush the area may allow full view of the RLN and the bleeding sites. Careful discrete bipolar cautery or specific clamping of the identified small bleeder is the best. Minimal oozing can be controlled with epinephrine soaked neurosurgical pledgets.

Lateral Approach

With an understanding that the RLN must be identified during thyroidectomy, we can divide its approach into three types (Figure 36.11 and Table 36.1). The first, the lateral approach, involves the identification of the RLN relatively high in the neck at the midpolar level. In the lateral approach to the RLN, the inferior and superior poles are initially dissected, and the entire lobe is subsequently retracted medially over the larynx and trachea. The medial traction of the thyroid and airway, along with lateral traction of the strap muscles, allows for wide exposure of the lateral thyroid region. The middle thyroid vein is divided to completely open this region. To fully retract the lobe medially, it is best to first dissect the inferior parathyroid off the inferior pole. In this lateral approach, the nerve is not uncovered inferiorly at the thoracic inlet. This helps to preserve parathyroid vascular supply, especially for the inferior parathyroid. Also, identification of the RLN higher in the neck through this lateral approach allows for a more limited segment of RLN dissection. Various landmarks during the lateral approach to the RLN can be used, including the inferior edge of the thyroid cartilage's inferior cornu and the RLN-ITA crossing.[150,159,160]

The lateral approach is ideal for routine thyroidectomy. In certain cases of goiter or in cases in which the TOZ is well developed, this area may not be adequately exposed to permit easy RLN identification. Also, this area tends to be obscured by dense scar in revision thyroidectomy. In such circumstances, the nerve is best identified inferiorly away from the region of previous dissection. Another disadvantage of the lateral approach is that at this relatively high level above its ITA crossing, the RLN may have extralaryngeal branches. Care must also be taken on the right side during the lateral approach to the nerve for a right NRLN, which will be traveling more or less at 90 degrees from the expected course of a normal RLN. This lateral approach for initial thyroidectomy is not the same as the so-called backdoor approach for revision thyroid and parathyroid surgery (see Chapter 9, Reoperation for Benign Disease; Chapter 50, Reoperative Thyroid Surgery; and Chapter 63, Reoperation for Sporadic Primary Hyperparathyroidism).[36]

Inferior Approach

The inferior approach, as introduced by Sedgwick and described by Lore (see Figure 36.11, *A*, and Table 36.1), involves identification of the RLN at the thoracic inlet/neck base, using the RLN triangle.[93,161,162] The RLN triangle, as described by Lore, has its apex inferiorly, in the thoracic inlet. The medial wall is formed by the trachea, the lateral wall by the medial edge of the retracted strap muscles, and the superior base by the lower edge of the inferior pole of the retracted thyroid gland.[93,161] The surgeon searches for the nerve in the lateral aspect of the thoracic inlet on the right and in the paratracheal position at the thoracic inlet on the left. Advantages of nerve identification here include the soft areolar bed in which the nerve lies in this region, which allows for atraumatic dissection. Unlike the fibrous LOB superiorly, here, the RLN would simply move away without injury if contacted by a dissecting hemostat during reasonably gentle spreading of soft tissue along a path adjacent to the nerve. Another advantage of finding the nerve in the thoracic inlet is that the nerve exists as a single trunk before extralaryngeal branching, which mainly occurs above the ITA crossing point.

This approach is especially suited for revision thyroidectomy, where the RLN can be initially identified and dissected inferior to the previous surgery's scar. It is also suited for large cervical goiters that preclude the lateral approach. Disadvantages of the inferior approach include the long segment of nerve that is dissected, the potential for parathyroid

TABLE 36.1 Approach to Recurrent Laryngeal Nerve (RLN) during Thyroid or Parathyroid Surgery

	When to Use	Advantages	Disadvantages
Lateral Approach Find RLN laterally at midpolar level with medial thyroid lobe retraction	Routine cases	Protects parathyroid vascular supply, especially inferior parathyroid; limits length of RLN dissection	Not available in some cases of large thyroid masses or scarring from previous surgery; extralaryngeal branches may occur at this level; nonrecurrence on the right must be considered with this approach
Inferior Approach RLN is identified at thoracic inlet in lateral thoracic inlet on the right and in the paratracheal thoracic inlet on the left	Revision or large cervical goiters	RLN is found in a loose areolar bed and usually exists as a single trunk before nerve branching; nerve can be found outside of previous surgery scarring; good for large cervical goiter for which lateral approach may not be possible	Long segment of RLN is dissected and may be associated with inferior parathyroid gland devascularization; must consider nonrecurrence on the right
Superior Approach RLN found at laryngeal entry point/ligament of Berry region	Large cervical or substernal goiters; when considering a nonrecurrent nerve; when other approaches fail	RLN most constant point in the neck; suited for large cervical and substernal goiters for which the nerve cannot be found inferiorly or laterally; inferior cornu of thyroid cartilage can be palpated to approximate location of nerve in this region	Ligament of Berry is fibrous and bleeds easily; superior pole must be taken down first so external branch and superior parathyroid should be reflected; technically more challenging with large superior pole and requires avoidance of the external branch of the superior laryngeal nerve

devascularization (especially inferior), and the lack of suitability for a right NRLN. Also, the inferior approach is not available with large substernal goiters.

Superior Approach

In the superior approach, the RLN is first identified at the LOB-laryngeal entry point (see Figure 36.11, *B*, and Table 36.1). Implicit with this approach is the initial dissection and lateral-caudal retraction of the superior pole to allow access to this segment of the nerve during the initial phases of lobectomy. The laryngeal entry point represents the most constant site in terms of RLN anatomy within the neck. The approach is ideal for large cervical or substernal goiters when their size and position make the lateral or inferior approach impractical. The nerve can be found after superior pole reflection within or deep to the LOB; it extends under the lower edge of the inferior constrictor. The inferior cornu of the thyroid cartilage can be palpated to assist in nerve location in this area.[150]

The disadvantage of the RLN identification through the superior approach is that the dissection occurs at the LOB, which is fibrous and bleeds easily. Also, the nerve at this region may be branched. Nerve stimulation can be very rewarding as the dissection proceeds in this relatively inhospitable segment. Minor bleeders often respond to brief tamponade with a pledget rather than indiscriminate cautery or clamping. The potential existence of a low-riding EBSLN, which can often be present with goitrous enlargement of the thyroid, makes this dissection additionally challenging. Because the superior pole must be dissected first with this approach, the surgeon must take care to avoid injury to the external branch. Moreover, he or she must avoid devascularization of the superior parathyroid gland, which can often receive vascular input from the superior thyroid artery. This approach is technically more challenging with large superior poles. The exposure of this superior pole region is dramatically increased by selective section of the upper (i.e., laryngeal) head of the sternothyroid muscle.

RLN SURGICAL DISSECTION TIPS AND PITFALLS

Through experience with neural anatomy and intraoperative neural monitoring (IONM), we offer the following practical points to consider while performing RLN dissection during thyroidectomy:

1. The "don't see, don't cut rule." During thyroidectomy, never cut any band of tissue in the distribution of the RLN that is not transparent without neural stimulation. If the VN has been identified and positively stimulated, then a band of nontransparent tissue that does not give neural stimulation as the stimulator probe is dragged over it can be safely divided.
2. If the nerve and a parathyroid compete for your surgical attention, the nerve wins. During thyroid lobar dissection, occasionally RLN dissection becomes problematic as one discovers parathyroid tightly adherent to the thyroid capsule in the area of nerve dissection. Certainly, all attempts should be made to lift the parathyroid gland off the thyroid gland on an adequate pedicle and then to completely dissected nerve. However, if this is not possible, exposure for the nerve becomes the main concern. The parathyroid gland can be autotransplanted.
3. As one is performing pretracheal dissection, one must confine the dissection to the anterior face of the trachea. One must avoid the temptation to extend the dissection or cautery into the paratracheal region on the lateral surface of the trachea because the RLN can be drawn up into this area and injured, especially in the distal-most portion of the nerve's course. This is true, especially on the left side where the nerve is typically in the adjacent tracheoesophageal groove.
4. Vagal stimulation, first and last, is a must. Vagal stimulation is required at the beginning of surgery to provide a positive EMG signal so that neural mapping and search for the nerve can be achieved. It is only in the presence of an initial positive vagal stimulation at the initiation of surgery that one can rely on negative stimulation as one searches for the nerve through RLN

paratracheal neural mapping (see the Monitoring section presented later in the chapter). Vagal stimulation can also be performed at the end of surgery and can provide full and complete segmental testing of the vagus and RLN that have been operated on.

5. Watch the nerve as you retract. Care must be taken in the final stages of RLN dissection at the LOB. At this time, the thyroid lobe is more fully dissected and retracted, so one must be mindful of lobar retraction and the effect that this retraction has on the RLN. Posterior leaflets of the LOB can result in appropriate lobar retraction being conveyed to the nerve, which results in neurapraxic nerve injury. Similarly, as the lobe is retracted there may be a feeding artery that may lift up and bowstring the nerve. In both circumstances, appropriate lobar retraction may be conveyed directly to the nerve. Neurapraxic nerve injury may occur especially in the setting of the nerve of reduced caliber, which is lifted off its surgical bed. In such circumstances, it is appropriate to identify such a specific neural variant before LOB dissection. In certain circumstances (e.g., especially when thyroid tissue is closely adherent to the final segment of the nerve and especially if the nerve is of reduced caliber or has been thoroughly dissected and lifted off its bed), a small focus of a nodular thyroid tissue that is away from any cancer may be left at the nerve entry site (see Figure 36.9, A and B).

6. Ventral delivery is risky until you see the nerve at the LOB. Be cautious of precipitous ventral delivery of the thyroid gland, because this may precipitate neural stretch at the LOB, especially with a posterior leaflet of the LOB. Such delivery is characteristic of some types of minimally invasive thyroid surgeries, so the anatomy of the LOB should be understood before such delivery of the gland.

7. As the nerve is operated on through all stages of surgery, especially as one operates on the LOB, one must always keep the nerve under direct visual controls so the maneuvers next to the nerve do not tent up or stretch the nerve.

8. The anterior arch of the cricoid cartilage in the midline is a superb landmark during thyroid surgery. The RLN is at risk until it dives underneath the inferior constrictor muscle at the lower edge of the cricoid cartilage laterally. At this nerve entry site, the nerve leaves the thyroid surgical field.

9. After the completion of surgery, the nerve may be injured (e.g., by imprudent suction, the use of gauze, or with small rolled peanuts that are aggressively applied with an instrument). Fingertips are better than instruments.

10. Bipolar cautery should always be applied in areas near the nerve with extreme caution and for limited time periods. We favor a fine jeweler's tipped cautery used transiently.

11. During goiter surgery, especially substernal, the RLN is the focus of attention throughout the initial portion of the case. Once such a goiter is delivered at later stages of the case, less attention may be directed toward the distal-most course of the nerve, and it may be injured in this segment. One must keep in mind that such a nerve may be redundant, and care of the nerve needs to be continued until it enters the larynx at the lower edge of the lateral cricoid cartilage.

12. If the distal nerve looks thin, then go back down and redissect it to exclude branching. If the nerve was initially addressed with the lateral approach and is found to be of quite small diameter, go back and dissect nerve retrograde to make sure you are not finding the only one of the RLN's branches in the distal course of the nerve.

13. Beware that you are being misled by a large posterior branch and then injure the unidentified anterior branch as you manage the LOB. The anterior branch is typically the motor branch and may be of smaller caliber, more tubular, and more sinuous than the flatter and sometimes wider posterior sensory branch. Neural stimulation allows definitive differentiation.

14. The SLN may not always be visualized, but its presence should be routinely excluded both visually and electrically in all tissue bands taken at the superior pole with EMG monitoring and assessment of cricothyroid muscle twitch. Care must be taken in the dissection of the cricothyroid muscle, as it is a thin muscle with a minimal fascia overlying. Injudicious cautery on the ventral surface of the muscle can lead to substantial muscle injury and postoperative laryngeal dysfunction. The laryngeal head of sternothyroid muscle is an excellent landmark for the EBSLN because it tracks along its descending path on the lateral aspect of the inferior constrictor muscle along the lateral larynx.

RLN MONITORING

"I am convinced the best management of RLN injuries is of a preventative character."

Lahey, 1938

Cranial nerve monitoring has been applied to head and neck surgery, especially in otology and neurotology, where it has become the norm.[42] EMG monitoring during skull base facial nerve surgery has been shown to improve outcomes.[163]

Vagal and RLN monitoring have now gained wide acceptance. It is estimated that IONM is used in approximately 80% of thyroid surgeries performed by head and neck surgeons, and over 65% of such surgeries performed by general surgeons in the United States, and has increased significantly over the last 5 years.[163a] Use is associated with being exposed to IONM in training. A survey of recently trained endocrine and head and neck surgeons reveals that the vast majority (95%) of these surgeons commonly use IONM during thyroid surgery. IONM was more commonly used by higher-volume surgeons. Routine users were more likely to modify surgery based on nerve integrity (i.e., not complete a total thyroidectomy if the nerve loses conduction signal).[163b] This suggests that IONM currently represents a useful tool to those most surgically experienced, rather than a substitute for knowledge of anatomy and surgical skill (see the categories of benefit, discussed later).[164-166] RLN monitoring can be considered not only for thyroid and parathyroid surgery but also for other neck surgeries, including Zenker's diverticulum, carotid endarterectomy, surgery for laryngotracheal stenosis, anterior cervical approaches to the cervical spine, and certain skull base, cardiac, and upper chest procedures.[167] During intracranial, glossopharyngeal, and upper vagal rhizotomy for refractive glossopharyngeal neuralgia, vagal motor rootlets are at risk for VCP (up to a 20% incidence).[167a] The endotracheal tube-based RLN monitoring system has been used for these procedures. The glossopharyngeal and three most cephalic vagal rootlets (sensory) in which vagal motor fibers could not be detected by evoked EMG were lysed. Postoperatively, glossopharyngeal pain was resolved, and bilateral normal cord motor function was preserved.

We feel that the benefit of this additional information should be distributed to all patients. This also substantially facilitates familiarity by both surgery and anesthesia with monitoring equipment. Laryngeal examination and vagal stimulation are necessary and informative elements of RLN monitoring for full understanding of the RLN dissection. For each patient, therefore, the necessary information includes preoperative laryngeal examination (L1), intraoperative initial vagal stimulation (V1), intraoperative RLN initial stimulation (R1), final RLN stimulation (R2), final intraoperative vagal stimulation (V2), and postoperative laryngeal examination (L2). This strategy is summarized by the following: L1, R1, V1 to R2, V2, L2. We feel that knowing these perioperative data is essential for all patients.

Guidelines and Current Standards for IONM in Thyroid and Parathyroid Surgeries

To serve the emerging field of neurophysiologic monitoring of laryngeal nerves in head and neck endocrine surgery, the International Neural Monitoring Study Group (INMSG), a multidisciplinary collaborative group was founded in 2006. The group has published several guidelines to do the following: promote a uniform and standard IONM technique, define standardized references of normative and pathologic RLN neurophysiology parameters, evaluate new technological developments, and to support standardized educational and research activities in the field of IONM for head and neck surgeries. It has published guidelines on basic RLN and EBSLN monitoring techniques and interpretations for monitored thyroid and parathyroid surgery.[168,169]

More recently, INMSG has published, a two-part consensus guideline discussing nerve monitoring for thyroid and parathyroid surgeries with specific focus of its application on intraoperative strategy and disease management. Part I extensively discusses monitoring loss of signal (LOS) and its application for of staging bilateral thyroid surgery, and Part II discusses optimal RLN monitoring for invasive thyroid cancer.[170,171]

The guidelines and advances in monitoring devices as well as the extensive research on IONM in thyroid and other neck surgeries have encouraged increasing organizational support for IONM in neck endocrine surgeries. The American Academy of Otolaryngology and Head and Neck Surgery (AAOHNS) guidelines on improving voice outcomes after thyroid surgery has acknowledged that IONM, when applied to thyroid surgery, can (1) reduce RLN identification time, (2) decrease temporary VCP rates, and (3) avoid bilateral VCP (through prognostication of postoperative vocal cord function). These guidelines have suggested that IONM is useful for (1) bilateral thyroid surgery, (2) revision thyroid surgery, and (3) surgery in patients with known RLN paralysis.[172] The ATA has recognized the utility of IONM in its 2015 Guidelines for Thyroid Nodules and Well Differentiated Thyroid Cancer as well as in the ATA Surgical Affairs Committee consensus statements on outpatient thyroid surgery and on optimal surgical management of goiters.[173-175] Additionally, guideline statements from the American Head and Neck Society (AHNS) on recurrent thyroid carcinoma, central neck dissection, and invasive thyroid carcinoma recognize IONM as an important adjunct.[176-178]

Evidence Based Discussion on Effect of IONM on Rates of RLN Paralysis

The analysis of the literature to assess the effect of neuromonitoring on rate of postoperative VCP requires that we take following information into consideration: (1) the measured end points—transient and permanent RLN injury—fortunately have an extremely low incidence, but that also means that a very large sample size is required for a study to obtain an adequate statistical power. This is demonstrated by Dralle et al.; they report that an adequately powered study performed to obtain a statistically significant difference would need 9 million patients per arm for benign goiter surgery and 40,000 patients per arm for thyroid malignancy surgery;[18] (2) there is lack of uniformity of application of monitoring uniformly in available literature; (3) studies do not take into account several, hard to isolate confounding factors (e.g., the surgeon's expertise, variable familiarity with neural monitoring, use of audio-based systems with audio signal rather than raw EMG data, multiple surgeon participation, the nature of the disease, and the type and extent of the surgical procedure); (4) many studies have a higher frequency of monitoring in selective surgeries, such as preoperatively perceived difficult surgeries; and (5) there is a lack of uniformity in performing preoperative and postoperative laryngoscopy to document vocal cord status; thus the only documentable measure of vocal cord status is missing in many studies.

It is of note that in Germany, Dralle noted that in most centers, surgeons are not willing to randomize to a non IONM group.[179] Neural monitoring, once implemented, has been reported to result in drastic changes in the surgical technique employed by surgeons.[180]

Several studies (i.e., Higgins et al., Pisanu et al., and Lombardi et al.) are of interest; in their separate meta-analyses, these studies did not show notable statistical benefit, especially as it relates to permanent RLN injury rate, between IONM versus visual identification alone during thyroidectomy.[181-183] However, they advised researchers to interpret these results with caution because they were largely based on nonrandomized observational studies. They note that multicenter, prospective, randomized trials based on strict criteria of standardization that are followed by clustered meta-analyses are required to make accurate inferences. Importantly, several studies have demonstrated benefit of IONM in specific high-risk thyroid surgeries, such as surgeries for thyroid cancer, revision surgeries, surgeries for large goiters, and surgeries performed by low volume surgeons.[184-186] The sole, randomized study by Barczyński, which compared nerve monitoring with visualization alone, showed statistically lower rates (nearly 3%) of temporary paralysis but not in permanent paralysis; the data pertained specifically to high-risk surgeries.[187] Two German reports documented large multicenter studies; the first involved 45 hospitals and 4382 patients using a multivariate analysis and showed statistically significant lower rates for VCP with IONM for benign goiter surgery. The second study involved 63 hospitals and nearly 30,000 nerves at risk; it demonstrated a significantly decreased incidence of VCP when IONM was used by lower-volume surgeons for primary thyroid surgery performed for benign conditions including Graves' disease and Hashimoto's thyroiditis (HT) in primary surgery.[18,184] Although these studies are criticized for their lack of randomization, it is of note that randomization was discussed thoroughly at the onset of the study but rejected by these surgeons who have previous experience with neural monitoring, remained committed to the routine application of neural monitoring in their patients.[188,189] Shindo et al. also found that neural monitoring resulted in significantly lower postoperative RLN paralysis rates in the benign subgroup.[190] Chan et al. showed a significantly lower rate of postoperative paralysis in patients undergoing high-risk reoperations; the rate decreased from 19% to 7.8%. Also, they found a trend toward lower rates of paralysis when nerve monitoring was used for cancer and retrosternal goiter.[191] Shin et al. have found a statistically significant decrease of RLN paralysis risk (by 87%) in a series of patients undergoing goiter surgery.[22] Barczyński et al. conducted a retrospective study of 850 patients with revision surgeries; they concluded that IONM significantly reduces the rate of transient RLN paralysis in revision surgeries.[187] Lower rates of permanent RLN paralysis with neural monitoring are noted in a study based on endocrine surgery quality data from the Scandinavian Endocrine Surgical Quality Registry.[10]

IONM Categories of Benefit

Regardless of the preceding discussion, the rates of nerve paralysis represent a single and relatively limited lens through which one can evaluate the benefit of neural monitoring to patients vis-à-vis the overall categories of benefit for neural monitoring, which include (1) neural mapping for nerve identification and aid for further dissection, (2) insight into pathologic states of the RLN, (3) identification of impending neural injury, and (4) detection of intraoperative injury and prognostication of postoperative neural function as it relates to postoperative glottic function. This information will affect intraoperative decision making as well as surgical plans to proceed with bilateral surgery These benefits become apparent when one appreciates nerve monitoring electrical information as additive and confirmatory to neural visual information. Visual information is deficient in the early portion of all cases and may be revealed to a limited degree during revision cases that may be encumbered by scar. When a nerve follows an unexpected course, such as a genu near the LOB, its presumptive course can be electrically confirmed even before dissection. Nerve monitoring also provides functional information that helps identify neurapraxic nerve injury as well as differentiate between motor versus sensory fiber content of the nerve branch. Such information is not available through visual assessment alone. The central doctrine behind neural monitoring is that a visually identified, surgically preserved, and morphologically intact nerve may not necessarily equal a functionally normal nerve. In thermal, traction, and compression injuries, RLN may appear morphologically intact; only a functional assessment of the nerve can identify the injury. Neural monitoring does not replace surgical skill and anatomic knowledge, instead, neural monitoring complements these things. IONM does not substitute the need for visual neural identification. IONM requires a strictly bloodless field. It also entails a period of learning curve, which can be shortened by following certain neural monitoring standards (discussed later). Neural monitoring equipment implies some added cost. We perceive this added cost as the price of added information and feel it is directly analogous to other added technological advances, such as the inclusion of standard pulse oximetry during anesthesia. With the initial introduction of pulse oximetry, the need for this added costly device was the subject of debate.

1. Neural Mapping for Nerve Identification and Aid in Nerve Dissection

The RLN can be mapped out in the paratracheal region through linear stimulation; the directed dissection helps in visual identification of the nerve (see the RLN monitoring video). A number of studies suggest such neural mapping is associated with the rates of nerve identification between 98% and 100%.[168] Chiang et al. reported a 100% RLN identification rate that included the identification of nerves (25% of the total), which were regarded as difficult to visually identify because of their complex anatomy.[192] The neural mapping through IONM is valuable in surgeries that involve distorted anatomy, such as revision surgeries with scar tissue, surgeries for large goiters, and surgeries for invasive malignancies.

After the nerve has been visually identified, intermittent stimulation of the nerve versus adjacent non-nerve tissue can be helpful in tracing the nerve and its branches through the surgical field; this is done in a way analogous to intermittent facial nerve stimulation during parotidectomy. Stimulation and accurate delineation of RLN can be very useful during LOB dissection. Snyder noted IONM aided dissection of the RLN in 9.2% of his initial patient series.[193]

2. Insight Into Pathologic States of the RLN

Sometimes a nerve invaded by malignancy can still demonstrate significant residual EMG response. Additionally, residual EMG activity can be present in the setting of preoperative VCP. We found that about one third of the patients with VCP due to nerve invasion revealed significant EMG activity.[9] When such a nerve is resected, the surgeon needs to be cognizant of the consequent functional issues attributable to the loss of residual electrophysiologic activity in the nerve. The patient may experience additional dysphagia and aspiration to some extent. Hence the presence of residual intraoperative EMG activity in such situations should be considered during surgical management of invaded nerves. Notably, IONM can provide important insights into the functioning of invaded nerves; these insights are not obtainable with visual identification alone.

3. Identification of Impending Neural Injury

EMG responses obtained during surgical manipulation of the RLN can help predict impending neuropraxia, which can afford an opportunity for modification of related surgical maneuvers. (Discussed later in Loss of Signal and Continuous IONM sections)

4. Detection of Intraoperative Injury and Prognostication of Postoperative Neural Function

One of the most important applications of IONM lies in its ability to predict the functional status of RLN with reasonable accuracy; it does this by aiding the surgeon in avoiding bilateral VCP.

Blunt and stretch injury to the nerve may not always be visibly detectable. As mentioned earlier, a nerve that appears structurally normal may not necessarily be functionally normal. The predictive ability of neural testing is extremely important in bilateral thyroid surgery because both nerves governing the laryngeal airway introitus are placed at risk with one surgery. Several studies have shown the surgeon is highly inaccurate at detecting intraoperative RLN injury. Several studies show that only 10% to 14% of injured nerves are identified as being injured by the operating surgeon.[5,194] Bergenfelz, in reviewing the experience of the Scandinavian endocrine quality register in more than 3660 cases, noted that the ability of the surgeon to recognize intraoperative injury occurred in only 11.3% of nerves injured, and when bilateral injury occurred, it was recognized intraoperatively in only 16% of bilateral injuries.[10] Recent work by Snyder et al. have also suggested that the majority of nerves injured are judged to be visually intact at surgery.[195] Thus visual examination is vastly insufficient to prognosticate postoperative RLN function; it identifies only about 10% of injured nerves. In comparison, existing studies show that postoperative neural function prediction with IONM is associated with uniform and high negative predictive values ranging between 92% and 100%.[179] In a large series, Goretzki et al. have shown that LOS on the first side allowed for rational change in operative strategy and the complete avoidance of bilateral nerve paralysis; however, when the second side was operated on after first side LOS, 19% of patients developed bilateral VCP. The positive predictive value of IONM is lower and can be variable; this is directly related to the use of accurate definition of LOS and implementation of equipment troubleshooting. Accurate standard definition of LOS and information of normative neural monitoring parameters can greatly augment prognostic function of IONM. Once it is confirmed that the LOS is due to neural injury, the injured nerve segment can be identified by retrograde testing of the affected RLN, starting from the laryngeal entry point and progressing proximally. This gives a chance to treat the injury and presents learning opportunities for the surgeon. In the setting of LOS, bilateral VCP can be avoided by postponing contralateral surgery. This concept of postponing contralateral surgery in the setting of nerve related LOS is possibly the utmost extension of neural prognostication function of IONM. This is also discussed in detail in the new INMSG guidelines and is described later in this chapter under the section "Loss of Signal." The prognostic power of neural monitoring is clear in the avoidance of the significant morbidity of bilateral VCP.[196] This significant advantage is not amenable to statistical testing but is likely one of the main reasons for IONM acceptance.

Past Techniques

Please see the Expert Consult website for discussion of this topic.

New Expanded Options for Surface Recording

A limitation of the clinical use of endotracheal tube-based surface electrodes is the need to maintain constant contact between the electrodes and vocal cords during surgery to obtain a high-quality recording.[74,199-202] A tube that is malpositioned during intubation (e.g., due to rotation, incorrect insertion depth, or incorrect tube size) or is displaced during neck extension or surgical manipulation can cause a decrease or frank loss of EMG signal upon neural stimulation.[199-205] Some examples of displacement during neck extension or surgical manipulation include lifting the patient to place a shoulder roll, rotating the patient's head, if the patient coughs or moves due to a light plane of anesthesia, or inadvertent pressure applied to the anesthesia circuit by a surgical assistant; all of these factors can cause the tube to rotate or migrate from optimal placement. The false-positive decline may result in inappropriate decisions by the surgeon. It also requires intraoperative verification or readjustment of the endotracheal tube position by the anesthesiologist, which can be complicated and time-consuming.

Alternative electrode systems that can circumvent the factors affecting endotracheal tube-based neural monitoring accuracy have been sought (Figure 36.12). Liddy et al. used endotracheal tube-based and postcricoid surface electrodes to record and compare evoked EMG responses in vocalis muscle and PCA muscle. The study shows that postcricoid surface electrodes reliably record PCA EMG waveforms and thus have utility as a complementary quantitative tool in IONM.[206]

The endotracheal tube-based electrode is used to detect the EMG activity of the vocalis muscles, which originate from the inner surface of the thyroid cartilage. Wu et al., therefore, hypothesized that needle or surface recording electrodes on thyroid cartilage or overlying neck skin should function like the endotracheal tube-based electrodes and enable access to the EMG response of the vocalis muscle elicited through RLN stimulation.[207] Theoretically, recording electrodes on the thyroid cartilage or neck skin should also be more stable than those on an EMG tube because the anatomic relationship is unaffected by surgical manipulation. A study by Chiang et al. compared EMG data from needle electrodes placed under the perichondrium of the thyroid cartilage to standard endotracheal tube-based electrodes during thyroid surgery.[208] Robust and stable EMG data was obtained from the thyroid cartilage electrodes and showed higher amplitudes for the vagus and RLN as well as more accurate detection of true LOS in comparison to endotracheal tube-based electrodes. Another recent study by Liddy et al.[209] evaluates normative EMG data using anterior laryngeal surface electrodes suturing to the perichondrium of the thyroid lamina compared with simultaneously recorded data from endotracheal tube-based surface electrodes for IONM during thyroid and parathyroid surgery. The study shows that the anterior laryngeal surface electrodes provide similar and stable EMG responses with equal sensitivity compared with the endotracheal tube surface electrodes for recording evoked responses during IONM. In addition, the anterior laryngeal surface electrodes offer significantly more robust monitoring of the EBSLN. Additionally, the surface electrodes on the thyroid cartilage are contained within the operative field; these are totally surgeon-controlled and are unaffected by potential endotracheal tube rotation or migration.

A recent experimental study using porcine model by Wu et al. further evaluated the feasibility, stability, and accuracy of the transcutaneous approach for EMG recording during IONM. Electrically evoked EMG obtained from surface electrodes on the endotracheal tube and from the adhesive pre-gelled surface electrodes on the anterior neck skin were recorded and compared. The study confirmed that the transcutaneous approach is feasible for recording typical evoked laryngeal EMG responses with vagus and RLN stimulation. The transcutaneous approach is stable during tracheal displacement and accurately depicts RLN stress. These findings suggest that the transcutaneous approach should be further studied for its potential application in future designs of recording electrodes for neural monitoring during thyroid and parathyroid surgery in humans.[207]

IONM SETUP AND STANDARDS

Introduction

Despite the increasingly broad use of IONM, a review of the literature and clinical experience suggests that there is great variability in the application of neural monitoring across different centers. Variation exists in the performance of pre- and postoperative laryngeal examination, in using different recording surface and stimulation electrodes, and in recording monitoring output; some of the methods depict laryngeal EMG waveform, but others provide only audio tone. Further, the standard algorithm for endotracheal tube placement and LOS troubleshooting algorithm are not followed. The literature suggests significant monitoring inaccuracies are derived from the nonstandard application of monitoring techniques with a number of recent series documenting significant equipment problems mostly relating to endotracheal tube malposition in 3.8% to 23% of monitored patients.[18,190,193,199,210-216] Dionigi et al. have shown that during initial exposure to neural monitoring, 10% of patients experience setup-related problems, 53% experience tube rotation, 33% have tube insertion of depth errors, 7% of patients have tube size error, and 1% of patients experience displacement of ground electrodes.[216] Initial experience with neural monitoring instructional courses suggests that before the course, trainees did not routinely apply standard neural monitoring protocols (Gian Dionigi, personal communication, 2011). Duclos et al. suggest the introduction of neural monitoring can significantly alter a surgeon's neural dissection technique and that the learning curve is mastered by the majority of surgeons in <100 cases.[180] Others have suggested the learning curve for neural monitoring is achieved after performance of 50 to 100 monitoring cases.[189,216] Chiang has shown a reduction in equipment-related problems, from 4.4% to 0%, with the routine application of IONM.[204]

The basic overarching standard essential elements for optimal IONM include (1) pre- and postoperative laryngoscopy (L1 and L2), as well as (2) presurgical and postsurgical vagal stimulation (V1 and V2) in all patients. Preoperative laryngoscopy provides us with essential functional status of the vocal cords before surgery. Although neural stimulation at the end of surgery and postoperative glottic function are highly correlated, our understanding of the relationship is still

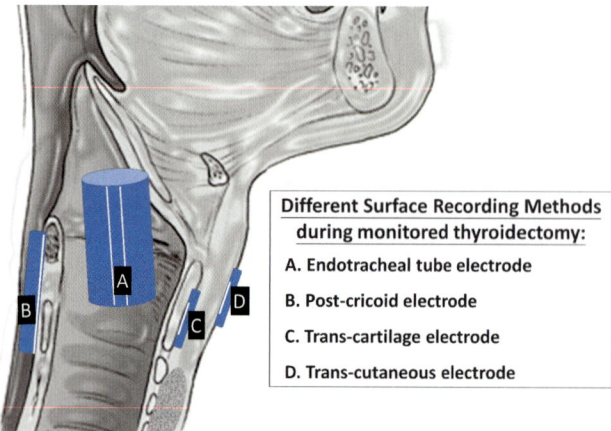

Fig. 36.12 New expanded options for surface EMG recording during intraoperative neuromonitoring.

Different Surface Recording Methods during monitored thyroidectomy:
A. Endotracheal tube electrode
B. Post-cricoid electrode
C. Trans-cartilage electrode
D. Trans-cutaneous electrode

emerging. Postoperative laryngeal examination is essential in all cases. However, IONM is still in the development phase to improve the prognostic correlation between the end of surgery neural stimulation and postoperative glottic function.

Presurgical dissection vagal stimulation allows for verification of system function and RLN mapping (i.e., a negative stimulation can be relied on as a true negative). Postsurgical vagal stimulation is the most accurate prognostic test available for postoperative glottic function and has been shown to have higher sensitivity, slightly higher specificity, higher positive predictive value, and slightly higher negative predictive value than does RLN stimulation in the prediction of VCP.[168,179] On the right side, a pattern of high vagal positive stimulation and lower vagal negative stimulation is the diagnostic for right NRLN.[217] The vagal stimulation can typically be performed successfully without direct vagal dissection by placing the stimulator probe between the jugular vein and carotid artery at a level of stimulation between 1 and 2 mA. The essential data elements for documentation of IONM can be codified as L1, V1, R1 and R2, V2, L2. Audio-only systems providing a tone rather than raw EMG data are problematic in that they do not offer information in terms of waveform morphology, threshold, amplitude, or latency. Exact determination of LOS as well as differentiation between signal and artifact may be challenging if not impossible with such audio-only systems.

Basic System Setup

Recording ground and nerve stimulator anode surface electrodes are placed on the patient's shoulders and are interfaced with the monitor through a connector box (Figure 36.13). Stimulating electrodes may be monopolar probe, bipolar probe, or stimulation dissectors. Most of the commercially available stimulating probes or dissectors have the entire shaft well-insulated and with only the tips exposed (Figure 36.14). The purpose of insulation is to prevent shunting of the electrical current and to offer more precise stimulation during IONM. Wu et al. performed experimental comparisons of stimulating electrodes including five monopolar probes, three bipolar probes, and two stimulation dissectors. The electrodes were compared in terms of EMG parameters, stimulus-response curve, and distance-sensitivity results for the EBSLN, RLN, and VN. The results showed that all the stimulation probes/dissectors can evoke typical EMG waveforms from all the laryngeal nerves with 1mA of stimulation. The stimulus current correlated positively with the resultant EMG amplitude. In monopolar probes and stimulation dissectors, maximum EMG was elicited by <1 mA.

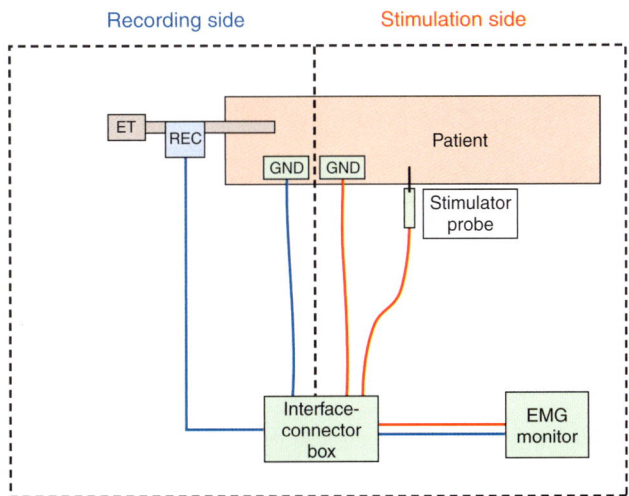

Fig. 36.13 Patient and monitoring endotracheal tube scheme.

In bipolar probes, maximum EMG required a higher current. In all electrodes, evoked EMG amplitudes decreased as the distance from the probe/dissector to the nerve increased. Evoked EMG amplitudes also decreased in stimulated nerves that had overlying fascia. Latency was unchanged in all stimulation probes/dissectors and in all trials.[218] Therefore given the previously-mentioned different stimulating characteristics, certain strategies may be employed when choosing stimulation probes/dissectors for optimal stimulation during monitored thyroid surgery:

1. Monopolar probes are most sensitive in neural depolarization at a distance from the nerve and with overlying fascia and so have the greatest utility in nerve detection during initial phases (neural mapping) of monitored thyroid surgery.
2. Bipolar probes are most specific and may be helpful for reduction of false-positive stimulation during IONM. However, they need to be close to the nerve and require higher stimulation current for maximal neural amplitude response. Therefore bipolar probe use has a potential advantage of focal nerve stimulation but may be less applicable than monopolar probe for initial neural mapping. In addition, they are suggested to be used with a correct probe–nerve orientation because the current flow is most effectively delivered when the cathode (-) electrode distal (i.e., closer to the laryngeal entry of RLN) on the nerve relative to the anode (+) electrode to avoid anodal block, which can elevate thresholds.
3. Stimulation dissector shares many of the attributes of monopolar probe and represents a viable alternative for surgeons. It provides dissection and stimulation in one instrument and offers surgeons real-time EMG feedback during nerve dissection without the need for repetitive exchanges between the surgical instrument and nerve stimulator.[219]

Anesthesia

Close partnership with anesthesiology is essential in a successful RLN monitoring program.[220] It is essential to discuss the anesthetic needs before initiation of the first case, because neural monitoring requires accurate and robust EMG response, and neuromuscular blockade must be avoided. Any neuromuscular blockade after induction could affect EMG activity. Therefore it is best after induction to allow intubation-related neuromuscular blockade to wear off. Aside from this, the anesthesiologist is free to choose the most appropriate anesthetic protocol for the patient, as other anesthetic agents (i.e., agents other than neuromuscular blockade) have very little effect on peripheral nerves and muscles. It should be noted that during the case, the anesthesia from nitrous oxide and other gas inhalational agents must be sufficiently deep to avoid any significant spontaneous activity of the vocal cords, which would make it difficult to differentiate between intentionally evoked stimulated activity and spontaneous activity; this level of anesthesia may be deeper than typically employed when a neuromuscular blockade is used.[168]

Our experience in more than 3000 cases has shown us that IONM is facilitated when a collaborative environment exists between the otolaryngology and anesthesia services leading to optimal IONM and better surgical outcomes as a result. A key element in the anesthetic technique is the avoidance of muscle relaxants or the use of muscle relaxants with a very short half-life for endotracheal intubation. Macias et al. have published an interdisciplinary collaborative protocol for administrating anesthesia for monitored neck surgery; the protocol is based on the published evidence and their clinical experience.[221]

Neuromuscular blockade management during monitored thyroid surgery can be accomplished in many ways.

1. No muscle relaxant use for entire perioperative period. It is possible to perform tracheal intubation without muscle relaxant in

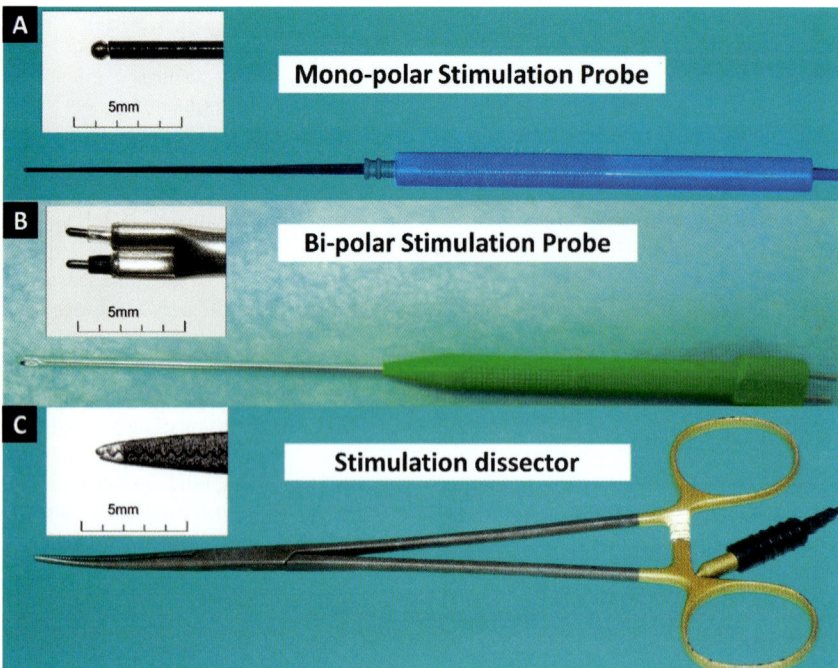

Fig. 36.14 Types of stimulating electrodes for monitored thyroid and parathyroid surgery.

experienced hands.[222] However, no muscle relaxant use is not suggested as a routine practice due to higher risk of airway injury at intubation.[223]

2. Succinylcholine or a small dose of nondepolarizing muscle relaxants can be used at intubation as long as normal muscle twitch activity can be recovered within several minutes subsequent to intubation. It is known that the larynx exhibits a shorter response time and recovers more quickly from neuromuscular blockade relative to systemic skeletal muscle including adductor pollicis.[220,224]

3. A single induction dose of nondepolarizing muscle relaxant such as rocuronium or atracurium is adequate for tracheal intubation and allows spontaneous recovery of neuromuscular transmission and positive EMG signals gradually.[225,226] Some prefer to use Rocuronium (0.6 mg/kg) at anesthesia induction with a subsequent reversal by Sugammadex (Merck & Co., Inc., Kenilworth, New Jersey). The regimen seems to meet both anesthesia (intubation) and surgery (monitoring) demands.[227,228] Sugammadex is also useful for rapid restoration of normal muscle twitch activity if a neuromuscular blockade agent has been inadvertently administered intraoperatively.[229] However, the high cost of Sugammadex restricts its use in many countries currently.[229,230]

Algorithm for Optimal Tube Placement and Function (Box 36.1)

Lidocaine ointment and other tube lubricants are avoided on monitoring endotracheal tube. Pooled saliva at the level of the vocal cords may result in altered signal, so the preoperative use of a drying agent and intraoperative suction may be helpful. At intubation, both the anesthesiologist and the surgeon should note the depth of insertion and the degree of rotation of exposed electrodes relative to the vocal cord. On average, 20 cm measured at the corner of the mouth was noted to be appropriate depth of insertion in an Asian population. Lu et al. found no relationship between depth of insertion and age or body mass index (BMI) but noted a positive trend with patient height, which has also been reported by Cherng et al.[231] In Lu's series, with great attention paid to initial tube placement, tube readjustment during subsequent surgery was required in only 5.7% of cases[2] (Figures 36.15 and 36.16). Some advanced airway devices have been designed to improve success rate of tracheal intubation and reduce intubation difficulty.[232-234] These devices are also helpful for the optimal placement of EMG endotracheal tube for IONM, the examples of these devices include (1) video-assisted *Laryngoscope*s (Figure 36.17) with a changeable blade (e.g., UESCOPE [UE Medical Devices, Newton, MA], GlideScope [Verathon Medical, Bothell, WA], and the Airway Scope [(Pentax-AWS® [Airway Scope;

BOX 36.1 Algorithm for Monitoring Tube Placement

1. Intubation with a short-acting, nondepolarizing paralytic agent with or without stylet. Note depth of insertion and rotation of exposed electrodes relative to vocal cord.
2. Position the patient (head extended, thyroid bag/shoulder roll), with anesthesia staff carefully holding the endotracheal tube stable in position.
3. After all patient positioning (i.e., after extension), confirm endotracheal tube electrode position by assessing the following:
   a. Respiratory variation of the baseline or
   b. glottic inspection
4. Secure tube in place with tape, and address support of tube as it exits the mouth. Tape surface ground electrodes in place on the skin.
5. Check monitor settings:
   a. Impedance values of less than 5 kOhm and impedance imbalance of less than 1 kOhm
   b. Event threshold, 100 μV
   c. Stimulator probe, 1 mA
6. In the surgical field:
   a. Test stimulator probe on muscle first; identify local muscle twitch and confirm that current is being received back on the monitor.
   b. Vagal stimulation: Before accepting tissue as being truly negative (in terms of recurrent laryngeal nerve [RLN]), identify the vagus and obtain a true, positive signal. You may now proceed with RLN neural mapping.

CHAPTER 36 Surgical Anatomy and Monitoring of the Recurrent Laryngeal Nerve

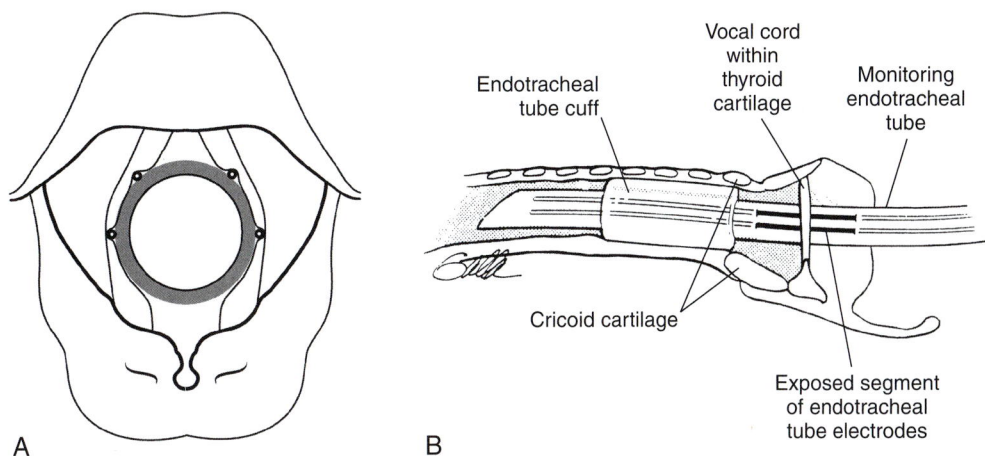

Fig. 36.15 A, Endoscopic view of monitoring endotracheal tube in correct position. **B,** Side cutaway view of the larynx and trachea, showing monitoring endotracheal tube in place. Endotracheal tube's cuff is in the subglottis; blackened lines on the side of the tube represent the exposed segment of electrodes that come into contact with the luminal surface of the vocal cord.

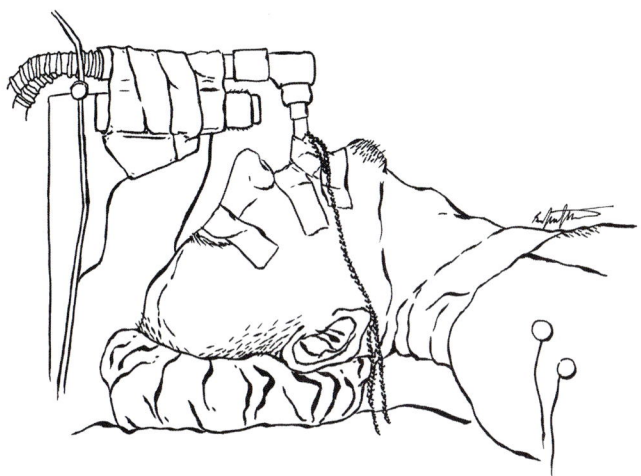

Fig. 36.16 Endotracheal tube support apparatus to prevent endotracheal tube shearing as the tube exits the mouth. Note surface grounding electrodes on the patient's right shoulder.

Hoya Corporation, Tokyo, Japan])]) that allow for direct visualization of glottis and enable proper surface electrode positioning to the vocal cords during tube placement;[235,236] and (2) intubating stylet with a rigid fiberscope for direct visualization (e.g., Trachway Video Intubating stylet [(Biotronic Instrument Enterprise Ltd., Tai Chung, Taiwan)] and the Bonfils fiberscope [Karl Storz Endoscopy, Tuttlingen, Germany]). The EMG tube can be placed via the device and further endotracheal tube position can be rechecked under fiberscopic visualization.

Recording and stimulator electrode grounds are placed through adhesive or subdermal needle electrodes at the level of the shoulder on the side of the monitor unit (Figures 36.13 and 36.16). Electrocautery units should be positioned greater than 10 feet away from neural monitoring units. Neural monitoring is not affected by the activity of cardiac pacemakers and will not affect their function; they are also compatible with both Harmonic (Johnson and Johnson, Cincinnati, OH) and the LigaSure (Medtronic, Mineapolis, MN) technologies.[74]

After intubation, the patient is positioned for surgery in the head extension. Yap et al. have found that the endotracheal tube may be displaced relative to a neutral intubating position up to 21 mm inward and up to 33 mm outward as the patient is moved into full neck extension, giving nearly 6 cm of possible endotracheal tube movement if the patient is taken from neutral to a fully extended position.[237] This implies that all tests for adequate endotracheal tube position, relative to vocal cord electrode contact, must be obtained after the patient is fully extended. The international IONM study group suggested two options. The first is to observe respiratory variation (Figure 36.18). Respiratory variation is the spontaneous waveforms varying from 30 to 70 µV present on the bilateral electrodes when they are in good position, which is observed after the paralytic agent from induction has worn off but before the inhalational plane of anesthesia is too deep. Respiratory variation is typically present as the patient starts to move spontaneously or "buck." If respiratory variation cannot be identified, then repeat laryngoscopy is recommended to visually assure adequate endotracheal tube positioning. A video-assisted Laryngoscope can be helpful in this postpositioning repeat laryngoscopy (see Figures 36.15 and 36.17). Chambers et al. reported that respiratory variation was identified in 91% of their patients, whereas the remaining 9% required a repeat laryngoscopy to adjust the endotracheal tube positioning.[238]

After the endotracheal tube is adequately positioned, the monitor setting should be assessed; impedance values, when low, suggest good electrode–patient contact. The monitor event threshold is generally set at 100 µV, and neural probe set at a value of 1 to 2 mA. At the onset of surgery, strap muscles can be stimulated to confirm gross muscle twitch showing lack of ongoing paralytic agent and intact stimulator function at the initiation of surgery. As has been discussed previously, before formal surgical dissection, predissection vagal stimulation is performed. It is only when the VN is stimulated and gives robust EMG activity that one is assured that the system is completely functional and that the RLN can be safely searched through neural mapping. With positive initial vagal stimulation, a subsequent RLN negative stimulation can be accepted (Box 36.1 and Figure 36.19).

Prognostic Testing Errors and How to Avoid Them

A surgeon using IONM during a neck surgery should be mindful of the following errors. We define EMG as a test, and postoperative RLN paralysis as disease state.

Test positive is defined as EMG LOS at the end of surgery (i.e., the test for postoperative RLN paralysis is positive), and test negative is

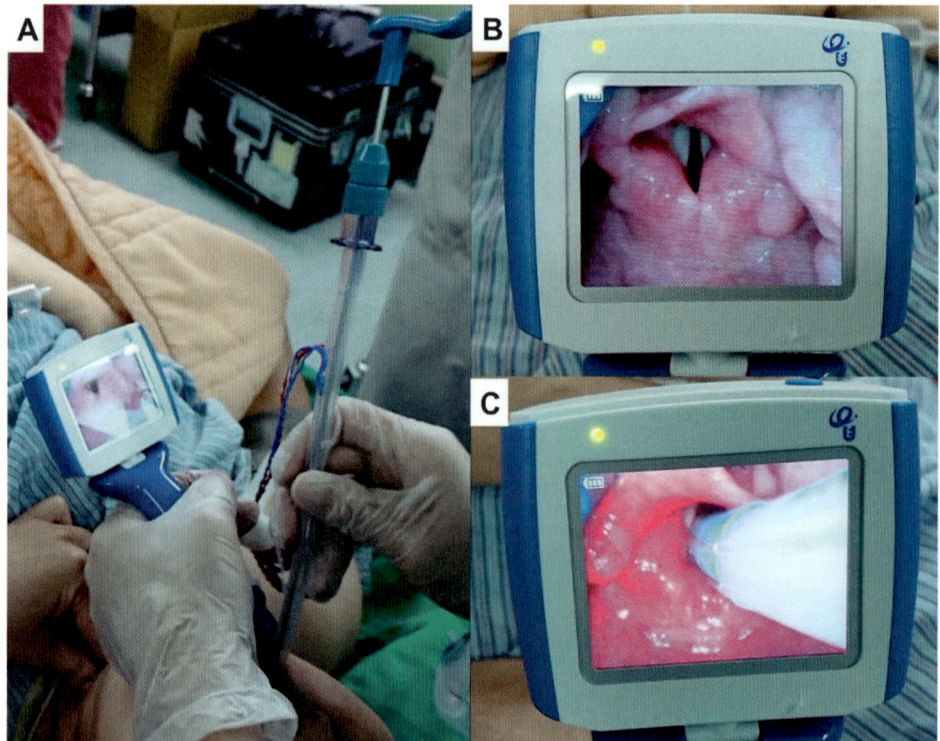

Fig. 36.17 Monitoring endotracheal tube intubation with video-assisted laryngoscope. **A,** The anesthesiologist performs the intubation. **B,** A portable color monitor, which attached on the top of the handle allows direct and clear visualization of glottis. **C,** The magnified airway images facilitate proper surface electrode positioning to the vocal cords. (Courtesy UE Medical Devices, Inc., Newton, MA.)

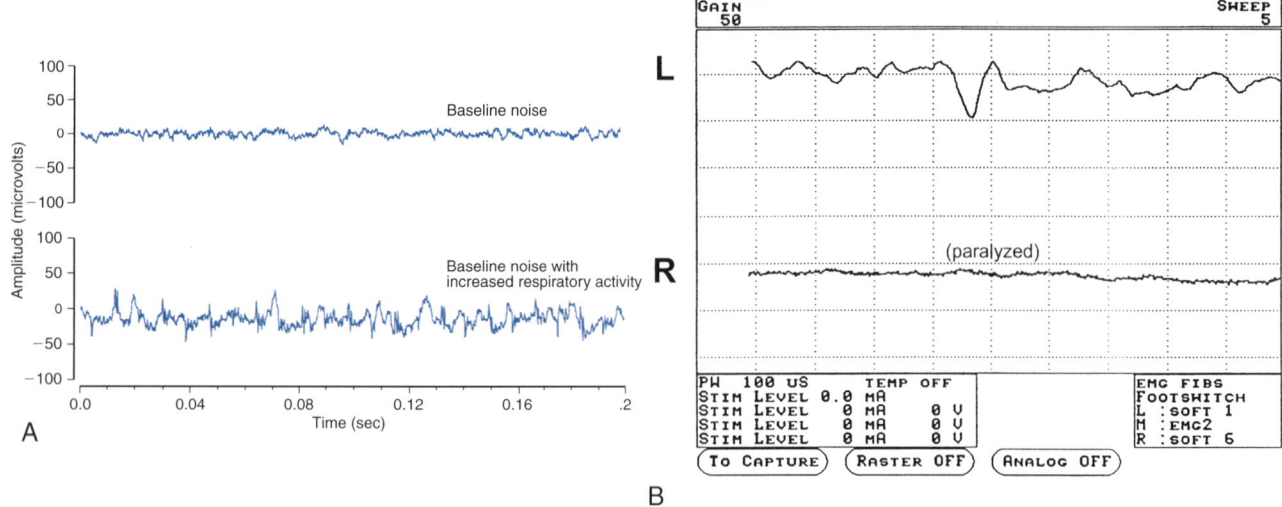

Fig. 36.18 A, Baseline noise, typically between 10 and 20 μV. *(upperline)* Coarsening of the baseline with intermittent amplitudes occurring in the 30- to 70-μV range, described as respiratory activity. This activity occurs when the patient is on the brink of bucking in the early anesthetic period *(lower line)*. **B,** Left and right baseline tracings in a patient with a known right vocal cord paralysis from past thyroid surgery. The left vocal cord demonstrates normal respiratory activity. The right cord is electrically silent.

defined as maintained EMG at the end of surgery (i.e., the test for RLN paralysis is negative).

Causes of False-Positive Tests (i.e., Loss of Signal With Intact Vocal Cord Mobility Postoperatively)

1. Endotracheal tube displacement (most common cause of false positive error)
2. Blood or fascia obscuring the stimulated nerve segment
3. Improper use of neuromuscular blockade or psuedocholinesterase deficiency
4. Ablation of early response though the stimulation suppression artifact period functionality of the monitor.
5. VCP with early neural recovery
6. Inadequate stimulating power or probe-current delivery malfunction

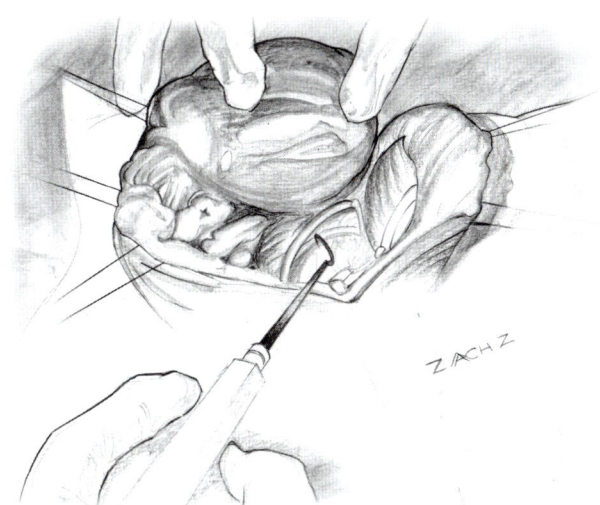

Fig. 36.19 The right thyroid lobe is retracted, and the nerve stimulator is placed on the recurrent laryngeal nerve for evoked stimulation.

Causes of False Negative Tests (i.e., Good EMG With Postoperative VCP)

1. Stimulation distal to the injured nerve segment. Performing vagal stimulation at the end of the surgery can offset this error.[168,170,204,205]
2. Injuries subsequent to the last stimulation test, such as during wound irrigation and closure.[168,170]
3. Delayed neurapraxia resulting from progressive edema affecting the RLN which may occur at an intralaryngeal location, such as the cricothyroid joint articulation.[168,170]
4. Posterior branch injury, potential posterior branch motor fibers may be disrupted despite ongoing glottic signal, and such patients may reveal an abduction defect postoperatively.[239,240]
5. Vocal cord immobility resulting from nonneural issues such as arytenoid cartilage dislocation.[168,170]
6. EMG activity is present, but is significantly reduced from initial level, or is still downsloping during final testing.[168,170]

Intraoperative RLN Stimulation Errors

A variety of stimulation errors may be experienced during intraoperative RLN stimulation. These can be segregated into three main groups[168]:
1. *Ineffective intraoperative stimulation of the RLN.* This includes insufficient current delivery because of blood fascia, insufficient probe nerve contact, probe malfunction, or insufficient stimulation current. Endotracheal tube malposition and a monitor event threshold set too high will give the impression of inadequate RLN stimulation. Given that the stimulation current is pulsed, it is best to "drag" the stimulator along tissue one desires to stimulate rather than "hopping" to avoid missing a stimulation pulse and assuming the tissue is nonneural.
2. *Intraoperative nonneural shunt stimulation.* Fluid or small vessels may shunt current from nonneural to neural tissue. In this scenario, it is best to turn the stimulation current down to a level where the false-positive stimulation is silenced but the true nerve continues to stimulate robustly. A second example of shunt stimulation is transtracheal stimulation, where stimulation on the side of the trachea directly shunts to the electrodes within the airway.
3. *Various anomalous responses to RLN stimulation related to either recording or stimulation side issues.* Electrocautery use silences the monitor and prohibits effective stimulation. Saliva pooling at the level of the glottis may be associated with reduced recording efficiency. False-positive responses may be seen when two metal instruments strike in the surgical field or when electrode and stimulator cables become tangled. Similarly, cold irrigation, heat from adjacent prolonged use of bipolar cautery, and patients who are in light planes of anesthesia may all be associated with a spontaneous train of EMG responses.

IONM Troubleshooting Algorithm

An important principle in RLN monitoring is that the surgeon must get satisfactory electrical confirmation during vagal stimulation before accepting that stimulation negative tissue can be divided. One should only regard tissue that does not respond to stimulation as not being neural after one has seen and electrically stimulated the true nerve and obtained a good response. A negative response should not be regarded as a true negative until a true positive has been identified. No tissue should be sacrificed based on a negative stimulation until a true positive has been identified.

The surgeon's first response to the absence of EMG activity when stimulating the nerve is to check for laryngeal twitch while stimulating the vagus (Figures 36.20 and 36.21). Laryngeal twitch is a simple method of intraoperative palpation of the poster cricoarytenoid muscle during stimulation of the RLN. This technique requires accurate placement of the finger on the posterior plate of the cricoid cartilage (see Figure 36.20). Laryngeal twitch correlates with postoperative vocal cord function with one study reporting a negative predictive value of 97.6%.[188] Laryngeal twitch is quite sensitive and can be identified as EMG activity first becomes detectable on the monitor.[241] The presence of laryngeal twitch indicates that the stimulation side of the monitoring system is working, that the current is being delivered adequately, and that the stimulated nerve is functional; if there is presumptive loss of EMG signal and laryngeal twitch is preserved it is the recording side of the equipment that is malfunctioning (see Figure 36.13). The majority of recording side problems relate to endotracheal tube malposition, though other recording side connection problems are also possible. The corrective maneuver is to stimulate the VN as the anesthesiologist repositions the endotracheal tube. An alternative to assessing laryngeal twitch would be to stimulate the contralateral vagus, which requires extra dissection; in unilateral surgeries, it is not feasible.

If the laryngeal twitch is absent when the nerve is stimulated, one should consider stimulation side issues such as improper strength or

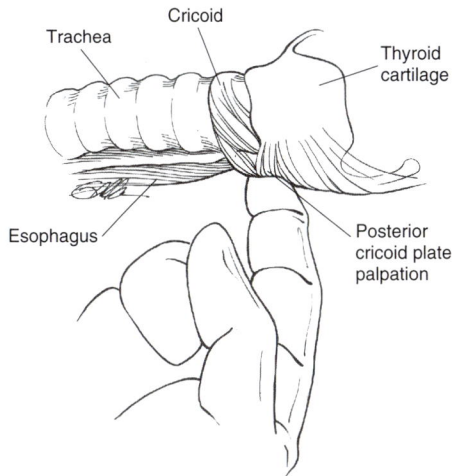

Fig. 36.20 Side view of the larynx, demonstrating the position of the finger to palpate laryngeal twitch.

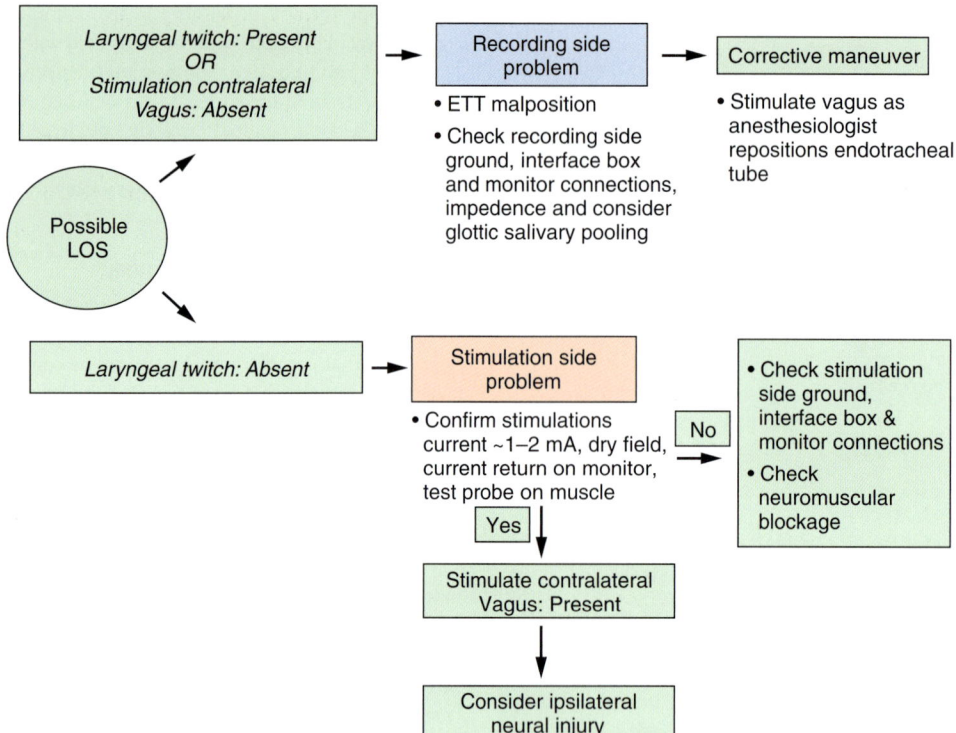

Fig. 36.21 Intraoperative loss of signal (LOS) evaluation standard.

delivery of stimulating current. The monitor screen can be assessed for current return. Neuromuscular blockade should be ruled out. If the strap or sternocleidomastoid (SCM) muscle responds to a stimulation by a current of 1 to 2 mA, then contralateral vagal stimulation should be attempted. If present, consider ipsilateral neural injury. If absent, then check stimulation side connections and also consider the status of the neuromuscular blockade.

Normative Human Monitoring Data
Standards in Waveform Definition and Assessment

Accurate interpretation of the IONM data during a surgery requires the knowledge of normative intraoperative monitoring data information. The definitions of amplitude, latency, and threshold for RLN and vagal intraoperative stimulations are defined, and normative values are reported in several studies.[242] The basic evoked waveform parameters for the human RLN or VN are defined in Figure 36.22.

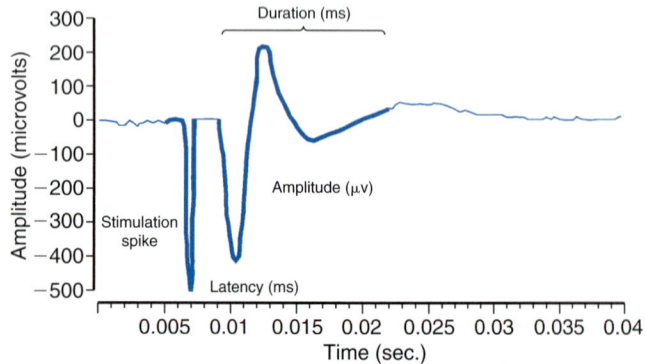

Fig. 36.22 Typical neural monitoring-evoked waveform with waveform parameters indicated.

Amplitude

The typically biphasic waveform represents the summated motor action unit potentials of the ipsilateral vocal cord muscle as recorded by cordal surface electrodes at the level of the glottis. Measures of amplitude may be correlated with the number of muscle fibers participating in the polarization during standard laryngeal EMG. Vocal cord depolarization amplitudes range from 100 to 800 µV during normal awake volitional speech.[242] Using existing standards in EMG monitoring physiology, we define monitoring waveform amplitude as the height from the vertical height of the apex of the positive waveform deflection to the lowest point in the opposite polarity phase of the waveform (i.e., peak to peak); however, it can also be defined from the baseline to the positive peak. Amplitudes during intraoperative monitoring may vary significantly within a patient and among patients. The substantial variability in the magnitude of the EMG amplitudes obtained during the course of thyroidectomy is likely caused by several major factors: (1) variation in nerve-stimulating electrode probe contact (this, in turn, may result from variation in contact pressure by the handheld probe); (2) variation in overlying soft tissue and fascia on the nerve; (3) variation in degree of moisture (blood and tissue fluid shunting) in the operative field; (4) variation in laryngeal electrode/endotracheal tube position; (5) Temperature and degree of nerve desiccation; (6) the variable exact position of motor fibers within the nerve relative to the position of the stimulating probe (i.e., eccentric position of motor fibers within the VN); and (7) sex, age, and other morphologic characteristics of the patient. Artifact waveforms are demonstrated in Figures 36.23 and 36.24.

Threshold

Threshold is defined as the current that, when applied to the nerve, first starts to trigger recognizable minimal EMG activity. The response amplitude that results at threshold stimulation is lower than the maximum amplitude achieved as stimulation current increases toward its maximum value, above which there is no further increase in EMG response. At this level of stimulation, all nerve fibers are being

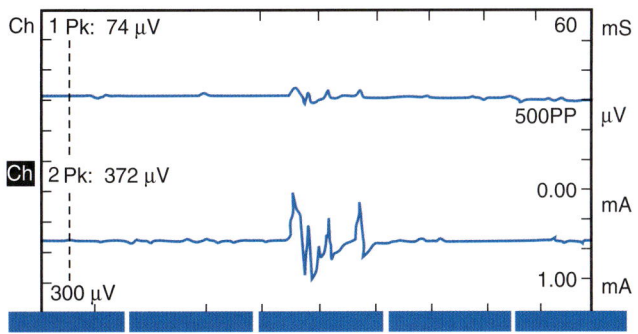

Fig. 36.23 Metal-on-metal artifact. Note sharp, discrete waveform, unassociated with a stimulus artifact.

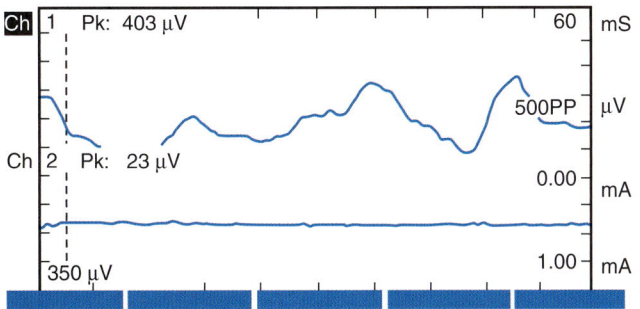

Fig. 36.24 Cuff leak artifact. Channel 1 represents broad deformation of baseline, prolonged over time and coincident with air leaking through the partially deflated endotracheal cuff.

depolarized, and maximal stimulation and resultant EMG are achieved. Beyond this point, increasing the stimulating current does not lead to further increases in recorded EMG. The human RLN maximally depolarizes at 0.8 mA. This is the rationale for stimulation during the bulk of the case at 1 mA, which represents a good and safe suprathreshold stimulation. The use of 2 mA does not get any higher EMG amplitude; however, it depolarizes a greater sphere of tissue around the probe tip and so has utility when one is initially searching/mapping out the RLN. Caragacianu et al. reported on normative values with special focus on amplitude range with definitive association with normal glottic function. They reported that amplitude >250 µV was highly predictive of a functioning RLN; despite the variations in normative amplitude values, they established a clinically useful normative range that can be used for surgical decision making[243] (Figure 36.25).

Latency

Latency is not uniformly defined in the surgical monitoring literature. Whereas amplitude is generally believed to represent the number of fibers participating in the depolarization event, latency is generally believed to be associated with the speed or ease of stimulation-induced depolarization and depends on the distance of the stimulation point to the ipsilateral vocal cord. Given the different length of the VN on both sides, latency is significantly longer at the left compared with the right side when the vagus is stimulated in the midneck during thyroidectomy (discussed later). There is no standard relating to the exact point on the waveform that is best used for calculating latency.

We define latency as the time from the stimulation spike to the first evoked waveform peak. Measuring latency to the first evoked waveform deflection from the zero baseline is a much more variable measure and requires agreement with each measurement as to exactly where the waveform first deviates from the baseline. However, German practitioners with significant monitoring experience have obtained significant data regarding monitoring latency using this definition (discussed later).

A recent study from our unit described normative EMG data and graphical waveforms generated from RLN, SLN, and left and right VN.[244] This data is described in Table 36.2 and Figure 36.26. Analysis

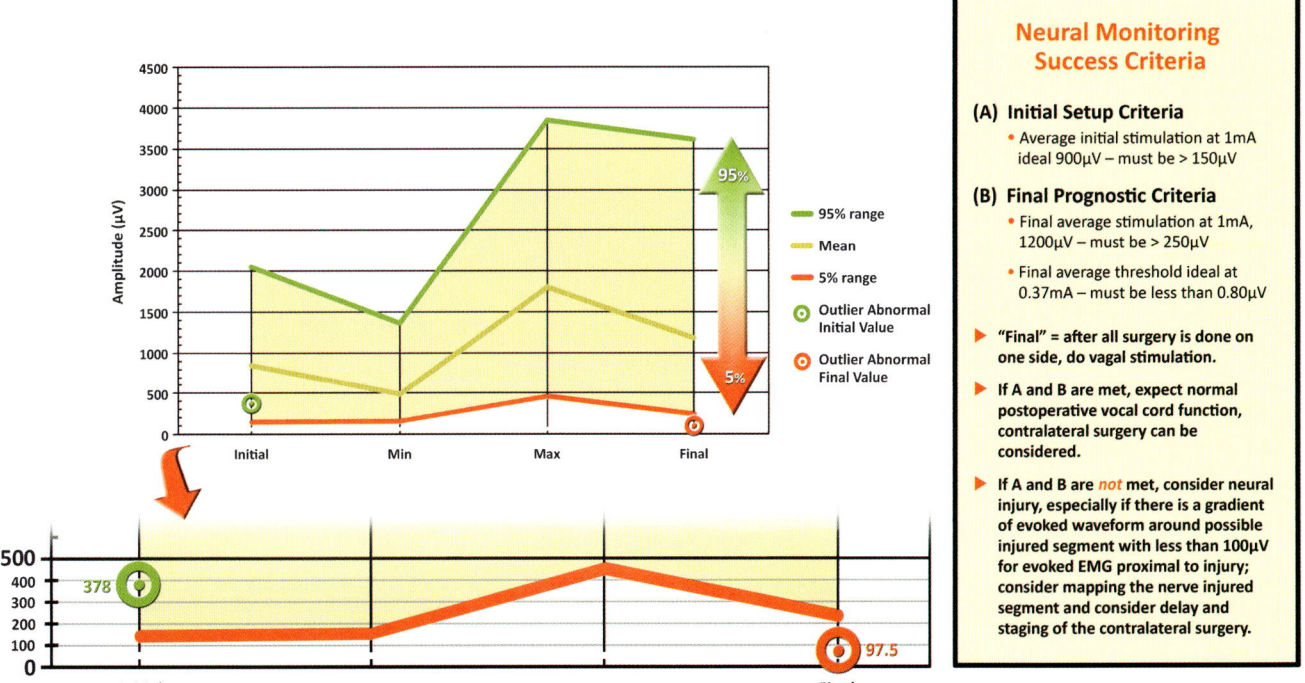

Fig. 36.25 Amplitude measures demonstrating normal range associated with normal glottis function. (From Caragacianu D, Kamani D, Randolph GW. Intraoperative monitoring: normative range associated with normal postoperative glottic function. *Laryngoscope*. 2013;123[12]:3026–3031.)

TABLE 36.2 Normative Human Monitoring Parameters*

	Amplitude (µV)	Latency (milliseconds)	Threshold (mA)
Right RLN	783 (+/-512)	3.19 (2.47–4.25)	0.51 (.025–1.4)
Left RLN	604 (+/-504)	3.7 (2.5–4.34)	0.61 (0.25–1)
Right vagus	717 (+/-479)	6.77 (4.25–9.5)	0.41 (0.25–0.85)
Left vagus	420 (+/-255)	7.67 (6.1–10)	0.41 (0.1–0.8)
SLN	269 (+/-178.6)		0.5 (+/- 0.1)

*Stimulation at 1–2 mA, parenthesis are +/- SD or ranges.

of this normative data shows that vagus and RLN latencies are significantly different. In addition, left vagal latency is higher than that of the right vagus. Latencies during intraoperative monitoring are discrete enough to distinguish artifacts from neural stimulated structures as well as to differentiate RLN, SLN, and VN, and, within vagal stimulation, to distinguish the left from right VN, easily. Interestingly, right vagal amplitude is significantly larger than left vagal amplitude. Further, we found no difference in RLN or SLN stimulation characteristics from the beginning of surgery to the end of surgery, implying that no electrical changes occurred from surgical dissection or repetitive neural stimulation during the case. Also, SLN amplitude on average represented 34% of the ipsilateral RLN amplitude. We found no significant differences in amplitude with stimulation at 1 or 2mA, and we found no differences between males and females.

These data are remarkably similar to the superb work of Lorenz et al.,[245] who reviewed a detailed analysis of nearly 2000 nerves in six German centers with stimulation at 2 mA. Their definition of latency diverged from ours, but the data are otherwise remarkably similar. Their work showed similar pattern of differences in latency between RLN and vagus and left vagus versus right vagus. They also found greater amplitude with right vagal stimulation. Interestingly, they found vagal amplitudes were greater in women than in men, and they found significantly longer latencies in women than men and in patients over 40 years of age.

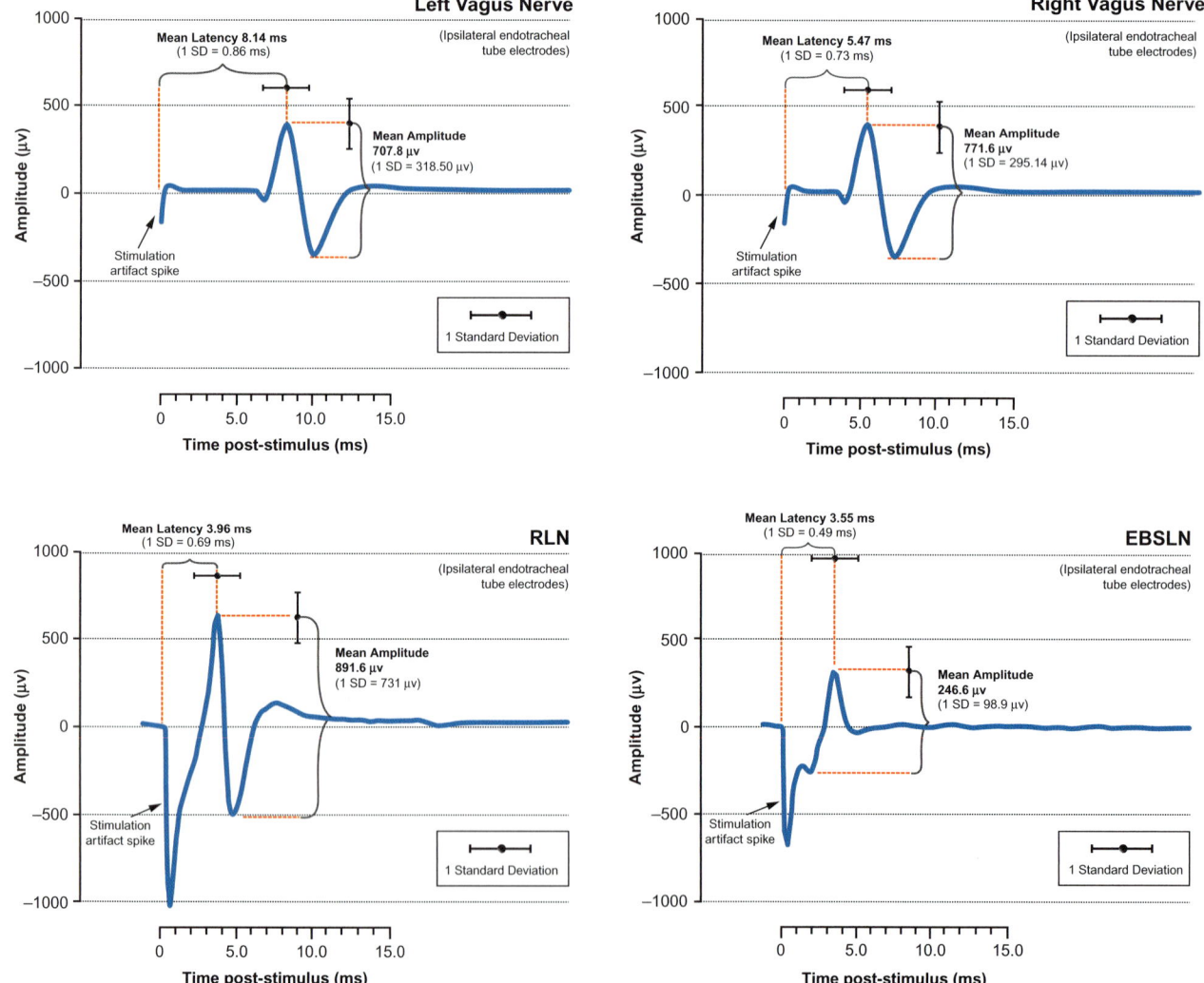

Fig. 36.26 Electromyography (EMG) waveforms recorded from ipsilateral endotracheal electrode for the left and right vagus nerve, pooled recurrent laryngeal nerve (RLN), and pooled external branch of superior laryngeal nerve (EBSLN) illustrating normal waveform morphology, latency, and amplitude standard deviation. (From Sritharan N, Chase M, Kamani D, Randolph M, Randolph GW. The vagus nerve, recurrent laryngeal nerve, and external branch of the superior laryngeal nerve have unique latencies allowing for intraoperative documentation of intact neural function during thyroid surgery. *Laryngoscope*. 2015;125[2]:E84–E89.)

Please see the Expert Consult website for more discussion of this topic.

Loss of Signal

In 2011, INMSG had proposed the definition of LOS as an EMG signal with amplitude ≤100 µV; however, recent studies have shown that good Negative predictive value (NPV) is obtained with a final amplitude of ≥250 µV.[243] With a final amplitude of ≥250 µV, the likelihood of normal cord function is extremely high, whereas VCP is more likely with amplitudes <250 µV.[5,248-252]

If there is LOS, a surgeon should first rule out setup related issues as described earlier in the section IONM problem troubleshooting: LOS algorithm.

To consider an event as true LOS, the following three conditions should be present:
1. Presence of a satisfactory EMG (V1 amplitude >500 µV) at the beginning of IONM.
2. No or low response (i.e., ≤250 µV) with stimulation at 1 to 2 mA in a dry field.
3. Absence of laryngeal twitch and/or glottis twitch on ipsilateral vagal stimulation.

When there is true LOS, with IONM the surgeon can identify the site of the injury and treat the nerve injury if possible. The surgical field must be checked to see as to whether a clip or suture may be compressing the nerve. If a focus of nerve entrapment is identified it may be corrected and the nerve damage may be reversible. Neural monitoring systems employing only audio tone response make the definitive definition of LOS problematic.[168] If the signal has been lost, the surgeon should start to stimulate the most distal point of the RLN's course (i.e., at the nerve entry site) and stimulate from this distal point serially and more proximately testing the entire nerve segment to determine whether a neurapraxic segment can be identified.[195] The identification of such a segment (termed type I RLN injury–segmental injury) can allow the surgeon to review the management of this portion of the nerve as it relates to excessive traction, compression, clamping, or other injury.[168] Should this retrograde mapping show the entire course of the RLN and vagus to be nonconductive, the injury is defined as a type II RLN injury–global injury. Though not completely understood, the type II RLN injury implies an intralaryngeal focus of dysfunction.[168] Most LOS injuries occur due to traction, especially around the LOB. However, few of these injuries will be visually evident intraoperatively. Part I of the recent two part INMSG guidelines extensively describes LOS, the interpretation of evolving changes, and application of LOS for staging bilateral thyroid surgery.[170] Bilateral VCP results in tracheostomy in approximately 30% of patients.[289]

For planned bilateral surgery, the INMSG recommends that neural monitoring information should be incorporated into surgical strategy. Preoperative patient counseling, informed consent, and discussion with endocrinologist should include discussion about decision to stage contralateral surgery in the setting of LOS. Further, when LOS occurs, the surgeon must consider the morbidity associated with bilateral VCP and tracheotomy; the surgeon must prioritize avoidance of bilateral VCP over his/her concerns about deviating from the surgical plan and over his/her concerns about the effect on one's reputation. The Part I document has defined a 'green-yellow-red-black' EMG model to represent the various stages of possible RLN injury as the LOS evolution takes place; it has recommended intraoperative management strategies for these events (Figure 36.27). EMG-Green represents stable normative EMG (relative to initial baseline with amplitude >50% of initial baseline and latency <10% of baseline) and is associated with no risk of VCP. EMG-Yellow reflects impending neuropraxia with amplitude decrease of ≥50% and latency increase of ≥10%, also known as "combined event." These changes are often reversible when associated surgical maneuver is modified. EMG-Red occurs as the EMG amplitude drops to ≤100 µV and reflects evolving neuropraxia with a further increase in the risk of developing VCP compared with the 'yellow' stage. The final EMG value is EMG-Black; this final prognostic EMG value can be obtained up to 20 mins after a prior adverse EMG value. Normal neural function is assured when this EMG, value is of at least 250 µV and that the EMG is >50% of baseline initial amplitude. Laryngeal twitch response to nerve stimulation may also be useful to support final LOS. Recovery lesser than this degree is considered to be consistent with high risk of postoperative VCP, and staged surgery is strongly recommended.

General Surgical Steps as It Relates to IONM and Algorithms for IONM Incorporation

The general surgical steps as it relates to IONM are listed in Box 36.2. Algorithms for intraoperative LOS management and staging of contralateral surgery are published by the INMSG to facilitate surgical decision making[170] (Figure 36.28). Incorporation of LOS into the surgical strategy by staging a planned bilateral thyroidectomy can dramatically reduce rates of bilateral VCP and tracheotomy. Al-Qurayshi et al. evaluated the cost-effectiveness of neural monitoring in relation to LOS and subsequently staged thyroidectomy; they found that IONM with LOS incorporated into the surgical strategy and leading to staged surgery was the most cost-effective algorithm for all rates of contralateral nerve paralysis (ranging between 1% and 17%).[253]

Timing of Completion Surgery

This is determined by the following:
1. Laryngeal recovery

    Laryngeal recovery is the primary determinant. Laryngoscopy should be performed initially within the time frame of 2 weeks and 2 months postsurgery and then performed intermittently every 4 weeks.
2. Safety in terms of surgical complications

    Based on available literature, completion surgery is considered safer when performed <3 days after the primary surgery or after 3 months of the primary surgery.[254-258]
3. Oncological safety

    Several studies have shown that there are no oncological implications for most thyroid cancers with no residual tumor or distant metastasis if the completion surgery is performed within 6 months of the first surgery.[254,257,259] Furthermore, our recent series on staged surgical management of extensive bilateral differentiated thyroid cancer showed that the delay did not affect oncological outcome if the second surgery was performed between 4 and 25 weeks.[259]

Mechanism of Injury

The exact mechanism of nontransection neurapraxic injury may vary and may include compression, stretch, or heating. IONM has been used to determine the mechanism of injury. Snyder et al., through postinjury mapping, have suggested that stretch at the LOB during lobar retraction is the most common mechanism for neurapraxic nerve injury. The nerve was most commonly injured in the distal 2 cm leading up to the laryngeal entry point. Other less common forms of injury include ligature and compression.[195] Chiang et al. used neural monitoring to elucidate the mechanism of injury in 16 patients with LOS and found one case of transection injury, one case of nerve constriction, two cases of nerve injury through compression, and 12 cases of traction injury at the LOB.[205] Serpell has recently found, through caliper measurement of

Initial EMG

☐ **I – EMG WHITE** -post patient position initial baseline V1 > 500 μV with appropriate latency (see normative EMG chart- figure 36.26) with good laryngeal twitch baseline assessment.

Normative baseline EMG

🟩 **G- EMG GREEN** -stable intraoperative normative EMG relative to initial baseline with amplitude >50% of initial baseline and latency < 10% of baseline. Isolated non-concordant amplitude or latency changes (i.e. amplitude changes without latency or latency changes without amplitude) suggest recording side anomaly requiring troubleshooting algorithm and likely tube repositioning. No risk of vocal cord paralysis.

Impending adverse EMG

🟨 **IA EMG YELLOW** - amplitude decrease of > 50% of initial baseline (with absolute amplitude > 100 μV) and latency increase of >10% of initial baseline. It should be understood that risk of vocal cord paralysis increases as amplitude decreases and latency increases as a bio-continuum. Significant risk escalation occurs at >70% amplitude decrease and >10% latency increase (if persistent for approximately 40 to 60 seconds or more with PPV 33%, NPV 97%) though with rates of intraoperative recovery of ~70 - 80% with inciting surgical maneuver modification.

IA EMG is designed to be a warning cut off *prior* to this initial adverse EMG event signaling the nerve is approaching EMG data consistent with impending neuropraxia.

Adverse EMG

🟥 **A EMG RED** -amplitude decrease to < 100 μV, typically associated with latency increase of >10% of initial baseline suggesting high risk of neuropraxia (PPV 83%, NPV 98%) with reduced potential for intraoperative recovery of ~17-25%.

Final EMG

⬛ **F EMG BLACK** -subsequent to IA EMG or A EMG (as defined above) – 20 minute intraoperative EMG recovery period should be given. Amplitude recovery of >50% of initial baseline and with absolute amplitude >250 μV suggests extremely low risk of vocal cord paralysis. Recovery of less than this degree of amplitude is consistent with high risk of vocal cord paralysis and staged surgery recommended (~PPV 75%, NPV 99%). Laryngeal twitch is an adjunctive assessment of maintenance of significant neural function.

Fig. 36.27 "Green-yellow-red-black" electromyography (EMG) model to represent the various stages of possible RLN injury. (From Schneider R, Randolph GW, Dionigi G, et al. International neural monitoring study group guideline 2018 part I: Staging bilateral thyroid surgery with monitoring loss of signal. *Laryngoscope*. 2018;128(suppl 3):S1–S17.)

BOX 36.2 General Surgical Steps Related to IONM

1. Preoperative discussion and informed consent: note IONM implementation, discuss possibility of staging as it relates to LOS
2. Operate on the dominant side first
3. Obtain, interpret, and respond to EMG information:
    - Adequate baseline IONM data
    - EMG throughout the surgery- "green, red, yellow, black EMG"
    - Final EMG data-
        ✓ If No LOS- perform total thyroidectomy as planned
        ✓ If LOS- troubleshoot, true LOS - give 20 minutes for recovery,
            ➤ if recovers—total thyroidectomy as planned
            ➤ if no recovery—consider staging second side, refer to points 4 and 5 below
4. Consideration of staged surgery
    - Disease process itself, patient wishes, endocrinologist opinion, second anesthesia candidacy of the patient, surgical judgment regarding type and intensity of nerve injury
5. Staged Completion Thyroidectomy
    - Performed only after laryngeal function is recovered
    - Reevaluate the necessity of the completion surgery/adjuvant therapy based on patient, endocrine, surgical and pathology information

---

the RLN at surgery, a postdissection diameter increase of 0.71 mm. This increase in diameter, possibly representing dissection-related edema, was not associated with an increased risk of paralysis and was associated with an EMG increase during the case.[260] Dionigi et al. also recently found that traction was the most common mechanism of injury in their study, with mechanisms of RLN injury in order of increasing frequency being the following: traction > thermal > compression > clamping > ligature entrapment > suction-related injury > transection. They also reported initial rates of RLN paralysis as well as permanent postoperative VCP rates (written in parenthesis) for different types of

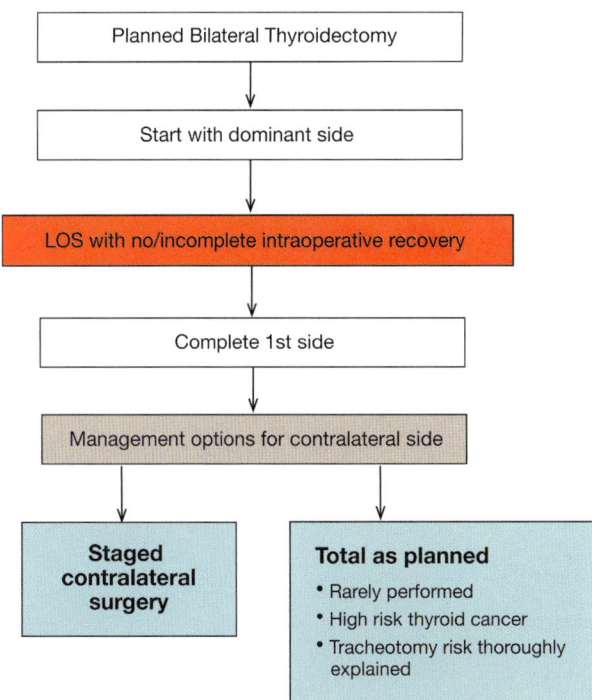

Fig. 36.28 Algorithm for intraoperative management of loss of signal with no/incomplete intraoperative recovery in bilateral thyroidectomy. (From Schneider R, Randolph GW, Dionigi G, et al. International neural monitoring study group guideline 2018 part I: Staging bilateral thyroid surgery with monitoring loss of signal. *Laryngoscope*. 2018;128(suppl 3): S1–S17.)

injury as follows: for traction 98% (1.4%), thermal 72% (28%), compression 100% (0%), clamping injury 50% (50%), ligature-associated injury 100% (0%), suction-related injury 100% (0%), and transection 100% (100%). This shows that thermal, clamping, and transection are the most consequential injuries when risk for long-term VCP is considered.[261] Several studies have shown that the RLN tolerates appropriate surgical dissection well.[32-35]

Passive EMG Activity During Thyroid Surgery

Please see the Expert Consult website for discussion of this topic.

Monitoring Safety

Multiple studies have demonstrated the safety of repetitive stimulation of the facial nerve in otologic and neuro-otologic surgery, assuming appropriate patient isolation and grounding.[237,265,267] Multiple practitioners have also demonstrated the safety of repetitive RLN stimulation during thyroidectomy.[142,239,268] In my experiments, we have seen that stimulation of individual RLNs can be performed hundreds of times with current-driven pulses in the 1- or 2-mA range (four pulses per second, with a stimulation duration of 100 µs) without ill effects. We agree with Hughes and Prass that pulsed constant current stimulation is safer than constant voltage stimulation.[269,270] Friedman found that in both dogs and humans, vagal and RLN stimulation in the 2- to 4-mA range at 10 to 25 Hz (with a pulse duration of 500 µs) was well tolerated without signs of laryngeal or cardiorespiratory symptoms.[270]

Leonetti has demonstrated the safety of vagal stimulation during human parapharyngeal space surgery.[271] Intermittent, prolonged vagal stimulation through permanent implantable vagal coil electrodes is now used to treat for some refractory forms of epilepsy and has been found to be well tolerated and safe. A short-duration, high-current stimulus is found to be safe in animal studies. A recent porcine study by Lu et al. reported on vagus nerve stimulation (VNS) with a high-current stimulus pulse (3, 5, 10, 15, 20, 25, and 30 mA, pulse width 100 µs, frequency 4 Hz, and duration 1 minute). All animals showed sinus rhythms, stable heart rates, and stable mean arterial pressure. Additionally, baseline EMG amplitude/latency in the vagus nerve-recurrent laryngeal nerve (VN-RLN) pathway proximal to the site of VNS remained stable after the high-current (3 mA to 30 mA) 1-minute stimulus was applied to the VN or RLN.[272] In clinical practice, a short-duration higher-current stimulus (e.g., 2 or rarely 3 mA) can be applied to facilitate neural mapping. After the VN and RLN are identified, the standard stimulus current (1 or 2 mA) should be used to minimize the potential for false shunting, artifact signals, nerve injury, or cardiopulmonary effects. Safety of continuous vagal stimulation is discussed in the later section of the chapter.

The INMSG, on the basis of its members' cumulative experience and review of the literature, has recently stated that repetitive stimulation of the RLN or VN is not associated with neural injury and has been applied safely in children and adults; the group noted that vagal stimulation is unassociated with bradyarrhythmias or bronchospasm.[168,273,274] There has been a report of neural monitoring associated with transient false elevation of bispectral index monitoring.[275]

Several studies have shown neural monitoring can be successfully performed with minimally invasive approaches.[276,277] A needle electrode placed through the cricothyroid membrane to monitor bilateral vocal cords has been described and has allowed vocal cord monitoring during local anesthesia.[198,206] Needle or surface recording electrodes placed or sutured to the perichondrium of the thyroid cartilage or overlying neck skin has also been described and have potential to be used as a complementary quantitative tool in IONM.[207-209] Recently, Zhang et al. reported the feasibility, safety, and advantages of using percutaneous probe stimulation for IONM during endoscopic thyroidectomy performed with a narrow operating space.[278,279]

Validity of Noninvasive Monitoring

See Figure 36.30.

Please see the Expert Consult website for discussion of this topic, including discussion of Figures 36.29, 36.30, and 36.31.

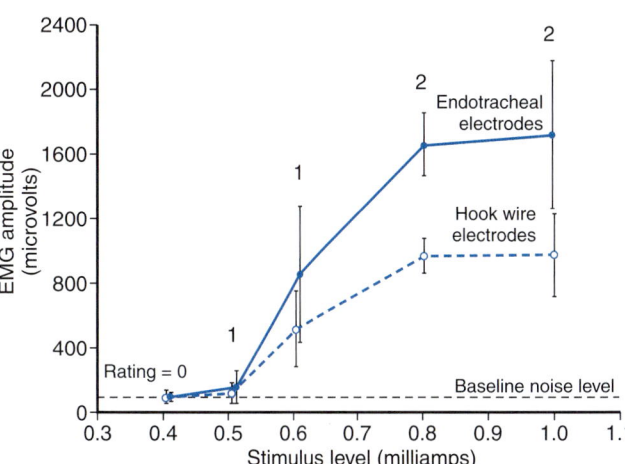

Fig. 36.30 Dose-response relationship as stimulus level is increased in EMG amplitude response. Rating (0 to 2) refers to palpation rating of laryngeal twitch. Note threshold for response occurs at approximately 0.4 mA and maximum response occurs at 0.8 mA.

Indications for Neural Monitoring

Monitoring, used appropriately, always adds advantage and should be considered for all cases. Certainly, cases that can be recognized preoperatively as likely having greater risk to the RLN should be monitored (discussed earlier). However, as all surgeons know, many cases lacking these preoperative features may well present significant intraoperative difficulties and may benefit from monitoring. Even if nerve monitoring yields the greatest advantage in difficult thyroid operations, routine application has been shown to steepen learning curves through greater experience and interpretation of signal and troubleshooting system malfunction.[216] The preceding information suggests that if the surgeon employs neural monitoring at all, one can consider applying neural monitoring to all patients.

Informed Consent and Patient Counseling as It Relates to IONM

With the increasing routine use of IONM and given its value in intraoperative surgical planning, it is important to discuss its use and implications on intraoperative decision making, especially in bilateral surgery. The other rationale for including this information in informed consent comes from the studies showing that most patients appreciate and wish to actively take part in shared decision making regarding management of their disease.[164,252,284]

Intraoperative Identification of Nonrecurrent Laryngeal Nerve

The NRLN represents an anatomic variant of RLN; it has no functional effect and is of importance only during surgery in related area due to its increased susceptibility to intraoperative injury by a surgeon unaware of its presence. The presence of right NRLN is reported as 0.5% to 1% of all RLNs; Left NRLN, which is always associated with situs invertus, is very rare, reported as only 0.04%.[59,285] Our series on NRLN monitoring has established an electrophysiologic algorithm; the presence of positive EMG response to proximal stimulation of vagus at the superior border of thyroid cartilage, and the absence of EMG response to distal stimulation of vagus below the inferior border of 4th tracheal ring reliably identifies a NRLN[64] (see Figure 36.4). This algorithm for NRLN identification is supported by Brauckhoff et al.[217]

CONTINUOUS NEURAL VAGAL MONITORING (C-IONM)

Although, intermittent intraoperative nerve monitoring (I-IONM) is extremely helpful, it may allow the nerve to be at risk for injury in between stimulations and may allow identification of such an injury once the damage has been done. With the introduction of continuous IONM (C-IONM) in the new millennium by Lamade, it is possible to obtain a real time intraoperative EMG data of VN and RLN constantly.[286] C-IONM uses an implanted vagal electrode and is useful not only during complex thyroid surgeries (especially in the settings of unusual anatomy) but also in routine thyroid procedures. In recent years, some device manufacturers have started to commercialize nerve monitoring equipment with various vagus electrode configurations, EMG displays, and/or alarm limits. Independent of electrode polarity, shape, size, and resilience, all stimulating electrodes represent a compromise between enhanced stability of the EMG signal, fewer electrode dislocations, greater flexibility for easier insertion, and better protection of the VN (Figure 36.32).[287]

The C-IONM technology enables a surgeon to (1) identify impending nerve injury as it unfolds, (2) release distressed nerves by reversing

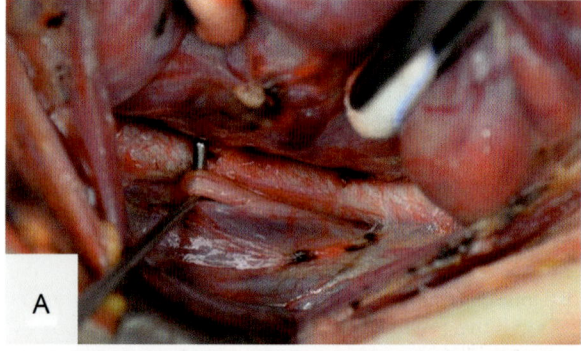
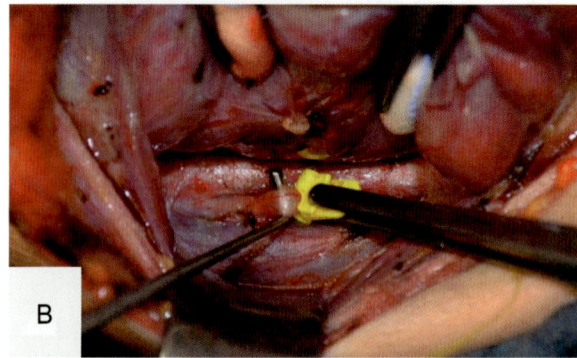
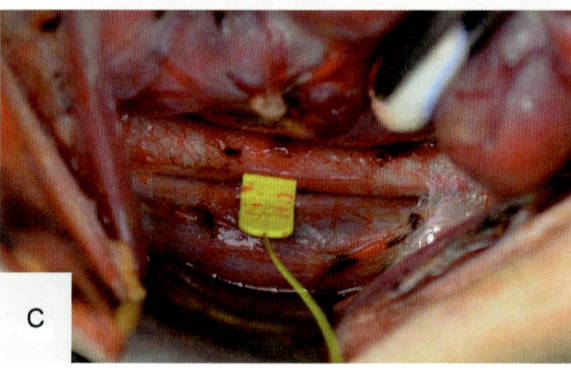

Fig. 36.32 Positioning of the APS (automated periodic stimulation) electrode on the right nerve. **A,** Dissected right carotid sheath with mobilized vagus nerve using a nerve retractor. **B,** Positioning of the electrode on the nerve from a 45-degree angle, keeping the enclosure tabs open with forceps. **C,** Resting the electrode on the vagus nerve in the perpendicular.

causative surgical maneuvers, and (3) verify functional nerve recovery after intraoperative loss of the electromygraphic signal.

For meaningful interpretation of signals, baseline amplitudes need to be ≥500 μV after suprathreshold stimulation (1 mA) of the ipsilateral VN, because (1) electrophysiological artefacts (featuring a reciprocal relationship between amplitude and latency) may be misconstrued when the baseline amplitude is <500 μV, and (2) receiver operating characteristic analysis for absolute LOS yielded an amplitude threshold of 259 μV to predict early postoperative VCP.[288,289] To become more familiar with the C-IONM technology, surgeons might have a steep learning curve because the operating surgeon needs to constantly monitor the electrophysiological response signals.

The possible advantage of a C-IONM format is that it has the potential to monitor the entire vagus and RLN functional integrity in real-time throughout surgery and could identify EMG signals associated with early-impending injury states.[200,290–292] The clinically important "combined electromyographic event" with specific concordant changes in both signal amplitude and latency (defined as >50% decreases in amplitude coupled with >10% increases in latency relative to baseline), indicative of impending RLN injury, prevents the majority of traction related injuries to the anatomically intact RLN, which enables modification of the causative surgical maneuvers in 80% of cases.[288,289,293] If corrective action is not taken, these EMG changes can progress to the loss of EMG signal with postoperative VCP. In a proof-of-concept study of 52 patients, unphysiological traction (1) where RLN courses through the LOB (2) or at the point where the RLN intersects the ITA led to RLN injury.[288] In another series of 102 patients, combined EMG events, 73% of which were reversible, yielded a positive predictive value of 33% and a negative predictive value of 97%.[250] In a recent series with 965 nerves at risk using I-IONM and 1314 nerves at risk using C-IONM RLN, dysfunction was significantly improved by C-IONM with diminished permanent VCP rate from 0.4% to 0% ($p = 0.019$).[293]

C-IONM can immediately identify RLN injury in almost real time, which may prompt instant release of the nerve so that it has the opportunity to recover intraoperatively or weaken the severity of injury. As an advanced innovation, C-IONM allows for early corrective action before permanent damage to the nerve sets in. Once LOS has been confirmed, a 20 minute wait period will allow the surgeon to know whether the affected nerve will recover fully or not and whether a staged thyroid surgery should be considered after the completion of the first side resection. Intraoperative functional nerve recovery with restitution of amplitude to ≥50% of initial baseline reliably predicts normal early postoperative vocal cord function and allows continuing of resection of contralateral side; this has been recently confirmed by an INMSG international multicenter study of 68 patients.[294] C-IONM's predictive accuracy (99.5%) is very high and represents a perfect basis for intraoperative decision making. The lower rates of false-positive and false negative with C-IONM compared with I-IONM (0.3 versus 0.5%; 0.2 versus 0.6%; n.s.) may further decrease the number of unnecessary staged procedures in false-positive, and of potential bilateral VCP in false negative findings (Figure 36.33) in particular when the concept of incomplete and complete amplitude recovery after LOS is incorporated in decision making in C-IONM guided thyroidectomy. Intuitively, one would expect (in the setting of an episode of gradual neural injury (such as retraction at the LOB) that an amplitude decrease and concordant latency increase would occur in the earliest forms of neurapraxic injury and perhaps even before more definitive durable injury. If traumatic surgical maneuvers are halted at the onset of these early electrophysiologic correlates of neurapraxic injury, such injury may be avoided. This, of course, may not be possible in certain forms of abrupt and significant nerve injury such as acute transection.

Chronic vagal stimulation has been employed for drug-resistant epilepsy, depression, and Alzheimer's disease. This has been done through indwelling vagal electrodes and has been found to be safe in terms of neural cardiac or pulmonary sequelae.[295-297] Multiple studies were conducted with a focus on the safety of C-IONM.[182,298] With rare anecdotal exceptions,[299,300] the totality of the clinical evidence argues against an adverse risk inherent in dissection around the VN or intrinsic to C-IONM stimulation (Table 36.3). Moreover, even pediatric patients and older patients with advanced atrioventricular (AV) block and/ or pacemaker can be monitored safely by C-IONM.[301,302] It is of the utmost importance to realize that 1 to 2 mA current for supramaximal stimulation used in the C-IONM technique does not activate thin demyelinated C-fibers responsible for the greatest autonomic effects.[297] This stimulation current does not engender concomitant or subsequent adverse vagal effect leading to central (headache, numbness), cardiac (arrhythmias, bradycardia), pulmonary (bronchospasm), or gastrointestinal (nausea, vomiting) symptoms.[250,288,291,303-305] Although

C-IONM augments vagal activity subclinically, this does not set off any counter regulation by the sympathetic nervous system. This increased parasympathetic activity had no appreciable effect on cardiac or hemodynamic parameters, nor on the level of proinflammatory cytokine tumour necrosis factor alpha (TNF-α).[306,307] C-IONM is safe if the established standards of IONM are heeded.

In especially complex cases, such as recurrent disease with numerous adhesions, tumor infiltrating adjacent structures, massive goiter with mediastinal extension or tracheal deviation, continuous monitoring changes from a simple support during traditional surgical procedures to an indispensable tool that assists the surgeon during risky and complex procedures. In these circumstances, early identification of the RLN and its pathway is not always possible. Despite that, once the vagal electrode is positioned, the EMG obtained during the C-IONM assists the surgeon constantly and in real time about the safety of every step.[294,308]

C-IONM is a recent but rapidly evolving technique, which is constantly being refined by various studies focusing on improvement in its implementation, interpretation, as well as on the elimination of the technical snags. Unlike I-IONM, which requires stimulation from a remote access, C-IONM can also be integrated more easily into robotic thyroidectomy.[309,310]

MANAGEMENT OF INFILTRATED NERVE

Locally invasive papillary thyroid carcinoma occurs in about 16% of cases.[311,312] Although overall local invasion tends to decrease 5-year survival through both increased local recurrence and distant metastasis, the exact site of invasion is important.[312-316] McCaffrey has shown that RLN invasion alone does not affect survival in papillary thyroid cancer.[312] The sites of malignant infiltration, in order of frequency for papillary carcinoma, are (1) muscle, (2) RLN, (3) trachea, (4) esophagus, (5) larynx, and (6) other (including carotid, jugular, and prevertebral fascia).[311,312,317] Much controversy exists regarding the management of invasive disease in well-differentiated thyroid carcinoma (see Chapter 37, Surgery for Locally Advanced Thyroid Cancer: Larynx, Tracheal Invasion and Esophageal).

Preoperative detection of RLN invasion is challenging, as RLN maybe functioning normally despite invasion. Additionally, patients with unilateral VCP may be asymptomatic; they may have normal voice. Sometimes, preexisting ipsilateral or contralateral VCP from an unrelated cause maybe present. Hence a clinician must perform vigilant clinical evaluation including laryngoscopy including comprehensive imaging to look for RLN compromise.

Several factors should be considered while deciding to resect or preserve an invaded nerve These factors include (1) overall disease type (e.g., benign, carcinoma, lymphoma), (2) preoperative vocal cord function (e.g., ipsilateral as well as contralateral), (3) intraoperative proximal stimulability of the nerve, (4) location and extent of neural infiltration. Multidisciplinary discussion and preoperative patient counseling are essential for effective management and successful surgical outcome.

First, one must exclude involvement of the nerve through a benign diseases such as Graves' disease, HT, viral thyroiditis, Riedel's thyroiditis, solitary nodule, multinodular goiter, benign thyroid cyst, parathyroid adenoma, and substernal goiter. This benign disease can infiltrate the nerve with or without paralysis. The incidence of VCP in patients with benign thyroid disease ranges from 0.96% to 1.15%.[318-325] Preoperatively malfunctioning nerves in a setting of benign disease may improve postoperatively. Falk described four out of seven patients who recovered nerve function postoperatively with benign disease.[317] Others have documented rates of VCP recovery after surgery for benign

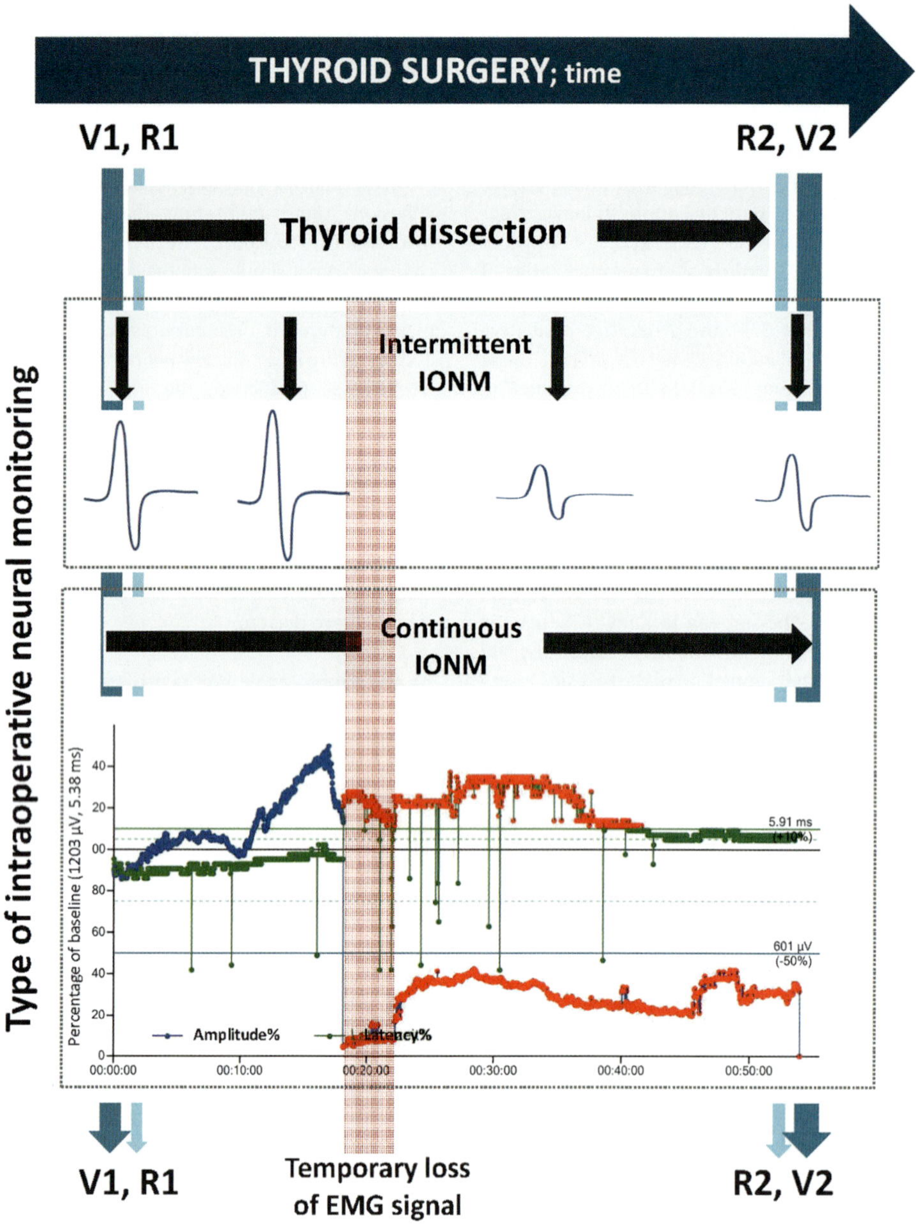

Fig. 36.33 Schematic example of superiority of C-IONM compared with conventional intermittent IONM regarding intraoperative identification of temporary loss of signal with incomplete (<50%) recovery of amplitude in relation to baseline in real-in-time electromyographic tracing, which is easily overseen in intermittent neural stimulation of the RLN with "intact" R2 and V2 at the end of thyroid dissection phase, but early postoperative vocal fold palsy. It might be misinterpreted as false negative result in intermittent IONM, but truly right positive after segmental loss of signal with incomplete recovery of signal amplitude with expected risk of vocal fold palsy of 95%.

disease ranging from 38% to 89% of cases.[319,321,323] The chance of recovery appears to be inversely related to the duration of paralysis.[314,318] Additionally, in considering the resection of a malfunctioning infiltrated nerve, one must also keep in mind the possibility of lymphomatous infiltration. VCP from lymphoma can improve after nonsurgical lymphoma treatment.[317]

In cases of differentiated thyroid carcinoma, it is agreed that infiltrated RLN associated with preoperative VCP should be resected. Controversy exists, however, as to RLN management if preoperative function is normal. It is important to recognize that RLN invasion does not independently influence survival. Whether an invaded nerve is resected or preserved appears to have little effect on prognosis.[317,326]

Please see the Expert Consult website for more discussion of this topic.

In general, if an RLN is invaded but has normal laryngeal function, if possible, attempts should be made to preserve the nerve with gross macroscopic tumor resection. Kihara et al. studied a series of 18 RLNs that were shaved/had partial layer resection, and they reported 83% rate of recovery of neural function.[327] When the invaded nerve is also the only functioning nerve, in an attempts to avoid bilateral VCP and tracheostomy, careful shave resection with consideration of adjuvant treatment should be seriously considered.[171]

Intraoperative proximal stimulation data provides useful information related to RLN function. Our study has demonstrated that 60%

TABLE 36.3 Review of Literature (Studies With More Than 40 Included Patients) Regarding Perioperative Parameters in Continuous Neural Monitoring Guided Thyroid Surgery

Reference	Year	Country	No. of Patients	No. of Nerves at Risk (NAR)	Type of Vagal Nerve Electrode	Stimulation Frequency (Hz)	Stimulation Current (mA)	Vagus Damage Through Traumatic Electrode Dislodgement	Cardiac or Pulmonary Adverse Effect	LOS; n (% of NAR)	Intraoperative Recovery; n (% of LOS)	Vocal Fold Palsy at 2nd Postop Day; n (% of NAR)	Permanent Vocal Fold Palsy; n (% of NAR)
Schneider et al.[291]	2009	Germany	45	78	Anchor	3.0	1.0	no	no	1 (1.3)	0	1 (1.3)	0
Jonas[375]	2010	Germany	100	188	V3	3.0	1.5-3.0	no	no	4 (2.1)	0	3 (1.6)	2 (1.1)
Schneider/Phelan et al.[250,288]	2013/2014	Germany, US	102	102	APS	0.2	1.0	no	no	6 (5.9)	1 (17)	6 (5.9)	0
Van Slycke[303]	2013	Belgium	100	180	S-shape	3.0	1.0	no	no	4 (2.2)	partially	4 (2.2)	1 (0.6)
Jonas and Boskovic[376]	2014	Germany	667	1184	V3	3.0	1.5-3.0	no	no	29 (2.4)	0	34 (2.9)	0
Schneider et al.[289]	2015	Germany	785	1291	APS	0.2 / 1.0	1.0	no	no	41 (3.2)	17 (41)	29 (2.2)	0
Brauckhoff et al.[300]	2016	Norway	55	87	APS	2.0	1.0	yes*	no	6 (6.9)	2 (33)	3 (3.4)	1 (1.1)
Xiaoli et al.[305]	2017	China	58	116	APS	0.2	1.0	no	no	n.d.	n.d.	1 (0.9)	0
Mangano et al.[304]	2016	Italy	211	400	APS	n.d.	n.d.	no	no	15 (3.8)	n.d.	15 (3.8)	0
Anuwong et al.[377]	2016	Italy	n.d.	626	APS	n.d.	n.d.	n.d.	n.d.	n.d.	n.d.	20 (3.2)	0
Kandil et al.[378]	2018	US	344	455	APS	0.2	1.0	no	no	15 (3.3)	0	15 (3.3)	0
Schneider et al.[294]	2018	Europe	68	68	APS, Delta, Saxophone	0.6-3.0	1.0-2.0	no	no	68 (100)	68 (100)	28 (41)	0
Schneider et al.[302]	2018	Germany	105**	175	APS	0.2 / 1.0	1.0	no	no	2 (1.1)	0	2 (1.1)	0

*Two patients: one with perineural bleeding and decrease of amplitude, and one with undetected torsion resulting in LOS but normal postoperative vocal fold function.
**Pediatric patients are <18 years of age.
n.d., not determined

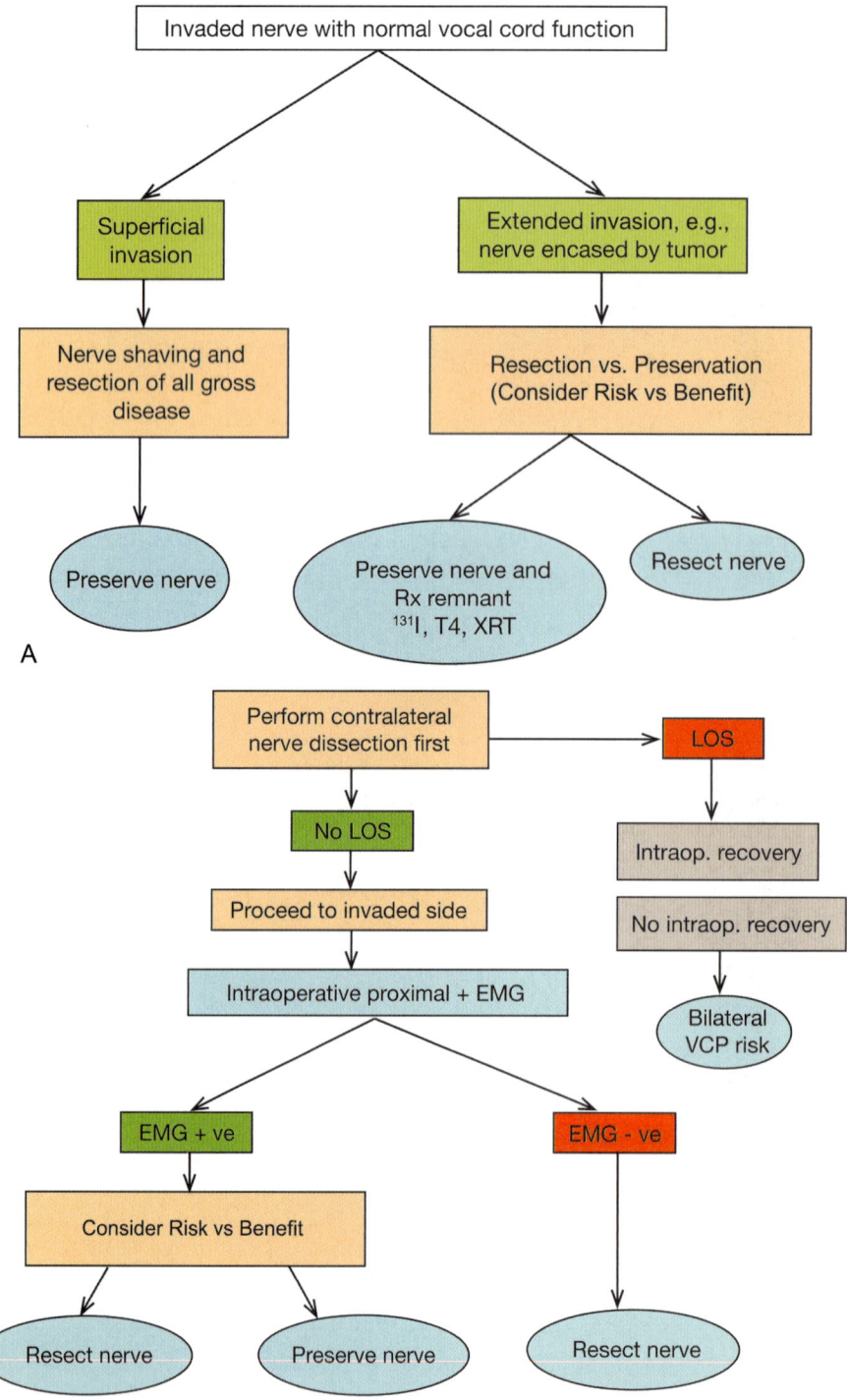

Fig. 36.34 **A,** Intraoperative management of invaded recurrent laryngeal nerve associated with normal preoperative laryngoscopy. **B,** Intraoperative management of invaded recurrent laryngeal nerve associated with ipsilateral preoperative vocal cord paralysis. (Modified From Wu CW, Dionigi G, Barczyński M, et al. International neuromonitoring study group guidelines 2018: Part II: optimal recurrent laryngeal nerve management for invasive thyroid cancer-incorporation of surgical, laryngeal, and neural electrophysiologic data. *Laryngoscope.* 2018; 128(suppl 3):S18–S27.)

of invaded nerves and about 33% of the nerves with preoperatively compromised glottic function can maintain electrical stimulability, which suggests the presence of some neural activity.[9] Intuitively, resection of such a nerve would lead to some worsening related to voice or swallowing function postoperatively. Notably, preservation of invaded nerves with preoperative VCP (but with intraoperative stimulability) has been shown to prevent postoperative development of vocal cord atrophy and worsening of vocal function.[24] INMSG has published algorithms for surgical management of nerve invasion incorporating EMG data; INMSG and has discussed intraoperative decision making in this setting in its recently published guidelines[171] (Figure 36.34).

The ability to achieve macroscopic removal of tumor while preserving the nerve depends on the extent of neural infiltration. Sometimes, the surgeon may consider leaving a small amount of macroscopic disease to preserve the RLN. However, in this scenario, adjuvant treatment is a must. If local recurrence or progression occurs, then a second surgery to resect the nerve may become necessary. It is important to note that when the nerve is invaded near its entry point into the larynx, resection of the nerve to achieve macroscopic tumor resection must be considered. The residual disease left at the laryngeal entry point has a potential to progress along its path into the larynx, which may require a more morbid and aggressive resection.

Besides the histologic types of the disease, other patient- and disease-related factors such as recurrent disease, iodine refractory disease, or cases where a patient has previously received external beam radiation therapy, necessitate an aggressive surgical approach. If a patient has distant disease or unresectable disease, resection of an invaded nerve may not add much benefit, and nerve preservation might be a better choice.

Lastly, patient discussion during preoperative counseling should include these decision scenarios along with their related postoperative expectations; these discussions should be considered while making intraoperative nerve management decisions.

Tumor should be dissected off the RLN with no gross disease left if that is possible. Microscopic disease should be treated with ^{131}I and T4 suppression. Should regional recurrence occur, aggressive reoperation can be performed (Figures 36.35 and 36.36). In the unfortunate scenario of bilaterally invaded nerves, one must consider single nerve resection on the side with greater invasion and careful follow-up and adjuvant therapy for the gross disease invading the contralateral nerve.

MANAGEMENT OF NEURAL INJURY

Severed Nerve

Please see the Expert Consult website for more discussion of this topic.

Although some isolated reports of normal glottic function after neurorrhaphy exist, most clinical neurorrhaphy and cross innervation studies show poor vocal cord function postoperatively, with two main features: (1) a strong adductor (over abductor) functional predominance and (2) abnormal vocal cord motion, described as synkinetic with paradoxical inward adductor motion with inspiration thought to result primarily from the misdirection of abductor and adductor fibers (see Chapter 42 Pathophysiology of Recurrent Laryngeal Nerve Injury).[105,136,281,321-323,337] The lack of success of RLN neurorrhaphy is in contrast to functional results with facial nerve reanastomosis.[333] The adductor functional predominance characterizing RLN neurorrhaphy is likely caused by adductor fiber predominance (over abductor fibers) in the RLN (approximately four to one) and to the substantially greater laryngeal adductor muscle mass (compared with abductor muscle).[31,48,56,71,72,89,217,326,332,338] Other factors leading to poor glottic function after neurorrhaphy, aside from misdirection of abductor and adductor fibers, may be a reduction of reinnervated motor units, failure of axonal sprouting to reach muscle fibers (secondary to scar, neuroma formation, or other factors), impaired muscle function (secondary to atrophy and scarring), and cricoarytenoid joint ankylosis.[333,336,339] Pitman et al., in a rat model, recently suggested that after RLN transection and anastomosis at the seventh tracheal ring, reinnervation is mature at 16 weeks.[340]

Arguments for primary neurorrhaphy with accidental nerve section include a more robust, less atrophic cord and a more normally positioned arytenoid (because of greater maintenance of inserting musculature). In patients having RLN transection at thyroidectomy, Ezaki believed that voice was better in patients after neurorrhaphy than in those suffering transection without neurorrhaphy.[341] Certainly, primary neurorrhaphy does not preclude subsequent static glottic treatment (Figure 36.37).

In those circumstances where transection injury is reoperated on to perform delayed nerve grafting or reanastomosis, one must keep in mind that the distal segment of the nerve may retain electrical stimulability for only a short period of time. Our studies in a canine model suggest distal RLN segment stimulability is maintained for only 5 days.[247] This has importance if nerve stimulation is going to be used to identify the distal segment during these reexplorations.

Segmental Loss of RLN

It is typically a segment of the RLN that must be resected when one is treating invasive carcinoma. Kanaji and Fujimoto reported that 12.5%

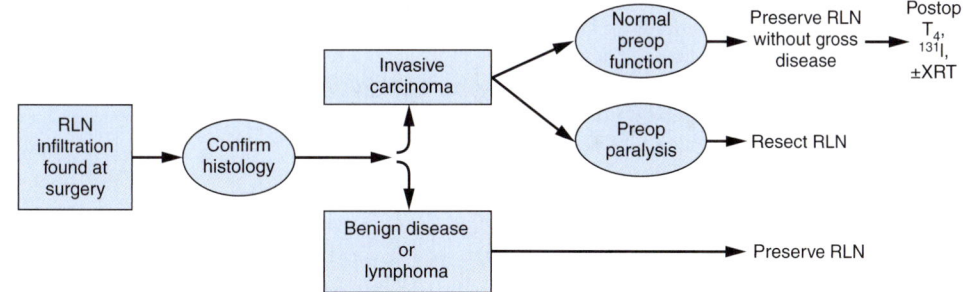

Fig. 36.35 Management algorithm of recurrent laryngeal nerve (RLN) infiltration. Preop, preoperative; Postop, postoperative; XRT, radiation therapy.

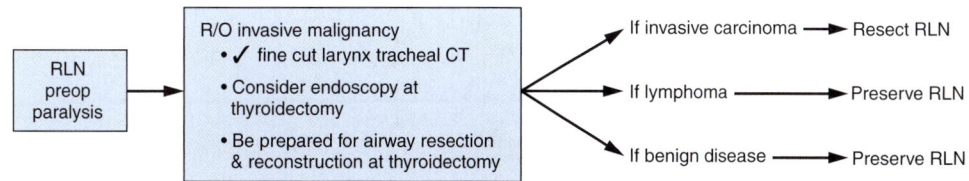

Fig. 36.36 Management of the recurrent laryngeal nerve (RLN) in preoperative RLN paralysis. CT, computed tomography; Preop, preoperative; R/O, rule out.

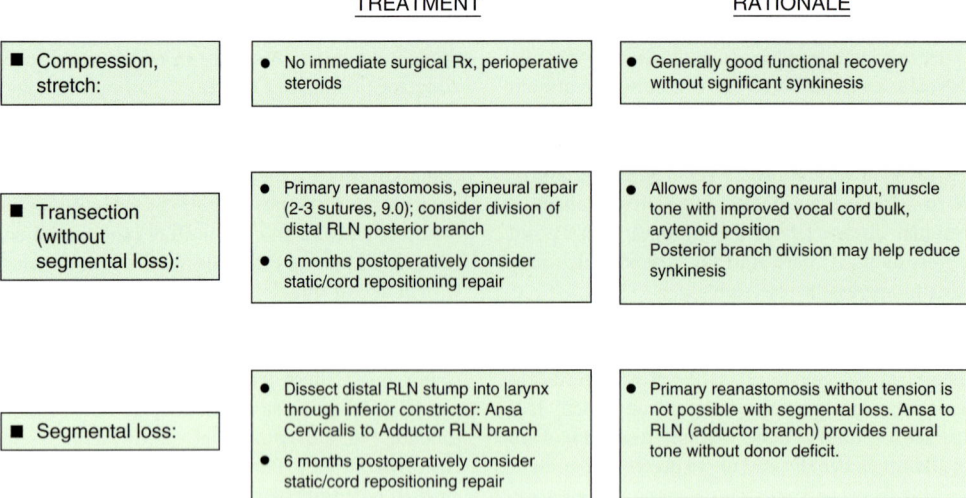

Fig. 36.37 Unilateral recurrent laryngeal nerve injury: intraoperative guide for blunt, transection, and segmental loss injuries.

of 320 patients required resection of the RLN in their series of patients with thyroid carcinoma (see Chapter 43 Management of Recurrent Laryngeal Nerve Paralysis).[325] With segmental RLN loss, primary anastomosis without tension may not be feasible. However, reinnervation is still desirable to have improved glottic tone (bulkier cord, improved arytenoid positioning) through ongoing neural input. With segmental loss, complete and normal glottic function is not recoverable. The best option to provide ongoing neural tone without neural donor deficit is the ansa hypoglossi, which has been described by Crumley.[337] The ansa can be anastomosed with the RLN trunk or its anterior branch. Ansa hypoglossi-anterior RLN branch anastomosis results in a good size match and may help to obtain primary adductor recovery. The goal is a medialized, immobile, but bulky cord with minimal synkinesis. Other options include split vagus, hypoglossal, or phrenic nerve donors. Functional deficit with ansa hypoglossi is insignificant. The sternothyroid and sternohyoid are active during respiration and phonation.[328] Such reinnervated patients can still be considered for static repair (i.e., thyroplasty) in the future.[126,322,329,337] Dissection of the distal RLN stump can be extended up through the lower inferior constrictor, gaining an additional 3 to 4 mm; this technique is reported by Miyauchi.[342] Crumley reported on 20 cases of ansa hypoglossi anastomosis to distal RLN. The distal RLN is identified using a microscope and confirmed through electrical stimulation. The ansa branch to the sternothyroid muscle, the longest and inferior-most branch of the ansa hypoglossi, is transected and reflected medially. Anastomosis is accomplished with 10-0 nylon under a microscope. Crumley combined this with a Gelfoam injection. He believes that voice results were excellent and noted no cordal atrophy and noted normally positional arytenoids. He believed that results were best if surgery was performed within 24 months of RLN injury (see Figure 36.37).[126,136,337] Su et al. reported on successful direct ansa hypoglossi implantation to the TA muscle through a thyroid cartilage window in 10 patients.[343] Miyauchi et al. have reported on 35 patients reconstructed with anastomosis, nerve grafting, or ansa hypoglossi to RLN anastomosis; they found significant improvement in patients reconstructed in maximum phonation time.[344] Similarly, Yoshioka et al. also reported that almost 90% of patients who required resection of the RLN showed phonatory recovery after RLN reconstruction. The recovery was not associated with gender, age, preoperative VCP, surgical method of reconstruction, or experience of the surgeon.[345] There is continued documentation of phonatory recovery, excellent long-term postoperative phonatory function and stroboscopic findings after nerve reconstruction, without any association with the method of reconstruction.[346-348] Feng et al. showed similar results in patients with nerve resection due to malignant invasion.[349]

Blunt, Nontransection Injury

Please see the Expert Consult website for discussion of this topic.

VOCAL CORD RECOVERY: TIMING AND ASSESSMENT

For more on RLN paralysis, evaluation, and treatment, refer to Chapter 42, Pathophysiology of Recurrent Laryngeal Nerve Injury and Chapter 43, Management of Recurrent Laryngeal Nerve Paralysis.

Please see the Expert Consult website for more discussion of this topic.

Hockauf et al. noted that many patients experiencing VCP after thyroid surgery, both unilateral and bilateral, had complete or partial recovery and recovery was more likely in surgery for benign disease.[331] Jatzko noted that VCP recovery is more likely when the nerve was identified during the case, compared with cases not involving RLN identification.[36] Several studies have shown that most neuropraxic RLN injuries generally recover within 2 to 6 months.[62,289,331,332,362] However, Woodson noted that among 35 patients with thyroid surgical injuries, none had normal recovery in her series.[333] The poor prognosis of the thyroidectomy-induced VCP found by Woodson has also been found by other practitioners.[334] On the other hand, Chiang recently studied 40 patients with VCP after thyroidectomy and found that, overall, 87% recovered with a mean time to recovery of 30 days with a range from 3 days to 4 months. Recovery was more likely if no intraoperative injury was appreciated during surgery. High rates of temporary paralysis ranging from 11% to 12% were seen for patients with Graves' and for reoperative patients; a permanent rate of 8% was noted for the reoperative group.[363]

Generally, transient paralysis is considered to be less than 6 months. Sinclair and others have noted that approximately 80% of those nerves will recover within 6 months.[14,46,100] Wagner noted recovery of VCP in 3 days to 9 months, whereas Karlan noted recovery from 1 week to 3 months.[18,98] Cricoarytenoid joint fixation has been shown to begin within 5 to 7 months of VCP onset.[364,365] Yet, Mundnich and several other practitioners showed that improvement is possible after 9 to 12 months, even after 18 to 19 months postoperatively.[24,335,366]

The role of EMG assessment in VCP is controversial, but the assessment is generally felt to be predictive of laryngeal outcome.[242] It appears most sensitive in the prediction poor recovery.[367] EMG activity, as noted earlier, may return without appropriate glottic function because of synkinesis (from misdirected RLN axonal growth, reinnervation from SLN, as well as from chronic cricoarytenoid joint abnormalities). It may be helpful in predicting recovery in the initial postoperative period (within 6 months), and it is optimally predictive if performed within 6 to 7 weeks from injury. The findings of positive sharp waves, fibrillation potentials, decreased recruitment, electrical silence, polyphasic waveforms, complex repetitive discharges, fasciculations, and synkinesis are associated with poor outcomes (see Chapter 42, Pathophysiology of Recurrent Laryngeal Nerve Injury and Chapter 43, Management of Recurrent Laryngeal Nerve Paralysis).[242,340,351,367-371]

SLN MONITORING

Please see Chapter 35 Surgical Anatomy of the Superior Laryngeal Nerve as well as the Expert Consult website for discussion of this topic, including Figure 36.38.

REFERENCES

For a complete list of references, go to expertconsult.com.

37

Surgery for Locally Advanced Thyroid Cancer: Larynx, Tracheal Invasion, and Esophageal

Mark L. Urken, John R. Sims, Eran E. Alon, Joseph Scharpf

Please go to expertconsult.com to view related video:
Video 37.1 Tracheal Resection for Locally Advanced Carcinoma of the Thyroid Gland.
This chapter contains additional online-only content, including exclusive video, available on expertconsult.com.

Invasive thyroid cancer is defined as a disease that extends outside of the thyroid gland or outside the capsule of metastatic nodes to involve adjacent structures. Several decades ago, the problem of invasive disease was more prevalent, as patients tended to seek medical care later in the course of their illnesses—when symptoms brought them to the attention of physicians. In the contemporary era, the increase in the prevalence of thyroid cancer in general is largely, but not exclusively, due to detection of the disease at an earlier stage.[1] This evolution has affected thyroid cancer care because clinicians who treat thyroid cancer often are lulled into complacency as to the complexity of the required surgery; they are not prepared to manage a more extensive disease that only becomes evident during the proposed surgical intervention that is not comprehensive enough for the appropriate management of the true invasive disease process. As such, clinicians also do not inform patients about the potential extent of the surgery required to achieve clear margins.

Invasion of the central compartment's visceral and neurologic structures has been reported in a number of articles dating to the publication by Frazell et al. in 1958.[2] The incidence of invasive thyroid cancer in a number of thyroid cancer series ranges from as low as 1% to as high as 23%.[3-5] The incidence of invasive disease may be affected by referrals to a particular center, as well as the era covered in the given series. In addition, the incidence of invasive disease can be affected by whether the series includes only well-differentiated thyroid cancer or poorly differentiated and anaplastic varieties as well.[6] The central compartment's visceral structures that may be involved include primarily the larynx, trachea, and esophagus. The neurologic structures include the superior and recurrent laryngeal nerves. Caudal extension of disease or metastatic nodes may lead to vascular involvement of the great vessels and extension to the mediastinum.

This chapter explores the management of invasive thyroid cancer involving the larynx, trachea, and esophagus. In virtually every series on invasive thyroid disease, the recurrent laryngeal nerve (RLN) is the most commonly involved central compartment structure. The incidence of RLN involvement was reported by Breaux et al. to occur in 47% of patients in their series.[7] The incidence varied in other series by Fujimoto (56%); McConahey (38%); McCaffrey (47%); Nishida (59%); and Nakao (61%).[5,8-11] Several authors group laryngeal and tracheal involvement together; therefore the true incidence of laryngeal involvement can be gleaned from only a handful of series. Incidence ranges from 0% reported by Nakao et al. to as high as 34% in the series by Breaux et al.[7,11] Tracheal invasion is far more common (37% to 60%) than laryngeal invasion, likely due to the proximity of the thyroid gland to the anterior and lateral tracheal walls. Esophageal invasion is also less frequent than tracheal invasion, with an incidence from 9% to 31%, with true transmural extension to involve esophageal mucosa on the lower end of that spectrum and outer muscular wall invasion on the higher end.

It is important to state at the outset that invasive thyroid cancer typically involves multiple structures within the central compartment, more often than it involves a single one. For example, in a given patient, disease may include the overlying strap muscles as well as the trachea and the esophagus (Figure 37.1).

In this chapter, we discuss signs and symptoms, mechanism for invasion, diagnosis of invasive disease, and surgical management of invasion of the larynx, trachea, and esophagus. As noted previously, combined visceral invasion is the norm rather than the exception. The role of postoperative ^{131}I and external beam radiotherapy (EBRT) will be discussed in subsequent chapters (see Chapter 49, External Beam Radiotherapy for Thyroid Malignancy).

SIGNS AND SYMPTONS OF INVASIVE THYROID CANCER

As noted earlier, a patient with invasive thyroid cancer is often asymptomatic. A patient may take the unsuspecting surgeon by surprise when the thyroid gland or paratracheal lymph nodes are mobilized away from the laryngotracheal complex.

One can identify five types of patients who may be recognized preoperatively as being at increased risk of having invasive thyroid cancer:
1. The patient with suspicious or biopsy-proven disease and an abnormal physical examination (PE) finding, such as vocal cord dysfunction, subglottic or tracheal mass, or asymmetry of the pyriform sinuses due to submucosal tumor extension in that location.
2. The patient with suspicious or biopsy-proven disease and such symptoms as dysphagia, dyspnea, hemoptysis, or a change in voice.
3. The patient who has biopsy-proven systemic metastasis.
4. The patient with recurrent thyroid cancer after a prior therapy.
5. The patient with biopsy-proven disease and preoperative cross-sectional imaging that demonstrates invasion of the visceral structures or extranodal extension from a metastatic lymph node.

All of the aforementioned patients should undergo more detailed imaging of the neck and mediastinum to better define the extent of their primary tumors. Even when cross-sectional imaging fails to show intraluminal extension by thyroid cancer, a surgeon may find involvement of the cartilaginous structure during the operation. Initial findings

CHAPTER 37 Surgery for Locally Advanced Thyroid Cancer: Larynx, Tracheal Invasion, and Esophageal

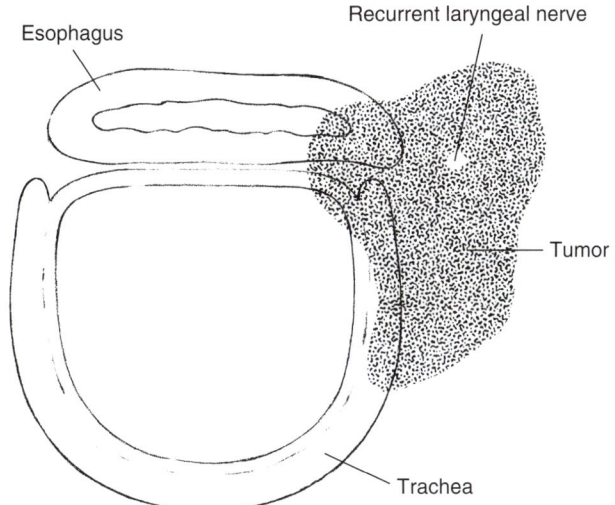

Fig. 37.1 Invasive thyroid cancer in the tracheoesophageal groove commonly involves the recurrent laryngeal nerve (RLN), the esophagus, and the trachea. Entry into the tracheal lumen may occur through the membranous trachea.

include a palpable neck mass (98% to 100%); hoarseness (18% to 22%); dysphagia (25%); hemoptysis (11% to 25%); or dyspnea (5% to 33%).[12,13] Patients with transmural tumor extension most likely experience symptomatic hemorrhaging or impending airway obstruction.[12] From 20% to 70% of patients with invasive thyroid carcinoma may have vocal cord paralysis.[12,14] However, Randolph et al. voiced a word of caution when they reported that only one third of patients with vocal cord paralysis had voice changes. Therefore the sensitivity of voice changes as a marker for vocal cord paralysis was surprisingly low at only 33%.[14]

Physical findings that may suggest invasion include a fixed cervical mass, a mass overlying the thyroid cartilage, or frank adherence or invasion of cervical skin. Because of the low sensitivity of voice changes as a marker for invasion, all patients must undergo either indirect or fiberoptic laryngoscopy to assess for true vocal cord paralysis or paresis, blood, pooling of secretions, submucosal changes, or distinct intramural invasion into the larynx, trachea, or hypopharynx. Office-based tracheoscopy and esophagoscopy may be performed to document the extent of invasion, to allow better surgical planning, and to provide for a more comprehensive discussion with the patient (Figure 37.2).[15,16]

It is important to realize that not everything visualized intraluminally in a patient with thyroid cancer represents invasive disease. The authors have presented their experience with several cases mistaken for invasive thyroid disease. The disease entities included in that series were a benign, intratracheal thyroid rest in a patient with thyroid cancer; a benign tracheal stenosis adjacent to a benign thyroid nodule; a collision tumor of the larynx and thyroid, involving papillary thyroid cancer (PTC) and a primary squamous cell cancer of the larynx; a large schwannoma of the recurrent laryngeal nerve with severe tracheal compression; and chondrosarcoma of the trachea and the larynx. In addition to these noted exceptions, even rare primary thyroid histologies can exhibit invasive behavior (Figure 37.3). The majority of patients with an intraluminal mass in the setting of biopsy-proven thyroid cancer have invasive disease; however, the surgeon should maintain a level of awareness of these other entities to ensure that the extent of the planned surgery is appropriate for the patient's actual disease process.[12]

IMAGING

Imaging modalities have become an integral part of the diagnosis and staging of thyroid cancer. Ultrasonography (US) is widely accepted as the first-line imaging tool. In skilled hands, high-resolution ultrasound is very sensitive and specific in detecting suspicious nodules in the thyroid and metastatic lymph nodes in the lateral neck. However, its role in evaluating extrathyroidal extension involving the trachea, larynx, and esophagus is limited. Several reports vary significantly regarding the sensitivity of US in detecting tracheal invasion, but no data exist as to the utility of US in laryngeal involvement. It may be of help in detecting tracheal invasion in 40% to 90% of individuals; however, this is highly operator dependent, and cross-sectional imaging is generally

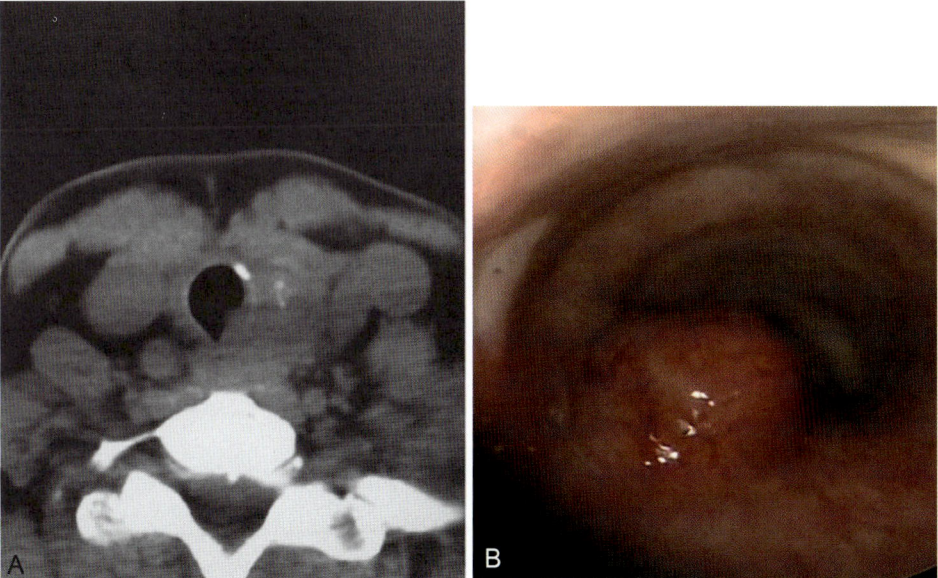

Fig. 37.2 **A,** Axial computed tomography (CT) showing a left thyroid mass with potential invasion into the tracheal lumen. **B,** Preoperative tracheoscopy was performed. It showed a submucosal tracheal mass consistent with invasive thyroid cancer.

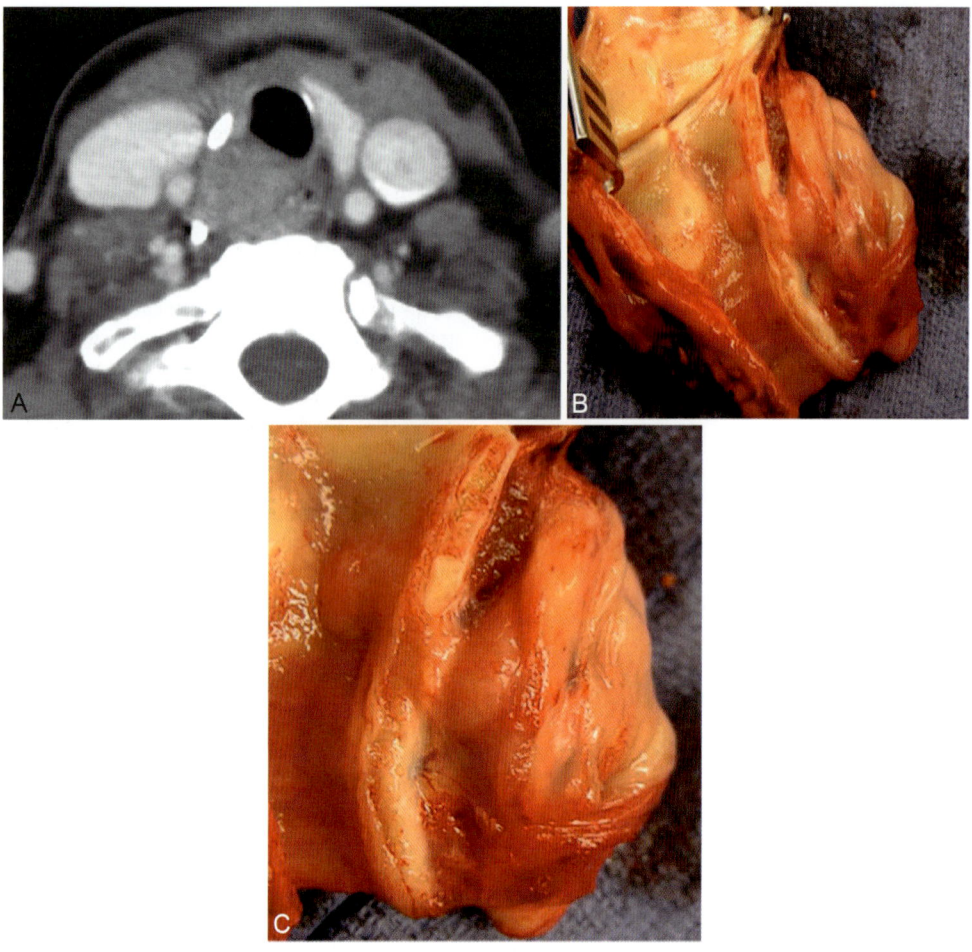

Fig. 37.3 A, Axial computed tomography (CT) showing an invasive malignant paraganglioma, a rare histology invading the laryngotracheal complex necessitating a total laryngectomy. **B** and **C,** The laryngectomy specimen, seen in sagittal orientation, demonstrates the invasion of the malignancy through the cricoid and thyroid cartilages.

more important.[17,18] Computed tomography (CT) has a higher sensitivity in detecting central and mediastinal lymph node metastases, as well as evaluating the anatomic extent of extrathyroidal extension.[19-21] The use of CT with iodine contrast may delay postoperative therapy with radioactive iodine, but lack of contrast CT may impede its overall sensitivity. The American Thyroid Association (ATA) recommends waiting 1 month after an iodine-contrasted CT to allow urinary levels of iodine to return to baseline before giving radioactive iodine. No evidence exists to suggest that waiting to give radioactive iodine for 1 month postoperatively negatively effects survival outcomes. Many patients with recurrent disease are in fact iodine nonavid. In some instances, magnetic resonance imaging (MRI) has proven useful in evaluating the scope of extrathyroidal extension to surrounding structures.[22-24]

Please see the Expert Consult website for more discussion of this topic.

MECHANISM FOR VISCERAL INVASION BY THYROID CANCER

Many parameters are important prognostic features in patients with well-differentiated thyroid cancer, including patient age, tumor size, histology, and distant metastases. (See Chapter 24, Dynamic Risk Group Analysis and Staging for Differentiated Thyroid Cancer.) Among the various staging systems proposed for differentiated thyroid cancer, the presence of extrathyroidal extension (ETE) is one of the few that is universally accepted.[27-34] In the eighth edition of the *American Joint Committee on Cancer Staging Manual*, extrathyroidal extension is divided between gross extension invading only strap muscles and more extensive invasion of the subcutaneous soft tissue; the larynx or trachea; esophagus; and RLN (T4).[35] The incidence of ETE rises as the primary tumor increases in size.[36] However, even micropapillary thyroid cancers, less than a centimeter in size, can extend outside the thyroid capsule in as much as 21% of cases.[37] The presence of ETE has been associated with an increased incidence of both recurrence and death resulting from disease.[38] Breaux and Guillamondegui reported on the institutional experience at the MD Anderson Cancer Center and noted an increased incidence of mortality from disease in invasive cancers greater than 4 cm in diameter. In addition, if more than four structures were involved by invasive disease, there were no survivors.[7]

Please see the Expert Consult website for more discussion of this topic, including Figures 37.5, 37.6, and 37.7.

Further classification of invasive thyroid cancer involving the trachea was delineated by Shin et al.,[43] who divided the disease into four stages. Stage 1 tracheal invasion involves tumor abutment of the outer perichondrium, but without invasion through the outer perichondrium. Stage 2 invasion involves cartilage erosion without transmural extension. In stage 3 invasion, the tumor invades through the cartilage but not through the mucosa. Finally, stage 4 disease is both transcartilaginous and transmucosal (Figure 37.4). In addition, the stage of

CHAPTER 37 Surgery for Locally Advanced Thyroid Cancer: Larynx, Tracheal Invasion, and Esophageal   363

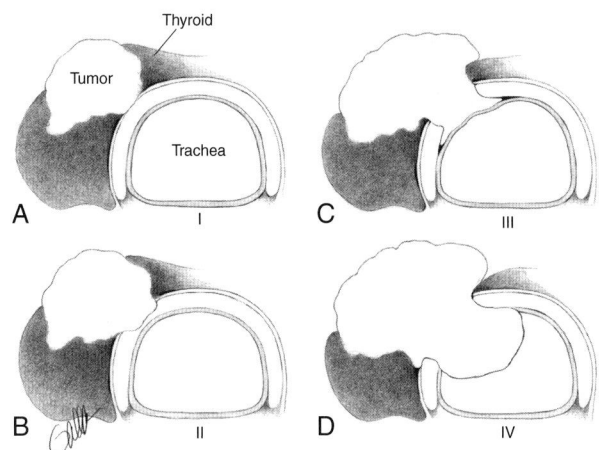

Fig. 37.4 Staging of papillary carcinoma of the thyroid invading the trachea, based on histopathologic extent of the invasion. **A,** Stage I tumor extends through the capsule of the thyroid gland and abuts external perichondrium but does not erode cartilage or invade between cartilaginous plates. **B,** Stage II carcinoma invades between rings of cartilage, or it destroys cartilage. **C,** Stage III carcinoma extends through cartilage or between cartilaginous plates into the lamina propria of tracheal mucosa but does not invade the epithelium. **D,** Stage IV tumor extends through the entire thickness of and expands tracheal mucosa. This is visible through a bronchoscope as a nodule or ulcerated mass. (Redrawn from Shin DH, Mark EJ, Suen HC, Grillo HC. Pathologic staging of papillary carcinoma of the thyroid with airway invasion based on the anatomic manner of extension to the trachea: a clinicopathologic study based on 22 patients who underwent thyroidectomy and airway resection. *Hum Pathol.* 1993;24[8]:866–870.)

invasion had prognostic significance. There was a clear distinction between those patients with stages 1, 2, and 3 disease in which none of the patients died of disease within the first 5 years after surgery, whereas 5 of 11 patients with stage 4 invasion succumbed during that time interval.[43] Although it seems apparent that the biologic aggressiveness of thyroid cancer leading to the various stages reported by Shin with regard to the trachea should apply to the larynx or esophagus, there has been no such classification of the depth of invasion of these structures by thyroid cancer.

There are three avenues for invasive thyroid cancer to affect the larynx. The first and most common is invasion of the RLN directly by the primary tumor or by a metastatic paratracheal lymph node. The second is by direct invasion of the larynx from the primary tumor with extension through the cricoid, the thyroid ala cartilage, or the paraglottic space around the posterior aspect of the thyroid cartilage. The last route of invasion is through a metastasis to the cartilage, which happens infrequently. Although infrequent hematogenous spread to cartilage is possible, an illustrative example is the thyroid ala cartilage, shown in Figure 37.5 (available on ExpertConsult.com).

McCaffrey et al. studied cases of invasive thyroid cancer treated at the Mayo Clinic from 1940 to 1990 and identified four routes of invasion of the laryngotracheal complex. In the first route, the disease extended from the superior pole around the posterior border of the thyroid ala to involve the paraglottic space. The second route entailed invasion of the trachea by a metastatic lymph node. For the third route, the authors described direct invasion of the thyroid ala by disease in the superior pole. Finally, the fourth route spread through direct invasion of the cricoid or trachea from a primary tumor in the isthmus[10] (Figure 37.6, available on ExpertConsult.com). The whole organ serial section of a patient with invasive papillary thyroid cancer necessitating a total laryngectomy demonstrates most of these pathways for disease spread into the laryngotracheal complex (Figure 37.7, available on ExpertConsult.com).

Dralle et al. classified their series of invasive thyroid cancer cases into six different varieties representing different sites of disease involvement. The site of involvement had implications for the extent of required laryngotracheal resection and reconstruction. As is typical of most cases of laryngeal invasion by thyroid cancer, the tracheal complex as well as the esophagus often become involved. Type 1 invasion involved a limited area of the lateral aspect of the cricoid cartilage and the first tracheal ring. The recurrent laryngeal nerve is typically also involved in type 1. Type 2 is similar to type 1 but is located more inferior in the trachea away from the larynx. The type 3 pattern included a larger portion of the laryngotracheal junction than Type 1 or type 2 more than 2 cm of longitudinal involvement or over a third of the circumference requiring resection. With regard to reconstruction, types 1 and 2 differed from type 3 primarily because type 1 and type 2 may be amenable to a patch repair with a sternocleidomastoid muscle flap, as opposed to type 3, which required a laryngotracheal resection and end-to-end repair. Type 4 is similar to type 3 with more than 2 cm of longitudinal involvement or over one third of circumferential involvement, but it is more inferior, only involving the trachea. Finally, type 5 invasion involves a much more significant portion of the laryngeal complex so that the opportunity for performing a partial laryngectomy with repair is not possible; a total laryngectomy is the only oncologically sound option. Type 6 invasion also requires a total laryngectomy, but it includes the esophagus or the hypopharynx.[44]

An additional route of laryngotracheal as well as esophageal invasion not previously described in McCaffrey's and Dralle's series travels via the tracheoesophageal common party wall.[45] Invasive thyroid malignancies near the tracheoesophageal groove or more superiorly near the cricothyroid articulation may spread along the thin connective tissue layer between the adventitia of the esophageal musculature posteriorly and the trachealis muscle anteriorly. Once access to the tracheoesophageal party wall is gained, the only anatomic barriers to intraluminal tumor spread is the thin smooth muscle of the trachealis and the relatively thicker muscular wall of the esophagus. Figure 37.8 demonstrates a case of common party wall invasion with intraluminal extension into the trachea and superior extension into the cricothyroid articulation.

This route of invasion may be even more important in the context of recurrent disease. The most challenging area of dissection during initial thyroidectomy is in the apex of the tracheoesophageal groove near the cricothyroid articulation because of the proximity of the RLN, which consistently enters the larynx in this area. Even primary tumors without significant extrathyroidal extension can be incompletely excised in this area during the initial resection in an effort to avoid significant dissection and compromising of the RLN. It is presumed that this is the likely etiology of recurrent disease in this region, which is at a high risk for invasion via the common party wall[45] (Figure 37.9).

As mentioned earlier, transmural mucosal involvement of the esophagus is rare, and the extent of involvement is usually limited to the muscular layer. The route of invasion typically involves direct spread from large or posteriorly based tumors or via the common party wall. Esophageal invasion is almost always accompanied by laryngotracheal complex and/or RLN involvement; it is almost never seen in isolation.

SURGICAL MANAGEMENT

The overarching goal of surgical management of gross macroscopic invasive thyroid cancer involving the larynx, trachea, or esophagus is to prevent disease progression in the central compartment that would

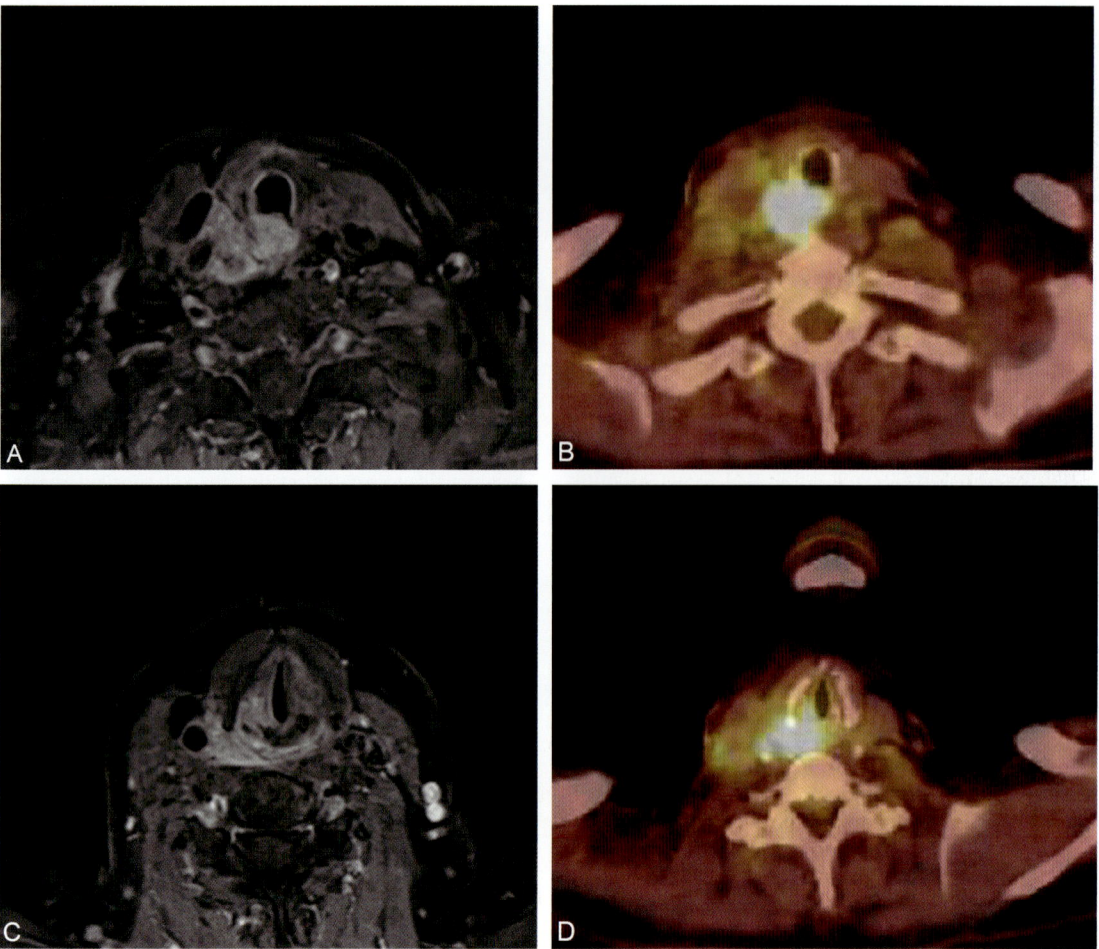

Fig. 37.8 Postcontrast T1-weighted magnetic resonance imaging (MRI) and positron emission tomography and computed tomography (PET/CT) scan of an aggressive papillary thyroid carcinoma recurrence invading the tracheoesophageal party wall **(A** and **B)** with intraluminal extension into both the trachea and the esophagus, superior extension through the cricothyroid articulation and into the right true vocal fold **(C** and **D)**, and lateral extension into the adventitia of the common carotid artery.

pose a threat to the patient's airway and hypopharynx and esophagus. In addition, the surgeon should strive to alleviate existing disease-related symptoms because of involvement of these structures. This is best accomplished through resection with negative margins and reconstruction of the central visceral structures in a manner that achieves a stable airway and alimentary tract and restores the patient's ability to speak.

Surgical approaches to invasive thyroid carcinoma range from limited procedures, such as shave resection, to total laryngopharyngectomy. The treating surgeon should be familiar with upper aerodigestive tract anatomy and the various surgical approaches available to achieve a cure while attempting to maintain function. The evaluation of the extent of disease entails a detailed PE with office-based or intraoperative esophagoscopy and bronchoscopy as well as appropriate imaging studies as previously described. Patients who are being considered for conservative laryngeal surgery should be evaluated carefully for underlying pulmonary disease because this may play a role in the decision-making process. In extreme cases, the extent of disease will require a multidisciplinary approach, including the assistance of vascular and thoracic surgical specialties.

Intraoperative frozen section pathology plays an important role in any surgical endeavor. In contrast to squamous cell carcinoma of the larynx, successful resection of well-differentiated thyroid carcinoma can be achieved with only a few millimeters of negative margins, and distant metastatic disease is not a contraindication for surgical management because patients with well-differentiated thyroid carcinoma may live many years with their underlying disease.[46] However, it is important to consider the histology of the tumor because certain histologic subtypes, such as tall cell, Hürthle cell, and insular or hobnail variant, may behave more aggressively and respond not as well to nonsurgical modalities, thus requiring more extensive resection. The surgeon must remember that when thyroid cancer is behaving in a more aggressive manner, it may not be iodine avid; as a result, the *complete* surgical management of the disease process is very important for achieving the goals noted earlier. Achieving grossly negative margins is mandatory before reconstruction. However, frozen section pathology has its limitations when cartilage is involved. For example, elderly patients with ossified thyroid cartilage may not be able to have their cartilaginous margins cleared with frozen section pathology; they may require permanent section analysis. Patients must be informed that final pathology results may necessitate further surgery. As previously discussed, Shin et al. attempted to stage tracheal invasion as a guideline for the extent of surgery required.[43] Controversy still remains as to the adequacy of shave resection with limited disease.[12,47-50] However, multiple studies have

CHAPTER 37 Surgery for Locally Advanced Thyroid Cancer: Larynx, Tracheal Invasion, and Esophageal 365

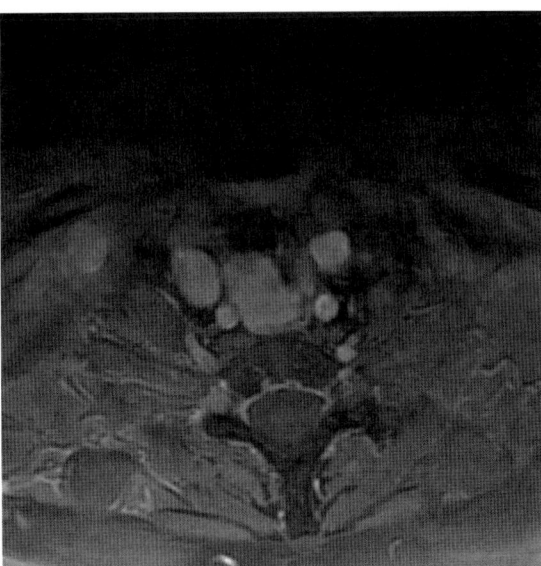

Fig. 37.9 Postcontrast T1-weighted magnetic resonance imaging (MRI) showing recurrent papillary thyroid carcinoma invading the tracheoesophageal party wall. The etiology of this recurrence was presumed to be from residual disease left in the tracheoesophageal groove near the recurrent laryngeal nerve (RLN).

cricoarytenoid complex must be preserved to allow adequate airway protection, a patent airway, and phonation.

MANAGEMENT OF THE RECURRENT LARYNGEAL NERVE IN INVASIVE THYROID CANCER

Please see the Expert Consult website for Figure 37.10.

As noted previously, hoarseness and evidence of vocal cord paralysis are often the first signs of invasive thyroid cancer (see Chapter 36, Surgical Anatomy and Monitoring of the Recurrent Laryngeal Nerve). Having said that, it is important for the surgeon to bear in mind that not all vocal cord paralyses with an associated thyroid nodule are due to invasive thyroid cancer. The senior author has encountered two cases of temporary vocal cord paralyses in patients with rapid substernal enlargement of a thyroid lobe caused by hemorrhaging into a nodule (Figure 37.10, available on ExpertConsult.com). The presumed etiology of those vocal cord injuries was a stretch of the RLN, which recovered in both cases after removal of the offending lobe. In addition, Riedel's thyroiditis as well as lymphoma also can cause vocal cord paralysis that may be temporary with treatment of the underlying condition (Figure 37.11). Hashimoto's thyroiditis also has been associated with vocal cord paralysis and *infiltration* of the RLN.[54] Hence benign or noninfiltrative malignancies may be associated with vocal cord dysfunction that should not lead the surgeon to sacrifice that nerve. The corollary to this statement is that surgeons should not sacrifice an RLN in a patient who has an ipsilateral vocal cord paralysis but does not have a diagnosis of thyroid cancer.

Management of the *involved RLN* varies. It depends on whether there is evidence of vocal fold dysfunction before surgery or whether the cords are freely mobile. In addition, knowledge of the status of the contralateral vocal cord innervation is vital to decision making. The implication of this statement is that the side of greater involvement in a case of invasive thyroid cancer should be operated upon first to determine the feasibility and safety of preserving the RLN at greatest risk. Several rules govern the surgeon's approach to managing RLNs in invasive thyroid cancer:

shown that survival will be significantly improved by removal of macroscopic disease followed by adjuvant therapy.[51]

When the depth and extent of laryngeal involvement are limited to the cartilage and overlying strap muscles, the surgeon may consider cartilage resection with preservation of the underlying soft tissue structures guided by principles similar to tracheal involvement. Usually, early disease involving the cartilage will be limited to one area, and cartilage resection will not impair function.[10,51,52] Often, one of the greatest challenges facing the surgeon is determining the extent of the disease invasion. Preoperative cross-sectional imaging is often very helpful (see Figure 37.1). However, the larger problem occurs when the unsuspecting surgeon encounters cricoid or thyroid cartilage involvement without imaging available. In these situations, it may be hazardous to attempt a more limited resection. The mechanism of tumor invasion and extent of disease will dictate the feasibility of laryngeal preservation surgery. Basic principles of partial laryngeal surgery as well as standard techniques that have been well defined in the management of squamous cell cancer involving the larynx should be employed in the management of patients with invasive thyroid cancer.[53] One functional RLN and at least one intact arytenoid with a functional

1. Every effort should be made to separate the RLN from the tumor, if the cords are mobile.
2. If the vocal cord ipsilateral to the involved RLN is indeed paralyzed, then that nerve can be resected in an effort to obtain clear margins.
3. The surgeon should not simultaneously sacrifice both RLNs in a patient with at least one functioning vocal cord. Delayed sacrifice is justified if the disease progresses after adjuvant therapy, including external beam radiotherapy.
4. Mobilization of the nerve at the entry point to the larynx should be performed if a resection of cartilage is required to obtain clear

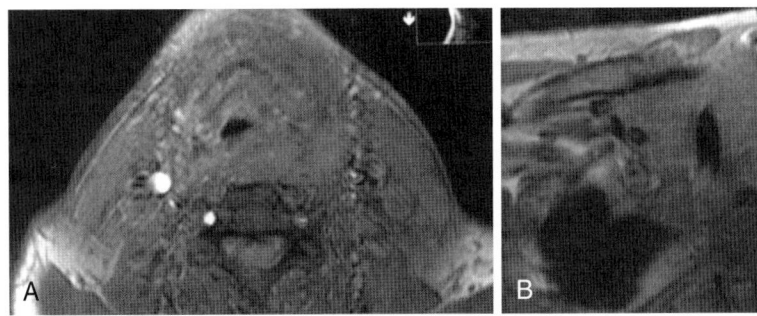
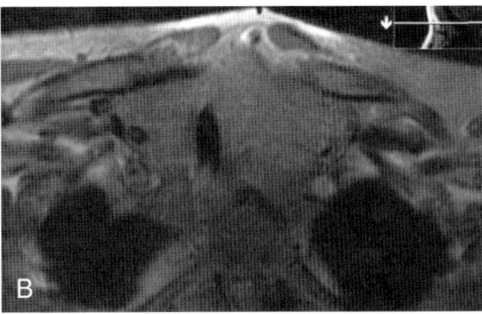

Fig. 37.11 **A** and **B**, Cross-sectional images demonstrate an infiltrative tumor arising in the thyroid gland with both preoperative vocal cord paralysis and Horner's syndrome. The final pathology revealed a B-cell lymphoma.

margins. Release of the inferior constrictor muscle provides the opportunity to lateralize the RLN near its entry point so that the cartilage can be safely resected.[55]

There is little controversy regarding the sacrifice of an RLN in the case of a patient who has an RLN affected by invasive disease in association with an ipsilateral vocal cord paralysis. The challenge comes when a nerve is found to be invaded, but preoperative assessment demonstrates normal vocal fold mobility. Hence there is an imperative to evaluate preoperatively vocal fold mobility in all patients undergoing surgery for thyroid cancer, not only to identify early mobility alterations, with or without hoarseness, but also to document the vocal fold function in the event that the nerve is found to be involved. Falk and McCaffrey evaluated a series of 262 patients with invasive thyroid cancer; the group included a cohort of 123 patients with RLN invasion. A subset of 24 patients was identified with RLN invasion either alone or in conjunction with muscle invasion. The authors had previously reported that muscle invasion did not affect patient prognosis, and thus they were included with this cohort. Five patients with vocal cord paralysis underwent complete excision of the ipsilateral RLN. Of the 19 patients with invaded RLNs but no vocal cord paralysis, 12 underwent complete excision with sacrifice of the nerve, whereas seven underwent incomplete tumor excision without sacrifice of the nerve. In these two groups of patients who underwent either complete or incomplete excision, the follow-up was an average of 19 years. All 24 patients underwent both radioactive iodine therapy as well as thyroid hormone suppression. There was no difference in survival when the RLN was sacrificed as opposed to when it was preserved (N = 17 and 7, respectively). Of note, the only patient in this series who died because of local or regional failure had undergone complete excision of the nerve. The authors concluded that complete excision through sacrifice of the RLN did not affect survival of the patient.[56] Although this study represents an important contribution to intraoperative decision making regarding management of the RLN, a word of caution is required because the number of patients was quite small and the number of patients with disease who demonstrated ^{131}I uptake was not reported. The authors noted the absence of any known recovery of vocal cord function after incomplete tumor excision and preservation of an RLN and treatment with radioactive iodine (RAI) and thyroid suppression.

Nishida et al. performed a retrospective review of 50 patients with normal vocal fold function who had thyroid cancer invading the RLN. Forty-five patients had papillary thyroid cancer, and the remaining 5 had follicular carcinoma. Twenty-seven cancers were deemed to be well differentiated; 23, poorly differentiated. Twenty-three patients formed the treatment group in which the RLN was preserved, whereas the remaining 27 patients underwent RLN sacrifice. These two groups posed significant challenges with respect to the percentage of patients with poorly differentiated cancer: 60% in the resected group and 30% in the preserved group. The incidence of local, regional, and distant recurrence was similar in both groups, leading the authors to conclude that the resection of the nerve to obtain a complete cancer extirpation did not confer any additional survival benefit. The problem with this study is similar to the problem with the Falk and McCaffrey study with respect to the size of the study and the lack of comparability regarding histology.[5]

In 2014, the American Head and Neck Society (AHNS) compiled a consensus statement for management of invasive thyroid carcinoma. In cases of intraoperative RLN encasement by tumor but preoperative normal true vocal fold function or contralateral paralysis or paresis, an attempt should be made to shave the tumor off the RLN while keeping the nerve intact. The society also recommended immediate reinnervation with a branch of the ansa cervicalis, when feasible, in cases where the nerve is sacrificed.

TRACHEAL INVASION

In cases of tracheal invasion, three different options exist for resection. They are dictated by the tumor size, location, and the extent of invasion.

1. *Shave resection* is removal of macroscopic disease from the surface of the trachea without a full thickness resection of the airway.
2. *Window resection* is full thickness resection of a portion of the airway and closure of that window using a variety of techniques. The general rule is that up to one third of the total tracheal circumference can be removed by a window resection without compromising the structural integrity of the airway.
3. *Sleeve resection* is circumferential resection requiring end-to-end anastomosis of the trachea. This is usually necessary when greater than a third of the tracheal circumference is resected.

A variety of reconstructive techniques exist; they depend on the type of resection required for invasive tracheal disease. Shave excisions do not usually require any reconstruction because the structural integrity and mucosal lining of the airway remain intact. Depending on the thickness of the shave excision, rotation of available strap muscle or sternocleidomastoid muscle can sometimes be performed to bolster the mucosa in the cartilaginous defect.

Variations of three techniques are used to reconstruct airway defects after window resection. The first is primary repair of the window defect, which sometimes requires excision of additional portions of the tracheal wall to allow for a tension-free closure. The second is to patch the defect with either an inferior- or superior-based sternocleidomastoid flap (Figure 37.12).

Sleeve resection defects are closed with end-to-end tracheal anastomosis (Figure 37.13). A tension-free, meticulous closure is critical for success of this operation. This can usually be achieved by mobilization of the anterior aspect of the distal trachea. Significant dissection of the lateral aspects of the trachea should be avoided to minimize disruption of the tracheal blood supply and to prevent ischemia. Removal of a shoulder roll and placing the patient's neck in some amount of flexion is another simple method to decrease tension on the anastomosis. Another technique that can be employed is suprahyoid or infrahyoid release of the larynx, which allows further inferior mobilization of the laryngotracheal complex.

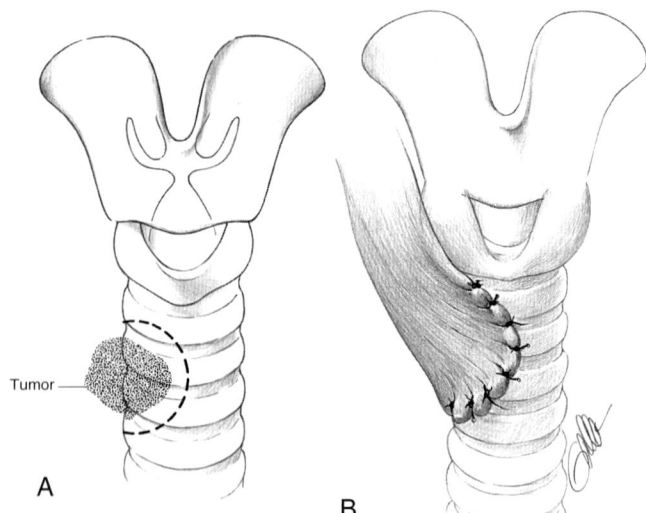

Fig. 37.12 Window resection of the trachea involving less than one third of the circumference with primary repair using a sternocleidomastoid muscle flap to patch the defect.

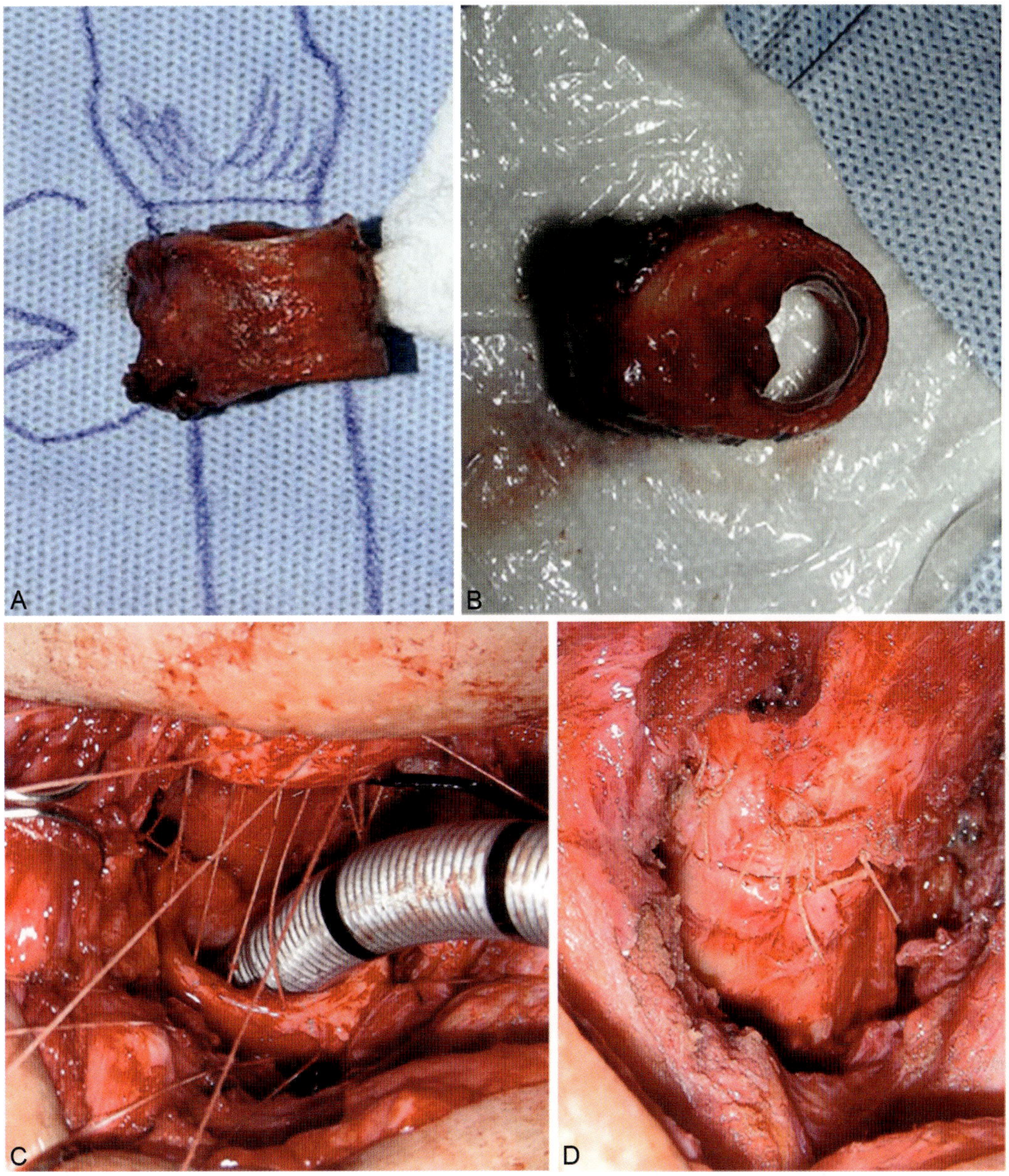

CHAPTER 37 Surgery for Locally Advanced Thyroid Cancer: Larynx, Tracheal Invasion, and Esophageal   367

Fig. 37.13 **A-D,** Sleeve resection of a segment of trachea and end-to-end anastomosis.

Please see the Expert Consult website for more discussion of this topic.

LARYNGEAL INVASION

Lateral Laryngeal Invasion

When there is lateral invasion of the hemilarynx with unilateral paraglottic space invasion, a vertical hemilaryngectomy or frontolateral hemilaryngectomy can be performed[58] (Figure 37.14). The surgical defect can be closed with local soft tissue, regional myocutaneous flaps, or various free flaps, depending on the defect size and the involvement of adjacent structures, such as the hypopharynx. If the unilateral thyroid ala is removed without the underlying soft tissue, then there is no need for reconstructive surgery (Figure 37.15). As demonstrated in the classic hemilaryngectomy for primary vocal cord cancer, reconstruction of the hemilarynx can be achieved with the overlying strap muscles, provided that they can be safely preserved (Figure 37.16).

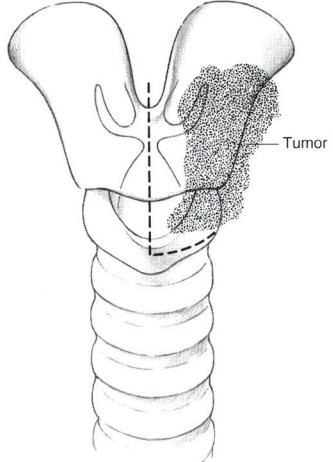

Fig. 37.14 Lateral invasion of the hemilarynx with dotted lines demonstrating the extent of the resection of both the cricoid and thyroid cartilage.

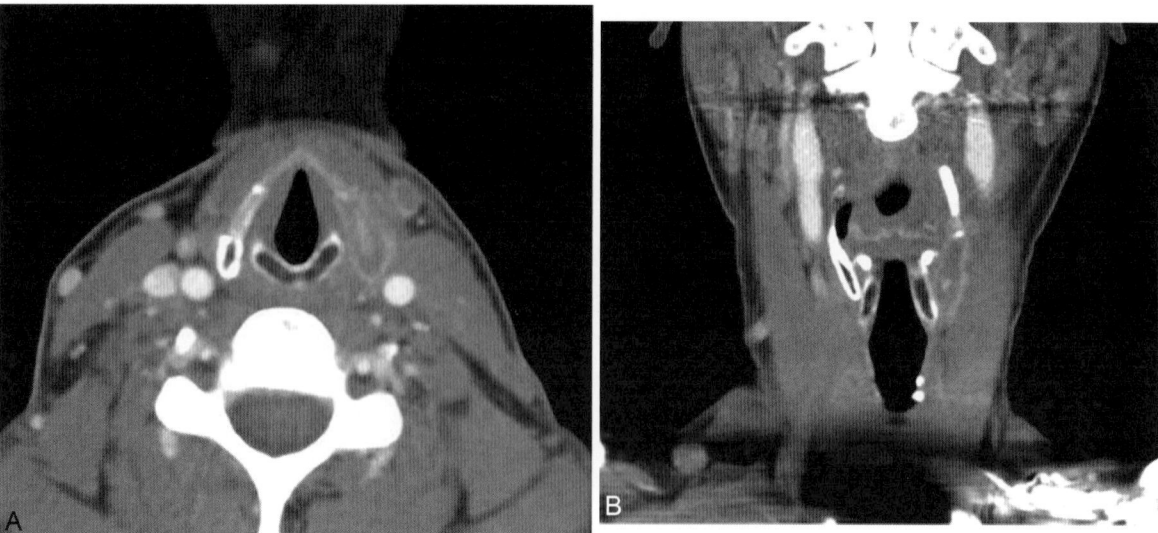

Fig. 37.15 A and **B,** Multiple recurrent thyroid cancer involving the thyroid cartilage. The majority of the left thyroid ala was removed, but no intraluminal invasion was present. No reconstruction was required for the defect.

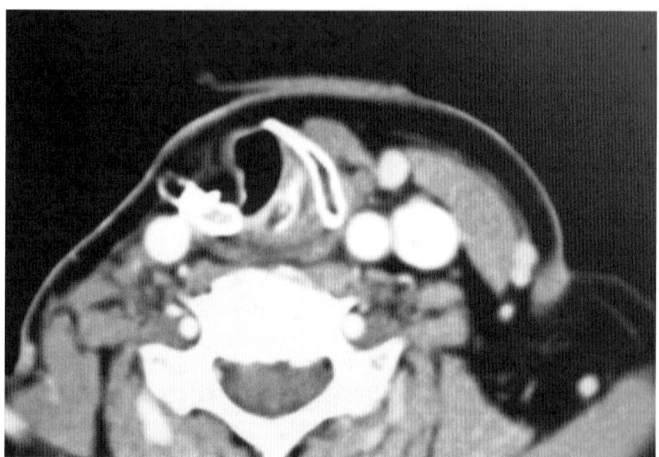

Fig. 37.16 Follow-up computed tomography (CT) image of the larynx in a patient who underwent a hemilaryngectomy for invasive thyroid cancer. Despite the loss of the laryngeal support of the hemilarynx, the airway was maintained.

Urken et al. described their experience in reconstruction of the hemilarynx and pharynx after hemicricoid and hemithyroid cartilage resection using a sensate, radial forearm free flap in combination with a free costal cartilage graft. This approach represents one option in reconstructing these more extensive defects where conventional methods of closure do not apply.[59]

Anterior Laryngeal Invasion

Anterior extension of disease to involve the lumen, although less common, poses a unique challenge because the surgery requires complex and sometimes staged reconstruction if laryngeal preservation surgery is attempted. This can be achieved only if at least one functional RLN is preserved. Most often, when anterior extension is seen, it will involve a significant portion of the cricoid, and often a laryngofissure is required to access the larynx. A staged reconstruction can be achieved in certain circumstances by creating a laryngostome. Initially, this will allow the surgeon to obtain a permanent pathology report before proceeding with definitive reconstruction. Multiple options can then be considered for reconstruction of the anterior wall, including laryngotracheoplasty with cartilage grafts or staged reconstruction with a titanium mesh. The titanium mesh reconstruction involves a three-stage procedure.[57]

The first stage involves the primary resection with the creation of a laryngostome for which healthy skin edges are sutured to the margin of the resected mucosa. The second stage of the reconstruction is performed 3 weeks later; it includes placement of a titanium mesh in a subcutaneous pocket created just adjacent to the laryngostome. The final stage involves raising a thick skin flap incorporating the titanium mesh. This flap is then rotated over the laryngostome to form the anterior laryngeal wall. Surrounding skin is then elevated to close the skin layer over the flap. In circumstances where the cervical skin is insufficient to achieve closure, a deltopectoral flap can be used as well.[60-62] Whenever possible, the ideal reconstruction involves the use of like tissue native to the upper airway, because this provides the combination of mucosal lining and cartilaginous support that is unique to this region and difficult to replicate using available reconstructive methods. Despite the replication of the cartilage and epithelial lining via use of a prefabricated radial forearm flap using implanted costal cartilage grafts implanted into subcutaneous pockets, the transplanted surface is skin, which may be hair bearing and which lacks the unique lubricating and cilial transport properties of native tracheal mucosa.[63]

CRICOID INVASION

When the cricoid cartilage is involved, superficial extension can be managed with shave resection. However, when partial cricoid resection is required due to intraluminal extension, no more than one third of the anterior cartilage can be resected without disrupting stability and putting the patient at significant risk for subglottic stenosis.[16,51,52] Various reconstructive techniques of the cricoid ring have been described. Friedman et al. described the use of a sternocleidomastoid myoperiosteal flap with clavicular periosteum for defects less than 25% in

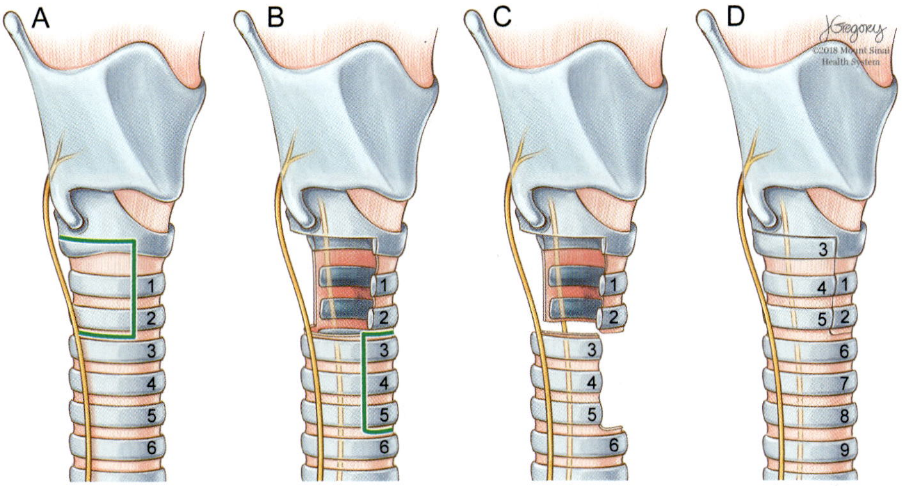

CHAPTER 37 Surgery for Locally Advanced Thyroid Cancer: Larynx, Tracheal Invasion, and Esophageal

Fig. 37.17 A-D, Stair-step reconstructive technique for partial cricotracheal resections. This allows the surgeon to avoid dissection of the contralateral recurrent laryngeal nerve at the level of the cricothyroid joint after ipsilateral RLN sacrifice or significant mobilization. (From Sims JR, Yue LE, Ho RA, Khorsandi AS, Brandwein-Weber M, Urken ML. A rare invasion route for differentiated thyroid carcinoma: the tracheoesophageal common party wall. *Laryngoscope.* 2019;129(12):E455–E459. © Jill Gregory, 2018 Mount Sinai Health System. Printed with permission from © Mount Sinai Health System.)

circumference. If more than one third of the anterior cricoid ring is resected, cartilage grafts may be used for reconstruction similar to those techniques used in laryngotracheoplasties. Sliding tracheoplasty techniques may be used when more than 60% of the anterolateral cricoid cartilage is resected.[64,65] One such technique is a stairstep resection that allows for contralateral RLN dissection to be minimized in cases of unilateral invasion or unilateral focal recurrences (Figure 37.17). Grillo et al. described various tracheal advancement techniques to reconstruct the resected cricoid and infraglottic larynx. Reconstruction of the cricoid cartilage with a vascularized osseous scapular free flap has also been reported.[6,16,66] The fundamental requirement for cricoid cartilage replacement is to provide lining and support. That lining must be well vascularized and thin to maintain luminal dimensions and avoid development of granulation tissue that will compromise the end result. It is rare that the vocal cord itself must be resected; therefore reestablishment of a fixed arytenoid cartilage atop the reconstructed cricoid provides an excellent glottic restoration against which the remaining mobile vocal cord can function. Primary repair through the advancement of trachea may require a laryngeal release to achieve a tension-free repair.[60] It is imperative that the surgeon be mindful of the potential necessity for external beam radiotherapy in the face of less well-differentiated invasive disease that may compromise the functional result that can be achieved in the early postoperative period. Some authors, however, advocate total laryngectomy when more than 50% of the cricoid is resected.[58]

ADVANCED LARYNGEAL INVASION

Total laryngectomy is required when there is significant bilateral intraluminal extension into the larynx and extensive involvement of the cricoid cartilage (Figure 37.18). Some authors advocate a total laryngectomy when more than 50% of the laryngeal framework is involved.[16,62,65,67] A laryngectomy should also be considered in circumstances when bilateral RLN involvement renders the larynx nonfunctional or after locoregional recurrent disease that follows previous resection or radiation.[67] Total laryngectomy defects can most often be closed primarily; however, when there is pharyngeal extension, additional soft tissue should be imported to augment the lumen for functional swallowing and avoidance of stenosis.

Total laryngectomy with partial pharyngectomy defects can be closed with regional myocutaneous flaps or pliable, soft tissue free flaps, such as a radial forearm or an anterolateral thigh flap. When there is a circumferential defect, the pharynx can be reconstructed with free flaps that may include tubed fasciocutaneous flaps, such as radial forearm and anterolateral thigh flaps; alimentary tissue, including jejunal and colonic free flaps; or a gastric pull-up that provides a reconstructive solution for defects that extend to the thoracic esophagus.[68,69] Finally, we routinely create a tracheoesophageal puncture for voice rehabilitation at the time of the initial reconstruction to provide access for placement of a tracheoesophageal speaking valve for alaryngeal speech.

The decision to perform conservation laryngeal surgery as opposed to a total laryngectomy must be balanced against the patient's underlying comorbidities. The loss of one vocal fold as well as the potential loss of laryngeal sensation will predispose many of these patients to airway penetration and frank aspiration. Patients with pulmonary disease and poor pulmonary function will not tolerate chronic aspiration, and they will face an increased risk for aspiration pneumonia. Their overall risk of complications should be carefully weighed against the potential benefits of extended conservation laryngeal surgery that avoids the necessity for a permanent tracheal stoma. Even when partial laryngectomy procedures are employed, temporary tracheostomies are usually required.

ESOPHAGEAL INVASION

Please see the Expert Consult website for discussion of this topic, including Figure 37.19.

370 SECTION 5 Thyroid and Neck Surgery

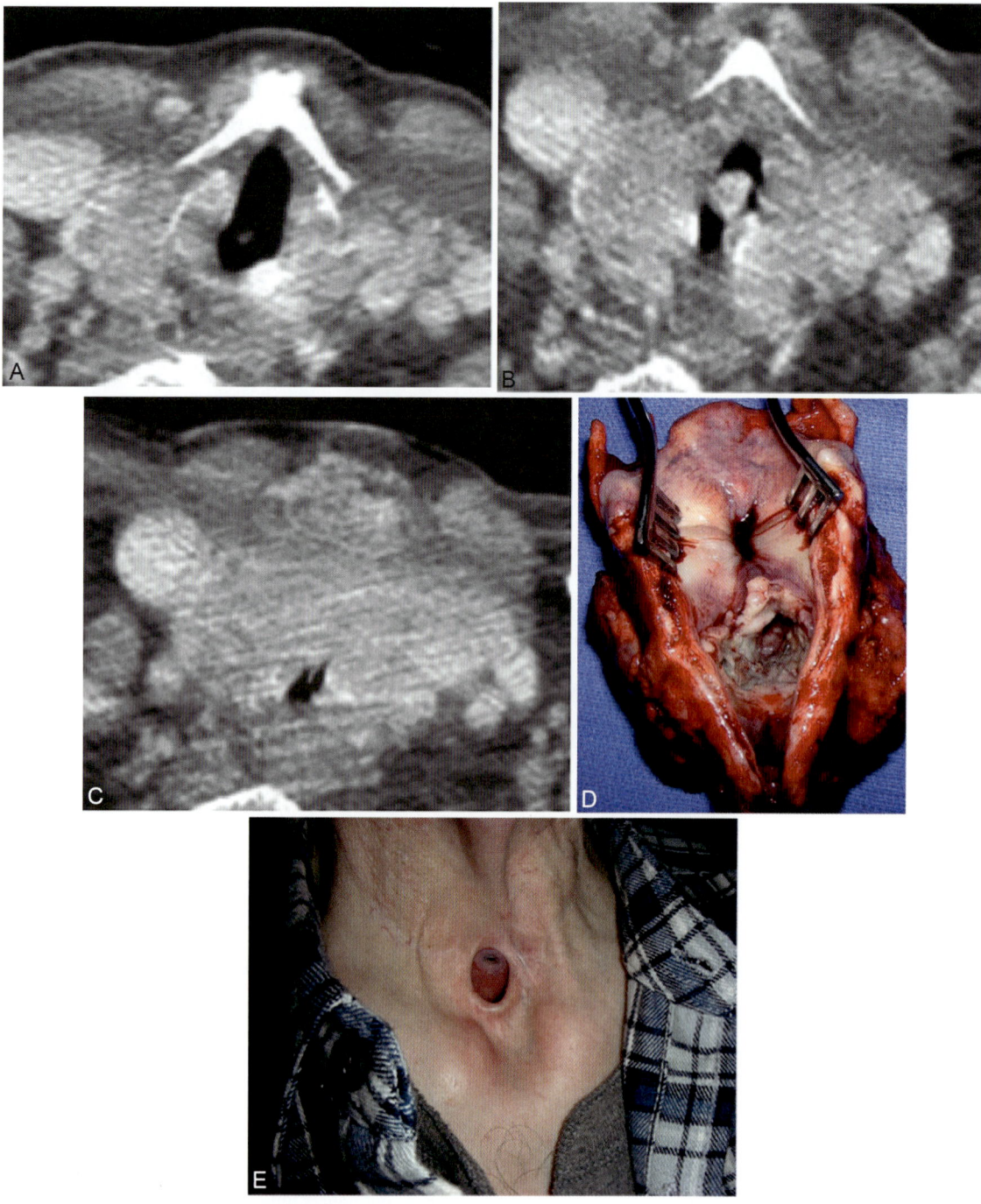

Fig. 37.18 A-C, Computed tomograph (CT) images showing extensive direct invasion of a primary papillary thyroid carcinoma, ultimately requiring a total laryngectomy. **D,** Posterior view of the laryngectomy specimen showing tumor invading directly through the cricoid and thyroid cartilage, extending superiorly to the level of the vocal folds. **E,** Postoperative photo of well-healed laryngectomy stoma. A tracheoesophageal puncture (TEP) was performed at the time of initial surgery.

CONCLUSION

The surgeon's high level of suspicion is the most important element in the management of patients with invasive thyroid cancer; this suspicion allows a low threshold for detailed preoperative radiographic evaluation. The initial management is the optimal time to achieve clear margins and to avoid complications. Understanding the various ablative and restorative surgical techniques is critical to yielding the optimal functional outcomes after tracheal resections and partial or total laryngectomies, with or without removal of the pharyngeal or esophageal wall. It is imperative that surgical training programs provide their trainees with the skill sets to accomplish these goals. As noted in the introduction of this chapter, the rapid increase in early stage thyroid cancer has the negative effect of lulling the unsuspecting surgeon into a state of complacency about performing uncomplicated thyroid surgery. Carefully compiling a patient's history and doing a complete physical and laryngeal exam as well as understanding the biology of recurrent disease, will help prepare the surgeon and importantly, the patient, for the possibility of a more extensive thyroid cancer that requires a more elaborate set of imaging studies and a more involved surgical procedure with the possibility of a prolonged recovery.

REFERENCES

For a full list of references go to expertconsult.com.

38

Central Neck Dissection: Indications and Technique

Alice L. Tang, Lisa M. Reid, Gregory W. Randolph, David L. Steward

> Please go to expertconsult.com to view the related video:
> **Video 38.1** Introduction to Chapter 38, Central Neck Dissection: Indications and Technique.
> **Video 38.2** Central Compartment Dissection.

INTRODUCTION

Central lymph node metastasis is very common in differentiated thyroid cancers, especially in papillary thyroid carcinomas (PTCs). Although therapeutic central neck dissection for cN1a is widely accepted, there continues to be ongoing debate regarding the role of elective/prophylactic central compartment dissection for cN0 necks.[1] In a 2016 meta-analysis that reviewed 37,655 patients with PTC, the incidence of occult metastasis in the central neck (pN1a) in cN0 necks was reported to be 26.4%.[2] Others have reported that occult or micrometastases may be present in up to 90% of well-differentiated thyroid cancer (WDTC).[3,4] This chapter outlines the pertinent surgical anatomy of the central compartment, the indications and ongoing debate for central neck dissection in differentiated thyroid cancer, and detailed surgical technique in performing a safe and comprehensive central neck dissection.

ANATOMY

The first echelon of lymph nodes in metastatic thyroid carcinoma are located in the central compartment of the neck and consists of four major nodal basins: prelaryngeal (Delphian), left paratracheal, right paratracheal, and pretracheal. Beyond these areas, parapharyngeal, retropharyngeal, retroesophageal, and superior mediastinal regions may also rarely be involved. The *central neck* lymph nodes include level VI and VII, which are based on the seven-compartment neck nomenclature; the *lateral neck* includes levels I to V. In level VI, the anatomic boundaries are the hyoid bone (superior), sternal notch (inferior), carotid sheath (laterally on each side), prevertebral fascia (posterior), and the undersurface of the sternothyroid muscle (anterior). Level VII lymph nodes are in the compartment inferior to level VI and are bordered by the innominate (brachiocephalic) artery (Figure 38.1). Inferiorly on the left side, the innominate artery does not extend into the paratracheal region; therefore the corresponding plane of the innominate crossing the trachea on the right defines the inferior border for the left side. Keep in mind that the sternal notch and the innominate artery have a variable relationship with the artery rising above the notch in 25% of cadaveric dissections; thus vigilance for high-riding innominate artery is needed, and variability in the definition and exact extent of the surgically approachable caudal central neck exists.[5] Mediastinal lymphadenopathy that is located caudal to the innominate vein adjacent to the tracheal bifurcation is rare and is significantly associated with poorly differentiated tumors.[6] The central neck and its major compartments are all readily available at primary thyroidectomy surgery.

The recurrent laryngeal nerves (RLNs) ascend the paratracheal spaces in different positions depending on the side of the neck and understanding this anatomy is vital when performing central neck dissections. Because of the different positions of the right subclavian artery and aortic arch relative to the midline trachea, the right RLN ascends the right paratracheal region obliquely extending from inferolateral to superomedial. The left RLN, however, ascends the neck in a more caudal-to-cranial direction in the tracheoesophageal groove. Furthermore, the right RLN is more *ventral* at the base of the paratracheal region than the left because of the relative ventral position of the subclavian artery compared with the aortic arch. Because of this ventral placement of the right RLN, nodes can be hidden deep to the nerve; therefore special attention should be paid in this region to ensure a thorough right paratracheal dissection. The number of nodes in the paratracheal nodal basins range widely from 3 to 30 in number[7] depending on a number of factors, but a central neck dissection specimen is typically associated with an average of eight nodes on pathologic examination[8] (Figure 38.2).

TERMINOLOGY

A multidisciplinary collaborative working group from the American Thyroid Association (ATA) published a consensus statement on central neck dissection terminology and classification for thyroid cancer in 2009.[9] In this statement, emphasis was placed on the importance of using consistent terminology for indications of central neck dissection (i.e., therapeutic versus elective/prophylactic), as well as for use in operative notes and publications. Therapeutic dissection involves removal of nodal metastases identified preoperatively or intraoperatively as containing metastases termed "clinically apparent" (clinically N1). Elective or prophylactic dissection involves removal of lymph nodes that do not appear to contain metastases (clinically N0).

Defining the extent of central neck dissection (i.e., unilateral or bilateral) was also clarified by anatomic terms in the consensus statement.[9] Unilateral central neck dissection involves comprehensive removal of pretracheal and prelaryngeal node-bearing tissue along with unilateral paratracheal node removal. Bilateral dissection includes removal of pretracheal, prelaryngeal, and bilateral paratracheal nodal basins (see Figure 38.1). Importantly, comprehensive central neck dissection, either unilateral or bilateral, is a compartmental dissection and is distinguished from node plucking (i.e., *berry picking*) of only the macroscopically involved nodes. This practice is associated with higher

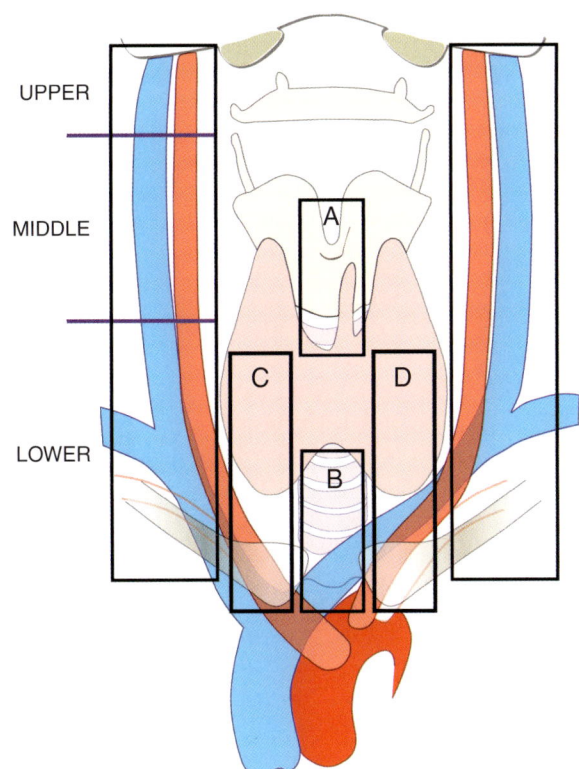

Fig. 38.1 The four major regions that constitute most important nodal-bearing regions within the central neck include prelaryngeal (Delphian) (*A*), pretracheal (*C*), and bilateral paratracheal (*B* and *D*).

However, this surgery results in a high clearance rate of structural disease and should be performed when the benefits are clear. At the time of thyroid surgery for PTC, metastatic lymph nodes often appear to have a dark blue or black appearance. This occasionally can be confused with anthracotic lymph nodes, which may have a similar look, but (upon close inspection) appear to have a powderily, specked, black, particulate, and charcoal-like material within. Frozen pathology at times of uncertainty may be helpful in these instances for surgical decision-making. Further clues to the presence of metastatic disease at the time of surgery include central lymph nodes that are larger than 1 cm; however, size can be considered less reliable in the setting of coexisting thyroiditis, for which frozen section can be helpful.

ELECTIVE/PROPHYLACTIC CENTRAL NECK DISSECTION

The indications for elective/prophylactic central neck dissection are generally (1) to provide accurate pathologic staging to plan adjuvant radioiodine (RAI) therapy; (2) to prophylactically remove occult metastasis to reduce recurrence, morbidity from reoperation, and mortality;[13,14] or (3) if there is a diagnosis of medullary thyroid carcinoma.[15]

Elective central neck dissection can provide accurate pathologic staging to guide the use of adjuvant RAI therapy. Confirmation of cN0 necks through pathologic staging may allow for avoidance of subsequent routine RAI therapy for cNx necks. Further, there may be a role for elective central dissection when used selectively in patients with higher-risk primary tumors, such as those with extrathyroidal extension (T3 or T4) or more aggressive histologies, such as diffuse sclerosing, insular, or poorly differentiated tumors.[2] Oh et al. demonstrated that young age (<40 years) and male sex were more frequently found to have large-volume lymph node metastasis even when preoperative work up revealed a cN0 neck.[16] A consensus report by the European Society of Endocrine Surgeons recommended prophylactic neck dissections for larger tumors (T3 or T4), patients >45 or <15 years of age, male patients, bilateral or multifocal tumors, or known lateral cervical neck disease.[17]

Another indication of elective neck dissection at the time of primary surgery is to decrease recurrence. A recent meta-analysis demonstrated that prophylactic central neck dissection with thyroidectomy appears to significantly lower locoregional recurrence compared with total thyroidectomy alone; this indicates that there may be a benefit in decreasing recurrence with elective central neck dissection.[13] However, small-volume microscopic disease (which are usually found as a result of prophylactic central neck dissections) may have little clinical relevance and electively removing these nodes may subject patients to greater harm than benefit.[10,18] Clear and consistent evidence demonstrates that there exists a higher morbidity when elective neck dissection is performed; specifically, there may be significantly higher rates of transient and permanent hypoparathyroidism.[13,19,20] Transient RLN injury is also seen to be higher in patients who undergo elective neck dissection.[13] Although there may be an increased risk of parathyroid and nerve injury, studies have shown that this surgery can be performed safely by experienced surgeons at high-volume centers, with low morbidity.[21]

Reoperative surgery for recurrent papillary thyroid cancer in the central compartment generally leads to greater morbidity to parathyroid glands and to the RLN compared with initial surgery.[22-24] Performing elective neck dissections could help a subset of patients who would benefit from avoiding the need for reoperative surgery. One study demonstrated that the number of patients needed to be treated with prophylactic central neck dissection to prevent one recurrence is 31.[25] Given that a significant number of patients would need to

rates of recurrence, which brings increased risk of morbidity given the need for reoperative surgery. Thus, when clinically apparent nodes are detected during surgery, a comprehensive central compartment dissection is warranted.

THERAPEUTIC CENTRAL LYMPH NODE DISSECTION

The risk of regional recurrence is higher in patients with palpable lymph node metastasis (cN1).[10] In patients with clinically apparent nodal disease, as evident on clinical examination, preoperative imaging or intraoperative findings, therapeutic central neck dissection (level VI and VII) is well accepted and indicated at the time of thyroidectomy. This comes as a strong recommendation by the 2015 ATA guidelines for management of differentiated thyroid cancer.[11] Therefore vigilance is required pre- and intraoperatively to accurately detect clinically evident nodal metastasis requiring central neck lymphadenectomy. The rationale for therapeutic central neck dissection at the time of thyroidectomy is relatively straightforward—namely to comprehensively remove all grossly evident nodal disease, along with any adjacent subclinical disease; this is done to minimize risk of recurrent/persistent disease and potential morbidity from reoperation for clinically evident disease initially undertreated. Detecting macroscopic disease and operative planning can be achieved by preoperative imaging using high resolution ultrasound (US) or computed tomography (CT) with contrast.[12]

The extent of therapeutic central neck dissection can be either unilateral or bilateral. Bilateral dissection is clearly required and indicated at the time of initial surgery when clinically apparent disease is present in both paratracheal regions. Bilateral central neck dissection definitely increases the risk of hypoparathyroidism and theoretically bilateral recurrent nerve injury resulting in potential airway complications.

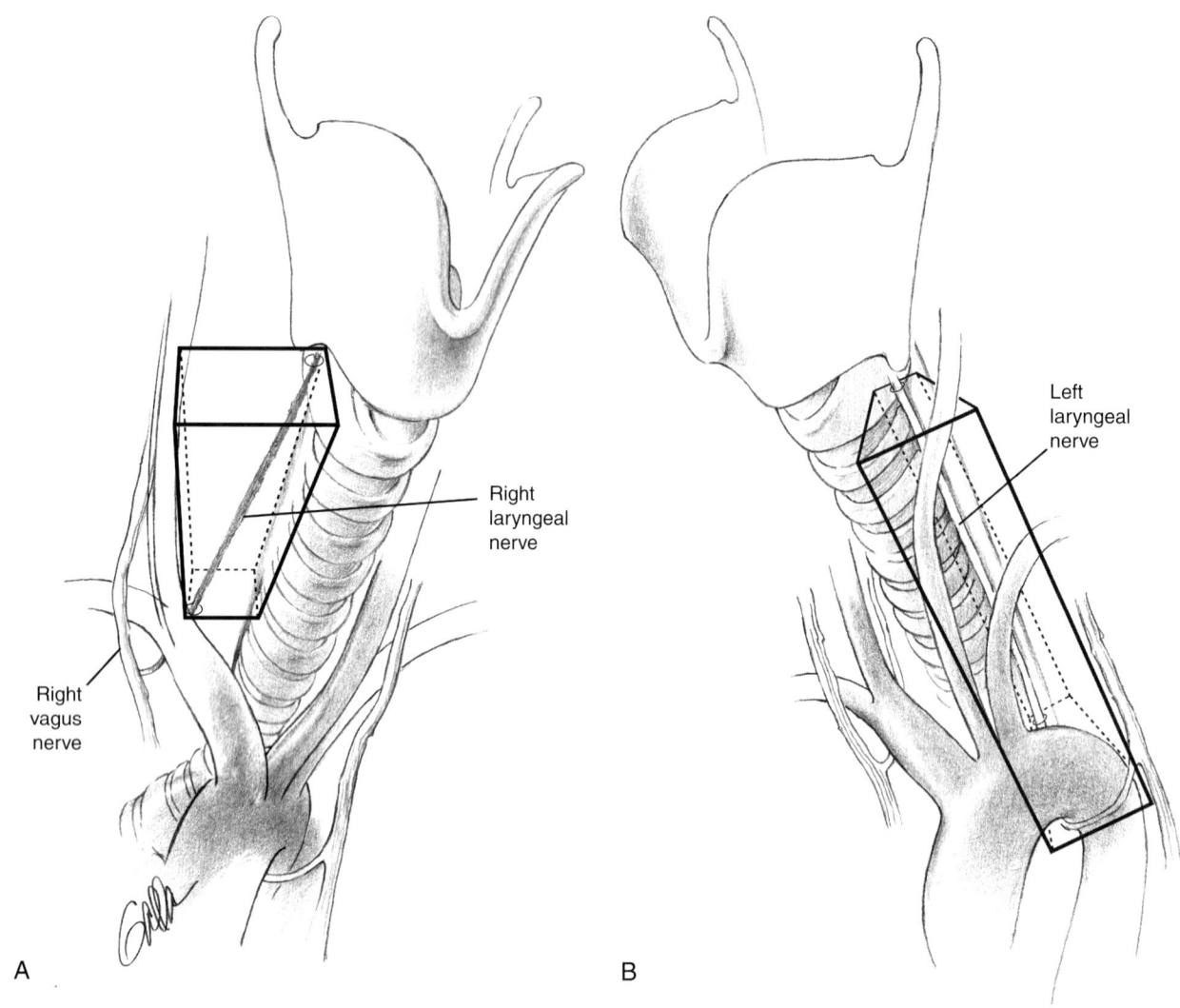

Fig. 38.2 Varying anatomy of the left versus right paratracheal regions. The nodal compartment on the left **(A)** has greater depth because the nerve enters more ventral underneath the bifurcating innominate artery, which lies ventral to the trachea. The right nerve then extends medially and descends to its laryngeal entry point at the right lateral inferior edge of the cricoid cartilage. The right paratracheal region can be divided into two triangles: an upper lateral triangle and a lower medial triangle. The nerve divides the compartment into an anterior and posterior compartment, and nodes may be deep to the right recurrent laryngeal nerve because of this increased depth of the right paratracheal region compared with the left. This may require a 360-degree dissection of the recurrent laryngeal nerve during right paratracheal dissection. The right paratracheal region **(B)** is flatter and more two-dimensional because of the tracheoesophageal groove location typical of the left recurrent laryngeal nerve as it traverses this region.

subjected to unnecessary surgery and that the estimated risk of recurrence in cN0 neck, which are unoperated is around 6%,[26] some practitioners have advocated that it may be better to forego routine prophylactic central neck dissections and refer the small subset of patients that do recur on to experienced centers for reoperative surgery. There is evidence that complication rates at experienced centers are similar when reoperative central neck surgery was compared with initial dissection.[27] Reoperative surgery involves the removal of persistent or recurrent nodal disease in a compartment-oriented fashion as outlined by recent guidelines.[9] Patients may present for surgery with preexisting hypoparathyroidism or RLN injury, which creates additional challenges in the reoperation setting.[28]

Although there is no consensus regarding absolute indications of elective neck dissections, the 2015 ATA guidelines published recommendations. Elective prophylactic dissection should be *considered* in patients with papillary thyroid cancer who have advanced primary tumors (T3 or T4) and/or clinically involved lateral neck nodes (cN1b); elective prophylactic dissection may also be considered if the information will be used in decision-making for adjuvant therapy.[11] A strong recommendation was given for thyroidectomy without prophylactic dissection for small (T1 or T2), noninvasive, cN0 papillary thyroid cancers, and most follicular cancers. If prophylactic dissection is planned, then it should be performed at initial surgical management for thyroid cancer.[11] Revision prophylactic central neck dissection after initial thyroidectomy is strongly discouraged. Similarly, the National Comprehensive Cancer Network (NCCN) also gives a recommendation for consideration of prophylactic neck dissection in the setting of T3 and T4 tumors (category 2B recommendation).

TABLE 38.1	Definition of Regional Lymph Node Staging for Differentiated/Medullary Thyroid Cancer (American Joint Committee on Cancer, 8th Ed)
N Category	N Criteria
NX	Regional lymph nodes cannot be assessed
N0	No evidence of locoregional lymph node metastasis
N0a	≥1 cytologically or histologically confirmed benign lymph node
N0b	No radiologic or clinical evidence of locoregional lymph node metastasis
N1	Metastasis to regional nodes
N1a	Metastasis to level VI or VII (pretracheal, paratracheal, or prelaryngeal/Delphian, or upper mediastinal) lymph nodes. This can be unilateral or bilateral disease
N1b	Metastasis to unilateral, bilateral, or contralateral lateral neck lymph nodes (levels I, II, III, IV, or V) or retropharyngeal lymph nodes

Used with the permission of the American College of Surgeons. Amin MB, Edge SB, Greene FL, et al. (eds.) *AJCC Cancer Staging Manual.* 8th ed. New York: Springer; 2017.

BOX 38.1	Indications for Central Neck Dissection
Therapeutic Central Neck Dissection	Elective/Prophylactic Central Neck Dissection
To remove clinically apparent disease (cN1)	To provide accurate pathologic staging to guide adjuvant therapy
To minimize risk of morbidity from reoperation from initially undertreated disease	To reduce regional recurrence
	To minimize risk of morbidity from reoperation for recurrent/persistent disease
	Medullary thyroid carcinoma

In light of the recently updated guidelines from the ATA, lobectomy/hemi-thyroidectomy is acceptable for tumors up to 4 cm with close surveillance of the contralateral lobe. In this setting, an elective ipsilateral central neck dissection (including ipsilateral paratracheal, pretracheal, and prelaryngeal nodal basins) can also be considered at the time of lobectomy to determine whether a second stage completion thyroidectomy would be necessary to allow for the use of adjuvant RAI treatment in patients who are found to have occult metastasis. Also to be considered, are patients with evidence of high-risk features based on histologic specimen (extranodal extension, ≥5 nodes involved). For patients undergoing total thyroidectomy and elective central neck dissection, unilateral ipsilateral dissection is preferred due to lower risk of hypoparathyroidism, unless the patient has clinical evidence of bilateral paratracheal nodal tumors or possibly multifocal bilateral primary tumors. If clinically detectable nodal metastasis is identified during elective/prophylactic central neck dissection, then conversion to therapeutic dissection is warranted.

Of note, the American Joint Committee on Cancer released its 8th edition on thyroid cancer staging in 2017, updating the classification of staging for differentiated and anaplastic carcinoma to provide optimal separation of disease-specific mortality. In this current edition, patients who have N1 disease and are <55 years old are classified as Stage I; patients who are ≥55 years of age are reclassified as Stage II. The rationale for this change stems from the data that reflect that lymph node metastasis may increase disease-specific mortality in all patients but most significantly in the elderly. Furthermore, the definition of regional lymph node status was refined to include N0a (one or more cytologically or histologically confirmed benign nodes) and N0b (no radiologic or clinical evidence of locoregional lymph node metastasis). Lymph nodes located in the central neck (level VI and VII) are still considered N1a; however, disease in the lateral cervical lymph node chains are N1b (Table 38.1).

SUMMARY OF INDICATIONS

There is little controversy that all clinically apparent nodal disease should be removed at initial operation via a compartment-oriented approach; thus a therapeutic central neck dissection is almost always indicated at time of thyroidectomy in the presence of clinically detectable nodal disease. The key then for the surgeon is to optimize preoperative and intraoperative recognition of nodal metastases so that they may be addressed appropriately at initial surgery.

The indications for elective central neck dissection are relative and more controversial. In general, they include (1) accurate pathologic staging for selective postoperative use of RAI in low-risk primary tumors and (2) prophylactic node dissection in high-risk primary tumors in hopes of reducing recurrence and subsequent morbidity from reoperation. Most surgeries (82%) for thyroid disease in the United States, including surgery for thyroid cancer, are performed by low-volume surgeons who perform as few as one or two thyroid operations per year.[29] Therefore prophylactic central lymph node dissection must be applied in light of available surgical expertise and must balance the risks of the disease and its treatment with any benefit to the patient. Though central lymph node dissection may be associated with higher morbidity, reoperative surgery is potentially more challenging and may create the possibility of further complications. A summary of indications for therapeutic and elective/prophylactic central neck dissections are listed in Box 38.1.

PREOPERATIVE EVALUATION

Surgical planning for management of papillary thyroid cancer involves preoperative evaluation of cervical lymph nodes. Preoperative neck US for cervical lymph nodes is recommended for all patients undergoing thyroidectomy for malignancy[11] and may reduce rates of recurrent or persistent disease by allowing adequate initial surgical treatment.[30] Cervical US is an accurate, noninvasive examination that can be performed by the operating surgeon or by another practitioner with a specific interest in node mapping; the procedure can be done as a part of a patient's initial evaluation and is the primary preoperative imaging modality (Figures 38.3 to 38.5). When used before initial operation, US has an 83.5% sensitivity and 97.7% specificity for nodal metastases[31] and may identify abnormal nodes not found on physical examination in up to 20% of patients.[32] Mazzaglia et al. illustrated the importance of preoperatively performed US by a provider focused on accurate mapping to permit lymph node dissection of the compartment containing the affected nodes.[33] Of note, central neck node detection is hampered by the poor sensitivity of US in the detection of nodes in this compartment when the thyroid is present (often less than 25%) or if the lymph nodes are microscopic.[34,35] Contrast-enhanced neck CT or magnetic resonance imaging (MRI) may be appropriate for the assessment of cervical nodal status as well,

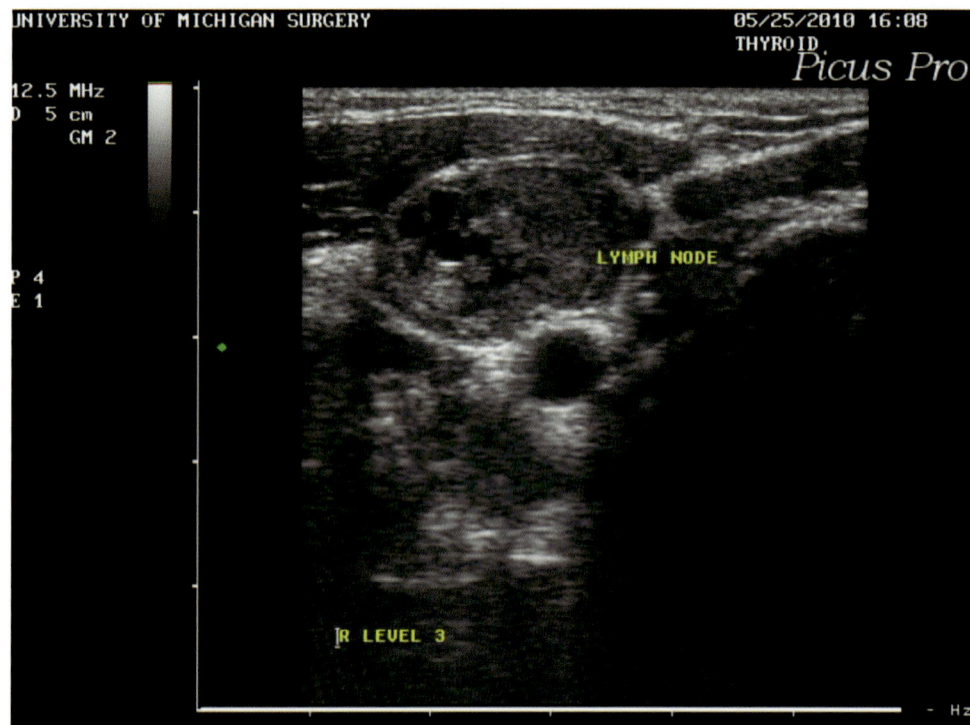

Fig. 38.3 Ultrasound image of level III malignant lymph node with partially cystic appearance.

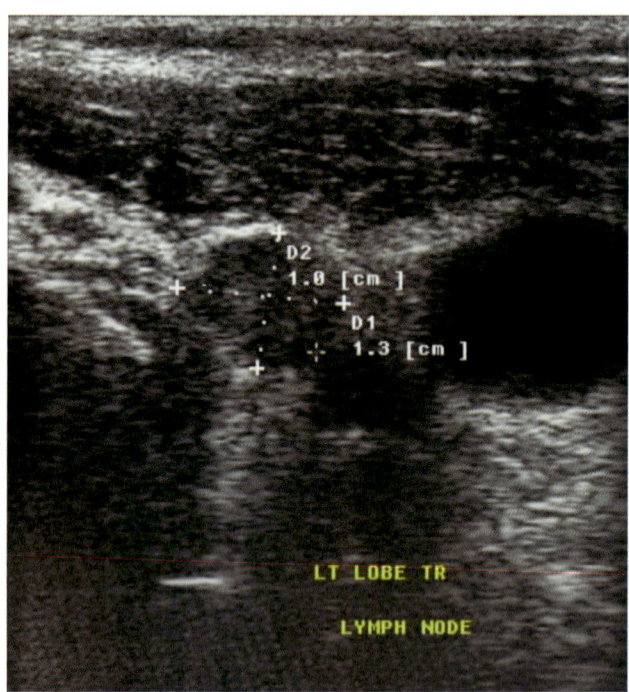

Fig. 38.4 Level 6 paratracheal lymph node.

US features of malignant lymph nodes include hypoechogenicity, hypervascularization, and loss of hilar architecture (hilar stripe) Figure 38.4. Cystic appearance, microcalcifications, absence of a hilum, and peripheral vascularization are considered major US criteria of lymph node malignancy. These findings were based on US done 4 days before surgery and correlated with surgical findings after lymph node dissection.[37]

Beyond imaging, a preoperative laryngeal examination should be performed to assess and document the integrity of the RLN. If the vocal fold is immobile, this may imply previous iatrogenic injury or tumor invasion. One can confidently resect the RLN in this scenario if it is found invaded by the thyroid primary or paratracheal nodal disease; this may enhance the oncologic outcome as long as contralateral nerve function has been determined. A more troubling situation is a scenario where the RLN is working but densely involved with tumor. The nerve may be invaded by the thyroid primary tumor, malignant paratracheal nodal disease, or recurrent thyroid cancer in a lobar remnant. Although most nodes can be carefully dissected from the nerve, the margin may be close. If a lymph node is significantly invading a working RLN, all attempts should be made to preserve the structural and neurophysiologic integrity of it while removing all gross disease as best as possible, especially in the setting of recurrent or persistent disease that is non-iodine avid. The surgeon should always endeavor toward complete gross disease resection. The reality is that the benefits of preserving the nerve must be weighed against the risks of leaving gross disease at this critical area. Observation, RAI, or external beam radiation can be considered in this setting should this be an only functioning nerve.

SURGICAL TECHNIQUE

Regardless of technique, the central neck dissection must incorporate the major regions that are most commonly involved in thyroid cancer: the prelaryngeal, pretracheal, and paratracheal nodal basins. The prelaryngeal compartment can be taken during the dissection of the

especially where experience with neck US for nodal disease is lacking. Kim et al. studied the combination of CT and US compared with US alone for detecting central lymph node metastasis; they found that the combination significantly had better sensitivity (48% versus 28%) and accuracy (69% versus 63%).[36] This objective radiographic map becomes part of the surgical plan and is preoperatively discussed with the patient and the endocrinologist.

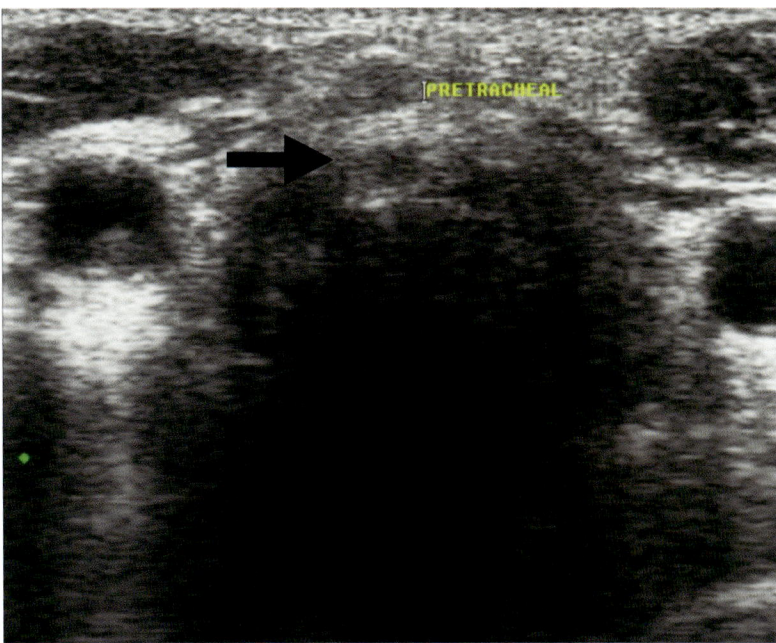

Fig. 38.5 Level 6 pretracheal lymph node.

pyramidal lobe and can be kept intact with the thyroid specimen or sent separately. The pretracheal and paratracheal compartments are generally dissected after completion of the thyroidectomy. The incision for central neck dissection is that of the standard thyroidectomy. Metastatic lymph nodes with extranodal extension strongly adherent to the thyroid should be kept on the specimen for en bloc removal. Skin flaps are raised upward to the level of the thyroid notch and downward to the sternal notch. Once opened, the median raphe of the strap muscles is identified and split vertically from the thyroid notch to the sternal notch. Incomplete opening of this raphe can later hinder exposure of the inferior pretracheal and paratracheal regions. There is some evidence that the use of magnification (loupes) is associated with a lower incidence of inadvertently removed parathyroid glands during thyroidectomy and paratracheal dissection.[38]

Step 1: Prelaryngeal Dissection (Delphian Nodes)

In the prelaryngeal compartment, the fibrofatty tissue containing lymph nodes is anterior to the cricothyroid muscle and extends superiorly to the thyroid cartilage. Soft tissue containing these lymph nodes are usually intimately associated with the pyramidal lobe. The pyramidal lobe can be dissected during this portion of the case and reflected down to be taken with the main thyroid specimen with care to avoid injury to the cricothyroid muscle, cricothyroid membrane, the perichondrium of the thyroid cartilage. The superior limit of this specimen is the hyoid/thyroid notch. Nodal tissue may be residing in the indented cricothyroid membrane, so dissection in the area of the cricothyroid membrane must extend deeply enough to recognize and excise such Delphian nodes.

Step 2: Pretracheal Dissection

Pretracheal dissection begins at the location the inferior extent of the isthmus on the anterior aspect of the trachea. The lower limit of this dissection is the innominate artery and palpating this landmark defines the inferior extent of the dissection. Care is also taken to not injure the vulnerable brachiocephalic vein on the left. If the pretracheal compartment is being performed separately from the paratracheal region, staying pretracheal will avoid injury to the RLNs. It is tempting to extend the dissection laterally; however, this tissue is best removed with the paratracheal dissection when both RLNs are identified and are in plain view.

Step 3: Paratracheal Dissection

During the thyroidectomy portion of the surgery, it is important to identify the parathyroid glands, which are at risk for inadvertent devascularization and/or removal while performing the paratracheal dissection. Superior parathyroids can generally be left in situ along with their vascular supply. The inferior parathyroid glands should be actively searched for and be reflected laterally with the vascular pedicle. Some surgeons advocate marking the inferior glands with clips to help identify and keep in plain view during the dissection; however these clips may result in scatter on subsequent CT or MRI scan assessment of the neck base in these patients. Occasionally, it is not possible to preserve the inferior parathyroid gland during the paratracheal dissection. If this is the case, then the gland should be removed, placed in cool saline, and autotransplanted at the end of the case. Because parathyroid glands can be similar in appearance to lymph nodes, verification with frozen section to protect from accidental implantation of pathologic lymph nodes is recommended. Parathyroid autofluorescence and angiography are new tools to optimally care for and preserve the parathyroid glands and their vascular supply (see Chapter 31, Principles in Thyroid Surgery).

The dissection begins at the cricoid with retrograde RLN dissection. The RLN is identified and must be kept in view during the entire dissection. The nerve is followed until its disappearance under the innominate crossing the trachea, signifying that the lower limit of the dissection has been reached. To help facilitate exposure in the paratracheal region, the trachea is retracted medially to expose the compartment. Nodes that are intimately associated with the RLN should be dissected gently without traction on the nerve itself.

In the right paratracheal resection, the RLN is followed obliquely toward the "corner" where the innominate makes its bend into the carotid artery. Because the subclavian artery crosses ventral to the trachea, this displaces the right nerve ventrally. Fibrofatty tissue is then dissected off the prevertebral fascia and the trachea.

The RLN in the left paratracheal compartment is less complex because the nerve usually traverses the tracheoesophageal groove from the ligamentum arteriosum in a more medial and two-dimensional caudal to cranial direction. The nerve is followed retrograde, but on this side of the neck, an arbitrary horizontal line from where the innominate artery crosses the trachea is used to limit the inferior dissection unless gross disease is evident. The thymus can also be used as a lower limit of dissection. Because the thymus rarely contains metastatic nodes and can have ectopic parathyroid tissue, it is generally left in situ.[39] The RLN should be dissected from the lateral cricoid cartilage inferiorly into the mediastinum below the clavicle. The lymphatic tissue is then dissected off the prevertebral and esophageal musculature and the trachea. Again, retraction of the trachea medially and carotid laterally can facilitate dissection.

BILATERAL PARATRACHEAL DISSECTION

Bilateral paratracheal dissection has the potential for substantial morbidity both in terms of parathyroid and bilateral nerve injury. To help offset these significant issues, one may offer bilateral paratracheal dissection with more aggressive ipsilateral paratracheal dissection; one might even consider sacrificing the inferior parathyroid on that side and performing a less aggressive contralateral paratracheal dissection as long as the pattern of nodal disease would permit this approach. This allows bilateral paratracheal specimens with a less aggressive and hopefully nerve- and parathyroid-preserving dissection in the contralateral paratracheal region. Of course, before the contralateral nerve is dissected, the ipsilateral vagus must be stimulated and shown to be robust in its electromyography (EMG) activity and laryngeal twitch. These imply good, ongoing function, and contralateral dissection should not be met with bilateral cord paralysis. Proximal RLN or vagal stimulation at the completion of one side of surgery for neural prognostication is an important and basic tenet in RLN monitoring.

At the conclusion of the case, the RLN should be checked for integrity by stimulating the nerve proximally or the vagus nerve within the carotid sheath. If autotransplantation of a parathyroid gland is to be performed, a small pocket in the sternocleidomastoid or anterior strap muscle can be made. Meticulous hemostasis is employed with vigilance to the location of the nerves and parathyroid glands. Hemostatic agents can be placed in the paratracheal compartments, particularly near the nerves where bipolar cautery is to be avoided. The remainder of the closure is similar to closure for a thyroidectomy alone. There is substantial and recent evidence including a prospective randomized clinical study suggesting that routine drainage for patients undergoing total thyroidectomy with or without central neck dissection is unnecessary, and that the absence of drains facilitates shorter overall hospital stays.[40,41]

REFERENCES

For a complete list of references, go to expertconsult.com.

39

Lateral Neck Dissection: Indications and Technique

Anastasios Maniakas, Amy Chen, Feng-Yu Chiang, Mark E. Zafereo

> Please go to expertconsult.com to view related video:
> **Video 39.1** Lateral Neck Dissection for Differentiated Thyroid Cancer.

The incidence of thyroid cancer has been increasing over the past few decades, and although the majority of cases are localized to the thyroid, the number of patients with lateral neck disease at first presentation has increased.[1-3] Although there is an abundance of literature on the patterns of metastasis for thyroid carcinoma, there remains some controversy surrounding the extent of neck dissection in patients presenting with suspicious or confirmed metastasis to the lateral neck. There is now more universal agreement that lateral neck dissection for metastatic thyroid cancer should follow principles of compartment-based neck dissection with resection of involved and at-risk neck levels, most commonly a level II through VB selective lateral neck dissection.

This chapter will address the indications and considerations of a lateral neck dissection for thyroid cancer, followed by the surgical approach for an oncologic resection of lateral neck disease. Details on thyroid cancer locoregional metastasis to the central compartment appear in Chapter 38, Central Neck Dissection: Indications and Technique, and postoperative management can be found in the chapters of Section 7.

ANATOMY OF THE NECK

Cervical and superior mediastinal lymph nodes are divided into seven levels delineated by anatomic boundaries (Figure 39.1). Level I, which is rarely involved with thyroid malignancy, includes both submental (level IA) and submandibular (level IB) lymph node groups. Level IA, which comprises the submental triangle, lies between the anterior bellies of bilateral digastric muscles, superior to the hyoid. Level IB is situated posterior to the anterior belly of the digastric muscle, superior to the posterior belly of the digastric muscle, and anterior to the posterior border of the submandibular gland.

Levels II, III, and IV represent the upper, middle, and lower thirds of the jugular chain, respectively, and they comprise the region most commonly involved in thyroid cancer nodal metastasis. Level II is bound by the submandibular gland anteriorly, the posterior border of the sternocleidomastoid muscle posteriorly, the skull base superiorly, and the carotid bifurcation or hyoid bone inferiorly. The spinal accessory nerve divides this level into anterior (level IIA) and posterior (level IIB) compartments. Level IIB is not commonly involved in thyroid cancer. Level III extends from the lateral limit of the sternohyoid muscle to the posterior border of the sternocleidomastoid muscle and from the inferior limits of level II superiorly (i.e., carotid bifurcation or hyoid bone) to the superior limit of level IV inferiorly, as marked by the junction of the omohyoid muscle with the internal jugular vein, or alternatively the cricoid cartilage. Level IV extends from the latter surgical or clinical landmarks superiorly to the clavicle inferiorly. As with level III, this level extends from the lateral border of the sternohyoid muscle to the posterior border of the sternocleidomastoid muscle.

Level V lies posterior to the posterior border of the sternocleidomastoid muscle, anterior to the anterior border of the trapezius muscle, and superior to the clavicle. The cricoid cartilage divides this level into superior (level VA) and inferior (level VB) compartments.

Levels VI and VII constitute the central compartment bounded on both sides by the carotid sheath. Level VI extends from the hyoid bone superiorly to the suprasternal notch inferiorly. Level VII, often referred to as superior mediastinal lymph nodes, extends from the suprasternal notch superiorly to the brachiocephalic vein inferiorly.[4]

In addition to understanding cervical lymphatic anatomy, it is important to know the cervical fascial planes. The superficial cervical fascia contains subcutaneous fat and sheaths the platysma muscle. The deep cervical fascia has three layers: superficial, middle, and deep. The superficial layer of the deep cervical fascia invests the posterior belly of the omohyoid muscle and the sternocleidomastoid and trapezius muscles. The middle layer of the deep cervical fascia envelops the strap muscles forming muscular subdivisions as well as the thyroid, larynx, trachea, and esophagus visceral subdivisions. The deep layer of the deep cervical fascia invests the deep paravertebral muscles of the neck. All three layers of the deep cervical fascia contribute to the carotid sheath.

THYROID GLAND LYMPHATICS

Thyroid gland lymphatics have been subdivided into three groupings. The lymphatics emerging from the inferior-medial aspect of the thyroid lobes follow the course of the inferior thyroid veins and drain to the primary echelon nodes in the pretracheal, paratracheal (also known as central compartment, level VI), and lower jugular and posterior neck regions (levels IV and VB). They drain secondarily into the nodes of the anterior-superior mediastinum (level VII) and less commonly into lower mediastinal nodes. The lymphatics emerging from the lateral aspect of the gland follow the middle thyroid vein and drain into paratracheal lymph nodes, as well as the jugular and posteroinferior lateral neck lymph nodes (levels II, III, IV, and VB). Lastly, the lymphatics from the superior aspect of the gland and the isthmus drain into the paratracheal lymph nodes, as well as the prelaryngeal and jugular lymph nodes, particularly to the midjugular nodes (level III).

Lymph node metastases from thyroid carcinoma tend to occur first in the prelaryngeal, para- and pretracheal nodes regardless of the location of the primary within the thyroid gland.[5,6] In a prospective study using sentinel lymphoscintigraphy in papillary thyroid carcinoma

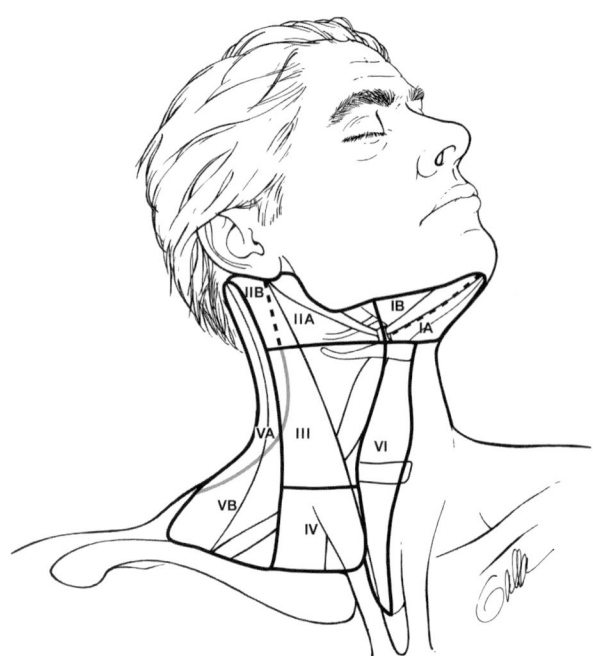

Fig. 39.1 Neck dissection levels.

(PTC), sentinel lymph nodes were located 83% to 88% of the time in level VI.[7,8] This drainage pattern is so reliable that the prelaryngeal lymph node found anterior to the cricothyroid membrane is often referred to as the Delphian node, named after the Greek oracle Delphi, because an enlargement of this lymph node often predicts the presence of thyroid cancer. Although it is safe to consider levels VI (and VII) lymph nodes as the primary echelon of drainage for all thyroid cancers, skip metastases to the nodes of the lateral compartment of the neck can occur in as many as 22% of patients with thyroid cancer.[9,10] Additionally, patients with superior thyroid tumors are at risk for skip metastases to lateral neck lymph nodes, most commonly level III.

This possibility of lateral-neck skip metastases further underlines the importance of rigorous preoperative screening for nodal metastases with preoperative high-definition ultrasound (US), including fine-needle aspiration (FNA) cytology for suspicious lymph nodes. Thyroglobulin washout measurements from lymph node biopsies can add value in cases where cytology is not conclusive. The 2015 American Thyroid Association Differentiated Thyroid Cancer Management Guidelines, hitherto referred to as 2015 ATA DTC [differentiated thyroid cancer] Guidelines, strongly recommended that all patients undergoing any thyroid surgery for malignant or suspicious nodules should have a neck US to evaluate central and especially lateral neck compartments (Recommendation).[11] Furthermore, for DTC, a therapeutic lateral neck dissection should only be considered if biopsy-proven metastatic nodes are found in the lateral neck (Recommendation 37) or if the biopsy-proven positive node is ≥10 mm in the smallest dimension in a previously opeated neck (Recommendation 71).[11] In patients with biopsy-proven lateral neck disease, a computed tomography (CT) scan of the head and neck region with contrast is generally also recommended. A CT with contrast can allow further lymph node mapping of the neck and provide the surgeon with an additional anatomic guide for the location of diseased node(s). Additionally, CT imaging can pick up retropharyngeal lymph nodes and superior mediastinal lymph nodes that cannot be seen on US.

Reported rates of metastases in the lateral neck compartments vary in the literature. Eskander et al.[12] have however demonstrated with their systematic review and meta-analysis that levels III (71%) and IV (66%) had the highest frequency of metastasis, followed in order by levels II (53%) and V (25%). Involvement of lymph nodes in the submandibular triangle (level I) is uncommon, occurring mainly with regionally advanced and/or poorly differentiated disease and with involvement of nodes at other levels of the neck, particularly at level II.[13]

Contralateral lymph node metastases occur in as many as 24% of patients, particularly in those patients with large tumors; those that involve the isthmus; with tumor recurrence[5,14]; or involving level VB lymph nodes.[15] For small unifocal and unilateral primary tumors, the risk of contralateral metastases is low.[16]

RISK FACTORS FOR LYMPH NODE METASTASES

Several important factors in the patient's history and tumor pathology are relevant to the rate of lateral neck metastases, including the patient's age, gender, tumor size, presence of lymphovascular invasion, extrathyroidal extension, and histologic subtype. More specifically, men and younger patients (<45 years old) are associated with significantly higher rates of locoregional metastases than women and older patients.[17] Multifocal disease[15,18] and large tumors (>4 cm)[19,20] in patients with well-differentiated thyroid carcinoma are also associated with increased risk for nodal involvement. Tumors that exhibit extrathyroidal extension or lymphovascular invasion can have more than two-fold or four-fold higher risk of lymph node metastases, respectively.[21-23]

PTC is associated with the highest rate of lymph node metastases, ranging from 40% to 50%, and the mean incidence in children and adolescents is even higher, approximately 80%.[9,24-28] A palpable lymph node metastasis may be the first clinical manifestation of a thyroid carcinoma in up to 30% of patients.[29,30] The follicular variant of papillary carcinoma is associated with a lower risk of lymph node metastases than the conventional papillary variant[31] and even less risk of lymph node metastasis if the tumor is fully encapsulated (see Chapter 23, Noninvasive Follicular Thyroid Neoplasm with Papillary-like Nuclear Features).[32] Follicular carcinoma has a propensity for hematogenous spread and a much lower risk of lymph node metastases (see Chapter 22, Follicular Thyroid Cancer).[33,34] Hürthle cell carcinoma has lower rates of nodal metastases than PTC, but higher than follicular thyroid carcinoma (FTC), occurring in approximately 15% of patients (see Chapter 25, Hürthle Cell Tumors of the Thyroid).[35,36] The tall-cell variant (TCV) of PTC is considered a more aggressive variant, with poor prognosis. Morris et al. undertook a matched-pair analysis, using the Surveillance, Epidemiology, and End Results (SEER) database, and they reported that rates of lymph node metastases of TCV did not significantly differ with conventional PTC.[37]

LYMPH NODE METASIS AND ITS EFFECT ON DISEASE OUTCOME

The presence of lymph node metastasis in thyroid cancer is associated with an increased risk of locoregional recurrence and may be associated with decreased disease-specific survival, as suggested in several large studies.[38-41] Mazzaferri and Jhiang[38] studied 1355 patients with papillary and follicular cancer and followed them for 10 to 30 years. They reported that survival was significantly decreased in patients with lymph node metastases, and certain disease-associated deaths occurred 20 to 30 years after primary treatment. Podnos et al.[42] completed a study of the SEER database in which they analyzed a cohort of 9904 patients with papillary thyroid carcinoma. Lymph node metastases, age >45 years, distant metastasis, and large tumor size were significant predictors of overall survival on multivariate analysis. Overall survival at 14 years was 79% for patients with lymph node metastases and 82% for patients without ($p<0.05$). In a subsequent study of the SEER database, Zaydfudim et al.[43] concluded that cervical lymph node metastases were independently associated with decreased overall survival, specifically in patients with follicular cancer or in patients with papillary cancer older than 45 years. Other studies have shown that the rate of regional recurrence is higher in patients with lymph node metastases, especially in patients with metastases in multiple lymph nodes or with extracapsular spread.[44]

MANAGEMENT OF THE N0 LATERAL NECK IN DIFFERENTIATED THYROID CANCER

In the past, elective lateral neck dissection of levels II to V was considered for thyroid cancer.[45-47] However, this practice is no longer recommended among contemporary high-volume thyroid surgeons for well-differentiated thyroid cancer.[11] Lateral neck compartment dissection should only be performed for well-differentiated thyroid cancer in the presence of clear-cut lateral neck metastases. If there is an ultrasonographically suspicious lymph node in level III, IV, or VB of the lateral neck that remains indeterminate after attempt(s) at FNA biopsy, consideration may be given to excisional biopsy with frozen section evaluation of the lymph node at the time of thyroid surgery, with concurrent compartment-oriented lateral neck dissection if frozen section is positive for metastasis. Some surgeons will offer empiric lateral neck surgery without FNA confirmation based on clear-cut suspicious nodal finding on nodal US and/or CT mapping studies.

MANAGEMENT OF THE N0 LATERAL NECK IN MEDULLARY THYROID CANCER

As described in the 2015 ATA Medullary Thyroid Cancer (MTC) Guidelines, controversy remains with regard to the question of elective lateral neck dissection for MTC.[48] Some surgeons base decision making only on the presence of disease on high-definition US. Others argue that elective ipsilateral lateral neck dissection (i.e., with negative imaging studies) can be pursued in patients with calcitonin levels above 20 pg/mL, and the contralateral lateral neck should be included if calcitonin levels are above 200 pg/mL.[49] One group has recently shown that there was no difference in locoregional disease control rates (98% versus 100%); biochemical cure rates (82% versus 85%); and 5-year overall survival rates (84% versus 100%) in patients having undergone observation versus elective lateral neck dissection.[50] We therefore continue to advocate US-based surgical decision making.

MANAGEMENT OF THE N+ LATERAL NECK

A therapeutic, compartment-oriented lymph node dissection is the mainstay of treatment in patients with clinically obvious and biopsy-proven lymph node metastases. Furthermore, when completed in the hands of highly experienced surgeons with significant thyroid surgery volume, locoregional control rates can be as high as 98%, even in necks that had previous operations.[51] A selective neck dissection levels of IIA, III, IV, and VB is most commonly performed while preserving important vascular structures, such as the carotid artery and internal jugular vein; nervous structures, such as the spinal accessory; hypoglossal, vagus, cervical rootlets, and brachial plexus nerves, and muscular structures, such as the sternocleidomastoid muscle, assuming these structures are free of disease. Preservation of these structures is generally possible and safe because well-differentiated papillary thyroid cancer nodal metastases most often tend to displace rather than infiltrate adjacent structures. This noninvasive nodal front is not always the case in higher-grade thyroid malignancies. In patients with significant extranodal disease extension with clear invasion (as opposed to displacement) of lateral neck structures (usually associated with poorly differentiated histopathology and bulky tumors), sacrifice of nerves, vessels, or muscles may be performed to achieve gross total resection of disease. Levels I, IIB, and VA do not require routine dissection because the rates of thyroid lymph node metastases in these levels are generally less than 5%.[13] Additionally, dissection of level IIB may be associated with higher rates of temporary or permanent shoulder dysfunction due to neuropraxia or injury to the spinal accessory nerve. Studies have shown that level IIB metastases generally occur in patients who also have level IIA metastases,[52] and therefore a reasonable strategy is to do a level IIB dissection only if there are clinically suspicious lymph nodes in level IIB or in the upper portion of level IIA. Similarly, routine dissection of level VA exposes the patient to increased risk of shoulder dysfunction, and it is unnecessary in the absence of clinical or radiological evidence of disease because these lymph nodes rarely harbor thyroid cancer metastases. Level VB lymph nodes, on the other hand, commonly harbor thyroid cancer metastases (approximately 20%), and removal of these lymph nodes does not typically require dissection of the spinal accessory nerve in level V.

RADIOACTIVE IODINE FOR NODAL METASTASES

Although radioactive iodine (RAI) may be effective for subclinical DTC nodal metastases, it should not be used as the primary treatment for clinically or radiographically apparent regional metastases,[27,53,54] and RAI should not substitute for an incomplete lateral neck dissection. If a patient has grossly metastatic DTC nodal disease in the lateral neck after a previous thyroid and/or lateral neck surgery, that patient generally should undergo lateral neck (or revision lateral neck) surgery before consideration for RAI. RAI ablation for patients with DTC thyroid cancer lymph node metastases in the absence of surgery may be considered for patients who cannot undergo surgery (e.g., severe comorbidities, inability to undergo general anesthesia, extreme age, and/or invasive inoperable disease), although such scenarios are very rare. RAI is not effective for medullary thyroid cancer.

TYPES OF NECK DISSECTION

The overwhelmingly most common type of neck dissection for DTC is a selective lateral neck dissection, most commonly levels IIA, III, IV, and VB. Omission of any of these four nodal levels in a selective lateral neck dissection increases likelihood of recurrence and revision surgery, and revision surgery is more challenging and associated with higher complication risk than primary surgery due to the presence of surgical scarring in the neck. Any lymph node level that is dissected should be completely dissected. Lymph node plucking (berry picking) is never recommended because this approach increases likelihood of regional recurrence and creates scar tissue, which makes future revision surgery more challenging. A modified radical neck dissection, rarely necessary for thyroid cancer, involves removing lymph node levels I to V, while preserving one or more of either the spinal accessory nerve, internal jugular vein, or sternocleidomastoid muscle. A radical neck dissection, very rarely necessary for thyroid cancer, includes the resection of the spinal accessory nerve, sternocleidomastoid muscle, and internal jugular vein, along with removal of lymph nodes in levels I to V.

Retropharyngeal and parapharyngeal lymph node metastases are rare in thyroid cancer. Although retropharyngeal nodal metastases

<2 cm may be observed or treated with RAI, larger lymph nodes should generally be removed because they ultimately may lead to such symptoms as dysphagia, hoarseness, pain, and trismus. Surgical excision is usually performed using a transcervical or transoral approach.[55] A thorough understanding of the anatomy of the neck and parapharyngeal space is required to undertake this approach safely.[56] The transoral approach can be performed either by direct excision if accessible,[57] or it can be robotically assisted.[58]

TECHNIQUE

Incision

Providing a cosmetically acceptable incision and ensuring adequate exposure for the intended procedure are important. When it is done with a thyroidectomy, the thyroid incision should be extended to the ipsilateral or bilateral lateral neck; in addition, the incision should be kept as low in the neck as possible and ideally in a natural neck crease. The extension of the incision to the lateral neck is best kept low in the neck (Figure 39.2). In some cases, this posterior vertical limb may need to be extended to the mid neck, but extension of the incision superiorly to the mastoid area is almost never required.

Flap Elevation

Flaps are elevated in the subplatysmal plane, remaining superficial to the anterior and external jugular veins and greater auricular nerve lateral to the platysma edge. At the midline platysmal dehiscence, the depth should approximate the subplatysmal plane. In rare cases where a formal dissection of level V is required, a posterior skin flap is elevated posterior to the sternocleidomastoid muscle in the subcutaneous tissue; great care is necessary to avoid injuring the distal spinal accessory nerve. The inferior flap is routinely elevated to the clavicle.

Level I

Metastases to level I of the neck are exceedingly rare in thyroid cancer; therefore this level is rarely included as part of a neck dissection for thyroid cancer. If there is level I disease, the superficial layer of the deep cervical fascia investing the submandibular gland is incised at its inferior border. One must consider this maneuver as soon as one has raised the flap to the level corresponding to the region of the thyroid cartilage notch cranially. Just superior to this will be the submandibular gland and digastric muscle. At this level, one incises the superficial layer of the deep cervical fascia, extending the dissection deeply to the undersurface of the submandibular gland. The fascia overlying the gland is then swept upward with the ramus mandibularis protected. Elevation of this fascia in a broad front to the mandibular body ensures protection of the marginal mandibular branch of the facial nerve. The facial vessels are then ligated at the level of the mandible, leaving a stump of vessel inferior to the mandible and retracting it over the mandible to protect the marginal mandibular nerve excluding facial lymph nodes (rarely involved with thyroid cancer) from the resection specimen.

Dissection of level IA begins at the medial border of the contralateral anterior belly of the digastric muscle. The fibrofatty lymph node packet of level IA is dissected off of the length of this muscle toward the ipsilateral side, continuing along the underlying mylohyoid muscle, with the hyoid bone serving as the inferior limit of dissection. The surgeon should be thorough and include lymph nodes just deep to the anterior bellies of the digastric muscles. As dissection continues laterally over the anterior belly of the ipsilateral digastric muscle, a small branch of the facial artery may be encountered, requiring ligation. As dissection proceeds over the lateral aspect of the mylohyoid muscle, great care should be taken to include fibrofatty tissue from the apex formed by the junction of the mandible, the mylohyoid muscle, and the anterior belly of the digastric muscle. The neurovascular bundle that pierces the mylohyoid muscle will be encountered, requiring ligation.

Once the lateral border of the mylohyoid muscle is identified, a loop retractor is introduced, retracting the mylohyoid muscle anteriorly. This reveals the lingual nerve with submandibular ganglion, the submandibular gland duct, and the hypoglossal nerve surrounded by its venae comitantes. The submandibular ganglion is ligated, which frees the lingual nerve. Likewise, the duct is ligated. Superiorly, the contents of level IB are dissected off the mandibular ramus in a supraperiosteal plane. Inferiorly, dissection continues posteriorly along the course of the digastric muscle. The facial vein is ligated as it passes over the posterior belly of the digastric muscle. The facial artery is encountered passing under this muscle and is ligated, freeing the contents of level I.

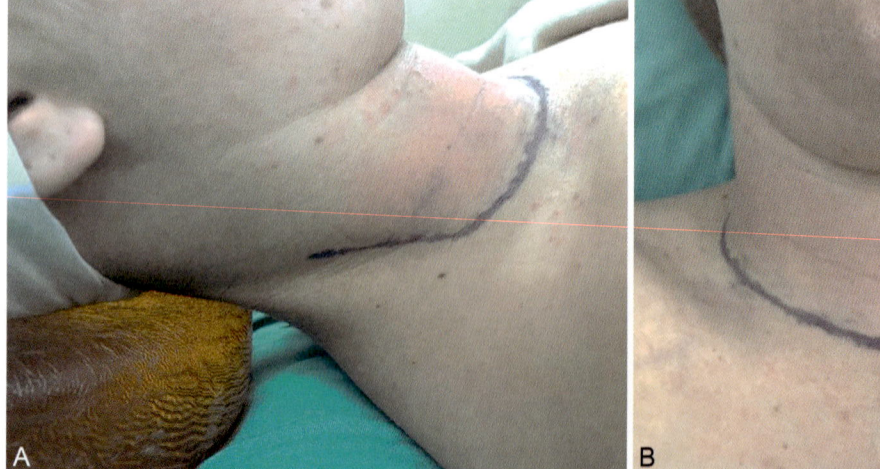

Fig. 39.2 Recommended incision for combined thyroid, central, and left lateral neck dissection with vertical limb placed behind the shadow of the sternocleidomastoid muscle. **A,** From the anterior view, the vertical limb hidden behind the sternocleidomastoid muscle cannot be visualized. **B,** The vertical limb extends about one third of the distance from the clavicle to the mastoid, allowing sufficient exposure of level II of the neck and minimizing the length of the incision.

Levels II, III, and IV

In most cases of thyroid cancer, no need exists to dissect level I, and the dissection is modified to exclude the structures in that level. After elevation of the neck flap, the superficial layer of the deep cervical fascia is incised at the lower border of the submandibular gland. The facial veins at the lower border of the gland may require ligation to permit elevation of the gland and exposure of the posterior belly of the digastric muscle and its tendon. This maneuver will delineate the superior limit of the dissection. The hypoglossal nerve will remain an important landmark to identify and preserve, even when excluding level I in the dissection (Figure 39.3). The superficial layer of the deep cervical fascia investing the sternocleidomastoid muscle is incised at the anterior border of the muscle along its length. The muscle is then unwrapped from its fascial envelope in a medial direction until the spinal accessory nerve is identified. The muscle is retracted posteriorly until the cervical roots are encountered (approximately 4 to 5 cm posterior to the internal jugular vein). Superiorly, the muscle is dissected free of surrounding fibrofatty tissue to the level of the posterior belly of digastric muscle. Just anterior to the spinal accessory nerve, the internal jugular vein is identified and dissected free of fibrofatty tissue on its lateral and posterior surfaces at the level of the digastric muscle. The limits of level IIB dissection are the digastric muscle superiorly, the posterior border of the sternocleidomastoid muscle posteriorly, and the fascia of the splenius capitis muscle medially. Dissection proceeds in an inferomedial direction until the specimen can be safely passed under the spinal accessory nerve, or the level IIB contents can be removed separately. Care should be taken to avoid injury to the occipital artery, which can be of variable caliber and location, and can thus potentially lead to significant bleeding in this area. The occipital artery travels below the posterior belly of the digastric muscle to the occipital region, and it is intimately related to the spinal accessory nerve, internal jugular vein, and vagus nerve (Figure 39.4).

Once the sternocleidomastoid muscle has been freed from its investing fascia, the superficial layer of the deep cervical fascia is then incised at the posterior extent of the sternocleidomastoid muscle retraction. The incision is deepened to the deep layer of the deep cervical fascia, which preserves the underlying cervical roots. Dissection then proceeds anteriorly along the floor of the neck, remaining superficial to the cervical rootlets. The omohyoid muscle may be isolated from surrounding tissue and retracted inferiorly to reach the lymphatics in level IV. If, however, this does not provide adequate exposure, the muscle may be divided. In level IV, dissection remains superficial to the transverse cervical vessels. Although the transverse cervical vessels can be preserved, the adjacent fibrofatty tissue must be included in the clearance of level IV, for these nodes are at risk for containing metastatic disease. Level VB lymph nodes can be resected from an anterior approach pulling these lymph nodes anteriorly and contiguously with level IV lymph nodes. Fibrofatty tissue in the inferior aspect of level IV posterior and immediately lateral to the internal jugular vein is meticulously ligated to avoid leakage from the thoracic duct, most notably on the left, although there are often chylous lymphatics on both sides. The compartment deep to the jugular vein and the common carotid artery must be carefully examined to avoid leaving involved lymph nodes in this area. A common site of surgical failure is metastatic lymph nodes deep to the inferior aspect of the common carotid artery and anterior to the vertebral artery. The phrenic nerve is identifiable beneath the deep layer of the deep cervical fascia overlying the anterior scalene muscle as the internal jugular vein is approached, and it should be left undisturbed. The specimen is then dissected off the lateral and anterior aspects of the internal jugular vein; the surgeon should ligate tributaries when encountered. Superiorly, the hypoglossal nerve is identified medial to the internal jugular vein and preserved. Dissection proceeds anteriorly; as surgeons proceed, they should identify and preserve the ansa cervicalis nerve. Often, surgeons may encounter anterior jugular veins, which require ligation. Figure 39.5 depicts the wound bed after removal of levels II through VB, and Figure 39.6 demonstrates the extent of level VB dissection, which can be achieved from an anterior approach.

If cervical metastases have extracapsular invasion involving the sternocleidomastoid muscle, the spinal accessory nerve, or the internal jugular vein, the surgeon sacrifices these structures during the course of dissection. However, such invasion is rare unless the tumor is high grade.

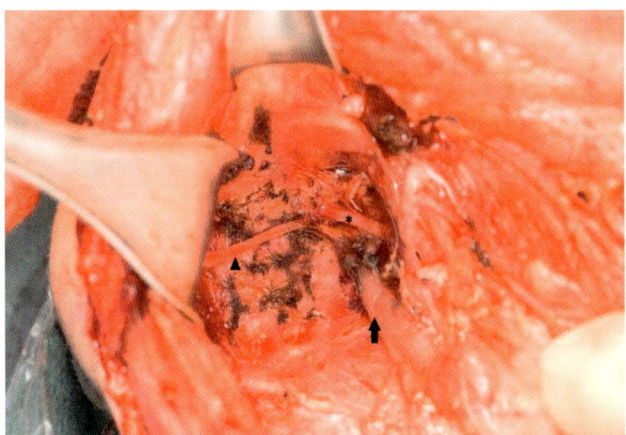

Fig. 39.4 Right neck level IIA and B with visualization of spinal accessory nerve *(arrowhead)*; internal jugular vein *(arrow)*; and occipital artery *(*)*. In this case the level 2B lymph nodes superior to the internal jugular vein have been removed.

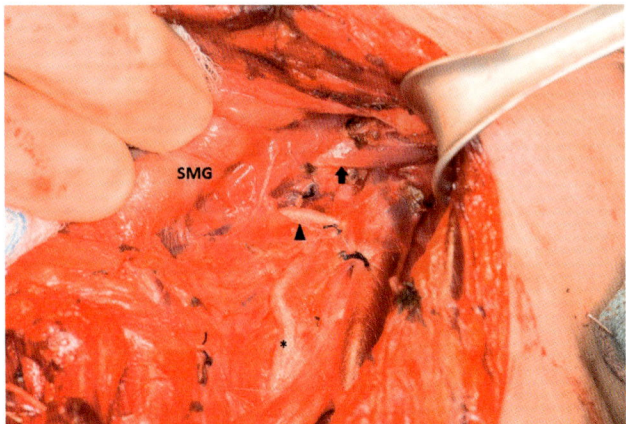

Fig. 39.3 View of dissected left neck with submandibular gland preserved and elevated *(SMG)*; hypoglossal nerve *(arrowhead)*; posterior belly of digastric muscle *(arrow)*; common carotid artery *(*)*; and internal jugular vein lateral to carotid. In the presence of metastatic thyroid cancer, it is important to remove lymph nodes inferior to the hypoglossal nerve (subdigastric lymph nodes) and medial to the internal jugular vein (including lymph nodes along the superior thyroid artery).

Level V

As mentioned in previous sections, formal complete dissection of level V is rarely necessary for thyroid cancer. Level VB lymph nodes are routinely removed from an anterior approach along with level II, III, and IV lymph nodes. However, in rare cases with aggressive histopathology

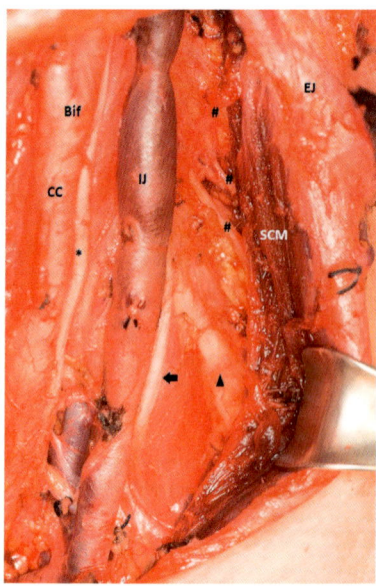

Fig. 39.5 Dissected left neck levels IIA, III, and IV, with visualization of the following key structures from left to right: common carotid artery *(CC)* with bifurcation *(Bif)*; vagus nerve *(*)*; internal jugular vein *(IJ)*; phrenic nerve *(arrow)*; cervical rootlets *(#)*; brachial plexus *(arrowhead)*; and sternocleidomastoid muscle *(SCM)*. The preserved external jugular vein *(EJ)* can also be seen over the sternocleidomastoid muscle. The deep layer of the deep cervical fascia overlying the phrenic nerve, scalene muscles, and brachial plexus is preserved.

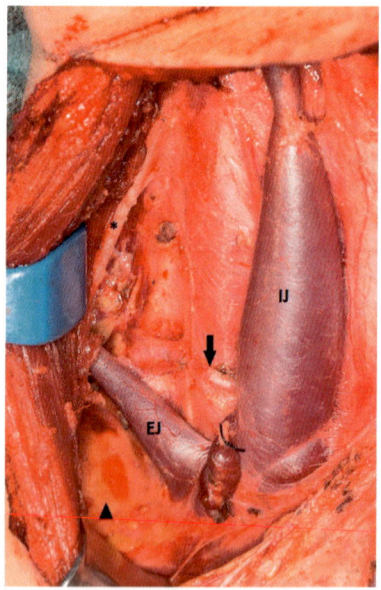

Fig. 39.6 Dissection of the left level VB *(arrowhead)* with visualization of a cervical rootlet *(*)*; transverse cervical artery *(arrow)*; internal jugular vein *(IJ)*; and the external jugular vein *(EJ)*, which in this patient has a direct drainage into the lower portion of the IJ, as opposed to the subclavian vein.

and regionally advanced disease, patients may have level VA metastases, which require a formal dissection of the entirety of level V.

In these cases, the spinal accessory nerve is identified along the posterior border of the sternocleidomastoid muscle, 1 cm superior and deep to Erb's point, i.e., the point where the superficial branches of the cervical plexus—including the greater auricular nerve—emerge from behind the posterior aspect of the sternocleidomastoid muscle. The spinal accessory nerve is then traced posteriorly until it dives under the anterior border of the trapezius muscle. The lateral aspect of the trapezius muscle is then released from the occiput, which allows access to the underlying lymphatics. Dissection proceeds inferiorly from the occiput. The occipital artery is identified and ligated. The deep resection margin is the deep layer of the deep cervical fascia investing the deep neck musculature, and the inferior limit of dissection is the clavicle. Dissection then proceeds medially along the floor of the neck toward the posterior border of the sternocleidomastoid muscle. The brachial plexus under the deep cervical fascia is preserved, and often the transverse cervical vessels can be preserved as well. Some of the cervical rootlets are generally sacrificed if levels VA and VB are formally dissected. However, it is important when dissecting the specimen anteriorly that the dissection is not too deep so that the deep cervical fascia and phrenic nerve are preserved. If a posterior triangle dissection accompanies the dissection of levels II to IV, the procedure may begin with level V dissection. This will keep the resection specimen contiguous.[13]

CLOSURE AND POSTOPERATIVE CARE

Drains have been shown to be unnecessary for most thyroid surgery.[59] In consideration of the extent of dead space, a drain can be placed after a comprehensive lateral neck dissection. Furthermore, if concern exists regarding a potential postoperative chyle leak, a drain should be placed. For a low-volume chyle leak encountered and controlled, a drain may exacerbate a postoperative leak and so may be omitted if it is in the surgeon's best judgment. Bulb suction or Hemovac drains are placed before closure and positioned and secured to drain the inferior-most gutters of dissection. Closure is performed in layers, reapproximating the superficial cervical fascia and platysma before skin closure. Patients generally stay overnight, during which time they are given shoulder exercises assuming level II dissection.

COMPLICATIONS

The complications associated with lateral neck dissection are dependent on the anatomy of the dissected level as discussed earlier in this chapter.

The hypoglossal nerve is at risk not only in a level I dissection, but also as the specimen is dissected off the anterior aspect of the carotid sheath in level II. Injury to this nerve will result in deviation of the tongue with eventual atrophy, which manifests itself as dysphasia and difficulty manipulating food in the oral phase of swallowing. Primary repair, or repair with a greater auricular nerve cable graft, if necessary, should be performed if transection is recognized intraoperatively. Also at risk during a level I dissection is the lingual nerve, which provides sensation to the tongue. Injury manifests as anesthesia of the tongue and, occasionally, a burning sensation.

The marginal mandibular nerve is at risk of injury during the approach to level I. Additionally, it is common for patients to experience some degree of temporary paresis of this nerve from retraction in a level II-VB dissection. Even in a level II-VB dissection, the surgeon should be careful to preserve the fascia immediately below the mandible where the marginal mandibular nerve courses, especially at the level of the mandibular gonial notch, where the marginal mandibular nerve descends to its lowest aspect. The rate of temporary paresis approximates 20%, with permanent paralysis in <1%. Paresis results in asymmetric movement of the mouth and may cause oral incompetence.

The spinal accessory nerve is most at risk for traction injuries, which present as shoulder weakness, particularly when a patient elevates the arm above the horizontal plane. If physical therapy is not initiated, adhesive capsulitis of the glenohumeral joint may result, causing a frozen shoulder. A report of complications resulting from neck dissection performed for thyroid cancer identified a temporary spinal accessory paresis of 27%.[15] The consequence of spinal accessory nerve transection is more pronounced, manifesting itself as a winged scapula. As with the hypoglossal nerve, the surgeon should perform primary repair, or repair with a greater auricular nerve cable graft as necessary, if transection is recognized intraoperatively.

The phrenic nerve lies between the anterior scalene muscle and the overlying deep layer of the deep cervical fascia. Injury to this nerve, which can be prevented by preserving the fascia, can result in up to a 25% reduction in lung capacity. However, most cases of paresis are transient.

The vagus nerve is at risk during dissection of levels II to IV as well as during ligation and transection of the internal jugular vein. The recurrent laryngeal nerve will be affected with any vagus injury, which manifests itself as vocal cord paralysis. If the injury is to the vagus in the superior neck (i.e., high vagal injury), this is coupled with the loss of supraglottic sensation through the superior laryngeal nerve. The dysphonia and dysphagia may be addressed with procedures that medialize the vocal cord; however, significant aspiration resulting from a high vagal injury may require a feeding gastrostomy.

The cervical sympathetic chain can be injured if dissection occurs posteromedial to the carotid sheath. This manifests as Horner's syndrome, typified by anhidrosis, enophthalmus, ptosis, and miosis.

Carotid exposure and rupture are extremely rare. The risk increases in an irradiated neck. The best management entails early recognition of potential carotid injury/exposure and repair, along with the potential placement of a locoregional fascio- or myocutaneous flap.

Hematoma formation can occur and should be promptly assessed and corrected with an open exploration of the surgical bed.

A chylous fistula occurs when branches of the thoracic duct in the left neck or the lymphatic duct in the right neck are interrupted. A higher chyle leak rate is expected as part of the lymph node dissection (LND) due to extensive dissection in level IV in the carotid/vertebral artery basin.[51] Carotid-vertebral lymph nodes must be considered a primary echelon of lateral neck metastasis in thyroid cancer, and therefore this area must be addressed. Intraoperatively, chylous fistula manifests as the pooling of viscous, milky fluid, which is augmented by positive pressure ventilation or the administration of propofol. The source of leaking should be identified and ligated. If the fistula is recognized postoperatively, it usually corresponds with the initiation of enteric feeding. The patient is at risk for infection, electrolyte imbalance, neutropenia, dehydration, and chylothorax. Conservative management entails the initiation of a medium-chain triglyceride diet, possibly supplemented by octreotide administration. If the leak does not respond to these measures, surgical re-exploration or transthoracic ligation of the thoracic duct may be necessary.

REFERENCES

For a complete list of references, go to expertconsult.com.

40

Incisions in Thyroid and Parathyroid Surgery

David J. Terris, Ahmad M. Eltelety

Please go to expertconsult.com to view related video:
Video 40.1 Introduction to Chapter 40, Incisions in Thyroid and Parathyroid Surgery.
This chapter contains additional online-only content, including exclusive video, available on expertconsult.com.

INTRODUCTION

Among endocrine surgeries, thyroidectomy remains a demanding procedure because of the specific patient population, the decreasing surgical morbidity, and increasing patient expectations. Patients now seek safe surgery with preservation of the laryngeal nerves and parathyroid glands, but increasingly, they also express interest in a better cosmetic outcome.[1-4] Thyroid surgical diseases disproportionately affect females more than males and younger individuals more than the elderly. This unequal representation has prompted research to develop more cosmetically favorable incisions. The proliferation of so-called *scarless* in the neck or remote-access approaches justifies the need for a separate chapter devoted to these innovative techniques (see Chapter 32, Robotic and Extra Cervical Approaches to the Thyroid and Parathyroid Glands). Therefore this current chapter will focus on incisions within the visible area of the cervical neck. These incisions will be seen by the public, so the specific characteristics have now been more precisely defined for surgeons than in the past. Length, width, location in the neck, pigmentation, and vascularization are the principal determinants of a scar appearance. Recent evidence demonstrates that patients of every age, gender, and race prefer a shorter and thinner thyroidectomy scar.[5]

Please see the Expert Consult website for more discussion of this topic.

HISTORICAL PERSPECTIVES

Please see the Expert Consult website for more discussion of this topic, including Figures 40.1 and 40.2.

GENERAL PRINCIPLES

Several important principles merit consideration when planning a thyroidectomy or parathyroidectomy, and these transcend the specific procedure that is anticipated.

Individualizing Incisions

The revolution driven by Paolo Miccoli and his team in the past two decades has led to a paradigm shift in consideration given to incision length and access to the thyroid compartment. Before his work, large incisions to access the front of the neck were thought to be uniformly necessary and were therefore completely unchallenged. A quantum shift occurred not only in the size of the incisions, but in our comfort level with the degree of overall access to the thyroid as a result of his seminal work introducing the concept of the minimally invasive video-assisted thyroidectomy (MIVAT). The popularity of this specific technique eventually subsided, and there has been a shift back to the realm of small (rather than very small) incisions.[2] His original disruptive innovations however resulted in nearly all surgeons now making thyroidectomy incisions substantially smaller than they once were without compromising quality and safety. The historic one-size-fits-all practice consisting of a standard length incision in a routine location for all patients no longer represents best practice.[9] The current convention has shifted toward customization of both the incision and the surgery to patients and their disease characteristics in the spirit of patient-centered care and personalized medicine.

Please see the Expert Consult website for more discussion of this topic, including Figures 40.3, 40.4, 40.5, and 40.6.

Location

Perhaps the most important element in optimizing access while maintaining good cosmesis is choosing the proper location for an incision. The fundamental and critical concept of using a skin crease and relaxed skin tension lines persists. It is nearly always preferable to identify and use a preexisting skin crease (if present), for this will result in the most optimally camouflaged scar. One must be cautious that normal creases may (especially in the more lateral portion of the neck) become asymmetric and even V-like in nature, rather than the more symmetric rounded creases of the lower central neck. For standard-length incisions, a good alternate choice, if a normal symmetric crease is unavailable, is a line parallel to a normal skin crease. All existing creases can be mapped to configure an incisional line parallel to a regional crease. The best way to identify the proper crease and overall location is with the patient sitting upright in the preoperative holding area rather than waiting until the patient is lying supine on an operating table (Figure 40.7). This previously identified principle is critically important, and it has emerged as a standard contemporary practice. Deploying the incision in a predetermined skin crease while the patient is in the upright position leads to the most predictable and consistent final scar location.[4] It is in this position that patients will be in public situations, such as dinner parties and cocktail receptions, and it is in this position that the suprasternal notch (and the depression created by the medial heads of the sternocleidomastoid muscle) can best be seen. In this way, the incision can be planned with the patient's input and awareness. New evidence exists that the anterior cervical skin shifts significantly from the upright position to the final surgical position when the patient is supine with a gentle neck extension.[10] Variation in the cranio-caudal incision location can lead to a scar either in an

CHAPTER 40 Incisions in Thyroid and Parathyroid Surgery

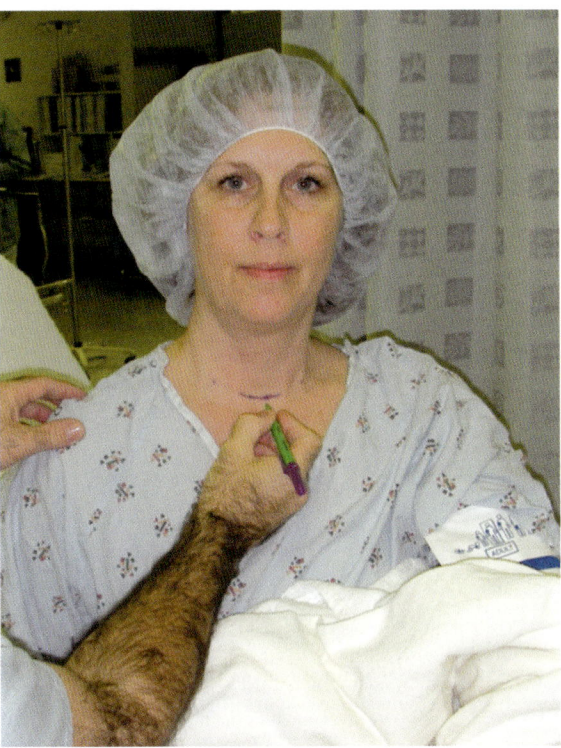

Fig. 40.7 The optimal position in which to mark the anticipated thyroid incision is with the patient seated upright in the holding area.

unfavorable vertical location that is difficult to conceal or to a scar in an area with a high risk of hypertrophic healing. The standard incision is best placed just above the suprasternal notch. Standard incisions placed too low—spanning this indented suprasternal notch region—may appear asymmetric, and they tend to be hypertrophic in their midsegment, unlike incisions placed higher in a more uniform, cylindrical region of the neck. Minimally invasive incisions might be placed in the hollow between the medial heads of the sternocleidomastoid

muscle. Consideration also should be given to breast size, especially in younger women, as over time the incision will be pulled downward if the breasts are large and pendulous. This information may influence the choice of the vertical height of the incision.

Please see the Expert Consult website for more discussion of this topic.

Skin Management

The contribution of the incision to the cosmetic outcome does not end with the making of the incision itself. It is important to minimize the amount of trauma to the skin edge either from retraction or from inadvertent instrument trauma (e.g., electrocautery and ultrasonic energy burns or gauze abrasion). We make every effort to eliminate the use of 4×4 gauze sponges during the operation, as the material is abrasive and behaves like sandpaper when it is placed into and retrieved from small incisions. However, despite careful technique, it is not uncommon to observe skin edges at the end of a procedure (particularly after minimally invasive surgery) that are ischemic and traumatized. Because of the risk of hypertrophic scarring, we recommend resecting a sliver of skin edge whenever and wherever this is recognized (Figure 40.8). This helps ensure proper wound healing in the postoperative period.

Drain Placement

Please see the Expert Consult website for more discussion of this topic, including Figure 40.9.

Skin Closure

Although fine monofilament sutures or staples can result in excellent wound healing and therefore better scars, we prefer to eliminate the risk of "railroad tracking," a particular risk in younger individuals (Figure 40.10). To eliminate the risk, the surgeon must remove the sutures or staples very early, usually on the fourth postoperative day, necessitating an early office visit, something that may be inconvenient for the patient and the surgeon. Although many surgeons advocate subcuticular sutures, it is difficult even in expert hands to accomplish perfect skin apposition with this method. We have found that the application of cyanoacrylate skin adhesives (LiquiBand and Dermaflex are

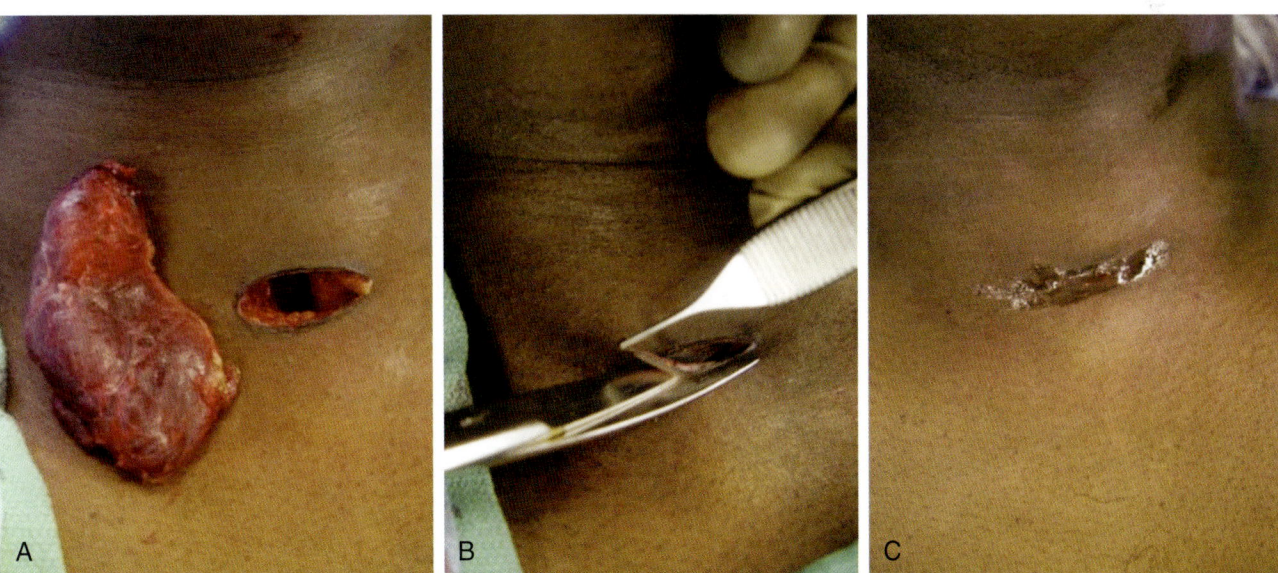

Fig. 40.8 A, When a large thyroid lobe is delivered through small incisions, it is not uncommon to observe evidence of an ischemic or traumatized skin edge. **B,** It is prudent to resect a sliver of skin edge on either or both sides of the incision. **C,** which leads to a more predictable healing result and minimizes the risk of hypertrophic scarring.

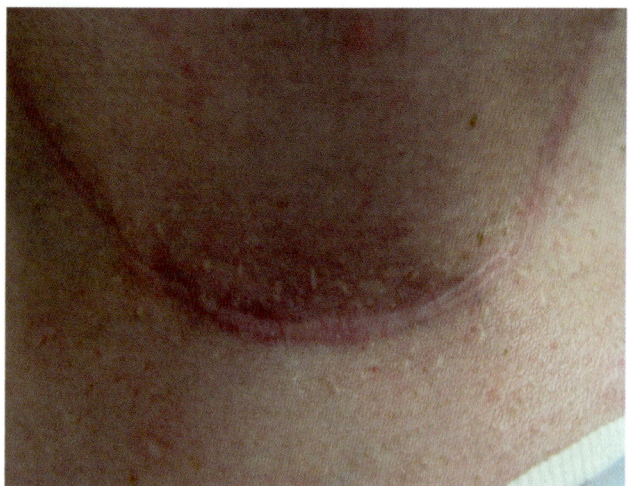

Fig. 40.10 The use of cutaneous sutures incurs the risk of "railroad tracking," which is completely eliminated when a liquid adhesive is used to seal the wound in lieu of sutures.

two suitable choices) is an optimal technique for approximating the skin after one or two subcutaneous absorbable sutures are placed (Figure 40.11, A). We have transitioned from Vicryl to Chromic absorbable sutures because of the lower propensity to extrude. A quarter-inch Steri-Strip placed horizontally on top of the adhesive serves the dual purpose of concealing any trace of blood and facilitating glue removal 3 weeks after surgery (Figure 40.11, B). An important advantage of this type of closure is that the patient does not need to return to the surgeon at a predetermined time for suture removal, making this convenient for both the patient and the surgeon.

SPECIFIC PROCEDURE CONSIDERATIONS
Standard Open Thyroidectomy

Open or conventional thyroidectomy remains a necessary approach in many patients, especially those with thick necks or large, substernal goiters (see Chapter 6, Surgery of Cervical and Substernal Goiter and Chapter 31, Principles in Thyroid Surgery). A 6- to 12-cm incision is placed in a natural skin crease with the specific length determined according to the patient and the disease characteristics. Subplatysmal flap elevation is not necessary; avoiding this step minimizes tissue trauma, the likelihood of both seroma formation, supraincisional flap edema, and the potential for skin to strap muscle tethering (with untoward skin movement with swallowing postoperatively).

Minimally Invasive Thyroidectomy

The most widely practiced version of minimally invasive thyroid surgery is the Miccoli video-assisted technique (see Chapter 34, Minimally Invasive Video-Assisted Thyroidectomy).[2] This method is best learned by high-volume thyroid surgeons,[12] and it has a number of compelling advantages. Incisional considerations for such video-assisted or minimally invasive open thyroidectomy are similar. (For information on non–video-assisted operations, see Chapter 57, Minimally Invasive Single Gland Parathyroid Exploration.) They are both performed through a small central anterior neck incision with no elevation of subplatysmal flaps. The strap muscles are separated in the midline and are retracted laterally to expose the thyroid compartment. The skin edges of these small incisions may suffer intraoperative trauma and stretch retraction-related ischemia. Because of the risk of hypertrophic scarring, we recommend resecting a sliver of skin edge whenever and wherever this is recognized (see Figure 40.8, A and B).

Thyroidectomy With Central Neck Dissection

Please see the Expert Consult website for more discussion of this topic.

Thyroidectomy With Lateral Neck Dissection

Previously, a classical thyroidectomy, when combined with a lateral neck dissection, often involved the use of a cervical collar incision extended up to the mastoid tip with a limb dropped laterally from the incision to the junction of the trapezius and the clavicle, referred to as either a Lahey or Schobinger incision. This would be accomplished on both sides if a bilateral neck dissection were anticipated. Alternatively, McFee incisions were sometimes used, with the advantage that they respect the principles of relaxed skin tension lines and yield improved cosmesis. An additional benefit is the elimination of trifurcated incisions (see Figure 40.2, available on the Expert Consult

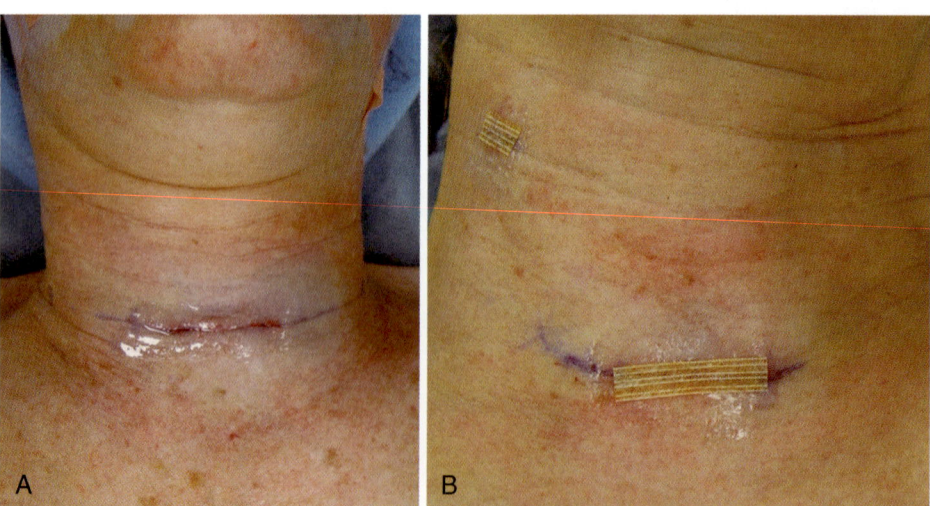

Fig. 40.11 **A,** Skin adhesive is used to seal the incision after placement of one or two subcutaneous absorbable sutures. **B,** A horizontal quarter-inch Steri-Strip serves the dual purpose of concealing the skin edge and providing an easy way to remove the adhesive 2 or 3 weeks after surgery.

website; see Chapter 39, Lateral Neck Dissection: Indications and Technique).

As the approach to the neck has evolved and the need for radical neck dissections has become infrequent, most surgeons now pursue a selective compartmental neck dissection, which can be accomplished through a single extended low cervical collar incision that does not cross the relaxed skin tension lines. Although curving the ends of the incision up toward the mastoid tip facilitates the elevation of flaps superiorly, it is possible to accomplish a thorough neck dissection incorporating levels II through VI by simply extending the incision laterally (Figure 40.12, *A* and *B*). This is the one procedure in which subplatysmal flaps are still routinely elevated to achieve adequate exposure. Drain placement is needed because of the wide-flap elevation required and the potential space created. Closure of the skin may still be accomplished with skin adhesives.

Parathyroidectomy

In cases where preoperative imaging reveals an isolated adenoma (usually via a Sestamibi scan or ultrasound), minimally invasive endoscopic parathyroidectomy may be performed through either a central or lateral incision (see Chapter 56, Standard Bilateral Parathyroid Exploration; Chapter 57, Minimally Invasive Single Gland Parathyroid Exploration; and Chapter 58, Minimally Invasive Video-Assisted Parathyroidectomy). A central incision allows bilateral access in the event the patient has a double adenoma or four-gland hyperplasia that was not anticipated preoperatively. Additionally, thyroidectomy may be more easily performed if the patient is noted to have suspicious thyroid disease. Laterally based parathyroid incisions have largely been abandoned because of increasing recognition of the prevalence of double adenomas in patients with hyperparathyroidism, which are often bilateral superior adenomas. In those cases, and if the abnormal gland is not in the expected location, more than one incision may be required.

Please see the Expert Consult website for more discussion of this topic.

Bilateral Parathyroid Surgery

Please see the Expert Consult website for more discussion of this topic, including Figure 40.13.

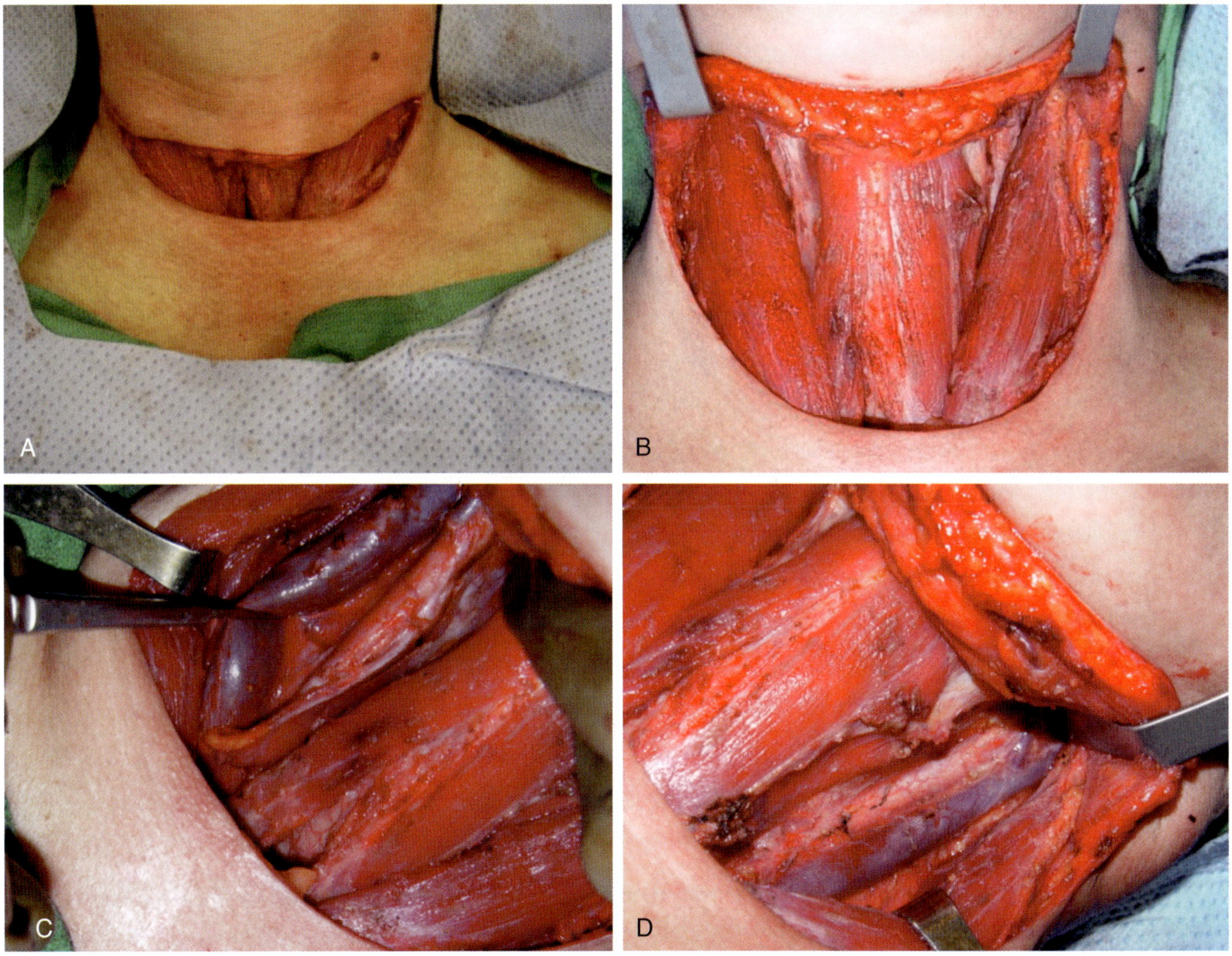

Fig. 40.12 A, An extended low cervical collar incision is used when a lateral neck dissection is indicated. **B,** With wide elevation of subplatysmal flaps, all levels of the neck are accessible. **C** and **D,** Both the right and the left neck may be thoroughly dissected with appropriate retraction assistance.

Novel Approaches

Please see the Expert Consult website for more discussion of this topic.

BEST PRACTICES

The public has become increasingly sophisticated in its acquisition of health care, and patients now demand not only a safe and adequate thyroidectomy but also one that optimizes functional and cosmetic outcomes as well. A number of pertinent cosmetic principles can help optimize the esthetic outcome. These are commonly understood fundamentals in the field of plastic surgery, and their application to thyroid surgery is logical and appropriate. The principles include the following:

- It is recommended to mark the patient's incision while he or she is conversant and upright in the holding area to optimize the location. A central incision assures symmetry.
- When possible, a skin crease should be identified and used to camouflage the incision.
- Drains are largely unnecessary during thyroid and parathyroid surgery with rare exceptions (renal parathyroidectomy and thyroidectomy associated with a lateral neck dissection).
- When a lateral neck dissection is necessary, the low cervical collar incision can simply be extended laterally as necessary to facilitate flap elevation sufficient to reach level II without incorporating limbs that cross relaxed skin tension lines.
- There should be a low threshold for trimming a sliver of skin edge before closure, which minimizes the likelihood of hypertrophic scarring.
- The risk of railroad tracking can be completely eliminated by use of cyanoacrylate skin adhesives, such as LiquiBand or Dermaflex.

REFERENCES

For a complete list of references, go to expertconsult.com.

Surgical Pathology of the Thyroid Gland

Zubair W. Baloch, Virginia A. LiVolsi

INTRODUCTION

Most surgical thyroid disease involves lesions that produce thyroid enlargement—sometimes diffuse but usually nodular. This chapter will discuss lesions of the thyroid that produce nodules. We will describe and discuss the pathologic features of these lesions as well as their differential diagnosis and prognostic features.

All neoplasms that arise from thyroid epithelial cells can have some functional capacities. They may respond to thyroid-stimulating hormone (TSH) and even produce excessive amounts of thyroid hormones, or if medullary carcinoma, they may release abnormal quantities of calcitonin or other peptide hormones.[1,2] Immunohistochemical localization of thyroid transcription factor-1 (TTF-1), thyroglobulin, or calcitonin aids in classifying unusual thyroidal tumors and in providing definite identification of metastatic thyroid carcinomas.[2]

BENIGN NEOPLASMS: ADENOMAS AND ADENOMATOUS NODULES

The definition of a follicular adenoma is controversial. Many pathologists believe that a follicular adenoma is a solitary, encapsulated lesion having a uniform internal architecture that is substantially different from the surrounding thyroidal parenchyma by both growth pattern and cytologic features.[1-4]

However, this definition of adenoma is too restrictive, especially the requirement that the lesion be completely encapsulated. In some instances, it is difficult to separate clearly hyperplastic/adenomatous nodules arising in the background of goiter or thyroiditis from adenomas; up to 70% of the hyperplastic nodules in goiter are clonal, thus representing neoplastic proliferations.[5-7] Therefore we propose that an adenoma should be defined as a follicular-derived and encapsulated (partially or completely) or circumscribed nodule with a distinct growth pattern limited to the confines of its capsule that is different from the surrounding thyroid parenchyma. These follicular lesions are rarely multiple; they arise in a background of a normal thyroid or in the setting of nodular goiter, toxic goiter, or thyroiditis.[8,9]

Grossly, adenomas and nodules are well circumscribed and often demarcated from adjacent tissue. Their size varies from about 1 mm in diameter to several centimeters. A classic adenoma is fleshy and pale; hemorrhage, fibrosis, and cystic change may be evident.[2,3,7] Long-standing lesions, especially in elderly patients, and calcifications (often multiple and centrally located in the lesion) may be seen.

Microscopically, an adenomatous nodule shows a varied pattern of large and small follicles, usually with abundant colloid. The cells range from flat to cuboidal or columnar with small, round nuclei with even chromatin pattern. The stroma of the nodule often appears edematous. Macrophages, lymphocytes, hemosiderin, fibrosis, and even calcification can be found. Cystic change is common, especially in adenomatous nodules, and it may frequently be accompanied by the formation of papillae. Occasionally benign lesions are hyperfunctional, or "hot"; usually this occurs in nodules arising in a multinodular goiter rather than with a classic adenoma. In adolescents, especially females, many of the hot, or toxic, nodules contain numerous papillae, often sufficient in number to cause a pathologist to suggest a diagnosis of papillary carcinoma.[10-12]

In the era of fine-needle aspiration (FNA), some cases of adenomatous nodules and adenomas, especially of oncocytic follicular (Hürthle) cell type, may exhibit prominent post-FNA changes, which include focal hemorrhage, fibrosis, endothelial proliferation, pseudovascular and capsular invasion, and even partial or total infarction.[13-15]

By immunohistochemistry, all adenomatous nodules and adenomas express TTF-1, thyroglobulin, and show cytokeratin expression similar to normal thyroid parenchyma.[16,17]

Several studies have suggested different biologic markers to differentiate between follicular adenoma and carcinoma. Via immunohistochemistry or molecular analysis, these studies have identified differences in expression of p53, PAX8 PPAR-gamma translocation, and RAS mutation in adenomas and carcinomas.[18,19] However, these differences are not sufficient or specific enough to allow definitive diagnosis, and hence one should rely on morphologic criteria alone to differentiate between follicular adenoma and carcinoma.

VARIANTS OF FOLLICULAR ADENOMA

Atypical Follicular Adenoma

The term atypical follicular adenoma refers to follicular lesions that exhibit some atypical features, including foci of necrosis, excess cellularity, mitoses, and lack of capsular and/or vascular invasion. This term has fallen into disuse in thyroid pathology, because many papers describing these lesions indicated incomplete sampling of the tumors, and some carcinomas were probably not identified.[20-22] The recent World Health Organization (WHO) classification includes the terms "Follicular Tumor Of Uncertain Malignant Potential" for encapsulated follicular pattern lesions with irregular tumor capsule interface, incomplete capsular involvement, and foci of mitoses. The great majority of such cases behave as benign adenomas.[23]

Hyalinizing Trabecular Neoplasm of the Thyroid AKA Hyalinizing Trabecular Adenoma (HTA)/Paraganglioma-Like Adenoma of the Thyroid (PLAT)

The hyalinizing trabecular adenoma is a follicular-derived lesion that has a distinctive histology.[24-26] Microscopically, these adenomas grow in nests surrounded by dense hyaline stroma. The histology is reminiscent of that seen in paragangliomas; however, the tumor is derived from the follicular epithelium. The nuclear features of the follicular cells are similar to those seen in papillary carcinoma. Through immunohistochemistry, the cells of hyalinizing trabecular adenoma stain positive for thyroglobulin and cytokeratin 19 and negative for calcitonin, although the presence of other neuroendocrine markers has been described.[27,28]

Recently, some authors propose that these adenomas actually represent a variant of papillary carcinoma.[29] This is due to similar nuclear cytology, immunoprofile, and RET-oncogene rearrangements in both tumors.[30] However, a benign behavior has so far been described in all cases of hyalinizing trabecular adenoma that show classic histology. Because of controversy regarding their nature and clinical behavior, these tumors have been designated as hyalinizing trabecular neoplasm by the WHO classification schema.[23,31]

Signet-Ring Cell Follicular Adenoma

This tumor is characterized by the presence of large vacuoles in the cytoplasm of follicular cells, causing peripheral displacement of the nucleus leading to signet-ring cell formation. A similar morphologic change also may be observed in hyperplastic nodules arising in the background of nodular goiter.[32,33] Rarely, widespread metastasis from an adenocarcinoma with signet-ring cell features can involve thyroid gland. Through immunohistochemistry, it has been shown that these vacuoles contain thyroglobulin, which is biochemically and physiochemically altered; in rare instances, the cytoplasm may also show mucicarmine positivity.[34]

Spindle-Cell Follicular Adenoma

This rare tumor shows a proliferation of spindle cells, which can comprise 1% to 99% of the tumor. The tumor cells are of follicular origin, being both TTF1 and thyroglobulin positive for immunostaining. The major differential diagnoses are medullary carcinoma and anaplastic carcinoma.[35] The immunoreactivity for thyroglobulin and negativity for calcitonin argue against C-cell origin, and the relative blandness of the spindle cells with rare mitotic figures and absence of necrosis and infiltrative growth argues against anaplastic carcinoma.[36]

Lipoadenoma (AKA Adenolipoma)

Some follicular adenomas contain clusters of benign adipose tissue. The edges of the normal thyroid, especially in the posterior aspects of the gland, can show intermingling of follicles and fat cells, so the diagnosis of adenolipoma must be reserved for tumors that lie within the gland and show complete capsules. Rarely may fat cells also be noted in adenomatous nodules in goiter.[2]

MALIGNANT NEOPLASMS

The most common malignant neoplasms that originate in the thyroid are well-differentiated carcinomas of follicular cell origin; most are papillary carcinomas.[2]

Most nonneoplastic diseases of the thyroid are not precursors of malignant diseases; autoimmune thyroiditis is an important exception, and it may predispose a patient to malignant lymphoma.[37,38] Rarely may an adenoma or adenomatous nodule contain a focus of papillary carcinoma.[3,39]

Anaplastic carcinomas can arise in goitrous thyroids, and careful examination of resected tissues may demonstrate benign tumors or well-differentiated carcinomas in close association with the carcinoma. Such findings suggest that the benign tumor or low-grade carcinoma has "transformed" into the anaplastic carcinoma.[40,41]

In modern endocrine practice, the initial approach to thyroid nodules is FNA; this technique can triage lesions, which must be removed surgically. However, about 30% of cases will yield an indeterminate diagnosis (see Chapter 10, The Evaluation and Management of Thyroid Nodules, and Chapter 11, Fine-Needle Aspiration of the Thyroid Gland–The 2017 Bethesda System).[42,43]

Frozen sections can be helpful in papillary cancer, but follicular and Hürthle cell tumors cannot be definitively diagnosed by frozen section.[44-47]

PAPILLARY CARCINOMA

When individuals receive sufficient iodine in their diets, about 80% of thyroid carcinomas are papillary carcinomas.[48] They occur more frequently in women than in men, and they are rarely familial.[43,48-50] In addition, most thyroid cancers in the pediatric population can be classified as papillary cancers.[51] The association of radiation, especially low-dose external radiation in childhood, with the development of adult papillary thyroid cancer is well documented.[52,53]

Grossly, papillary cancers have various sizes and forms. These tumors are predominantly solid, although small cystic foci may be present. Cystic cancers can occur with one or more cystic spaces occupying most of the neoplasm. Bits of calcified material and crystals may be present in the cyst fluid. Papillae may be so numerous that the cut surface appears granular.[2-4,54]

Papillary carcinomas can infiltrate the surrounding gland, and their margins often are poorly defined; however, about 10% to 20% of papillary cancers appear grossly encapsulated.[39] Encapsulation of the primary carcinoma is associated with a lower frequency of lymph node involvement.[2,55,56]

Fibrosis is common in and around papillary carcinomas, and it may be distributed in an extremely irregular fashion, grossly and microscopically. Occasionally, fibrosis is so extensive that almost no neoplastic cells can be found. Nonlamellated calcification is also common.[57-60]

Small papillary carcinomas—microcarcinomas—are defined as 1 cm in diameter or less.[31] The prevalence of these lesions ranges from 6% to 36%, depending on the population studied and how the thyroid was sectioned and examined for pathologic examination. When visible on gross examination, they appear as small, irregular, firm scars; as soft foci of discoloration; or as tiny calcified lesions. Occasionally, the tumor manifests itself as a metastatic focus, usually as an enlarged cervical lymph node; often the node is cystic and clinically mistaken for a branchial cleft cyst. Microscopically, microcarcinomas contain neoplastic follicles or papillae, with the smallest ones showing a predominance of follicular pattern.[61-63] They may be encapsulated or infiltrative.[64]

Histologically, most papillary cancers contain papillae; however, papillae may constitute only a small part of the neoplasm. Papillary cancer may show a solid pattern, may consist of follicles (follicular variant), or may be almost entirely papillary (Figure 41.1, *A*). The papillae contain well-developed fibrovascular cores and are covered with a single layer of the epithelial cells.[2-4,65]

In papillary carcinoma, the epithelial cell is usually cuboidal to low columnar, and it contains a distinctive nucleus. The latter is relatively large and irregular in shape, with folds or grooves, indentations, and cytoplasmic inclusions (Figure 41.1, *B*). The nucleolus is often inconspicuous and eccentric in location, lying near the nuclear membrane.[65,66] The nuclear heterochromatin tends to be concentrated near the nuclear membrane, causing the central portion of the nucleus to appear relatively pale and empty or look like "ground glass."[66,67] When the cells form papillae or follicles, often most of the cytoplasm is concentrated in the apical or basal portions of the cells, thereby causing neighboring nuclei to appear to overlap one another.[68]

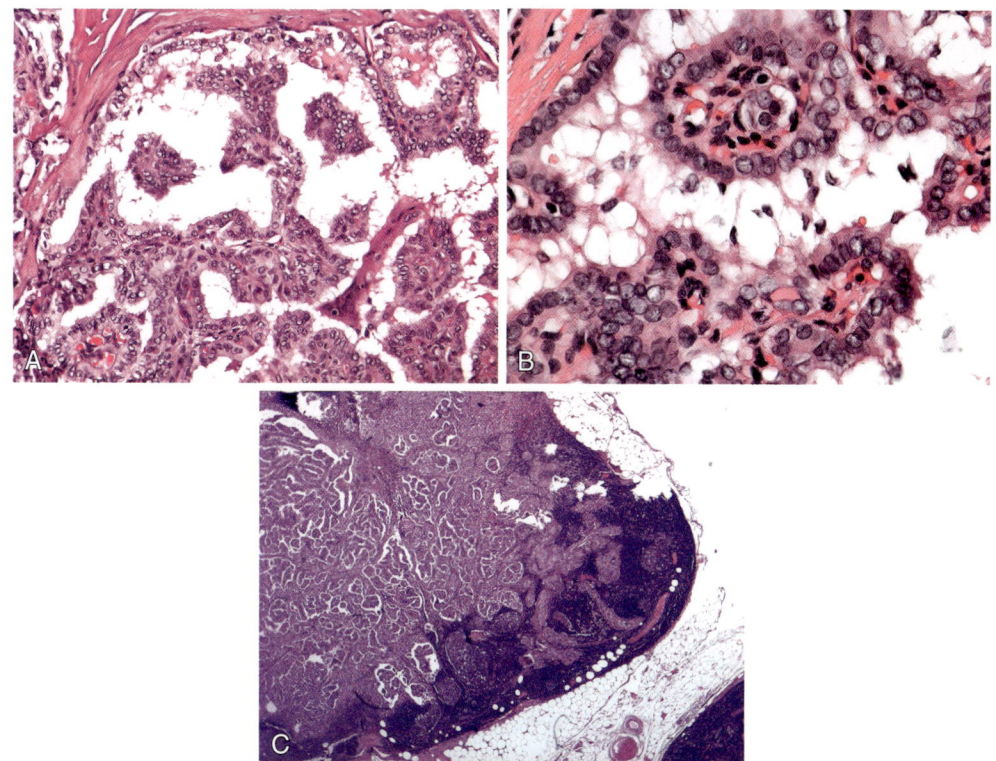

Fig. 41.1 A, Low-power view of classic variant of papillary thyroid carcinoma showing encapsulated tumor with papillary growth pattern. **B,** High-power view showing papillae lined by tumor cells with nuclear features of papillary carcinoma. **C,** Lymph node metastasis from a papillary thyroid carcinoma.

About one third to one half of papillary carcinomas form laminated calcific spherules, known as psammoma bodies. They measure 5 to 100 mm in diameter, appear in stroma or lymphatics, and probably begin in damaged or dying cells of papillary carcinomas. Anytime a psammoma body is found in normal thyroid tissue; cervical lymph nodes (Figure 41.1, C); or perithyroidal soft tissue, a physician should search for papillary thyroid carcinoma.[69,70] Structures resembling psammoma bodies are occasionally found within the colloid of follicles in adenomas or adenomatous nodules, especially those composed of oxyphilic cells, where they seem to arise from calcification of inspissated colloid; these structures should not be equated with psammoma bodies.[71,72]

Lymphocytic infiltration is often present within and around papillary carcinomas.

Multiple intrathyroidal foci of tumors and metastasis to cervical lymph nodes are common and are probably a direct result of lymphatic invasion by tumor.[73,74] Occasionally, cervical nodal enlargement is the presenting sign of metastatic papillary; this is especially found in young males.[75] If a nodal metastasis is cystic, it must be differentiated from a branchial cleft cyst.[76] The nuclear features of papillary carcinoma may not be present in differentiated follicular-patterned metastases.

Blood vessel invasion by papillary carcinoma is uncommon, and metastatic foci in distant sites are unusual (about 5% to 7% of cases), with the lungs most frequently involved.[39,77,78]

VARIANTS OF PAPILLARY CANCER

Follicular variant of papillary thyroid carcinoma (FVPTC) is the most common histologic variant of papillary carcinoma after the usual or classic variant; it is characterized by formation of follicles lined by cells with nuclear features of papillary carcinoma. FVPTC clinically behaves similarly to conventional papillary carcinoma.[64,79,80] At least four distinct variants of FVPTC have been described. The first of these is a tumor that is unencapsulated and infiltrative, thus resembling the growth pattern of classic papillary carcinoma. The difference is that the tumor is totally composed of follicles; these have the appropriate nuclei for the diagnosis of papillary cancer (Figure 41.2). These neoplasms spread and behave as ordinary papillary carcinoma, with multifocal involvement of the gland and lymphatic and nodal metastases. Indeed, in the nodal metastases, a papillary pattern may be found.

The ***diffuse follicular variant*** leads to total replacement of thyroid by tumor. Both lymph node metastases and distant metastases (pulmonary) are common in this variant.[80,81] The *encapsulated variant* usually behaves in indolent fashion. The encapsulated follicular variant refers to the follicular variant, which is characterized by the presence of a capsule around the lesion. These lesions are associated with an excellent prognosis.[55,56] In some cases, the diagnosis of this particular variant of papillary carcinoma can be difficult due to presence of multifocal rather than diffuse distribution of nuclear features of papillary thyroid carcinoma.[7] Because of this peculiar morphologic presentation, these tumors can be misdiagnosed as adenomatoid nodule or follicular adenoma.[7] Some authors have suggested that these tumors be classified as *"tumors of undetermined/uncertain malignant potential"* due to excellent prognosis;[82] however, others have shown that some cases belonging in this category can lead to distant metastasis.[83]

In 2015, a multidisciplinary panel—the Endocrine Pathology Society (EPS) Working Group—including thyroid pathologists, endocrinologists, and endocrine surgeons, was established to address the issues and controversies in the diagnoses of encapsulated and invasive follicular variant of papillary thyroid carcinoma. This panel evaluated a large cohort of FVPTC with clinical follow-up ranging from 10 to 26 years; the evaluation confirmed that noninvasive encapsulated

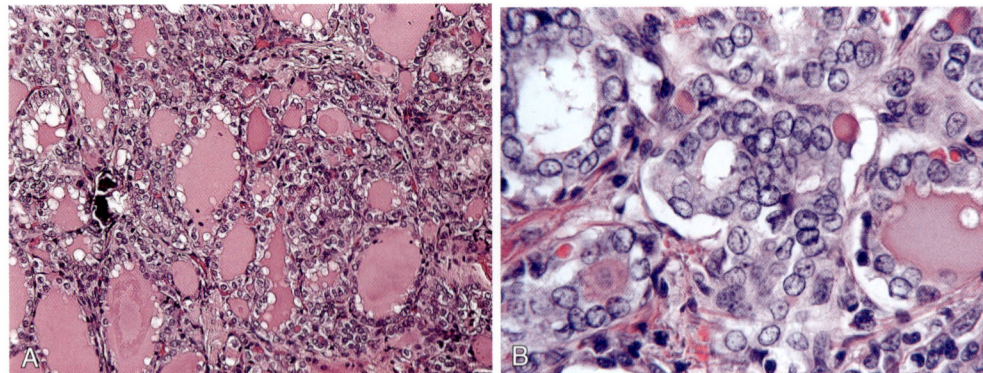

Fig. 41.2 Follicular variant of papillary thyroid carcinoma showing the **(A)** presence of follicles filled with thick colloid **(B)** lined by cells with nuclear features of papillary carcinoma.

FVPTC were free of recurrences and any metastatic involvement.[84] The EPS suggested removing the word "carcinoma" for noninvasive encapsulated FVPTC and renaming it "noninvasive follicular thyroid neoplasm with papillary-like nuclear features" (NIFTP). This entity was defined by a set of histopathologic features, including a noninvasive follicular-patterned neoplasm with nuclear cytology of papillary thyroid carcinoma (PTC), lack of any necrosis, and papillary architecture.[84,85] This new diagnostic paradigm would significantly affect the future classification and management of thyroid neoplasms, but, as can be easily forecasted, would be associated with significant downstream effects on cytologic diagnosis and classification of thyroid nodules as well as on the surgical follow-up of the nodules.[86,87]

An occasional FVPTC can be composed almost entirely of distended, colloid-filled follicles of moderately uniform size and shape, thereby closely resembling the common pattern of an adenomatoid nodule; such tumors are called *macrofollicular variants* of papillary carcinoma. In this variant of FVPTC, rare papillae, an occasional focus of infiltration at the periphery, and the characteristic nuclei confirm the diagnosis.[88,89]

Although FVPTC is a variant of papillary carcinoma (based on cytology and clinical behavior), it does share some morphologic and clinical features with follicular carcinoma. These include follicular growth pattern, encapsulation, capsular and vascular invasion, and distant metastases to lung and bone. Gene expression profiling studies have shown that some cases of FVPTC will show a profile similar to follicular carcinoma.[90,91] Comparative genomic hybridization analysis and *TCGA* analysis showed that the presence and pattern of chromosomal aberration in FVPTC were significantly different from those in classical PTC but more comparable to follicular adenoma and follicular carcinoma.[92] RAS gene mutations, abnormalities seen in follicular adenoma and carcinoma, are exclusively seen in FVPTC and not in classic PTC.[90,93] Similarly, RET gene translocations and BRAF mutations, which are common in classic PTC, are rare in cases of FVPTC.[90,94,95] Therefore in view of morphologic features, clinical behavior, and genetic analysis, it is not unreasonable to hypothesize that FVPTC cases, especially of the encapsulated type, may represent a hybrid of papillary carcinoma and follicular adenoma or carcinoma. What does this hybrid theory mean? If one agrees, then this reclassification would have significant prognostic and therapeutic implications. Encapsulated FVPTC without any capsular and vascular invasion (if the tumor is well sampled) now classified as NIFTP will behave more as a follicular adenoma and the ones with capsular and vascular invasion as follicular carcinoma.

Papillary carcinoma may be largely or exclusively solid and is termed **solid variant**. In young people, it is not known if this pattern may affect the prognosis. In middle-aged and elderly patients, a solid growth pattern may be associated with a loss of differentiation that suggests an aggressive neoplasm. Follicles or papillae may be rare or nonexistent in the primary focus, although they may be present in lymph node metastases.[96]

Rarely PTC involves all lymphatic channels of one lobe or of the entire thyroid and is accompanied by severe lymphocytic thyroiditis with interstitial fibrosis. Psammoma bodies are numerous. A primary mass lesion (epicenter) may not be identified. This **diffuse sclerosis variant** (DSV) occurs more often in young people. It is virtually always accompanied by lymph node metastases, and it often has pulmonary metastases.[97-99] DSV is an unusual histologic variant of PTC.[100] Most reported cases of DSV affect young children and young adults with a reported prevalence of 0.7% to 6.6%. This tumor shows diffuse involvement of one or both lobes of the thyroid gland with extensive calcification and sclerosis.[97,101-104] By light microscopy, DSV-PTC is characterized by classic papillary nuclear features with dense sclerosis, extensive squamous metaplasia, focal to diffuse lymphocytic infiltration, numerous psammoma bodies, and small papillary to solid tumor deposits within intraglandular lymphatics. The background thyroid shows well-developed chronic lymphocytic thyroiditis.[98,99,105]

The **tall cell variant** is an unusual type of papillary carcinoma (about 10%) that appears to be more aggressive than the usual variety (some authors dispute the aggressive behavior of this tumor). The cells in this type are narrow and elongated (three times as long as they are wide), and they often are oncocytic (Figure 41.3, A). These oncocytic tumors often show extrathyroidal soft tissue extension and vascular invasion (20% to 25%). Most occur in older patients, an average of 20 years older than those with usual papillary cancer. A mortality rate of 25% is reported.[106-109] **Columnar cell variant** is a rare tumor composed of clear cells with marked nuclear stratification. Although original reports indicated an aggressive clinical behavior, recent studies of tumors confined within the thyroid indicate a more indolent course.[110-112]

Rarely, a papillary carcinoma is composed of oxyphilic cells (oncocytes, Hürthle cells) and arises in a thyroid altered by lymphocytic thyroiditis. These lesions may show central cystic change. Morphologic resemblance to a benign parotid lesion led to designating this lesion as "**Warthin-like papillary carcinoma.**" This variant appears to have the same spectrum of behavior as the conventional variety[113-115] (Figure 41.3, *B*).

Papillary carcinoma on occasion can demonstrate easily found mitotic figures; enlarged or hyperchromatic nuclei; abnormal DNA content; necrosis; and regions of nondescript neoplastic cells often growing in sheets (loss of differentiation). These characteristics may indicate that more aggressive behavior is likely.[116] These features occur most often in cancers diagnosed in older people and in those tumors that are extrathyroidal.[116,117] **Hobnail variant** of PTC is a rare and

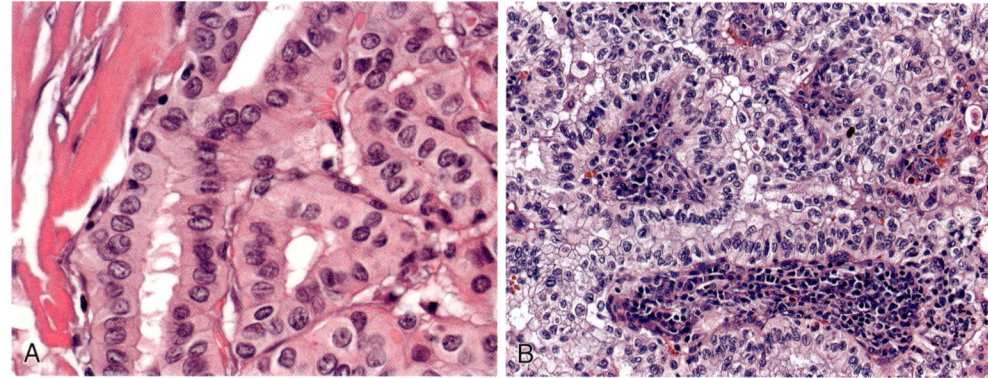

Fig. 41.3 A, High-power view of tall cell variant of papillary thyroid carcinoma showing tumor cell height three times the width. **B,** Warthin-like variant of papillary thyroid carcinoma demonstrating papillary fragments lined by oncocytic tumor cells with nuclear features of papillary carcinoma and lymphoplasmacytic infiltrate in the core *(center)* of the papillae.

clinically aggressive variant of PTC characterized by a micropapillary growth pattern, similar to that encountered in tumors in other biopsy sites: ovary, peritoneum, breast, bladder, kidney, and lung.[118-123]

IMMUNOHISTOCHEMISTRY OF PAPILLARY CARCINOMA

Almost all papillary cancers express TTF-1 and thyroglobulin. Papillary cancers show a different cytokeratin profile than a normal thyroid and other follicular lesions. It has been shown that immunostains for cytokeratin-19 can be helpful in the diagnosis of papillary carcinoma. A mesothelial-derived marker HBME-1 can be expressed in up to 68% of PTCs.[17,124,125] The other antigens studied in papillary cancers include Galectin-3, S-100, neuroendocrine markers, CD44, CD57, CA-125, and more. However, despite these extensive studies, morphology remains the single most important tool for the diagnosis of this tumor.[16,17,124-126] (See Chapter 18, Molecular Pathogenesis of Thyroid Neoplasia.)

FOLLICULAR CARCINOMA

Follicular carcinoma accounts for about 5% or less of all thyroid carcinomas in the United States. It is more common in women than in men, and it occurs more frequently in patients older than 30.[4,127] This tumor is more often found where iodine deficiency occurs.[128,129]

Follicular carcinoma is an expansile neoplasm that is nearly always encapsulated; it grossly resembles follicular adenoma. It presents as a fleshy, solid, encapsulated mass, sometimes with focal fibrosis and calcification. The capsule is usually well developed, but in some examples, extensions beyond the capsule may be noted. Sometimes, invasion of veins can be appreciated in or outside the tumor capsule (Figure 41.4).[4,127,130]

Upon microscopic examination, follicular carcinomas most often have a microfollicular pattern and resemble a cellular follicular adenoma; rarely, the tumor may exhibit a macrofollicular growth pattern. Trabecular or solid patterns are also fairly common. The cells of follicular carcinoma are slightly to moderately larger than those present in most adenomas and adenomatous nodules, but otherwise they are similar. Mitotic figures range from rare to easily identified.[64,127,131]

Follicular carcinomas have been divided traditionally into (1) localized, minimally invasive cancers and (2) more widely invasive cancers.[64,132] Because follicular carcinomas are nearly always encapsulated, the distinction between adenoma and minimally invasive carcinoma may be difficult to ascertain.[7,127] Carcinoma is recognized by its penetration into and through the capsule that surrounds it; by its extension into vessels at its periphery; and (occasionally) by the presence of distant metastasis. Even a minimally invasive carcinoma can present as a metastatic lesion.[133-135] Multiple sections of the periphery of the neoplasm may be necessary to find the invasion, although most follicular cancers will be diagnosed on examination of 10 different

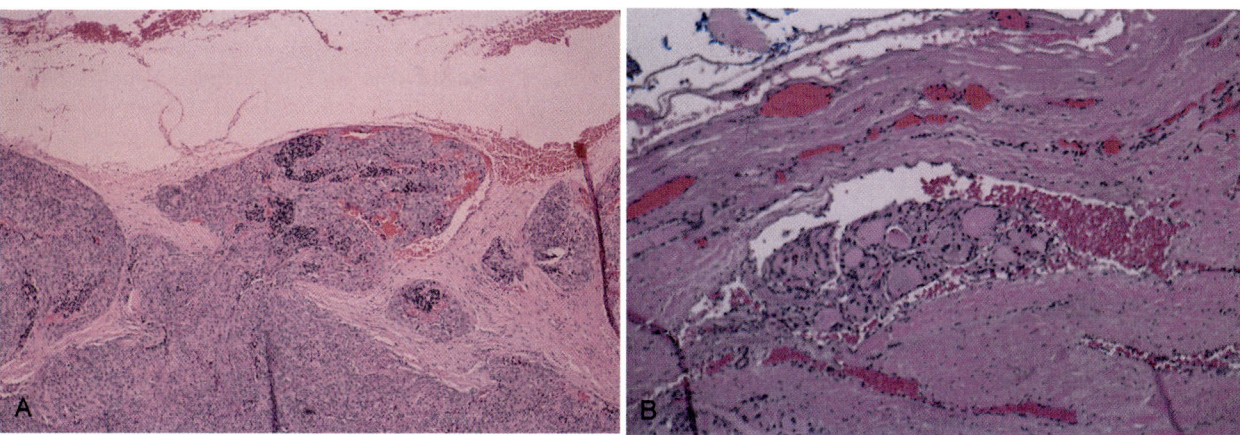

Fig. 41.4 A case of follicular thyroid carcinoma showing thickly encapsulated tumor with **(A)** multiple foci of tumor invasion into the tumor capsule and **(B)** into a capsular vessel.

sections of the capsule-tumor interface. Whether the number of invaded veins can be correlated with outcome is unclear.[127,136,137]

In our practice we divide follicular carcinomas into the following:
- Lesions that penetrate or invade their capsules but do not show vascular invasion. These are termed **minimally invasive.**
- Follicular neoplasms that invade veins in or adjacent to the tumor capsule. These should be called **encapsulated angioinvasive carcinoma.**

"Invasive adenoma" does not exist; all these lesions are malignant. We feel those lesions, which are extensively invasive within the gland or even in the perithyroidal tissues, should be diagnosed as widely invasive follicular carcinoma.[23]

Minimally invasive neoplasms rarely recur or spread to distant sites, so the outlook for most patients is good.[138] However, data on long-term prognosis for minimally invasive follicular carcinoma are not available because much of the clinical literature fails to differentiate the encapsulated form of FVPTC from follicular carcinoma. Follicular carcinoma has little tendency to invade lymphatic vessels and to spread to lymph nodes. Hematogenous spread to the skeleton, lungs, brain, liver, and other tissues occurs.[139,140]

Some follicular carcinomas that are not localized or minimally invasive have been called widely invasive; these include examples in which multiple fingers of neoplastic cells extend into the surrounding thyroid or in which there is extensive replacement of the thyroid gland and soft tissues of the neck noted on gross pathologic examination.[140]

Capsular "invasion" and "penetration" may be mimicked by post-FNA effect. Histologic clues to differentiating between true invasion and pseudoinvasion include the geographic linear pattern of FNA-induced pseudoinvasion as well as the presence of granulation tissue; macrophages (many containing hemosiderin); cholesterol clefts; fibrosis; and rarely, well-formed granulomas.[13]

MOLECULAR PATHOLOGY OF FOLLICULAR CARCINOMA

A specific translocation t (2;3) leads to the expression of *PAX8-peroxisome proliferator-activated receptor-gamma (PPAR-gamma)* chimeric protein; initial studies by Kroll et al. demonstrated that this translocation is specific to follicular carcinoma.[141] However, follow-up studies employing immunohistochemistry and molecular biology have shown that PPAR-gamma expression can occur in some cases of follicular adenoma, follicular variant of PTC, and even in benign thyroid parenchyma.[142,143] Ras mutations are more frequent in follicular carcinoma compared with follicular adenoma; some authors have found an association between ras mutations and clinically aggressive follicular carcinomas.[18,91,92,144,145] Loss of heterozygosity on chromosome 10q and 3p can be seen in follicular carcinoma, suggesting a role of tumor suppressor genes in its pathogenesis.[146,147]

It has been postulated that follicular carcinoma (or at least some examples) derive from follicular adenomas. The finding of RAS mutations in some adenomas and many follicular carcinomas has been suggested as proof of this. Based on clinical and pathologic studies this concept has not definitively proven however.[91,92]

WELL-DIFFERENTIATED FOLLICULAR "TUMORS OF UNDETERMINED/UNCERTAIN MALIGNANT POTENTIAL"

This designation has been proposed in thyroid pathology for follicular patterned and encapsulated tumors that have been controversial and difficult to diagnose because of (1) questionable or minimal nuclear features of PTC or (2) questionable or one focus of capsular invasion that is confined to the tumor capsule, does not traverse the entire thickness of the capsule, and lacks any nuclear features of PTC.[23,82]

The concept of such lesions has been recently accepted by the WHO in 2017.[23] There are two types: follicular tumor of uncertain malignant potential (FTUMP) and well-differentiated tumor of uncertain malignant potential (WDTUMP). FTUMP is defined as a thyroid tumor in which the nuclei are not of PTC, but there is partial capsular invasion. WTUMP shows partial capsular invasion and abnormal nuclear features, not completely characteristic of papillary carcinoma nuclei. This terminology may be extremely helpful to pathologists in the diagnoses of certain follicular patterned lesions; however, these terms are proposed on the basis of data that lack complete clinical follow-up. Therefore clinicians may find it problematic to establish treatment strategies.[7]

HÜRTHLE CELL / ONCOCYTIC FOLLICULAR TUMORS

Hürthle cell, or oncocytic, follicular neoplasms are still the subject of debate (see Chapter 25, Hürthle Cell Tumors of the Thyroid).[148] However, many studies from numerous institutions throughout the world have shown that oncocytic, or Hürthle cell, tumors can be divided into benign and malignant categories by adhering to strict pathologic criteria. More important, these pathologic distinctions predict clinical behavior.[23,31,149,150]

Most oncocytic (Hürthle cell) neoplasms behave as follicular carcinomas; that is, pathologically the capsule or vessels should be assessed for invasion.[149,150] However, some papillary carcinomas show oncocytic cytology and appropriate nuclear features; these behave as typical papillary cancers.[151]

Oncocytic follicular (Hürthle cell) carcinomas should be separated as a category of thyroid neoplasms different from true follicular cancers. They can metastasize to regional lymph nodes as well as spread hematogenously; in addition, histologic evidence of invasive characteristics is found more frequently in oncocytic cancers than in nononcocytic follicular tumors.[21] Approximately one third of oncocytic thyroid tumors show invasion (i.e., are cancers) compared with 2% to 5% of nononcocytic follicular tumors. Hence the finding of oncocytic (Hürthle cell) cytology in a fine-needle aspiration sample of a thyroid nodule should lead to surgical resection of the lesion to assess malignancy.[152] Size is an important feature because large oncocytic (Hürthle cell) tumors (4 cm or greater) have an 80% risk of malignancy.[149,152,153]

It has been shown that oncocytic follicular (Hürthle cell) tumors are biologically different than other follicular-derived tumors. H-ras mutations are more frequent in oncocytic follicular (Hürthle cell) carcinoma than follicular carcinoma.[154,155] Maximo et al. studied the relationship between mitochondrial DNA alterations and thyroid tumorigenesis. This study showed that oncocytic follicular (Hürthle cell) tumors display a relatively higher percentage of deletions of mitochondrial DNA compared with other follicular-derived tumors. In addition, oncocytic follicular (Hürthle cell) tumors also showed germline polymorphisms of *ATPase 6* gene, which is required for the maintenance of mitochondrial DNA.[156]

"HIGH-GRADE" THYROID CARCINOMAS

The categorization of *"high-grade thyroid carcinoma"* includes malignant tumors of the thyroid that show recognizable architectural and cytologic patterns of differentiated thyroid cancer, usually papillary, but also have certain histologic and cytologic features that place the lesions in the "high-grade" category.[157,158] It should be noted that the "high-grade" term has not been endorsed by the 2017 WHO classification of thyroid tumors.[23] Tumors defined as such may have a classic papillary carcinoma, but in some foci, demonstrate marked nuclear pleomorphism, unequivocal tumor necrosis, and numerous mitotic figures. These lesions often large and show multifocal vascular invasion as well as a grossly identifiable extrathyroidal extension; they are associated with regional and distant metastases.[80,120,158,159] By next-generation sequencing, a subset of these tumors show RAS mutations, TERT promoter BRAFV600e mutations.

POORLY DIFFERENTIATED CARCINOMA

Poorly differentiated thyroid carcinomas consist of a heterogeneous group of tumors between well-differentiated follicular or papillary carcinomas and anaplastic carcinomas. They have been included in the 2017 *WHO classification of thyroid tumors*;[23] *however, a controversy still exists* regarding their nature, morphologic diagnostic features, clinical significance, and management.[160,161] Studies of thyroid carcinomas classified as "poorly differentiated carcinoma" have often included examples of tumors that can be more definitely classified as originating from follicular epithelium (often with evidence of coexistent papillary or follicular carcinoma), but with some notable differences: moderate to high rates of mitotic activity; composition of solid masses or trabeculae of relatively uniform epithelial cells; tiny follicles present in varying numbers; regions of acute necrosis; and greater aggressiveness than the usual well-differentiated carcinomas[162] (Figure 41.5). Included among these lesions are insular carcinoma; columnar cell, tall cell, and trabecular types of papillary cancer; and poorly differentiated carcinoma of Sakamoto.[162] These tumors generally lack the usual histologic features and exceptional aggressiveness of anaplastic carcinomas, but they are neither typical follicular nor papillary carcinomas.[56,157] At present most experts agree that the common pathologic features of poorly differentiated carcinomas include solid, trabecular, or insular growth; large size; frequent extrathyroidal extension; extensive vascular invasion; presence of necrosis; and increased mitotic activity. They may be associated with well-differentiated components of either follicular or papillary type, and less frequently, with anaplastic carcinoma.[116,159,160] A study from Memorial Sloan Kettering Cancer Center in New York identified a group of encapsulated tumors with features of poorly differentiated carcinoma; in this small subset the survival was better than expected for patients with poorly differentiated thyroid cancer. This suggests that gland-confined encapsulated lesions may not *harbor* the serious prognosis of those tumors with extrathyroidal extensions even in the presence of aggressive morphologic features.[163] Literature data, although limited, have shown a distinct molecular pathway in poorly differentiated carcinomas, almost exclusively involving RAS gene alterations.[164]

ANAPLASTIC CARCINOMA

Fewer than 5% of thyroid carcinomas may be classified as anaplastic or undifferentiated.[165] They are most common in regions of the world where iodine is deficient. Traditionally, these tumors include spindle-cell and giant-cell cancers as well as the rare small-cell carcinomas. However, most lesions originally classified as small-cell anaplastic carcinomas represent medullary carcinoma, insular carcinoma, or small-cell malignant lymphoma.[165,166] The possibility of a metastatic carcinoma from another organ always has to be considered.

Most anaplastic thyroid carcinomas are spindle-cell and giant-cell tumors.[167] These aggressive neoplasms usually occur in elderly people, more often women than men. The patient may have a thyroid nodule that, after many years of stability, suddenly begins to grow rapidly. Some patients are known to have had low-grade thyroid carcinoma, and others have low-grade thyroid carcinoma discovered at the time of diagnosis of the anaplastic tumor.[165,168-170]

Careful pathologic examinations of thyroids that contain anaplastic carcinomas have demonstrated a high incidence (50% to 70%) of remnants of well-differentiated follicular or papillary carcinomas or sometimes adenomas or adenomatoid nodules, thus confirming clinical impressions that anaplastic carcinomas arise out of tumors of a low grade.[171]

In general, a hard, pale infiltrative mass with soft foci of necrosis and hemorrhage is seen. These tumors invade the cervical soft tissues and involve the regional lymph nodes, often by direct extension.

Microscopic examinations reveal varied histologic patterns, many mitotic figures, and regions of tumor necrosis.[165]

Anaplastic carcinomas are pleomorphic; they can consist of medium to large cells with a vaguely epithelial appearance. There may even be squamous cell differentiation (or a tendency toward this pattern).[172] Others appear sarcomatous, resembling malignant fibrous histiocytoma, fibrosarcoma, or angiosarcoma. The giant-cell carcinomas often have bizarre giant cells, frequently multinucleated, and containing abnormal mitotic figures. Less commonly, some giant cells resemble osteoclasts[173] (Figure 41.6).

Ultrastructural studies support an epithelial phenotype.[174] Immunohistochemical evidence of thyroglobulin has been found in a few anaplastic carcinomas. It is likely that in most of these cases, the thyroglobulin staining represents diffusion of thyroglobulin cells from destroyed neighboring thyroid follicles; 50% to 100% of these tumors

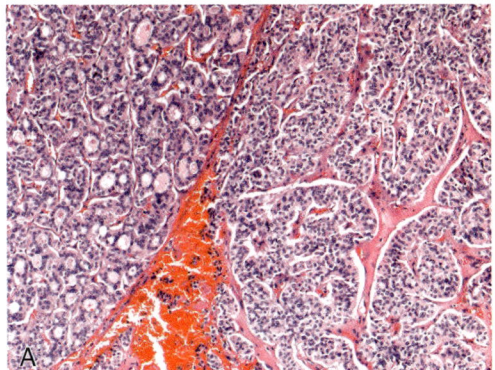
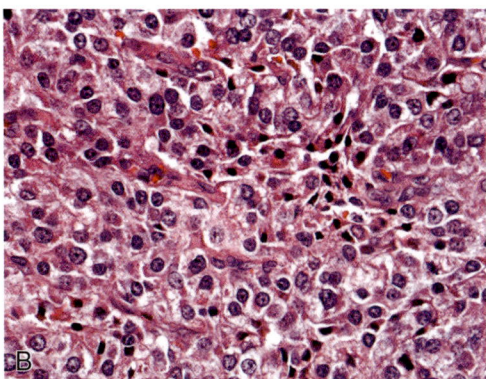

Fig. 41.5 A, A case of poorly differentiated carcinoma *(right)* arising from a well-differentiated carcinoma *(left)*. **B,** The poorly differentiated component showing a solid growth pattern.

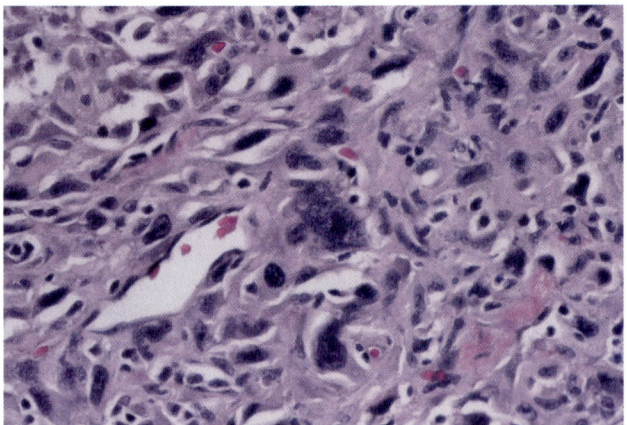

Fig. 41.6 Anaplastic carcinoma of the thyroid showing marked nuclear pleomorphism, oval- to spindle-shaped cells, and multinucleated tumor cell.

contain keratin.[175,176] Carcinosarcoma of the thyroid has been described; most contain malignant bone and/or cartilage.[177]

In rare cases, a small focus of anaplastic carcinoma will be found incidentally within a differentiated thyroid carcinoma, where it is confined.[166,171] Even less common is the finding of an anaplastic focus in a lymph node metastasis of a differentiated thyroid cancer.[166] Such tumors are the only anaplastic cancers that may be "cured" by surgery. These unusual lesions must be distinguished from post-FNA spindle cell nodules, which can appear in the center of aspirated thyroid nodules and represent exuberant granulation tissue. The latter lesions are mesenchymal in origin, which can be documented by immunochemical staining; they do not contain keratin positive cells as do anaplastic carcinomas.[13]

It should be noted that in some patients with multiply recurrent and metastatic low-grade carcinomas, anaplastic transformation may occur only in a metastatic site. In our experience, this is usually in the bone.

FOLLICULAR-DERIVED FAMILIAL TUMORS

The frequency of follicular cell–derived tumors as familial events is not known but is estimated to be between 1% and 5% of all thyroid tumors.[178,179] This group can be conveniently divided into two main categories: familial nonmedullary thyroid carcinoma (FNMTC) or associated with syndromes having extrathyroidal manifestations[180] (see Chapter 30, Familial Nonmedullary Thyroid Cancer).

Thyroid papillary carcinomas of classic or follicular variant type may occur in multiple family members. To be considered familial cancer, at least three first-degree relatives should be affected. The histology of these tumors can be no different from classic or follicular variant of papillary carcinoma with or without oxyphilia although multifocal and bilateral lesions are found. Some series indicate that clinically these tumors behave more aggressively than sporadic tumors, including extensive lymphatic invasion, lymph node metastases, and frequent recurrences.[181] In some of these, chromosomal abnormalities have been found, however, specific genes need to be identified.[178]

Papillary thyroid carcinomas and other follicular-derived thyroid tumors can be seen in other familial syndromes; these include familial adenomatous polyposis syndrome, PTEN hamartoma syndrome, McCune-Albright syndrome, Carney complex, Peutz-Jeghers syndrome, Werner syndrome and MEN (Types 1 and 2A) syndromes.[178,180,182-184] Recent studies have also shown strong associations between DICER1 mutations and differentiated thyroid carcinomas in these familial syndromic thyroid lesions.

MEDULLARY CARCINOMA

Medullary carcinomas constitute about 5% of thyroid carcinomas and originate from C cells; they may be sporadic or familial, and they may be associated with disorders of other endocrine glands (see Chapter 26, Sporadic Medullary Thyroid Carcinoma, and Chapter 27, Syndromic Medullary Thyroid Carcinoma: MEN 2A and MEN 2B).[185-190]

On gross examination, most medullary carcinomas present as firm and white or yellow with circumscribed nodules; some are infiltrative. The encapsulated ones have a better prognosis.[191] On light microscopic examination, the cells appear rounded, polygonal, or spindle shaped (Figure 41.7, A). They are arranged as a diffuse solid mass; as islands separated by fibrous tissue (usually dense or hyalinized); as trabeculae or ribbons of cells; and (uncommonly) as glandular structures.[191-193] Pseudopapillary formations and even true papillary and follicular patterns have been reported.[194] The carcinomas may consist of small cells (in the past confused with small-cell anaplastic carcinoma); may contain numerous giant cells; and like some anaplastic carcinomas, may have large cells with eosinophilic cytoplasm, resembling oncocytic follicular cells; these carcinomas can also contain glands.[195,196] Clear cell medullary carcinomas have been reported.[197] Cells producing mucus may be present in varying numbers.[198] Rarely do these carcinomas produce melanin.[199]

The nuclei are rounded or elongated; occasional nuclei are large and irregular. Cytoplasmic inclusions in nuclei may occur. Some authors described the nuclear chromatin as stippled or like salt and pepper (pattern).[191,200,201] Amyloid is frequently present, both in the primary neoplasms and in the metastatic foci (about 75% of cases) (Figure 41.7, B). Both tumor stroma and the amyloid may undergo calcification.[202,203]

Medullary carcinomas nearly always produce calcitonin (Figure 41.7, C), although a few may lack this peptide. Other substances detected include Chromogranin A; calcitonin gene-related peptide; carcinoembryonic antigen; and other peptide hormones.[203,204] If only a few tumor cells reveal calcitonin through immunostaining, the prognosis appears worse. In some series, necrosis, squamous changes, and oxyphilic tumor cells are also associated with a worse outcome.[204-206]

The tumors can invade both lymphatic and blood vessels; cervical nodes metastases are common.[207,208] A few patients develop widespread disease and die in 2 or 3 years.[209,210] A few have extraordinarily indolent tumors (these encapsulated lesions were initially misdiagnosed as adenomas) that persist for as long as 30 years.[211] Some reports indicate familial medullary carcinomas (especially patients with Sipple's syndrome, MEN type 2A) have a better prognosis.[212,213] Several authors indicate that patients with MEN type 2B have tumors that are particularly aggressive.[214-217]

Most cases of medullary carcinoma are sporadic, particularly in patients over 40 years old; they may involve only one lobe and may not be associated with other endocrine lesions.[218,219] A considerable number of cases are familial, however, especially in younger patients. Such cancers may be associated with bilateral pheochromocytomas or adrenal medullary hyperplasia and with parathyroid hyperplasia (Sipple's syndrome, MEN type 2A).[190,207,223]

Some patients have a variant syndrome with mucosal and cutaneous neuromas and with skeletal abnormalities (MEN type 2B).[220,221] The familial medullary carcinomas are usually bilateral and multicentric. Other family members may have C-cell hyperplasia and medullary carcinomas of microscopic size, some of which may have already spread to lymph nodes. In this situation, the so-called C-cell hyperplasia is premalignant.[49,221-225]

A few medullary carcinomas are discovered incidental to thyroid operations for other conditions, during an autopsy, or through an elevated serum calcitonin.[226,227] The so-called micromedullary carcinomas have an excellent prognosis if they are confined to the thyroid gland.[228,229]

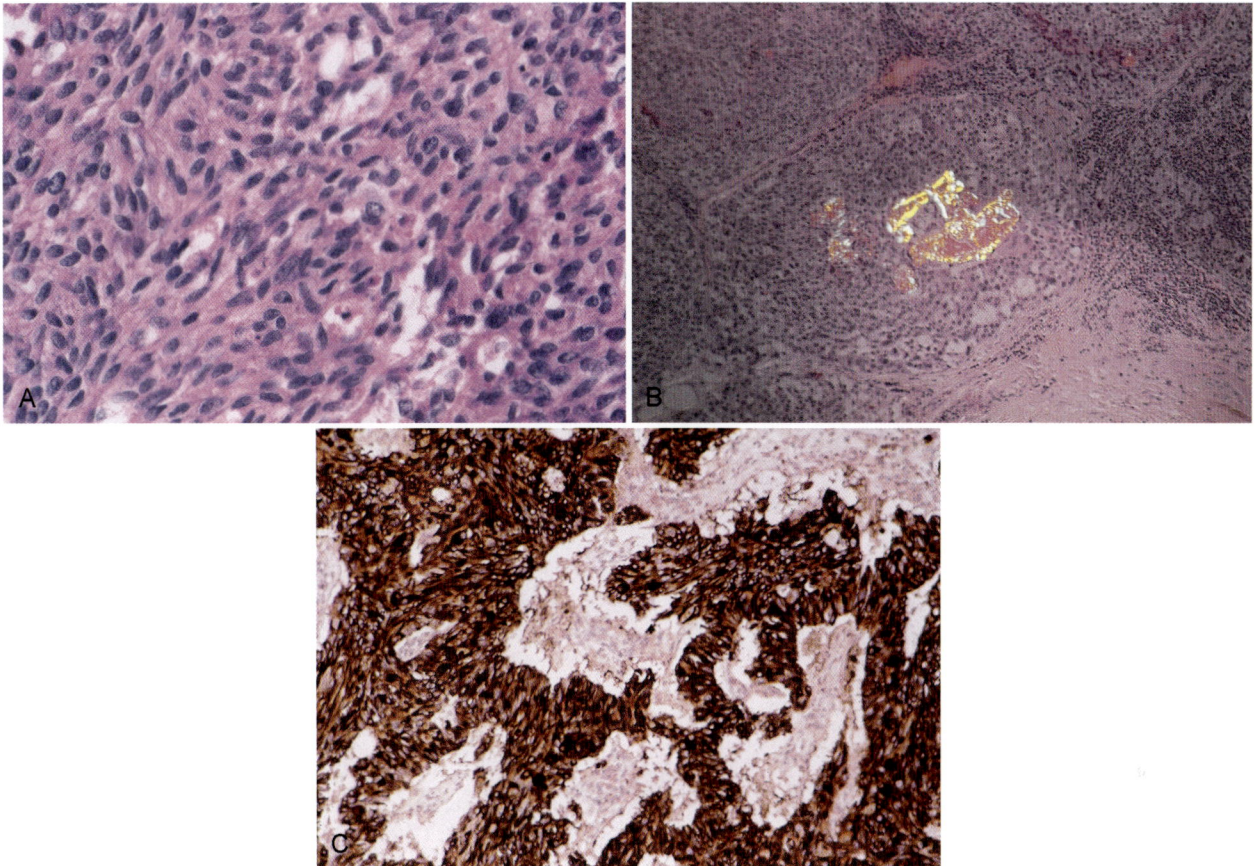

Fig. 41.7 A, A case of medullary thyroid carcinoma showing oval- to spindle-shaped tumor cells; **B,** presence of amyloid (Congo red stain); and **C,** calcitonin (immunoperoxidase stain for calcitonin).

Some medullary carcinomas grow sufficiently slowly to allow them to trap thyroid follicles. A few neoplasms have been reported that appear to represent joint C-cell and follicular-cell proliferations, but these are rare. A putative example must be evaluated critically because of the possibility of collision tumors.[230,231]

TUMORS WITH THYMIC OR RELATED BRANCHIAL POUCH DIFFERENTIATION

This category of primary thyroid tumors includes lesions that by morphology, immunohistochemistry, and electron microscopy show thymic or related branchial pouch differentiation.[232]

Thymic remnants can be in 1.8% of thyroid glands. Rarely may tumors form in these rests and give rise to *intrathyroidal thymoma.*[232,233]

Spindle epithelial tumors with thymus-like differentiation (SETTLE) are commonly seen in children and young adults; the tumors exhibit slow growth, late recurrences, and distant metastases. These tumors usually present as solitary circumscribed masses, and on histology show a mixture of bland spindle and epithelial cells. Occasionally squamous differentiation reminiscent of Hassall's corpuscles can be seen. The spindle cells stain positive for cytokeratins and smooth muscle actin but stain negative for thyroglobulin and calcitonin.[232,234-236]

Carcinomas showing thymus-like differentiation (CASTLE) usually appear in the middle to lower thirds of the thyroid in adults 40 to 50 years old. By histology these tumors appear similar to lymphoepithelioma-like carcinomas found in the thymus and nasopharynx. However, no association between this tumor and Epstein-Barr virus has been demonstrated.[237,238]

MUCOEPIDERMOID CARCINOMA OF THYROID GLAND

This is a rare thyroid tumor; two tumors fall under this heading: *mucoepidermoid carcinoma (MEC) and sclerosing mucoepidermoid carcinoma with eosinophilia (SMECE).*[239-241]

MECs are common in women, and they behave in an indolent fashion. These tumors usually present as solitary solid thyroid nodules with areas of cyst formation. Microscopically, the tumors resemble MECs of salivary glands and show squamous and glandular differentiation with mucin production. Most tumors stain positive for thyroglobulin.[239,242-244]

SMECEs are similar in their clinical presentation and biologic behavior to MECs. However, they can be separated from MECs on the basis of both morphology and immunohistochemistry. The tumors show both squamous and glandular differentiation in backgrounds of prominent hyaline stromas and mixed inflammatory infiltrates with prominent eosinophilia. Almost all SMECEs arise in glands with lymphocytic thyroiditis. The tumor cells are usually negative for thyroglobulin and calcitonin but positive for cytokeratin.[234,239,240,245] So far no BRAFV600E mutations have been detected in these tumors.[240]

PRIMARY NONEPITHELIAL TUMORS OF THYROID

The tumors described this category include mesenchymal tumors and lymphoma.

Mesenchymal tumors of the thyroid are extremely rare; they include smooth muscle tumors (leiomyomas and leiomyosarcomas);[246,247]

solitary fibrous tumors;[248] and vascular tumors (hemangiomas, epithelioid hemangioendotheliomas, and angiosarcomas).[249,250]

Secondary involvement of the thyroid by malignant lymphomas has been reported in 20% of patients dying from generalized lymphoma.[251-254]

Malignant lymphoma presenting as a primary neoplasm in the thyroid is uncommon but not rare. Its apparent rarity in older literature reflects diagnoses of lymphomas as anaplastic carcinomas (small-cell type). Most patients may have a history of diffuse goiter (probably the result of autoimmune thyroiditis) that has suddenly increased in size.[37,251-254]

Grossly, the tumor is firm, fleshy, and pale. Evidence of previous lymphocytic thyroiditis is present in most cases in which some thyroid parenchyma persists.

Most thyroid lymphomas are of diffuse type. Virtually all examples are B-cell types; many are extranodal lymphomas that arise in mucosa-associated lymphoid tissue (MALT). The latter show characteristic lymphoepithelial lesions, which represent colonization of the thyroid follicles by lymphoma cells.[37] Some patients have typical plasmacytomas; these have a good prognosis. Hodgkin's disease is extremely rare.[254,255]

CARCINOMA IN THYROGLOSSAL DUCT CYST AND ECTOPIC THYROID TISSUE

Neoplasms that arise in thyroid tissue associated with the thyroglossal duct have been mostly papillary carcinomas. Remnants of the duct should be identified to document the site of origin of the lesion. If no ductal remnants are found, it may represent papillary carcinoma arising in the pyramidal lobe of the gland; therefore it is a primary thyroid lesion.[256-261]

Morphologically, thyroglossal duct-associated papillary carcinomas are usually classic papillary cancers, but they tend to show extensive sclerosis of the papillary core connective tissue and to have many psammoma bodies. Because of this, FNA or core biopsy can be frequently diagnostic.[260,262] Only rarely are the tumors follicular variants of papillary carcinomas; we have seen two such cases out of about 25 thyroglossal duct carcinomas we have studied. About 20% of the patients studied have papillary cancer in the cervical thyroid gland. Whether the two tumors are separate clonal proliferations or whether they represent metastases remains unclear.[260,261] About 15% to 25% of patients with papillary carcinomas of the thyroglossal duct thyroid show cervical node metastases.[263]

Rare examples of follicular, Hürthle, or even anaplastic carcinomas have been reported in ectopic thyroid tissues;[264,265] however, as one would expect from embryologic considerations, medullary carcinoma has not been reported. In contrast to thyroglossal carcinomas, neoplasms of sublingual and lingual ectopic thyroid tissue can resemble the various types encountered in the main gland.[265-267]

PATHOLOGIST AND THYROID

The pathologist plays a key role in the management and diagnosis of thyroid nodules. Pathologists select patients requiring surgery on the basis of neoplastic, indeterminate, suspicious, or malignant FNA diagnoses as well as on histopathologic examinations of surgically excised nodules to provide information for appropriate staging and postoperative management.[1,4,54] In this section, we will review the role of intraoperative assessment in surgical management of thyroid nodules; suggested criteria for gross pathologic examinations of thyroid nodule; and essentials of the histopathologic reporting of thyroid tumors.

INTRAOPERATIVE ASSESSMENT OF THYROID NODULES

In the majority of cases, the surgical management of thyroid nodules can be planned on the basis of the preoperative FNA diagnosis. Patients with definite diagnoses of malignancy can undergo total or near-total thyroidectomies; whereas those diagnosed with follicular neoplasm can undergo a lobectomy, and upon completion of the histopathologic examination, a completion thyroidectomy can be performed if the nodule removed is diagnosed as a carcinoma.[268-270] A similar scenario can also be seen in cases diagnosed as suspicious for malignancy or indeterminate for neoplasm. However, this two-step procedure—that is, lobectomy followed by completion thyroidectomy—does expose the patient to a second surgical procedure and its associated risks as well as increased costs.[271,272]

Several authors have suggested the use of frozen section in the definite surgical management of thyroid nodules.[273-275] In general, the primary role of frozen section in surgical pathology is to establish a diagnosis (i.e., to differentiate between benign and malignant tumors); to identify tissue types (e.g., parathyroid versus lymph node); and to assess the extent of surgical resection.[276,277] In some cases of surgical resection, frozen sections can deliver this information and guide surgery; however, in some instances, the pathologist may not be able to provide a definite diagnosis, which leads to deferral of frozen section diagnosis to final histopathologic examination. In such cases, the surgeon usually delays the definite procedure and waits for the final diagnosis.

Several authors have discussed the use of intraoperative assessment of thyroid lesions in the literature. Some have found that this procedure is of limited utility; whereas, others have reported it to be of more or equal diagnostic value compared with FNA.[46,275,276]

Arguments against the use of frozen sections in thyroid nodules include the following:
1. FNA can diagnose papillary carcinoma in more than 90% of cases; therefore it is not cost effective to perform frozen section in cases diagnosed as definite for malignancy via FNA.[278,279]
2. Frozen sections are known to produce artefactual nuclear changes, which can mimic nuclear changes of papillary thyroid carcinoma, leading to a false-positive diagnosis.[276]
3. Frozen sections are of limited value in the diagnosis of follicular or Hürthle cell carcinoma, because to differentiate between benign and malignant follicular and Hürthle cell lesions, one must demonstrate true capsular and/or vascular invasion, which requires a thorough and detailed examination of the lesion's capsule.[7,280] Therefore due to limited sampling at the time of the frozen section, it is likely that a majority of lesions diagnosed through FNA as follicular neoplasm will be deferred to final histopathologic examination.[7]

The latter is one of the major arguments used by many authors to prove the limited utility of frozen section in thyroid nodules. Montone and LiVolsi in their report of thyroid frozen sections found that 50% of the frozen sections were deferred to permanent sections, and of those, 22% were diagnosed as malignant on final histology; they required additional surgery.[281] Chen et al. studied 125 patients with follicular thyroid lesions, and from these, 87% were deferred to permanent sections on intraoperative assessment. In addition, 5% of cases were misdiagnosed, leading to inappropriate excision of the entire thyroid.[282]

In addition, to the deferral on frozen section examination, it is also possible that some of the malignant follicular lesions may be interpreted as benign due to limited sampling.[282] Kingston et al. in their study of 198 follicular neoplasms, found that 21% of the lesions were incorrectly diagnosed benign on frozen section.[283] In a similar study,

Crowe et al. found that 6% of the malignant lesions were underdiagnosed as on frozen section.[284]

In the era of FNA of thyroid nodules, one must also be aware of the histologic alterations that can be induced by this procedure. The most notable of these that can be problematic on frozen section is post-FNA pseudocapsular and vascular invasion; such lesions can be mistaken for foci of true tumor invasion on frozen section. In our experience, the post-FNA foci of pseudoinvasion are usually linear, and they are surrounded by areas of hemorrhage and granulation tissue. However, in our view, such distinction between true and false post-FNA foci of invasion is only possible through detailed examination of permanent histologic sections.[13,285]

Among the proponents of frozen sections in thyroid lesions, the most commonly quoted report is from the Mayo Clinic in Rochester, Minn.[275] The authors studied 1023 patients undergoing surgery due to a diagnosis of follicular and Hürthle cell thyroid neoplasms; 78% of cases were diagnosed as malignant on frozen section, thus leading to definite surgical management instead of a two-step procedure (lobectomy followed by completion thyroidectomy). However, in our view, this study reflects experience from a unique pathology laboratory, where the majority of surgical specimens is diagnosed on the basis of multiple frozen sections (sometimes requiring up to 15 frozen sections). Therefore if we consider the working environment of the usual pathology laboratory in community practices and academic centers, it seems practically impossible to perform multiple frozen sections to distinguish between benign and malignant follicular and oncocytic follicular (Hürthle cell) tumors.

In view of the studies mentioned earlier, one can deduce that frozen sections are of limited value in the diagnoses of follicular and oncocytic follicular (Hürthle cell) tumors. The frozen sections do not provide additional information compared with preoperative FNA. Therefore is there any role of intraoperative assessment examination in the surgical management of thyroid nodules?

Despite extensive discussion and evidence provided in the literature for and against the use of frozen section in surgical management of thyroid nodules, some authors have proven by both retrospective and prospective analyses that intraoperative evaluation of thyroid nodules can be useful in cases diagnosed as suspicious for PTC via FNA.[286-288] Rodriguez et al. investigated the value of frozen section in cases diagnosed as benign, suggestive, or malignant. They found that frozen section analysis is useful in cases with a "suggestive" cytology diagnosis, whereas there was no significant effect in cases with benign or malignant diagnosis.

Basolo et al. reported the use of intraoperative cytology as an adjunct to frozen section analysis of resected thyroid specimen.[286] Scrape rather than touch preparations may be useful adjunct to the frozen sections; which sometimes has led to completion thyroidectomy on the basis of intraoperative diagnosis in cases diagnosed as suspicious for PTC through FNA.[277,288] Interestingly, a majority of cases diagnosed as suspicious for PTC represents follicular variant of PTC; most of these are follicular-patterned encapsulated nodules without any obvious capsular and/or vascular invasion. Therefore one can easily mistake these cases as follicular adenoma or neoplasm through frozen sections alone because the diagnostic nuclear features of PTC are usually not seen in frozen sections.

We believe that in view of the evidence presented in favor and against the use of intraoperative consultation in thyroid nodule, one can draw few major conclusions. They include the following:
1. Intraoperative consultation is not indicated in cases diagnosed as definite for malignancy through FNA.
2. The diagnosis of follicular or Hürthle cell carcinoma cannot be rendered on frozen sections because the histologic characterization of these lesions requires detailed analysis of the tumor capsule for demonstrating capsular and/or vascular invasion.
3. Intraoperative consultation is most effective in cases diagnosed as suspicious for PTC through FNA. The sensitivity of frozen sections in such cases can be enhanced with the addition of intraoperative cytology.

GROSS EXAMINATION OF THYROID SPECIMENS

A detailed gross examination of the surgical specimen is as important as the microscopic diagnosis. It serves as the foundation upon which the final histopathologic report is built; it includes type of resection as well as tumor location, size, and appearance (Box 41.1). It is prudent that the gross examination be performed on the fresh specimen received in the pathology laboratory and that tumor size and appearance be documented before sections are taken for frozen section or other studies.[270]

As part of the macroscopic assessment of thyroid resection specimens, pertinent clinical and historical data should be provided to the pathologist. This information includes age and sex of the patient; relevant history (previous treatment, history of head and neck radiation, and family history of thyroid disease); and identification of the procedure type (lobectomy and near-total or total thyroidectomy). Appropriate functional and laboratory data, if pertinent, should be included. Examples include data from thyroid function tests; radiologic studies (ultrasound, thyroid scan); and laboratory studies (thyroid antibodies, serum calcitonin).

The specimen should be oriented spatially by the surgeon. Gross examination of the specimen should cover weight and measurement (in three dimensions) of the specimen as well as description of the external surface and the cut surface (color, consistency). If nodules are present, each should be described (size, location and characteristics [solid, cystic, calcified, hemorrhagic]). If a solitary or dominant nodule is identified, its location; size; encapsulation; surgical margins; and characteristics (color, cystification, hemorrhage, FNA tracks, necrosis), should be inked with India ink, and the presence of extrathyroidal extension should be noted.[270]

If the specimen contains regional lymph nodes, description of levels and characteristics of any grossly involved nodes should be given. Presence of parathyroid gland(s) should be documented. After a careful and complete gross examination, and appropriate fixation, sections should be submitted for histologic examination. The macroscopic findings determine the number of sections to be taken to diagnose inflammatory lesions of the thyroid, such as thyroiditis or Graves' disease. Without any obvious nodules, up to three sections should be submitted from each lobe and one from the isthmus. In the case of a solitary or dominant encapsulated nodule, it is recommended that the entire circumference of the nodule be sectioned. Each section should include a tumor

---

BOX 41.1 Gross Examination of Thyroid Tumors

Features to be included:
1. Weight
2. Measurement in three dimensions
3. External surface (nodular/diffuse enlargement)
4. Cut surface (color/consistency)
5. If nodules, size and characteristics
6. Surgical margins
7. Presence of nodes, parathyroid glands

capsule and the main tumor mass with a margin of normal surrounding parenchyma, if present. Lang et al. have shown that an increase in the number of sections from the tumor capsule increases the chances for identification of foci of vascular invasion.[289] In a study by Yamashina, total circumferential evaluation of the tumor capsule was found to be necessary to differentiate between follicular adenoma and follicular carcinoma.[136] For a nonencapsulated nodule, one section per 0.5 cm should be submitted.

HISTOPATHOLOGIC REPORTING OF THYROID TUMORS

The final histopathologic report is important in determining patient prognosis and treatment; it should be comprehensive, and it should include all known prognostic parameters, which help the treating clinician devise a thorough postoperative treatment plan. The final pathology report for thyroid tumors should describe the tumor by histologic type, number or multicentricity, size, encapsulation, presence of tumor capsule, and extrathyroidal invasion. By extension, the report should also share information about any disease in the contralateral lobe as well as about blood or lymphatic vessel invasion (vessels at the periphery or beyond tumor not within the main tumor mass; Box 41.2).[270]

If lymph node sampling or dissection was performed, the presence of lymph node metastases—number and size—should be recorded. The identification of extranodal extension into soft tissues is also recognized as an important prognostic finding.

The number of parathyroid glands, if any, removed during surgery should be documented and their location given, if possible. Additional pathologic findings in the thyroid, such as nodular goiter, thyroiditis and benign tumors, should be described. Additional (optional) sections to include in the report include correlation with FNA findings (especially in discrepant cases) and correlation with intraoperative diagnosis and clinical information. The results of special studies—special stains (Congo red for amyloid, elastic stain for vessels) and immunostains (calcitonin, thyroglobulin, endothelial markers for vascular invasion), or flow cytometry— should be added as appropriate.

It is also important in some cases that specific variants of a main tumor category, which clinically behave in a different manner, should be identified in the pathology report. This is more commonly seen in the papillary carcinoma category; the variants, which have been shown to behave in a more aggressive fashion than usual papillary carcinomas, include tall cell variant, diffuse sclerosing variant, and columnar cell variant. Besides prognostic value, description of a specific variant in the final pathology report may also help explain some unusual findings observed with FNA; for example, tall cell variant of papillary carcinoma can show oncocytic cytoplasm and prominent nucleoli on FNA smears and can be mistaken for oncocytic follicular (Hürthle cell) tumors. Follicular variants of papillary carcinoma, due to their follicular growth pattern, can be underdiagnosed as follicular neoplasm.

Capsular and/or vascular invasion: Controversy still exists over whether capsular invasion alone justifies a diagnosis of carcinoma in encapsulated follicular lesions. Some authors have suggested that the term minimally invasive carcinoma should be used for tumors with minimal vascular invasion and the term widely invasive should be used for tumors with extensive vascular invasion.[127] However, others have shown that tumors with capsular invasion only can lead to distant metastases.[290] At our institution, we restrict the term "minimally invasive carcinoma" for tumors that show only capsular invasion and lack vascular invasion; whereas, tumors with vascular invasion are termed as angioinvasive carcinomas.

> **BOX 41.2** **Histologic Features of Thyroid Tumors to be Defined in Pathology Report**
>
> 1. Tumor type and subtype
> 2. Tumor size
> 3. Capsule
> 4. Multicentricity
> 5. Invasion
>   - Into tumor capsule (in encapsulated tumors)
>   - Into normal thyroid
>   - Into extrathyroidal tissues
>   - Vascular invasion
>   - Perineural invasion
> 6. Presence of tumor in contralateral lobe
> 7. Nontumoral-associated conditions: goiter, thyroiditis, etc.
> 8. Lymph nodes examined and involved by tumor
>   - Size of the largest lymph node involved
>   - Size of the metastatic deposit
>   - Extranodal extension
> 9. American Joint Committee on Cancer (AJCC) Staging

REFERENCES

For a complete list of references, visit expertconsult.com.

Postoperative Considerations

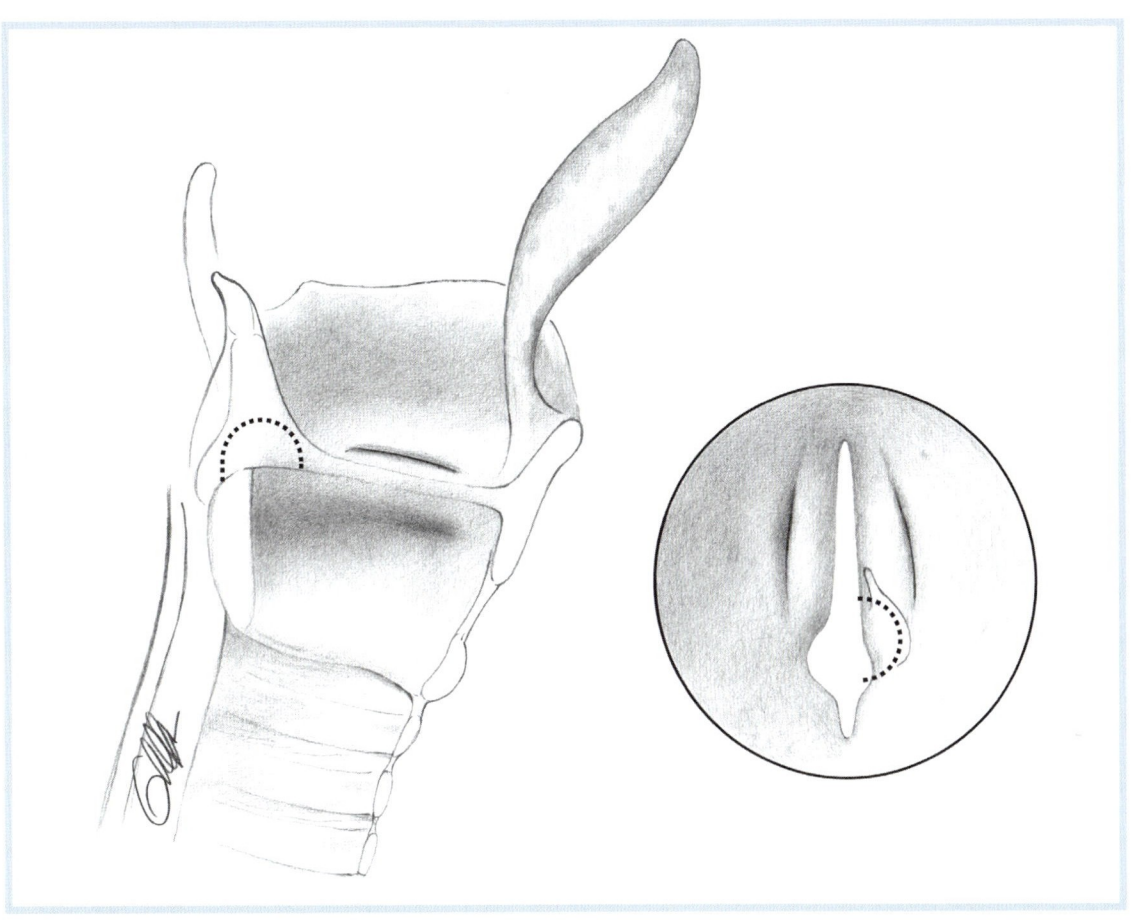

Pathophysiology of Recurrent Laryngeal Nerve Injury

Gayle Woodson

INTRODUCTION

Laryngeal nerve injury is a serious complication of thyroid surgery. Unilateral injury impairs the voice and, occasionally, swallowing. Bilateral injury can result in life-threatening airway obstruction. Symptoms vary greatly over time and between patients, depending on the site and severity of the lesion and the biology of the healing process. This chapter deals with the pathophysiology of recurrent laryngeal nerve (RLN) injury and the biology of nerve regeneration (see Chapter 43, Management of Recurrent Laryngeal Nerve Paralysis).

VARIATIONS IN SYMPTOMS

Unilateral laryngeal paralysis can be completely asymptomatic, an incidental finding during the course of a routine laryngeal examination in a patient with a normal voice. Patients with acute laryngeal nerve injury virtually always have some voice impairment, ranging from mild vocal fatigue to severe hoarseness, depending on the degree of nerve damage. In the most severe cases, the glottis is incompetent, resulting in aphonia and even aspiration during swallowing. Laryngeal paralysis can impair all functions that require tight glottal closure, such as cough, defecation, and stabilization of the thorax for heavy lifting. Unilateral paralysis can cause stridor in infants. Otherwise, one mobile vocal fold usually provides an adequate airway. But some patients experience episodic airway obstruction due to laryngospasm.[1] In some cases, the paralyzed vocal fold adducts during inspiration, resulting in stridor or even warranting a tracheotomy.[2]

It has long been observed that vocal function can improve, even if a vocal fold remains immobile. The position of the paralyzed vocal fold tends to shift toward the midline over time.[3] It is now apparent that this change in position is due to reinnervation of adductor muscles.[4]

When both RLNs are injured, vocal symptoms take a back seat to respiratory issues. Acute bilateral paralysis can require emergent tracheotomy or intubation. Other patients may have a marginal but adequate airway. As in unilateral paralysis, symptoms change over time due to reinnervation of laryngeal muscles (Figure 42.1). A weak and breathy voice may become stronger as the airway becomes worse. Patients frequently have some appropriate adduction with phonation, but abductor function is rare. Inappropriate adduction with inspiration can also occur, sometimes because of a passive inward collapse of flaccid paralyzed musculature during inspiration (e.g., the Bernoulli effect), sometimes as a result of inappropriate contraction from synkinetic reinnervation (Figure 42.2).

CONFIGURATION OF THE PARALYZED VOCAL FOLD

The severity of vocal symptoms is related to the distance of the paralyzed vocal fold from the midline. The voice is weak when the glottis cannot close completely during phonation, and it becomes breathy or aphonic when the glottic gap is large. Surgical procedures such as thyroplasty and vocal fold injection move the anterior portion of the paralyzed vocal fold nearer the midline. This effectively restores vocal function in patients with a paramedian vocal fold position. But when the arytenoid is externally rotated, the paralyzed vocal process is too far lateral to permit approximation by the mobile contralateral vocal process (Figure 42.3). In such cases, adequate closure of the glottis requires surgery that addresses the posterior portion of the vocal fold as well.

The terms *median* and *paramedian* have traditionally been used to describe a paralyzed vocal fold that lies at or near the midline. A more abducted position is referred to as *cadaveric*. An alternative to using the terms *paramedian* or *cadaveric* is to measure the angle formed between the vocal folds during inspiration. A line is drawn from the anterior commissure to the vocal process on each side. Together these lines form the anterior glottic angle. This parameter is a quantitative measure that is useful in preoperative assessment and in tracking the results of treatment. Figure 42.4 illustrates the glottic angle in two patients: one with a vocal fold paralyzed in the paramedian position and the other in a more lateral position.

Over the years, many explanations have been postulated for the variation in the appearance of the larynx in unilateral paralysis and the shift in position over time. The two theories with the most historical significance are *Semon's law* and the *Wagner-Grossman hypothesis*. Semon postulated that in the progression of nerve injury, nerve fibers to the abductor muscles were affected first, so that the glottal opening would be impaired first.[5] Later, adductor muscles would also become paralyzed, and the vocal fold would move laterally. However, Semon's law actually predicts that the affected vocal fold will shift laterally over time. This is exactly opposite to the gradual adduction that has been so widely observed for many years. The Wagner-Grossman hypothesis asserts that after an RLN injury, the vocal fold is adducted by the cricothyroid muscle, the only intrinsic laryngeal muscle that is not supplied by the RLN. After a high lesion of the vagus nerve injury, both the recurrent and superior laryngeal nerve fibers are affected. Therefore the Wagner-Grossman hypothesis predicts that without the adductor force of the cricothyroid, the vocal fold would lie in the cadaveric position.[6] Because it is more consistent with clinical observations of the vocal fold position in RLN and vagus nerve injuries, the Wagner-Grossman hypothesis has been widely accepted for many years.[7]

But the preponderance of experimental evidence has dispelled the notion that the cricothyroid muscle adducts the vocal fold.[8-13] Although it is true that the cricothyroid muscle behaves as an accessory muscle of inspiration, recruited by increased inspiratory effort, blockade of the nerve to the cricothyroid muscle has no influence on glottic area or transglottic resistance, even during stimulated breathing with maximal cricothyroid activity.[9-11] Simulated cricothyroid muscle

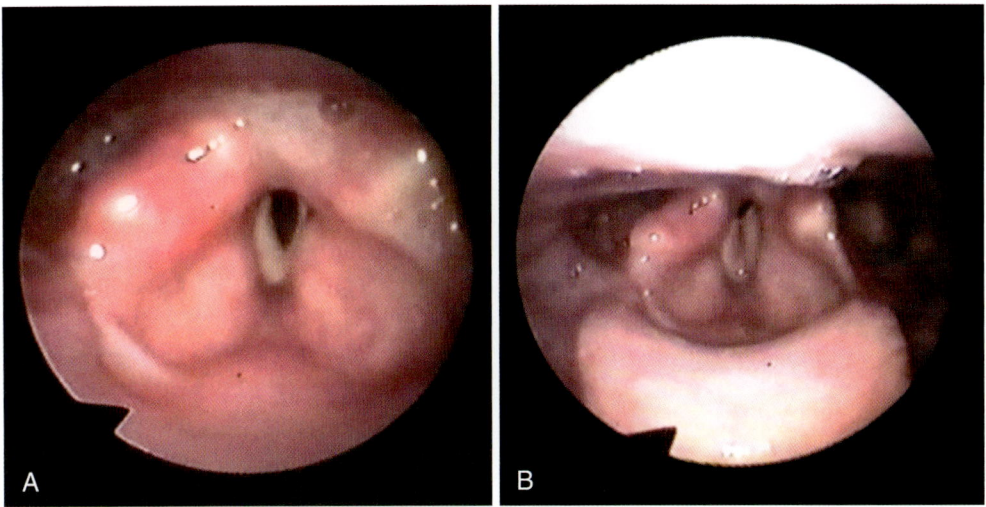

Fig. 42.1 Bilateral laryngeal paralysis resulting from a thyroidectomy for cancer involving both recurrent laryngeal nerves. **A,** Immediately after surgery: vocal folds are partially abducted. **B,** Six months later: vocal folds have shifted toward the midline.

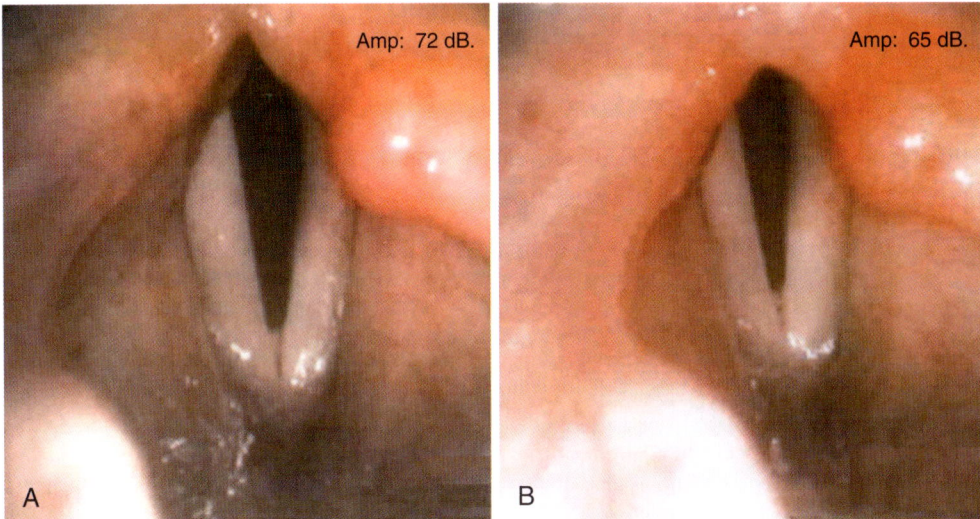

Fig. 42.2 Paradoxical motion of the vocal folds in bilateral laryngeal paralysis after total thyroidectomy. **A,** Quiet breathing. **B,** Deep breathing.

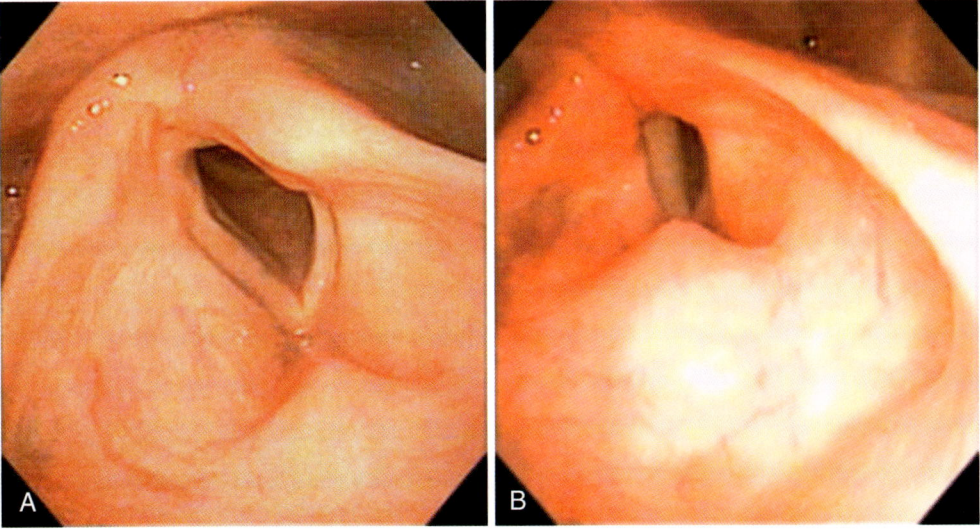

Fig. 42.3 Limitation of glottic closure in flaccid laryngeal paralysis. Note how the vocal process is rotated laterally so that the body of the arytenoid precludes closure.

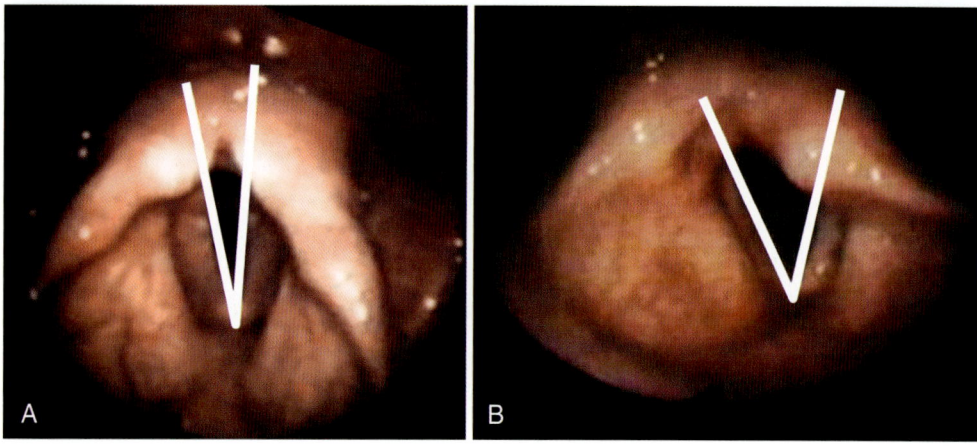

Fig. 42.4 Anterior glottic angle, measured during deep inspiration, is defined by lines connecting the anterior commissure with each vocal process. **A,** Paramedian vocal fold position. **B,** Lateral, or "cadaveric," vocal fold position.

contraction in cadaver larynges results in vocal fold lengthening but no adduction.[9] A three-dimensional model of vocal fold motion supports this finding.[14]

Many clinical series have failed to confirm a correlation between the position of the vocal fold and innervation of the cricothyroid muscle.[8,15-17] Instead, vocal fold position is determined by the forces of reinnervated (or residually innervated) muscles. In a study of 114 patients with a fixed vocal fold, Hirano found electromyographic (EMG) activity in 65%. Vocal fold position correlated with the number of motor units detected in the thyroarytenoid muscle by EMG and not with the status of the cricothyroid muscle.[8] In another study of patients with laryngeal paralysis, resulting from known sites of nerve injury, the position of the paralyzed vocal fold was quantified by measuring the angle formed by the vocal folds during prephonatory inspiration. A narrower glottic angle (i.e., a medial position of the paralyzed vocal fold) was observed in patients with greater EMG activity of the thyroarytenoid muscle.[15] In addition, the arytenoid tilts forward in patients with little or no detectable EMG activity.[15,17] This anterior tilt has been attributed to loss of tonic support from the posterior cricoarytenoid (PCA), a muscle that is not often sampled in EMG studies.

The PCA muscle is regarded as the sole abductor muscle in the larynx, but computer modeling suggests that the interarytenoid muscle participates in abduction. Further, the PCA muscle does not function solely as an abductor. It is also active in phonation, providing posterior support to the arytenoid and counterbalance to the anterior tipping forces exerted by the adductor muscles and the cricothyroid muscle. Indeed, in total laryngeal paralysis, the arytenoid tips forward due to the loss of this support.

EMG activity in a clinically paralyzed vocal fold can represent residual innervation after an incomplete original injury. It may also represent reinnervation of the muscles, either from a regenerated RLN or by sprouting from other nerve sources.

BIOLOGY OF NERVE INJURY AND REGENERATION

Peripheral nerve injuries provoke a complex biologic response that involves not only local tissues but also the central nervous system (CNS).[18] Within hours after transection, Wallerian degeneration begins, ultimately involving the entire length of the nerve distal to the injury. The proximal stump degeneration back to the first node of Ranvier. Both axons and surrounding myelin degenerate and are cleared away by proliferating Schwann cells and mast cells. Injured axons sprout new daughter axons that regenerate at a rate of 1 to 3 mm/d.[19] Regeneration through the distal nerve stump depends on the function of Schwann cells in the distal nerve, which begin to secrete neurotrophins, such as nerve growth factor (NGF), brain-derived nerve growth factor (BDNF), and NT4/5. These growth factors are taken up by the proximal axon stumps to be transported to the central nerve cell body where they promote neuron survival and axon regeneration.[20] The neural tubules in the distal nerves guide the axon to the target; however, the tubules contract over time.

With nerve transaction, each involved motor neuron initially undergoes chromatolysis. The nucleus migrates to the edge of the motor neuron, and Nissl granules break up and disperse. These changes herald the shift of the axon from neural transmission to repair. With time, the motor neuron returns to the center of the cell, Nissl bodies reorganize, and the neuron begins to synthesize proteins and lipids that will be transported to reconstruct the distal axon. Not all motor neurons survive after transaction of a nerve. In the spinal cord, 20% to 50% of motor neurons die after axonotmesis.[21] Survival is inversely correlated with the distance of the lesion from the neuron, presumably because after a proximal injury there is a long segment that must be regenerated. It has been reported that cell death is more frequent after injury to a cranial nerve. However, an experimental study in rats of transection and repair of an RLN animal studies documented survival of most motor neurons.[22] Other rat studies found no loss of neurons after nerve crush injury and no loss of neurons for up to 1 month after avulsion of the RLN.[23,24] The brain contains neural stem/progenitor cells that migrate toward a variety of CNS tissue injuries and may result in generation of new neurons and glia in response to injury and inflammatory disease.[25] Research has documented the migration of neural progenitor cells from the fourth ventricle of the brain to the nucleus ambiguus after RLN avulsion in rats.[26]

Injured neurons whose axons fail to make target connections in a timely fashion are said to be subjected to chronic axotomy.[19] Retrograde labeling studies in rat hind limbs found that after 1 year of chronic denervation of the distal nerve stump, <10% of motoneurons regenerated their axons when reconnected to the distal nerve stump. Motor units were enlarged, as regenerating axons branched to support more muscle fibers. A novel cross-suturing technique was used to independently control the times of axotomy, denervation of distal nerve sheaths, and muscle denervation. Results indicated that chronic denervation of the distal stump plays a key role in reduced functional recovery after delayed nerve repair, but denervated muscle is also a contributing factor.

Immediately after transection of a motor nerve, muscles begin to atrophy. Within days, satellite cells become activated, and neurotrophic and myogenic regulatory factors are upregulated. In this early phase, the muscle may lose up to 90% of its mass, yet it can regain normal strength with reinnervation. In the second stage of atrophy, the sarcoplasmic reticulum becomes disrupted, acetylcholine receptors proliferate along the muscle fiber, and spontaneous fibrillation activity appears. In the terminal phase, there is marked atrophy and minimal capacity to regain function. Slow muscle fibers undergo atrophy more quickly than fast fibers. In the rat hind limb, the first phase lasts 2 months, and the terminal phase is reached after 7 months. The time intervals have not been determined for human muscle, but at roughly 2 years, the success of reinnervation is sharply diminished.[27]

Although motor nerves regenerate, functional recovery is poor. A nerve is a complex collection of axons that supplies specific muscular targets not a simple power cord that can be "unplugged" and then "plugged back in." Axons are organized into fascicles, and if this structure is disrupted, regenerating axons can lose direction and reinnervate the wrong sites. This is termed *synkinesis*.[28] The risk of synkinesis increases with the degree of nerve injury. Sunderland's classification of the degree of nerve injury is based on histologic structure, recognizing the differential vulnerability of different tissues in the nerve.[29] A first-degree injury interrupts impulse conduction in axons, without anatomic disruption. This can be caused by compression or perhaps ischemia. In a second-degree injury, the endoneurial tube remains intact, but the axon loses continuity. This is possible because the endoneurium is more elastic than the axon itself and therefore more resistant to disruption by traction. During recovery from the injury, intact endoneurial tubules guide regenerating axons back to their original targets. But in third-degree injury, the intrafascicular structure is disorganized. Thus regenerating axons, though confined to the same fascicle, are no longer constrained by endoneurium to the original course within that fascicle and may reinnervate the wrong target. Further, scarring within the fascicle can block axonal regeneration. In fourth-degree injury, the fascicles themselves are disrupted so that there is even more disorganization of regenerating axons and a greater propensity for scarring that blocks nerve regeneration. In fifth-degree injury, the nerve trunk is completely transected so there is no longer a conduit to guide regeneration.

Sunderland's degrees of nerve injury are widely accepted. However, it should be noted that the degree of injury to individual axons within a nerve is not necessarily uniform. Some axons may be interrupted, whereas others may be merely compressed. Myelin may be preserved in some areas and destroyed in others. It seems logical that such mixed lesions would be more common in injuries which may be heterogeneous that may occur during thyroidectomy.

MECHANISMS OF INTRAOPERATIVE LARYNGEAL NERVE INJURY

Often, the cause of surgical injury cannot be identified. Stretching, without visible disruption, is the most commonly cited reason for laryngeal paralysis after thyroid surgery.[30,31] Intraoperative neural monitoring has been used in several animal studies to study specific mechanisms of nerve injury, including traction, clamping, crush, thermal, cautery, and transection.[32] In pigs, loss of signal was documented at a traction power of 2.83 MPa. All these animals sustained RLN paralysis that recovered within 7 days and did not result in structural nerve damage.[33] Other studies have indicated that amplitude and latency of the signal are important indicators of nerve damage.[34,35] Increased latency is the first sign of injury. Signal loss with traction is usually recovered unless the amplitude dropped more than 50%.

Thermal injury, from the use of hemostasis devices, has also been implicated.[30,31] Animal experiments indicate that the critical temperature for RLN injury is in the range of 60° C.[36] Other animal studies have compared the effects of various coagulation devices on the RLN to inform safe use.[32] Ultrasonic, bipolar, and integrated energy devices cause loss of RLN injury when fired within 1 mm from the nerve, but not when distances of ≥2 mm.[37]

The resilience of the RLN and its ability to recover from compression is evident in reports of laryngeal paralysis due to compressive goiter that recovers after thyroidectomy.[38,39] The nerve can also withstand partial resection. Kihara and colleagues reported on 18 patients (out of 4585 thyroidectomies for cancer) in whom tumor involved the nerve and only 50% was preserved. Fifteen of these patients ultimately regained function.[40]

Loss of continuity of the RLN is a severe injury, but the strong propensity for regeneration of the RLN is well documented in the literature. Animal studies have documented consistent regeneration of the RLN, even across a several centimeter gap.[4,41] In spasmodic dysphonia patients with recurrent symptoms after RLN section, the nerve has been found to regenerate, even after removal of a large segment and ligation of the stumps.[42] Surgical exploration in 29 patients with chronic laryngeal paralysis after thyroidectomy revealed that the nerve had been transected in 25.[43] Every transected nerve had regenerated to some degree, even if it had been ligated. But despite significant reinnervation of laryngeal muscles, normal motion never returns to a transected RLN, even if that nerve is precisely realigned and repaired.[44]

WHY ARE VOCAL FOLDS IMMOBILE DESPITE REINNERVATION?

The ultimate result of RLN injury is usually dysfunctional motion or spastic immobility. Even if the nerve is not repaired, nerve regeneration and muscle reinnervation always occur to varying degrees, but misdirected reinnervating nerve fibers result in opposing and inappropriate muscle contractions and no net movement. As Crumley stated, "Hence it appears that aberrant and poorly functioning reinnervation, rather than denervation, is the most common laryngeal problem in patients after RLN injury."[28] Synkinesis is also observed after nerve damage at other anatomic sites, such as the face or the limb.

Retrograde neurotracer research in rats has confirmed the inappropriate reinnervation of laryngeal muscles by the wrong brainstem neurons after nerve transection and repair.[45] Loss of somatotopy has also been reported after partial freezing nerve injury or crush injury.[23,46] Crumley proposed the classification of synkinesis as "favorable" or "unfavorable." With favorable synkinesis, muscles do not have adverse motions. Instead, muscle reinnervation holds the vocal fold in a favorable position and maintains muscle bulk so that the vocal fold is not thin and atrophic. With unfavorable synkinesis, there is adverse muscle activity, such as paradoxical adduction with inspiration, or spasms that disrupt speech. Unilateral paralysis can cause chronic upper airway obstruction due to hyperadduction. Rarely, RLN injury leads to recurrent severe airway obstruction as a result of such unfavorable synkinesis.[1] Synkinetic adduction with inspiration has been clearly documented in rat models of unilateral nerve transection.[47]

Laryngeal synkinesis clearly occurs; however, complete immobility as a result of synkinesis would require that opposing forces exactly cancel each other. This implies precisely orthogonal vectors with exactly equal strength—not the most likely outcome of a random process of reinnervation, particularly given the degrees of freedom of motion within the cricoarytenoid joint. Joint ankylosis has been suggested as a factor in chronic changes in the paralyzed vocal fold. However, histologic evaluation of 10 human laryngeal specimens with a history of chronic laryngeal paralysis revealed no evidence of ankylosis.[48] Moreover, exploration of the joint for arytenoid adduction in patients with paralysis as long as 25 years did not disclose such ankylosis.[49] The arytenoid rotated easily, but the vocal fold remained foreshortened, suggesting that soft tissue contraction was limiting motion.

Another explanation for immobility despite reinnervation is preferential reinnervation of adductor muscles, with poor or no reinnervation of the PCA muscle.[50] The adductor muscles pull the vocal fold medially, and the vocal fold remains in that position because of inadequate abductor muscle force. This is similar to a flexion contracture of a limb.

Vocal fold immobility is only one possible outcome of a RLN injury. The vocal fold may be mobile but weak, or it may have paradoxical adduction during inspiration. The vocal fold may be shrunken because of atrophy of the vocalis muscle. Sometimes the problem is a difference in the rostrocaudal level of the vocal folds. Variations in laryngeal posture after RLN injury can be accounted for by the complex action of laryngeal muscles and their compartments.[14]

MUSCLE COMPARTMENTS AND LARYNGEAL MOTION

The vocal folds do not merely open and close in one plane, like windshield wipers, but move and change shape in three dimensions. Each vocal fold has two distinct portions. The anterior portion is soft and pliable, composed of muscle covered by flexible mucosa. The posterior portion is cartilaginous, formed by the medial portion of the arytenoid. All the intrinsic laryngeal muscles (except the cricoarytenoid muscle) attach to the arytenoid cartilage. All vocal fold motion is affected by active rotation or translation of the arytenoid cartilage; the membranous fold is passively displaced by arytenoid motion.

The arytenoid cartilage articulates with the cricoid cartilage in a shallow ball-and-socket joint, which allows a wide range of motion. The larynx is opened by the PCA muscle, which pulls the arytenoid up and out of the glottis, displacing the vocal process laterally and superiorly.[51] The lateral cricoarytenoid (LCA) muscle closes the larynx by bringing the vocal process medially and caudally. Although these appear to be orthogonal motions when observing the larynx from above (particularly with two-dimensional video imaging), PCA abduction and LCA adduction involve rotation about different axes[52] (Figure 42.5). The thyroarytenoid and interarytenoid muscles also have distinctly separate vectors of force and axes of rotation. The thyroarytenoid and cricothyroid muscles control the shape of the membranous vocal fold. The cricothyroid lengthens, tenses, and thins the vocal fold, whereas the thyroarytenoid shortens and thickens it. Moreover, intrinsic laryngeal muscles appear to be divided into functional compartments with different functions. For example, the human PCA muscle has two bellies with different vectors of force on the arytenoid cartilage and separate nerve branches.[51,53] The thyroarytenoid muscle can be divided into two distinct anatomic compartments. The medial portion is commonly referred to as the vocalis, and the lateral portion is the muscularis. The compartments vary significantly in myosin content and concentration of muscle spindles.[54] A three-dimensional model of laryngeal motion demonstrates muscularis adduction of the vocal folds, whereas vocalis contraction causes slight abduction.[14] The varied and complimentary actions of intrinsic laryngeal muscles provide fine control of the glottis. Normal phonation involves precise coordination of this complex system. The vocal processes must be precisely approximated. The length, tension, and bulk of the vocal fold must be just right

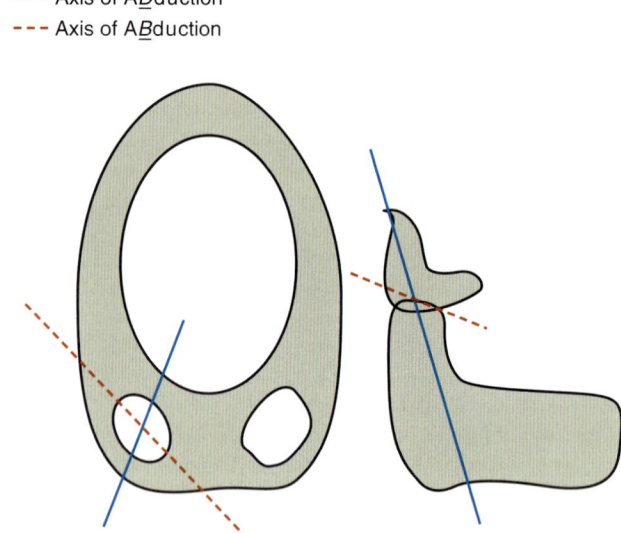

Fig. 42.5 Motion of the arytenoid cartilage in cadaver larynges. The axis of rotation is different with simulated contraction of the lateral cricoarytenoid and posterior cricoarytenoid muscles.

so that the vocal folds can be easily set into vibration, at the intended frequency of vibration, and so that the two sides vibrate synchronously. Control of pitch and vocal quality in professional singers requires even more precise adjustments in glottic configuration. This complex function is profoundly impaired when regenerating axons become scrambled and do not restore the normal connections between the brain and the larynx. Thus it is not surprising that even a slight disruption of nerve supply can have profound effects, particularly on the professional singer.

PREFERENTIAL REINNERVATION

Spontaneous RLN regeneration predominantly results in a vocal fold that is immobile in an adducted position. This is beneficial for the voice in unilateral paralysis but restricts the airway in bilateral paralysis. Understanding the processes that guide nerve fibers to denervated muscles could lead to therapeutic approaches for improving function after nerve injury.

Paniello developed a mathematical model to simulate synkinesis.[55] The model predicts that after complete transection of the RLN, about 75% of the fibers that reinnervate the PCA muscle will be adductor muscle fibers, but it does not address the lower overall number of axons reaching that muscle.

It is possible that the PCA and adductor muscles differ in the capacity to attract reinnervation axons. Research in rats has documented that rat hind limb muscle differs in the expression of some neurotrophic factors after denervation.[56] Research has also found significant differences in growth factor expression between the denervated PCA and adductor muscles.[57-59] In particular, Netrin-1 has been found to be upregulated in the rat PCA muscle during nerve regeneration.[60] As mentioned earlier, the PCA does not compete well for reinnervation, which is more robust in adductor muscles. Injection of high concentrations of Nitri1-11 into the PCA significantly reduced motor end plate reinnervation.[60] In vitro studies show promising evidence that neurotrophic factor-secreting muscle stem cells could be used therapeutically to selectively promote and direct laryngeal reinnervation after RLN injury.

ACUTE MANAGEMENT OF THE TRANSECTED NERVE

For many years, there was a widespread reluctance to repair an acutely transected nerve. Many investigators repeatedly observed that in both patients and experimental animals repair of the RLN did not restore normal motion. In fact, aberrant activity and airway obstruction were observed after RLN repair. It has also become apparent that there is a very strong propensity for the RLN to regenerate without any therapeutic intervention. Therefore the fundamental question to be answered is this: Are functional results better with spontaneous regeneration or surgical repair?

There are conflicting reports in the literature of clinical experience and animal experiments. Several authors have reported some return of function after immediate repair of a transected RLN.[61-66] Many, however, have noted adverse functional results, including airway obstruction resulting from paradoxical motion, return of adductor but not abductor function, and poor voice.[66-72]

The potential for dysfunction, due to synkinetic reinnervation, has led many to recommend against repairing the acutely transected nerve. This would be a valid recommendation if the unrepaired nerve resulted in flaccid paralysis and no inappropriate motion. However, the literature indicates that whether or not the nerve is repaired, aberrant nerve regeneration can occur. At present, the prevailing consensus is that an acutely transected nerve should be repaired because this will maximize the amount of reinnervation. If there is a large gap that precludes primary repair, reinnervation can be accomplished with another nerve, such as a branch of the ansa cervicalis, could be warranted. This approach should restore tonic activity and hopefully block reinnervation by synkinetic fibers (see Chapter 43, Management of Recurrent Laryngeal Nerve Paralysis).

SUMMARY

Laryngeal paralysis is a serious complication of thyroid surgery. Unilateral paralysis primarily affects the voice, whereas bilateral paralysis impairs the airway. The injured RLN has a very strong propensity to regenerate and reinnervate laryngeal muscles, even if the nerve is transected or ligated. But despite regeneration, normal motion is not recovered. This is synkinesis, with abductor fibers supplying adductor muscles and vice versa. Laryngeal motion is complex, requiring coordinated action by muscles with varied vectors of force. A reinnervated larynx is generally immobile, in a relatively adducted position, due to preferential innervation and inadequate reinnervation of the abductor muscle, the PCA muscle. Synkinetic reinnervation can sometimes result in inspiratory stridor or episodic laryngospasm. Recent research indicates that laryngeal muscles differ in molecular response to denervation. Such differences could prove useful in improving the specificity of reinnervation. Continued research is essential to develop better means of treatment, with the goal of restoring normal function (see Chapter 43, Management of Recurrent Laryngeal Nerve Paralysis).

REFERENCES

For a complete list of references, go to expertconsult.com.

43

Management of Recurrent Laryngeal Nerve Paralysis

Simon Brisebois, Andrew M. Vahabzadeh-Hagh, Fermin Zubiaur, Albert Merati

Please go to expertconsult.com to view related video:
Video 43.1 Vocal Fold Augmentation Using Transcricothyroid Membrane Submucosal Approach.
This chapter contains additional online-only content, including exclusive video, available on expertconsult.com.

INTRODUCTION

Alteration in the function of the recurrent laryngeal nerve (RLN) is an unfortunate and sometimes unavoidable consequence of thyroid surgery. It may result from errors in surgical technique or judgment or from the disease process itself. Injury to the RLN may yield vocal fold hypomobility or frank immobility. Preoperative counseling on the risks of transient or permanent vocal fold paralysis is important with typical figures reporting a rate of permanent vocal fold paralysis after thyroid surgery to be about 1% or less, whereas rates of transient impaired vocal fold mobility may range from 1.8% to 2.6%.[1] Risk factors for RLN injury include total thyroidectomy, revision surgery, and cases in which the RLN was not identified intraoperatively.[2] Patients with vocal fold paralysis after thyroidectomy have significantly increased morbidity as well as postoperative health care expenses.[3] Persistent dysphonia can have a major effect on the patient's quality of life and is the leading cause of litigation after thyroidectomy.[4] The surgeon must ensure that patients are well informed of the risks before surgery, and they must do everything they can to mitigate those risks while taking appropriate care of the patient's primary thyroid problem. In the event of vocal fold paralysis, they should be aware of the clinical presentation and be able to implement or direct the patient toward rehabilitative measures.

UNILATERAL VOCAL FOLD PARALYSIS

Evaluation

The classic presentation seen in clinical care is altered voice with or without some level of swallowing difficulty due to unilateral vocal fold paralysis (UVFP) after thyroid surgery. This may happen even despite an intact RLN and confirmatory intraoperative neural monitoring (IONM) findings at the completion of surgery. Sahli et al. found this rate to be as high as 18.8% with age ≥50 years as an independent risk factor for postoperative dysphonia and/or dysphagia.[5] Although RLN injury may seem like the first logical culprit, thoughts should be given to alternative diagnoses. The chart should be reviewed for preoperative evaluation to ensure that there was no preexisting dysfunction before surgery. Otherwise, an intubation-related injury by compression of the nerve microcirculation may be considered but is probably a rare occurrence with a reported incidence of 0.08%.[6]

UVFP after thyroidectomy most commonly presents with a breathy, weak voice. Projection is limited, and the voice is easily fatigued; there may be a subjective sense of shortness of breath during phonation. In addition to dysphonia, patients may also experience dysphagia with or without aspiration.[7] One should therefore inquire about issues of choking or coughing while eating or drinking as well as any history of interval pneumonia. The voice is evaluated by both the clinician and the patient. The clinician performs a perceptual voice assessment most commonly using the GRBAS scale (grade, roughness, breathiness, asthenia, strain) or CAPE-V (consensus auditory perceptual evaluation of voice) tool to determine voice quality.[8] Additionally, acoustic measures, such as jitter, shimmer, and noise-to-harmonic ratio, may be collected.[9] The patient is asked to complete a voice handicap assessment survey, most commonly the Voice Handicap Index-10.[10] These tools help establish a baseline from which progress can be tracked and the success of interventions can be measured. A comprehensive head and neck examination should follow. This includes assessment of cranial nerve function with special attention to the vagus nerve. The neck should be palpated for any lymphadenopathy, neck masses, or laryngotracheal malformations.

Videolaryngoscopy

Videolaryngoscopy is essential for the examination of the larynx in the dysphonic patient. Updated clinical practice guidelines published by the American Academy of Otolaryngology—Head and Neck Surgery state that laryngoscopy should be performed on any patient for which dysphonia does not improve or resolve within 4 weeks.[11] For the postsurgical candidate in whom vocal fold paralysis is predicted, more expeditious laryngoscopy is warranted. Flexible laryngoscopy allows examination of the larynx in its physiologic position and during respiratory and phonatory tasks while providing magnified, high-resolution images of the larygopharyngeal mucosa. Videolaryngoscopy with the addition of stroboscopy provides further insight into vocal fold mobility and vibratory function as well as symmetry and completeness of glottic closure.

Please see the Expert Consult website for more discussion of this topic.

Laryngeal Electromyography

Laryngologists have reported the diagnostic inaccuracy of pure visual assessment of the larynx to diagnose neuromuscular dysfunction to be as high as one-third of cases.[17] This is in comparison to laryngeal electromyography (LEMG), a technique to directly and objectively assess the integrity of laryngeal nerves and muscles. LEMG is a useful tool used as an adjunct to videostroboscopy, helping distinguish between neurologic causes of vocal fold immobility or hypomobility and mechanical causes, such as cricoarytenoid joint fixation. It is also

410

a tool that can help prognosticate return of function in cases of paresis or paralysis and help predict whether patients will respond well to voice therapy alone or will require procedural intervention. The utility of LEMG has been a topic of much debate with sparse evidence-based support. In 2016, a consensus statement on the utility of LEMG for diagnosis and treatment of vocal fold paralysis after recurrent laryngeal neuropathy was published. It concluded that LEMG should be used if prognostic information is sought in a patient with vocal fold paralysis for more than 4 weeks but less than 6 months. In such patients, if they have active voluntary motor unit potential recruitment and polyphasic motor units potentials, recovery is anticipated.[18] Furthermore, use of LEMG in the clinical algorithm led to a change in clinical management by better understanding the diagnosis in 48% of cases reviewed by Munin et al.[18] LEMG in practice may take on a variety of forms from an individual to a team-based approach. Often an electrodiagnostic physician and an otolaryngologist work together to complete this office-based procedure.[17]

MANAGEMENT OF UNILATERAL VOCAL FOLD PARALYSIS

Treatment of vocal fold paralysis often has two main goals: namely to provide efficient, effortless, and intelligible phonation and to provide a safe swallow free from aspiration. With newly diagnosed vocal fold paralysis, conservative measures are the frontline and first choice to help manage voice and swallowing issues. If vocal fold paralysis is secondary to a known transection of the RLN or meaningful recovery of function is not anticipated, then more definitive procedural intervention is offered. Here we will begin with a discussion of more conservative interventions and progress to more invasive and definitive treatment options.

Voice and Swallow Therapy

Patients with vocal fold paralysis and dysphonia are best served by a team effort between the otolaryngologist and a speech language pathologist. Speech language pathologists' early evaluation and treatment of such patients is critical. They can implement potentially useful compensatory strategies for the patient while identifying and eliminating behaviors that might be counterproductive. Although vocal fold paralysis is by definition a hypofunctional disorder, patients may exhibit a compensatory hyperfunctional behavior, such as muscle tension dysphonia. This can make an already poor voice quality potentially worse and compound the perceived phonatory effort.[19] Early voice therapy is aimed at improving phonatory efficiency, vocal ease, and endurance. Such techniques may include control of hyperfunctional behaviors, pitch modification, abdominal support for breathing, and exercises to improve intrinsic laryngeal muscle strength. A comprehensive review of such techniques can be found in Miller 2004.[20] Heuer et al. found that of 41 patients with UVFP, 68% of female patients and 64% of male patients did not elect to have surgical intervention after voice therapy and that outcome satisfaction was similar among conservatively and surgically treated patients. It is therefore always reasonable to send patients into voice therapy regardless of the anticipated likelihood of future procedural interventions.[19]

Vocal fold paralysis results in glottal insufficiency, reduced subglottal pressures, and less airway protection during swallowing. This may result in aspiration, which can be identified by history or the development of an aspiration pneumonia. When there is concern for aspiration, a formal swallow evaluation must take place, which often includes a fiberoptic endoscopic evaluation of swallowing (FEES) and/or modified barium swallow (MBS). These tests can be used to confirm aspiration, risk stratify different liquid consistencies or foods, and test postural or behavioral adjustments to reduce the likelihood of aspiration. Swallow therapy often includes the observation of meals and the teaching of techniques to obtain a safer swallow. Such techniques may include head turn to the paralyzed side, chin tuck, effortful swallow, and the supraglottic swallow technique.[21] Swallowing techniques are taught and are often followed by a repeat MBS and/or FEES. In cases of persistent aspiration, early vocal fold medialization procedures may be offered to improve glottal closure and to achieve a stronger cough.

Vocal Fold Augmentation for Unilateral Vocal Fold Immobility

Few interventions have dramatically affected the way voice disorders are currently managed more than vocal fold augmentation for RLN paresis and paralysis. Wilhelm Brünings initially introduced injection laryngoplasty in 1911 to correct the problem of glottic insufficiency resulting from unilateral vocal fold immobility.[22] In this procedure, a material is injected into the true vocal fold in an attempt to add bulk and medialize the edge of the vocal fold. Over the years, however, the procedure suffered some setbacks because of complications from injectable materials such as paraffin and polytetrafluoroethylene paste (Teflon).[23,24] Since the introduction of flexible indirect laryngoscopy in the 1970s, in office procedures regained popularity and vocal fold augmentation became one of the most widely performed procedures in laryngology.[25] Indeed, the development of distal chip cameras and the use of transoral angled rigid telescopes for routine laryngeal examinations have made laryngeal visualization one of superb quality. Furthermore, the development of U.S. Food and Drug Administration (FDA)-approved injection materials has allowed the increased use by otolaryngologists with fewer concerns regarding legal issues or payments by insurance companies. All this combined with the emergence of laryngology as a subspecialty in the 1990s led to an expanded range of indications. Nowadays, vocal fold augmentation can be used routinely for vocal fold atrophy, hypomobility, immobility, and scarring, and more recently as a promising alternative for chronic cough.[26,27]

Please see the Expert Consult website for more discussion of this topic.

Five main approaches are used for in office injections: (1) transorally using a long, curved injection needle guided by either rigid endoscopy or flexible nasolaryngoscopy (Figure 43.1, line 1); (2) percutaneous transthyrohyoid injection entering the lumen of the airway at the petiole of the epiglottis (see Figure 43.1, line 2); (3) percutaneous transthyroid cartilage injection with needle insertion through the ala of the thyroid cartilage at the approximate level of the vocal fold (see Figure 43.1, line 3); (4) percutaneous transcricothyroid injection where the needle is inserted below the inferior margin of the thyroid cartilage and angled superolaterally into the vocal fold (see Figure 43.1, line 4). The approach can be performed 3 to 7 mm off the midline entering the vocal fold submucosally or medially entering the airway in the subglottis to then angle the needle laterally toward the posterior aspect of the vocal fold. Finally (5) the transnasal endoscopic approach, using a 23- to 25-gauge flexible needle through a working channel laryngoscope. All the percutaneous techniques are usually performed with visual guidance using flexible laryngoscopy, but rigid transoral endoscopy is also possible. The different needles used can be bent proximally and/or distally according to surgeon preference and patient anatomy. Simultaneous live endoscopy and injection projected on a monitor in front of the patient is useful as it allows immediate feedback that, along

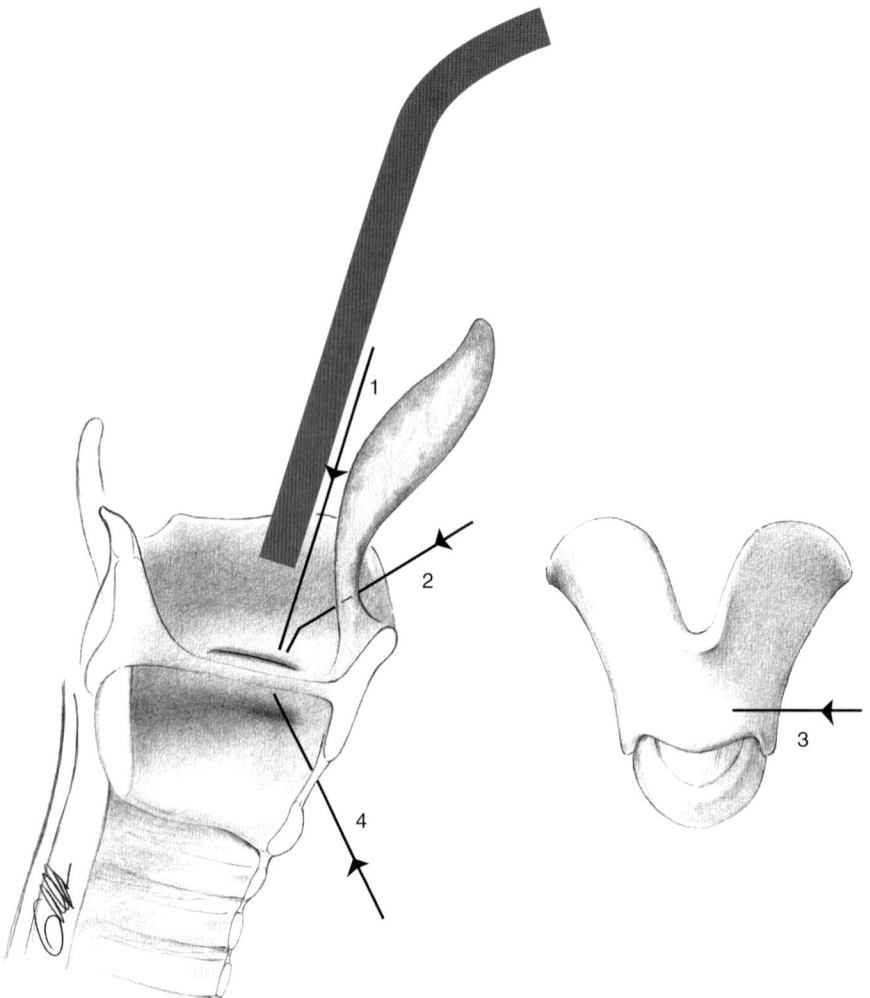

Fig. 43.1 **Approaches for Awake Vocal Fold Augmentation.** The thicker line entering the larynx from above represents the flexible nasolaryngoscope that is used for visual guidance. Approach (1) is the transoral route, using a curved needle. The second (2) is the transthyrohyoid approach where a 25-gauge 1½-inch needle is introduced over the thyroid notch and pierces the petiole of the epiglottis to access the superior surface of the vocal folds, the ventricles, and the false vocal folds. Approach (3) is the transthyroid cartilage that gives direct access to the paraglottic space but is hampered by the needle becoming clogged with a cartilage plug. The fourth (4) approach is the transcricothyroid, allowing excellent access to the inferior vocal folds.

with constant verbal communication from the surgeon, can also aid with the natural anxiety that is generally experienced. These techniques require different degrees of topical anesthesia in the airway, beginning in the nasal cavity for the flexible endoscope followed by the oropharynx, hypopharynx, and the larynx. Proper and effective anesthesia is a relatively simple task to perform and can usually be done in a few minutes. There are many ways to apply topical laryngeal anesthesia, but this becomes the key step toward obtaining adequate visualization to then perform a precise injection. A laryngeal lidocaine gargle, lidocaine dripping through a flexible endoscope working channel or a flexible catheter and/or a transtracheal injection, results in a quick and efficient way to anesthetize the vocal folds. Vocal fold augmentation transorally in the operating room and under general anesthesia through a direct microlaryngoscopy is a valid alternative in selected patients, but performing injections in the awake patient is not only faster, more cost-effective, and results in less morbidity, but also permits auditory feedback from patient phonation during the procedure. This allows fine-tuning of the injection volume in an attempt to obtain the best possible voice outcome.

Please see the Expert Consult website for more discussion of this topic.

The best time to inject after RLN injury depends on a variety of factors, including vocal, respiratory, and airway protection needs. It is not necessary to wait for nerve recovery when any of these factors becomes an issue in the patient's everyday needs, considering that early injection has been demonstrated to be safe and useful, helping the patient resume daily routine activities that involve voice use while eliminating symptoms of dyspnea and vocal fatigue.[29] Early vocal fold augmentation is warranted in cases where airway penetration and/or aspiration is suspected.

Swallowing alterations that accompany some RLN lesions should be considered a priority in the decision-making process of when to augment a paralyzed vocal fold. A vast number of materials have been used over the years for injection laryngoplasty; however, the ideal material has yet to be discovered. Among the characteristics of the ideal material would be biocompatibility, low viscosity for easy injectability, similar biomechanical properties to native vocal fold tissue, ready availability, resistance to resorption and migration, and ease of removal.[30] Each material has different properties, and the choice for injection is made

TABLE 43.1 Most Common Materials Currently Used for Vocal Fold Augmentation*

Material	Duration	Preparation	Advantages	Drawbacks
Hyaluronic acid (Restylane, Juvederm)	3–6 months	Very easy	Safety and efficacy supported by clinical studies	Can have unexpected rapid absorption
Carboxymethylcellulose (Prolaryn Gel)	2–3 months	Very easy	Low viscosity	Very rapid absorption
Calcium hydroxyapatite (CaHa) (Prolaryn Plus)	1–3 years	Easy. Warm CaHa offers less resistance during injection.	Minimal inflammatory response. No evidence of toxicity.	Superficial injection may need surgical removal
Bovine-based collagen (Zyplast, Zyderm)	3–4 months	Easy	Viscoelastic properties	Hypersensitivity reactions
Human-based collagen (Cymetra – micronized cadaveric dermis) (Cosmoplast, Cosmoderm – tissue engineered)	2–3 months	Moderate	Facilitates fibrous in-growth and angiogenesis	Requires reconstitution
Autologous fat	One to several years/ permanent	More complex/time consuming	Abundant availability, viscoelastic properties	Requires fat harvest and general anesthesia. Unpredictable duration.

*Consider saline for "trial injections."

based largely on the desired duration of effect and surgeon preference. The use of Teflon is fairly limited these days because of the necessity of injecting it through a large-gauge needle and the risk of granuloma formation.[31]

A comparison of the most common materials used for vocal fold augmentation is shown in Table 43.1. Hyaluronic acid (HA), carboxymethylcellulose, and calcium hydroxyapatite are used in many institutions as primary alternatives as they are easy to use, do not require special preparation, and can be adapted to a variety of injection needles. In case of an accidental superficial injection resulting in increased hoarseness, excess HA can be partially eliminated with an intralesional injection of hyaluronidase, but it should be used judiciously to avoid alteration of the naturally occurring extracellular matrix glycosaminoglycan found in the vocal fold lamina propia.[32]

Over the years, other popular materials have included collagen (bovine and autologous), Cymetra (micronized human dermis), autologous fat, and gel foam. These require more time for preparation and involve some degree of hypersensitivity risk in the case of bovine collagen.

Almost all injection materials require overinjection, as initial partial reabsorption and substance accommodation during phonation is expected, which is why it is important to warn the patient that a strained voice is a normal immediate result (Figure 43.2).

Laryngeal Framework Surgery

Laryngeal framework surgery was described by Payr in 1915 and popularized in the 1970s by Nobohiko Isshiki of Kyoto University. Dr. Isshiki refined this technique as a way to alter vocal fold position and tension without ever touching the "sanctuary" of the vocal fold itself. These techniques have been implemented to treat dysphonia from UVFP, vocal fold atrophy with presbylarynges, and pitch-related dysphonia.[33] The most widely used techniques for UVFP include the type I thyroplasty and arytenoid adduction, which will be further discussed here. These techniques seek to recreate the prephonatory posture of the vocal fold that would naturally be achieved by activation of the intrinsic laryngeal muscles, namely, the thyroarytenoid and the lateral cricoarytenoid muscles. Whereas injection laryngoplasty

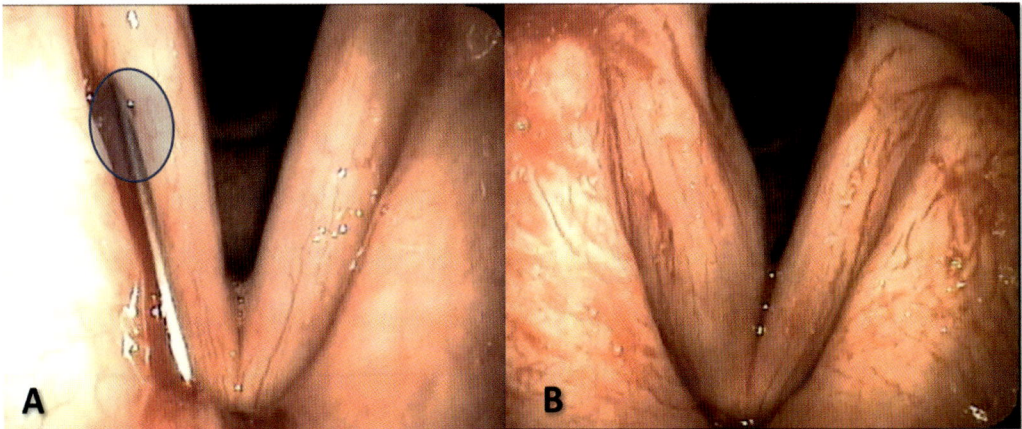

Fig. 43.2 Indirect laryngoscopy during right vocal fold augmentation with transthyrohyoid approach using hyaluronic acid. **A,** Ideal area of needle insertion (posterior third and lateral); **B,** Immediate result after the recommended overinjection.

seeks to improve glottal competence, laryngeal framework surgery considers many variables that contribute to the complex nature of vocal fold motion and prephonatory posture. These include the position of the arytenoid, the shape of the vocal fold medial surface, the height of the membranous vocal fold and the vocal process, the length and tension of the vocal fold, and the vocal fold mass and viscoelastic properties.

A type I thyroplasty is the most widely used technique to rehabilitate the paralyzed vocal fold. Since being refined by Isshiki in 1975, the technique and materials used have taken on various forms. The technique involves cutting a window in the thyroid lamina at the level of the paralyzed vocal fold. The vocal fold is then medialized by placing an implant in the paraglottic space, most often using a carved silicone block or Gore-Tex that is then secured in place. Carving of the silicone implant has taken on various forms but is most often performed with medium to firm softness and roughly approximates the shape of the sail of a sailboat. Netterville et al. provide a discussion of one such preparation.[34] In 1997, Montgomery published his experience using the Montgomery Thyroplasty Implant System (Figure 43.3, A), a procedural kit with medialization implants of varying sizes for male and female patients, a measuring device, and surgical instruments meant to provide a standardization to type I thyroplasty surgery.[35] Improvement in the majority of clinicians' perceptual voice analysis and patients' overall satisfaction with use of the Montgomery Thyroplasty Implant System has been demonstrated.[36] In 1998, Hoffman and McCulloch introduced the use of expanded polytetrafluoroethylene (ePTFE; Gore-Tex®) for thyroplasty as a uniquely simple technique that allows for adjustments and does not require special instrumentation.[37] The medical use and biocompatibility of ePTFE is well documented. It comes in the form of a thin sheet that can be cut into strip(s) and layered through the thyroplasty window into the paraglottic space until the desired phonatory outcome is achieved (see Figure 43.3, B). It is favored by many surgeons because precision is not required in making the cartilage window or shaping the implant, the position and size of the implant is easily adjustable, and it can be easily removed or modified in revision surgery. Nouwen et al. compared the voice outcomes and morbidity of treating 57 patients with unilateral vocal cord paralysis with either the Montgomery or ePTFE type I thyroplasty implants. They found that implant selection did not influence the success of the procedure or the associated morbidity but did lead to significant improvements in speech and voice outcome metrics.[38] Although a type I thyroplasty can achieve closure of the membranous vocal fold, it alone cannot effectively address a large posterior glottal chink nor the position of the arytenoid. For this, Isshiki described the arytenoid adduction.

Arytenoid adduction surgery is designed to recreate the action of the lateral cricoarytenoid muscle, rotating and medializing the cartilaginous vocal fold, or vocal process, into a permanent prephonatory posture, closing a posterior glottal chink and reestablishing a more symmetric height or level of the vocal cords. It is accomplished by affixing a permanent suture to the muscular process of the arytenoid and then pulling the muscular process in an anteromedial direction to rotate the arytenoid inferomedial.[39,40] This can be done under local anesthesia and intravenous sedation so that the degree of arytenoid adduction may be adjusted in real time to produce the best voice, or it can be done under general anesthesia with the use of a small-caliber endotracheal tube as more experience is obtained in the ideal tension on the arytenoid adduction stitch, which is minimal. An arytenoid adduction is technically more demanding and requires more experience and skill to prevent injury to the pyriform sinus, which must be mobilized to

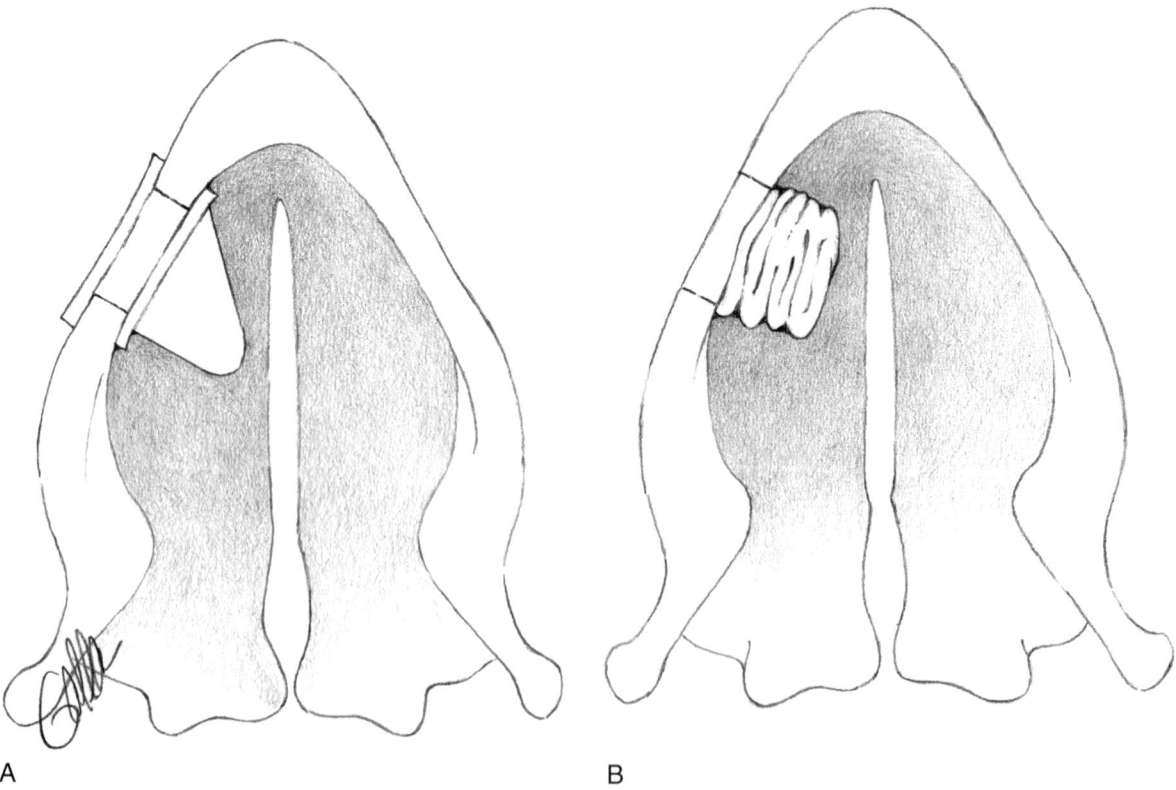

Fig. 43.3 Type I thyroplasty can be performed using many different materials, including a **(A)** solid implant (e.g., Montgomery or silastic) or **(B)** Gore-Tex®.

reach the muscular process of the arytenoid. Arytenoid adduction may exaggerate the medial rotation of the vocal process and result in suboptimal outcomes. Another approach, the adduction arytenopexy, involves opening the cricoarytenoid joint; the arytenoid is manually medialized along the cricoid facet, and a single suture is placed through the posterior cricoid and the muscular process of the arytenoid. This provides for lengthening of the membranous vocal fold and a more normally contoured arytenoid (Figure 43.4).[41] Combined arytenoid adduction with type I medialization thyroplasty has been and continues to be a much-debated topic. Many argue that the added morbidity of arytenoid adduction is not worth the potential improvements in voice outcome. Mortensen et al. performed a retrospective review of patients who underwent medialization laryngoplasty (ML) alone or in combination with arytenoid adduction (ML-AA). They found that patients in the combined ML-AA group had worse preoperative function and better postoperative function in terms of acoustics and aerodynamic measures.[42] As such, for the properly selected and counseled patient, a combined ML-AA may provide the best functional outcome.

Framework surgery is truly at the juncture of art and science in the field of otolaryngology. Its outcomes are highly reliant upon clinical expertise and judgment. Complication rates have been shown to be higher in surgeons who performed fewer than 2 procedures per year or have done less than a total of 10 cases. As arytenoid repositioning procedures are associated with manipulation of the posterior glottis and greater postoperative edema, one must always consider the potential for postoperative airway issues. The rate of tracheotomy with arytenoid adduction has ranged from 1.7% to 3.5%, with most airway issues occurring 9 hours postoperatively.[43] In a 10-year follow-up to a

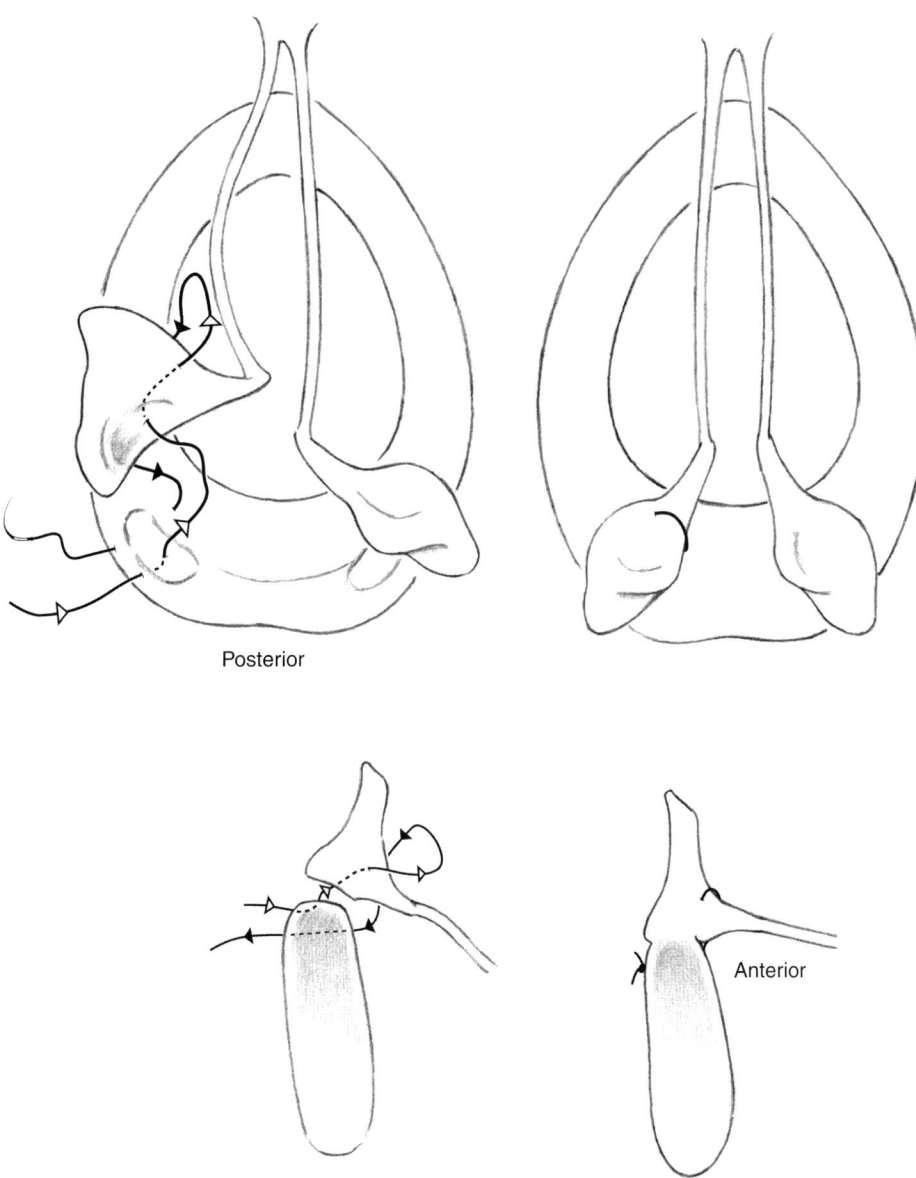

Fig. 43.4 Adduction Arytenopexy. The suture repositions the arytenoid in the midline, pulling posteriorly (up the cricoid) on the cricoarytenoid joint into its normal phonatory position. A 4-0 Prolene suture passed through the lateral cricoid exits the medial/posterior cricoarytenoid joint. The suture is then passed through the arytenoid cartilage from the articulating surface (undersurface) of the arytenoid cartilage and passed from the inner cortex to outer cortex of the cricoid cartilage, under the cricoarytenoid joint where it is pulled taut and tied.

national survey by Young et al. on the incidence, success, and complication rates of laryngeal framework surgery, medialization thyroplasty, and arytenoid adduction were being performed with increasing frequency. Use of silastic for thyroplasty implants decreased over time in lieu of other materials. The overall complication rate was 15%; the revision rate was 6%, most commonly for replacement with a larger implant; airway compromise requiring intervention occurred 2.2% of the time; and suboptimal voice outcomes were seen 4% of the time.[44]

Laryngeal Reinnervation

Reinnervation of a paralyzed vocal fold by repair of an injured RLN is, in theory, the most appealing way to restore function. The first description of RLN reanastomosis is from Horsley in 1910, when he reported on a patient with left UVFP after a gunshot wound to the neck, which was reanastomosed primarily. He then reported almost complete recovery of motion a little more than a year after the surgery. However, we know today that direct anastomosis or any other type of laryngeal reinnervation (LR) of a transected RLN does not restore normal motion but usually results in a vocal fold fixed in a favorable median or paramedian position. In 1982, Ezaki et al. reported vocal improvement in seven thyroid cancer patients after primary anastomosis, even though the vocal folds were immobile. They surmised that though normal motion was not restored, the reinnervated muscles recovered from atrophy, and tension improved during phonation.[45] After that, many studies have also shown favorable outcomes on objective and subjective voice-related measures.[46-51]

The RLN consists of adductor and abductor fibers without spatial segregation of the fibers within the nerve. In 1963, Siribodhi et al. reported nerve fiber regeneration after direct anastomosis of the transected RLN, albeit with the mixing of adductor and abductor fibers.[52] This phenomenon is called misdirected regeneration. The RLN contains two to four times as many adductor fibers as abductor fibers, and adductors are stronger than abductors. Therefore reinnervated vocal folds are usually positioned toward the median position. This situation is better described as synkinesis, simultaneous contraction of adductors and abductors, rather than paralysis.[53] The presence of minimal or no glottic gap during phonation, symmetric shape and mass of the vocal folds and adequate tension of the folds are essential for good phonation. It is possible to achieve all these results after reinnervation. In cases showing extreme misdirection in reinnervation, however, paradoxical motion of the vocal folds may occur.

The purpose of LR is to restore tone, bulk, and positioning of the vocal fold.[54,55] In comparison with medialization interventions, such as injection laryngoplasty or thyroplasty, reinnervation may provide active resting tone to the reinnervated muscles, resistance, and thus prevent vocal atrophy.[56] The procedure is considered safe[57] and offers good voice outcomes.[50] Still, even though it is considered as being an effective and reliable surgical procedure, it is not as widely performed as other medialization techniques, such as framework surgery, for the treatment of UVFP.

Indications and Timing of Reinnervation Surgery

The most common indication for LR is a unilateral neurogenic injury to the RLN with no expectation for recovery. This can be confirmed by knowledge of the status of the nerve, for example, if it has been transected, or after an adequate period of observation for recovery. Reinnervation could thus be applied intraoperatively in cases where nerve sacrifice is expected or unavoidable. In other cases, when the status is unclear, LEMG can potentially help confirm the complete absence of efference before deciding to proceed with surgery. Interestingly, a study by Jun Lin et al. has shown that LEMG at least 6 months after RLN injury only infrequently showed complete denervation (11%).[58] Thus a lot of patients may still have some neural activity in the nerve from their nerve, and a different surgery may be sought.

Even though there is one report of successful reinnervation after more than 20 years postinjury,[61] it is potentially more successful if the procedure is performed within 2 years after nerve injury.[47] Age may also play a role, and it is suggested that the surgery can be more successful in patients less than 60 years old.[46] Other comorbidities that may affect proper healing, like diabetes, may be considered as relative contraindications.

Various techniques have been described in the literature to deal with reinnervation, such as primary anastomosis, free nerve grafting, ansa cervicalis-to-RLN (possibly combined with cricothyroid muscle-nerve-muscle pedicle), ansa-to-thyroarytenoid neural implantation, ansa-cervicalis-to- thyroarytenoid neuromuscular pedicle, or hypoglossal-to-RLN. The combination of these techniques with injection laryngoplasty can help improve the patient's symptomatology quickly, while waiting for the reinnervation, as this may take place over the course of many months. Framework surgery, such as type I thyroplasty or arytenoid adduction, can also be combined to potentially improve voice outcomes and has been reported to be feasible and safe.[57,62]

Ansa Cervicalis-to-Recurrent Laryngeal Nerve Anastomosis

LR using ansa-to-RLN anastomosis was first reported by Frazier in 1924 in patients with bilateral vocal fold paralysis after a thyroidectomy.[63] In 1986, Crumley and Izdebski published their surgical technique, which served as the basis for contemporary work on reinnervation.[64] It is the most commonly studied technique for LR.[50]

For RLN-Ansa anastomosis the presence of a distal RLN stump and ansa cervicalis is necessary to proceed with the ansa-to-RLN anastomosis. In the absence of an ipsilateral ansa, the contralateral one can be used by passing between the branch between the trachea and esophagus.[59] Also, in cases of absent RLN stump, other techniques, such as an ansa neural implantation or ansa neuromuscular pedicle technique, can still be used. It is important to consider, when choosing this treatment approach, that the time to recovery may be close to 9 months or more.[60] Thus the patient must be willing to wait. A patient who is not expected to survive this long should not be a candidate for the procedure.

A cervical incision of about 4 cm is made in a skin crease at the level of the cricoid and placed off midline on the side to be reanastomosed. If a scar is already present from prior thyroid surgery, it can be used. Subplastymal flaps are raised superiorly and inferiorly. The fascia between the strap musculature and the sternocleidomastoid muscle is opened, and the jugular vein is exposed. The ansa cervicalis should be found looping over it. The loop and branches can then be followed and dissected free. The main distal branch is usually used to provide length. It is divided and flipped inside the tracheoesophageal groove. The RLN can either be found distally at its insertion at the cricothyroid joint and followed in a retrograde fashion or found more proximally in the tracheoesophageal groove. Enough of the nerve should be released to allow for tension-free anastomosis. Under microscopic magnification, neurorrhaphy is performed using 8-0 nylon and placing two to four epineural sutures around the anastomosis.

Results

Miyauchi et al. reported on 51 patients who had either direct anastomosis, free nerve grafting, or ansa-to-RLN anastomosis for thyroid cancer invading the RLN. They used maximum phonation time (MPT), defined as the sustained phonation of the vowel "a" at the loudness of usual conversation voice after maximum inspiration at a sitting position, as well as the phonation efficiency index (PEI), defined as the MPT over vital capacity ratio (s/L), which should indicate vocal cord function by converting a unit volume of exhaled air to a certain duration of phonation. Both values were improved after LR in their cohort after 1 year of follow-up.[65]

Long-term outcomes from a prospective cohort of 237 patients diagnosed with UVFP after thyroid surgery, and operated on for ansa-to-RLN anastomosis, was provided by Wang et al. in 2011. Overall, their analysis demonstrated postoperative improvement in glottic closure, vocal fold edge, vocal fold position, phase symmetry, and regularity of the mucosal wave. Perceptual and acoustic analysis and MPT were also improved, and no significant difference was found compared with matched controls. Postoperative LEMG demonstrated improved recruitment.[66]

A systematic review by Aynechi et al. on the various LR techniques reported improvement in perceptual analysis and electromyography findings for all reviewed studies. The first sign of reinnervation is reported to be around 4.5 months. Furthermore, glottic gap based on visual analysis was closing, with the greatest mean improvement from ansa-to-RLN technique, changing from 2.25 mm before to 0.75 mm after surgery. Finally, acoustic analysis also demonstrated favorable outcomes, which was greater with neural reimplantation. The mean MPT changed from 7 to 16 seconds.[50]

A prospective clinical trial compared 19 patients who underwent LR for intraoperative RLN resection versus 43 patients undergoing injection laryngoplasty for diagnosis of permanent vocal fold paralysis, all after thyroid surgery. It reported steady improvement in subjective and objective voice measures over a follow-up period of about 3 years. The time to voice improvement was significantly quicker with injection laryngoplasty at 1.4 months versus 4.3 months for reinnervation. However, compared with reinnervation, injection laryngoplasty did show some deterioration at the 3-year mark.[49]

A multicenter randomized clinical trial comparing ML with LR was published by Paniello et al. in 2011. Twenty-four patients were randomized between the two groups. Ultimately, after 12 months of follow-up, both groups showed improvement in the ratings by untrained listeners, blinded speech pathologist GRBAS scores, and voice-related quality of life scores, without significant differences between groups. Interestingly, they looked at each group using the median age of 52 from their study population as a cutoff point to compare younger versus older patients. Doing so, they showed improved performance of the younger subgroup of LR patients compared with improved performance in the older subgroup of ML patients. As such, they suggested taking age as a factor in the decision-making process between those two interventions.[67]

BILATERAL VOCAL FOLD IMMOBILITY

Bilateral vocal fold immobility (BVFI) is a very different entity from unilateral dysfunction in the sense that it affects breathing more than voice. It can occur secondary to many etiologies: paralysis, cricoarytenoid joint fixation, or interarytenoid scar formation. In cases of thyroidectomy, the underlying process will be neurogenic in the majority of cases, secondary to an injury to both RLNs. This surgery has been reported as the etiology of the dysfunction in 17% of cases of a small cohort.[68]

Bilateral RLN injury will result in flaccid paralysis of the bilateral vocal fold. In addition, a certain amount of laryngeal edema from the intubation and procedure is to be expected. Thus this combination may create a restriction of airflow, especially if the vocal folds are fixed in a median or paramedian position. This phenomenon can be compounded by the increased work of breathing as patients are waking up from their anesthesia, creating a Venturi effect with the flaccid vocal fold paradoxically moving in during inspiration.

In postthyroidectomy BVFI, the patient would typically wake up from surgery in the operating or recovery room and demonstrate acute, persistent, and worsening inspiratory stridor, increased work of breathing, and respiratory failure. These patients will usually require urgent airway management, either intubation or surgical. In some cases, if the presentation is mild, they can be supported with positive pressure ventilation until they fully wake up and are able to better control their breathing. BVFI can be confirmed on-site using laryngoscopy (direct or indirect) while the patient is in spontaneous ventilation. Other patients may be diagnosed later on as they present for routine postoperative follow-up or because they show signs of breathy dysphonia or dyspnea on exertion. Again, the diagnosis can be made on-site using flexible laryngoscopy. If in doubt about the exact etiology of the bilateral immobility, LEMG can be used to confirm a neurogenic process.

Treatment

The treatment of BVFI will be guided by the symptomatology of the patient and prognosis for recovery. Unless transected, the RLN holds potential for recovery over the next 6 to 12 months. Thus in selected cases, observation could be acceptable for patients with minimal symptoms. Otherwise, tracheotomy can be an acceptable solution for a subset of patients as a permanent or transient option while waiting for nerve recovery. The advantage is that it is very effective at correcting airway obstruction while maintaining any residual voice function once fit with a speaking valve. However, the presence of a tracheotomy requires constant care and also represents, for many patients, a social stigmatization. It has been shown to negatively affect the quality of life in patients.[69] Vocal fold or arytenoid lateralization (or laterofixation) has also been described as a reversible approach to enlarging the airway in cases of temporary BVFI. This procedure is useful in the acute setting after injury to the RLNs when a return of function might be expected over 6 to 12 months. Róvó et al. reported success using vocal fold laterofixation in managing 15 consecutive patients with bilateral RLN paralysis after thyroid surgery.[70]

More definitive surgical options include medial arytenoidectomy (MA), described by Crumley, which attempts to improve airway size by creating a concavity along the glottic edge of the body of the arytenoid cartilage, leaving the vocal process and attachment of the vocal ligament intact (Figure 43.5).[71] Transverse cordotomy (TC), as described by Kashima, is performed by making a transverse cut through the vocal fold just anterior to the vocal process without exposing cartilage.[72] Bosley et al. conducted a retrospective review comparing MA and TC and found that both procedures were efficacious for improving the airway with minimal negative effect on phonatory and swallowing function and no statistical difference between the two procedures.[73]

Novel treatments exist, including adductor botulinum toxin injection, selective bilateral LR, and laryngeal pacing, but the evidence is still scarce, and the research is ongoing. Still, these may hold great promises for the future.

SUMMARY

Management of RLN paralysis and paresis requires a detailed laryngeal examination to determine the degree of immobility to adequately offer the best treatment alternatives. Management of unilateral versus bilateral immobility differs greatly, but the goal for both should be to give balance to the main laryngeal functions: protection of the airway, ventilation, and phonation. Achieving adequate balance among the three is easier with unilateral vocal fold immobility, but correct planning and a

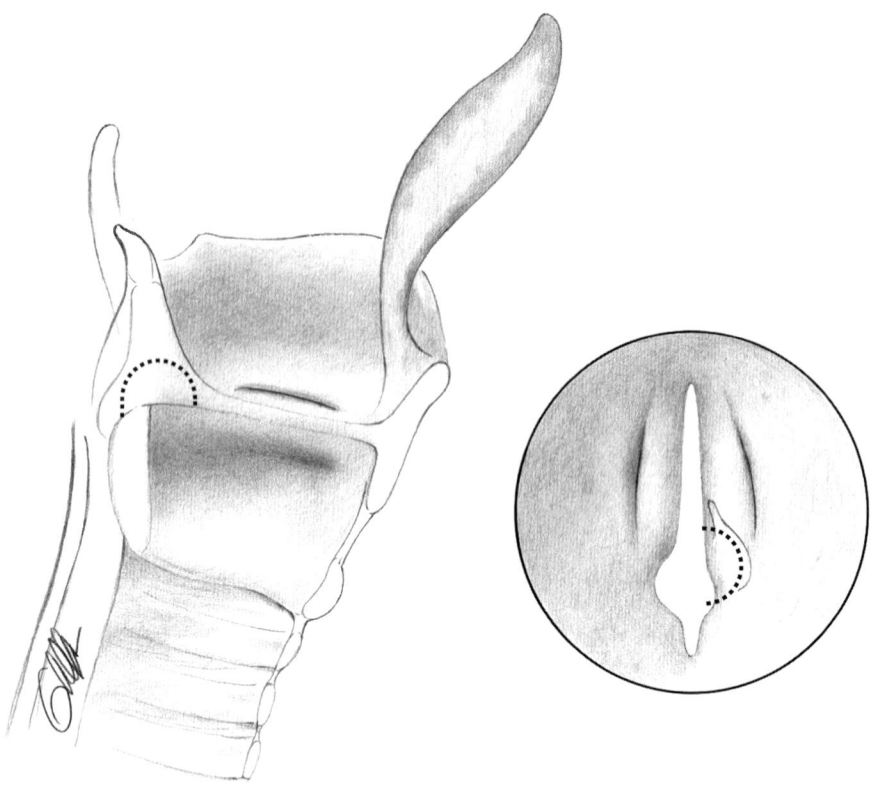

Fig. 43.5 Medial Arytenoidectomy. With the larynx exposed via suspension microlaryngoscopy, a CO_2 laser is used to remove a piece of the medial arytenoid, preserving the vocal process but carving out an airway from the body of the arytenoid. This allows the vocal fold to maintain its tension and shape to preserve voice and increases the posterior airway enough for the patient to breathe better.

thorough clinical evaluation may give the surgeon and the patient the best possibility for successful results. Key factors to consider for improving laryngeal function after RLN injury include etiology, possibility of spontaneous nerve function recovery, elapsed time from onset of paralysis/paresis, age and comorbidities, vocal fold position, and respiratory and vocal needs.

Finally, early intervention, including therapy and/or vocal fold augmentation, is justified whenever protection, respiratory, and phonation needs affect a patient's quality of life. Waiting several months for spontaneous recovery is only recommended when the patient decides to pursue no specific treatment and after a detailed informed consent of all therapeutic alternatives is well understood.

REFERENCES

For a complete list of references, go to expertconsult.com.

Nonneural Complications of Thyroid and Parathyroid Surgery

William B. Inabnet, III, David Scott-Coombes, Erivelto Volpi

INTRODUCTION

Thyroid and parathyroid operations rank among the most common procedures performed by endocrine surgeons and are generally considered low-risk procedures. Yet, complications occur even when surgery is performed by experienced surgeons. Endocrine neck surgery mandates adherence to certain core principles of surgery, such as absolute hemostasis, distinct identification and preservation of the relevant surrounding tissue, clear illumination and visualization of the operative field, and staying in the correct dissection plane. A firm understanding of embryology and anatomy are obligatory (see Chapter 31, Principles in Thyroid Surgery). The importance of teamwork in preventing complications cannot be overemphasized.[1] It is also essential that the modern-day endocrine surgeon stay abreast of ancillary technology that may assist the him or her with intraoperative decision making, such as intraoperative nerve monitoring or the use of immunofluorescence to assess the viability of parathyroid glands. These surgical adjuncts do not necessarily prevent complications from occurring but may help improve outcomes by providing the surgeon with actionable information at the point of care. Thyroid and parathyroid complications can be divided into two broad categories: neural complications and everything else. This chapter will address the latter category, nonneural complications.

HYPOPARATHYROIDISM

Permanent hypoparathyroidism is a devastating outcome after thyroid and parathyroid surgery and is associated with significant morbidity, reduction in quality of life, and increased risk of death.[2-4] The true incidence is unknown as the definition of hypoparathyroidism varies around the world, but most authorities would agree that patients with an undetectable intact parathyroid hormone (PTH) level 6 months after surgery who require ongoing calcium supplementation can be classified as having permanent hypoparathyroidism. The signs and symptoms of hypocalcemia can be subtle and include perioral or digital paresthesias, muscle cramping, or anxiety. Furthermore, Chvostek sign, facial twitching when the facial nerve is tapped, and Trousseau sign, ischemia-induced carpal spasm, highlight the state of neuromuscular excitability during hypocalcemia. Importantly, Chvostek sign may be positive in up to 20% of normocalcemic individuals. More overt and alarming signs and symptoms include tetany, altered mental status, seizures, prolonged QT interval, heart failure, bronchospasm, and laryngospasm. Patients who experience tetany often describe the inability to move as nothing short of terrifying, leading to anxiety and in some extreme cases posttraumatic stress syndrome.

Identifying patients who are at increased risk for postoperative hypoparathyroidism *before* surgery is important because preventive measures can be undertaken to minimize the occurrence and/or clinical severity after surgery. For example, patients with Graves' disease have a much higher incidence of temporary hypoparathyroidism after total thyroidectomy due to the increased vascularity and firm texture of the thyroid gland.[5] These findings create challenges in preserving the blood supply of the parathyroid glands during parathyroid gland dissection. Moreover, the inherent hypermetabolic state of hyperthyroidism exacerbates postoperative hypoparathyroidism. Parathyroid gland preservation is also challenging in patients with Hashimoto's thyroiditis due to the "woody" texture of the thyroid gland. Patients with thyroid cancer may require ipsilateral and/or bilateral level 6 and 7 central lymph node dissection, which may compromise parathyroid gland function after surgery due to a shared blood supply. In the era of routine ultrasound imaging before thyroid cancer surgery, the surgeon often has a good sense of who will require a central node dissection before the skin incision is made. For patients with hyperparathyroidism, four groups of patients have an increased risk of postoperative hypoparathyroidism: reoperative cases, familial cases (especially multiple endocrine neoplasia type 1 patients), pediatric patients (due to the high bone turnover and uniform hungry bone syndrome), and patients with secondary/tertiary hyperparathyroidism, all of whom require a multigland excision. The surgeon should consider commencing oral calcium supplementation with Rocaltrol 5 to 7 days *before* surgery in these patients.

The best treatment for hypoparathyroidism is prevention; a firm understanding of parathyroid blood supply is mandatory to minimize the risk of injury to the parathyroid blood supply. In most patients, the parathyroid glands derive their blood supply from small arteriolar branches from the inferior thyroid artery; collateral blood supply also arises from the superior thyroid artery, the thyroid ima, and other small neighboring vessels. During thyroidectomy, careful attention and the utmost care should be given when dissecting the parathyroid glands, taking every precaution to avoid dissection near the pedicle of the parathyroid gland. Many surgeons commence gland dissection with a top-down approach, gently sweeping the parathyroid glands from the thyroid gland in a posterolateral direction. Suction should be used judiciously, as parathyroid glands can easily be aspirated into the suctioning tubing.

During the course of surgery, parathyroid glands that appear to be devascularized should be reimplanted into neighboring musculature.[6] This is recognized by a gland that becomes dusky or even black throughout the course of surgery. After thyroidectomy, a thorough examination of the surgical specimen should be undertaken to identify any parathyroid glands that have been inadvertently removed. Any glands that are identified should be considered for autoimplantation.

Autoimplantation is accomplished by sectioning the gland with a sharp scalpel into 1-mm pieces and placing it into a pocket of strap musculature or in the sternocleidomastoid muscle.[7] Another technique involves suspending the tissue in saline and injecting it with a syringe

TABLE 44.1 Elemental Calcium by Preparation

	Percentage of Elemental Calcium
Calcium carbonate	40
Calcium citrate	21
Calcium lactate	13
Calcium gluconate	9
Calcium glubionate	6.6

and needle into the muscle. These maneuvers have been shown to decrease rates of permanent hypoparathyroidism.[6]

Surgical adjuncts and point-of-care testing can assist the surgeon with intraoperative decision making. Immunofluorescence imaging and parathyroid gland angiography are relatively new techniques that can be used to assess gland viability during thyroid (and parathyroid) surgery. In a randomized control trial assessing the utility of indocyanine green (ICG) fluorescence in predicting parathyroid gland function after thyroid surgery, the authors demonstrated that ICG imaging can reliably predict postoperative gland function and obviate the need for laboratory testing and oral supplementation (see Chapter 31, Principles in Thyroid Surgery).[8] This technology can be extremely helpful in determining parathyroid remnant viability when performing subtotal parathyroidectomy in patients with known or suspected multigland disease (multiple endocrine neoplasia type 1 [MEN 1] and secondary/tertiary hyperparathyroidism).[9] Intraoperative PTH testing has been shown to identify patients who are at risk for postoperative hypocalcemia.[10] During thyroid surgery, rapid PTH levels less than 15 mg/dL correlate with a higher incidence of postoperative hypoparathyroidism.[4]

Treatment for hypocalcemia is determined by its degree and duration. The goal is to maintain a low-normal calcium level, thereby controlling symptoms while stimulating gland function. The first line of treatment is oral calcium supplementation with or without calcitriol to improve calcium absorption. Oral calcium supplementation is commenced, administering 2 to 10 g daily in divided doses. It is important to note that different calcium preparations provide different levels of elemental calcium (Table 44.1).[11] Severe cases of symptomatic hypocalcemia are treated with intravenous calcium gluconate. Calcium chloride may be used when a central venous catheter is present.

HYPOTHYROIDISM

The requirement of levothyroxine after total or partial thyroidectomy is used to restore thyroid function or during suppressive hormone therapy. After partial, less-than-total thyroidectomy, clinically apparent hypothyroidism arises in 11% to 50% of patients.[12,13] This wide variation in literature may be due to different definitions of hypothyroidism, and differences in follow-up, surgical techniques, and the timing of commencing levothyroxine supplementation among other reasons.[14] As hypothyroidism after total thyroidectomy is a consequence and not a complication, we will discuss only the occurrence of hypothyroidism after partial thyroidectomy. The need of hormone therapy should be an important issue when deciding the best surgery for the patient because in some situations even partial or total thyroidectomy can be acceptable options. Many factors have been described as predictors for the development of postoperative hypothyroidism, such as age, gender, the presence of microsomal antibodies, thyroiditis, multinodular goiter, preoperative thyrotoxicosis, and a thyroid remnant volume measuring <6 mL.[14,15]

In a systematic review and meta-analysis of patients who underwent partial thyroidectomy, Verloop et al. showed that 1 in 5 patients will develop some form of hypothyroidism (subclinical or clinical, definite or transient) and 1 in 25 will have clinical hypothyroidism.[14] In this study, as in many others, the most important preoperative predictors of hypothyroidism are thyroid-stimulating hormone (TSH) in the high-normal range and positive anti-thyroperoxidase (TPO) status.[13] Generally, it is important to discuss with the patients preoperatively the possible eventual need for hormone replacement after partial thyroidectomy.

THYROTOXIC STORM

Thyrotoxic storm or crisis is a rare but life-threatening complication of thyroid surgery that is unfamiliar to most surgeons due to its infrequent occurrence. Typically, a precipitating event such as surgery, trauma, infection, myocardial infarction, and other systemic events will transform thyrotoxicosis into thyroid storm. Also, this can be precipitated with excess iodine intake such as with iodinated contrast agents or amiodarone exposure. The physiology surrounding this event is the sudden dissociation of thyroid hormone from its binding proteins. This increase in free thyroid hormone can then lead to the constellation of signs and symptoms as it affects the neurologic, cardiopulmonary, gastrointestinal, and other systems. Common signs and symptoms include fever, tachycardia, cardiac arrhythmias, and, in extreme cases, cardiovascular collapse, hepatic failure, and death.[16]

The best treatment of thyroid storm is prevention. Antithyroid medications are administered before surgery, and beta-blockade is commonly used to control the systemic cardiac effects. In those with poorly controlled thyrotoxicosis requiring urgent thyroidectomy, preoperative iopanoic acid (500 mg bid), dexamethasone (1 mg bid), propylthiouracil or methimazole, and beta-blockade have been shown to decrease the likelihood of thyroid storm.[17] In spite of these preventive measures, a small number of patients will develop thyroid storm. Treatment involves decreasing thyroid hormone synthesis, decreasing its release from the thyroid gland, preventing conversion of Tetraiodothyronine (T4) to Triiodothyronine (T3), managing systemic effects, and supportive care. When recognized intraoperatively, manipulation of the thyroid gland should cease and the operation terminated. First-line pharmaceutical treatment includes beta-blockade and administration of corticosteroids. Propranolol (4 to 10 mg/kg) is administered to reduce sympathetic activity and to block peripheral conversion of T4 to T3. Hydrocortisone (100 to 300 mg) ameliorates the toxicity associated with thyrotoxicosis by reducing fever, iodine uptake, TSH levels, and the inhibition of the peripheral converseion of T4 to T3. Thioamides such as methimazole are also used acutely to block thyroid hormone synthesis, and propylthiouracil inhibits the peripheral conversion of T4 to T3. Sodium iodine (1.0 to 2.5 g) also reduces thyroid hormone synthesis and release. Temperature reduction is achieved with cooling blankets and acetaminophen.

Postoperatively, the thyrotoxic storm patient may have altered mentation including confusion, agitation, and anxiety in addition to fever and tachycardia. Early recognition and prompt intervention are required to prevent cardiovascular and hepatic decompensation. Thyrotoxic storm is rare but potentially lethal, and its successful management relies on early diagnosis and prompt appropriate therapy.

HEMORRHAGE AND HEMATOMA

Hemorrhage and hematoma formation after thyroid and parathyroid surgery can be life threatening. Fortunately, these complications occur in less than 2% of thyroid and parathyroid surgeries in developed countries, but some studies show an incidence up to 4.39%.[18] Recently, there has been a trend for outpatient surgery in which the risk of postthyroidectomy hemorrhage will increase hospital stay and medical expenses and even threaten life in patients discharged.[18] Predicting those patients who are at risk for these complications is difficult. Liu et al., in a recent meta-analysis,[18] pointed out that older age, male sex, Graves' disease, antithrombotic agent use, bilateral operation, neck dissection, and previous thyroid surgery are significant risk factors for postthyroidectomy hemorrhage. Suzuki et al.[19] include the risk factors of obesity and blood transfusion on the day of surgery. Multiple studies have shown that postoperative hemorrhage and hematoma rates are equivalent in patients who have and have not undergone wound drainage.[20,21] Therefore the need for wound drainage should be determined by the surgeon on a case-by-case basis, and a drain should not be relied on to prevent hematoma formation.

Prevention of hematoma begins preoperatively with attention to native and acquired coagulopathies, although routine coagulation studies are not performed. A detailed history of personal or familial bleeding should be ascertained. Additionally, the use of prescription and over-the-counter medicines, including herbal supplements, that may promote hemorrhage, should be ascertained and discontinued before surgery.

Intraoperatively, meticulous hemostasis should be maintained. Any bleeding encountered near the recurrent laryngeal nerve should be treated with judicious use of bipolar electrocautery. Additionally, fibrin sealants, cellulose-based hemostatic agents, or microfibrillar collagen may be useful adjuncts when electrocautery is deemed unsafe, although the efficacy of these hemostatic agents is still controversial in the literature.[22-26] At present, newer vessel-sealing devices have not been shown to decrease hematoma rates, although more recent studies have shown a decrease in surgical time and intraoperative bleeding.[26-29]

Before closing the wound, the Valsalva maneuver can be performed repetitively or the patient can be placed in the Trendelenburg position, and any identified bleeding sites can be identified and controlled. Cervical pressure dressings, such as the Queen Anne dressing, have been advocated in the past. These dressings, however, are cumbersome and may delay the recognition of a hematoma. These dressings do not prevent hematoma formation[30] and therefore are not recommended. The patient should be awakened from anesthesia in a manner to avoid coughing. Recent studies has shown that the use of prophylactic dexamethasone before induction of anesthesia can reduce the incidence of postoperative nausea and vomiting in thyroidectomies.[31,32] Perioperative antiemetics are also used to decrease the risk of emesis, but they have not been shown to affect hematoma rates.[18,19,33,34] Taking these precautions and using meticulous surgical technique will decrease the risk of hemorrhage.

The timing of postoperative hematomas can range from immediate to several days postoperatively. The majority of hematomas, however, occur within the first 24 hours of surgery.[19,35] The signs and symptoms of hematomas include neck swelling, pain, oozing from the suture line, ecchymosis, dysphagia/odynophagia, stridor, and respiratory distress. Hematomas are classified as superficial or deep depending on their relationship to the strap muscles.[36] Deep hematomas are thought to cause respiratory distress and airway compromise by causing venous congestion and subsequent laryngopharyngeal edema. Time is essential as the longer the hematoma is present, the greater the resultant airway edema and difficulty in intubation. It has been advocated that the strap muscles be reapproximated loosely or incompletely to allow for egress of any accumulating deep neck hematoma.

When recognized, symptomatic hematomas should be decompressed immediately (Figure 44.1). The wound is opened and the hematoma is evacuated. The airway should be controlled in cases with respiratory distress. Endotracheal intubation may be difficult depending on the degree of laryngopharyngeal edema. Therefore emergent tracheostomy may be necessary. Tracheotomy access is usually straightforward because of the ease of accessing the exposed trachea. Once the airway is secure, the patient is returned to the operating room for a formal wound exploration and control of hemorrhage. The wound is irrigated and closed as described previously.

Postoperative bleeding complications are rare but potentially life threatening and are associated with increased economic burden and resource utilization.[37] Standard techniques are used to control any bleeding at the time of surgery, paying careful attention to any mediastinal vessels that are in the field. Hematomas are often discovered by floor nurses who are educated on the signs and symptoms of a cervical hematoma. A protocol for the management of this complication should be written and widely available to all members of staff responsible for the patient's postoperative care. A regular examination of the neck (palpation and visualization) should be performed postoperatively at regular intervals.[38]

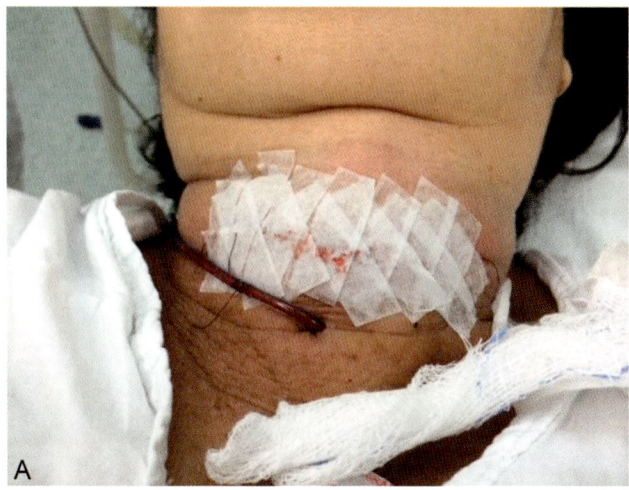 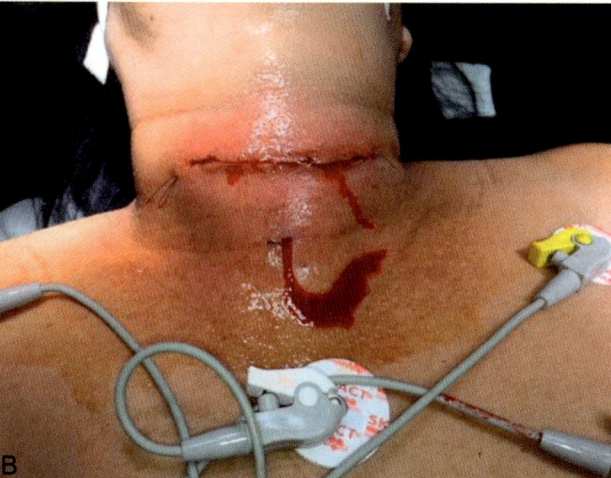

Fig. 44.1 A and **B,** Female patient with 2 h postoperative hematoma with respiratory distress needing reoperation. The use of drain did not prevent the hematoma. (Courtesy Dr. Emerson Favero.)

HYPERTROPHIC SCAR

A scar is not typically classified as a complication; however, the negative effect of hypertrophic scars and keloid formation on a patient's well-being cannot be underestimated. To expand on this concept, the psychosocial consequences of scar formation is a challenging outcome measure to study due to the wide variation in validated methodology (surveys and scar scores), heterogeneous patient populations, and differing cultural bias. It is safe to say that no patient desires an unfavorable scar on his or her neck.

The surgeon can undertake certain strategies to minimize or disguise scar formation. Placing the incision in a natural skin crease can help hide a scar. The length of a scar can be minimized by placing the incision in the higher skin crease; by doing so, the relatively fixed superior pole vessels can be divided early in the procedure, permitting the surgeon to elevate the relatively mobile inferior pole through the incision. Energy devices and/or excessive traction can lead to an abrasion or burn of the skin edge, which can exacerbate scar formation. If the skin edges are traumatized during the operation, reexcision of the skin edge should be considered before closure. Remote access endoscopic thyroid and parathyroid surgery, including the transaxillary, breast and transoral approaches, avoid a scar on the neck altogether by strategically placing the incision(s) in a remote location (see Chapter 32 and Extra Cervical Approaches to the Thyroid and Parathyroid Glands). Out of these options, the transoral route provides the most inconspicuous scar as the incisions are placed in the oral vestibule where the oral mucosa rapidly heals in a genuinely hidden location (see Chapter 33 Transoral Thyroidectomy).[39]

Several precautions in the postoperative period will reduce hypertrophic scarring and keloid formation. If permanent skin sutures are used, the sutures should be removed in a timely fashion to avoid permanent markings. The wound at that point can be reinforced with Steri-strips. Over-the-counter wound products may help minimize scar formation. Additionally, the patient is counseled to avoid sun exposure, which may cause scar pigmentation. In women, breast support is encouraged to avoid any undue tension on the healing wound. Despite these measures, some patients will develop hypertrophic scars or form keloids. Initial management consists of intralesional steroid injection with triamcinolone acetonide. If this fails, scar revision can be performed. Importantly, keloid scar revision can lead to a worse outcome. Recently, laser therapy for the prevention of thyroidectomy scars has been studied and found to be efficacious.[40]

SEROMA

Wound seroma formation can be defined as a collection of fluid clinically identifiable within a surgical cavity in the postoperative period; it is uncommon and occurs in up to 7% of cases.[41] Wound drainage does not significantly decrease the incidence of seroma formation,[41,42] but factors like older age, increased body mass index (BMI), and decreased postoperative ionized calcium are factors related to seroma formation in thyroidectomies.[42] The use of fibrin sealants seems to be a useful tool to avoid this complication.[43] Seroma management includes observation, serial needle aspirations, or placement of a suction drain. With conservative management, the fluid collection will gradually resolve but can be a source of anxiety and slight discomfort for the patient. If the decision to drain the seroma is made, it is important to use sterile technique to avoid contamination of the wound.

INFECTION

Thyroid and parathyroid surgery is clean and surgical site infections rarely occur. The frequency ranges between 0.5% and 3.0%.[44] Perioperative antibiotics have not been shown to reduce the incidence of wound infections and are not routinely used.[45] Although infection is rare, it is associated with higher health care costs resulting from prolonged hospital stays and increased readmission rates.[46] Infections present either as cellulitis requiring oral antibiotics or as an infected seroma necessitating drainage and culture-directed intravenous antibiotics (Figure 44.2). Deep infections should raise the suspicion of an injury to the aerodigestive tract. At the time of incision and drainage, the esophagus and trachea should be explored and identified injuries managed accordingly.

There are two principal specific risk factors for surgical site infection in thyroid surgery. The use of drains and concomitant lymph node dissection are independent risk factors for infection.[47] Drains neither prevent postoperative bleeding nor do they facilitate early diagnosis of bleeding,[48,49] and their use in routine nonmalignant thyroid surgery should be discouraged.[47] Infection associated with modified lymph node dissection occurs in 13% to 20% of patients.[50,51] Consideration should be given toward antibiotic prophylaxis in patients undergoing lymph node surgery with drain placement.[47]

AERODIGESTIVE TRACT INJURY

Preoperatively, tumor involvement of the trachea and esophagus should be anticipated based on clinical, radiographic, and endoscopic findings. Procedures requiring the resection of these structures during extended thyroidectomy are discussed separately in this text. Inadvertent injury to the aerodigestive tract in thyroidectomy is almost unheard of[52] and should not occur in parathyroid surgery. A recognized esophageal injury should be closed with inverting, absorbable sutures and the wound copiously irrigated before closing a suction

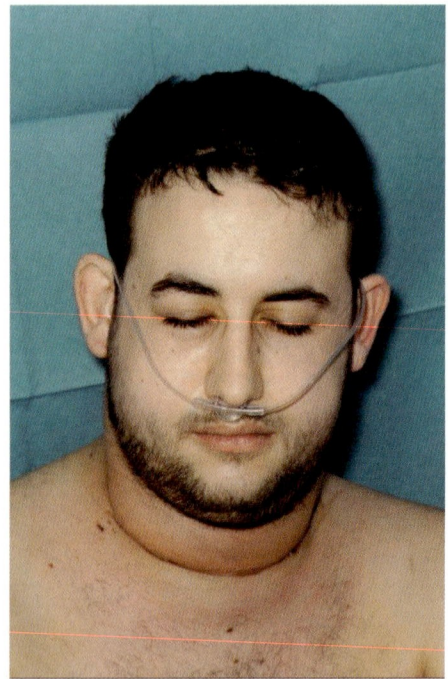

Fig. 44.2 Patient presenting with cellulitis from occult tracheal injury.

CHAPTER 44 Nonneural Complications of Thyroid and Parathyroid Surgery

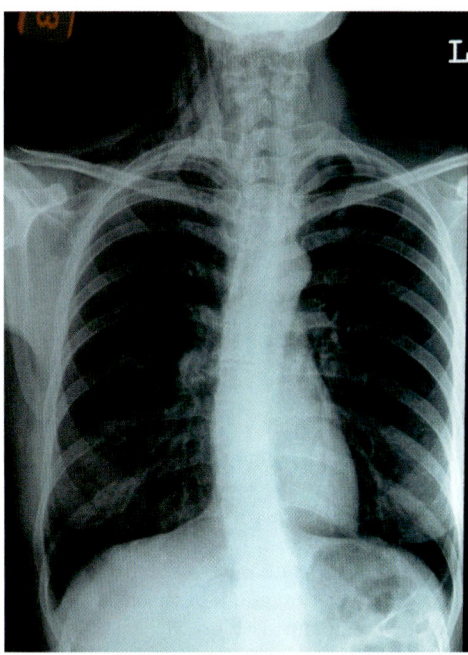

Fig. 44.3 Chest x-ray showing surgical emphysema from a tracheal injury.

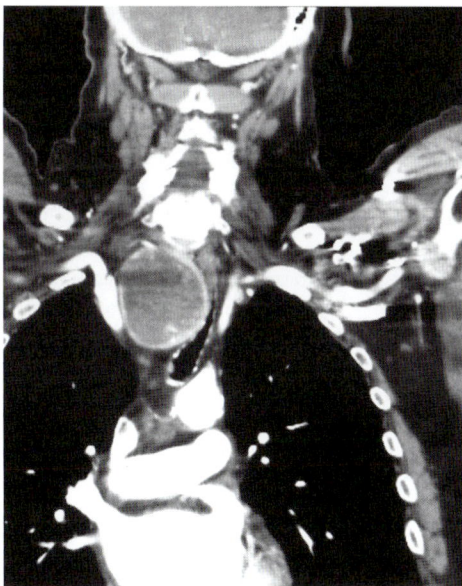

Fig. 44.4 Computed tomography (CT) coronal reconstruction demonstrating substernal goiter with tracheal compression.

drain. Unrecognized injury may present with neck pain, dysphagia, subcutaneous emphysema, fever, leukocytosis, or systemic signs of sepsis. The diagnosis is confirmed by a Gastrografin swallow, and the management can either be conservative (drainage and antibiotics) or require surgical repair with drainage.[53] The patient is kept nil per os (NPO) for several days.

When a tracheal injury is identified at the time of surgery, this should also be closed primarily with absorbable sutures; a drain is placed and antibiotics prescribed. When primary closure is not possible, placement of a tracheotomy tube or segmental resection of the trachea may be necessary (see Chapter 37, Surgery for Locally Advanced Thyroid Cancer: Larynx, Tracheal Invasion, and Esophageal). With both types of injuries, the strap muscles may be used to buttress the surgical closure. On occasion a patient may present a few days after surgery with neck swelling. The physical hallmark is surgical emphysema that can be confirmed with a plain x-ray (Figure 44.3). This can either result from an occult injury or occur after primary closure when the platelet plug on the mucosal surface of the trachea detaches and initiates a fit of coughing, which in turn forces air out through a tiny breach in the trachea. Management is conservative: admission for observation, reassurance, and antibiotics. In extreme cases, the wound may need to be reexplored, lavaged, and drained.

AIRWAY COMPLICATIONS

Difficult Intubation

Difficulty with intubation can result from either compression and/or deviation of the larynx and trachea by a goiter. The surgeon and anesthesiologist should communicate preoperatively and anticipate those patients who might pose a challenge for airway management. An anesthesiologist with a subspecialty interest in the "difficult airway" is a key ally in these situations. The surgeon should be present at the time of intubation in the event that assistance with airway control is needed or if a surgical airway is required.

The incidence of difficult intubation in the general surgical population has been estimated to be 1.8%, and this rises to 4% to 11% for goiter surgery.[54-57] Risk factors for difficult intubation can be generalized or goiter-specific. Generalized risk factors for a difficult intubation include neck thickness,[58] reduced mouth-opening,[58,59] and older age.[60] Older age is associated with reduced neck mobility, thyromental distance, and interincisor gap.[58-61] Thyroid-related risk factors include malignancy,[54] large goiter (>40 g), and reduced thyromental distance (<6.5 cm).[62] Interestingly, radiologic signs of tracheal compression are not associated with difficult intubation.[60] For thyroid-related risk factors, a computed tomography (CT) scan with three-dimensional reconstruction will aid the anesthesiologist in preoperative planning (Figure 44.4).

Patient-related factors such as age and health status, rather than the size of the goiter, should be the focus when determining the appropriate intubation approach.[60] Despite the potential for difficult intubations, mask ventilation is not typically impaired.[56,63] The site of airway obstruction or distortion related to goiters is typically the trachea (see Chapter 6, Surgery of Cervical and Substernal Goiter). Thus routine direct laryngoscopy and transoral intubation can usually be accomplished. The endotracheal tube will usually pass through the narrowed tracheal segment without difficulty. Endotracheal tubes of different sizes should be available, and the use of a stylet may be of assistance. Rarely, the larynx is also displaced, making routine intubation with direct laryngoscopy challenging. Fiberoptic intubation should be considered in this setting and has the advantage of allowing visualization of any invasive component of thyroid carcinoma within the lumen of the airway but requires advanced anesthesiology skills. Videolaryngoscopic devices have been reported to aid in these difficult cases as well.[63] Lastly, decompressive surgery under local anesthesia[64,65] and even the use of extracorporeal membranous oxygenation have been reported in exceptional circumstances.[64]

Tracheomalacia

Tracheomalacia occurs when the cartilaginous trachea becomes weak from long-standing pressure and subsequently narrows with the negative inspiratory force of inhalation.[66] The incidence of this problem varies from 0% to 10% and is related to long-standing goiter and significant retrosternal extension.[66,67] Most of the experience of tracheomalacia comes from outside the Western world, often in areas of endemic goiter.[68,69] Tracheomalacia can be recognized intraoperatively as a soft, collapsible trachea upon palpation. In the majority of cases, this condition does not have any clinical significance. Rarely, however, it can lead to postoperative airway obstruction.[69,70] When anticipated, the patient is kept intubated overnight and the endotracheal tube cuff is deflated the next morning. If there is a good air leak, the patient can then be extubated. Repeat airway obstruction at that time will necessitate either tracheostomy or a longer period of endotracheal intubation. The latter approach will allow the endotracheal tube to serve as a stent while paratracheal fibrosis occurs and supports the airway extrinsically.[66,69,70] Alternatively, tracheopexy, miniplate fixation, mesh splinting, or tracheal resection can be performed, depending on the degree of tracheomalacia. It is important to rule out bilateral vocal cord paralysis as a cause for the airway obstruction.

METHYLENE BLUE

Various localizing studies and techniques have been described to assist with parathyroid identification at the time of surgery. One technique uses intravenous methylene blue to stain the parathyroid glands and has been used since the 1970s.[71] Within the hour before incision, methylene blue is injected intravenously at a dose of 5 to 7.5 mg/kg in 100 mL of 5% dextrose in water. This will cause the patient to appear cyanotic and hypoxic, but these signs are artifactual.

There is mounting evidence that methylene blue usage in those patients who use selective serotonin reuptake inhibitors (SRIs) puts them at increased risk for altered mental status on the spectrum leading to serotonin syndrome.[71,72] Methylene blue is a competitive inhibitor of monoamine oxidase A and, when given to those already taking a serotonin agonist, it leads to excess levels of serotonin and, thus, serotonin syndrome. This syndrome is characterized by altered mental status, neuromuscular hyperactivity, and autonomic dysfunction. It may be difficult to diagnose signs and symptoms in all three areas in a given patient considering that a spectrum of altered neurologic function exists. The treatment for serotonin syndrome related to methylene blue is supportive.[72] To avoid this complication, these patients should stop taking their SRIs for 2 weeks or more preoperatively to allow for an adequate washout period. Fluoxetine has a longer half-life and requires a longer washout period. Methylene blue can be avoided in these individuals and other parathyroid localization strategies used.

RARE COMPLICATIONS

Horner's Syndrome

This arises as a result of injury along the cervical sympathetic chain, which is most at risk during nodal dissection. It results in partial ptosis, enophthalmos, miosis, and anhidrosis (Figure 44.5). Occasionally, there may be ipsilateral facial flushing due to capillary vasodilation. The incidence is reported to be in the region of 0.2%.[73]

If secondary to hematoma/seroma, it may be reversible by prompt drainage. Permanent injury may arise from division, ischemia, or stretching from lateral retraction. When suspected, patients should be referred to an ophthalmologist. The diagnosis is confirmed with the application of alpha-agonist apraclonidine to both eyes, whereby an increased mydriatic effect is observed on the affected side. Corrective surgery may be indicated if the ptosis is severe.

Chyle Leak

This complication results from inadvertent injury to the thoracic duct or one of its branches, usually on the left side of the neck, during lymph node dissection. The thoracic duct typically drains into the venous system within 1 cm of the confluence of the left internal jugular and subclavian veins.[74] However, the wide variability in its location makes it more prone to injury that is often not recognized during the operation. The incidence of this complication ranges from 0.6% to 1.4% for central node dissection and 4.4% to 8.3% for lateral dissection.[75]

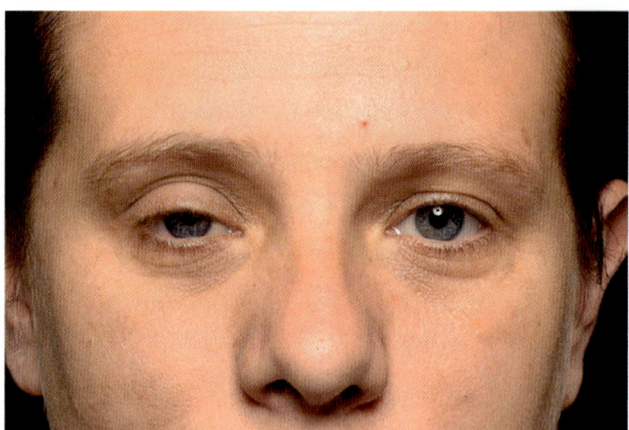

Fig. 44.5 Horner's syndrome showing ptosis and miosis.

In those with surgical drains, the leak manifests as milky-white fluid. For those patients without drains, it presents later as a fluctuant swelling under the wound. Chyle leak impairs wound healing, can lead to laryngeal edema, and prolongs hospital stays. Chyle contains fat, protein, electrolytes, and lymphocytes, and its loss can result in severe nutritional, metabolic, and immunologic disorders.[76]

Conservative methods of treatment are used first as they allow a cure rate of 58% to 100%.[77,78] The mainstay of conservative treatment is modifying the diet to a content of medium chain triglycerides which are absorbed directly into the bloodstream rather than via the thoracic duct. This is often successful for low-to-medium volume leaks and may take up to 3 weeks to resolve. Alternatively, patients may remain fasting and receive total parenteral nutrition.

Somatostatin analog (octreotide) reduces chyle formation by decreasing splanchnic blood flow and is a promising alternative therapy that increases the success of conservative management.[77]

When conservative methods fail or in the presence of a high-volume fistula (>700 mL/day), thoracic duct ligation is the typical surgical intervention via a transcervical approach.[75] Oversewing the duct is the favored maneuver, but other options include clips, glues, and muscular flaps. If these measures fail, thoracoscopic duct ligation can be considered.[79] Alternatively, embolization of the thoracic duct has been described.[80]

MORTALITY

Thyroid Surgery

Historically, thyroid surgery was associated with such a high mortality rate (40%) such that in 1850 it was forbidden by the French Academy of Medicine.[81] At the end of the 19th century, contributions from Billroth, Kocher, and Halsted combined to transform the outcomes of thyroidectomy to a safe procedure.[81,82] Nowadays, national data reveals the in-hospital (30-day) mortality of thyroidectomy to be in the region of 0.6%.[83,84] Most deaths are associated with a combination of older age, large goiters, and airway complications. Postoperative hemorrhage is a potentially life-threatening complication of thyroidectomy. A review of publications containing large cohorts of more than 1000 patients from single centers found reexploration rates for hemorrhage of 0.3% to 1.2%.[85] The main risk factors are old age, male gender, and bilateral surgery. In a large series of thyroidectomies, the overall mortality rate related to postoperative hemorrhage was 0.01% overall and 0.6% for patients who had surgery for postoperative bleeding.[85]

Permanent hypoparathyroidism is the most common adverse outcome after total thyroidectomy and necessitates lifelong supplementation with vitamin D. A recent study from the Scandinavian Endocrine Surgery Registry has demonstrated that permanent hypoparathyroidism is associated with a twofold increased risk of death.[3] The reason for this increased mortality is not clear.

Parathyroid Surgery

Mortality in parathyroid surgery differs according to the underlying pathology. Data from both national and unit series reveal that mortality in primary hyperparathyroidism is in the region of 1 per 1000 operations.[86,87] However, there is a significantly higher mortality of parathyroidectomy in secondary hyperparathyroidism, which approaches 1%.[86,87] As would be expected, predictive factors of poor outcomes include hypertension and elevated creatinine and alkaline phosphatase.[86]

REFERENCES

For a complete list of references, go to expertconsult.com.

45

Quality Assessment in Thyroid and Parathyroid Surgery

Eric Monteiro, Carolyn Seib, Julie A. Sosa, Jonathan Irish

> Please go to expertconsult.com to view related video:
> **Video 45.1** Introduction to Chapter 45, Quality Assessment in Thyroid and Parathyroid Surgery.

Increasing focus has been placed on the quality of care physicians and hospitals provide to ensure excellent health outcomes for their patients. Thyroid and parathyroid operations are often performed in the outpatient setting with overall low morbidity and rare mortality, but variation in care and outcomes between institutions and providers suggests there is opportunity for quality improvement in perioperative care.[1] "Quality assurance" (QA) refers to the overall systems in place to ensure that quality standards are being met. For QA to be effective in health care, an acceptable definition of quality is required (Figure 45.1). In addition, feasible and robust methods for measuring quality are needed to facilitate targeted improvement efforts.[2]

QA in surgical specialties is inextricably linked to economic considerations and the value of surgical care. "Value" in health care is defined as the quality of outcomes divided by the costs associated with achieving them. The cost of health care in the United States continues to rise faster than inflation, and health care spending as a percentage of gross domestic product is significantly more than that of other industrialized nations.[3] However, the U.S. has been shown to underperform in comparison to 11 other high-spending nations with respect to access, equity, and health care outcomes based on recently published data from The Commonwealth Fund.[3] In an effort to curb health care spending, policy reform has shifted reimbursement from traditional fee-for-service models to focus on the quality of care and its associated cost. This has been achieved through the initiatives of pay-for-performance, value-based purchasing, and bundled payments via Medicare and private insurers.[4] Given that the costs attributed to surgery and perioperative care are estimated to account for as much as 40% of all hospital and physician spending,[5] increasing scrutiny is being placed on providing high-value surgical care.

Within this economic and regulatory backdrop, surgeons performing thyroid and parathyroid surgery must be familiar with ways to assess if they are providing high-quality care. Therefore in this chapter we will review (1) the history of quality improvement in medicine and surgery, (2) how to define and measure quality surgical care in thyroid and parathyroid operations, and (3) methods for implementing quality improvement initiatives to improve health care outcomes through targeted system-level changes.

HISTORY OF QUALITY IMPROVEMENT IN MEDICINE

Institute of Medicine Reports and Policy Outcomes

In 1999 the newly established Institute of Medicine (IOM), now called the National Academy of Medicine (NAM), published *To Err is Human: Building a Safer Healthcare System*, a report highlighting the toll of medical errors on patients and the health care system.[6] In this document the authors reported that up to 98,000 patients died annually due to medical error and charged the medical field as being woefully behind other high-risk industries, such as aviation, in reducing preventable harm. This report received wide media attention and led to a call for reform to ensure patient safety, energizing the movement for surgical quality assessment. A follow-up report published in 2001, titled *Crossing the Quality Chasm*, focused attention on six domains needed for a safer and more effective health care system: safety, effectiveness, patient-centeredness, timeliness, efficiency, and equity.[7]

In the wake of these publications, concerted efforts were made by hospitals, academic and professional societies, and accrediting bodies to prevent medical errors and improve patient safety. Figure 45.2 highlights the important events in the quality of care movement in medicine and surgery. In 1999 the U.S. congress passed the Healthcare Research and Quality Act, which started the Agency for Healthcare Research and Quality (AHRQ) with a mandate to support research focused on identifying the causes of preventable errors affecting patient safety and to track disparities in health care. In 2003 the AHRQ published its first annual National Healthcare Quality Report, which measures trends in quality metrics, such as patient safety, timeliness of care, and access to care.[8] The AHRQ remains a leader in efforts to systematically collect and analyze health care outcomes to guide improvement in patient care with the support of federal funding. In 2008, the National Quality Forum convened the National Priorities Partnership (NPP), which included 28 organizations representing consumer groups, employers, governments, private insurers, health care professionals, accrediting and certifying bodies, and quality alliances, to align health care reform with a set of National Priorities and Goals decided upon by all parties.[9] The coordination of all stakeholders in health care administration is essential to the quality improvement movement.

Pioneers of Surgical Quality and Morbidity & Mortality Conferences

One of the most notable early champions of surgical quality improvement was Ernest Amory Codman (1869–1940), a surgeon at Massachusetts General Hospital. Codman devoted much of his career to his "end result idea," which he described as "the common-sense notion that every hospital should follow *every* patient it treats, long enough to determine whether or not the treatment has been successful, and then to inquire 'if not, why not' with a view to preventing a similar failure in the future."[10] Through this idea, Codman emphasized both documenting surgical outcomes and analyzing the root cause of variations in outcomes, which at the time was a novel and controversial topic. As a founding member of the American College of Surgeons (ACS), he participated in the establishment of the Hospital Standardization

CHAPTER 45 Quality Assessment in Thyroid and Parathyroid Surgery

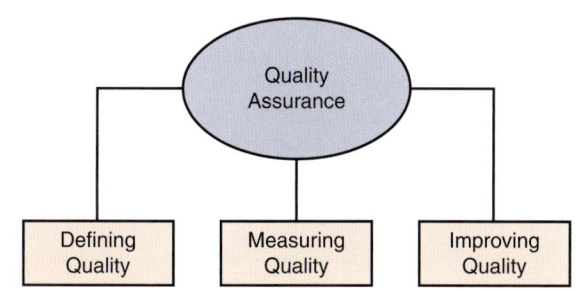

Fig. 45.1 Three pillars of quality assurance.

Program, which was the precursor to the Joint Commission on Accreditation of Health Care Organizations.[11] He also contributed to the drafting of the ACS Minimum Standard for Hospitals in 1919, in which the ACS charged hospitals with ensuring staff "review and analyze at regular intervals their clinical experience in various departments of the hospital" and set the standard for the recording of patient data.[12]

A direct result of Codman's work was the establishment of what would become The Anesthesia Study Commission by Henry Ruth in Philadelphia in 1940.[13,14] This group was composed of anesthesiologists, surgeons, and internists from multiple institutions who would review fatalities and adverse outcomes related to anesthesia and surgical care, with a key focus on medical errors, for the purpose of education and system improvement. These tenets formed the basis for the modern Morbidity and Mortality (M&M) conferences.[13] In 1983, the Accreditation Council for Graduate Medical Education (ACGME) mandated that all training programs institute regular M&M conferences,[15] which to this day are focused on review of complications and deaths for the purpose of quality improvement. However, there is little standardization in how these conferences are run or the methodology to implement change. Although the tradition of M&M conferences in surgery has focused on addressing adverse events and errors, focus on the responsibility of individual decision making often underemphasizes the need for addressing system deficiencies.[16,17] In addition, the M&M system has been shown to underreport complications and deaths compared with more rigorous methods of documenting perioperative outcomes.[11] Focused effort is required to structure M&M conferences to be effective for quality assessment and improvement.[18]

Multidisciplinary Cancer Conferences/Tumor Boards

Unlike the retroactive approach to systems improvement employed through M&M conferences, the formation of multidisciplinary cancer conferences (MCCs) or tumor boards represented a proactive approach to improving patient outcomes by focusing on providing up-to-date and comprehensive cancer care. Given surgery was the mainstay of cancer care in the early 20th century, the ACS also led the charge to improve cancer care by establishing the Committee on the Treatment of Malignant Diseases in 1922, which became the ACS Commission on Cancer in the mid-1960s.[19] This group established the standards for dedicated "cancer clinics" that were accredited to provide consistent diagnostic and cancer treatment services. To this day, the Commission on Cancer recognizes cancer care programs that are voluntarily compliant with standards that ensure quality, multidisciplinary, and comprehensive cancer care delivery. One aspect of care that is required of these institutions is documentation of MCCs/tumor boards. Given that there is evidence transdisciplinary cancer care improves adherence to guidelines, timeliness of treatment, and patient outcomes,[20-23] MCCs/tumor boards are seen as important tools to facilitate this interaction to coordinate patient care. There is also evidence that surgeons find participation in MCCs/tumor boards important for their professional development.[24] Although there is no definitive documentation that MCCs/tumor boards on their own function as tools of quality assessment, they are a component of multidisciplinary cancer care that likely facilitates the improved outcomes seen with the participation of practitioners from medical, surgical, and radiation oncology, among others, in treatment planning.[25,26]

DEFINING QUALITY

Developing Quality Indicators

In 2001, the IOM defined quality of health care as "the degree to which health services for individuals and populations increase the likelihood

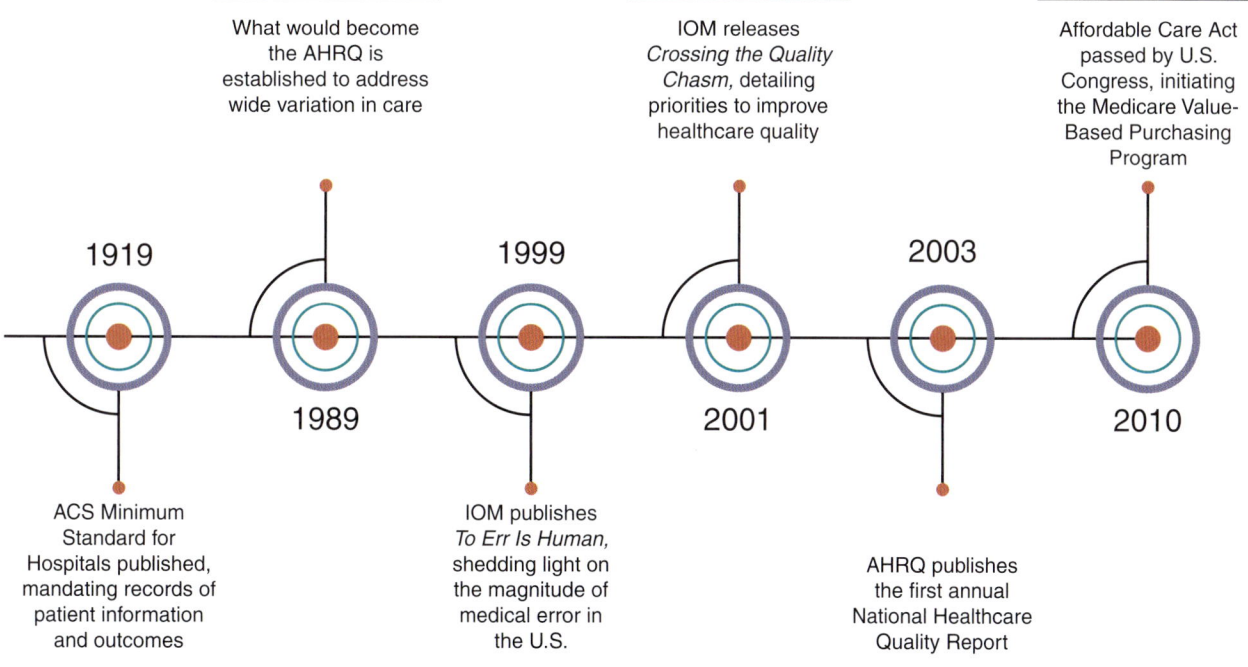

Fig. 45.2 Timeline of quality of care movement in medicine and surgery.

of desired health outcomes and are consistent with current professional knowledge."[7] To determine whether a high quality of care is being delivered to patients, measures of quality, called quality indicators (QIs), need to be defined and developed. QIs have been defined in numerous ways. Stelfox and Straus adopted the definition put forth by the National Library of Medicine, which defines QIs as "norms, criteria, standards and other direct qualitative and quantitative measures used in determining the quality of health care."[27]

QIs can serve multiple purposes, including documenting the quality of care; comparing institutions and providers; prioritizing quality improvement initiatives; supporting accountability, regulation, and accreditation; assisting patients in the process of choosing their providers; and establishing pay-for-performance initiatives.[28]

In thyroid and parathyroid surgery, there is a paucity of literature pertaining to the rigorous development of QIs, which will be discussed in more detail later in this chapter. When choosing a topic for the development of QIs, there are numerous factors requiring consideration. Stelfox and Straus argue that a needs assessment and a consideration for measurement frameworks are required to help guide QI development. Development of QIs, the authors argue, should be prioritized when a large burden of illness exists, where evidence suggests either variable or substandard care, where opportunity for improvement exists, when evidence suggests that improving quality will lead to patient benefit, and for clinical problems where QIs have not been previously developed.[29] Thyroid and parathyroid surgery meet many of these prerequisites, and both are great examples of areas where rigorous and relevant QI development are essential. Furthermore, the known variation in the management of thyroid and parathyroid disorders further supports the effort to define relevant measures of quality, so that appropriate, evidence-based care can be measured, implemented, and improved.[30,31]

There are various methods for developing QIs. Kotter et al. performed a review assessing the development of QIs from published guidelines.[32] The authors highlight several advantages to this approach, including increased efficiency and decreased resource utilization. This method is preferred by the authors when possible. In addition, this method is an excellent approach for thyroid and parathyroid surgery given the numerous, high-quality guidelines that are currently available in the literature, particularly those from the American Thyroid Association (ATA).[33] The most common approach used for QI development involves a combination of a formal literature review and a separate consensus process. Mainz was one of the first authors to propose an approach to QI development and testing.[28] After topic selection and team assembly, the author recommends beginning by performing a literature review to provide an overview of existing practice and evidence, and to select candidate indicators.[28] The next step involves selecting the final set of QIs from the literature review, using the Research ANd Development Corporation/University of California Los Angeles (RAND/UCLA) method or a modification thereof. Patient representatives are becoming more frequently involved in QI development; however, a systematic approach involving patients is lacking.[34] Patient-reported outcome measures (PROMs) are additional measures of quality that are gaining popularity in health care. PROMs are already being incorporated in value-based purchasing programs.[35] PROMs remain controversial as a surrogate measure of surgical quality, as surveys measuring the patient experience fail to capture the quality of the technical aspects that occur in the intraoperative setting. Notwithstanding, evidence is emerging that hospitals who score well on PROMs also perform well on measures of surgical quality, including length of stay, readmission rates, and surgical mortality.[35] In a study by Zanocco et al., The Patient-Reported Outcomes Measurement Information System (PROMIS) of the National Institutes of Health was used to assess changes in physical and mental health after parathyroidectomy in patients with hyperparathyroidism.[36] The authors found that several validated measures of physical and mental health improved after parathyroidectomy, suggesting that PROMIS can be a practical means of measuring patient-reported outcomes. PROMs will likely become more widely used as measures of quality, and further evaluation of the relationship between PROMs and surgical quality is essential.

Perhaps the most detailed and informative attempt at outlining the process of QI development comes from the AHRQ. A report published in 2011 outlines the agency's recommended steps for QI development.[37] QIs are defined by four components: a health care concept, a point of view or perspective of measurement (e.g., patient, clinical, health care system), a method for collecting data (data source, risk adjustment, etc.), and an application of use.[37] Furthermore, the report describes four phases: QI measure development, QI implementation, QI maintenance, and QI retirement. The process involves selecting candidate indicators from a systematic review of the literature, followed by using the RAND/UCLA appropriateness method for selecting the final set of QIs. After QI finalization, it is crucial to perform a rigorous risk adjustment analysis, especially for outcome indicators, which can be influenced by other factors such as patient comorbidities or disease severity.[37] The process of risk adjustment is crucial for the QIs to provide meaningful comparisons between individual clinicians and institutions.

QI mapping is another critical component of quality measurement and QA. The most commonly reported method for mapping QIs is the Donabedian framework, which subclassifies QIs into structural, process, or outcome measures[38] (Table 45.1). Structural QIs represent the environment in which health care is delivered, whereas process measures analyze the way in which health care is delivered.[29] Outcome measures assess the consequences of the delivered health care, such as surgical complications. Surgical QIs are also commonly mapped as preoperative, perioperative, and postoperative QIs. As an example, Cancer Care Ontario (CCO) maps QIs into the following areas: effectiveness, appropriateness, integration, efficiency, access, and patient-centeredness.[39]

Most authors recommend QI validation through pilot testing. This involves defining the population, defining both the numerator and the denominator of the QI, determining inclusion and exclusion criteria, performing risk adjustment (especially for outcome measures), and identifying both methods of data collection and available data sources. This step is crucial in determining the content, construct, and criterion validity of the QIs, which is necessary before any broad scale implementation.[28,40,41]

There are numerous challenges in implementing QIs into practice. First, sufficient supporting evidence for a QI may be lacking, and often QIs are selected based on expert opinion alone.[42] Second, efficacious treatments under controlled experimental settings do not necessarily

TABLE 45.1 Donabedian Model

Quality Indicator Type	Definition	Example(s)
Structural	Measures reflecting the environment in which health care is delivered, including capacity and standards	Surgeon volume/experience
Process	Measures reflecting the delivery of health care (i.e., what a health provider does to improve or maintain health)	Preoperative time out; Case discussion at multidisciplinary tumor board
Outcome	Measures reflecting the outcome of health care delivery on patients/populations	Postoperative complications; Survival

translate into effective treatments under "real-world" conditions.[42] In addition, a lack of adequate risk adjustment is problematic, allowing critics to use the old adages of "my patients are different," or "my patients are the most difficult." Third, QI measurement at a macrosystem level with administrative data is often challenging, especially when it pertains to data granularity. Measuring QIs on a small-scale microsystem level (i.e., a single practice or hospital setting through chart review and practice audits), although time consuming, allows most areas of care to be accurately measured. However, on a large-scale macrosystem level, data collection is often expensive, and the available measurement systems may not be sufficiently comprehensive.

Defining Quality in Thyroid and Parathyroid Surgery

One common method for improving quality and reducing treatment variation is to develop and disseminate evidence-based clinical guidelines. There is no shortage of excellent, high-quality, clinical practice guidelines for thyroid and parathyroid diseases. The National Comprehensive Cancer Network (NCCN) has published guidelines for thyroid cancer, and the ATA has multiple guidelines for the management of different types of thyroid cancer in specific patient populations.[33,43-46] There are also multidisciplinary consensus guidelines for management of thyroid and parathyroid disease by the American Academy of Otolaryngology Head and Neck Surgery (AAOHNS), the American Association of Endocrine Surgeons (AAES), and the American Head and Neck Society (AHNS) Endocrine Section.[47-52]

There are several important differences between clinical practice guidelines and QIs. First, whereas guidelines provide evidence-based best practices, they are management suggestions, with varying levels of supporting evidence. QIs, on the other hand, are calculable rates, with a defined numerator and denominator. Second, whereas treatment suggestions in a guideline often have different levels of evidence, from expert opinion to randomized control trials, appropriate QIs require a high degree of supporting evidence to be both appropriate and accepted. With the current economic implications of quality assessment, evidence for and consensus agreement upon QIs in thyroid and parathyroid surgery is essential.

QIs in thyroid surgery have been proposed by several authors. Both generic indicators and thyroid surgery-specific indicators have been proposed. Liu and Wiseman proposed several disease-specific QIs for thyroid surgery.[53] The indicators proposed include remnant thyroid tissue uptake of radioactive iodine (RAI), metastatic lymph node ratio (MLNR), and postoperative thyroglobulin (Tg) level. Although these indicators may seem reasonable, there are some challenges and limitations. First, the majority of the studies supporting the use of these indicators are retrospective in nature.[53] The lower the quality of evidence supporting a quality metric, the less likely it will be broadly accepted by those it seeks to evaluate. Second, MLNR is affected not only by lymph node yield but also by the burden of metastatic disease.[53] This makes its utility in measuring surgical quality very limited. Third, postoperative Tg level, although seemingly a reasonable QI, has numerous problems as a measure of surgical quality. Patients with antithyroglobulin antibodies, distant metastatic disease, high disease burden, and undifferentiated malignancies would all be inappropriate for use of Tg levels postoperatively as a QI. Furthermore, remnant RAI uptake is becoming less practical with more and more patients and surgeons choosing less-than-total thyroidectomy for the management of low-risk differentiated thyroid cancer. In addition, the increased use of active surveillance for papillary microcarcinomas and low-risk differentiated thyroid cancer (currently only in clinical trial settings) makes this QI even less appropriate.[54] Furthermore, with any QI, balancing measures need to be considered.

Balancing measures refer to any negative effects that arise from implementation of a specific QI. One concern is that the three aforementioned indicators may persuade surgeons to be more aggressive surgically, which may not be necessarily appropriate or evidence-based in all circumstances. In other words, those who propose or use QIs need to strongly consider the effect they will have on surgeon behavior, including creating any unintended consequences that may arise with the implementation of the QI.

Most thyroid surgeons would agree that rates of recurrent laryngeal nerve paralysis and postoperative permanent hypocalcemia are the most practical QIs, assuming appropriate risk adjustment is carried out. However, measuring these QIs can be difficult at a macrosystem level. CCO recently has proposed numerous QIs for thyroid surgery, and although rates of recurrent laryngeal nerve paralysis and permanent hypoparathyroidism were considered by the surgical expert panel as very important, accurately measuring these indicators at a macrosystem (provincial or state) level was deemed currently not possible.[39] This speaks to the difficulties that are often faced when trying to track QIs on a large scale, as current measurement frameworks, including administrative data sets, often lack the necessary degree of data granularity. Table 45.2 refers to the QIs currently measured by CCO.

One interesting and controversial structural QI that has been proposed in thyroid and parathyroid surgery is surgeon volume. Using a statewide hospital discharge database, Sosa et al. performed a cross-sectional study of patients undergoing thyroidectomy between 1991 and 1996.[55] In this study, high-volume surgeons were more likely to have shorter length of stay rates and a lower rate of complications.[55] Similarly, Meltzer et al. assessed thyroid surgical efficiency, outcomes and resource utilization between high- (>40) and low- (<20) volume

TABLE 45.2 Cancer Care Ontario Quality-Based Procedure Indicators

Quality Domain	Generic QIs	Thyroid Specific QIs
Effectiveness	Reoperation rate within 30 days after resection	*
	30- and 90-day mortality rate after resection	
Appropriateness	Discipline participation in a high-quality Multidisciplinary Cancer Conference (MCC)	Proportion of patients who received a partial thyroidectomy for low-risk disease
		Proportion of patients found to have benign disease after thyroidectomy
		Lymph node retrieval after central neck dissection
Integration	30-day unplanned hospital visit rate after resection (readmission or ER visit)	*
Efficiency	Average length of stay after resection	*
Access	Proportion of patients who received surgery within appropriate malignancy-specific, predefined time frame	*
Patient-centeredness	*	*

*No indicators currently available.

surgeons. Compared with low-volume surgeons, high-volume surgeons had shorter operative times, shorter lengths of stay, more outpatient procedures, and fewer readmitted patients in hemithyroidectomies.[56] In total thyroidectomies, high-volume surgeons had lower rates of complications, shorter lengths of stay and operative times, and performed more outpatient procedures compared with low-volume surgeons.[56] Al-Qurayshi et al. assessed outcomes and costs after thyroidectomy performed by low- (1 to 3 cases per year), intermediate- (4 to 29 cases per year), and high-volume surgeons (>30 cases per year).[57] Compared with high-volume surgeons, low-volume surgeons had a higher risk of complications and higher costs associated with thyroidectomy. The same effect was not seen between intermediate- and high-volume surgeons.[57] Despite these findings, there are challenges with using surgeon volume as a structural QI. Understanding the minimum number of surgeries required is an evolving area of study. Adam et al. used an administrative data set to try and answer this difficult question. Their study found that the likelihood of a patient experiencing a complication after total thyroidectomy decreased with increasing surgeon volume up to 26 cases/year.[58] Although the literature seems to support the concept that increasing surgical volume is associated with decreasing complications and costs, moving patients to "experienced surgeons" can be challenging, particularly in geographically isolated areas. Furthermore, although surgeon volume is important, one cannot discount the confounding effect that hospital volume has on the interpretation of this data.[59] Future studies and analysis are required before surgeon volume can be considered a QI at a macrosystem level.

Although no formal QIs have been proposed for parathyroid surgery, many of the aforementioned QIs in thyroid surgery would similarly apply. Biochemical cure and surgical complications become relevant outcome indicators of interest. In addition, measuring adherence to predefined processes of care, such as discussion at a multidisciplinary conference or compliance with evidence-based guidelines, needs to be given further consideration in the future. Process measures are more readily modifiable compared with structural and outcome measures, and therefore lend themselves more appropriately to quality improvement initiatives.

MEASURING QUALITY

Accurate data collection is essential for measuring and evaluating the quality of surgical care. There are many different forms of data collection that have advantages and disadvantages related to assessing quality in different episodes of care. Data collection focused on large health systems or population-level health care often involves leveraging administrative data, which refers to data collected for the purposes of billing for medical care; these are often based on clinical encounters rather than individual patients. Advantages of administrative data are that they are abundant, do not require additional infrastructure to collect, and can document surgical outcomes for a nationally representative patient population. However, longitudinal patient follow-up is not always available; coding errors affect data quality; and the granularity of clinical information is often lacking, including the intent of care, limiting the applicability of results. Patient-level information is often collected via retrospective chart review at single centers or prospective, single institutional or multiinstitutional data registries. Review of patient charts via the electronic medical record allows collection of clinically relevant information that can be used for risk adjustment in quality assessment. However, this data collection process can be labor intensive and requires focused effort to ensure all information relevant to QA is collected. The advantages and disadvantages of each data source must be considered in relation to the QIs that are relevant in thyroid and parathyroid surgery.

Administrative Data

An administrative database that is commonly used in the assessment of outcomes after thyroid and parathyroid surgery is the National Inpatient Sample (NIS), which is a publicly available health care database that contains administrative data on a 20% stratified sample of all-payer inpatient hospitalizations through a Federal-State-Industry partnership sponsored by the AHRQ. Researchers, health economists, and policymakers use NIS to assess the encounter-level outcomes of surgical procedures, disparities in surgical care, regional health care utilization, and hospital charges. NIS has been used to document associations between surgeon volume, patient age and race, and extent of operation with outcomes in thyroidectomy[58,60-62] and outcomes in pregnant and pediatric patients and risks factors for neck hematoma after parathyroidectomy.[63-65] With the use of representative data sampling, NIS allows researchers to estimate the national prevalence and incidence of surgical conditions, such as thyroid cancer and primary hyperparathyroidism, and short-term outcomes after thyroidectomy and parathyroidectomy. However, coding systems used for billing purposes lack specificity to assess disease severity and information about intraoperative factors that affect outcomes.[66] For example, using NIS, Hauch et al. found that the risk of perioperative complications after total thyroidectomy was higher than that of unilateral thyroidectomy performed both by high- and low-volume surgeons, with the conclusion being that this increased risk should be considered when offering total thyroidectomy for benign disease or low-risk thyroid cancer.[62] However, the authors noted that limitations of the study were that the NIS does not include information about thyroid cancer stage or extent of disease and does not allow follow-up beyond inpatient hospitalization, resulting in underreporting of true 30-day perioperative complications. In addition, the NIS only provides data on inpatient hospitalizations. Given that the majority of thyroid and parathyroid surgery is now being performed in the outpatient setting, it is likely the population captured in the NIS is not representative of all patients undergoing these procedures nationally. Therefore the absence of detailed clinical information from administrative data limits our ability to assess the quality of specific aspects of surgical care.

American College of Surgeons National Surgical Quality Improvement Program (ACS NSQIP)

The ACS developed NSQIP to allow the collection of robust, accurate, and clinically rich data to measure and improve surgical quality.[67] NSQIP began in the early 1990s as a Veterans Affairs (VA) data collection program and now represents the most robust and frequently used method for documenting risk-adjusted surgical outcomes across multiple surgical specialties for the purpose of quality measurement. It contains prospective, multiinstitutional information about preoperative risk factors, intraoperative variables, and 30-day morbidity and mortality outcomes for a systematic sample of major inpatient and outpatient surgical procedures at participating institutions. Dedicated and specifically trained surgical clinical reviewers examine medical records and obtain complete 30-day follow-up on all selected patients, rather than using information related to billing codes, and the quality of collected data is regularly audited for completeness and accuracy with an interrater reliability audit of participating institutions.[68] Participating hospitals receive biannual risk-adjusted surgical outcomes benchmarked against other hospitals' performance (in a blinded fashion), allowing identification of areas to target for improvement. Individual sites are responsible for implementing change to improve outcomes, but the ACS NSQIP provides guidance with successful interventions, best practice guidelines, and other support to reduce complications. With this infrastructure, multiple institutions have reported improved patient outcomes and cost savings with participation.[69,70] Although participation in NSQIP requires resources to establish and maintain it, there is evidence to support the economic benefit of the program over time. Hollenbeak et al. reported reduced postoperative complications and, importantly, an improvement in the cost-effectiveness of NSQIP with longer duration of participation.[70] The authors found that the incremental cost of the total NSQIP program per patient and the cost to avoid one postoperative event decreased from $832 and $25,471 in the first 6 months of participation to $266 and $7319 in the second year of enrollment, respectively, demonstrating quality improvement initiatives through NSQIP became more cost effective over time through a reduction in adverse events.[70]

A number of studies have used NSQIP to evaluate risk factors for adverse outcomes after thyroidectomy and parathyroidectomy, and this body of work has affected perioperative patient management. For example, Roy et al. documented that the risk of neck hematoma requiring reoperation was 10 times greater than the risk of deep vein thrombosis and pulmonary embolism in patients undergoing thyroid and parathyroid operations in the 2005 to 2007 NSQIP, providing information regarding the threshold for administering venous thromboembolism prophylaxis in this patient population.[71] The NSQIP program has also developed a risk calculator to help predict the risk of complications and surgical outcomes based on patient/disease factors.[72] However, in thyroid and parathyroid surgery, the NSQIP risk calculator may be inaccurate in predicting postoperative surgical complications.[73] In a study of 436 patients undergoing thyroid and parathyroid surgery, Margolick and Wiseman found that the NSQIP surgical risk calculator did not accurately predict rates of reoperation, emergency room visits, or unplanned readmissions. Only 17% of patients who experienced a postoperative complication scored above average on the NSQIP risk calculator, whereas 71% of these patients actually scored below average risk.[73] Although the NSQIP is an excellent platform to collect postoperative quality data for many types of operations, the current risk calculator does not seem to be able to accurately predict the likelihood of postoperative complications in thyroid and parathyroid patients. This intuitively makes sense, as measures such as surgical site infection, mortality, ED visits, and readmission are uncommon occurrences in thyroid and parathyroid operations.[73]

Over time, NSQIP has refined its analytic methods to allow more detailed and accurate evaluations of hospital performance.[74] To improve the granularity of data collection and, as a result, the ability to assess quality within specific procedures, the NSQIP developed a "Procedure-Targeted" program in 2011. Data collection for a thyroidectomy-specific NSQIP database began on a trial basis in 2013 and is now available as a full data set starting in 2016, in which there are data from 5871 cases from 93 participating institutions. Using thyroid specific indicators, including recurrent laryngeal nerve injury, severe hypocalcemia, and hematoma, Liu et al. demonstrated a lower rate of nerve injury and hypocalcemia in the "best" versus the "worse" performing hospitals (based on their overall NSQIP performance).[1,75] Processes of care also varied, with patients more likely prescribed calcium and vitamin D and being less likely to have parathyroid hormone levels measured at the "best" performing hospitals.[1] The increased use of a thyroid specific NSQIP data set will likely increase the utility and relevance of this powerful measurement tool, making it more useful as a mechanism of measuring quality in thyroid surgery.[75]

Collaborative Endocrine Surgery Quality Improvement Program

Subspecialty academic societies have been proactive in establishing platforms with which to assess quality. The Collaborative Endocrine Surgery Quality Improvement Program (CESQIP) was formed in 2012 by members of the AAES to serve as a quality improvement platform focused on thyroid, parathyroid, adrenal, and neuroendocrine pancreas and gastrointestinal operations. Patient data related to patient complexity, preoperative workup, intraoperative management, and postoperative endocrine-specific complications are entered by surgeons and their care teams to track outcomes and identify areas for quality improvement. In addition, surgeons can view their performance in comparison to that of other participating surgeons, allowing real time feedback for performance improvement, which is important given that surgeons' self-assessment of complication rates tends to be lower than those observed.[76] The program was recently approved by the Centers for Medicare & Medicaid Services (CMS) as a Qualified Clinical Data Registry, allowing it to fulfill requirement of the Merit-based Incentive Payment System (MIPS), one additional way of encouraging participation by subspecialists. Early reports from CESQIP are just now being published. Contributions to the literature include documentation of patients at high risk of readmission and neck hematoma after thyroidectomy and parathyroidectomy and outcomes of patients undergoing remedial parathyroidectomy.[77] Kazaure et al. published a retrospective cohort study of outcomes from 367 remedial parathyroidectomies and found that 24.8% of patients only had a single localization study before surgery, and 21.1% were not cured postoperatively.[78] In addition, less than half of patients undergoing remedial parathyroidectomy underwent preoperative laryngoscopy to evaluate for recurrent laryngeal nerve injury from the prior operation. Therefore the authors suggested a potential need for additional preoperative imaging to improve surgical cure rates and focus on standardizing preoperative evaluations of patients undergoing remedial surgery.[78] An assessment of CESQIP use as a quality assessment and improvement tool has not yet been documented. As with all quality registries, data collection methods will need ongoing recalibration in response to feedback from providers.

IMPROVING QUALITY

Additional Tools for Surgical Quality Assurance

There are several current strategies of QA in surgery. These include Maintenance of Certification (MOC) and the use of surgical checklists. The development of MOC represented the engagement of physicians in the quality movement. Although a focus on MOC predated *To Err is Human: Building a Safer Healthcare System,* after its publication new momentum was instilled in documenting to the public that surgeons were committed to maintaining an up-to-date knowledge base and improving patient care.[79] In 2018, the American Board of Surgery (ABS) transitioned to continuous certification focused on providing high-quality, practice-related assessment of general surgeons, who now are often subspecialists. As of now, there is no endocrine surgery-specific MOC assessment available through the ABS, but this is likely on the horizon with the documented benefits of high-volume, specialized surgical care in thyroid and parathyroid surgery. Surgical checklists were developed after it was noted that other high-risk fields had established standard practices to minimize the risk of human error to achieve a higher standard of error reduction than in health care.[7] This required a shift in practice from blaming individuals for medical error and to concentrate on systems improvement to prevent medical error. Checklists allow users to enhance and use existing knowledge when they may be impaired by fatigue or overwhelmed by the number of required actions.[80] The World Health Organization (WHO) Surgical Safety Checklist was an evidence-based and expert-approved initiative developed to ensure that safety standards in surgery were met worldwide.[81] Van Klei et al. documented that implementation of the checklist in clinical practice resulted in a decrease in 30-day mortality and that this association was strongly related to completion of all items in the checklist.[82] It is important to recognize that although checklists can be useful tools, their implementation and success in improving outcomes can be affected by other factors, such as resource allocation, the adequacy of team training, and the institutional safety culture.[83,84] The use of checklists was highlighted as an important component to ensure the safety and efficiency of implementing new techniques of thyroidectomy, with a focus on robotic thyroidectomy.[85] With the recent increase in use of remote access thyroidectomy, including transoral thyroidectomy, checklists and other methods for procedural standardization will be important to reduce adverse events and improve quality, but attention must be paid to the method with which they are developed and implemented.

Evidence-Based Methods for Improving Quality

The most important component of QA is improving quality. Although effectively defining and accurately measuring quality are both crucial, the main purpose for performing these activities is to use this information to improve the care provided to patients. The field of quality improvement is growing rapidly, and it is important for clinicians to have a basic understanding of the various methodologies and principles.

In 1996 Berwick proposed the central law of improvement, which argues that every system is designed to achieve the results it achieves.[86] He further argued that we need to reframe our view of performance from one of effort to one of design. One common QI methodology for achieving system-level change and improvement is The Model for Improvement.[86] This model asks three basic questions:

1. What are we trying to accomplish?
2. How will we know that a change is an improvement?
3. What change can we make that will result in an improvement?

A fourth component, called plan, do, study, act (PDSA) cycles, describes a method for designing, testing, and implementing change.[86]

The first question pertains to the importance of having a specific, definable aim for any improvement effort. The second question speaks to the importance of measurement to learn how our efforts are affecting the system (both positively and negatively). Finally, the third question relates to changes that can be made to the system, as opposed to changes focusing on individual behavior, such as asking providers to "try harder." PDSA cycles are then used to test the changes that are introduced, initially on a small scale. Continuous cycles of PDSA thus provide an opportunity of inductive learning, with each cycle generating knowledge through change and also providing an opportunity to reflect on the changes made.[86]

One common measurement approach in QI is statistical process control. Control charts are a method of data collection in time series format and are an effective way of displaying system performance.[87] They also provide an excellent way of distinguishing normal system variation (common cause variation) from abnormal system variation (special cause variation).[88] Common cause variation is a component of any stable process/system, and efforts to reduce common cause variation usually require system design changes. On the other hand, special cause variation (variation unlikely due to chance alone) requires investigation, and if appropriate, actions to eliminate it or maintain it are instituted.[88] Duclos et al. used control charts for QA in thyroid surgery.[87] Recurrent laryngeal nerve paralysis and hypocalcemia were monitored using control charts. During the study period, special cause variation was identified in the proportion of patients experiencing complications during the third quarter of 2007. *This signal was observed on the control charts*, allowing the team to investigate the special cause variation, which, in this case, was secondary to operating room changes and surgeon scheduling.[87] Control charts are an excellent and effective QA tool, and it is likely that their use will continue to increase in the future.

Another common QI methodology is applying the Lean System. Lean was initially introduced in manufacturing by Taiichi Ohno in the Toyota Production System.[89] Lean methodology uses the customer's perspective as to what are "value-added" and "non-value added" steps in a system. In other words, nonvalue added components of a system are considered as waste. Lean methodology seeks to continually eliminate waste and improve the efficiency of a system to deliver a service or a product.[89] Matt et al. used Lean to improve the efficiency of ultrasound-guided needle biopsy in the head and neck.[90] Using Lean principles, the authors reduced the time from decision to perform a biopsy to an actual biopsy date from 37.6 days to 4.8 days ($p < 0.00001$). In addition, time from biopsy to diagnosis also was reduced from 6 days to 2.3 days ($p < 0.03$). Lean methodology achieved these results by eliminating waste, allowing the authors to reduce the number of steps in the process from 17 to 9.[90]

FUTURE DIRECTIONS

One certainty in the search for quality care in thyroid and parathyroid surgery is that it will continue to evolve with clinical practice. What will define quality care in thyroid and parathyroid surgery 5 and 10 years from now is dependent on the products of rigorous and innovative research and quality assessment today. The current epidemic of opioid abuse and documentation of persistent narcotic use in more than 5% of patients 90 days after thyroid and parathyroid surgery suggests that quality care will include the routine use of nonnarcotic pain regimens in opiate-naive patients undergoing these operations.[91,92] In addition, as research on the optimal use of molecular testing in the workup and management of indeterminate thyroid nodules increases, standardized protocols to guide the implementation of selective molecular testing will likely emerge with the goal of improving quality by avoiding unnecessary surgery and allowing patient-centered surgical decision making. With the establishment of protocols for active surveillance of papillary microcarcinomas or clinical trials for the active surveillance of low-risk papillary thyroid carcinoma,[93] QA will have to extend beyond the confines of the operating room to include nonoperative treatment strategies.

CONCLUSION

QA in thyroid and parathyroid surgery will continue to grow in the future. Properly defining quality and accurately measuring quality are crucial steps in the process of QA. Proper risk adjustment, especially for outcome indicators, is especially important to make sure that providers and institutions are accurately and fairly evaluated. Most important, when gaps in quality are identified, quality improvement methodologies are a useful way for designing and implementing system-level changes to improve the care delivered to patients. Finally, we need to continue to promote an open QA dialogue in thyroid and parathyroid surgery, refraining from punitive and exclusionary measures, instead focusing on continuous quality improvement at a system level.

REFERENCES

For a complete list of references, go to expertconsult.com.

46

Ethics and Malpractice in Thyroid and Parathyroid Surgery

Peter Angelos

> Please go to expertconsult.com to view related video:
> **Video 46.1** Introduction to Chapter 46, Ethics and Malpractice in Thyroid and Parathyroid Surgery.

ETHICAL ISSUES

Optimizing Informed Consent

One of the central ethical challenges for surgeons is to ensure that patients have given adequate informed consent before having an operation. Certainly, informed consent for surgery is much more than just a patient's signature on a consent form. In fact, informed consent for surgery is best thought of as a process whereby the surgeon informs a patient of the risks, benefits, and alternatives of a particular operation and the patient then freely agrees to undergo the procedure.[1] Years ago, surgeons made choices for their patients based on the surgeon's judgment about what was in the patient's best interest. Today, the paternalism of the past has been supplanted by the important principle of respect for patient autonomy.[2] In the current era of shared decision-making, surgeons must approach the informed consent process as a means of educating the patient about his or her condition so that the patient can participate in the decision about whether to have surgery or not. In an era where there are many approaches to thyroid and parathyroid surgery, it is essential for patients to play a significant role in decision making.

The quality of the interchange between a surgeon and a patient is dependent on the relationship between the parties. Although much has been written analyzing the doctor-patient relationship, little has been written about the significant challenges that surgeons face in engendering the level of trust required by patients to consent to surgery. In few other areas of medical care are patients asked to put themselves in such a vulnerable position as when they enter the operating room for surgery under general anesthesia. Patients must be willing to place enough trust in their surgeons that they are willing to risk disfigurement and potentially permanent disability or even death at the hands of the surgeon. This is not only a deep level of trust but also something that must be developed in a relatively short period of time in a preoperative visit. Rather than getting to know a patient over months or years, as many primary care physicians are able to do, surgeons must develop a rapport with patients in one or more relatively short preoperative visits.

As noted previously, the informed consent process for surgery involves the surgeon explaining to the patient the risks of the operation. It is critical that patients undergoing thyroid and parathyroid surgery understand the risks of recurrent laryngeal nerve (RLN) injury and permanent hypocalcemia, which are always present with these procedures. This explanation by the surgeon of these risks should be thought of as an opportunity to teach the patient and gain the patient's trust. Some surgeons find it very helpful to give the patient diagrams or other written materials that describe not only the operation being recommended but also the risks. Others refer patients to appropriate websites, but it is essential that the surgeon give a thorough verbal explanation with ample opportunity for the patient to ask questions. It is more important that the surgeon document that such a discussion took place than to rely on the type of standard consent form required by all hospitals and frequently obtained by staff.

The legal standard of informed consent requires the surgeon to give the patient the opportunity to receive the information that a reasonable person would want to know to make an informed decision. In particular, the surgeon should offer the patient information about complications that might deter a reasonable person from undergoing surgery. As such, every consent discussion with a patient undergoing thyroidectomy or parathyroidectomy must include information about the risks of nerve injury, hypoparathyroidism, and bleeding. Although national rates may be valuable, surgeons should endeavor to know their own rates of complications so that surgeon-specific information can be provided to patients whenever possible. The detail of information that each individual patient needs to make an informed decision varies; therefore surgeons should strive to engage in a dialogue with patients about risks, adding more detail as directed by the patient's desire for such detail.

Ethical Issues in Surgical Innovation and New Technology

Unlike new drugs, which in the United States are regulated by the Food and Drug Administration, surgeons who develop new or innovative surgical procedures have very little oversight or regulation. Not only is there little oversight of surgical innovation, but the lack of regulation is seen by many as essential to allowing surgeons to continually question how they can make an operation better.[3] Although surgical research certainly must abide by all of the regulations for all research on human subjects—namely, oversight by institutional review boards (IRBs)—most commonly, innovation occurs in surgery outside of formal surgical research. This informal approach to innovation has led to many improvements in how contemporary surgery is performed. To see just one example of such improvements in surgical care, consider the change in the safety of thyroid surgery from the mid-19th century to the early 20th century. In 1866, the influential surgeon, Dr. Samuel Gross, wrote about thyroidectomy, "Thus whether we view this operation in relation to the difficulties which must necessarily attend its execution, or with reference to the severity of the subsequent

433

inflammation, it is equally deserving of rebuke and condemnation. No honest and sensible surgeon, it seems to me, would ever engage in it."[4] In contrast, Dr. Theodor Kocher, who was awarded the Nobel Prize in Medicine in 1909, had been able to reduce operative mortality in benign goiter surgery from 13% in his first 101 cases to 2.4% in his subsequent 250 cases. By 1917, Kocher reported a mortality rate of 0.5% in approximately 5000 operations.[5]

Unfortunately, there are many examples of surgical innovations that seemed promising to the surgeons who tried them but ultimately proved to have no benefit for patients. Consider the following surgical "innovations" that were either not helpful or actually harmful to patients. Prefrontal lobotomy was used to treat many psychiatric problems, even though it was not effective for any of them.[6] Internal mammary artery ligation was performed on thousands of patients to treat angina, yet it had no affect on patient survival.[7] As recently as 50 years ago, significant research and technological advancements were undertaken to refine gastric freezing for ulcer disease, but the technique ultimately proved to be ineffective.[8] These "innovative" attempts at treating significant medical and psychiatric problems were all ineffective. Any consideration of how to approach the regulation of surgical innovation today must find the middle road between too much regulation so that patients are prevented from getting the latest and potentially best operations and too little oversight so that patients are harmed by overly enthusiastic surgeons who push innovative surgical techniques without data to show the benefits.

Given the mixed record of surgical "innovation" throughout history, what are the criteria for deciding whether a new technology or approach is better? For a new surgical technique to be accepted as surgical progress, it should be safe and effective in solving the surgical problem for the patient. As straightforward as this sounds, it is often difficult to determine whether a new technique or technology is truly safe and effective. Often, studies to assess safety are underpowered, and effectiveness can frequently only be determined with long-term follow-up. In addition, the determination of what outcomes are even considered important to assess becomes a value judgment and therefore a moral question.[9]

If we turn our attention specifically to innovations in thyroid and parathyroid surgery, the difficulties noted earlier in deciding whether a new technique is an improvement are readily apparent. The risks of permanent RLN injury are in the 1% to 2% range in most series. Therefore to show even a doubling of the risk of permanent RLN injury, a study would need to be quite large. In addition, if the concern is over the long-term efficacy of a new technique for thyroidectomy for papillary cancer, given the biology of the disease, one would need to follow a very large number of patients for many years to show any difference in the outcome.

In recent years, many of the innovative techniques applied to thyroid and parathyroid surgery have focused on the attempt to improve the cosmetic results, shorten the convalescence, or reduce the morbidity of the procedure.[10] Certainly, many authors have shown that thyroids can be removed through very small incisions[11-13] or even without incisions visible on the neck.[14-18] However, with the exception of a few widely used procedures such as the video-assisted thyroidectomy by Dr. Paolo Miccoli[12] and the "scarless" transoral thyroidectomy by Dr. Angkoon Anuwong,[18] it remains to be determined whether these new techniques can duplicate the safety of the conventional approaches. If the safety of the "minimally invasive" technique can be shown, then the additional question that will need to be addressed is how important a smaller or nonvisible scar is to the well-being of the patient. In other words, what is the improvement in quality of life that a smaller scar or nonvisible scar has for patients. Most surgeons accept that there is a benefit to patients by having smaller, less noticeable scars. However, it will be important to carefully assess patient-reported outcomes to determine whether the assumed improvements in quality of life are really seen when actual patients are carefully studied. We must be certain that the purported improvements that a new technique brings are truly beneficial to patients rather than being solely attempts by surgeons to increase their practices by suggesting that these new techniques are "better" for patients.

Some attempts at new surgical procedures are made to treat previously untreatable medical problems. Although the Vineberg operation (direct implantation of the internal mammary artery into the left ventricle) was ultimately considered a failure,[19] the concept of myocardial revascularization was proven valid as the effectiveness of coronary artery bypass grafting was established. Although laparoscopic abdominal surgery and video-assisted thoracic surgery certainly result in smaller scars, the major advantage of these procedures is not cosmetic but rather fewer wound and respiratory complications as well as less pain, shorter hospitalization, and more rapid return to normal activity. Can the same be said about video-assisted, transaxillary robotic thyroidectomy and transoral thyroidectomy? At best, we anticipate that the surgical complication rates will be the same as conventional thyroidectomy. At best, the oncologic outcomes will also likely be the same. Recovery after surgery may be related in a minor way to the size of the incision, but many patients now undergo conventional thyroidectomy and parathyroidectomy and are discharged on the day of surgery. The only real benefit to the patient is a smaller or inconspicuous scar. The procedures may take longer to perform than the traditional operation and certainly have a substantial learning curve. Is it reasonable to consume scarce health care resources and possibly risk an increased incidence of complications for a small cosmetic benefit? This is a question for which the answer may become increasingly important in upcoming years and for which surgeons and patients may have less input in the future.

Ethics and Advertising

Before recent decades, advertising by physicians was thought to be unprofessional and unethical. In fact, until 1981, the American Medical Association (AMA) specifically banned advertising by doctors.[20] In 1975, using the Sherman Antitrust Act of 1890, the United States Federal Trade Commission brought a lawsuit against the AMA challenging the ban on advertising. The premise was that a ban on advertising by physicians prevented competition and encouraged monopolistic practices.[21] Ultimately, the case was taken to the U.S. Supreme Court, which in 1981 forced the AMA to change its policy. As a result of this change, advertising by physicians in the U.S. is legal and widely used. False advertising is illegal, but it is rare that anything other than misstating one's credentials is actually seen as false advertising. From a *legal* perspective, therefore, almost anything goes.

However, not all advertising is considered to be *ethically* acceptable. The AMA requires that advertising by physicians "regardless of format or context, is true and not materially misleading" (AMA Code of Ethics, 5.02 Advertising and Publicity: American Medical Association, 2009). As one might imagine, the question now focuses on what is "materially misleading?" The difficulty is that many of the words commonly used in advertising, such as "best," "leading," and "outstanding" cannot be exactly defined or quantified.[22] As a result, it is very difficult to prove that an advertisement that uses such indefinite adjectives is actually misleading. For example, for many years, one of the prominent cancer hospitals in the U.S. used the advertising slogan, "The best cancer care - anywhere." Such a statement is impossible to prove to be false although many might not agree that it is true.

In an attempt to promote ethical advertising, some commentators have emphasized the differences between advertising that is informative from that which is persuasive.[23] Medical advertising is considered ethically acceptable if it informs patients about a treatment, a physician, or an institution. In this manner, informative medical advertising is seen as respecting the autonomy of the patient.[24] In contrast, persuasive medical advertising is ethically problematic because it seeks to override autonomy by manipulating subconscious desires, associations, and vulnerabilities.[25] The ethical challenge for every surgeon is how to inform patients without misleading or trying to unduly influence them.

The popularity of the Internet has created further concerns when it comes to ethical issues in marketing. Often, an Internet site that appears to be focused on informing the public can shift into the promotion of a single institution, a single practice, or a single physician. Although it is not unethical for a surgeon to make factual statements about his or her own experience or results on the Internet, one should not make unsupported claims or make claims of excellence that denigrate other practitioners. Every advertisement or statement, either on the Internet or in other media, should be thought of as the initiation of the informed consent process and should therefore be balanced.[20] Surgeons should use this standard to judge whether their own advertising or websites are ethical, and they should encourage their patients to use the same standard when evaluating the claims made by others.

In addition to the aforementioned ethical considerations, surgeons must be careful to not expose themselves to legal risks by the statements made in advertising in mass media or on the Internet. The primary legal risk is to overstate the benefits of certain techniques while minimizing the risks. For example, if an advertisement or website were to claim that "scarless" transoral thyroidectomy through the lower lip results in reduced risks of RLN injury, the surgeon might be at risk of a suit for false advertising if there is not sufficient data to support such a claim. Such claims are readily seen in advertising, and often it is not the surgeon who is writing the text but rather a marketing department that may be accustomed to the usual hyperbole seen in advertising. Unfortunately, although it is not unusual to see advertisers playing fast and loose with the facts when promoting many products, when it comes to promoting a surgeon or an operation, the exact statements must be grounded on the actual evidence, and surgeons should be proactive to ensure that patients are not being misled.

THE SURGEON'S RESPONSIBILITY

The code of professional ethics of the American College of Surgeons states,

> Since a team of specialists undertakes much of modern patient care, physicians who are not surgeons may often do the initial evaluation of patients. However, the surgeon bears the ultimate responsibility for determining the need for and the type of operation. In making this decision, the surgeon must give precedence to sound indications for the procedure over pressure by patients or referring physicians, or the financial incentive to perform the operation. The surgeon is responsible for the patient's safety throughout the preoperative, operative, and postoperative period ... The surgeon's responsibility extends throughout the surgical illness.

In patients referred for thyroid and parathyroid surgery, the most important decisions are made before the skin incision. Patients are frequently referred "for surgery." This does not free the surgeon from making an independent assessment of the patient's need for surgery. Such an assessment requires a thorough understanding of the indications for surgery as well as alternative treatment options and how these options might affect the patient's goals. To make such assessments, the surgeon must endeavor to establish a relationship with the patient that emphasizes the patient's best interests. The surgeon may have a better understanding of the potential risks and complications of surgery than the referring physician and should use this information in deciding whether or not to recommend surgery for a specific patient. The surgeon who independently evaluates each patient referred and makes a recommendation based on the patient's interests will establish the reputation of someone who is objective and willing to recommend nonsurgical treatment when appropriate. Such a surgeon will ultimately be busier than the surgeon who operates on everyone who comes through the door.

A suspicious fine-needle aspiration biopsy (FNAB) is the most common indication for thyroidectomy. Not all cytologists are equally experienced in the interpretation of these biopsies. In spite of efforts to standardize the descriptive terms used to categorize these biopsies,[26] different cytologists may use the same term to indicate different things. For example, the likelihood of malignancy in an FNAB interpreted as "suspicious for malignancy" is estimated to range from 50% to almost 100% in different series. The term "atypia" has a wide variety of meanings.[27] If an FNAB has been evaluated by a cytologist or in a laboratory with which the surgeon is not familiar, it is helpful to have the slides reviewed by a cytologist familiar to the surgeon to avoid making surgical decisions based on a misunderstanding of the cytology report. In fact, many hospitals require that outside slides be reviewed before surgery.[28]

Not all surgeons are equally experienced in performing thyroid and parathyroid surgery. Studies have shown that surgeons who perform a large number of thyroidectomies each year have fewer complications than those who perform fewer operations.[29,30] Such data do not mean that low-volume surgeons should not perform these operations. However, before undertaking a difficult operation, the surgeon should consider whether that patient might be better served by referral to a specialized institution for care. A less experienced surgeon might consider asking a more experienced colleague to be available for intraoperative consultation when a difficult procedure is performed.

The extent of involvement in the long-term management of patients varies among surgeons, particularly in the care of patients with thyroid cancer. For some, their relationship ends after the first postoperative visit. Others, with a particular interest and extensive experience in the treatment of thyroid cancer, may choose to follow their patients indefinitely and collaborate with their endocrinology colleagues in the therapeutic decision making and surveillance of these patients. Many of the major advances in the understanding of thyroid cancer, particularly those related to risk stratification, were made by surgeons who followed their patients for many years. It is always the surgeon's responsibility to ensure that patients are referred to an appropriate physician for follow-up and consultation when needed, before they are discharged from his or her care.

MALPRACTICE ISSUES

Although unethical behavior may not lead to a malpractice suit and a complication leading to a malpractice suit may not be unethical, there is nevertheless a relationship between ethics and risks of malpractice. All surgeons strive to limit the complications that their patients may suffer from; to do otherwise would be unethical. In the U.S. the concerns about malpractice lawsuits are magnified by the possibility of surgeons having a malpractice lawsuit brought against them even when a complication does not occur. However, one must not forget that malpractice suits are possible in most countries in the world. In many countries, the concerns of surgeons may be even greater because legal risks are not limited to civil proceedings as in the U.S. but may actually involve criminal prosecution.

Even the most experienced, careful surgeons occasionally have complications, and some of these complications can result in permanent injury to patients. Although many technical errors in the operating room result in complications, the fact that a complication has occurred is not evidence that an error has been made. Surprisingly, many technical errors involve routine operations performed by experienced surgeons within their area of expertise.[31] With regard to thyroid and parathyroid surgery, malpractice suits are most frequently related to recurrent nerve injury or hypoxic brain damage due to airway obstruction resulting from bilateral nerve injury or hematoma.[32] The most common nontechnical cause for malpractice suits related to the thyroid is the delayed diagnosis of cancer.[32] Although most malpractice cases list lack of informed consent in the legal complaint, informed consent issues alone are rarely the cause of action.

It is therefore difficult to develop a strategy to protect surgeons from malpractice suits that are based on data rather than anecdotes and personal opinion. In the remaining sections of this chapter we will explore the available data regarding the risks of malpractice suits in thyroid and parathyroid surgery. We will focus primarily on this issue in the U.S. where the risks of malpractice lawsuits are the greatest.

Determining the actual number of malpractice lawsuits related to thyroid and parathyroid operations that are filed in the U.S. is virtually impossible. Many lawsuits are either dropped completely or settled out of court, and frequently the terms of the settlement are sealed and not available as public record. However, a review of the literature on the topic allows a rough estimate of the scope of the problem.

One method of identifying malpractice lawsuits is to study the number of jury verdict awards, as these are matters of public record. Kern examined jury verdict reports from U.S. civil court cases between 1985 and 1991 and found that there were a total of 62 cases related to endocrine diseases.[33] Of these cases, 32 jury awards were related to complications of thyroid surgery and only two related to complications of parathyroid surgery. In 22 of the 62 cases analyzed, a delay in the diagnosis was the basis of the verdict of which 11 cases were related to thyroid cancer and two were related to hyperparathyroidism.

More recently, in 2003 Lydiatt reported on jury verdicts related to cases involving thyroid surgery between 1987 and 2000 by searching the Westlaw computerized legal database.[32] He found 33 cases total, of which 10 (30%) were related to surgical complications, all but one of which was due to RLN injury. In a third of these cases of RLN injury, bilateral nerve injuries had occurred.

In 2010, Abadin and colleagues used a different computerized legal database (Lexis/Nexis Academic) to study U.S. cases between 1989 and 2009 related to thyroid disease.[34] These authors identified 143 cases; however, individual case reviews revealed that only 33 cases involved alleged negligence after thyroid surgery. Of these 33 cases, 15 cases (46%) involved RLN injury, 3 cases (9%) claimed inadequate surgery, and the same number alleged unnecessary surgery. Of the 15 cases related to RLN injury, 7 cases were decided in favor of the patient, whereas eight favored the surgeon. The jury awards ranged from $150,000 to $3.7 million.

In 2009 Shaw and Pierce used a different method to study malpractice claims.[35] By studying closed claims involving vocal cord paralysis that were reported by 16 of the largest malpractice insurers between 1986 and 2007, these authors were able to identify 112 claims of which only 28 (25%) actually went to trial. Of the 112 claims reviewed, 39 (35%) were related to thyroid or parathyroid surgery. A full 60% of the 112 closed claims were settled before trial. Overall, in 15% of the 112 filed cases, no settlement or jury trial was ever pursued. In their analysis, of the 28 cases that went to trial, only 2 (7%) were found in favor of the plaintiff. In contrast to the high jury awards seen in the Abadin study, Shaw and Pierce noted the largest payment to be $875,000 (although adjusted for inflation the number would be approximately $1,575,000).

The numbers of cases noted by all of these authors is really quite small when one considers that the number of thyroidectomies estimated to have been performed in the U.S. in 2016 was approximately 150,000.[36] Although there is no way to quantify exactly how many malpractice claims involving thyroidectomy are filed, informal discussions with many experienced thyroid and parathyroid surgeons who have reviewed medical records as expert witnesses suggest that many more than the few cases noted per year in the aforementioned studies are actually considered or filed in the U.S. annually. It appears that the malpractice cases reported in these studies are only the tip of the iceberg of malpractice cases related to thyroid and parathyroid surgery.

Legal Basis of Malpractice

The legal basis of any malpractice suit rests on four components. The surgeon has entered into a relationship obligating provision of care to the patient. The surgeon violated the relevant "standard of care." The "substandard care" resulted in an injury to the patient. This resulted in compensable damages to the patient.[37] The essence of the case is usually the question "Did the surgeon deviate from the standard of care?"

The "standard of care" is not an absolute algorithm or set of guidelines. In legal terms it is the level at which the average, prudent provider in a given community would practice. It is how similarly qualified practitioners would have managed the patient's care under the same or similar circumstances. The standard of care is essentially redefined in each case based on the testimony of expert witnesses. It does not imply the highest standard of care and might even represent "a course of treatment advocated by a considerable number of recognized and respected professionals" even if this is a minority of practitioners.[38]

Of note, the legal doctrine that is most commonly used by plaintiffs in malpractice cases involving RLN injury is *res ipsa loquitur* which translated from Latin means, "the thing speaks for itself." According to this view, the proof of negligence is in the actual complication itself. For example, if a patient is found to have an infection secondary to a retained sponge, no proof of negligence is required as the event itself is the proof. Many malpractice attorneys make a similar argument about RLN injuries after thyroid or parathyroid surgery. However, surgeons and defense attorneys will uniformly disagree with this concept. Surgeons maintain that an RLN injury is a known complication of surgery that may occur regardless of the great care that may have been taken by the surgeon. As such, the occurrence of an RLN injury is an unfortunate, but known, complication of surgery but not necessarily a result of negligence.[34]

The Standard of Care

Numerous professional organizations have published guidelines that are relevant to the surgical treatment of patients with thyroid and parathyroid diseases. Perhaps the most commonly discussed in the U.S. are those developed by the American Thyroid Association (ATA).[39] These guidelines were developed using the principles of evidence-based medicine. Guidelines are not absolute rules and the authors of the ATA guidelines state "it is not the intent of these guidelines to replace individual decision making, the wishes of the patient or family, or clinical judgment."[40]

Although guidelines are not synonymous with the legal concept of standard of care, they can be used to help establish the standard of care and their use in litigation appears to be increasing.[41] Most often, they are used to demonstrate that there was a deviation from a presumed standard treatment, but they also can help exculpate a physician rendering care consistent with recognized guidelines. To protect oneself in the event of a malpractice suit, and potentially to avoid suits, the surgeon should provide care consistent with published guidelines when it is in the best interest of the patient. When unique situations or the patient's informed wishes require substantial deviation from published guidelines, the reason for these deviations should be carefully documented in the medical record.

Permanent injury to the RLN occurs in approximately 1% of patients undergoing thyroidectomy[42] and less often during parathyroidectomy.[43] Actual transection of the nerve during surgery is less common.[44] Some data suggest that exposure of the entire nerve is less likely to result in nerve injury than simple identification of a portion of the nerve.[45] It is our opinion that identification of the nerve during thyroidectomy represents the standard of care in the U.S. today. There may be situations where the nerve cannot be identified, such as during operations on advanced cancers or very large thyroid glands, or when performing reoperations. The standard of care cannot mandate that the nerve actually be identified but rather that every reasonable attempt should be made to do so and that these attempts should be documented in the operative report. If the nerve cannot be identified, the reasons for this and whatever other strategies were employed to minimize the risk of nerve injury should be similarly documented. Many surgeons do not routinely identify the RLN during parathyroid surgery, particularly during focused, minimally invasive, single gland exploration. This can be acceptable, as long as appropriate care is taken and documented to avoid the nerve in such a focused operation.

Preoperative laryngoscopy obviously does not influence the incidence of nerve injury during surgery. However, this practice could possibly protect a surgeon from litigation if a paralyzed vocal cord had been identified preoperatively. Some experts believe that every patient undergoing thyroidectomy should have a preoperative laryngoscopy to help plan the operation and appropriately counsel the patient about the risks of the surgery, which would protect the surgeon from litigation.[46,47] There are situations wherein such information may be valuable for operative decision-making. However, its utility in asymptomatic patients without malignancy has been questioned.[48] Patients undergoing thyroidectomy, particularly those with cancer, who have symptoms suggesting vocal cord paralysis or invasion of the larynx, hypopharynx, trachea, or esophagus, should be appropriately evaluated using whatever techniques or imaging studies are necessary, including fiberoptic laryngoscopy. Based on these considerations, it is difficult to define a standard of care for laryngeal examination other than in patients with prior surgery at this time (see Chapter 15, Pre- and Postoperative Laryngeal Examination in Thyroid and Parathyroid Surgery).

Intraoperative RLN monitoring is being used with increasing frequency[49] and is discussed in detail elsewhere in this book (see Chapter 36, Surgical Anatomy and Monitoring of the Recurrent Laryngeal Nerve). Several studies do not demonstrate a decrease in RLN injury when this technique is used.[50] There is at least a suggestion that the incidence of nerve injury may be lower in reoperations when nerve monitoring is used[51] and that temporary nerve injury rates are lower when a nerve monitor is used.[52] We believe that surgeons should be aware that this technique is gaining greater acceptance and appears to be used with greater frequency among younger as well as higher-volume thyroid surgeons.[49]

Although the use of neuromonitoring has not been shown to result in a statistically significant reduction of RLN injuries, it does accurately predict a nerve that will not likely work at the end of an operation despite the nerve being visually intact. The knowledge that the RLN on the first side of a planned total thyroidectomy is not likely to work at the completion of the operation is valuable because a surgeon may (depending on the specific clinical scenario) choose not to proceed to the second side. In this fashion, neuromonitoring is likely to result in lower rates of bilateral RLN injury.

The clear ethical imperative of neuromonitoring is similar to the ethical imperative of all technology. If a surgeon is going to use the technology, he or she should ensure that there has been appropriate education and training in the use of the technology so that patients garner the greatest benefit from its use.

Some have argued that the use of nerve monitoring could potentially help in the defense of a surgeon sued for injuring a nerve during thyroidectomy by demonstrating that he or she used every possible precaution to avoid nerve injury. Given the conflicting evidence on rates of vocal cord paralysis and the difficulty in quantification of the benefit of neural monitoring, we feel it is difficult to define the standard of care relative to neuromonitoring at this time.

Malpractice Claims and the Parathyroid Glands

Permanent hypoparathyroidism is a recognized complication of thyroidectomy,[53] but it alone is rarely a reason for a malpractice suit.[34] The risk of parathyroid injury can be decreased by identifying the glands during surgery, avoiding injury to their blood supply, and autotransplanting glands that cannot otherwise be preserved. As mentioned earlier, the occurrence of this complication does not mean that there has been a deviation from the standard of care. The operative report should carefully detail whatever techniques the surgeon employed to avoid parathyroid injury. Failure to mention the parathyroids and the attempt to preserve them in the operative report of a patient who ends up with permanent hypoparathyroidism is a difficult case to defend.

Malpractice suits resulting from parathyroidectomy are less common than after thyroidectomy.[33] Some of the possible causes for action are similar to those during thyroidectomy, including RLN injury and airway obstruction. Issues unique to parathyroid surgery include the role of preoperative imaging and intraoperative parathyroid hormone (PTH) measurement. Preoperative imaging can identify the abnormal parathyroid in most cases of primary hyperparathyroidism[54] and is discussed extensively elsewhere in this book (see Chapter 59, Intraoperative PTH Monitoring during Parathyroid Surgery, and Chapter 54, Guide to Preoperative Parathyroid Localization Testing). Although preoperative imaging may be helpful when conventional bilateral exploration is performed, there is little evidence that the success rate is improved when imaging is performed. Some sort of preoperative imaging must be performed if limited, single gland exploration is planned. Preoperative imaging, frequently with more than one modality, is mandatory if reexploration for recurrent or persistent hyperparathyroidism after previous exploration is planned.[55] Although there may be situations where parathyroid exploration without preoperative imaging is not a deviation from the standard of care, we believe that a failed parathyroid exploration would be easier to defend in court if preoperative imaging had been performed.

Intraoperative PTH measurement to assure the adequacy of parathyroidectomy is being employed with increasing frequency, particularly when limited, single gland exploration is planned.[56] Although radioguided surgery may be used instead of intraoperative PTH measurement,[57] it is not as sensitive.[58] Strategies have been proposed to minimize the risk of persistent hyperparathyroidism without the use of intraoperative PTH or radioguidance.[59] In most cases, intraoperative PTH measurement should be used if limited, single gland exploration is planned. If intraoperative PTH is not available, after careful explanation of the risks and benefits of limited exploration compared with bilateral exploration, including the increased risk of persistent hyperparathyroidism, performance of a limited operation might be defensible in the event of a malpractice suit. As with so many special circumstances in the care of individual patients, this discussion with the patient should be carefully documented. Referral to an institution where these techniques are available might also be considered if the surgeon cannot offer the appropriate modalities. Although measurement of intraoperative PTH in conventional bilateral exploration may be helpful, particularly if all four parathyroids cannot be identified, we do not believe that failure to use this technique is a deviation from the standard of care.

CONCLUSIONS

Although ethical issues and malpractice considerations certainly do not completely overlap in thyroid and parathyroid surgery, there is clearly a relationship between these sets of concerns. The ethical issues primary revolve around the surgeon-patient relationship, informed consent, and the development of trust by a patient in his or her surgeon. The considerations in malpractice primarily revolve around reducing complications and ensuring adequate disclosure of risks to patients. Despite the differences in these topics, there is clear overlap in that it is well-known that patients who trust their surgeons are less likely to bring a malpractice suit even in the face of a complication. Thus attention to the ethical dimension of the surgical care of the thyroid and parathyroid patient can have both intrinsic and extrinsic value to the surgeon.

REFERENCES

For a complete list of references, go to expertconsult.com.

Postoperative Management

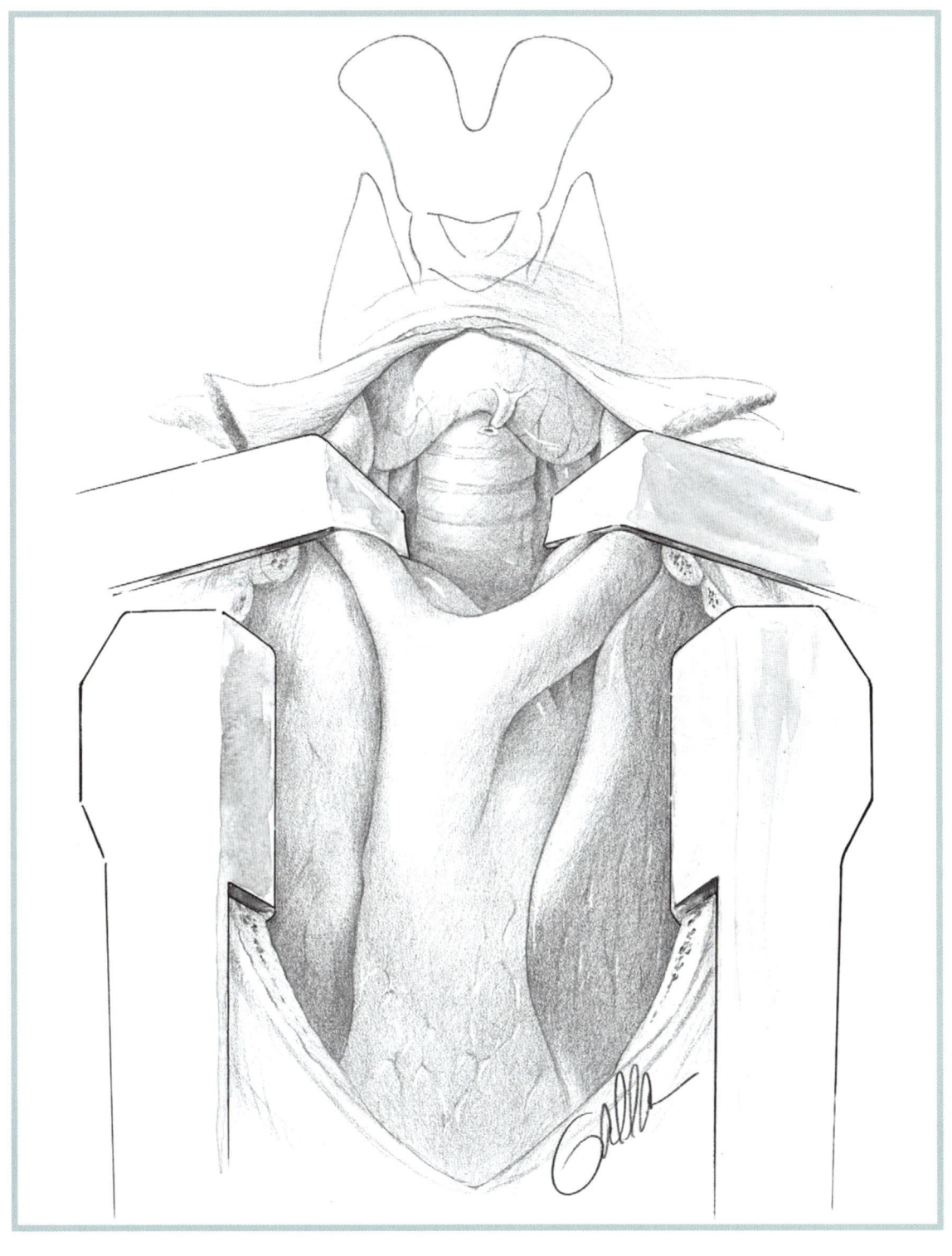

47

Postoperative Management of Differentiated Thyroid Cancer

Dana Hartl, Sophie Leboulleux, Julien Hadoux, Amandine Berdelou, Ingrid Breuskin, Joanne Guerlain, Martin Schlumberger

GOALS OF POSTOPERATIVE MANAGEMENT

Differentiated thyroid cancer (DTC) is being diagnosed with increasing incidence, but the mortality rate has remained low.[1,2] The vast majority of these tumors are low-risk cancers, limited to the thyroid gland, which have a 20-year disease-specific survival rate close to 100%. Current recommendations aim to best adapt adjuvant therapy and follow-up to each patient and each cancer, avoiding overtreatment and oversurveillance of indolent disease while escalating therapy for cancers with a high risk of recurrence and/or death. Current treatment paradigms will avoid unnecessary acute toxicity and long-term side effects associated with radioactive iodine (RAI) and thyroid hormone replacement therapy while effectively diagnosing and treating patients with distant metastases (DM) with appropriate techniques and drugs, improving quality of life and progression-free survival. Current classifications divide patients into risk groups that determine the extent of recommended adjuvant therapy and follow-up.

TREATMENT ACCORDING TO RISK OF CANCER RECURRENCE

Certain clinical, preoperative, and postoperative histopathological tumor and patient characteristics enable physicians to evaluate risk factors for recurrence and classify patients into groups according to the estimated risk of tumor recurrence. Table 47.1 enumerates these characteristics for each risk group, according to the American Thyroid Association (ATA) Guidelines published in 2015.[3]

The American Joint Commission on Cancer classification evaluates the risk of death from thyroid cancer, which is based on the extent of disease, tumor size, location of regional lymph node metastases, and the presence of DM.[4,5] The stage grouping according to age illustrated the excellent outcomes of treatment for patients <55 years old, even with DM, compared with older patients (Boxes 47.1 and 47.2).

In clinical practice, the indications for adjuvant treatment after surgery are currently based on the risk grouping as described in the ATA guidelines. For epidemiologic purposes and prognostication, the tumor, node, metastases (TNM) classification is employed.

Adjuvant treatments include RAI, external beam radiation therapy (EBRT), thyroid hormone replacement or suppression therapy, localized treatment of individual metastatic lesions, and systemic therapies mainly with orally administered tyrosine kinase inhibitors (TKIs).

Radioactive Iodine (^{131}I) Therapy

RAI is employed to (1) destroy any normal remnant thyroid tissue and render thyroglobulin (Tg) assays highly sensitive; (2) to destroy local or regional recurrent/persistent disease and DM; and (3) to perform whole-body imaging for diagnostic purposes (see Chapter 48 Postoperative Radioactive Iodine Ablation and Treatment of Differentiated Thyroid Cancer).

RAI is administered orally after stimulation with recombinant human thyroid-stimulating hormone (rhTSH) (1 injection per day on the 2 days preceding ^{131}I administration) or after thyroid hormone withdrawal for 4 weeks, with or without temporary substitution with liothyronine (LT3), which also should be withdrawn for at least 2 weeks before ^{131}I administration.[3] Thyroid-stimulating hormone (TSH) should be >30 mUI/mL at the time of ^{131}I to optimize uptake. A whole-body scintiscan, often coupled with computed tomography (SPECT-CT), is performed 3 to 5 days after ^{131}I administration to determine isotope distribution.

The destruction of normal remnant thyroid tissue is generally referred to as "ablation." In patients with a low risk of recurrence, two prospective randomized trials have shown that low doses of ^{131}I (1.1 GBq versus 3.7 GBq) and the use of injectable rhTSH, as opposed to thyroid hormone withdrawal, are effective for remnant ablation, defined by undetectable serum Tg in the absence of antibodies and normal (i.e., negative) imaging.[6,7] It is thus currently recommended to use the lowest possible activity (1.1 GBq or 30 millicuries) and rhTSH for ablation in low-risk patients if it is performed.[3] For known or suspected locoregional disease or DM, and for patients with high-risk disease, higher doses of ^{131}I are recommended (3.7 to 5.5 GBq) with thyroid hormone withdrawal (see later). The benefits and risks of RAI administration must be weighed for each patient according to risk factors for recurrence and mortality[3] (Table 47.2).

Toxicity

Immediate effects of treatment, such as gastric radiation exposure, may be responsible for transient nausea and vomiting. Colon irradiation should be mitigated by laxative treatment, and bladder and gonadal irradiation should be reduced by abundant hydration and frequent urination.

RAI is concentrated in salivary glands and may cause dose-related acute and late effects on salivary function. Acute sialadenitis causes swelling, pain, and loss of or distorted taste. The parotid glands are most often affected uni- or bilaterally, and the symptoms resolve spontaneously in several days or more rarely, weeks. Chronic sialadenitis also most often affects the parotid glands bilaterally, but it is not related to the occurrence of acute sialadenitis. It manifests with pain, swelling, and xerostomia due to salivary duct stenosis and generally resolves within 1 year with the atrophy of the salivary gland parenchyma.[8-11] Xerostomia can lead to an increased risk of dental caries. Lacrimal

TABLE 47.1 Risk Grouping According to the American Thyroid Association Guidelines

ATA Risk Group	Tumor Characteristics	Estimated Risk of Recurrence
Low-risk papillary carcinoma	Intrathyroidal micropapillary carcinoma (single or multifocal, including BRAFV600E mutated) or Papillary carcinoma with *all* of the following characteristics: No local or distant metastases All macroscopic tumor has been resected No tumor invasion of locoregional tissues or structures No aggressive histology No vascular invasion Clinical N0 or N1 with ≤5 micrometastases all <2 mm in largest dimension No RAI-avid metastatic foci outside the thyroid bed on the first posttreatment whole-body RAI scan (if ^{131}I is given)	≤5%
Low-risk follicular carcinoma	Intrathyroidal, well-differentiated follicular thyroid carcinioma with capsular invasion and <4 foci of vascular invasion	
Intermediate risk	Papillary of follicular cancer with *any* of the following: Microscopic invasion of perithyroid soft tissues Aggressive histology Papillary thyroid cancer with vascular invasion Clinical N1 or >5 N1 all <3 cm in the largest dimension RAI-avid metastatic foci in the neck outside the thyroid bed on the first posttreatment whole-body RAI scan	5%–20%
High risk	Papillary of follicular cancer with *any* of the following: Macroscopic invasion of perithyroid soft tissues and/or structures N1 with any metastatic node > or = 3 cm in the largest dimension Incomplete tumor resection Distant metastases Follicular cancer with extensive vascular invasion (>4 foci) Postoperative serum thyroglobulin suggestive of distant metastases	>20%

RAI, radioactive iodine; ^{131}I, iodine-131.

BOX 47.1 TNM Classification

T—Primary Tumor
T1a: intrathyroidal tumor ≤1 cm
(m) multifocal tumor
T1b: intrathyroidal tumor >1cm but ≤2 cm
T2: intrathyroidal tumor >2 cm but <4 cm
T3a: intrathyroidal tumor > or = 4 cm
T3b: tumor of any size with gross extrathyroidal extension invading strap muscles
T4a: extrathyroidal extension with invasion of any of the following: subcutaneous soft tissues, larynx, trachea, esophagus, recurrent laryngeal nerve
T4b: tumor invades prevertebral fascia or mediastinal vessels or encases carotid artery

N—Regional Lymph Nodes
Nx: regional lymph nodes cannot be assessed
N0a: no regional lymph node metastasis on cytology or pathology of at least one lymph node
N0b: no regional lymph node metastases on palpation and ultrasound
N1a: metastases to the central compartment (level VI) and/or upper mediastinal lymph nodes (level VII)
N1b: metastases in other unilateral, bilateral, or contralateral cervical lymph nodes (levels I, II, III, IV, or V) or retropharyngeal lymph node

M—Distant Metastases
M0: no distant metastases
M1: distant metastases

BOX 47.2 TNM Stage Grouping

Patients <55 Years of Age
Stage I: any T, any N, M0
Stage II: any T, any N, M1

Patients 55 Years of Age and >55
Stage I: T1–T2, N0, M0
Stage II: T1–T2, N1, M0, and T3, any N, M0
Stage III: T4a, any N, M0
Stage IVA: T4b, any N, M0
Stage IVB: M1

gland dysfunction with ocular dryness and lacrimal duct stenosis with epiphora has not been shown to be dose related.[12] Patients with salivary or ocular symptoms should be referred to an otolaryngologist, head and neck surgeon, or ophthalmologist.

Tumors in certain locations, such as the brain, spinal cord, and paratracheal region, may swell in response to TSH stimulation or after ^{131}I therapy, causing compressive symptoms that should be prevented by corticosteroid therapy at high doses for a few days. The use of rhTSH does not eliminate and may even increase the possibility of rapid swelling of metastatic lesions.[13-15] Pneumonitis and pulmonary fibrosis are rare complications of high-dose RAI treatment given at short intervals of time. Dosimetry studies with a limit of 80 mCi whole-body retention at 48 hours and 200 cGy to the bone marrow should be considered in patients with diffuse ^{131}I pulmonary uptake.[16] In most patients with diffuse lung involvement, there are no respiratory side effects of RAI treatment.[17] Mild pancytopenia may occur after repeated ^{131}I therapy, especially in patients with bone metastases who are also treated with external radiotherapy.

RAI administration is contraindicated in cases of pregnancy or lactation and should be postponed in these cases. Temporary infertility and a temporary increase in miscarriages have been reported after RAI administration. In female patients pregnancy should be avoided

TABLE 47.2 Tumor Characteristics Guiding Use of RAI Administration

ATA Risk Group	Specific Characteristics	Evidence for Improvement in Disease-Specific Survival	Evidence for Improvement in Disease-Free Survival	Indication for Postsurgical [131]I
Low risk	Tumor < or = 10 mm Uni- or multifocal	No	No	No
	T1bT2 N0Nx	No	Conflicting data*	Not routine, may be considered on a case-by-case basis, 30–100 mCi with rhTSH
Low/intermediate risk	Tumor >4 cm	Conflicting data	Conflicting data	May be considered 30–100 mCi with rhTSH
	Microscopic extrathyroidal extension	No	Conflicting data	Generally favored 30–100 mCi with rhTSH (unless other unfavorable characteristics) but may not be needed for small tumors
	N1a	Possibly for patients 45 years or older	Conflicting data	Generally favored Dose and method of stimulation according to number and size of lymph node metastases
	N1b	Possibly for patients 45 years or older	Conflicting data	Generally favored Dose and method of stimulation according to number and size of lymph node metastases
High risk	Gross extrathyroidal extension	Yes	Yes	Yes High doses of RAI and thyroid hormone withdrawal
	Distant metastases	Yes	Yes	Yes High doses of RAI and thyroid hormone withdrawal

*A prospective randomized study is currently underway (the "Estimabl2" study, NCT01837745), comparing low-dose (1.1 GBq) radioiodine ablation with no ablation in low-risk (T1a(m)T2N0) differentiated thyroid cancer.
RAI, radioactive iodine; ATA, American Thyroid Association; ^{131}I, iodine-131, rhTSH, recombinant human thyroid stimulating hormone.
Modified from Haugen BR, Alexander EK, Bible KC, et al. 2015 American Thyroid Association management guidelines for adult patients with thyroid nodules and differentiated thyroid cancer: the American Thyroid Association Guidelines Task Force on Thyroid Nodules and Differentiated Thyroid Cancer. *Thyroid.* 2016;26(1):1–133.

during the 6 to 12 months after the administration of [131]I. Premature menopause (an average of 1 year) may occur. In males ^{131}I may result in decreased sperm count and it may be recommended to avoid procreation for 3 to 6 months after ^{131}I administration. Cumulative activities of >14.8 GBq (>400 mCi) are correlated with a risk of permanent male infertility, and male patients should be counseled and sperm banking proposed for patients likely to receive repeated doses of [131]I.[3]

The relative risk of second primary malignancies—leukemia, breast, colon, kidney, salivary, and bone/soft tissue tumors— in patients treated with RAI was reported in a meta-analysis of two multicenter studies to be 1.19. This risk is dose related and higher with cumulative doses of 500 to 600 mCi. There is no direct evidence, however, that one administration of 30 to 100 mCi carries a significant risk for developing a second primary cancer.[3,18]

External Beam Radiation Therapy

EBRT may be used in the adjuvant setting in selected cases but is not recommended routinely (see Chapter 49, External Beam Radiotherapy for Thyroid Malignancy).[3,19] Patients >45 years old with locally invasive gross residual or unresectable disease, particularly if [18]FDG-PET-avid, may benefit from a locoregional response after EBRT. It may also be considered in selected patients >45 years old after complete resection of locally invasive disease but with a high risk of harboring microscopic residual RAI-refractory disease.[19,20] It should not be used routinely after complete surgery for all locally advanced tumors, however, but only in these selected cases. Cervical lymphadenopathy alone is not an indication for adjuvant EBRT but may be considered in older patients with RAI-refractory neck disease with multiple neck recurrences and reoperations.[3]

DYNAMIC RISK ASSESSMENT

After initial therapy (lobectomy or total thyroidectomy, and/or RAI), new measurements of serum Tg and neck ultrasound are used to redetermine the "response to therapy," which is again correlated to the risk of recurrence (see Chapter 24 Dynamic Risk Group Analysis and staging for Differentiated Thyroid Cancer). This dynamic risk stratification enables clinicians to determine which patients require further treatment and/or close follow-up and which patients have a low risk of recurrence and thus may be followed-up with a longer interval between visits.[3,21,22] Table 47.3 proposes a definition of each type of response and the implications for further management.[22]

Thyroid Hormone Replacement Therapy

The goal of thyroid hormone replacement therapy after total thyroidectomy for low- to intermediate-risk patients is to maintain normal physiologic function and quality of life. For these low- to intermediate-risk patients before remnant ablation or response to therapy evaluation, the ATA recommends TSH levels in the 0.1 to 0.5 µUI/mL range. This is, however, a weak recommendation based on low-level evidence.[3]

TABLE 47.3 Dynamic Risk Assessment

Response to Therapy Category	Definition: Patients Treated With Total Thyroidectomy and RAI Ablation	Expected Risk of Recurrence	Proposed Definition: Patients Treated With Total Thyroidectomy *Without* RAI Ablation	Proposed Definition: Patients Treated With Thyroid Lobectomy	Management Implications
Excellent response	Negative imaging *And* Tg with L-thyroxin treatment <0.2 ng/mL *or* TSH-stimulated Tg <1 ng/mL *And* no thyroglobulin antibodies	<1%–4%	Negative imaging *And* Tg with L-thyroxin <0.2 ng/mL *or* TSH-stimulated Tg <2 ng/mL *And* no thyroglobulin antibodies	Negative imaging *And* Tg <30 ng/mL *And* no thyroglobulin antibodies	Should lead to decreased intensity and frequency of follow-up and less TSH suppression (TSH 0.5–2 ng/mL)
Biochemical incomplete response	Negative imaging *And* Tg with L-thyroxin treatment > or = 1 ng/mL *Or* stimulated Tg > or = 10 ng/mL *Or* rising thyroglobulin antibodies	May evolve spontaneously to excellent response 20% develop structural disease	Negative imaging *And* basal Tg >5 ng/mL *Or* stimulated Tg >10 ng/mL *Or* rising Tg levels over time with stable TSH *Or* rising thyroglobulin antibodies	Negative imaging *And* basal Tg >30 ng/mL *Or* rising Tg levels over time with stable TSH *Or* rising thyroglobulin antibodies	Tg stable or declining: continued observation Tg or Tg antibodies rising: consider additional investigation and therapy
Indeterminate response	Nonspecific findings on imaging *And* basal Tg 0.2–1 ng/mL *Or* stimulated Tg 1–10 ng/mL *Or* stable or declining Tg antibodies over time	15%–20% will develop structural disease	Nonspecific findings on imaging *And* basal Tg 0.2–5 ng/mL *Or* stimulated Tg 2–10 ng/mL *Or* stable or declining Tg antibodies over time	Nonspecific findings on imaging *And/or* stable or declining Tg antibodies over time	Continued observation with repeated imaging of nonspecific lesions and Tg monitoring
Structural incomplete response	Evidence of disease on imaging	100%	Evidence of disease on imaging	Evidence of disease on imaging	Additional treatment or observation (depending on lesion size, location, growth rate, RAI/[18]FDG avidity, pathology subtype)

RAI, radioiodine; Tg, thyroglobulin; TSH, thyroid-stimulating hormone; [18]FDG-PET, 18-Fluorodeoxyglucose Positron Emission Tomography.
Data from Haugen BR, Alexander EK, Bible KC, et al. 2015 American Thyroid Association management guidelines for adult patients with thyroid nodules and differentiated thyroid cancer: the American Thyroid Association Guidelines Task Force on Thyroid Nodules and Differentiated Thyroid Cancer. *Thyroid.* 2016;26(1):1–133.

Once an excellent response has been established, TSH levels for these patients should be maintained between 0.5 and 2 µUI/mL. TSH suppression will not decrease the already low recurrence rate but may cause adverse effects such as cardiac arrhythmia, osteoporosis, anxiety/nervousness, or insomnia.[22]

After lobectomy for low-risk patients, the suggested goal for TSH levels is also 0.5 to 2 (ATA) mUI/L, based on low-quality evidence, however. Recent data suggests that as many as 73% of patients treated by lobectomy will need thyroid hormone supplementation to maintain the TSH level within this range.[23]

For high-risk patients, thyroid hormone suppression with a TSH below 0.1 mUI/L is recommended based on moderate-quality evidence showing improved disease-specific survival in advanced disease.[3]

FOLLOW-UP

As for adjuvant treatment, follow-up should be tailored to the initial risk group and then to the response to therapy dynamic risk assessment, thus avoiding oversurveillance of patients with a very low risk of disease recurrence.

Serum Thyroglobulin

Serum Tg is the most sensitive means of determining disease-free status for DTC. After total thyroidectomy and RAI ablation, a low to undetectable serum Tg (ultrasensitive Tg <0.2 ng/mL if measured under levothyroxine suppression and Tg <1 ng/mL, if measured after TSH stimulation) in the absence of Tg antibodies and a normal neck ultrasound in the context of an excellent response for patients initially in the low- and intermediate-risk groups is indicative of a subsequent risk of recurrence <2%. In these patients ultrasound should not be repeated annually, but instead at a longer interval, as long as annual Tg measurements remain low in the absence of anti-Tg antibodies due to the high rate (8% to 67%) of false-positive images that can be found on routine neck ultrasound.[22]

After total thyroidectomy without RAI, the evaluation of serum Tg is more difficult because some patients will have a significant thyroid remnant, the size of which depends on the extent of surgery and the experience of the surgeon. Patients treated in high-volume thyroid surgery centers can have undetectable (<0.2 ng/mL) Tg levels postoperatively in up to 60% of cases, however, and these patients can be followed in the same manner as mentioned earlier. In the presence of detectable Tg postoperatively, Tg should be monitored to ensure that the level remains stable over time and is not increasing and that anti-Tg antibodies do not increase or do not appear if absent initially. These biological modifications may alert the clinician and suggest administering RAI at that time.[22] RAI administration should be considered in cases of serum Tg (while taking levothyroxine treatment) above 2 ng/mL. The optimum absolute values of Tg after thyroid lobectomy remain to be more fully elucidated, but rising Tg and/or antibodies or the appearance of initially absent anti-Tg antibodies should alert the clinician as to the possibility of recurrent disease.

In low-risk patients Tg measured while taking levothyroxine treatment is sufficient in most cases, and the use of rhTSH-stimulated Tg measurements (rhTSH/Tg) can be reserved for patients with Tg between 0.2 and 1 ng/mL.[24] In patients with intermediate- to high-risk tumors, less data is available, but Tg measured under levothyroxine treatment also currently tends to replace rhTSH/Tg measurements.

Neck Ultrasound

A neck ultrasonography (US) should be performed in all patients at initial workup, and 6 to 18 months after RAI administration to determine the type of response to therapy. Patients with suspicious lymph nodes should be assessed with fine-needle aspiration biopsy (FNAB), cytology, and Tg measurements in the needle washout fluid if any treatment would be considered after the diagnosis of locoregional persistent/recurrent disease. The latest ATA guidelines suggest performing FNAB in cases of suspicious central compartment lymph nodes measuring 8 mm or more in the smallest diameter and suspicious lateral compartment lymph nodes measuring 10 mm or more in the smallest diameter.[3] In cases of indeterminant lymph nodes, FNAB or follow-up can be advised depending on Tg levels and the ATA risk classification.

The time frame at which a neck US should be repeated is not clearly defined. It should be adapted to the risk of relapse based on Tg levels, ATA risk stratification, and response to therapy. In low-risk patients with an excellent response (see Table 47.3), it is suggested that follow-up with a neck US is not necessary before 3 to 5 years after the initial treatment.[22] Intermediate-risk patients with an excellent response may benefit from a routine neck US at more frequent intervals (12 to 24 months), whereas in high-risk patients it is suggested to perform neck US every 6 to 12 months. Imaging is also performed according to Tg and Tg antibody assessment, and biological suspicion of recurrence should prompt an earlier neck US.

18-Fluorodeoxyglucose Positron Emission Tomography ([18]FDG-PET)

FDG-PET/CT should not be performed in all patients with DTC. It has demonstrated its usefulness in patients with suspected recurrence and in patients with DM. In a large meta-analysis, the sensitivity of FDG-PET/CT was found to be 83% (ranging from 50% to 100%) and the specificity 84% (ranging from 42% to 100%) for non-RAI-avid DTC.[25] Its sensitivity is increased in cases of poorly differentiated tumors and in cases of high-tumor volume, whether locoregionally or metastatic. It is therefore recommended to perform FDG-PET/CT in patients with elevated Tg levels (above 10 ng/mL), a threshold that should be lowered in cases of poorly differentiated tumors that may produce less Tg. In cases of suspicious neck lymph nodes with FDG uptake, cytology should be performed if possible to exclude PET false-positive inflammatory lymph nodes, especially if surgery is planned. In patients with known DM, FDG-PET/CT is useful for the detection and localization of DM. It has a prognostic value as well, and patients with high FDG uptake will not, in most cases, be cured by RAI alone. Performing FDG-PET/CT after stimulation with rhTSH slightly improves the sensitivity and the number of metastatic lesions found, but the therapeutic implications of finding more lesions has been shown to be minimal (affecting only 6% of patients in the main study of this technique).[26]

Other Imaging Modalities

Neck CT scans can be helpful in case of local relapse, especially before a surgical procedure. Before initial surgery in cases of invasive disease and before surgery for persistent/recurrent neck disease, CT allows clear delimitations with neck vessels, the trachea, and the esophagus. In cases of suspicion of local invasion, laryngeal, tracheal endoscopy, and esophagoscopy may be necessary.

PROGNOSIS

Only 1% to 7% of patients have DM at diagnosis. Only a fraction (~15%) of patients are likely to experience relapse of disease, which most commonly manifests as a cervical lymph node(s). Spread to mediastinal nodes is usually associated with extensive nodal involvement in the neck. Eighty percent of recurrences occur during the first 5 years of follow-up. Few patients (~ 5%) have a lethal outcome. Among those with lethal DTC, 20% of deaths occur in the first year after diagnosis, and 80% of the deaths occur within 10 years.[27-31]

Multivariate analyses have been used to identify variables predictive of cause-specific mortality. Increasing patient age and the presence of extrathyroidal invasion are independent prognostic factors in all studies. The presence of initial DM and a large size of the primary tumor are also significant variables in most studies, and some groups have reported that histopathologic grade (degree of differentiation) is an independent variable. The completeness of initial tumor resection (postoperative status) is also a predictor of mortality. The presence of initial neck lymph node metastases, although relevant to future nodal recurrence, does not influence cause-specific mortality. Several scoring systems based on these significant prognostic indicators have been devised and provide prediction of postoperative events comparable to that of the internationally accepted TNM staging system. Each system allows one to assign the majority of patients (80% or more) to a low-risk group, in which the cause-specific mortality at 25 years is less than 2%, and the others (a small minority) to a high-risk group, in which almost all the cancer-related deaths are observed.

Cox model analysis and stepwise variable selection has led to a final prognostic model that includes five variables: DM, age, completeness of resection, local invasion, and size (MACIS). The final score is calculated as follows: 3.1 (if age 39 years or younger) or 0.08 (if age 40 years or older) × age + 0.3 × tumor size (in centimeters) + 1 (if tumor not completely resected) + 1 (if locally invasive) + 3 (if DM are present). The MACIS scoring system permits identification of groups of patients with different risks of dying from DTC. Twenty-year cause-specific survival rates for patients with MACIS scores of less than 6, 6 to 6.99, 7 to 7.99, and 8 + were 99%, 89%, 56%, and 27%, respectively ($p < .0001$). When cumulative mortality from all causes of death was considered, approximately 85% of patients with MACIS scores below 6 had no excess mortality over rates predicted for control subjects in the general population.[28]

Thus the prognosis of differentiated thyroid carcinoma is generally excellent, and even for metastatic tumors, is better than most other solid tumors. Disease-specific survival at 20 years for the low-risk group

(T1T2N0) is estimated at 99%, for intermediate-risk patients at 87%, and for high-risk patients at 57%.[32] Patients <55 years old without DM have an estimated 10-year disease-specific survival of 98% to 100% versus 85% to 95% for those in the same age group with DM. For patients >55 years, 10-year disease-specific survival is 98% to 100% for stage I disease, 85% to 95% for stage II, 60% to 70% for stage III, and <50% for stage IV.[33,34]

TREATMENT OF DISTANT METASTASES

Radioactive Iodine

For the treatment of RAI-avid DM, high doses of ^{131}I are recommended (>3.7 GBq) after thyroid hormone withdrawal (see Chapter 48, Postoperative Radioactive Iodine Ablation and Treatment of Differentiated Thyroid Cancer). In patients with DM, retrospective data showed no difference between the efficacy of a standardized dose (3.7 GBq or 100 mCi) and that of a personalized dose based on dosimetry; both approaches may be used.[3,35] Several treatments may be necessary to eradicate disease. If necessary, ^{131}I can be repeated every 6 months for 2 years then yearly up to a cumulative dose of 22.2 GBq (600 mCi). Higher cumulative doses may be warranted in very select cases.

RAI therapy for lung metastases leads to remission (normal imaging and the absence of residual ^{131}I uptake) in 45% of patients with tumors showing RAI uptake with no significant side effects. Almost all complete responses are attained with cumulative activities equal or less than 22 GBq, with few recurrences (7%) and few tumor-related deaths (3%) after remission. In case of bone metastases, remission is achieved in only 9% of cases, however. In one study the reported 10-year survival rate was 92% in metastatic patients with ^{131}I uptake who showed complete remission after treatment. In comparison, the 10-year survival rate was only 29% in patients with ^{131}I uptake but who had persistent imaging abnormalities and only 10% in those without any initial ^{131}I uptake. Remission was achieved in >90% of patients younger than 40 years with small metastases (<1 cm in diameter) who had high RAI uptake. In contrast, remission was achieved in <15% of older patients with metastases >1 cm. Finally, remission was achieved in half of patients who were either younger than 40 years with large metastases or older with small metastases[17] (Box 47.3).

RAI-refractory DTC is defined as follows:
1. ^{131}I uptake is absent in all target lesions (initially or during treatment).
2. Uptake is present in some lesions but not in others.
3. Progression within 12 months after ^{131}I treatment
4. Some centers also consider persistent disease after the administration of a cumulative activity of 600 mCi ^{131}I to be RAI-refractory.

RAI-refractory tumors are thus not amenable to repeated administrations of RAI, and metastatic lesions should be managed with other modalities—TSH suppression, focalized treatments, and/or systemic agents—always taking into consideration the rate of disease progression and symptoms and the risk of morbidity of these treatments.

Despite DM, patients have a highly variable life expectancy, with a high survival rate in younger patients with slowly progressive disease and with a limited tumor burden. These patients can often be followed conservatively on TSH-suppressive therapy with minimal evidence of radiographic or symptomatic progression. For select patients, however, other palliative treatment options need to be considered for symptomatic intrathoracic lesions, such as metastasectomy or radiofrequency ablation, endobronchial laser ablation, stenting or EBRT for obstructing or bleeding endobronchial masses, and pleural or pericardial drainage for symptomatic effusions. Palliative local treatment may also be considered for symptomatic bone or brain lesions. However, the majority of metastases will progress, and referral for participation in clinical trials or systemic therapy should be considered.

> **BOX 47.3 Recommendations for Radioiodine Treatment in Patients With Structurally Persistent/Metastatic Disease**
>
> 1. Only patients with significant uptake benefit from radioiodine treatment.
> 2. Treatment should be administered after TSH stimulation; withdrawal of thyroid hormone treatment should be preferred to rhTSH injections in patients with metastatic disease. Iodine contamination and pregnancy should be excluded before treatment.
> 3. The activity per treatment is either standard (3.7 to 7.4 GBq or larger) or based on dosimetry. Treatment based on individual dosimetry has not shown better efficacy compared with a standard dose of 3.7 GBq.
> 4. A total body scan performed several days after the administration of radioiodine is mandatory and may guide further treatment in case of residual disease.
> 5. Pulmonary micrometastases may be treated with an interval of 6 to 12 months, during which patients are treated with thyroxine at suppressive doses (TSH <0.1 µU/mL).
> 6. Treatment may be repeated as long as radioiodine uptake is present in all metastases, and as long as disease does not progress (tumor is not radioiodine-refractory, see text). After a high cumulative activity, the decision to give further radioiodine treatments should be made on an individual basis.

TSH, thyroid-stimulatin ghormone; rhTSH, recombinant human thyroid stimulating hormone.

Localized Treatments

Localized treatments aim at destroying lesions located within the lungs, liver, bones, or other organs or soft tissues. Surgery and/or EBRT are employed for localized bone lesions that are symptomatic (painful), at risk of fracture, or at risk of other complications such as neural compression. Minimally invasive image-guided techniques performed by interventional radiologists include chemo- and radioembolization,[31,36] radiofrequency ablation,[37] vertebroplasty and cement injection, and cryotherapy.[38-42] Treatment of bone metastases with bisphosphonates may delay progression and relieve symptoms.[41,42]

Systemic Treatments

Patients with symptomatic, RAI-refractory, progressive (according to RECIST criteria), or metastatic disease should be considered for referral to participate in clinical trials or, if ineligible or in the absence of an appropriate trial, considered for systemic treatment with currently approved TKIs (see Chapter 52, Medical Treatment Horizons for Metastatic Differentiated and Medullary Thyroid Cancer).[3] Patients with stable, asymptomatic disease need not be treated actively as long as the disease remains stable, asymptomatic, and nonmenacing to vital structures.

The two currently U.S. Food and Drug Administration (FDA)-approved TKIs for differentiated thyroid carcinoma are lenvatinib[43] and sorafenib.[44] Sorafenib is an orally administered multikinase inhibitor targeting VEGFR2 and 3, RET, BRAF, and c-KIT. Sorafenib was the first small-molecule kinase inhibitor to be approved as systemic therapy in patients with progressive RAI-refractory metastatic DTC by showing efficacy in improving progression-free survival in a large multicenter, randomized, double-blind, placebo-controlled, phase III clinical trial evaluating 417 patients.[44] Progression-free survival was improved by 41% in the sorafenib-treated group with a median progression-free survival of 10.8 months compared with 5.8 months in the placebo group. Grade-3 adverse events occurred in 42% of the patients treated with sorafenib compared with 20% for the placebo group.

Lenvatinib is also an orally administered multikinase inhibitor targeting VEGFR 1-3, FGFR 1-4, PDGFR alpha, RET, and KIT, subsequently approved in this indication in light of the results of another phase III placebo-controlled trial randomizing 392 patients.[43] The median progression-free survival in the lenvatinib-treated group was 18.3 months compared with 3.6 months for the patients receiving a placebo, with an overall response rate of 64.8% in the lenvatinib group compared with 1.5% in the placebo group. Grade-3 adverse events occurred in 76% of the patients treated with lenvatinib compared with 10% for the placebo group.

Several adverse effects of these drugs derive from their antiangiogenic effect, with risk of cardiovascular events, gastrointestinal bleeding, and the risk of fistula and bleeding from advanced metastatic lesions in the neck, thorax, and mediastinum.[45] These two drugs are both anti-VEFG. There is a higher rate of skin toxicity and diarrhea for sorafenib and a higher rate of hypertension and proteinuria for lenvatinib. Poor candidates for TKIs include patients with recent cardiovascular events, poorly controlled high blood pressure, cardiac arrhythmia, or prolonged QTc interval, recent bleeding, liver disease, chronic gastrointestinal inflammation, cachexia, untreated brain metastases, and severe depression.[3] Other side effects include fatigue, diarrhea, hypertension, and skin toxicity (hand-foot skin lesions). In addition, serum TSH levels should be frequently controlled because thyroxine requirements frequently increase with these drugs.

Cytotoxic chemotherapy may be warranted in patients with symptomatic progressive disease who are not amenable to other approaches.[3] The few prospective cytotoxic chemotherapy trials so far reported have not included sufficient numbers of patients to demonstrate benefits. Because of the absence of demonstrated benefits and the significant toxicity of chemotherapy, many physicians enrolled only rare DTC patients with large tumor burden and rapidly progressive metastatic disease refractory to RAI treatment in these trials. None of the studies used response criteria in solid tumors (RECIST), and many trials included heterogeneous cohorts of DTC, anaplastic, and medullary thyroid cancer patients grouped together.[46] Of the drugs administered to patients with metastatic differentiated thyroid carcinoma, the most frequently tested agent is doxorubicin. Tumor response rates range from 0% to 22%, with all responses being partial and only lasting a few months. Very few trials have been reported with other cytotoxic agents.

Current clinical trials aim at (1) specifically treating tumors with mutations or other alterations using specific kinase inhibitors targeted to these alterations; (2) administering redifferentiating agents with the aim to reactivate the NIS transporter at the tumor cell membrane rendering it susceptible to RAI uptake and treatment; (3) immunotherapy, which aims at altering the tumor-host immune relationship and eliminating mechanisms of immune tolerance induced by the tumor; (4) combining TKIs with each other or with conventional cytotoxic agents or immunotherapy (see Chapter 52, Medical Treatment Horizons for Metastatic Differentiated and Medullary Thyroid Cancer).

CONCLUSION

Treatment of DTC today should be tailored to the extent of disease as defined by risk groups based on specific tumor and patient characteristics. The majority of thyroid cancers today are low-risk cancers with a disease-specific mortality rate close to 0%, for which therapy and follow-up should not add morbidity or decrease quality of life. RAI treatment and TSH suppression should be reserved for patients with adverse tumor characteristics. Many metastatic tumors, particularly small lung metastases in young patients, remain curable with repeated administrations of RAI with low morbidity. RAI-refractory tumors often grow slowly over a period of several years, and initial management of these slowly growing, asymptomatic lesions should be watchful waiting combined with TSH suppression and local therapies for appropriate lesions. For progressive symptomatic disease, local treatments combined with systemic therapy with TKIs palliate symptoms and improve progression-free survival. Clinical trials aimed at improving these outcomes with combination therapy, redifferentiation protocols, and immunotherapy are currently underway.

REFERENCES

For a complete list of references, go to expertconsult.com.

48

Postoperative Radioactive Iodine Ablation and Treatment of Differentiated Thyroid Cancer

Mona M. Sabra

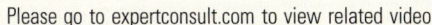

Please go to expertconsult.com to view related video:
Video 48.1 Introduction to Chapter 48, Postoperative Radioactive Iodine Ablation and Treatment of Differentiated Thyroid Cancer.

INTRODUCTION

The role of radioactive iodine (RAI) therapy in the postoperative management of patients with newly diagnosed differentiated thyroid cancer (DTC) is a highly controversial topic. Endocrinologists and nuclear medicine physicians strongly differ in their opinions regarding the diagnostic and therapeutic uses of RAI therapy in the postoperative setting. This has resulted in vastly different guidelines and position statements from the groups' respective societies.[1,2]

RAI therapy aims to improve the disease-specific survival, decrease the disease-specific recurrence risk, facilitate the initial staging, and allow for highly sensitive follow-up of patients with DTC.[1] The difference in opinion is in the selection of patients that would most benefit from RAI therapy.[3] The first position advocates using RAI therapy on all patients except those presenting with intrathyroidal papillary thyroid microcarcinoma without aggressive features. The second position advocates selective use of RAI, thus reserving RAI therapy for those patients who are most likely to benefit from it. Selection of patients who are candidates to be treated with RAI therapy is based on the (1) assessment of disease-specific risks for recurrence and mortality, (2) assessment of postoperative disease status, (3) likelihood of clinical benefit with RAI therapy, (4) likelihood of adverse effects with RAI therapy, (5) need for postoperative staging, (6) need for highly sensitive follow-up, (7) treatment philosophy of the treating multidisciplinary team, and (8) patient wishes and values.[1,2,4]

The main reason for the controversy is that most of the evidence regarding the use of RAI therapy in the postoperative setting is largely gathered from retrospective, observational studies that vary greatly in their enrollment criteria, risk assessment models, definition of the RAI therapy role, clinical response criteria, and results.[5] Outside of the two multicenter prospective randomized prospective clinical trials studying the role of RAI ablation in low-risk DTC patients, there are no well-conducted multicenter randomized control trials (RCTs) that support one position over the other.

WHY RAI THERAPY FOR THYROID CANCER MANAGEMENT?

RAI therapy has been used in the management of DTC since the 1940s. Its use is based on the unique ability of thyroid cells to concentrate RAI through the activity of membrane sodium iodide symporter.[6] Compared with normal thyroid tissues, tumors of follicular cell origin are less likely to concentrate RAI due to their lower membrane expression of transporter.[7] Also, different histologies of DTC vary in their ability to express the membrane transporter with some tumors unable to concentrate enough RAI for an effective treatment response.[8,9]

The two most commonly used RAI isotopes in thyroid cancer are ^{123}I and ^{131}I. These isotopes have different emitted radiation particles released from their decay, with gamma rays mostly emitted with ^{123}I and beta mostly emitted from the decay of ^{131}I.[10] If absorbed in thyroid tissues after thyroid-stimulating hormone (TSH) stimulation, both gamma and beta rays can be visible on a gamma camera. Although gamma rays are high-energy particles that provide a good image resolution, their tissue absorption/concentration is low, making them less effective in thyroid cancer therapy. Thus ^{123}I is mostly reserved for diagnostic imaging.[11] On the other hand, beta rays (emitted by ^{131}I) are moderately high energy particles with short median path length in human tissues, allowing them to penetrate tumoral tissues about 2 to 5 mm on average. They also interact with the surrounding tissues.[12] This results in DNA injury and damage. In general, DTC cells can repair minor DNA damage through the activation of p53 pathways; however, more extensive DNA damage results in cell death (apoptosis).[13,14] Because tumor cells lack efficient ways to repair double stranded DNA damage, they are more susceptible to the ionizing radiation effects than normal tissues. Due to low tissue penetrance, it is not to be expected that RAI therapy would destroy persistent disease exceeding 1 cm in the longest diameter.

Role of RAI Therapy

Whereas past definitions of RAI therapy regarded the treatment of locally persistent thyroid cancer or distant metastasis, the current consensus is that RAI therapy encompasses all the intended roles of RAI administration in patients with DTC.[3] These roles are divided into (1) ablation, (2) adjuvant therapy, or (3) treatment of persistent thyroid cancer in the neck and/or distant metastatic disease[1] (Table 48.1).

RAI Ablation

RAI ablation's role is to eliminate normal thyroid tissue that is left behind after a total thyroidectomy. When electing to administer RAI for ablation, it is implicitly recognized that the patient is already cured of thyroid cancer and is at low risk of future recurrence and mortality from his or her disease. In this setting, RAI therapy is administered with the aims to facilitate the initial staging and allow for easier long-term patient follow-up with the elimination of postoperative thyroglobulin (Tg) level and/or any interfering antibodies and the eradication of thyroid remnant tissues that otherwise could be detected on follow-up sonogram and/or diagnostic whole-body scans.

447

TABLE 48.1 Aims of RAI Therapy

	Goals	Assumption	Potential Benefits
RAI ablation	Eliminate persistent normal thyroid tissue	Patient is cured without persistent thyroid cancer	Improve staging Facilitate follow-up
RAI adjuvant therapy	Destroy persistent microscopic thyroid cancer deposits	Some patients are cured, whereas others have persistent subclinical disease	Achieve cure Decrease recurrence Improve disease-specific survival
Treatment of persistent thyroid cancer	Eliminate locally persistent or distant metastatic thyroid cancer	All patients have persistent disease that can be detected clinically by imaging or elevated thyroglobulin level	Achieve cure or stable disease Improve progression-free survival Improve disease-specific survival.

RAI, radioiodine.

Adjuvant Therapy

RAI adjuvant therapy's role is to eliminate subclinical microscopic tumor deposits that may be present. The patients selected for adjuvant therapy are generally at intermediate or high risk for thyroid cancer recurrence but do not have clear evidence of persistent thyroid cancer on postoperative disease assessment. It is implicitly recognized that (1) many of these patients are already cured by the initial surgery and may not benefit from further therapy, but (2) other patients may still have microscopic tumor deposits in the neck, lungs, or elsewhere, which, left untreated, would increase their risk for recurrent thyroid cancer. Therefore the perceived benefit from adjuvant therapy is to hopefully decrease the risk for disease-specific recurrence, improve the progression-free survival (PFS) and the disease-specific survival, and achieve a cure for thyroid cancer.

Therapy of Persistent Thyroid Cancer

Some patients present with persistent disease in the neck and/or distant metastatic site after initial surgery. In general, RAI administration is not recommended in patient with persistent bulky metastatic nodes in the neck. In these situations, patients are referred to surgery for complete neck resection of their thyroid cancer before RAI therapy. However, in some cases, patients present with low-volume neck metastasis that can be detected by postoperative neck sonography and/or diagnostic whole-body scans. RAI therapy is administered in this setting with the aim to decrease PFS and improve disease specific survival and achieve a cure.

About 10% of patients with DTC present with distant metastasis at diagnosis.[15,16] RAI therapy is recommended for the patients who are deemed to have RAI-avid disease. However, the tumor's ability to concentrate RAI is often not known after initial surgery and empiric RAI therapy is advocated at least once. The potential benefit from RAI therapy in distant metastatic thyroid cancer is to decrease the disease progression and improve the overall prognosis.[1] Although cure is not expected with RAI therapy in many patients with distant metastatic thyroid cancer, partial response with significant tumor shrinkage and/or stable disease is achievable.[17]

SELECTIVE USE OF RAI THERAPY

Before 2009, almost all patients presenting with DTC were treated with RAI therapy. The only exception was patients presenting with isolated papillary microcarcinoma without other aggressive features. In 2009, the American Thyroid Association (ATA) Management Guidelines for Adult Patients with Thyroid Nodules and Differentiated Thyroid Cancer introduced the concept of a risk-adaptive approach to the management of DTC patients.[18] Using this approach, the decision to treat with RAI is dependent on the estimation of the patient risk for recurrence and mortality from thyroid cancer, the assessment of the postoperative disease status, the need for postoperative diagnostic scanning and highly sensitive Tg level, the potential benefit to risk ratio from the proposed RAI therapy, and the patient's wishes.

Assessing Future Risk for Disease Specific Recurrence Using ATA Classification

In 2009, the ATA guidelines introduced the ATA risk assessment classification for estimation of future risk for recurrence based on presenting clinicopathologic features.[18] (see Chapter 24 Dynamic Risk Group Analysis and staging for Differentiated Thyroid Cancer). Under this classification, patients were classified as having ATA low-risk thyroid cancer if they had classic papillary thyroid cancer smaller than 2 cm, with no evidence of local or distant metastasis, having undergone a complete resection of their disease. On pathology, extrathyroidal extension or vascular invasion were not noted. If a postoperative diagnostic whole-body scan is obtained, uptake outside the thyroid bed is not noted. Patients with ATA high-risk thyroid cancer included those with gross extrathyroidal extension, those with incomplete resection of their disease after initial surgery, those with distant metastatic thyroid cancer, and those with inappropriately elevated Tg level. All other patients were grouped under the ATA intermediate risk classification. This included patients with minimal extrathyroidal extension to surrounding tissues and/or with aggressive histologies and/or vascular invasion and/or nodal involvement. In general, due to the lack of a perceived benefit, RAI therapy was not recommended for patients with ATA low-risk thyroid cancer. RAI therapy was strongly recommended for those patients in the ATA high-risk category due to moderate quality of evidence showing improved overall outcomes with RAI therapy. Selective use of RAI was recommended for those patients in the ATA intermediate-risk category because the evidence was not strong enough to support or circumvent RAI use. The treating physician and patient were left to decide whether to use RAI based on perceived potential benefit, potential risk for RAI therapy, and the patient's wishes.[18]

In 2015, the guidelines committee recognized that thyroid cancer risk for recurrence is not boxed into categories but rather follows a continuum of risk that can be assessed based on presenting histopathologic presentation (Figure 48.1).[1] Under the 2009 modified ATA risk classification system, many patients who were previously classified as intermediate risk are now classified as ATA low risk thus expanding the proportion of patients for whom RAI therapy is not generally recommended after initial surgery. Similarly those patients with estimated risk for recurrence exceeding 30% have now been reclassified as ATA high risk, making them eligible for RAI therapy.

It is important to note that the ATA risk classification system is not the only available risk assessment classifier in DTC patients. There are 16 different classification systems, making the decision to treat or withhold RAI more complex.[5]

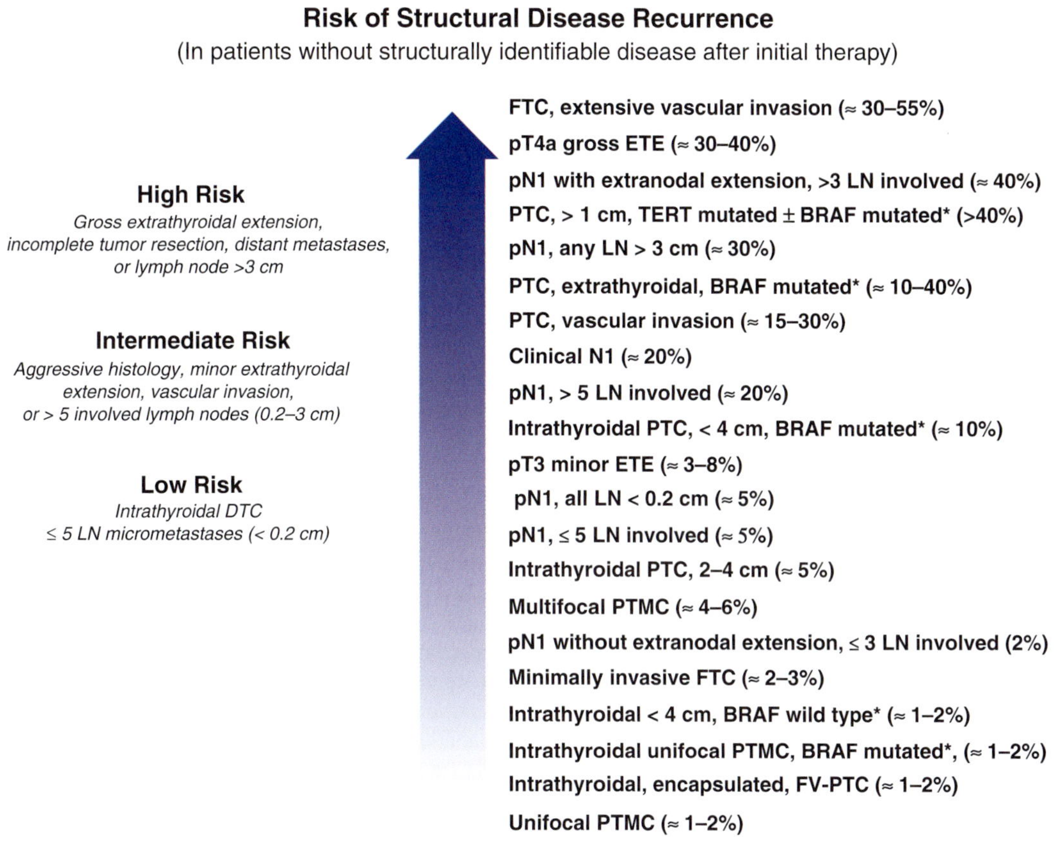

Risk of Structural Disease Recurrence
(In patients without structurally identifiable disease after initial therapy)

High Risk
Gross extrathyroidal extension, incomplete tumor resection, distant metastases, or lymph node >3 cm

Intermediate Risk
Aggressive histology, minor extrathyroidal extension, vascular invasion, or > 5 involved lymph nodes (0.2–3 cm)

Low Risk
Intrathyroidal DTC
≤ 5 LN micrometastases (< 0.2 cm)

- FTC, extensive vascular invasion (≈ 30–55%)
- pT4a gross ETE (≈ 30–40%)
- pN1 with extranodal extension, >3 LN involved (≈ 40%)
- PTC, > 1 cm, TERT mutated ± BRAF mutated* (>40%)
- pN1, any LN > 3 cm (≈ 30%)
- PTC, extrathyroidal, BRAF mutated* (≈ 10–40%)
- PTC, vascular invasion (≈ 15–30%)
- Clinical N1 (≈ 20%)
- pN1, > 5 LN involved (≈ 20%)
- Intrathyroidal PTC, < 4 cm, BRAF mutated* (≈ 10%)
- pT3 minor ETE (≈ 3–8%)
- pN1, all LN < 0.2 cm (≈ 5%)
- pN1, ≤ 5 LN involved (≈ 5%)
- Intrathyroidal PTC, 2–4 cm (≈ 5%)
- Multifocal PTMC (≈ 4–6%)
- pN1 without extranodal extension, ≤ 3 LN involved (2%)
- Minimally invasive FTC (≈ 2–3%)
- Intrathyroidal < 4 cm, BRAF wild type* (≈ 1–2%)
- Intrathyroidal unifocal PTMC, BRAF mutated*, (≈ 1–2%)
- Intrathyroidal, encapsulated, FV-PTC (≈ 1–2%)
- Unifocal PTMC (≈ 1–2%)

Fig. 48.1 Risk of structural disease recurrence in patients without structurally identifiable disease after initial therapy. *Although analysis of BRAF and/or TERT status is not routinely recommended for initial risk stratification, these findings have been included to assist clinicians in proper risk stratification in cases where this information is available. FTC, follicular thyroid cancer, FV, follicular variant, LN, lymph node, PTMC, papillary thyroid microcarcinoma, PTC, papillary thyroid cancer. (Redrawn from Haugen BR, Alexander EK, Bible KC, et al. 2015 American Thyroid Association management guidelines for adult patients with thyroid nodules and differentiated thyroid cancer: The American Thyroid Association Guidelines Task Force on thyroid nodules and differentiated thyroid cancer. *Thyroid.* 2016; 26[1]:1–133.)

ROLE OF POSTOPERATIVE DISEASE ASSESSMENT

Although the initial risk assessment is an important step in determining whether RAI therapy is needed after the initial total thyroidectomy, it is not the only factor to consider.[4] It is thus crucial to determine whether the patient has persistent disease after the initial surgery as this information will influence whether RAI therapy is given and what activity of RAI to administer. Postoperative disease status can be estimated by measuring postoperative Tg level, antithyroglobulin antibody level, and obtaining postoperative neck sonogram and/or diagnostic whole-body scans. The problem is that there are no uniform guidelines detailing proper postoperative disease assessment in DTC patients upon which to make these RAI treatment decisions.

The 2015 ATA Management Guidelines for Adult Patients with Thyroid Nodules and Differentiated Thyroid Cancer addressed the role of postoperative testing in recommendation 50. It states that postoperative disease status "should be considered in deciding whether additional treatment (e.g., RAI, surgery or other treatment) may be needed."[1] This was based on strong recommendation, but with a low quality of evidence. The guidelines committee recommended measuring Tg level at least 4 weeks after surgery allowing for the level to reach the nadir. However, they recognized that uncertainty remains regarding the proper postoperative Tg measurement, with lack of consensus and insufficient evidence for an optimal cutoff point for postoperative Tg and the state in which it should be measured (after TSH stimulation or on thyroid hormone therapy). Furthermore, although diagnostic whole-body scans can be potentially useful in postoperative disease testing, strong supportive data is lacking regarding the isotope to be used, the timing of RAI scanning after isotope administration, and how these factors influence the results.[1]

In the absence of clear guidelines for postoperative testing, it is generally advised that each center come up with its own acceptable guidelines for the estimation of persistent disease after initial surgery for DTC.

POSTOPERATIVE USE OF RAI THERAPY USING A SELECTIVE USE APPROACH

As clinicians, the decision to use or delay RAI therapy in the postoperative setting is easy to make in ATA low-risk patients where there is no clear evidence for benefit from such therapy and in the intermediate to high and high-risk patients where RAI therapy is shown to decrease recurrence and improve overall survival. When considering the patient with low to intermediate and intermediate-risk thyroid cancer patients, the decision to use RAI postoperatively is more complex. It is much easier to give the patient the benefit of the doubt and treat with a low activity of RAI, hoping to decrease the recurrence risk and improve outcomes. The decision is hardest when deciding not to give RAI for the same patient, delaying its use to if and when the patient presents with future recurrent thyroid cancer.

2015 Modified ATA Low-Risk Thyroid Cancer

Assuming there are no other factors that influence the decision to use RAI (such as Tg or Tg antibody status, patient comorbidities, patient wishes), RAI therapy is generally not recommended for the low risk patient. This is especially true for those patients with papillary thyroid cancers up to 4 cm, without local or distant metastasis, with complete disease resection, without evidence of extrathyroidal extension or vascular invasion, lacking aggressive histologies (such as tall cell variant or columnar variant, etc.), and without nodal involvement or with low-volume nodal involvement (fewer than 5 nodes, <0.2 cm in largest dimension). In these patients, the risk for recurrence is estimated to be less than 5%, and these patients, are at low risk for disease-specific mortality.[1]

There is also consensus despite weak evidence that patients with unifocal papillary thyroid microcarcinoma without other adverse features are at very low risk for future recurrence and would not benefit from RAI. The consensus does not extend to those patients with multifocal papillary thyroid cancer without other adverse features where the estimated risk for recurrence is about 5%.[19]

There are no studies that specifically addressed RAI efficacy in follicular thyroid cancer or follicular variant of papillary thyroid cancers. However, patients presenting with encapsulated intrathyroidal follicular variant of papillary thyroid cancer or intrathyroidal follicular thyroid cancer without significant vascular invasion have been demonstrated to have very low risk for recurrence (<2%).[1,20] Thus in these situations the risk from RAI therapy outweighs any potential benefit and RAI therapy is generally not administered.

2015 Modified ATA Intermediate to High- and High-Risk Patients

RAI therapy is strongly recommended in the management of patients with intermediate to high or high-risk thyroid cancer for adjuvant therapy and for the treatment of persistent nodal or distant metastatic disease. Recommendation 51D of the ATA guidelines is based on moderate quality of evidence demonstrating decreased recurrence risk and increased change for cure in the adjuvant setting, improved disease specific survival, and improved PFS for those patients with distant metastatic thyroid cancer.[1] This includes patients presenting with either tumors >4 cm, large volume nodal metastasis, with vascular invasion, those with poorly differentiated thyroid cancer, with gross extra-thyroidal extension, with distant metastasis, with inappropriately elevated TSH level, and/or with structural evidence of persistent low-volume disease of postoperative imaging (Table 48.2).

2015 Modified ATA Intermediate-Risk Patients

Recommendation 51D of the ATA guidelines states that "radioactive iodine adjuvant therapy should be considered "in these patients, based on low quality of evidence.[1] It is difficult to estimate the degree of subclinical microscopic foci that may have been left behind after total thyroidectomy and their influence on overall recurrence risk, hampering the decision to treat with RAI. In these instances, it is important to examine other clinical features that may sway the clinician one way or another such as Tg level after surgery, postoperative antithyroglobulin antibody level, patient's comorbidities, and risk for long adverse effects with RAI preparation and/or administration. In some instances, patients present with many clinicopathologic features. While each clinical feature on its own is not enough to administer RAI, the co-existence of these features in one patient presentation would justify administering RAI therapy.[4]

TABLE 48.2 Clinical Indications for RAI Therapy

Clinical Indication	Rationale	Administered Activity
Primary tumor >4 cm	Likely to decrease recurrence, decrease disease-specific mortality, and may facilitate initial staging/follow-up	30–75 mCi with normal postoperative Tg** 100–150 with elevated postoperative Tg
Gross extrathyroidal extension	Likely to decrease recurrence, decrease disease-specific mortality, and may facilitate initial staging/follow-up	100–150 mCi
Distant metastases	Likely to decrease recurrence, decrease disease-specific mortality, and may facilitate initial staging/follow-up	150–200 mCi
Large volume cervical lymph node metastases*	Significant risk of recurrence and distant metastases, RAI may facilitate initial staging and follow-up. Conflicting data regarding effect on risk of recurrence	75–100 mCi with normal postoperative Tg 100–150 with elevated postoperative Tg
Papillary, follicular, or Hürthle cell thyroid cancer with vascular invasion	Significant risk of distant metastases, RAI may facilitate initial staging and follow-up	30–75 mCi with normal postoperative Tg 100–150 with elevated postoperative Tg
Poorly differentiated thyroid cancer with or without vascular invasion	Significant risk of recurrence and distant metastases, RAI may facilitate initial staging and follow-up. Inadequate data regarding effect on risk of recurrence	30–75 mCi with normal postoperative Tg 100–150 with elevated postoperative Tg
Inappropriately elevated postoperative Tg without structural evidence of disease	RAI may facilitate initial staging and follow-up. Inadequate data regarding effect on risk of recurrence	75–100 mCi
Nonspecific findings on radiology imaging that could represent metastatic disease	RAI may facilitate initial staging and follow-up	30–75 mCi with normal postoperative Tg 100–150 with elevated postoperative Tg

*Clinical N1 disease defined as more than 10 involved nodes if all are less than 5 mm, more than 5 involved nodes if the majority are 5 to 15 mm, or any single lymph node more than 15 mm.
**Normal postoperative Tg defined as nonstimulated Tg <5 ng/mL or stimulated Tg <10 ng/mL and negative anti-Tg antibodies.
RAI, radioiodine; Tg, thyroglobulin.
From Tuttle RM, Sabra MM. Selective use of RAI for ablation and adjuvant therapy after total thyroidectomy for differentiated thyroid cancer: a practical approach to clinical decision making. *Oral Oncol.* 2013;49(7):676–683.

Often, the decision to treat with RAI is made by patients based on their general health risk aversion and anxiety levels. Some patients may be minimalists when confronted with health issues, preferring to avoid unnecessary therapies and potential complications, being quite comfortable with a delayed therapy approach. Other patients are maximalists in their approach and not willing to take any risk for disease recurrence, preferring to take potentially ineffective therapy on the off chance it may improve their prognosis.[21]

THYROID HORMONE WITHDRAWAL VERSUS RECOMBINANT THYROID-STIMULATING HORMONE

Preparation of patients for RAI therapy includes avoidance of high iodine load a month before RAI therapy,[22] low iodine diet for 1 to 2 weeks,[23] and TSH stimulation. TSH stimulation will stimulate the sodium iodine symporter expression, allowing for better incorporation of iodine into tumor cells. TSH stimulation (TSH >30 mIU/L) can be achieved either with a few weeks of thyroid hormone withdrawal (THW) before RAI therapy or through intramuscular injection of recombinant TSH (rhTSH) the week of RAI therapy. If the recombinant human thyroid stimulation hormone (RhTSH) route is chosen, the patient will be maintained on thyroxine replacement therapy thus avoiding hypothyroid symptoms. The duration of TSH stimulation is shorter with rhTSH, with less of a risk of promoting cancer growth.

When RAI is administered for ablative purposes, rhTSH was found to be equivalent to THW with noninferiority in ablation efficacy, no difference in long-term outcomes, and an overall better patient short-term quality of life.[24,25] Thus rhTSH is recommended for RAI ablation.[1] In RAI adjuvant therapy, there are no RCTs that compared clinical response and outcomes based on the preparation method (rhTSH versus THW). Thus although rhTSH is often used in this setting and considered an adequate alternative to THW, this recommendation is based on low quality of evidence.[1] Furthermore, there are no data examining the clinical outcomes of patients treated for persistent disease under rhTSH stimulation versus THW. In fact, rhTSH is not Food and Drug Administration (FDA) approved in the U.S. for the RAI preparation of patients with metastatic thyroid cancer. However, it can be used in special situations, such as patients with severe comorbidities who cannot withstand prolonged hypothyroidism. At our institution, rhTSH has been routinely used for RAI therapy of metastatic disease over the past 20 years. In our retrospective studies on metastatic thyroid cancer, we do not see a difference in RAI therapy response after rhTSH or THW. However, randomized clinical trials are needed to prove the noninferiority of one preparation method or the other.

CHOICE OF ADMINISTERED RAI ACTIVITY BASED ON CLINICOPATHOLOGIC PRESENTATION

The choice of administered activity varies depending on intent of RAI therapy (see Table 48.2). In general, physicians aim to use an activity that is high enough to achieve the best clinical response but low enough to minimize the potential adverse effects. The risk for adverse effects with RAI becomes significant when activities exceeding 70 mCi are administered. For RAI ablation, there is very good evidence that 30 mCi is enough to ablate a thyroid remnant and eliminate low-volume nodal metastasis.[1,24,25] However, there is no true consensus regarding the appropriate RAI adjuvant therapy activity, which can range between 30 to 150 mCi.[1] We have previously shown that in younger patients (≤ 45 years of age) with N1b disease, clinical outcomes did not differ based on the activity of RAI administered, with a chance of cure similar in those treated with a median activity of 100 mCi, 150 mCi, or 200 mCi. In older patients, the risk for a structurally incomplete response was lower in those treated with a median 150 or 250 mCi activity as opposed to those treated with a median 100 mCi activity ($p = 0.03$). For this reason, our approach has been to use a 100 mCi administered activity for most patients eligible for adjuvant therapy, reserving a higher activitiy (150 mCi) for older patients presenting with aggressive features including bulky nodal involvement, those at risk for pulmonary metastasis, or those with known distant metastatic disease.[26] In recent years, we have preferred to avoid using activities exceeding 200 mCi in patients with metastatic thyroid cancer who were treated outside of clinical trials. This is based on evidence demonstrating noninferiority of lower empiric activities of RAI as opposed to higher blood dosimetry-based administered activities. The latter achieved higher lifetime cumulative RAI-administered activities with comparable clinical responses and a higher risk for serious adverse effects (increased risk for salivary gland cancer, lung cancer, myelodysplastic syndromes, etc.).[27]

CONCLUSION

RAI therapy encompasses all the roles of RAI, including ablation, adjuvant therapy, and treatment of locally persistent or metastatic thyroid cancer. In the absence of randomized clinical trials, there remains controversy regarding the selection of the patients who will benefit from therapy, the proper estimation of postoperative status, the choice of RAI preparation, and the choice of RAI-administered activity. Efforts are underway to bridge the gaps in expert opinions in the field, with hopes that this will lead to significant breakthroughs in the years to come.

REFERENCES

For a complete list of references, go to expertconsult.com.

49

External Beam Radiotherapy for Thyroid Malignancy

Meredith E. Giuliani, Richard W. Tsang, James D. Brierley

INTRODUCTION

Surgery is, with the exception of lymphomas described in this chapter, the mainstay of therapy for all types of thyroid cancer. However, if there is an increased risk of recurrence, further additional treatment may be warranted. In differentiated thyroid cancer (DTC), also described elsewhere, this is often in the form of radioactive iodine. However, in DTC, if the risk of locoregional recurrence is high and it is determined that radioactive iodine will be insufficient to minimize the risk of such recurrence, there is a potential role for external beam radiotherapy (EBRT), akin to a situation with surgically unresectable disease. Similarly, in both anaplastic thyroid cancer (ATC) and medullary thyroid cancer (MTC), if the cancer is unresectable or if there is a high risk of locoregional recurrence, postoperative EBRT may be an important part of the patient's management.

This chapter will describe the evidence for a role for EBRT in management of unresected and resected DTC, ATC, and MTC, as well as in the role of palliating symptoms from metastatic disease, and will describe the role of EBRT in the treatment of thyroid lymphoma. It will discuss technical aspects of delivering EBRT and its potential side effects.

DIFFERENTIATED THYROID CANCER

Unresectable Disease

One of the earliest reports on the use of EBRT in DTC comes from the 1960s and reported that just over 50% of patients with unresected tumor had long-term control of the disease in the neck.[1] Much more recently, our group reported a 90% local relapse-free rate at 10 years in 40 patients with gross residual disease after surgery. However the 10-year cause-specific survival was 48%; a lower rate of survival was observed because of the number of patients who went on to have distant metastases.[2] Another important series with a large sample size consists of 217 patients with post surgical residual disease from Hong Kong. In the 70% of patients who had EBRT, the 10-year local control rate was 64% compared with only 24% who did not receive EBRT.[3] The cause-specific survival at 10 years was 74% with EBRT and 50% without EBRT. Both differences were statistically significant. As in all the retrospective reports discussed in this chapter, concern however, about potential biases, especially case selection, must be acknowledged. There are other small series that also show a benefit to EBRT in controlling neck disease. For instance, the Christie Hospital group in Manchester, U.K., reported local control rates of 69%, and the MD Anderson Cancer Center group in Houston, U.S., reported a 60% local control rate.[4,5]

Given how devastating uncontrolled disease in the neck can be, it is important all patients who have unresectable DTC be considered for EBRT. For patients who have had a thyroidectomy, we consider giving radioactive iodine (RAI) before EBRT, as there is a theoretical risk of blunting the uptake of RAI if EBRT is given first. However, if because of the local extent of disease, thyroidectomy is not performed, we proceed with EBRT. It is important to ensure the airway is sufficiently patent for EBRT, including accounting for possible swelling from EBRT. If there is a risk of obstruction, a tracheotomy should be discussed, and if required, inserted before simulation for EBRT. Our usual practice is to give 66 Gy in 33 fractions over 6.5 weeks or, as in the case in Figure 49.1, in a patient with small-volume lung metastases, 50 Gy in 20 fractions. If the patient's performance status is poor, upfront palliative radiotherapy may be considered to protect the airway. The recent American Head and Neck Society guidelines endorsed the value of EBRT in gross residual disease and recommend EBRT for patients with gross residual or unresectable locoregional disease, except for patients less than 45 years old with limited gross disease that is radioactive iodine-avid.[6]

Resected Disease

It is well recognized that age and extrathyroid extension are two of the most import prognostic features for local recurrence in thyroid cancer. The American Joint Committee on Cancer (AJCC) and International Union Against Cancer (UICC) 8th edition of the tumor, node, metastases (TNM) classification of cancer have recently recognized that both the extent of local invasion and the age cutoff at which the risk of recurrence increases needed to be revised.[7,8] In the 8th edition of the TNM, the respective age cutoff and definitions of high-risk extrathyroid extension were changed. The age cutoff for defining a poor prognostic group was increased to 55 years of age having previously been 45. The definition of T3 was changed so that minimal extrathyroid extension is no longer a definition for T3 and that only gross extrathyroid extension is recognized. T3a is reserved for lesions with a largest diameter over 4cm and T3b for gross strap muscle invasion. T4a disease is defined as (tumor extends beyond the thyroid capsule and invades any of the following: subcutaneous soft tissues, larynx, trachea, esophagus, recurrent laryngeal nerve) and T4b disease (tumor invades prevertebral fascia, mediastinal vessels, or encases carotid artery). T4b disease is invariably unresectable and benefits from radiotherapy (Figure 49.2). It is these older patients with gross extrathyroid extension who are at risk of recurrence after surgery and may benefit from EBRT (Table 49.1, Figure 49.3).

Although the evidence for a role of EBRT in the management of unresectable DTC is well established, the role in the adjuvant management after the resection of all gross disease is more controversial. There

CHAPTER 49 External Beam Radiotherapy for Thyroid Malignancy

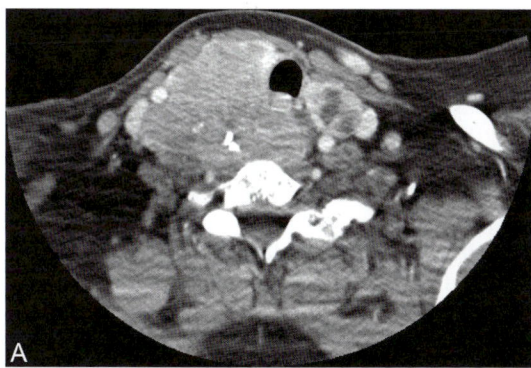

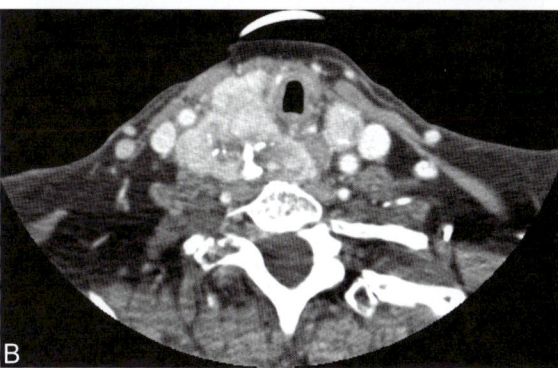

Fig. 49.1 A 72-year-old woman presented with a 6-cm thyroid mass. Biopsy showed differentiated thyroid cancer with focal poor differentiation (**A**). There was tracheal compression and carotid artery involvement. The tumor was considered unresectable. She had a tracheostomy and was treated with 66 Gy in 33 fractions. **B,** Mass 4 years later with stable partial response. CT thorax, not shown, shows slowly progressing lung metastases.

TABLE 49.1 Outlining Recommendation on the Use of External Beam Radiotherapy for Differentiated Thyroid Cancer

Disease Extent	Stage	Radiotherapy	Exception
Unresectable or gross residual	T4b	High dose radical radiotherapy and RAI if thyroidectomy performed	Young patients with small-volume residual disease and RAI uptake in the thyroid bed
Gross extrathyroid extension Microscopic residual	T4b	High dose radical radiotherapy and RAI	Consider even in patients <55 years old
Gross extrathyroid extension Microscopic residual (see Figure 49.3)	T4a	High dose radical radiotherapy and RAI	Young patients <55 years old
Gross extrathyroid extension No residual disease, negative margins	T4a	RAI only radiotherapy not required	Older patients ≥55 with tall cell or insular changes may benefit
Minimal extrathyroid extension and positive margins	T1-3	RAI only radiotherapy not required	Older patients with tall cell or insular changes may benefit
Recurrent nodal disease after surgery and repeated RAI or extracapsular nodal disease with positive margins (see Figure 49.4)	N1b	Adjuvant radiation	

RAI, radioactive iodine.

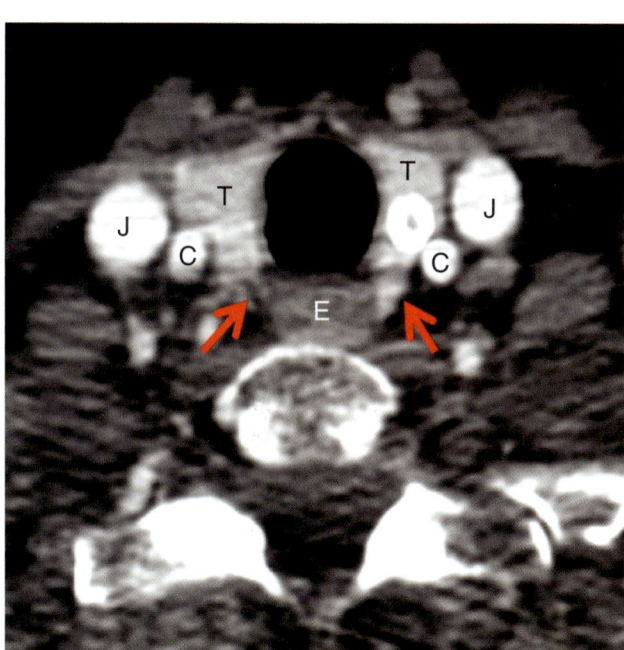

Fig. 49.2 *Arrows* demarcate location of right and left tracheoesophageal grooves. C, common carotid artery, E, esophagus, J, internal jugular vein, T, thyroid gland.

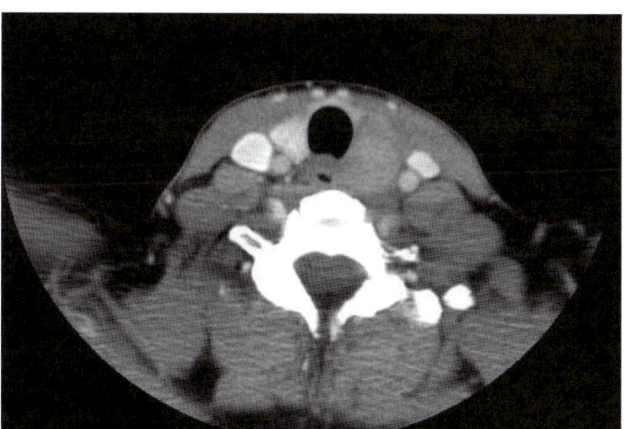

Fig. 49.3 A 67-year-old man presents with hoarseness for 2 months. On examination he has a 3-cm left thyroid mass, no palpable lymphadenopathy but left recurrent laryngeal palsy. Image shows a CT scan with contrast. He undergoes a thyroidectomy and central node dissection. He has extensive extrathyroid extension, tumor is dissected of left RLN and trachea, and microscopic residual disease left behind. Pathology reveals a 3.5-cm papillary thyroid cancer with 30% tall cell changes and extrathyroid extension. All identified nodes are negative. He has 150 mCi RAI, with uptake in central neck, his stimulated TSH is 67, and thyroglobulin is 11.2 with negative antibodies. RAI is followed by external beam radiotherapy 60 Gy in 30 fractions, to thyroid bed and 54 Gy to low-risk nodal volume.

TABLE 49.2 Local Recurrence Rates After Adjuvant External Radiotherapy for High-Risk Disease: Resected Differentiated Thyroid Cancer Compared With Surgery Without External Beam Radiotherapy

		TREATMENT	
First Author	Years of Follow-Up	Surgery With Radioactive Iodine	Surgery and Radioactive Iodine With Radiotherapy
Tubiana[65]	10	21%	14%
Phlips[66]	10	21%	14%
Farahati[9]	10	50%*	3%
Ford[67]	5	63%	7%
Kim[68]	5	37.5%	18%
Brierley[10]	10	34%	4.8%
Keum**[69]	10	89%	14%
Tamm***	5	82%	18%

*Includes distant failures
**All had tracheal invasion
***All had T4a disease

have been numerous single institution retrospective studies that indicate improved outcome after EBRT in high-risk DTC; these are summarized in Table 49.2. Most of these studies are flawed due to uncertain case selection biases and inconsistent use of RAI. In the study of Farahati et al., probably the study with the most consistent case selection and treatment, all patients were treated with RAI and all were defined as high risk in that they were all over the age of 40 and all had extrathyroidal extension.[9] They report that there was a reduction in local and regional recurrences in 85 patients who had EBRT and RAI compared with 52 patients who only had RAI. Our own study defined high-risk patients as those over 60 who had extrathyroidal extension but no gross residual disease after surgical resection. We reported an overall 10-year local control rate of 86.4% after EBRT compared with 65.7% if no EBRT was given.[10] There was also a small but significant improved local control rate (95.9% versus 85.4%, $p = 0.03$) but not an improved rate of survival in patients between the ages of 45 and 60 years. More recent single institutional studies have not compared patients treated with and without EBRT but have reported the local control rate in patients considered at high risk of recurrence. For example the MD Anderson group reported a regional local control rate of 86% and 82% cause-specific survival at 4 years in patients with microscopic residual disease after resection.[5]

Ideally, to prove a role for EBRT, a randomized controlled study should be performed, but unfortunately there has not been one due to the difficulty in recruiting sufficient patient numbers and the length of follow-up required. One was attempted in Europe, but it failed to recruit and was closed. In our opinion, it was flawed as patients we would consider to be low risk of local relapse (young patients and patients with only minimal extra thyroid extension) were included.[11]

In a systematic review, 16 articles were thought to be appropriate after a comprehensive literature review of the role of EBRT that initially identified 821 articles. This resulted in a pooled population of 5114 patients. There were no randomized studies and only one prospective study identified. In the 13 studies that reported local regional recurrence, the recurrence rate was 20% without EBRT and 13% with EBRT. The authors concluded that there was an improvement in locoregional control after EBRT in high-risk patients over 45.[12] In another report, which reviewed the English and French literature on the role of EBRT in DTC, French authors proposed a scoring system that they acknowledged requires validation. In this system, various prognostic factors are assigned a score. For instance, less than 45 years of age is 0 points, 45 to 60 years is 1 point, and greater than 60 years is 2 points. They conclude any patient with a score of 6 or more should be recommended EBRT. For example a patient over 60 (2 points), with extrathyroid extension (2 points) and microscopic residual (2 points) scores 6 points and would be recommended EBRT.[13]

In a study of patients in the U.S. National Cancer Database (NCDB) with stage IV DTC and who had primary surgical treatment between 2002 and 2012 in a multivariate analysis, the addition of RAI to surgery significantly improved 5- and 10-year survivals in stages IVA, IVB, and IVC. EBRT was associated, however, with a higher mortality and in Stage IVB (T4b, any N, M0), this was statistically significant. However, the authors conclude that the clinical indications to treat with EBRT were associated with poorer survival and that it would be a misinterpretation of the data to conclude that EBRT treatment resulted in the poorer survival.[14]

Although the American Head and Neck Society has stated that after complete resection EBRT may be considered in select patients greater than 45 years old with a high likelihood of microscopic residual disease and a low likelihood of responding to RAI, it may be that a higher age cutoff of 55 would be more appropriate.[12] The 2009 American Thyroid Association (ATA) guidelines recommend that EBRT should be considered in patients over age 45 with grossly visible extrathyroidal extension at the time of surgery and a high likelihood of postoperative microscopic residual disease.[15] The authors also state that although after complete resection, cervical lymph node involvement alone should not be an indication for EBRT, EBRT may be considered if there is extensive extracapsular spread with high risk of microscopic residual disease (Figure 49.4). The more recent 2015 ATA guideline does not address the situation of adjuvant radiotherapy but comments that for tumors that invade the upper aerodigestive tract, surgery combined with additional therapy such as ^{131}I and/or EBRT is generally advised.[16] The U.K. guidelines recommended in addition to RAI that EBRT should be considered in unresectable tumors and when there is residual disease after surgery, even if the residual disease concentrated RAI.[17]

All patients having high doses of EBRT should have treatment with modern radiotherapy techniques such as intensity-modulated radiotherapy (IMRT) or a variation of IMRT such as volumetric-modulated arc therapy (VMAT). IMRT has been shown to reduce toxicity and in some cases improve disease control in head and neck cancers although data does not exist specifically for thyroid cancer patients. In our institution, 60 Gy in 30 fractions is usually prescribed to the thyroid bed and areas of surgical dissection, and a lower dose of 54 Gy in 30 fractions to undissected areas at risk of microscopic disease (see Figure 49.4). In patients with gross residual disease, a higher dose of 66 to 70 Gy in 33 to 35 fractions is given to the disease with 56 Gy in 33 fractions to the areas at risk of microscopic disease. The volume to be treated in this setting is controversial, and one must balance the risk of microscopic disease versus the risk of toxicity. The volume we treat in our institution is usually the surgical thyroidectomy bed and levels III, IV, VI, and part of level V. The volumes typically extend from the hyoid bone superiorly to the aortic arch inferiorly but are adjusted depending on the clinical findings. It is important before proceeding with any EBRT to have a discussion with the patient and the surgeon to confirm the high risk of locoregional recurrence and in determining the anatomic volume of tissues at high risk. If possible, the placement of

CHAPTER 49 External Beam Radiotherapy for Thyroid Malignancy

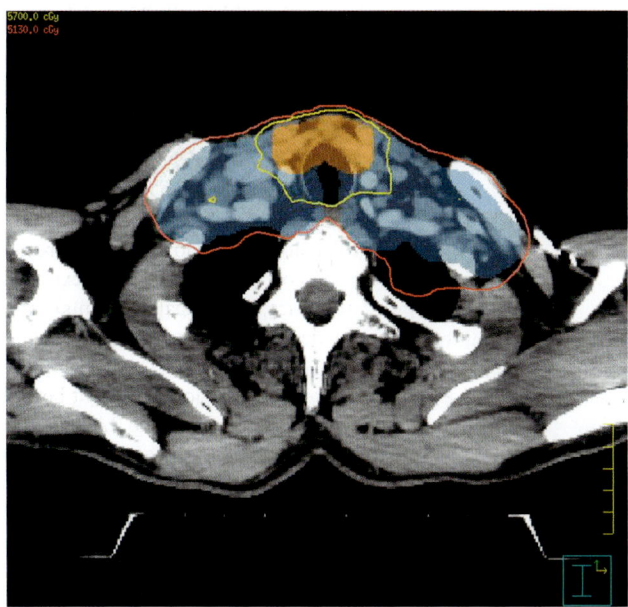

Fig. 49.4 A 57-year-old man presented with a thyroid mass; biopsy showed papillary carcinoma. He had central compartment nodes. A thyroidectomy and ipsilateral central compartment dissection were performed. The pathology showed a 4.5-cm papillary carcinoma with angioinvasion and eight nodes involved. He had 100 mCi iodine with no significant uptake. Follow-up 2 years later showed a paratracheal node. He had resection. There was significant extra nodal extension into the tracheoesophageal groove and the tumor was dissected off the trachea with residual microscopic disease. Given the lack of previous RAI uptake, he was offered external beam radiotherapy. Six years later he is asymptomatic and free from disease. He received 60 Gy in 30 fractions to high-risk volume and 54Gy to lower-risk volume. The orange shaded volume presents the area considered to be at high risk of recurrence and the blue shaded volume the lower-risk adjacent lymph node volume. The yellow line represents the 95% isodose volume; all the tissue inside the line received 95% of the prescribed 60Gy (i.e., 57 Gy). The outside brown line represents the 95% isodose volume for the lower-risk volume of 51.3 Gy.

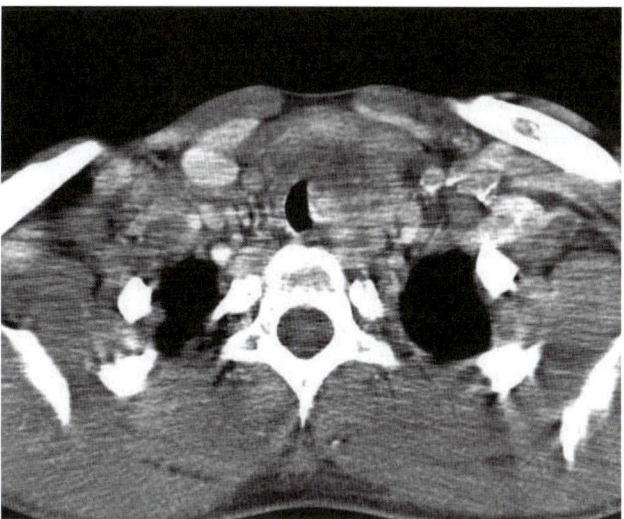

Fig. 49.5 A 29-year-old man presents with a 3-month history of increasing shortness of breath. He has a 6-cm left thyroid mass with tracheal displacement and left vocal cord paralysis. He undergoes bilateral neck dissection, total thyroidectomy, tracheal resection and anastomosis, and resection of esophageal muscle with complete gross resection. The pathology is reported as a 6-cm medullary thyroid cancer with lymphatic, venous, and arterial invasion. There is extrathyroid soft tissue and tracheal invasion, and positive margins. There is no C cell hyperplasia. 34 out of 78 bilateral II, III, IV,VI nodes are positive but with no extracapsular extension. There is no evidence of metastatic disease. He receives radiotherapy, 66 Gy in 33 fractions, to thyroid bed and trachea, 56 Gy in 33 fractions to bilateral cervical lymph nodes.

markers such as surgical clips in the areas of greatest concern at the time of surgery can aid in delineating the boost volumes for EBRT. In addition, ensuring there is a computed tomography (CT) scan of the extent of disease before surgery is important to allow this to be fused to the postsurgical CT simulation to aid in delineation.

MEDULLARY THYROID CANCER

Surgery is the main curative treatment modality for medullary thyroid cancer (MTC). Because regional lymph nodes are involved in approximately 50% of sporadic patients, meticulous neck and superior mediastinal dissections are often required. For those who have normal calcitonin and carcinoembryonic antigen (CEA) levels after surgery, the prognosis is excellent.[18,19] Additional factors that predict for a poorer prognosis include extrathyroidal invasion, postoperative gross residual disease, and clinical stage (Figure 49.5).[20] In these patients, further investigation to locate regional and/or metastatic disease is required, with CT scans, somatostatin and bone scans, and other appropriate radionucleotide scanning.

Because RAI has no role in MTC, EBRT may be used to control residual or potential residual disease in the neck. The evidence in support of EBRT in MTC is less strong than for DTC but if first principles are applied, then it may be assumed that in patients at high risk of local regional recurrence after surgery, maximizing local regional therapy with the addition of EBRT may improve local regional control further. This is supported by retrospective reviews. The one from our institution reported improved local control but not survival with the addition of EBRT to surgery in high-risk patients defined as having extensive extrathyroidal extension with or without nodal involvement. The 10-year local/regional relapse-free rate was 86% in those who received EBRT and 52% in those who did not ($p = 0.049$). The MD Anderson group and the Royal Marsden group in the U.K. have reported similar results in the past.[21,22] However, these studies are old and before the era of extensive lymphadenectomy or, more recently, the use of targeted molecular therapy.[23,24] An analysis of the U.S. Surveillance, Epidemiology, and End Results (SEER) program data reported that for patients treated between 1988 and 2004 EBRT resulted in improved overall survival in node-positive patients, but this was not demonstrated in the multivariable analysis.[25] Given the limitations of the available data, local regional relapse for which EBRT would probably be of importance was not analyzed.

We recommend postoperative EBRT to patients with locally advanced MTC and a high likelihood of recurrence. These are usually patients with unresectable disease or resected T4a disease with microscopic residuum, or extensive nodal disease with extra nodal extension. We counsel patients that although the aim is to improve local control, it will not improve the overall chance of cure as locally advanced disease almost invariably is associated with a high risk of distant recurrence of disease (Table 49.3). This is in keeping with the ATA guidelines that "Postoperative adjuvant EBRT to the neck and mediastinum should be considered in patients at high risk for local recurrence (microscopic or macroscopic residual MTC, extrathyroidal extension, or extensive

TABLE 49.3 Outlining Recommendation on the Use of External Beam Radiotherapy for Medullary Thyroid Cancer

Disease Extent	Stage	Radiotherapy	Exception
Unresectable or gross residual	T4a or T4b	High-dose radical radiotherapy	Palliative if widespread metastases
Gross extrathyroid extension and microscopic residual (see Figure 49.5)	T4a or T4b	High-dose radical radiotherapy for local control	Widespread metastases
Widespread nodal disease	N1b	Adjuvant radiotherapy may improve local control but not survival	Widespread metastases

lymph node metastases), and those at risk of airway obstruction."[26] The U.K. guideline supports the use of EBRT stating that "is of use in controlling local symptoms in patients with inoperable disease and improving the relapse free rate after surgery where residual disease is present macroscopically or microscopically."[17]

The doses we prescribe are similar to that described earlier for DTC. However, given the natural history of MTC and the propensity for nodal metastatic disease, the volumes to the nodal areas are usually larger, extending to cover the whole of the cervical nodal chains (excluding levels IA and IB), and include the superior mediastinum.

ANAPLASTIC THYROID CANCER

The prognosis after a diagnosis of ATC is usually dismal, particularly in an elderly person (see chapter 28 Anaplastic Thyroid Cancer and Thyroid Lymphoma). It accounts for about 50% of all thyroid cancer deaths though less than 5% of all thyroid cancers. This is because it is often inoperable at presentation due to extensive invasion of adjacent tissues, and even if surgically resectable, it often has metastases at presentation. Multimodality therapy is the mainstay of treatment in patients with resectable disease who wish for aggressive treatment. Given the poor outcome of most patients and the potential toxicity from aggressive treatment, it is even more important than for other thyroid malignancies that the wishes and directives of the patient are developed in accordance with their goals of care.

As with other thyroid malignancies, there is a lack of randomized controlled studies in the management of ATC, and most data come from retrospective reviews with a few phase II studies usually involving chemotherapy. The best outcomes in terms of both local control and survival based upon consistent results from multiple studies appear to be associated with complete/near-complete surgical resection followed by radiotherapy, often administered in combination with chemotherapy. As always with retrospective studies, there is an element of case selection bias; invariably, patients with better performance status, younger age, and less extensive disease receive more treatment. Nevertheless, unselected SEER data detailing 516 patients revealed in a multivariate analysis that, along with age, only the combined uses of surgical resection and radiotherapy were identified as independent predictors of survival.[27] These results, supported by data from single institutions, led to the 2012 ATA guidelines recommending surgery if grossly negative margins can be achieved without extensive ablative surgery.[28] In patients with good performance status and no evidence of metastatic disease who wish for an aggressive approach, surgery should be followed by high-dose radiotherapy with or without concurrent chemotherapy. For patients with unresectable disease, a similar approach with definitive radiotherapy with or without concurrent chemotherapy is recommended. These guidelines are in the process of being revised and readers should review the next update when available.

The recommendations in the 2012 ATC guidelines have been supported by three analyses of the NCDB data obtained from U.S. cancer centers. In one analysis of 1288 patients, both high doses of radiotherapy and an intermediate dose (defined as 45 to 59.9 Gy) were associated with better survival.[29] In a second analysis of NCDB data with 2742 patients, a small survival benefit was found from trimodality treatment. In stage IVB patients median survival was 5.9 months with surgery and radiotherapy and 9.9 months with surgery, radiotherapy, and chemotherapy. For stage IVC patients, it was 3.5 months and 5.9 months, respectively.[30] In the largest analysis of 3552 patients who had unresected disease, longer survival was associated with doses of radiotherapy greater than 59.4 Gy.[31] In this analysis, although the addition of chemotherapy resulted in improved survival, this advantage was lost after a condition landmark analysis but total thyroidectomy and radiation dose greater than 59.4 Gy remained significant factors for prognosis. At present, although there may be advantages of concurrent chemotherapy and radiotherapy, the data is conflicting.

Dose escalation and accelerated hyperfractionation (multiple small fractions given over a shorter overall time period) may help offset the rapid proliferation and radioresistance of anaplastic disease. In a series from Princes Margaret Cancer Centre of radiotherapy for patients treated with hyperfractionation (60 Gy in 40 fractions over 4 weeks; Figure 49.6) the median survival was 13.6 months compared with 10.3 months for those treated with conventional fractionation (both approaches without concurrent chemotherapy).[32] An alternative to altered fractionation that is commonly used in North America is

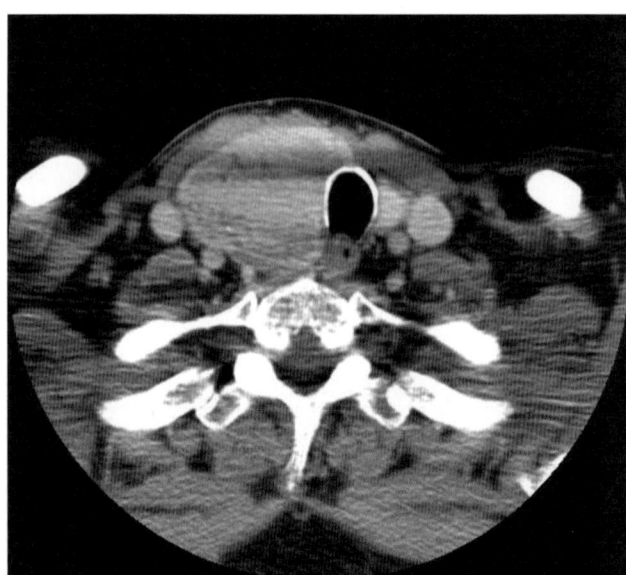

Fig. 49.6 A 71-year-old healthy woman presents with a rapidly enlarging thyroid mass which is initially diagnosed by fine-needle aspirate with papillary thyroid. A total thyroidectomy and central compartment dissection are performed. The right lobe mass is adherent to the trachea. Final pathology is reported as a 6.5-cm anaplastic carcinoma. A PET/CT scan reveals no metastases. She is treated with IMRT 60 Gy in 40 fractions, twice daily over 4 weeks to the thyroid bed and adjacent lymph nodes with 52 Gy in 40 fractions to the bilateral cervical neck up to level of the hyoid and down the superior mediastinum.

concurrent chemoradiation, the addition of cytotoxic chemotherapy to hyperfractionated radiotherapy, has resulted in significant toxicity so radiotherapy is usually conventionally fractionated with single daily fractions. With conventional fractionation a variety of different cytotoxic agents have been used. In 30 patients treated by the Mayo Clinic with IMRT and concurrent chemotherapy after surgical resection when possible, the median survival was 9 months, with a 1-year survival of 42%, compared with 3 months and 10%, respectively, for those treated with palliative intent only. A variety of different chemotherapy regimens were used, but the most common were doxorubicin and docetaxel (66%). Carboplatin and paclitaxel in combination or doxorubicin, cisplatin, or paclitaxel as single agents were also used.[33] For a subgroup of 22 patients with stage IVB disease, the median survival was 22.4 months after multimodality treatment and only 4 months after palliative intent treatment. It should be noted that the authors describe the treatment as "highly toxic," with 60% requiring hospitalization. The benefit-to-cost ratio of triple modality therapy to the patient has yet to be accurately determined.

Given the toxicity and shortcomings of conventional chemoradiotherapy, the development of novel biologically targeted approaches is of increasing importance. Published data have demonstrated single agent activity in mixed study populations with radioiodine-refractory differentiated or undifferentiated thyroid disease for multitargeted tyrosine kinase inhibitors.[34,35] For tumors with BRAF V600E mutation, the combination of a BRAF inhibitor (dabrafenib) and a MEK inhibitor (trametinib) gave a 69% response rate, and this combination received U.S. Food and Drug Administration (FDA) approval in early 2018 for the treatment of ATC.[36] Exploring better targeted drug combinations and the role of combined EBRT and targeted drugs, is important so that patients with a limited life expectancy, are spared the significant toxicities associated with a multimodality therapy. Strategic patient selection for such combined multimodal treatment plans is of central importance.

Currently, at our institution, we recommend hyperfractionated radiation to a dose of 60 Gy in 40 fractions, 1.5 Gy per fraction delivered twice daily, over 4 weeks, to motivated patients with good performance status and no evidence of distant disease. For patients with known metastases but disease in the neck requiring control, we consider 50 Gy in 20 fractions, 2.5 Gy per fraction once daily, over 4 weeks. For patient with poor performance status who wish to proceed with radiotherapy rather than just comfort measures, we consider 20 Gy in 5 fractions over 1 week which can be repeated 4 weeks later with sparing of the spinal cord, depending on response, performance status, and patients' wishes (Table 49.4). As discussed in the first section, close collaboration with the surgical team around the patency of the airway is essential. If a tracheostomy is required, it should be performed before simulation for EBRT.

TREATMENT OF METASTATIC DISEASE

EBRT has an important role in the management of metastatic disease in patients with all types of thyroid cancer. For many years it has been acknowledged that EBRT can relieve the symptoms of metastatic disease: pain in bone metastases, shortness of breath due to distal lung collapse and hemoptysis in localized symptomatic lung metastases, and brain metastases. It has been reported that up to 42% of patients dying from thyroid cancer have bone metastases.[37] To palliate these metastases, single fraction radiation such as 8 Gy or multiple fractions (20 Gy in 5 fractions) of radiotherapy are used. Similar doses are used to palliate symptomatic lung metastases.

The role of EBRT in the treatment of metastatic thyroid cancer is expanding since the development of stereotactic body radiotherapy (SBRT), which allows for very high doses of radiotherapy, usually given with large fraction size, over a small number of fractions or treatments (often 1 to 6 fractions) with great precision. SBRT can be used to treat brain, lung, and bone metastases in highly selected patients and clinical scenarios. Examples of stereotactic radiotherapy given for brain, lung, and bone metastases are shown in Figures 49.7 to 49.9). The application of the oligometastatic paradigm in thyroid cancers is evolving. The central principles of oligometastatic cancer management is the aggressive treatment of limited metastases to prolong survival, disease-free periods, and in some cases, long-term disease control.[38] Given that most thyroid carcinomas have a propensity to disseminate widely, it remains uncertain whether the introduction of stereotactic radiotherapy to treat unifocal or oligometastatic disease will make a significant difference to the natural history of the disease and result in cure. However, given the toxicity and the often short time to progression with currently available systemic therapies, treatments such as stereotactic radiation may find a definite role if it can delay the start of systemic therapies in patients with MTC.

Patients with DTC and limited brain metastases may have a more prolonged survival than many other patients with metastases from other solid cancers, and the benefit of SBRT sparing patients the potential of the long-term side effects of whole-brain radiotherapy is important.

LYMPHOMA

Lymphomas of the thyroid gland can present in the gland itself and/or in cervical lymph nodes. In a large U.S. study, lymphomas presenting in the thyroid accounted for 1.2% of all lymphomas during the years 2001 to 2009.[39] In all cases, a philosophy of functional preservation without resorting to surgical thyroidectomy should be followed. The need for chemotherapy and/or radiotherapy is not diminished after surgical excision of lymphoma. Surgery is required to procure adequate tissue for diagnosis, and not infrequently when the thyroid tumor mass is bulky and causing airway compromise, surgical management with a tracheostomy may be required. Fine-needle aspirate biopsy is generally inadequate to obtain an accurate lymphoma diagnosis. Optimal pathology interpretation involves immunophenotypic and sometimes molecular studies. A special fixative and fresh tissue are often necessary, and therefore specific protocols for tissue retrieval and processing are required. Standard staging investigations involve cross-sectional and functional imaging Such as [18]fluoro-2-deoxy-d-glucose positron emission tomography([18]FDG-PET), assessment of blood indices, and in most cases, a bone marrow biopsy.

TABLE 49.4 Outlining Recommendation on the Use of External Beam Radiation for Anaplastic Thyroid Cancer

Disease Extent	Stage	Radiotherapy	Exception
Regional disease (see Figure 49.6)	IVA or IVB	Radical radiotherapy +/- chemotherapy	Patient choice Poor performance status. Consider palliative radiotherapy
Metastatic disease	IVC	Palliative radiotherapy	Consider radical if good performance status and well-motivated and small-volume metastases

458 SECTION 7 Postoperative Management

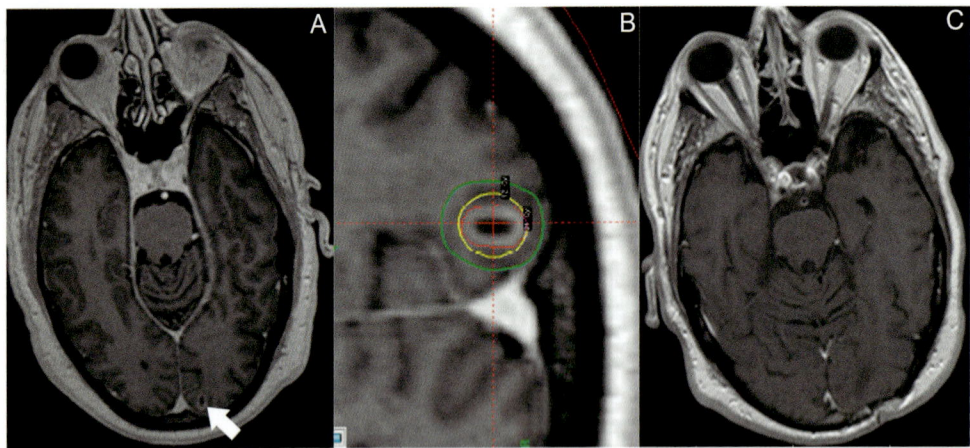

Fig. 49.7 A 59-year-old man who has locally advanced differentiated thyroid cancer is treated by surgery, radioactive iodine, and external beam radiotherapy. Follow-up CT of his head and neck shows an occipital lesion, magnetic resonance imaging (MRI) shows the lesion (**A**, *arrow*) and an additional frontal metastases but no other lesions. He has the frontal lesion excised, and metastatic thyroid cancer is confirmed. He undergoes stereotactic radiation, 21 Gy in 1 fraction (**B**) to the occipital lesion after whole-brain radiotherapy. Follow-up 5 years later shows no evidence of persistent disease (**C**).

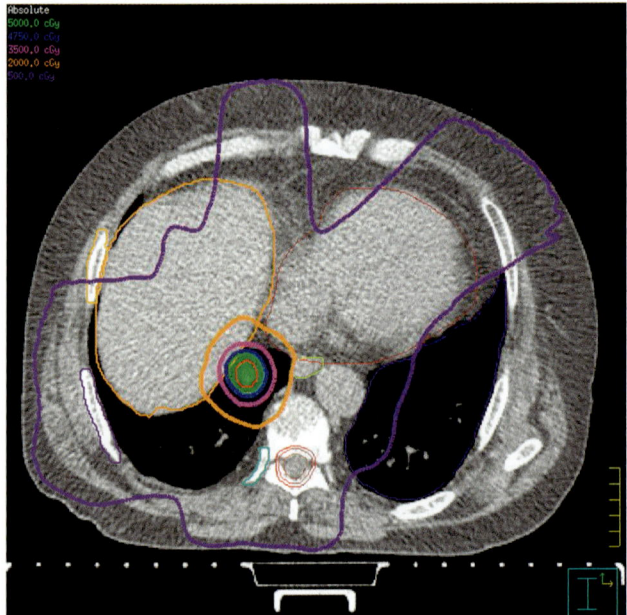

Fig. 49.8 A 66-year-old man has a total thyroidectomy, right neck dissection, and mediastinal resection in April 2015 for T4a, N1b papillary carcinoma with 50% tall cell variant. He is given 150 mCi radioactive iodine ablation. A known right lower lobe lung nodule did not pick up radioactive iodine. A year later the nodule is stable with no new nodules. A biopsy confirms metastatic papillary carcinoma. He has stereotactic body radiation therapy, 50 Gy in 5 fractions, in August 2016. CT August 2018, post radiation changes only. The green shaded area represents the planning target volume (PTV). The green line is the 100% isodose so that all tissue within the green line receives 50 Gy. The pink line is the 70% isodose line, so that all tissue within the line receives 35 Gy. The orange line is the 40% (20 Gy) isodose line.

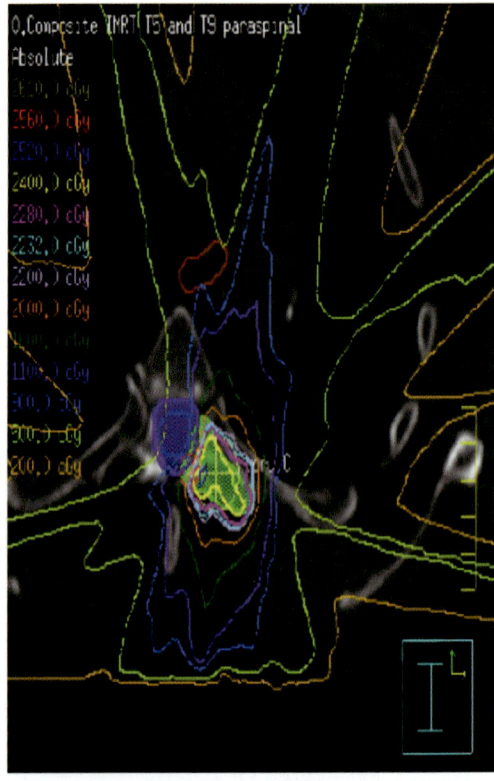

Fig. 49.9 A 62-year-old man presented with back pain. He was found to have a bone metastasis. He had resection, thyroidectomy, radioactive iodine, and external beam radiotherapy. Subsequently he had a recurrence and underwent minimal invasive decompression and partial excision followed by stereotactic radiotherapy, 24 Gy in three fractions.

The management is primarily influenced by histology and the Ann Arbor stage, as endorsed in the TNM system, modified in the Lugano classification.[7,8,40] Treatment strategies can be addressed in two broad categories: for indolent (low-grade) lymphoma and the contrasting group with aggressive histology (intermediate or high grade, most commonly diffuse large B-cell) lymphoma. Advanced stages (stages III and IV) of lymphoma are treated primarily with chemotherapy and will not be further discussed. For stages I and II presentations in the thyroid gland, the treatment approach involves radiotherapy alone, or combined modality therapy (CMT), with chemotherapy followed by consolidation radiation, with a curative intent.

INDOLENT (LOW-GRADE) LYMPHOMAS

The most common indolent lymphomas presenting in the thyroid gland are the mucosa-associated lymphoid tissue (MALT) type followed in incidence by follicular lymphoma.[41] Both are B-cell lymphomas with indolent biologic behavior and a low proliferation rate. MALT lymphomas present with localized (stage IE-IIE) disease in 70% to 90% of cases and is associated with preexisting Hashimoto's thyroiditis as a predisposing factor to its development.[42] Patients tend to present in the sixth and seventh decade of life, and there is a female predominance of 3:1. In contrast, follicular lymphoma often involves lymph nodes and the bone marrow and is widely regarded as a systemic disease. However, up to one-third of patients at the time of presentation have localized (stages I and II) nodal disease after standard staging investigations, although the addition of FDG-PET in staging assessment reduced this to 15% to 20%.[43-45] Stage IE presentation of follicular lymphoma in the thyroid gland is rare.[46,47]

Stages I and II indolent lymphomas are treated with involved-site radiotherapy.[48,49] Both MALT lymphoma and follicular lymphoma are known to be radiation-sensitive diseases. Because of this, low to moderate doses (25 to 35 Gy, fractionated over 3 to 4 weeks) have been the standard approach, with a long-term disease-free survival of 50% to 70% and a local control rate exceeding 95%. Short-term toxicity is mild and serious long-term toxicity is rare in virtually all the perithyroidal neck tissues irradiated.[49-52] A significant risk of hypothyroidism is expected after external radiotherapy and thyroid function should be monitored regularly and replacement hormone therapy instituted, when necessary. Relapse of lymphoma happens rarely for treated MALT lymphomas, but it can develop in up to 50% of patients with follicular lymphoma, typically occurring in other lymph node regions; when this happens, the treatment required is chemotherapy or radiotherapy for palliation of symptoms.[41,47,49]

AGGRESSIVE HISTOLOGY LYMPHOMAS

Aggressive lymphomas are actually more common than the indolent lymphomas and can arise in the thyroid gland and have the potential for systemic disease.[53] The most common histology is diffuse large B-cell lymphoma (DLBCL), for which standard therapy has been well established based on phase III clinical trials. Other rare aggressive lymphomas (e.g., T-cell lymphomas, Burkitt's lymphoma, and Hodgkin's lymphoma) are based on a similar philosophy of therapy with CMT specific for the histology.[54,55]

For early stage presentations (stages I and II), the recognition of the high risk for occult systemic disease mandates the use of anthracycline-based chemotherapy to achieve the best cure rates.[52,56-58] Patients are treated with CMT, with chemotherapy delivered first for three to six cycles, followed by moderate-dose involved-site radiotherapy (30 to 40 Gy) 3 to 6 weeks later.[48] In general, a cure rate ranging from 60% to 80% is achieved, depending on age, tumor burden, and other prognostic factors such as performance status and LDH level. For B-cell lymphomas, the addition of immunotherapy with anti-CD20 antibody (rituximab) in combination with chemotherapy improves the clinical outcome.[59,60] The most common regimen is CHOP-R (cyclophosphamide, doxorubicin, vincristine, prednisone, and rituximab).[55,59] Because of the moderate radiation doses required (30 to 40 Gy), short-term toxicity is mild and serious long-term toxicity is rare, particularly with current precision radiotherapy techniques (IMRT or VMAT) with improved ability to further reduce the dose to uninvolved normal tissues, such as the larynx, salivary glands, and the spinal cord (Figure 49.10). In general, thyroid lymphomas have a better prognosis than comparable lymphomas arising in other anatomic locations.[39]

EXTERNAL BEAM RADIOTHERAPY TECHNIQUE

The challenging location of the thyroid bed plays a key role in determining the efficacy and therapeutic ratio of radiotherapy. Treatment of unresected disease must frequently encompass a bulky, primary and nodal tumor, which surrounds or infiltrates critical structures, such as the larynx, esophagus, trachea, and mediastinal structures. In the case of postoperative treatment, geometric challenges are further complicated by a wide distribution of surgical dissection requiring large, irregularly shaped treatment volumes which can encompass the central neck compartment and superior mediastinum. The geometry of the thyroid bed has historically led to undesirable dose reductions and/or treatment morbidity with older radiotherapy techniques. Historically, a number of conventional 2D and 3D planning techniques have been employed, but these have fortunately become outdated with the

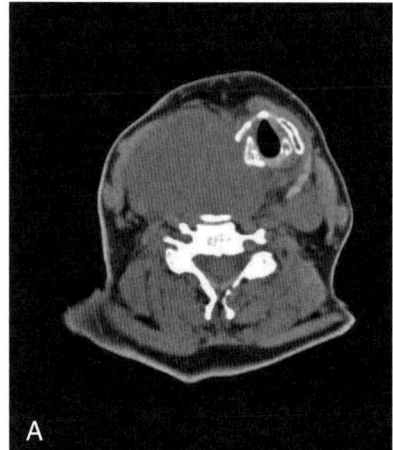
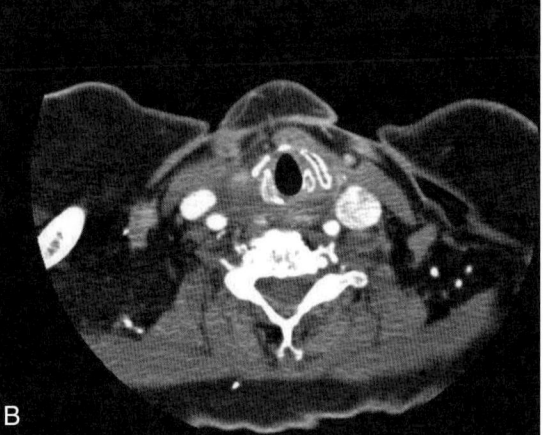

Fig. 49.10 An 80-year-old woman presented with a rapidly enlarging right neck mass, shortness of breath, and dysphagia. She has an 8-cm mass in right thyroid gland displacing trachea to the left **(A)**. Biopsy showed diffuse large B-cell lymphoma. Investigations showed no dissemination (stage IAE). She started on chemotherapy (cyclophosphamide, doxorubicin, vincristine, prednisone, rituximab—CHOPR regimen) urgently, followed by radiotherapy, 35 Gy in 20 fractions. Complete remission was obtained **(B)**. She is alive and well 10 years after treatment.

advent of IMRT. Advances in imaging, with readily available magnetic resonance imaging (MRI) and functional imaging with PET, aid the accurate definition of the target volumes.

When EBRT is indicated, IMRT or VMAT techniques should be used as they enable high-dose, high-precision radiotherapy to be delivered to a target while minimizing doses to adjacent organs at risk (OARs). There are no randomized data on the role of IMRT specifically for thyroid cancers; however, the data from other head and neck cancers show that IMRT can ensure a greater dose of radiotherapy delivered to the target(s) while keeping doses to OARs at a reasonable level.[60] This has, for instance, resulted in improved local control of nasopharyngeal cancer control and reduced salivary gland dysfunction.[61,62]

In addition to ensuring safe radiation OARs, in particular the spinal cord, salivary glands, and the mandible, IMRT also facilitates the delivery of differential doses to different areas at risk. Typically, as indicated earlier, at our institution we recommend two distinct volumes, 66 Gy in 33 fractions to gross residual disease and 56 Gy in 33 fractions to elective adjacent volume and nodal areas. If there is no gross residual disease but the patient is being treated for potential microscopic disease, 60 Gy in 30 fractions is prescribed to the higher risk volume and 54 Gy in 30 fractions to the elective nodal areas. (see Figure 49.2).

Although IMRT facilitates sparing of OARs, the esophagus is the OAR that is responsible for a significant component of toxicity in EBRT of the thyroid bed, with both acute esophagitis and esophageal stenosis, which can occasionally require a gastrostomy tube. This is because for those with extrathyroid extension into the region of the tracheoesophageal groove, there is the greatest concern for potential or actual residual disease at or near the esophagus after surgery resulting in the recommendation for EBRT. This results in the esophagus frequently being in the clinical target volume (CTV) to be treated and therefore appropriately not spared. However, after careful delineation of the volume at risk for residual disease IMRT can reduce the length and volume of the esophagus getting high-dose radiation. In one series, the incidence of esophageal stenosis requiring dilatation with non-IMRT planned treatments was 12% compared with only 2% after IMRT planned treatments.[5]

In our institution, the elective nodal CTV includes levels III and VI, with levels II and IV partially included judiciously. These volumes are extended to ensure a minimum of 0.5 to 1 cm on any gross nodal disease. We have reported our patterns of failure after IMRT using restricted elective neck volumes and found few out of field failures.[63] When the extent of elective nodal coverage is being considered, the clinician must carefully balance the risk of regional failure for that nodal zone, the potential salvage options, and the radiation-related toxicity.

TOXICITY FROM EXTERNAL BEAM RADIOTHERAPY

Serious complications are not common after radiotherapy and it is important to be aware that even aggressive radiotherapy may not preclude future surgical intervention in the hands of experienced head and neck surgeons. Acute skin toxicity is common given the need to cover surgical incisional lines, and depending on the volume being treated, mucositis of the esophagus, trachea, and larynx typically occur toward the end of the course of radiotherapy but resolves shortly thereafter. More serious late toxicity, such as esophageal or tracheal stenosis, is less common but can occur, particularly in patients who have undergone tracheal resection with reconstruction. Tsang et al. reported no grade IV toxic effects (using the Radiation Therapy Oncology Group scale) and Farahati et al. observed no irreversible late toxic effects in patients given high-dose EBRT in addition to RAI.[9,64] A report from MD Anderson Cancer Center suggested less frequent severe late radiation morbidity after IMRT than for conventional three-dimensional radiotherapy (3DRT) techniques.[5]

REFERENCES

For a complete list of references, go to expertconsult.com.

50
Reoperative Thyroid Surgery

Jeremy L. Freeman, Andrew B. Sewell, Nathan W. Hales, Gregory W. Randolph

> Please go to expertconsult.com to view related video:
> **Video 50.1** Introduction to Chapter 50, Reoperative Thyroid Surgery

INTRODUCTION

Approximately one-third of patients with differentiated thyroid cancer (DTC) have tumor recurrence, and most are diagnosed within 10 years of initial treatment.[1-3] Locoregional recurrences may arise in the thyroid bed, the central or lateral neck, the mediastinum, or, rarely, invasive to the trachea or the muscle overlying the thyroid bed. The mortality from locally recurrent DTC varies from 4% in low-risk group patients (according to the Age, Metastases, Extent, and Size [AMES] prognostic index) to as high as 27% in high-risk group patients, such as males and those older than 45 years of age.[4] The 2015 American Thyroid Association (ATA) thyroid cancer guidelines advocate for a new risk-adapted continuum model that provides patients and clinicians with continuously updated risk stratification based on response to therapy during routine follow-up. Patients are initially staged in the classic low-, intermediate-, and high-risk classification to determine initial treatment options. After the initial treatment, patients are restratified based on their response to their treatment-based serial thyroglobulin (Tg) levels and ultrasound (US) imaging to evaluate for persistent and recurrent disease. Clinicians then adapt treatment and follow-up algorithms specific for each patient (see Chapter 24, Dynamic Risk Group Analysis and Staging for Differentiated Thyroid Cancer).

Although the standard treatment for most recurrent disease remains reoperative thyroid surgery, several nonoperative options are available for select patients. Low-risk patients with low-volume persistent/recurrent disease can be followed closely with long-term active surveillance. A significant majority of these patients will have stable disease without progression and can avoid any reoperative surgery. Additionally, nonsurgical treatment options, including US-guided percutaneous ethanol ablation, have been shown to be safe and effective in treating small foci of recurrent or persistent disease, especially in patients who are at high risk for surgical complications (see Chapter 51, Nonsurgical Treatment of Thyroid Cysts, Nodules, Thyroid Cancer Nodal Metastases, and Hyperparathyroidism: The Role of Percutaneous Ethanol Injection.

Revision or reoperative thyroid surgery is often technically challenging because of anatomic changes and reparative fibrosis after primary surgery, especially in the central neck (see Chapter 9, Reoperation for Benign Thyroid Disease). Consequently, reoperative surgery is associated with high rates of complications in inexperienced hands.[5,6] However, with experience and appropriate preparation, the risk of permanent hypoparathyroidism or injury to the recurrent laryngeal nerve (RLN) after reoperative surgery is reported to be low (less than 3% and 1%, respectively).[7-9] Surgeons contemplating revision thyroid surgery must possess the essential reoperative surgical skills and an intimate knowledge of regional anatomy to achieve such a low morbidity for what can often be a tedious and difficult procedure.

INDICATIONS FOR REVISION SURGERY

Approximately 10% of low- to intermediate-risk patients with DTC who undergo thyroid lobectomy have high-risk histologic features on final pathology, necessitating completion thyroidectomy before adjuvant radioactive iodine (RAI) ablation.[10-14] Around 30% to 40% of patients with DTC treated with total thyroidectomy will have persistent or recurrent structural disease, and many of these patients require reexploration of the thyroid bed, central compartment, and/or lateral neck compartments. Surgery in these patients should be limited to disease identifiable on imaging, >8 mm in the central neck or >10 mm in the lateral neck, and confirmed with fine-needle aspiration (FNA) biopsy.[10,15,16] Additionally, cancer may arise in a thyroid remnant in patients treated with a subtotal thyroidectomy for Graves' disease or symptomatic goiter.

Definitions

In 2015 the ATA recommended a risk-adapted stratification model for recurrence risk based on response to initial therapy. Patients are initially stratified using traditional low-, intermediate-, and high-risk groups based on clinicopathologic features known during the initial treatment (presence of locoregional or distant metastases, invasion, and aggressiveness of histologic subtype). This initial stratification is critical in guiding primary treatment and early surveillance decisions, but it is a static measurement of recurrence risk, which does not reflect the patient's response to treatment, a significant factor affecting recurrence risk.

Initially proposed by Tuttle and modified in the 2015 ATA guidelines, the "response-to-treatment restratification model" acknowledges that recurrence risk is on a continuum and employs a dynamic model based on an individual's actual response to therapy during surveillance. After definitive treatment, patients are categorized into one of four groups based on biochemical and structural response to therapy. "Excellent response" indicates no clinical, biochemical, or structural evidence of recurrence. "Biochemically incomplete response" describes a patient with rising Tg or stable anti-Tg autoantibody (TgAb) levels in a patient without evidence of structural recurrence. "Structurally incomplete response" denotes a patient with a persistent or newly identified locoregional or distant metastasis. "Indeterminate response" is used in patients with nonspecific imaging findings and equivocal biochemical profiles. By definition, "recurrence" is reserved for patients previously staged as an "excellent response" without biochemical or structural evidence of disease after initial treatment; otherwise the patients disease would be termed persistent.[10,15,17]

Recurrence Rates and Patterns

Approximately 30% to 40% of patients with DTC will have persistent disease and 1.2% to 6.8% of patients will have structural tumor recurrences during their surveillance, as determined by Tg levels and high-resolution US.[18] Long-term survival in patients with only biochemical evidence of disease is nearly 100%, and decreases to 85% for patients with evidence of structural recurrence during surveillance.[19] Given that only a fraction of these patients will develop adverse outcomes related to their persistent or recurrent disease, it is important to understand structural disease progression and its clinical implications.

Studies looking at metastasis rates in prophylactic lateral and central neck dissections in patients with normal preoperative ultrasonography (cN0) demonstrated that up to 90% of patients with PTC <1 cm have metastatic central neck nodes and up to 40% have metastatic lateral neck lymph nodes.[10,20,21] Despite the high incidence of occult lymph node metastasis, the observed clinical locoregional recurrence rate for patients with DTC is significantly lower.[10] Although most patients with DTC present with clinically negative (cN0) nodal disease by examination and imaging, approximately 35% of patients will have clinically evident disease at presentation. In these patients, high-risk features associated with increased rates of recurrence and persistent disease include lymph node metastases >3 cm (27% to 32% risk of recurrence), extranodal extension, and metastases in >5 lymph nodes (19% risk of recurrence).[22]

In one of the largest prospective cohort studies looking at sites of recurrences, Mazzaferri et al. found that most recurrences localized to the cervical and mediastinal lymph nodes (74%), whereas 20% involved the thyroid remnant and 6% involved the trachea and adjacent muscle. In addition, 21% of patients had distant metastases, with 63% isolated to the lungs alone. In this study, the time interval from detection of distant metastasis and death was less than 5 years in 49% of cases, 5 to 9 years in 38%, 10 to 14 years in 20%, and 15 years or more in 8% of cases.[3]

Shah and colleagues retroactively reviewed 86 patients who underwent revision central compartment surgery with or without lateral neck dissection. 43% of patients had recurrent disease confined to the central neck, whereas 12% had disease limited to the lateral neck and 35% of patients had involvement of both the central and lateral neck compartments.[9]

A large study by Merdad et al. looked at patterns of nodal involvement in 185 patients undergoing 248 selective neck dissections of levels II-Vb for biopsy-proven DTC metastatic to cervical lymph nodes. 73% of patients had metastatic disease in multiple levels, with 9% demonstrating skip lesions. The patterns of nodal involvement were as follows: level II, 49%; level III, 76%; level IV, 61%; and level Vb, 29%.[23] A subsequent meta-analysis by Eskander et al. looked at 18 studies in 1145 patients undergoing 1298 neck dissections for well-differentiated thyroid carcinoma to determine patterns of disease spread within the lateral neck with similar rates of nodal spread, leading the authors to recommend that a comprehensive selective neck dissection for recurrent DTC should encompass levels II, III, IV, and Vb.[24]

ROUTINE POSTOPERATIVE SURVEILLANCE

According to the 2015 ATA guidelines, standard posttreatment surveillance in patients who undergo total thyroidectomy with postoperative RAI ablation includes following serum Tg measurements and high-resolution US scanning to stratify for risk of recurrence (see "Definitions" section). Patients with DTC staged as low-risk who undergo thyroid lobectomy alone, or total thyroidectomy without RAI ablation should also be followed with surveillance neck USs and Tg levels, though Tg levels may be insensitive in predicting low-volume locoregional recurrences in these patients.[10]

Patients initially staged as high-risk may have Tg levels checked more frequently than the usual 6- to 12-month intervals recommended for low- to intermediate-risk patients. Additionally, they may need additional diagnostic imaging, including computed tomography (CT) or magnetic resonance imaging (MRI), to evaluate their response to therapy after initial treatment. Radioiodine whole-body scanning (WBS, single-photon emission computed tomography [SPECT]/CT) and FDG-PET/CT scans may be indicated in select cases but generally do not provide sufficiently accurate anatomic imaging data upon which to base surgery. An FNA biopsy performed under US guidance may be carried out on suspicious lesions found on physical examination, radiologic examination, or radioiodine scan. FNA should be sent for cytology as well as Tg rinsing.

Serum Thyroglobulin Levels

Serum Tg measurement is the most widely used method for early detection and monitoring of persistent or recurrent thyroid cancer. Tg is produced by thyroid epithelial cells in response to thyroid-stimulating hormone (TSH) stimulation. As such, it is highly specific for the presence of thyroid epithelial cells, but serum Tg is only a reliable marker in the setting of a total thyroidectomy. It has a half-life of 65 hours and should be undetectable within weeks of a total thyroidectomy without any remnant thyroid tissue. Persistently elevated Tg after surgery suggests residual tumor burden (residual or recurrent tumor, regional nodal disease, or distant metastases) or residual functioning benign thyroid tissue. By following the trends of serum Tg levels, one can determine the doubling time of Tg, and by inference, thyroid/cancer burden. A doubling time of <1 year has been shown to portend a poorer prognosis for disease recurrence and possibly aggressiveness.[25-27]

Older Tg tests were less sensitive in detecting small increases of Tg, especially in patients undergoing TSH-suppression therapy with levothyroxine [T4] therapy. These patients usually have undetectable or very low basal Tg levels. However, upon levothyroxine withdrawal (hypothyroid state), or administration of recombinant thyrotropin (rhTSH), serum Tg increases 10-fold. Furthermore, comparing stimulated-Tg titer to suppressed-Tg titer estimates the tumor's sensitivity to TSH. Normal thyroid and well-differentiated thyroid carcinomas should display >10-fold increase in the stimulated-Tg titer, whereas poorly differentiated thyroid carcinomas only modestly respond to TSH stimulation (less than threefold increase in Tg). Although a useful adjunct in complex cases, stimulated-Tg testing has some disadvantages; levothyroxine withdrawal can take weeks and is associated with decreased quality of life in patients, and rhTSH is expensive and may be less sensitive than levothyroxine-withdrawal.[28]

Newer second-generation, high-sensitivity immunometric assays (Tg^{2G}IMA) have detection sensitivities <0.1 ng/mL, a full magnitude of power more sensitive than the first-generation tests. Previously "undetectable" Tg levels may now be detectable, necessitating a new definition of biochemical cure, suppressed-Tg <0.2 ng/mL or stimulated-Tg <1 ng/mL. The increased sensitivity of the second-generation tests has obviated the need for routine TSH-stimulated Tg testing.[10,28]

Approximately one-third of patients with DTC have detectable levels of anti-TgAb or heterophilic antibodies (most commonly

HAMA) at some point during treatment, with 12.7% of patients clearing the antibodies after successful treatment (positive to negative). Tg antibodies invariably interfere with the measurement of Tg to some degree, regardless of testing methodology. Therefore current guidelines mandate concurrent testing of TgAb titers to validate each Tg test. To variable extents, failure of TgAb levels to fall, rising TgAb titers, and de novo TgAb appearances are all highly predictive of an increased risk of recurrence.[8,29]

One important caveat to trending Tg and TgAb levels during long-term surveillance is that levels can only be compared if the same testing methodology is used, and ideally within the same laboratory on the same machine. Each manufacturer uses different immunoassays to test various epitopes with different reagents, making between-method testing variability too high to compare results.

Ultrasonography

Ultrasonography is a highly sensitive and specific imaging modality used to monitor patients for recurrent thyroid carcinoma. With detection limits as small as 3 to 4 mm, preoperative US mapping improves the detection and assessment of occult lymph node metastasis. Stulak et al. reviewed almost 1000 patients who underwent preoperative US scans before thyroid surgery (primary and revision) and showed that in reoperative patients, nonpalpable disease was detected with US in 64% of patients. In patients with palpable neck disease, US altered the extent of planned operation in 43% of reoperative cases, with reported sensitivity, specificity, and positive predictive values of 90%, 79%, and 94%, respectively.[30]

US's advantages include its portability, ease of use, lack of ionizing radiation, and physiologic evaluation with Doppler mode. It has a key role in the standard posttreatment surveillance algorithm, and can detect recurrences in nonradioiodine-avid lesions and when Tg measurements are compromised by the presence of autoantibodies. All pretreatment and surveillance scans should encompass both the central compartment and lateral necks in a comprehensive fashion. Intraoperative US can be used during revision surgery when thick scar tissue hinders localization of recurrent disease (see "Adjunctive Techniques in Revision Surgery" section).

Despite the clear-cut utility of surveillance US imaging in patients with thyroid cancer, it has a few specific limitations when working up patients with suspected recurrent disease. US is limited in evaluating retropharyngeal, retrotracheal, and mediastinal disease, and has poor sensitivity for tracheal invasion and extranodal extension of disease. Any patients with suspected recurrent disease should be further evaluated using either contrast-enhanced CT or MRI for accurate assessment of these areas and features.

CT Axial Imaging With Contrast

Contrast-enhanced CT imaging is commonly used in the head and neck in the evaluation of nodal metastases (see Chapter 14, Preoperative Radiographic Mapping of Nodal Disease for Papillary Thyroid Carcinoma). CT is not operator dependent but is highly repeatable, obtained with 1.5 mm axial cuts, and has a very fast acquisition time. CT images are familiar to surgeons and give detailed anatomic information. They image lymph node regions that are less accessible or less accurately seen by US, such as the central neck, mediastinum, and retropharynx, and is the test of choice for evaluating laryngeal or tracheal cartilage invasion in thyroid cancer. CT imaging also remains the most sensitive modality for detection of multiple small lung deposits from thyroid cancer, which are often missed on whole body scan (WBS) and PET/CT.

Although it had previously been recommended to avoid iodinated contrast because of the delay in RAI ablation by 8 weeks, this is no longer recommended.[10] RAI ablation is not typically given until 6 to 8 weeks after surgery, and any delay resulting from iodinated contrast is minimal. Furthermore, data has shown that even significant delays in RAI administration do not have an adverse effect.[31] Given the small size of most residual or recurrent thyroid masses, the benefit of contrast on localizing locoregional disease and evaluating soft tissue invasion outweighs the delay for RAI ablation. Communication is important when patients are administered iodinated contrast so that appropriate modifications to any planned RAI scanning or ablation can be made.

The combined use of US and contrast-enhanced CT is extremely useful in surgical planning to map out the location of suspected metastases and structural invasion. The surgical planning map amalgamates the preoperative localization studies allowing the surgeon to create a three-dimensional map of nodal targets to minimize the risk for persistent and recurrent disease.

Other Imaging Modalities

MRI

MRI is often used as a second-line imaging modality for further evaluation of a suspicious lesion after US and CT. Advantages of MRI include lack of radiation exposure and avoidance of iodinated contrast. It is useful for delineating the extent of muscular invasion, particularly within the esophagus and is indicated for patients with possible distant metastases within the central nervous system presenting with neurologic symptoms, especially before receiving RAI ablation.[10,32] However, its role in preoperative imaging is limited reduced sensitivity for detecting small-volume disease secondary to respiratory motion artifact, especially in the lower neck and chest.

Radioiodine Nuclear Imaging

Radioiodine nuclear imaging has historically held a large role in DTC surveillance, though its indications have narrowed since the introduction of surveillance USs, serial Tg measurements, and the decreased use of RAI ablation. Furthermore, about one-third of DTC tumors do not concentrate ^{131}I, which significantly decreases the sensitivity of these imaging modalities.[33] Traditional planar gamma camera WBS using ^{131}I had sensitivities as low as 50% to 60%, but with relatively good specificity (80% to 90%). Newer SPECT imaging acquires data in three dimensions and can be combined with CT (SPECT/CT) for anatomic coregistration and attenuation. The specificity of SPECT/CT with either ^{123}I- or ^{131}I-avid lesions is 100% in several studies, but its use is still limited by the fact that approximately one-third of lesions do not concentrate iodine. In cases with increasing Tg levels without clear evidence of metastasis, SPECT/CT may be useful in detecting iodine-avid lesions, both in the neck and distant metastases, and can be complementary to FDG-PET/CT when noniodine-avid lesions are present.[10,34,35]

PET/CT Scanning

^{18}FDG-PET (positron emission tomography with 18-fluoro-2deoxy-D-glucose) is primarily indicated for use in high-risk patients with biochemical evidence of recurrence (usually with Tg levels >10 ng/mL) with negative RAI imaging.[36] The sensitivity of PET/CT has been shown to be optimal in bulky diseases associated with high Tg levels. Some believe ^{18}FDG-PET can be enhanced further with rhTSH stimulation.[37] Two-thirds of DTC recurrences and metastases maintain ^{131}I-avidity, and most of these are FDG-negative.[38] The remaining one-third of metastases are ^{131}I-negative and typically demonstrate FDG uptake, which provides important prognostic information. FDG-avidity correlates with rapid tumor growth and is associated with poorly differentiated carcinomas. The combination of ^{131}I-WBS and ^{18}FDG-PET/CT detects more than 90% to 95% of recurrences and metastases.

However, [18]FDG-PET/CT scans have a high false-negative rate compared with other modalities. It is less useful in detecting low-volume recurrent disease, particularly in small metastatic nodal deposits where US and CT remain superior. It also has poor sensitivity in detecting lung metastases. Therefore negative imaging must not stop further investigations when clinical suspicion or other evidence of recurrence prevails.[39] Additionally, FDG-avidity is not limited to malignancy, and false-positive results are seen in foci of inflammation, a unilateral functioning vocal cord, and in the normal thymus.

Fine-Needle Aspiration and Thyroglobulin Washout

The ATA guidelines have strongly recommended that suspicious lesions should be at least 8 mm in the central neck or 10 mm in the lateral neck before performing a biopsy or surgical resection.[10,15] Although these measurements are typically measured in the short axis, some authors have recommended that a threshold of >8 mm or >10 mm in any diameter can signify disease and is sufficiently large enough to be targetable for surgical localization. Lesions that are smaller than 8 mm/10 mm should be closely followed for progression, but generally should not be biopsied until they reach the threshold size limits.

US-guided FNA allows for an accurate evaluation of suspicious lesions within the thyroid bed. In one study, the reported sensitivity of US-guided FNA for diagnosing recurrent carcinoma in the thyroid bed after total thyroidectomy was 100%, with a specificity of 85.7%.[40] However, inconclusive and false-negative results occur. By evaluating Tg measurements in fine-needle aspirate washouts (FNAC-Tg) of suspected metastatic lymph nodes and disease recurrence, the diagnostic accuracy and sensitivity of FNA increased significantly, with Cuhna et al. reporting 100% sensitivity and accuracy.[41,42] Furthermore, this relatively simple and inexpensive assay is valid even in the presence of TgAbs.[43]

MANAGEMENT OPTIONS

The management of recurrent and persistent locoregional metastatic disease is fundamentally different than the management of the disease at the initial surgery. Although the decision for surgery in the primary setting is usually straightforward, there is a myriad of factors that must be accounted for when deciding on treatment options for recurrent disease.[16]

- Patient-specific factors
  - Demographics (age, gender, history of radiation exposure, ethnicity[44,45])
  - Family history (thyroid cancer, Cowden syndrome,[46] familial adenomatous polyposis[47])
  - Comorbid conditions (Hashimoto's thyroiditis, high-risk surgical candidates, immunosuppression, RLN and parathyroid status)
  - Prior treatments (extensive neck surgery, history of external beam radiation therapy, number of attempts to clear locoregional recurrences)
  - Patient anxiety and ability for close surveillance
- Tumor-specific factors
  - Histologic subtype (tall cell, columnar or diffuse sclerosing variants[48])
  - Disease at initial presentation (size, extrathyroidal extension [ETE], multifocality of primary and regional metastases, lymphovascular invasion[10])
  - Tg levels (absolute levels, rate of change, doubling time <1 to 3 years)
  - Iodine avidity and/or FDG avidity on PET/CT
  - Response to initial treatment (excellent, biochemically incomplete, structurally incomplete, indeterminate[17])
  - Stability or growth of known distant metastatic lesions ("pacemaker lesions")
  - Molecular markers (BRAF^{V600E}, TERT, PAX8/PPRG)
- Anatomic factors
  - Radiographic features (microcalcifications, irregular margins, ETE)
  - The number, position, and size of metastatic nodes (ability to follow on routine examinations, accessible and amenable for percutaneous ethanol ablation)
  - Evidence of invasion of vital structures (including the larynx, trachea, esophagus, carotid artery, internal jugular vein (IJV), and vagus nerve)
  - Proximity to the RLN (especially if ipsilateral to the only functioning vocal cord)
  - Curative or palliative intent of surgery

Many patients will present with strong indications for surgical treatment of their disease, whereas other patients present with equally strong indications for observation. However, some patients will fall into a gray zone of management decision making. Appropriate therapy must be tailored to the individual patient scenario with a detailed multidisciplinary discussion regarding the risks and benefits of all options. To help clinicians incorporate increasingly complex decision-making algorithms, a multidisciplinary panel of thyroid cancer experts have created a web-based series of clinical decision-making modules (CDMM) based on current guidelines. It is important to provide a rationale behind the various treatment options and actively involve patients and their families in the decision-making process.[16]

Active Surveillance

Active surveillance with close serial follow-up using Tg, US, and possibly CT/MRI is a valid option for patients with low-volume disease. A study by Tuttle et al. found that small (<11 mm) postoperative thyroid bed nodules occur in approximately one-third of patients undergoing total thyroidectomy, with and without adjuvant RAI ablation. Of these, less than 10% of these nodules were found to be malignant lymph nodes, and even fewer demonstrated progression over time.[49] A second study by Robenshtok et al. showed that lateral neck lymph nodes also demonstrated a low potential for disease progression, even among nodes with imaging suspicious for malignancy. Over a median of 3.5 years during surveillance, only 9% of nodes increased by more than 5 mm.[50] In both studies, delay of surgical resection until disease progression was not associated with local invasion or distant metastases. In the absence of suspicious US characteristics and stable Tg levels, the majority of subcentimeter thyroid nodular disease will remain stable over a 5-year period. In contrast, a Tg doubling time of less than 1 year is a negative prognostic indicator that should prompt discussion for possible intervention. Therefore in the setting of low-volume disease, active surveillance may serve as a viable option. Many patients will be pleased with this option to avoid further surgery if they have an understanding that this is a safe and reasonable alternative.

Medical Therapies

There is growing evidence in the safe and effective use of selective treatment such as US-guided percutaneous ethanol ablation, radiofrequency ablation (RFA), and laser ablation therapies in select patients with persistent/recurrent disease (see Chapter 51, Nonsurgical Treatment of Thyroid Cysts, Nodules, Thyroid Cancer Nodal Metastases, and Hyperparathyroidism: The Role of Percutaneous Ethanol Injection). The Mayo Clinic has more than 25 years of experience with percutaneous ethanol ablation and has reported excellent outcomes in lymph node response rates based on size and Doppler blood flow.[51] In one study of 109 patients, Lewis et al. found that 93% of patients demonstrated decreased nodal volume, and they reported successful treatment of nodal disease up to 3 cm as well as treatment of lesions in close proximity to the IJV, carotid artery, and RLN.[52] A second study by Heilo et al. looked at 64 patients who received ethanol ablation and found that 84% of lymph nodes responded completely to ethanol ablation based on imaging.[53] These techniques often require multiple administrations to obtain satisfactory results but may confer significant health system cost savings compared with surgery and postoperative hospitalizations.

RFA under US guidance is a similar nodule-directed technique for nonsurgical ablation. RFA typically uses a 1 to 2 cm active tip probe placed under local anesthesia within the center of a nodule and heated to 90° C for 2 minutes, creating a coagulative necrosis of the thyroid nodule.[54] Some have argued that the heat generated may cause damage to the RLN, parathyroid gland, carotid, or IJV, though many studies have demonstrated the safety and efficacy, albeit in limited cohorts of patients.[55,56] Currently, the ATA guidelines state a general consensus, but no formal recommendation, that both ethanol ablation and RFA should be considered in patients who are poor surgical candidates. Most studies that describe this technique are limited in sample size, had a relatively short follow-up, and consisted of lymph node disease smaller than a centimeter.[10]

Although surgical resection continues to be favored in the ATA guidelines for recurrent structural disease management, RAI may be an option in certain situations, including patients with rising Tg levels in the absence of radiographic disease, those with surgically unresectable disease, such as disease involving a single functioning RLN, and distant metastatic disease where surgical resection may not provide a cure. However, the ATA guidelines recommend against the use of RAI in cases with iodine-refractory masses on scintigraphy or persistently elevated Tg levels despite RAI administration.[10] Important side effects and complications of RAI, including xerophthalmia, xerostomia, and radiation-induced malignancy to breast, bone, and stomach, must be discussed with the patient and weighed into the risk-benefit analysis (see Chapter 48, Postoperative Radioactive Iodine Ablation and Treatment of Differentiated Thyroid Cancer).[57,58]

SURGICAL MANAGEMENT

The two main indications for reoperation are completion thyroidectomy for thyroid cancer diagnosed after initial lobectomy, and reexploration of the central compartment and superior mediastinal dissection for recurrent disease after prior total thyroidectomy. Additional indications include locoregional metastasis to the lateral neck requiring therapeutic lateral neck dissection with elective central neck dissection for occult disease, and oligometastatic lesions in the mediastinum that are amenable to surgery with curative intent.

The 2015 ATA guidelines recommend that surgical treatment should be reserved for structurally persistent or recurrent lesions that are of sufficient size (defined as >8 mm in the central neck, >10 mm in the lateral neck). Under no circumstances should an exploration be undertaken if a lesion cannot be localized on anatomic imaging using either US or CT scan.[10,15]

Reoperation can be associated with significantly increased risks, particularly with respect to the RLNs and parathyroid glands.[5,59] Prior injury to these structures during the initial surgery may have significant implications after revision surgery, and these risks should be discussed with the patient thoroughly, including tracheostomy. However, reoperative surgery has been shown to have low morbidity in experienced hands, and many studies have reported rates ranging from 0.4% to 4% of permanent hypocalcemia or RLN injury (see "Complications" section).[7,9,60] Each surgeon should know his or her individual operative risk rate, and if the volume of reoperative surgery is low, then referral to a more experienced surgeon may be in the patient's best interest.

Preoperative Documentation

Careful review of the primary surgery operative note (and subsequent operative notes, if any) and all pathology reports is essential for planning revision surgery. Factors associated with increased surgical difficulty include the need for resection of the strap muscles, extensive IJV dissection, and cases associated with sternotomy, as these scenarios cause potentially dangerous distortion of venous anatomy in the lower neck. The status of the parathyroid glands may be discerned from the operative note, but in many cases, it can be more helpful to look for the presence of parathyroid tissue in the pathology reports as it is not uncommon to have unrecognized parathyroid gland removal.

The status of the RLN should be noted in the initial operative report, and its functional status should always be tested and documented preoperatively with the use of indirect laryngoscopy or stroboscopy. Unrecognized RLN injuries occur during thyroid surgery, and clinical symptoms alone are not reliable for documenting RLN function. Recognizing RLN dysfunction preoperatively is essential for surgical planning, especially in circumstances where there is risk of injury to the last functioning RLN, as this may alter the extent of surgical resection or increase the likelihood of a tracheostomy postoperatively. Reoperation on the last functioning nerve should only be performed after a thorough discussion with both the patient and the referring endocrinologist because this can dramatically alter the quality of life after surgery, and the surgical risk may be higher than other nonsurgical options.

Anatomic Changes After Thyroidectomy

A thorough knowledge of the normal anatomy of the neck and its common variations, especially within the central visceral compartment, provides the fundamental basis for considering both primary and reoperative surgery. Changes in cervical anatomy after primary thyroidectomy provide increased challenges to the surgeon. Scar tissue and subsequent scar contraction may cause increased difficulty in identifying and dissecting important structures. The carotid sheath is an important landmark in revision thyroid surgery as it provides a constant lateral boundary of dissection is also important when identifying the RLN.[61] The great vessels of the neck may medialize after thyroidectomy and may be directly adjacent and adherent to the trachea. If the strap muscles were excised because of tumor involvement, the great vessels may be superficial and medial, and the scarring in the central neck is typically dense. The IJV may become superficial and adherent to the undersurface of the anterior border of the sternocleidomastoid (SCM) muscle, particularly if a tumor was peeled off the IJV during a prior surgery. These venous structures in reoperative surgery are perhaps the most difficult to manage, primarily because of their tendency to scar to adjacent musculature. The brachiocephalic artery may be drawn high in the lower central neck because of scar contracture.

Within the central neck compartment, the RLN is often difficult to identify and dissect because it is buried in scar tissue. Scarring under the strap muscles may lead to a superficial RLN becoming adherent to the undersurface of the muscles. On occasion, RLNs have been described on the anterior wall of the trachea due to scarring and wound contracture. During revision central neck dissection, the RLN is frequently scarred to the upper cervical trachea over a span of the first several tracheal rings and lateral cricoid cartilage and is most commonly injured in this segment (see Chapter 36, Surgical Anatomy and Monitoring of the Recurrent Laryngeal Nerve). The tracheoesophageal groove itself may be scarred and distorted, making the identification of the esophagus almost impossible. Placement of a bougie may help prevent inadvertent esophageal perforation during dissection. The location of preserved parathyroid glands will often be grossly distorted. Parathyroid and RLN identification during revision central neck dissection require a bloodless field.

General Principles of Reoperative Thyroid Surgery

The use of surgical loupes and a headlight may be of benefit in the identification of critical structures and aid in safe disease removal. Hemostasis is critical for reoperative procedures. Traditional techniques rely on bipolar cauterization and vascular suture ligation, but newer devices (such as Ligasure, Harmonic scalpel, and Thunderbolt) have shown similar rates of success with potentially narrower thermal transfer and shorter operative times.[62] Surgical clips can result in scatter artifact, complicating subsequent cross-sectional imaging (CT or MRI) during follow-up.

An important surgical technique in the reoperative setting is to first work in areas more distant from the prior dissection to safely identify neural and vascular structures and then safely transition into the previously dissected areas. The carotid artery is the key landmark that allows global orientation in the reoperative field.

Recurrent Laryngeal Nerve Identification

In 1938, Lahey and Hoover reported their techniques of microdissection of the RLN in more than 3000 thyroidectomies, showing a fivefold reduction in clinically evident RLN injuries at only 0.3%. Lahey advocated for complete exposure of the nerve using 2.5× magnification loupes with the surgeon standing on the ipsilateral side of dissection and immediate end-to-end reanastomosis of the RLN if it is divided. Lahey demonstrated that avoidance of RLN injury is best achieved by identifying the nerve early in the dissection and maintaining positive visualization, thus protecting the entire length of the nerve throughout the surgery.[63] As a general principle, the RLN should be identified in a previously undissected area and then followed into the dissected area. In this way, the reoperative surgeon goes below the former surgeon's scar.

Many surgeons routinely use intraoperative neural monitoring (IONM) to provide a functional assessment of the RLN during surgery. In 2010 the International Intraoperative Monitoring Study Group published guidelines for safe and effective use of IONM in thyroid surgery.[64] The use of IONM can be valuable in maintaining the functional integrity of the RLN, particularly in reoperative thyroid surgery, as the location of the RLN is less constant and embedded in scar tissue (see Chapter 36, Surgical Anatomy and Monitoring of the Recurrent Laryngeal Nerve).[65-68] A large study evaluating the use of IONM on 1000 RLN-at-risk patients showed that the postoperative RLN palsy rate in reoperative patients was significantly higher in the control group compared with the neuro-monitored group (19% versus 7.8%).[67]

RLN Invasion

New guidelines exist for the management of RLN invasion with thyroid cancer.[69,70] Invasive disease should be dissected sharply free from the nerve if at all possible. On rare occasions, this may not adequately remove gross disease and the nerve must be sacrificed (see Chapter 36, Surgical Anatomy and Monitoring of the Recurrent Laryngeal Nerve). However, there are several important considerations that the surgeon must weigh before nerve resection. The first is to confirm that the diagnosis is carcinoma and that the nerve has been thoroughly dissected both above and below the invaded region and cannot in any way be preserved. The preoperative function of both nerves is also important. A nonfunctioning RLN discovered preoperatively and found to be invaded at surgery should be sacrificed. Invasion of the last functioning RLN deserves special consideration, and ideally, should be discussed preoperatively with the patient and referring endocrinologist. The surgeon must weigh alternative treatment options, including thyroid hormone suppression, RAI ablation, alcohol ablation, or external beam radiation therapy. In patients with distant metastasis, one should also consider the location of the "pacemaker" of the disease and be less aggressive at the neck if there is distant disease that is progressing.

If a segment of the RLN is necessarily sacrificed because of disease involvement, a tension-free end-to-end anastomosis is the best option for improving vocal quality. If a tension-free end-to-end anastomosis is not possible between the distal and proximal ends, an ansa cervicalis-to-RLN anastomosis has been shown to provide acceptable laryngeal reinnervation with favorable synkinesis providing excellent functional results.[71] Care should be taken to preserve the ansa cervicalis during initial jugular dissection. The SCM is mobilized laterally to expose the omohyoid muscle. The ansa cervicalis is then identified deep to the SCM overlying the IJV. A sufficient length of the ansa is mobilized to the cut end of the RLN to allow a tension-free anastomosis using 9-0 nylon with interrupted epineural stitches. In circumstances where the distal stump of the RLN is too short for ansa-to-RLN graft, or the ansa cervicalis is injured, a bridging cable graft using the great auricular nerve between the RLN-to-RLN or ansa-to-RLN anastomosis can be considered with favorable voice outcomes.[72]

Parathyroid Gland Preservation

Permanent hypoparathyroidism can be a disabling complication. Preservation of all parathyroid tissue at the first operation helps decrease the incidence of hypoparathyroidism in reoperative surgery. However, many times the parathyroid glands have not been seen or been commented on in the original operative report. Further, the persistent function of all the parathyroid glands documented to have been preserved and deemed viable at the end of the primary surgery cannot be relied on when undertaking completion or revision thyroid surgery.

Despite the risk of hypoparathyroidism in the reoperative setting, the literature has demonstrated that in experienced hands, transient hypocalcemia may occur in up to 30% of cases, but permanent hypoparathyroidism remains less than 3% to 4%.[6,7,9] Careful immediate extracapsular dissection of the thyroid and autotransplantation of devascularized parathyroid tissue are believed to be important contributory factors to achieving such a low complication rate.

Knowledge of the normal anatomic locations and the common variations of the parathyroid glands is a prerequisite in the identification and preservation of these structures in both primary and revision surgery. Revision surgery poses more of a challenge because the normal anatomic location of the parathyroid glands has been invariably disrupted and there is scarring, making it difficult to visually locate the glands. When reoperative surgery is done in the clinical setting of central neck recurrences after a previous total thyroidectomy, any remaining parathyroid glands are sometimes removed en bloc with the tumor dissection specimen. If the parathyroid glands can be safely separated from the dissection mass and confirmed to be uninvolved with the tumor, then the remaining parathyroid tissue should be reimplanted.

Parathyroid Autotransplantation

Parathyroid glands left in situ should be carefully inspected upon completion of resection to ensure that they are viable. When the vascularity of the gland is questionable, it should be removed and placed in normal saline solution immediately to prevent desiccation and a nonviable autograft. A small biopsy may be sent for frozen section (FS) to confirm parathyroid tissue and exclude tumor involvement, as lymph node metastases can closely mimic parathyroid tissue. After histologic confirmation, the gland is finely minced with scissors or scalpel. A small pocket is created within a well-vascularized muscle bed, typically the SCM. The minced parathyroid gland is inserted in the muscle pocket, which is closed with a figure-of-eight suture using absorbable suture. We mark the implant site with titanium ligation clips for future identification in the unlikely event that the patient requires a subtotal parathyroidectomy for secondary hyperparathyroidism. There are other methods of autotransplantation, and the site of implantation varies with the surgeon's preference, including forearm, pectoralis muscle, and trapezius.

Some authors have questioned the value of autotransplantation when other normal/viable parathyroid glands are seen in situ. Lo et al. showed that autotransplantation significantly reduced the risk of permanent hypoparathyroidism compared with patients who did not undergo autotransplantation.[73]

REOPERATIVE SURGERY: COMPLETION THYROIDECTOMY

Indications

In patients with a solitary, cytologically indeterminate nodule, the 2015 ATA guidelines strongly recommend performing a thyroid lobectomy as an initial surgical approach for patients who would otherwise be at low-risk for malignancy. Completion thyroidectomy should be offered to patients who would have been recommended to undergo a total thyroidectomy if the diagnosis had been known before the initial surgery (multicentric disease, size >4 cm, high-risk histologic subtypes, ETE). A completion thyroidectomy can allow for better postoperative surveillance with Tg levels and is strongly recommended in patients requiring RAI ablative therapy.[10,12]

Surgical Pearls

The best way to minimize the complication risk of revision surgery is to avoid it altogether with appropriate patient selection. Surgeons should ensure that any unavoidable need for reoperation be facilitated by employing good surgical principles in the initial surgery to reduce associated morbidity.

Adequate Treatment of Disease at Primary Surgery

For all thyroid nodules, the minimal operation should be a total lobectomy, which entails the complete removal of one lobe along with the isthmus. This helps eliminate the need for revision surgery on the ipsilateral side in the event of recurrence. Reoperation in the invariably scarred ipsilateral thyroid bed because of a recurrence after a partial lobectomy puts the patient at an unnecessarily high risk for injury and is avoidable by performing a total lobectomy at the initial surgery. Additionally, clearance of all prelaryngeal and pretracheal nodes at the first surgery serves to limit completion surgery to removal of the contralateral lobe only.

Avoidance of Contralateral Lobe Palpation

Unnecessary exposure and dissection of the contralateral lobe increases scarring and thus morbidity. Reoperation on the contralateral lobe will be easier when the tissue plane between the sternothyroid muscle and the thyroid capsule is not disturbed during primary surgery. Therefore intraoperative assessment of the contralateral lobe should be performed without disrupting this plane by palpating the lobe superficial to the sternothyroid muscle. Given that palpation is known to be less accurate than ultrasonography, an intraoperative examination is generally unnecessary, because ultrasonography is widely performed preoperatively.

Timing of Completion Surgery

Once the need for completion thyroidectomy has been established, the completion thyroidectomy should be performed at an interval from the original surgery that may decrease the risk of surgical complications. However, this timing is controversial. Some authors state that the completion thyroidectomy should optimally be performed within 7 days before the development of scarring. Other authors say that 6 weeks to 3 months after the initial operation is the optimal time, after the resolution of perioperative inflammation.[74] Still other authors state that the timing of reoperation has no effect on the development of complications.[75,76] We generally prefer to wait 2 months after the first surgery to offer completion surgery.

REOPERATIVE SURGERY: CENTRAL NECK DISSECTION-PARATRACHEAL AND SUPERIOR MEDIASTINAL DISSECTION

General Principles

Reoperation of the central compartment and thyroid bed after a prior total thyroidectomy calls for meticulous dissection of the resultant scar tissue to identify the RLN and preserve remaining parathyroid tissue (see Chapter 38, Central Neck Dissection: Indications and Technique).[77]

Anatomic and Surgical Boundaries of Central Neck Compartment Surgery

The 2008 Consensus Statement on the classification and terminology of neck dissection by the American Head and Neck Society describes the medial border of the sternomastoid muscles to delineate the lateral boundary of level VI from levels III and IV.[78] However, this landmark is not easily discerned radiographically, and radiologists typically use the medial aspect of the common carotid artery as the radiologic landmark separating levels III and IV from level VI. Level VI extends from the level of the hyoid bone superiorly to the level of the suprasternal notch inferiorly. Superior mediastinal lymph nodes, designated level VII, are paratracheal lymph nodes below the suprasternal notch extending to the innominate artery inferiorly. In 2009, the ATA provided its consensus statement on central neck dissection and described the central neck compartment as representing levels VI and VII together, extending from the hyoid bone superiorly to the innominate artery level inferiorly. Four nodal basins are described within the central neck compartment: prelaryngeal (Delphian) nodes located centrally between the hyoid bone and cricoid cartilage; pretracheal nodes located centrally between the cricoid cartilage and the innominate artery; and bilateral paratracheal nodes located between the trachea and carotid arteries bilaterally, the cricoid cartilage superiorly, and the innominate artery inferiorly. Clinically evident nodal disease in the supracricoid prelaryngeal basin is infrequent and dissection is usually only undertaken if clinically evident nodes are present.[79]

Indications for Lateral Neck Dissection

Approximately 30% to 40% of patients will present with metastatic DTC in lateral neck nodes during routine surveillance (see "Recurrence

Rates and Patterns" section). The 2015 ATA guidelines strongly recommend therapeutic neck dissection for biopsy-proven lateral neck metastases. Approximately 73% of these patients will have disease in multiple levels, and current literature supports the selective neck dissection of levels II to Vb, though some authors propose dissection of levels II to IV alone.

In patients who present with disease limited to the lateral neck, the authors advocate for an elective ipsilateral central neck dissection based on high rates of occult central neck nodes. Roh et al. reviewed patients who underwent therapeutic lateral and elective central neck dissections for lateral cervical recurrence of papillary thyroid cancer (PTC) and found a high incidence (86%) of positive central nodes in patients with only clinically evident lateral neck disease.[80]

When performing a lateral neck dissection, we prefer to begin our procedure with the lateral neck dissection before performing the revision central neck dissection.

Revision Central Neck Dissection Operative Technique

Step 1: Preparation and Positioning

The patient is intubated with a nerve-monitoring endotracheal tube. A shoulder roll is placed to slightly hyperextend the neck, and the function of the nerve monitor is verified. The patient is placed in reverse Trendelenburg position to facilitate venous drainage and minimize bleeding.

Step 2: Planning the Incision

In patients with recurrent/persistent disease, the incision line is usually dictated by the patient's prior surgical procedure(s). A 4 to 5 cm incision length can adequately provide access and visualization for a reoperative total thyroidectomy and central compartment dissection. Further extension laterally (paralleling the collar line into level V) can be used for those patients requiring a selective lateral neck dissection of levels II to V as well.

Step 3: Excision of Scar and Flap Elevation

Many surgeons use local anesthesia, commonly 1% lidocaine or 0.5% bupivacaine with 1:200,000 epinephrine, for both postoperative pain management and incision hemostasis.

The previous incisional scar is excised down to the subplatysmal level and sent for routine pathology. Monopolar electrocautery is used to develop subplatysmal flaps to the level of the laryngeal prominence superiorly, and the sternal notch and clavicles inferiorly. The platysma is frequently dehiscent in the midline and scar tissue may obscure the proper level. Care is taken to avoid injury to the underlying anterior jugular veins. The flaps are retracted with either six 1-0 silk sutures placed at the base of the elevated flaps or using self-retaining retractors.

Step 4: Management of Strap Muscles

The strap muscles are divided in the midline with monopolar cautery using fingertip retraction to help identify the midline raphe. This division continues to the intervening soft tissue inferiorly at the sternal notch to as inferiorly as possible, with care to avoid damage to the anterior jugular veins. Given that optimal exposure is mandatory, we divide both the ipsilateral sternohyoid and sternothyroid strap muscles horizontally midway between the cricoid cartilage and the sternal notch, using mosquito forceps and monopolar cautery. The superior and inferior slips of muscle are then carefully reflected from the underlying soft tissue using bipolar cautery and blunt dissection with a Kittner/pusher/peanut sponge. The strap muscles can easily be reapproximated at the end of the procedure if they do not need to be resected for oncologic reasons.

Some surgeons prefer to dissect the lateral margin of the strap muscles and then retract the strap muscles medially. Other surgeons choose to release the infrahyoid strap musculature at the most inferior extent of their sternal and clavicular attachments. Some surgeons routinely resect the strap muscles in recurrent cases out of concern that they are implanted with carcinoma. This may be important to consider in high-risk patients or those who have undergone more than one surgical procedure in this area, but with retraction of these muscles usually provides satisfactory superior mediastinal access. The lateral or backdoor approach can avoid midline scarring and provide carotid sheath orientation and vagal stimulation and has great utility in revision central neck surgery (Figure 50.1).

Step 5: Exposure of Common Carotid Artery

The key to anatomic identification in this operation is the extensive dissection of the common carotid artery (see Chapter 38, Central Neck Dissection: Indications and Technique; Figure 50.2). The carotid arteries act as a "shield" to protect the RLN, which lies deep to the carotid artery.

Dissection begins with identifying the carotid superiorly at the level of the thyroid cartilage. The soft tissue overlying the anterior surface of the carotid is dissected with a fine mosquito hemostat and microbipolar cautery using the "pinch-burn" technique. Dissection proceeds inferiorly to the level of the innominate artery in the upper mediastinum. The "pinch-burn" technique employs grasping a small amount of tissue to be divided, applying energy to cauterize the tissue, and then firmly pinching the tissues with a light flick of the wrist to cut the tissue.

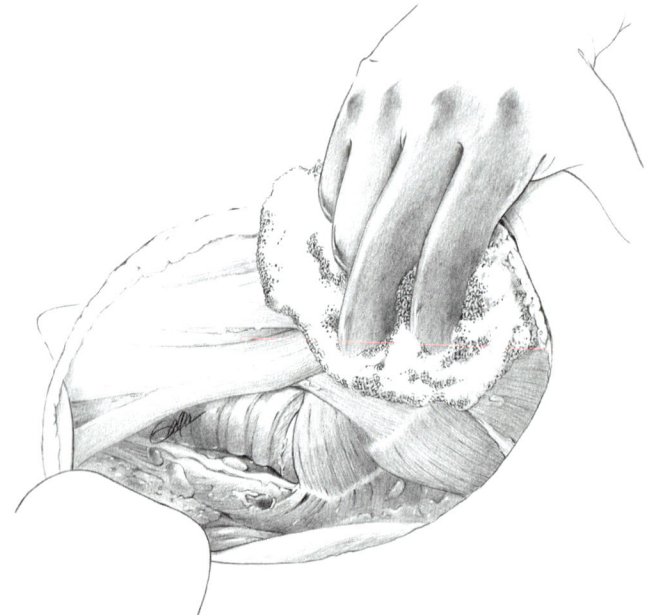

Fig. 50.1 Lateral or backdoor approach to recurrent laryngeal nerve exposure during revision central neck surgery.

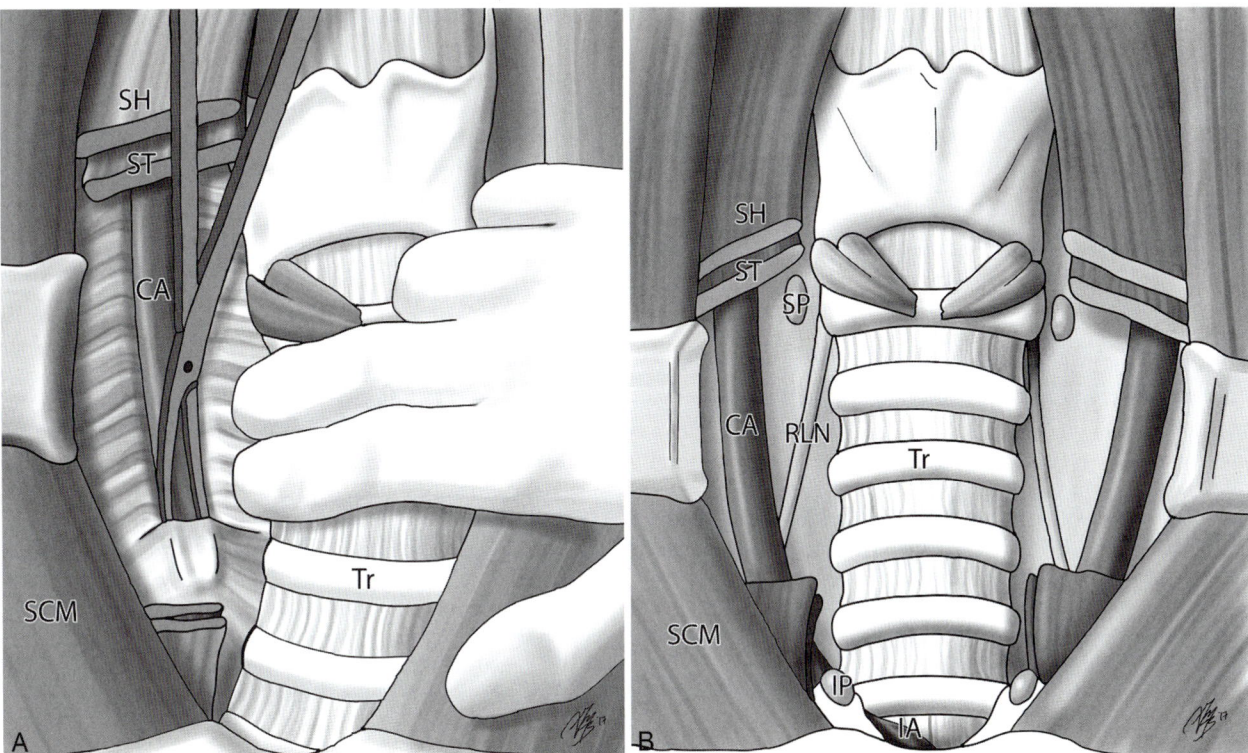

Fig. 50.2 Unsheathing the anterior aspect of the carotid artery (CA). Note the previous division of the sternohyoid (SH) and sternothyroid (ST) muscles. Tr, trachea, SCM, sternocleidomastoid muscle. **(B)** Final view of a revision bilateral central neck compartment dissection. IA, innominate artery, IP, inferior parathyroid gland, RLN, recurrent laryngeal nerve, SP, superior parathyroid gland. (From Busato GM, Freeman J. Revision central neck dissection. *Oper Tech Otolaryngol Head Neck Surg.* 2018;29[1]:24–29.)

The insulated, nonstick ophthalmic microbipolar forceps focus energy at the tip, allowing for effective cauterization and efficient division of tissue.

When operating within the superior mediastinum, we lower the patient's head to a near-flat or even Trendelenburg position, raise the bed, and the primary surgeon repositions to the head of the bed. This provides an important vantage point in visualizing and dissecting the superior mediastinum.

Step 6: Identification of the RLN

Once the carotid artery is exposed along its length down to its origin, the RLN is identified inferiorly using blunt dissection with a Kittner/pusher sponge. The technique of neural mapping can be used to localize the RLN before visualization (see Chapter 36, Surgical Anatomy and Monitoring of the Recurrent Laryngeal Nerve). Identifying the RLN in its inferior-most extent has two benefits: first, the nerve tends to have a more constant position in this area in a previously operated neck; and second, this area is less likely to have been violated during the initial procedure with less fibrotic tissue to dissect over the nerve. Gentle teasing of the fascia away from the lateral surface of the nerve along its long axis with dissecting mosquito forceps and blunt dissection with cotton pushers provides safe identification of the nerve.

Microdissection of the nerve continues from an inferior to superior direction, up to the nerve's insertion under the cricothyroid muscle, with care to preserve any small branches along its course. Great care must be taken to avoid stretching the nerve or using the bipolar cautery too close to the nerve, as there can be collateral thermal damage 1 to 6 mm from the site of contact.[62]

Step 7: Dissection of the Parathyroid Glands and Thymus

The inferior parathyroid glands are usually situated at the superior aspect of the thymus. As such, the thymic tissue along with the inferior parathyroid gland is dissected away from the pretracheal tissues with bipolar cauterization and blunt dissection. This tissue is reflected anteriorly out of the central compartment in continuity with the thymus, usually preserving the blood supply and thus decreasing the risk of hypoparathyroidism. The superior glands are usually found just lateral and posterior to the insertion of the RLN as it passes deep to the cricothyroid muscle. It is always preferable to positively identify the parathyroid glands before completing the central neck dissection (see "Parathyroid Gland Preservation" section).

Step 8: Paratracheal Dissection

At this point in the dissection, all relevant anatomic structures within the central neck compartment should be exposed—from the thyroid cartilage to innominate artery and from carotid to carotid laterally. To dissect the paratracheal tissues, the operating surgeon should reposition to the ipsilateral side of dissection. The lymphatic tissue can now be carefully microdissected around the RLN as necessary. Dissection medial to the nerve is always required. The contents medial to the RLN are freed from their fascial attachments to the nerve and elevated toward the midline. In patients with more extensive disease burden, it may be necessary to dissect out the fibrofatty tissue lateral or deep to the RLN. Dissection of tissue lateral to the RLN can increase the risk of damage to the nerve and the blood supply to the parathyroid glands and is not necessary if there is no disease noted here. Metastatic nodes lateral to the nerve and lying on the esophagus are not infrequent, and removing these as a separate specimen rather than as an en bloc resection is safe and may be preferable to trying to pass them under the nerve.

Nodal disease may be found associated with thyroid superior pole structures. Less frequently, lymph nodes around the constrictors of the pharynx and esophagus are found. Rests of residual disease can be found both lateral and medial to the RLN at its insertion point, usually because of incomplete primary resection at Berry's ligament. The superior mediastinal, pretracheal, and paratracheal contents are then stepwise freed from the pretracheal fascia. Monopolar electrocautery in the pretracheal fascial plane can be safely used as long as the RLNs are maintained at least 1 cm from the cautery.

Step 9: Check Dissection Specimen for Parathyroid Tissue

Identified parathyroid glands should be checked for viability on their natural pedicle. Any signs of devascularization should prompt removal and autotransplantation (see "Parathyroid Gland Preservation" section). The dissected specimen is then examined ex vivo for potential parathyroid tissue. Parathyroid tissue may be difficult to differentiate from metastatic nodes, which may necessitate frozen-section pathology before reimplantation. Parathyroid tissue that is intimately associated with involved nodal tissue should not be transplanted (see "Parathyroid Autotransplantation" section).

Step 10: Final Hemostasis and Surgical Bed Preparation

After the return of normotension, a Valsalva maneuver is performed to evaluate for bleeding, which is controlled with bipolar cautery if the bleeding is not near critical structures. The wound bed is then irrigated, and a second Valsalva maneuver is performed to check for final hemostasis. Troublesome bleeding frequently occurs close to the recurrent nerves.

If healthy and unresected, the previously divided sternohyoid strap muscles are repaired with absorbable suture horizontally and reapproximated in the midline to provide coverage of the great vessels, RLNs, parathyroid tissue, and bare trachea from the overlying skin flaps. If the strap muscles have been excised because of disease involvement, soft tissue coverage of the trachea and great vessels can be achieved using a unilateral or bilateral SCM muscle rotation flap. A sufficient amount of the anteromedial portion of the SCM is divided with monopolar cautery and rotated into the midline while maintaining either a lower or upper pedicle attachment to the rest of the muscle belly and centrally apposed to its opposing muscle flap covering the bare trachea and adjacent carotid sheaths.

Step 11: Wound Closure

We do not routinely place surgical drains for our thyroidectomies and central neck dissections without lateral neck dissection. Closure is performed in an esthetic fashion with platysmal plication using a running absorbable suture and a running subcuticular skin closure with absorbable monofilament suture. Steri-Strips are placed over the incision.

Postoperative Management

Most patients are discharged the morning after surgery with appropriate wound care instruction. Many studies have shown that postoperative parathyroid hormone (PTH) levels predict hypocalcemia (although lacking 100% accuracy) and thus allow early implementation of calcium replacement therapy and calcitriol to reduce the incidence and severity of hypocalcemia and the duration of the patient's hospital stay.[81,82] Stable or improving serum calcium levels are verified in all patients before discharge.

Complications

Because of scarring in the thyroid bed, several studies have reported the incidence of transient and permanent RLN injury and hypoparathyroidism after reoperative thyroid surgery to be significantly higher than that of primary thyroid surgery. However, more recent studies report that, in experienced hands, the incidence of permanent hypoparathyroidism and permanent RLN injury is in the range of 0.4% to 4%, and overall morbidity after reoperative surgery is comparable to that for primary surgery of the same extent. Lefevre et al. reported on a large series of patients operated on for recurrent benign and malignant disease with a permanent RLN paralysis rate of 1.5%, and they found a permanent hypoparathyroidism rate of 2.5%. In this series, significant hematomas occurred in 0.9% and wound infections in 0.2% of patients.[6] Two recent series demonstrate low rates of RLN paralysis and variable rates of up to 6% of permanent hypoparathyroidism.[83,84] To achieve such low morbidity, adherence to a well-established revision surgery algorithm and ongoing auditing of performance is required. If the local complication rates are significantly higher than general reported figures from experienced centers, the patients must be appropriately counseled about the institutional morbidity rates and consideration must be given for external referral.

Adjunctive Techniques in Revision Surgery

Preoperative and Intraoperative Investigations

Pre- and intraoperative investigations may be used to reduce the need for re-operative surgery and unnecessary overtreatment for benign and low-risk disease. US guidance has significantly augmented the success of FNA examinations and is the gold standard for all thyroid nodules in many institutions. However, a significant number of indeterminate FNAs and the inability to differentiate malignant Hürthle cell and follicular lesions from benign nodules remains a challenge for the surgeon. Some centers employ intraoperative FS analysis to delineate some of these lesions.[85] The clinical utility of FS is highly variable, and the value of FS must be carefully assessed at each center.

Ultrasound-Guided Revision Thyroid Surgery

Intraoperative localization of small recurrent disease, clinically undetectable (palpation or visually), can be very challenging and result in a failed exploration. Several adjunctive methods using US imaging intraoperatively may be used to improve the successful excision of small-volume disease and lesions obscured by thick scar tissue. Several studies have described US-guided techniques to inject dye or radioactive material into the diseased tissue to aid intraoperative visualization or localization using gamma probes. These studies have reported favorable outcomes.[86,87] Also, given that relative anatomy alters with head positioning on the operating room table, preincision "tattooing" of the recurrent disease has been described to offer benefit in accurate location of small-volume disease.[88]

Radioguided Revision Thyroid Surgery

Radioguidance surgery with ^{131}I or ^{123}I radioisotopes has gained attention in reoperative thyroid surgery, both in the management of residual thyroid tissue (thyroid remnant), and recurrent or persistent iodine-avid DTC.[89] Salvatori et al., in their series of 10 patients, were able to locate and remove the foci of disease using ^{131}I-guided surgery with high sensitivity and specificity.[90] For noniodine-avid DTC, ^{99m}Tc–sestamibi scanning has been successfully used for radioguided surgery.[91]

In a series of 58 patients with iodine-negative locoregional recurrent DTC, Rubello et al. found that ^{99m}Tc–sestamibi-guided radiosurgery was helpful in locating tumors intraoperatively, especially when those tumors were located in fibrotic tissue or hidden behind blood vessels.[92] Others have used ^{18}FDG isotope in noniodine-avid recurrences and have shown benefit in disease localization.[93] A combined technique using US-guidance for the injection of radioisotope into the lesion preoperatively has also been described. Although the feasibility of radioguided surgery has been established and may help decrease the morbidity of reoperative surgery, its utility in treatment and benefit in survival has yet to be proved in large prospective studies.

Outcomes of Revision Thyroid Surgery for Recurrent Disease

Al-Saif et al. examined their outcome of surgical resection of recurrent thyroid cancer and demonstrated biochemical complete remission (undetectable stimulated Tg [sTg] levels) in 27% of patients, and a further 46% of patients achieved a significant reduction of sTg levels <2 ng/mL.[94] Schuff et al. reported that 41% of cases achieved complete biochemical remission and a further 31% achieved more than a 50% reduction in sTg levels after revision surgery for recurrent disease.[95] Palme et al. researched the outcome of revision surgery in 73 patients with recurrent DTC and demonstrated a 20-year disease-specific survival of 94% in those with a single recurrence and 60% in those with multiple recurrences, with an overall 20-year survival of 83% and 58%, respectively.[96] Multivariate regression analysis demonstrated that male gender, advanced stage at presentation, and ETE were most predictive for multiple treatment failures/recurrences. This study reaffirmed the importance of close surveillance with patients after surgery, with worse survival in patients presenting with clinically evident disease. It also demonstrated that patients with only one recurrence had similar survival rates as those without recurrence, but multiple recurrences significantly decrease disease-specific and overall survival rates.

CONCLUSION

- Routine surveillance with Tg and neck US should be performed on all patients with thyroid carcinoma.
- The workup of concerning findings should include CT with intravenous (IV) contrast and FNA biopsy with Tg washout of sufficiently sized lesions (>8 mm in the central neck, >10 mm in the lateral neck).
- Nonoperative management options include active surveillance, US-guided percutaneous ethanol ablation or RFA, RAI ablation, or external beam radiation therapy.
- Surgical risks due to anatomic changes after primary surgery are best managed with appropriate patient selection, careful preoperative planning, and meticulous surgical techniques.

Reoperative thyroid surgery for recurrent and persistent differentiated thyroid carcinoma presents multiple challenges for clinicians from surveillance, diagnosis, and management options to intraoperative decisions involving at-risk structures, including the RLN and parathyroid glands. Clinicians must remain up to date on current practice guidelines so that they can have informative discussions with affected patients.

REFERENCES

For a complete list of references, go to expertconsult.com

51

Nonsurgical Treatment of Thyroid Cysts, Nodules, Thyroid Cancer Nodal Metastases, and Hyperparathyroidism: The Role of Percutaneous Ethanol Injection

Devaprabu Abraham, Nikita R. Abraham

> Please go to expertconsult.com to view related video:
> **Video 51.1** Floating Debris
> **Video 51.2** Percutaneous Ethanol Injection: Cyst Injection
> **Video 51.3** Percutaneous Ethanol Injection: Toxic Adenoma
> **Video 51.4** Percutaneous Ethanol Injection: Metastasis
> **Video 51.5** Ultrasound Cord Check

INTRODUCTION

Thyroid neoplasms and cysts are common in the general population.[1] The primary intervention offered to these patients in the United States is surgical removal. Despite the advances in surgical training and techniques, surgery carries a 2% to 10% risk of complications, even when performed in large-volume surgical centers.[2] The wide availability of high-resolution ultrasound (US) equipment and the ever-increasing interventional expertise among practicing clinicians enables the use of novel US-guided percutaneous interventional procedures during office visits, in particular, percutaneous ethanol injection (PEI).[3,4] The equipment costs and the needed materials are minimal for PEI compared with radiofrequency ablation (RFA) or LASER therapies. Although the use of percutaneous interventions has potential cost-saving benefits with fewer side effects, they are still not offered widely or as first-line therapies, particularly in the U.S.[5] The head and neck lesions amenable to PEI, the techniques involved, and its efficacy, will be reviewed in this chapter.

GENERAL PRINCIPLES OF US-GUIDED PERCUTANEOUS ETHANOL INJECTION OF CYSTS AND TUMORS

Injection of chemical agents with nonspecific tissue destructive properties poses risks to patients; therefore acquiring expertise and training a team of skilled assisting staff are prerequisites. A thorough understanding of the US anatomy and recognizing the danger areas are needed to avoid procedure-related complications. A thorough explanation of the procedure, purpose, alternatives, and the risks involved with PEI should be disclosed to patients. Nervous patients who cannot be reassured verbally may require pretreatment with a suitable anxiolytic. Intravenous or conscious sedation is generally not needed for PEI. If desired, lidocaine infiltration is an acceptable form of anesthesia for PEI. During PEI, if a patient encounters unusual pain, voice changes (recurrent laryngeal nerve [RLN] or vagus nerve injury), or breathing difficulties, the procedure should be stopped immediately.

Several organic and inorganic chemicals have been tried as sclerosants in clinical practice for inducing tissue destruction and fibrosis. The agents that have been used for sclerotherapy are ethyl alcohol, talc, tetracycline and bleomycin, acetic and hydrochloric acids, and attenuated strains of bacteria.[5,6] Even though various agents have been tried for the injection of thyroid cysts and tumors, the use of ethanol has become the mainstay for percutaneous injection sclerotherapy.[5-9] In higher concentrations (>95%), ethyl alcohol is very effective at inducing tissue destruction and sclerosis. Ethanol is not tissue specific in its destructive potential; therefore, whenever possible, only the minimal amount of alcohol required for therapeutic success is administered, using the thinnest gauge needle for any given tumor. This may even mean that submaximal treatment is administered over many sittings with reassessment and reinjections based upon response. A large-volume ethanol injection in any one sitting is best avoided because the diffusion of alcohol is unpredictable as the injected volume increases. Ethanol in high concentration destroys any type of tissue given sufficient duration of contact. Therefore a clear understanding of the anatomy and accurate needle placement under imaging guidance is crucial for preventing collateral tissue destruction during PEI.[10] Ethanol-mediated tissue destruction is attributed to several mechanisms. Immediate functional impairment results from acute tissue dehydration and protein denaturation.[6] The main effect is due to acute arteriolar and small vessel coagulation leading to gradual necrosis and fibrosis. Alcohol injection into recurrent cystic lesions results in the destruction of the epithelial lining and promotes inflammatory obliteration of the cavity leading to elimination of the dead space. Other agents such as hydrochloric acid, bleomycin, tetracycline, and talc are not typically used in the ablation of cysts or solid tumors of the neck in the adult population.[5,6] The blood level of alcohol elevates transiently and drops within 1 hour after the procedure. Signs and symptoms of alcohol toxicity are encountered if the injected volume approaches or exceeds 100 mL.[6] The volume typically required for PEI of head and neck tumors is much lower than this limit; therefore alcohol toxicity is not seen during PEI of thyroid cysts or nodules.

ULTRASONOGRAPHY IMAGING ANATOMY OF HEAD AND NECK

Understanding the US imaging-specific human anatomy of the neck is sine quo non for effective and safe PEI. Detailed discussion of US findings is discussed in chapters elsewhere in this textbook (see Chapter 13, Ultrasound of the Thyroid and Parathyroid Glands). The most relevant anatomic correlation for PEI is described here. The thyroid gland is located anterior to the larynx and posterior to the strap muscles, with a ground glass echo appearance and flanked bilaterally by the great vessels. The location of the RLN, vagus nerve, and the great vessels are as depicted in Figure 51.1, A. The cervical portion of the vagus nerve is typically located within the carotid sheath, posterolateral to the common carotid artery (CCA) in 80% of the subjects (see Figure 51.1). Less commonly it can be located anterolateral to the CCA. It can be seen during neck ultrasonography as a hypoechoic 2 to 3 mm thick, linear, avascular structure with echogenic striation. The location can be altered by the presence of metastatic lymphadenopathy or a large, laterally protruding nodular goiter. The right and left RLN nerves arise from the respective vagus counterparts in the lower part of the neck and course within the tracheo-esophageal (TE) grooves to supply the muscles of the larynx. (see Figure 51.1). The RLN cannot be reliably visualized with present-day US equipment. Alcohol injections performed on thyroid nodules or cysts located within the posteromedial aspect of the thyroid lobes, medially located central compartment thyroid cancer recurrences, and parathyroid adenomas carry risk of injury to RLNs. Attempted PEI of metastatic lateral compartment lymphadenopathy poses risks to vagus nerves, sympathetic ganglia, and accidental intravascular injection-related complications.[10]

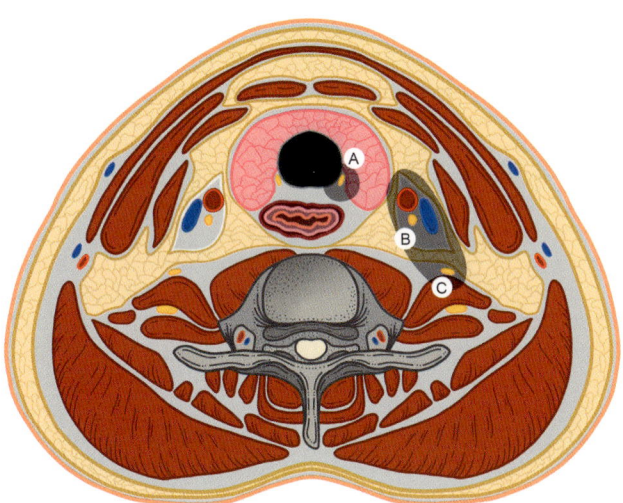

Fig. 51.1 Cross section of the neck at the level of mid-thyroid gland. A, Recurrent laryngeal nerve; B, vagus nerve; C, sympathetic ganglia. (Illustration courtesy Ms. Nikita Abraham, BS.)

ETIOLOGIES AMENABLE TO PEI IN HEAD AND NECK ENDOCRINE TUMORS

The following are the list of conditions most commonly subjected to outpatient PEI:
1. Cystic thyroid nodules and thyroglossal cysts
2. Toxic thyroid adenomas and nonfunctional benign thyroid nodules
3. Malignant metastatic thyroid cancer lymph nodes
4. Parathyroid adenomas and parathyroid hyperplasia

Thyroid Cysts and Cystic Thyroid Nodules

About 15% to 25% of thyroid nodules are cystic or predominantly cystic.[1] Most thyroid cysts in adults are a sequelae of acute and spontaneous degeneration of solid nodules or gradual development of colloid cysts. The cyst cavities formed after acute cystic generation are often unlined with epithelium; therefore they are pseudocysts that perhaps acquire an epithelial lining (Figure 51.2). Large simple colloid cysts can arise in the thyroid and are likely lined with epithelium. If cysts are lined with an epithelial layer, it may increase the risk for recurrence

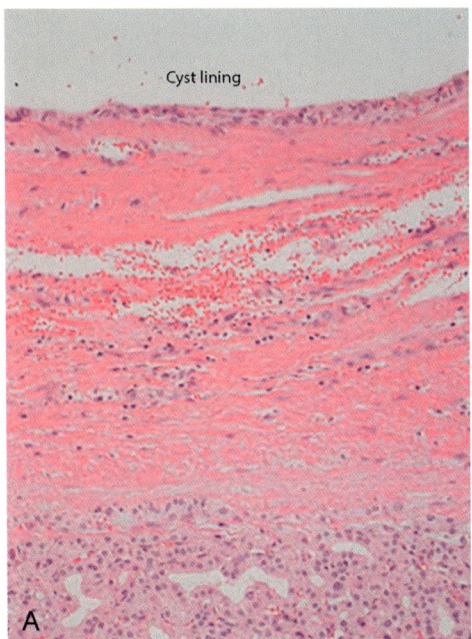
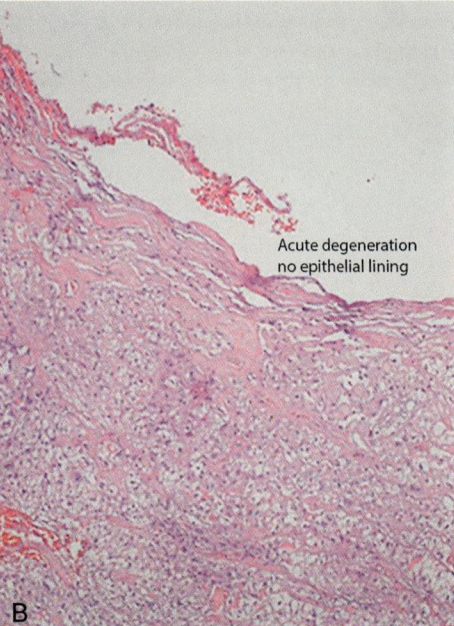

Fig. 51.2 A, Cyst. **B,** Pseudocyst.

after aspiration and PEI, but this has not been systematically studied with histologic correlation. Most thyroid cysts are benign, and the risk of malignancy is about 6%.[11,12] Therefore all cysts should be aspirated first and the cyst contents submitted for cytologic assessment to rule out malignancy before PEI. If a mural mass is encountered in a complex, even though it may be a predominantly cystic nodule, fine-needle aspiration (FNA) should be conducted based upon the individual US findings and malignancy should be ruled out before PEI. This also applies to thyroglossal cysts in adults.

THE PROCEDURE OF CYST INJECTION

If anesthesia is desired, US-guided infiltration with lidocaine up to the thyroid capsule using 27- to 30 G-needles is all that is required. Some interventionists do not use or recommend any form of anesthesia.[13] If anything at all, local anesthesia helps calm the patient who anticipates pain with the procedure. There are considerable variations with pain perception and procedural tolerance among patients, which should be taken into consideration. After establishing infiltration anesthesia and observing aseptic precautions, a suitable size needle is inserted under US guidance to form a "Z-track." The Z-track technique is a widely accepted practice that reduces leakage of administered medications after intramuscular (IM) injections.[14] In the authors' observation, this is an excellent technique that can be adopted for PEI to prevent alcohol leakage and reduce pain. The skin and the underlying soft tissue are gently but deliberately pulled away from the proposed site of needle entry before insertion of the needle. This leads to the formation of a "Z" track, and a built in "seal" develops upon withdrawal of the needle after completion of the injection (Figure 51.3).

The selection of a suitable size needle makes the procedure brief and reduces pain. This, however, involves calculated guesswork and even trial and error and is influenced by the variable viscosity of the cyst contents. (see Video 51.1). The visualization of a flat or shifting fluid level within a cyst implies acute or subacute bleeding and separation of blood components. At least a portion of the cyst contents should be aspirated. Uniformly anechoic cysts can contain fluid consistency ranging from watery, thin colloid to the thickness of pine tar. The presence of fixed and immobile reverberation artifacts indicates highly viscous cyst contents. Cysts can also contain loose debris or mural masses that can clog the needle tip during aspiration. These can be dislodged under guidance by injecting a small amount of sterile saline or by the repositioning of the needle with gentle plunging of the piston or partial withdrawal followed by aspiration. When performing these maneuvers, it is important to stabilize the hub of the needle to make sure that the needle does not come out of the cyst. Reinsertion of the needle into a collapsed cyst cavity may not always be successful, particularly if the cyst cavity is mostly or completely empty. Attaching extension tubing between the syringe and needle is used to stabilize the needle tip from dislodgment from the cyst cavity during aspiration (Figure 51.4). Modified percutaneous transhepatic cholangiography needles with side ports or "windows" have been shown to be effective in aspiration of cysts with viscid contents, but these needles are not available in the US.[15] The goal is to use the smallest gauge needle for effective aspiration and injection. Access to a wide selection of needles of various gauges and lengths is desirable to handle the different situations that may be encountered. The amount of alcohol required for successful injection depends upon the completeness of aspiration, thin-floppy walls vs thick walled cyst, presence of mural mass, aspirated volume and the viscidity of cyst contents.

Zingrillo and others use a fixed volume of alcohol for injection, 2 mL of ethanol for cysts <20 mL, 3 mL for 20 to 30 mL cysts, and 4 mL for larger cysts, and reported good outcomes.[16] Shu et al. injected 50% of the aspirated cyst volume with ethanol but also removed the alcohol after a cyst wall contact time of 2 to 5 minutes; the needle was left in place for the entire duration of the procedure.[17] The thinner the walls and more complete the cyst collapses after the aspiration, the lesser the volume of alcohol that needs to be injected. If there is doubt that the needle tip has penetrated the posterior capsule or accidentally withdrawn outside of the cyst, then it is advisable to not proceed with alcohol injection in that session. Reinsertion of the needle into a collapsed cyst is not always successful. If the needle is reinserted, the positioning of the needle tip within the cyst cavity should be confirmed by injecting a small amount of sterile saline under guidance, which can be reaspirated before completion of PEI. If the position of the needle tip cannot be confirmed with confidence, it is prudent to reassess the cyst a few weeks or months later when the procedure can be repeated as needed. Thyroglossal (TG) duct cyst aspiration and injection is similar to the one we have described. The limiting factor of PEI in TG duct cysts is the presence of very thick fluid that can thwart complete aspiration. PEI of a thyroid cyst is demonstrated in Video 51.2.

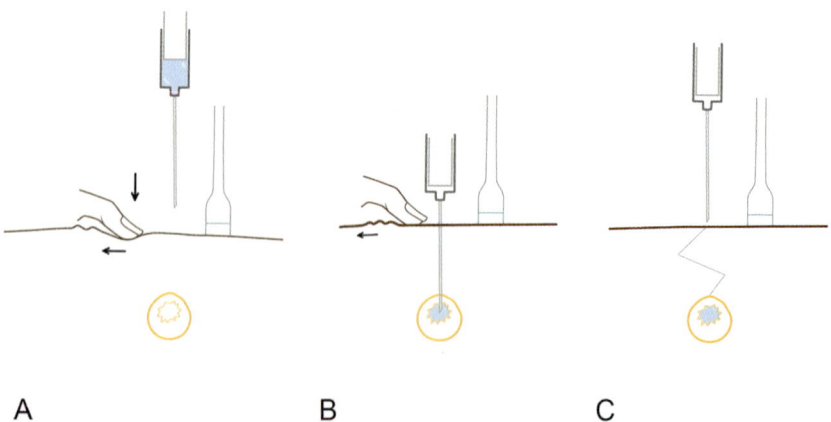

Fig. 51.3 A to C, Z-Track injection technique to prevent alcohol leak and reduce pain. (Illustration courtesy Ms. Nikita Abraham, BS.)

CHAPTER 51 PEI in the management of diseases of the thyroid and parathyroid glands

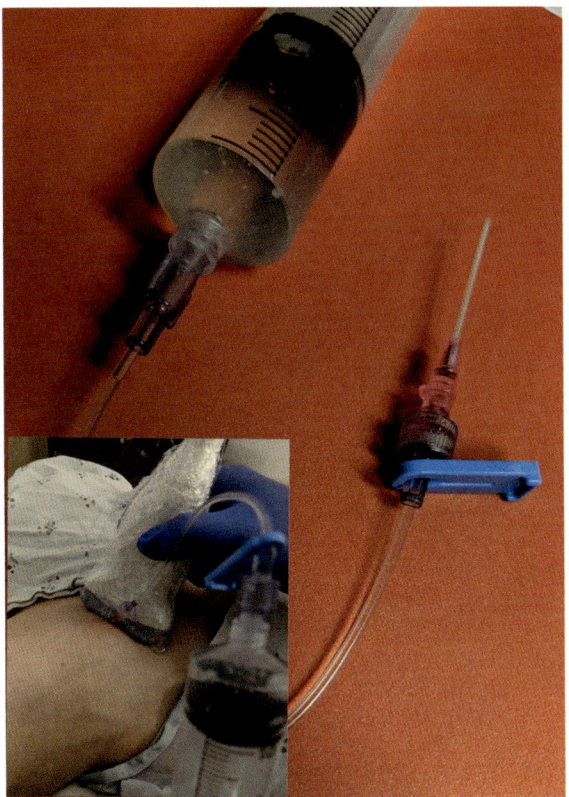

Fig. 51.4 Cyst aspiration using intravenous (IV) cannula and extension tube.

OUTCOMES OF PEI IN CYSTIC AND PREDOMINANTLY CYSTIC NODULES

Nodules that are >50% to 90% cystic in nature are amenable to alcohol injection. Since the early 1990s, several interventionists have reported their short- and long-term patient outcomes, universally corroborating the effectiveness of PEI.[16-21] A double-blind controlled study by Bennedbaek and others used alcohol as the sclerosant and saline as the control. The superiority of alcohol injection was established after the observation of 100% cyst volume reduction. However, it should be mentioned that the "inert" saline injections performed in the placebo arm were effective in up to 68% cyst volume reduction.[21] Valcavi and Frasoldati reported a randomized study on 281 patients receiving simple aspiration versus PEI. A remarkable 86% reduction of cyst volume was seen in the PEI group versus 7% in the aspiration-only group.[18] Some interventionists drain the injected alcohol after a contact time of 2 to 5 minutes with the cyst wall.[20,22] In the latter study, the total recurrence rate was 38.3%, with a short-term recurrence of 18.7% and a delayed recurrence of 24.1%.[22] Kim did not find any difference in the outcomes between leaving the alcohol in versus subsequent removal after a stipulated contact time with the cyst walls.[23] Therefore we feel reaspiration of the introduced alcohol may affect outcomes adversely.[5,23] One of the problems encountered during attempted PEI of cysts is that the cystic nodules may contain very thick and viscid contents, preventing complete aspiration. Zieleznik et al. reported that the initial introduction of a small amount of alcohol facilitates liquefaction of the contents, enabling a more complete aspiration and introduction of larger amounts of alcohol.[24]

The predictors for recurrence of cysts after PEI were a size greater than 10 mL and the presence of mural mass.[22] The presence of vascularity within the mural mass was also observed to be an independent predictor for PEI failure.[25] The other possible mechanism is needle tip-related trauma to the mural mass resulting in bleeding into the cyst cavity. When highly vascular mural mass is encountered, the authors recommend the use of an intravenous soft tip cannula in place of hypodermic metal needles. After the insertion of the cannula, the trocar is removed; the procedure of aspiration and injection is accomplished through the soft cannula connected to an extension tube and syringe (see Figure 51.4).

PEI for Functional and Nonfunctional Solid and Predominantly Solid Thyroid Tumors

PEI can be performed for both functional and nonfunctional thyroid nodules. About 5% to 10% of thyroid nodules are functional.[26] Toxic adenomas (TAs) are particularly suited for PEI because they are almost never malignant, and the recovery of low or suppressed thyroid-stimulating hormone (TSH) allows biochemical monitoring, indicating successful sclerotherapy. The reduction in volume over time by US is used for both functional and nonfunctional nodule monitoring after injections. The risk of hypothyroidism is negligible with PEI in the absence of underlying autoimmune thyroiditis. PEI in TA results in "functional volume reduction" of the nodule; in other words, the therapy makes the nodules subclinical. Therefore, there is a risk of delayed recurrence because the destruction of the nodule is never total. This has led to the leaders in this field to recommend radioactive iodine (RAI) over PEI for larger TAs.[3]

THE PROCEDURE OF ALCOHOL INJECTION INTO SOLID NODULES

There are procedural differences between cyst- versus solid-nodule PEI. The needle is inserted into solid portions of the nodule under guidance using small gauge needles usually under pressure, which leads to unpredictable diffusion and a risk of collateral tissue injury.[26] Rarely does one need to use needles thicker than 25 G in the authors' observation. The typical volume of alcohol injected ranges from 0.5 to 2 cc per injection. The use of small-bore needles using the previously described Z-track method for needle insertion reduces the risk of alcohol leakage and to some extent reduces discomfort (see Figure 51.3). The injection occurs under pressure which leads to dispersion of alcohol and stretching of the thyroid nodule and capsule leading to pain that is almost universal, even if adequate local anesthesia is achieved by lidocaine infiltration. This visceral pain is often referred to the ipsilateral jaw, upper neck, or the ear, and very rarely, to the tooth. Pretreatment with acetaminophen is also a useful strategy to reduce pain. The referred pain usually settles within 10 to 15 minutes with observation and reassurance. Pain can be reduced by patient education, lidocaine infiltration anesthesia, use of small-bore needles, and slower injection. Visible bruising can be controlled using ice packs.

Efficacy of PEI for Toxic and Pretoxic Adenomas

Preliminary PEI outcomes with TA reports emerged from Italy during the late 1980s and early 1990s. Goletti and Livraghi published early data in 1990, followed by Papini and others.[3,7,27-29] Both TAs and toxic multinodular goiter (MNG) were included in a larger study reporting 5 years outcome and follow-up of 117 patients who had undergone PEI.[29] In this study, 26 males and 91 females were included. Seventy-seven patients had solitary TAs, 17 with MNG and 40 with solitary pretoxic adenoma (PTA). No anesthesia was used and 20- to 22-G needles were used for the injection. Complete cure was achieved in 77.9%, partial cure in 9.1%, and failure in 13% of the subjects. During the 5 years of follow up period, no regrowth was observed in TAs with a volume of >40 ml. Also, the use of methimazole (MMI) did not affect the outcome of PEI therapy.[29] In an Italian multicenter study from 1996, by Lippi and others, 429 patient outcomes were reported, of which 242 (56%) were TA and the rest were PTA. Different sites with multiple interventionists were involved in conducting the procedures. Patients underwent 2 to 12 sessions of PEI under guidance with a median injection of 4 sessions. One and one half ml of alcohol per each cubic ml of the calculated nodule volume was injected. The administered volume ranged from 1 to 8 ml of ethanol per session. The total volume of alcohol injected was 2 to 50 mL and the follow-up duration was 12 months. Biochemical and imaging monitoring was conducted every 3 months. Treatment success was observed in 66.5% of patients with TA and 83.4% in patients with PTA. They also observed the best results in nodules that were less than 15 cc^3 with the least favorable outcomes for nodules >30 cc^3. These observations led to their conclusion recommending RAI and surgery for the treatment of larger TA. Minor complications such as burning or radiating pain were observed in 90% of the patients. Transient hyperpyrexia was seen in 8%, hematoma in 3.9%, and thrombosis of the internal jugular vein (IJV) in one patient, with subsequent self-resolution without permanent sequela in any of the patients.[30] In 1997 Monzani and others reported a 5-year follow-up study on 117 patients who underwent PEI. Twenty- to 22-G needles were used to inject 1 to 5 cc of alcohol without anesthesia. Burning pain was reported by patients for 30 to 60 minutes after the injection. This duration is longer than what has been reported when local anesthesia is used.[29]

Bennedbaek, compared the efficacy of alcohol injection of solid nonfunctioning nodules versus L-thyroxine suppression. In this prospective randomized study, 50 euthyroid patients with a single nodule were administered one alcohol injection (n = 25) versus suppressive doses of thyroxine (n = 25), and the outcomes were analyzed for 12 months. The nodules in the PEI group underwent a 47 volume reduction versus a 9% volume reduction in the thyroxine group.[31]

A summary of the available studies suggests that pretoxic adenomas respond best to PEI, whereas larger TAs require more alcohol and higher number of injections to control biochemical hyperthyroidism, and they also carry a higher risk for recurrence. At the 2018 Annual American Thyroid Association (ATA) meeting, a novel vascularity-targeting approach was reported. Doppler interrogation is conducted first, the highly vascular areas are mapped, and blood vessels within the adenoma are targeted for injection (see Video 51.3). Preliminary results of this targeted approach require a lower volume of alcohol injection and fewer sessions are required for therapeutic success. Ongoing long-term follow-up is anticipated to provide answers regarding durable control of hyperthyroidism using a vascularity-targeted injection technique.[32]

ALCOHOL ABLATION OF MALIGNANT METASTATIC LYMPHADENOPATHY IN THYROID CANCER

Papillary thyroid cancer (PTC) is the most common endocrine cancer encountered in practice, with outstanding survival and outcomes despite lymph node metastasis.[33] In a Mayo Clinic study, 38% of patients had lymph node metastasis thyroidectomy surgery.[34] Lymph node metastasis within the central compartments and mediastinum is encountered in as high as 82% of subjects undergoing prophylactic neck dissections.[35] True postoperative recurrence or residual cancers is seen in about 20% to 40% of patients during surveillance imaging.[36,37] The easy availability of sensitive thyroglobulin (Tg) assays coupled with the use of high-resolution US equipment and ever-increasing expertise among practitioners has led to the identification of small residual locoregional disease that may not pose mortality risks or morbidity to patients.[38] Several studies report that in a majority of low-risk patients, small-scale lymph node metastasis does not progress or cause morbidity.[39,40] The 2015 ATA guidelines allow watchful waiting of these lymph nodes in select patients as a management strategy.[38] However, clinicians are faced with the conundrum of addressing these small-scale metastatic lymph nodes because the management policies thus far have been surgical excision when disease is identified. Observation is not an appealing option to most patients, particularly once they are made aware of its presence or if FNA confirmation of metastasis has occurred.

The use of US-guided PEI for the intended nonsurgical destruction of metastatic lymph nodes raises several questions. Short-term successful injection (based upon Tg normalization or even a meaningful drop in TG) has not been proven to have positive long-term survival benefits or a reduction of recurrences. The Mayo Clinic investigators, Hay and Charboneau, observed no recurrence of targets subjected to PEI. However, 6 subjects (24%) developed 18 "recurrences" that were previously unobserved and were amenable to treatment without causing morbidity.[41] Berry picking surgeries have been universally condemned in the management of thyroid cancer metastasis for both PTC[38] and medullary thyroid cancer (MTC) due to incomplete resection.[42] Presurgical US mapping has its limitations due to underestimation as to the extent of metastatic lymphadenopathy.[43] The ATA guidelines committee bluntly state their position regarding PEI as follows (page 75, Rec 71, C-20): "Focal PEI treatment does represent a nonsurgical form of berry picking."[38] Nevertheless, several studies by Hay, Heilo, Monchik, and others have all shown good therapeutic and patient safety outcomes.[41,44-48] A meta-analysis performed by Fontenot and others comparing PEI and surgery for the management of locally recurrent PTC suggests that they are equally effective, with similar outcomes of 88% versus 95% efficacy, respectively.[49] It is apparent from several studies that a subset of patients with localized disease can benefit from PEI with substantial cost saving and the complete elimination of surgical risks. Careful case selection appears even more critical in the PEI treatment of patients with cervical metastasis because only the US-apparent lymph node or nodes are treated. Heilo and others reported outcomes on 69 PTC patients with lymph node metastasis who received PEI during a 5-year period (2004-2009) in 2011. All patients received prior surgery and RAI yet presented with residual lymph node disease in the neck during follow-up. Three patients underwent surgery due to disease progression; the rest (n = 63) received PEI, and a total of 109 lymph nodes were injected after FNA confirmation. Forty-six of these lymph nodes were located within the central compartments and 37 within the lateral compartments. The criteria used for successful treatment includes disappearance of lymph nodes, reduction in AP measurement by more than 4 mm, less visible vascularization, and negative FNA cytology and TG washout. The pretreatment lymph node volumes varied from 0.01 to 3.56 mL, and the injected ethanol volumes ranged from 0.1 to 1 mL of these 92 nodes; 72 lymph nodes disappeared during follow-up after PEI. The authors conclude that PEI should replace berry picking surgeries.[45] Refer to Video 51.4 for an injection demonstration.

The more obvious and readily applicable indications include the following:

1. Proven low volume lymphadenopathy in subjects who have already undergone initial surgery and RAI with a curative intent
2. Those patients who refuse further surgery
3. Small lymph nodes that are <2 cm in maximal dimensions
4. Older subjects or patients with comorbidities that preclude surgery
5. Palliation in a patient who is troubled by a visible or palpable lymphadenopathy

The following situations wherein PEI is not an ideal option or considered high risk are as follows:
1. Multilevel disease by US or as a primary therapy for biopsy-proven lymphadenopathy
2. Bilateral lymph node disease in young individuals
3. Bulky lymph nodes >2 cm in size
4. Patients with obvious distant metastasis proven by imaging, unless PEI is performed for palliation
5. Injection of ipsilateral level VI or thyroid bed disease in a subject who has preexistent contralateral RLN injury

TECHNIQUES, MATERIALS USED, AND PRACTICAL CONSIDERATIONS

The use of infiltration local anesthesia is desirable in most situations, particularly if patients are allowed to participate in the decision and lidocaine infiltration is offered before the procedure. The Mayo Clinic group reported using lidocaine routinely in all patients; moreover, several patients required intravenous midazolam sedation.[44] Helio et al. report that in their series only 1 of 63 patients who underwent PEI using the same technique as Lewis et al needed local anesthesia.[45] Sequential injection into the posterior aspect of the target lesion first, followed by injecting into the anterior areas, ensures visualization of the needle tip throughout the procedure. Injecting anteriorly can impair visualization of the needle tip if injection of a posterior area is attempted during the same sitting.[45] Intentional undertreatment of medial "danger areas" is quite acceptable during injection of central compartment disease. The opacification of the metastatic lymph node indicates successful injection. If preprocedure Doppler interrogation reveals blood flow, commensurate disappearance of flow can also be observed with successful injection.[41] Refer to Video 51.4 for an injection demonstration.

COST EFFECTIVENESS OF PEI FOR METASTATIC LYMPHADENOPATHY

Hay and others have done cost projection analysis on patients undergoing PEI for metastatic thyroid cancer. In the 25 patients who underwent PEI, a projected 40 neck dissections were avoided. This resulted in an anticipated average cost savings of $61,440.[41]

PERCUTANEOUS ETHANOL INJECTION OF PARATHYROID ADENOMA AND HYPERPLASIA

Primary hyperparathyroidism (PHPT) is a common condition that occurs in the general population. The vast majority of PHPT are incidentally identified during routine serum calcium testing as a part of yearly primary care evaluations. Surgery is the first-line recommended therapeutic intervention. PEI is an option for patients who have had a failed surgery or those subjects considered poor surgical candidates.[50-52] The procedure of PEI for parathyroid adenoma was described by the Mayo Clinic.[50] After FNA parathyroid hormone (PTH) confirmation,[53] alcohol injection is conducted under guidance as described earlier, similar to PEI of metastatic lymph nodes. Accurate injection results in opacification of the adenoma with reduction of disappearance of vascular flow during Doppler interrogation. In a series from the Mayo Clinic, patients with multiple endocrine neoplasia type 1 (MEN 1) who recurred after initial surgical intervention were treated successfully with PEI under US guidance.[54] Patients with chronic renal failure develop secondary hyperparathyroidism (SHPT). In a study from Japan, 321 subjects with SHPT were subjected to PEI, which resulted in reduction of PTH levels in 201 patients (62.6%).[55]

RISKS AND SIDE EFFECTS OF ALCOHOL INJECTION

PEI carries general side effects of any percutaneous procedures such as pain and bruising.[7,13,20,27-30] The side effects and risks that are unique to alcohol injection are due to the nonspecific destructive properties of alcohol. This is almost always a consequence of extravasation. Tissue necrosis and RLN damage are the most notable consequences of misdirected injections.

The greatest risk of alcohol injection is extravasation. The risks are highest in the following situations:
1. Large-bore needle being used, usually to drain thick cyst contents
2. Large volume of injection of alcohol (greater than 5 cc) into solid nodules
3. Injection under pressure into thick-walled, noncollapsible cysts or solid nodules
4. Accidental puncture of posterior capsule and injection outside of the nodule or cyst
5. Inexperienced operator

Due to the small volume (<1 cc) of alcohol being injected into lymph nodes and solid nodules (thyroid and parathyroid adenomas), the risk of extravasation is lower compared with cyst injections. The pain that is almost universally perceived by patients undergoing solid nodule injection is likely due to capsular distension of the target undergoing injection. Awareness of the presence of critical nerves and vessels in the immediate vicinity of the target undergoing injection is most important. This is particularly true of targets located near the TE groove (RLN) and lateral compartments (vagus nerve and sympathetic ganglia). To avoid injury to critical nerves, deliberate undertreatment of targets in these critical areas is quite acceptable.[10] Other uncommon side effects include precipitation of Graves' disease and eye diseases after PEI.[56,57] Massive tissue necrosis requiring a major reconstructive procedure was reported in one subject.[58] Cutaneous implantation of thyroid cancer has been observed as a complication of PEI.[59]

STRATEGIES FOR REDUCING RISK OF ETHANOL EXTRAVASATION AND RELATED TISSUE DAMAGE

1. Avoid injecting large volumes of alcohol. Typical volumes include about 30% to 50% of the cyst volume and 0.1 to 1 cc for malignant lymph nodes and 1 to 2 cc for TA.
2. Needle tip location awareness throughout the procedure is crucial to prevent extravasation.
3. Avoiding injection or intentionally undertreating lesions located within the danger areas of the neck (see Figure 51.1).
4. Abort procedure if patient experiences unusually severe pain or visible extravasation by US.
5. Using the smallest gauge needle for a given situation.
6. Use of a "Z" or zig-zag track as the needle is inserted into the target.

PROCEDURE SUITE SAFETY POLICIES, COMPLICATION RECOGNITION AND MITIGATION

A small amount of alcohol leakage is inevitable and is without dangerous consequence. The most morbid side effect reported is after the extravasation of a large volume of alcohol into the soft tissues of the neck, leading to skin and cartilage necrosis.[58] This could be a result of a lack of expertise with the procedure or a result of confusion between lidocaine and alcohol, which are both clear and colorless liquids. Therefore every effort should be taken by the operator not to confuse alcohol with lidocaine as they are indistinguishable once loaded into a syringe. The authors recommend avoiding the

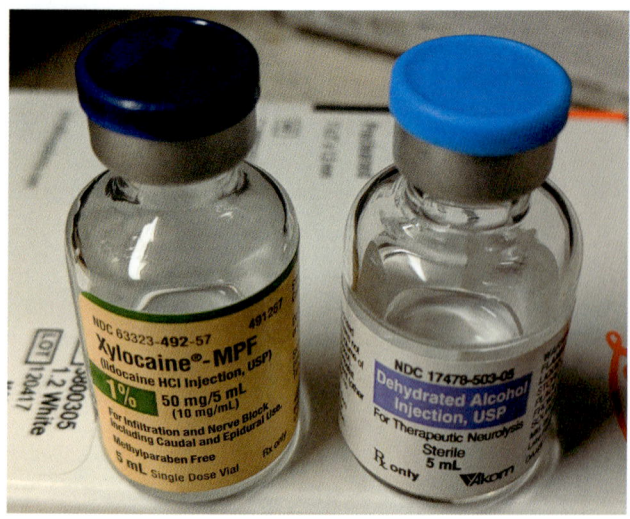

Fig. 51.5 Similar appearing vials containing alcohol and lidocaine should be avoided to prevent medical error.

use of vials of similar size or appearance to avert this regrettable "mix-up" (Figure 51.5). Preloading syringes without accurate labeling should be avoided altogether. In fact, the operator self-loading syringes just before injections and adhering to appropriate procedural time-outs are both sound and safe practice patterns that can prevent accidental injury to patients. Permanent RLN injury during PEI is rare. In more than 110 consecutive injections, two patients developed dysphonia that resolved over time.[60] The authors practice and recommend a meticulous pre- and postprocedure US-guided vocal cord function assessment as described by Cheng and others.[61] Video 51.5 demonstrates a US-guided, noninvasive evaluation of vocal cord function.

SUMMARY AND CONCLUSIONS

PEI is an acceptable and effective procedure. When performed well by skilled interventionists, it yields very favorable and cost-effective outcomes in the management of cystic and solid thyroid nodules. On a case-by-case basis, PEI is also an excellent adjunctive therapy for the management of recurrent thyroid cancer, locoregional metastasis, and parathyroid adenomas. As with most US-guided procedures, there is considerable operator variability and unique skill sets that can be enhanced with structured training programs. At present, there is no consensus on the number of observed procedures required to determine competency.

REFERENCES

For a complete list of references, go to expertconsult.com.

52

Medical Treatment Horizons for Metastatic Differentiated and Medullary Thyroid Cancer

Jean G. Bustamante Alvarez, Lori J. Wirth, Manisha H. Shah

> Please go to expertconsult.com to view related video:
> **Video 52.1** Introduction to Chapter 52, Medical Treatment Horizons for Metastatic Differentiated and Medullary Thyroid Cancer.

INTRODUCTION

Metastatic differentiated thyroid cancer (DTC) and medullary thyroid cancer (MTC) are rare tumors with limited treatment options and an overall poor response to cytotoxic chemotherapy. Oral small molecule inhibitors targeting several different oncogenic pathways relevant to thyroid cancers have emerged over the past decade. Development of such kinase inhibitors has revolutionized the treatment of DTC and MTC, leading to sorafenib, lenvatinib, vandetanib, and cabozantinib becoming new standard therapies in advanced thyroid cancer. However, these multikinase inhibitors have off-target side effects that can take a toll on the patient's quality of life (QoL). Thus the overall benefits must be weighed against the potential downsides in therapeutic decision making. The advent of genomic analysis and identification of specific driver alterations have spurred the study of more potent and highly selective therapies intended to treat subgroups of patients harboring targetable alterations more effectively and with less drug-related adverse events.

DIFFERENTIATED THYROID CANCER SUBTYPES

Who and When to Treat With Systemic Therapy

Metastatic DTC often presents as a relatively slow-growing and asymptomatic cancer. As long as there is response to radioactive iodine (RAI), these malignancies carry a good prognosis even when metastatic disease is present. Tumors that have de novo resistance to RAI or become RAI-refractory have a considerably worse prognosis.

In general, locoregional therapy, such as surgery and external beam radiation, is considered for localized tumor burden, whereas systemic treatments are reserved for more widespread metastatic disease, especially when disease progression occurs. Because kinase inhibitors are not curative and can cause side effects that affect QoL, deciding when to initiate therapy can be challenging. Factors to be taken into account include the pace of tumor growth and symptoms. Thyroid cancers that progress slowly over time, are asymptomatic, and of a low burden may be appropriately followed under active surveillance, whereas systemic treatment should be considered in progressive disease, especially if bulky or symptoms are thought to be imminent. Other factors to consider when deciding on systemic treatment initiation include the anatomic location of the disease (such as brain, proximity to airway, spinal cord, or risk for pathologic fracture from bone metastasis), side effects from systemic therapies, the patient's performance status and comorbidities, and the patient's desire for treatment after discussion and risk-benefit assessment.[1]

RAI-Refractory DTC

Patients with RAI-refractory DTC fall into four categories: (1) those with malignant disease that has never concentrated RAI, (2) patients with tumors with prior RAI uptake that subsequently lost the ability to concentrate RAI, (3) patients with RAI uptake in some but not all sites of disease, and (4) disease progression despite RAI uptake.[2–4]

Current Standard of Care

In RAI-refractory progressive DTC, lenvatinib and sorafenib are the current standard of care therapies approved by regulatory bodies.

Lenvatinib

Lenvatinib is an oral multikinase inhibitor that blocks vascular endothelial growth factor receptors (VEGFR) 1-3, fibroblast growth factor receptors (FGFR) 1-4, platelet-derived growth factor receptor alpha (PDGFR-α), KIT, and RET. Lenvatinib became an established standard treatment for locally recurrent unresectable and/or metastatic, progressive, RAI-refractory DTC based on the Study of E7080 (Lenvatinib) in Differentiated Cancer of the Thyroid (SELECT).[5,6] This was a phase 3, randomized, double-blind, multicenter international study of lenvatinib versus placebo. 261 patients were randomized to receive lenvatinib (at a dose of 24 mg daily in 28-day cycles), and 131 patients to placebo. Progression-free survival (PFS) was the primary endpoint of this study, and secondary endpoints included response rate (RR), overall survival (OS), and safety. At the time of disease progression, patients were unblinded, and those found to have been initially randomized to placebo were offered crossover to open-label lenvatinib. The median PFS was 19.4 months in the lenvatinib group and 3.6 months in the placebo group (hazard ratio [HR] for progression or death, 0.21; 99% confidence interval [CI], 0.14 to 0.31; $P < 0.001$). 65% of the patients in the lenvatinib group had a response, of which 4 cases were complete responses, and responses were durable, lasting a median of 30 months. The median OS could not be reached by the time of data cutoff as more than 50% of patients remained alive in both arms, though the study's crossover design can make detection of an OS benefit impossible.[7] Indeed, 88% of patients on placebo did cross over to receive open-label lenvatinib after disease progression on placebo. Updated analysis of the elderly patient population enrolled in SELECT did, however, show that patients greater than 65 years of age did experience an OS benefit with lenvatinib compared with placebo.[8] In additional subgroup analyses, all subgroups of patients had a PFS benefit with lenvatinib compared with placebo, including patients who had received a prior VEGF-targeted therapy, patients with all histologic subtypes, and all anatomic sites of metastasis, including bone. Treatment-related side effects related to lenvatinib were seen frequently, including hypertension in 68% of patients, diarrhea in 59%, fatigue in 59%, anorexia in 50%, weight loss in 46%, and nausea in 41%. Side effects were generally manageable with supportive care, dose holds, and dose reductions, but lenvatinib was discontinued due to toxicity in 37 patients (14%). Two percent of deaths out of the 261 patients who received lenvatinib were attributed to treatment by the investigator, though it is important to note that the rate of death on study was significantly higher in the placebo arm, and the majority of deaths were due to disease progression.[6]

Sorafenib

Sorafenib is another oral multikinase inhibitor that targets VEGFR 1-3, RET, RAF, and PDGFR-β and has been established in the treatment of progressive RAI-refractory DTC based on the DECISION trial.[9] This was a phase 3, international multicenter, randomized, double-blind, placebo-controlled trial that investigated sorafenib versus placebo, also with a crossover design and PFS as the primary endpoint. 417 patients were enrolled. 207 were randomized to sorafenib (400 mg twice a day) and 210 to placebo. The median PFS was 10.8 months on sorafenib versus 5.8 months on placebo (HR 0.59; 95% CI, 0.45 to 7.6; $p < 0.0001$). Twelve percent of patients on sorafenib responded, with a median duration of response lasting 10.2 months. Ninety-nine percent of patients receiving sorafenib had adverse events, most of which were grade 1 or 2. The most common adverse events seen in the sorafenib group included hand-foot syndrome (76%), diarrhea (69%), alopecia (67%), and desquamation or rash (50%). One death was attributed to sorafenib (myocardial infarction). At the time of analysis, median OS could not be reached by the time of data cutoff as more than 50% of patients remained alive in both arms, though no separation of survival curves was seen.

QoL was also studied in the DECISION trial using the Functional Assessment of Cancer Therapy General Survey, which considers physical, social, familial, emotional, and functional well-being of individuals receiving cancer treatment. The results of this survey indicated that patients in the sorafenib group had an overall lower QoL compared with those who received placebo, especially early on in therapy. In light of the potential effect on QoL, a discussion addressing potential side effects and the benefits of therapy must take place before starting any therapy.[10]

BRAF-MEK Targeted Therapies

The *BRAF*V600E mutation is present in approximately 58% of all papillary thyroid cancers (PTCs),[11] whereas 40% to 50% of follicular thyroid cancers (FTCs) harbor *N* or *H RAS* mutations.[12] BRAF is a serine-threonine kinase that binds to RAS and triggers downstream activation of the MAP kinase signaling cascade. *RAS*-mutated thyroid cancers are prone to distant metastases to lung and bone. Given the limited therapeutic options for RAI-refractory DTC, the identification of BRAF and RAS as potential therapeutic targets has been of interest.

Vemurafenib

Vemurafenib is a kinase inhibitor initially designed as a specific inhibitor of the mutated BRAF kinase frequently present in melanoma. A retrospective analysis of the efficacy and tolerability of vemurafenib in patients with advanced *BRAF*V600E mutated PTC showed efficacy and tolerability.[13] Of the 17 patients identified, 7 had a partial response and 8 had stable disease. Duration of response was more than 6 months, and the median time to treatment failure was 13 months. Vemurafenib was also studied in a phase 2, open-label, clinical trial for patients with RAI-refractory recurrent and/or metastatic PTC harboring a *BRAF*V600E mutation. Participants were enrolled into two cohorts, one treatment-naïve, and the other for patients who had received one prior VEGFR multikinase inhibitor.[14] In the first cohort 10 of 26 patients (38%) experienced a partial response, a median PFS of 18.2 months, and a median duration of response of 16.5 months. In the second cohort 6 is the actual number instead of 10, hence 27% is correct 10 of 22 patients (27%) had a partial response, with a median PFS of 8.9 months and median duration of response of 7.4 months. The most commonly reported adverse events included rash, fatigue, weight loss, taste alteration, and alopecia. Seventeen patients in each cohort had grade 3 to 4 side effects, including cutaneous squamous cell carcinoma, keratoacanthoma, dyspnea, pneumonia, and hypotension.

Dabrafenib

Dabrafenib and trametinib combination. Dabrafenib is a BRAF inhibitor and trametinib inhibits MEK. BRAF and MEK are components in the same signaling pathway that ultimately activate tumor proliferation and growth. In a phase 1 study of dabrafenib in patients with solid tumors, 3 of the 9 evaluable patients achieved a partial response.[15] Subsequently, the combination of dabrafenib and trametinib compared with dabrafenib monotherapy was studied in patients with RAI-refractory PTC. This randomized phase 2 study enrolled 53 patients, of whom 25% had received 1 to 3 prior multikinase inhibitors. Patients in arm A (N = 26) were treated with dabrafenib monotherapy (150 mg twice a day), and those in arm B (N = 27) received combined dabrafenib and trametinib (dabrafenib 150 mg orally twice a day plus trametinib 2 mg orally daily). Preliminary data analysis showed an overall response rate (ORR) of 50% for arm A and 54% for arm B, median PFS was 11.4 months and 15.1 months, respectively, and median duration of response was 15.6 months and 13.3 months, respectively. Unlike in melanoma, in which combined BRAF plus MEK inhibition is both better tolerated and has greater activity than treatment with BRAF-directed monotherapy, this study showed no statistically significant difference in ORR, median PFS, or duration of response between the two arms; however, monotherapy and combination therapy were both tolerable.[16]

Selumetinib to reverse RAI resistance in DTC. Small molecule inhibitors of MEK were found to restore the expression of the sodium iodide symporter and uptake of iodine in preclinical thyroid cancer mice models.[17] Based on this finding, a clinical trial with selumetinib, a MEK inhibitor, was done to assess if reacquisition of RAI uptake was possible in human subjects.[18] Twenty-four patients were screened, and 20 were evaluated. Twelve of 20 patients had increased uptake of RAI 4 weeks after starting selumetinib but only 8 had a predicted RAI adsorption in target lesions of 2000 cGy or more. Five of 8 treated patients had partial responses and 3 stable disease. No grade 3 adverse events attributable to selumetinib occurred, but one patient did develop myelodysplasia and acute leukemia 51 weeks after RAI. Findings of the ASTRA trial, a phase 3 study comparing the addition of selumetinib to adjuvant RAI compared with placebo, showed no improvement in outcomes among patients with high-risk nonmetastatic DTC when treated with Selumetinib.[19] Complete remission rates (CRRs) were not statistically significant among the 157 evaluable patients. The selumetinib arm had a CRR of 40% compared with 38% in the placebo arm (odds ratio [OR], 1.07; 95% CI, 0.61 to 1.87; $p = 0.82$). There is currently an ongoing phase 2 multicenter clinical trial (NCT02393690) of RAI with and without selumetinib in patients with recurrent or metastatic thyroid cancer being conducted by the International Thyroid Oncology Group (ITOG).

Second-Line Options
Cabozantinib

Cabozantinib is an oral kinase inhibitor with multiple targets, including MET and VEGFR. c-MET upregulation has been implicated as a mediator of resistance to VEGFR kinase inhibitors. Cabozantinib showed objective responses in 5 of 8 patients with DTC previously treated with VEGFR inhibitors in a phase 1 trial. A multicenter phase 2 clinical trial of cabozantinib in individuals with RAI-refractory DTC who had progressed on prior VEGFR kinase inhibitors was conducted by ITOG (Table 52.1).[20] This trial is the only prospective study that addresses the unmet need for patients are refractory to prior VEGFR inhibitors. Twenty-five patients were enrolled of which 10 (40%) had a partial response and 13 (52%) had stable disease. Median PFS was 12.7 months and median OS was 34.7 months. The most common adverse events included fatigue, weight loss, diarrhea, palmar-plantar erythrodysesthesia, and hypertension. There was one treatment-related death due to CNS bleeding in a patient on enoxaparin for pulmonary embolism. Cabozantinib showed clinically significant and durable response in this population of patients.

Immunotherapy
Pembrolizumab Monotherapy
Given the broad activity of checkpoint immunotherapy across multiple malignancies seen recently, the potential role for immunotherapy in advanced thyroid cancer has been of interest. Pembrolizumab, a monoclonal antibody that blocks the inhibitory signal of the program cell death inhibitor 1 (PD-1) protein on cytotoxic T cells, has been evaluated as monotherapy in a basket trial (KEYNOTE-028, NCT02054806.) in patients with advanced PTC or FTC who failed prior standard therapy. PD-L1 expression by immunohistochemistry of more than or equal to 1% was required for enrollment. Of the 22 patients enrolled, 68% had PTC and 32% had FTC. Two patients experienced a PR for an ORR of 9%. Twelve patients (55%) had stable disease. The OS at 6 months was 100% and PFS 59%. Further phase 2 studies are ongoing with pembrolizumab monotherapy.[21]

Pembrolizumab and Lenvatinib Combination
Given the modest single agent activity in DTC with pembrolizumab, an ongoing phase 2 multicenter trial by ITOG is studying the combination of pembrolizumab with lenvatinib in RAI-refractory DTC based on preclinical evidence of synergy between VEGFR inhibition and immune therapy (NCT02973997). The primary objective of this trial is to investigate if pembrolizumab added to lenvatinib can yield better clinical benefit by improving on the complete RR seen with lenvatinib alone (see Table 52.1). Patients are enrolling in two cohorts: cohort one is composed of lenvatinib-naïve patients with progressive RAI-refractory DTC, and cohort two is composed of patients with progressive disease on lenvatinib, who will remain on lenvatinib and have pembrolizumab added to their treatment regimen.

Other Targets for DTC
Anaplastic Lymphoma Kinase Driven DTC
Anaplastic lymphoma kinase (*ALK*) translocations have been found in PTC in 11 of 498 (2.2%) PTCs and 3 of 23 (13%) patients with diffuse sclerosing variant PTC. The 14 patients with *ALK* translocations were females, and ages ranged from 38 years old to 48 years old. *ALK* translocations are mutually exclusive with other driver mutations. Crizotinib is a tyrosine kinase inhibitor that targets *ALK* translocations and has been reported in animal models, in vitro, and some case reports to have antitumor activity in thyroid carcinoma harboring *ALK* translocations. Prior studies have shown *EML4*, *STRN*, *TGF*, and *GTF2IRD1* as translocation partners.[22]

Neurotropic Tyrosine Receptor Kinase (NTRK) Driven DTC
The *NTRK* 1-3 genes encode for the Trk A-C proteins. Fusions in *NTRK* have been found in a small subset of thyroid cancers. Overall approximately 2% of PTCs harbor *NTRK* fusions, but somatic rearrangements of *NTRK* have been found in up to 14.5% of patients exposed to radiation.[23,24] An ongoing basket trial is studying entrectinib for the treatment of patients with *NTRK1/2/3*, *ROS1* and *ALK* gene rearrangements, including locally advanced unresectable or metastatic PTC. Larotrectinib, a specific and potent inhibitor of Trk alone, is also being investigated in a phase 2 clinical trial in patients with advanced cancers harboring *NTRK1/2/3* gene fusions (NCT02576431) with ORR as the primary endpoint.[25] Of 55 patients receiving larotrectinib reported thus far, 7 of the patients had thyroid cancer, including 1 patient with anaplastic thyroid cancer. All 7 patients responded to larotrectinib, even the patient with anaplastic thyroid cancer.[26]

TABLE 52.1	Ongoing Clinical Trials for DTC			
Drug	Mechanism of Action	Condition	Phase	NCT
Selumetinib	MEK1 and MEK2 inhibitor	RAI-avid recurrent/metastatic thyroid cancers	2	NCT02393690
Vemurafenib	BRAF inhibitor	BRAF-mutated papillary thyroid cancer	2	NCT01286753
Dabrafenib/trametinib versus dabrafenib alone	BRAF and MEK inhibitors	BRAF-mutated papillary thyroid cancer	2	NCT01723202
Cabozantinib	MET and VEGFR inhibitor	RAI-refractory differentiated thyroid cancer who progressed on prior VEGFR-targeted therapy	2	NCT01811212
Cabozantinib	MET and VEGFR inhibitor	RAI-refractory DTC in the first-line setting	2	NCT02041260
Pembrolizumab and lenvatinib	PD-1 checkpoint inhibitor and multikinase receptor inhibitor (including VRGFR1,2,3, PDGFRα, KIT, and RET)	RAI-refractory DTC in the first- and second-line setting	2	NCT02973997
Nivolumab plus ipilimumab	PD-1 checkpoint inhibitor and CTLA-4 inhibitor	RAI-refractory DTC	2	NCT03246958
Pembrolizumab monotherapy	PD-1 checkpoint inhibitor	Rare thyroid cancer including DTC (papillary, follicular, Hürthle cell, poorly differentiated thyroid carcinoma), medullary, and anaplastic thyroid carcinoma	2	NCT03012620 NCT02628067 NCT02054806 (phase 1)
Pembrolizumab in combination with intratumoral injection of clostridium novyi-NT	PD-1 inhibitor	Treatment refractory solid tumors including thyroid cancer	1b	NCT03435952

Rearranged During Transfection-Driven DTC

The first oncogenic events identified in PTC were the chromosomal rearrangements that resulted in the expression of fusion proteins involving the *rearranged during transfection* (*RET*) proto-oncogene, playing an oncogenic role in about 20% of the PTCs. 72% of the analyzed PTCs of patients living in the proximities of Chernobyl's nuclear facility, hence exposed to ionizing radiation, revealed *RET/PTC* fusions.[27] *RET* fusions are also enriched in pediatric and young adult thyroid cancers.[28,29] LOXO-292 and BLU-667 are two novel, highly specific, and potent drugs against *RET* mutations.

Potential Effect of Genotyping in RAI-Refractory DTC and Targeting Driver Alterations

Our current systemic therapies for RAI-refractory DTC are primarily multikinase inhibitors that target multiple kinases, including VEGFRs. Although these agents can yield durable anticancer benefits, they can cause significant side effects, limiting the doses that can be used or tolerated. Side effects commonly reported include hypertension, fatigue, diarrhea, anorexia, and weight loss. Rare but serious related adverse events include thrombosis, impaired wound healing, risk of fistula formation, and hemorrhage. Ideally, treatment with less toxicity and even greater efficacy will become available for patients with advanced thyroid cancer. Given the frequency of driver alterations in thyroid cancers that are detectable by next-generation sequencing (NGS) and potentially druggable with current and emerging cancer therapies, practice may be changing to incorporate NGS profiling in routine clinical decision making. Taking driver alterations in advanced thyroid cancer as a whole, including mutations in *BRAF, N/H RAS, and PTEN*, and fusions involving *RET, NTRK 1&3, BRAF, PPARγ, ALK,* and *ROS1*, the majority of patients with advanced thyroid cancer in need of treatment will be found to have an actionable alteration on NGS testing. In fact, PTCs harbor the highest rate, 12%, of recurrent oncogenic kinase fusions seen in all solid tumors analyzed in The Cancer Genome Atlas (TCGA) program,[30] and targeting such oncogenic kinase fusions has led to major breakthroughs in the field of oncology. A new paradigm for genotype-phenotype-treatment approaches in advanced thyroid cancer is thus on the horizon.

MEDULLARY THYROID CARCINOMA

Medullary thyroid carcinoma (MTC) is a neuroendocrine tumor arising from parafollicular C cells of the thyroid gland. Although it accounts for only 1% to 2% of all thyroid cancer cases, MTC is responsible for a disproportionally large number of thyroid cancer deaths, with a 50% survival at 10 years. Approximately 25% of MTC cases are hereditary, occurring as part of multiple endocrine neoplasia type 2 syndromes (MEN 2A, MEN 2B, and familial MTC) as a result of germline activating mutations in the *RET* proto-oncogene. Importantly, of the 75% of MTC cases that are sporadic, approximately 60% harbor somatic mutations in *RET*.[31–33]

RET is located on chromosome 10q11.2 and encodes for a transmembrane tyrosine kinase receptor that dimerizes after ligand binding. Tyrosine residues are autophosphorylated by the dimerized receptor, activating several downstream pathways, including the RAS/MEK/ERK pathway that promotes cell cycle progression, and the P13K/AKT/NF-κB pathway that increases cell motility, survival, and also progression through the cell cycle. p38, MAPK, JAK/STAT, and protein kinase C are also stimulated by RET activation and lead to cell growth, differentiation, and survival.[34]

Hereditary MTC

MEN 2A, MEN 2B, and Familial MTC are autosomal dominant syndromes with nearly 100% penetrance. To date, more than 100 different *RET* mutations and other genomic alterations have been described in hereditary MTC. The MEN 2 syndromes are characterized by varying phenotypes based on the specific *RET* genotype, which increase not only the aggressiveness of the MTC, but also increase the risk for pheochromocytoma, hyperparathyroidism, cutaneous lichen amyloidosis (CLA), and Hirschsprung's disease. This genotype-phenotype correlation is summarized well in the most recent American Thyroid Association (ATA) MTC guidelines[4] and is important in the management of the syndrome as the specific mutation governs the age at which prophylactic thyroidectomy is indicated as well as determines the need for screening for pheochromocytoma and hyperparathyroidism. When an index case of MEN 2 is identified, screening of at-risk family members is critical, as early thyroidectomy prior can cure affected family members of an otherwise life-threatening malignancy. MEN 2A mutations, the most common of which is *RET* C634R, typically occur in the extracellular cysteine-rich domain of the RET protein, leading to homodimerization and constitutive activation of the receptor tyrosine kinase. In addition to MTC, patients with MEN 2A are at risk for pheochromocytoma, primary parathyroid hyperplasia and, rarely, CLA. MEN 2B is most frequently associated with the *RET* M918T mutation in the kinase domain, leading to autophosphorylation of the intracellular tyrosine residues, which results in constitutive kinase activation. In MEN 2B, MTC is typically highly aggressive, arising early in life. Pheochromocytomas are seen in approximately 50% of affected patients, and marfanoid features, intestinal ganglioneuromas, and mucosal neuromas are characteristic. Familial MTC, which many consider a variant of MEN 2A, presents usually between 20 and 40 years of age and is characterized by MTC without other MEN 2A or B diagnoses. All newly diagnosed patients with MTC should undergo testing for germline *RET* mutation, even in the absence of family history suggestive of a hereditary syndrome, in part due to the importance of prophylactic thyroidectomy in related carriers, but also given that de novo germline mutations in the absence of family history have been identified in up to 75% of MEN 2B and almost 10% of MEN 2A patients.[35,36]

Sporadic MTC

Sporadic MTC most commonly presents in the fourth to sixth decade of life, with approximately half of patients presenting with early stage disease limited to the thyroid alone, whereas nodal with or without distant metastases are present at diagnosis in the other half. Metastases are seen most commonly in regional and distant lymph nodes, bones, lungs, and the liver where a military pattern of numerous small metastases can be difficult to detect on routine imaging. Less common sites of metastases include the brain and skin.

MTC patients may present with or develop symptoms such as dysphagia due to esophageal compression, hoarseness with or without signs of aspiration due to involvement of the recurrent laryngeal nerve, or systemic symptoms resulting from tumor of calcitonin secretion causing diarrhea and/or flushing.[31,37]

Variable Natural History, CT, and Carcinoembryonic Antigen Doubling Times

The natural history of MTC is dependent on whether or not the MTC is sporadic or inherited and the specific mutation carried. Sporadic MTCs have a variable clinical behavior, with some patients living for years even with distant metastases, whereas other cases progress more rapidly.

Hereditary MTC classically progresses from C cell hyperplasia to MTC to locoregional lymph node invasion to distant metastatic disease in the span of months to years. The ATA defines moderate-, high- and highest-risk designations, characterizing the specific *RET* mutations and the associated aggressiveness of the resulting MTC case. Patients with MEN 2B harboring *RET* M918T fall into the highest-risk category of disease, which develops early in childhood and has a high propensity to metastasize. As a result, infants identified to carry germline *RET* M918T should undergo prophylactic thyroidectomy before 1 year of age. The ATA high-risk category includes patients with *RET* C634 and A883F mutations. Carriers of these germline mutations should undergo thyroidectomy before 5 years of age or earlier if indicated by calcitonin levels. The ATA moderate-risk category includes patients with *RET* mutations other than M918T, C634, and A883F. Carriers of moderate-risk *RET* mutations should begin neck ultrasound and calcitonin monitoring by 5 years of age, with the timing of prophylactic thyroidectomy individualized based upon findings and other factors that may be relevant to the particular case.[31] In patients with hereditary MTC, the rate of 5-year survival is 93% for stages I through III; however, 5-year survival drops dramatically to 28% for stage IV disease.[38]

Serum calcitonin levels correlate with tumor burden in both sporadic and familial cases of MTC and should be measured preoperatively when MTC is suspected. Not all newly diagnosed patients require initial assessment for distant metastasis, but patients with bulky cervical adenopathy, symptoms suggestive of distant metastasis, or serum calcitonin greater than 500 pg/mL should be evaluated for distant metastasis.[39,40] Both calcitonin and carcinoembryonic antigen (CEA) also provide important information about disease status postoperatively. When serum calcitonin remains greater than 150 pg/mL postoperatively, the likelihood of metastatic disease is high and systemic radiographic evaluation is warranted. Moreover, calcitonin and CEA followed over time are not only sensitive markers for disease progression, their doubling times are also prognostic for survival. Meta-analysis of several studies evaluating the prognostic value of calcitonin and CEA doubling times indicates that when the calcitonin doubling time is less than 1 year, the 5- and 10-year survival rates were 36% and 18%, respectively, whereas a calcitonin doubling time greater than 1 year predicts 5- and 10-year survival rates of 98% and 95%, respectively.[41] Similarly, a CEA doubling time of less than 1 year predicts 5- and 10-year survival rates of 43% and 21%, respectively, versus 5- and 10-year survival rates of 100% and 100%, respectively, when CEA doubling time is greater than 1 year.[42] Furthermore, CEA and calcitonin levels can be indicative of tumor differentiation. CEA elevated out of proportion to calcitonin or low levels of both tumor markers in the setting of bulky disease suggests dedifferentiation of the tumor and typically heralds rapid disease progression.[31]

In addition to secreting calcitonin and CEA, MTCs also occasionally produce other hormones, including adrenocorticotropin hormone and corticotropin-releasing hormone, which can lead to ectopic Cushing's syndrome. When Cushing's syndrome emerges in MTC, the prognosis is poor. Still, treatment, including medical therapy to combat hormonal production, tumor debulking, bilateral adrenalectomy, and systemic MTC treatment, can be effective at mitigating this otherwise serious and debilitating syndrome.

Systemic Therapy

The surgical management of MTC is addressed elsewhere in this text (see Chapter 26 Sporadic Medullary Thyroid Carcinoma, and Chapter 27 Syndromic Medullary Thyroid Carcinoma: MEN 2A and MEN 2B). Focal approaches to metastatic MTC, such as palliative radiotherapy to painful bone metastases or radiofrequency ablation to a solitary liver metastasis, are occasionally indicated. At present, two systemic therapies, vandetanib and cabozantinib, are available and approved by health regulatory agencies specifically for the treatment of unresectable locoregionally recurrent and or distant metastatic MTC, and new agents are well along in development.

Current Standards of Care
Vandetanib

Vandetanib is an oral multikinase inhibitor of VEGFR-2 and 3, epidermal growth factor receptor (EGFR), and RET. The central role of RET in MTC led to vandetanib preclinical studies with promising activity in MTC cell lines,[43] which ultimately led to the phase 3 clinical trial (ZETA) in which patients with measurable, unresectable locally advanced or metastatic sporadic or hereditary MTC were randomized in a 2:1 fashion to vandetanib or placebo.[44] At the time of disease progression, patients were unblinded, and those on the placebo arm were offered treatment with open-label vandetanib. The primary objective of PFS prolongation was met with vandetanib versus placebo, with median PFS in the vandetanib arm not reached by the time of analysis predicted to reach 30.5 months versus a median PFS of 19.3 months in the placebo group (HR, 0.46; 95% CI, 0.31 to 0.69; $p < 0.001$). At the time of analysis, there was no difference in OS, though 93% of patients who progressed on placebo went on to receive open-label vandetanib. The ORR per RECIST with vandetanib was 45%, with a disease control rate of 87%, and biochemical responses were seen in more than half the patients on vandetanib. Common side effects for vandetanib included diarrhea, rash, nausea, and hypertension and occurred in 30% or more of patients on vandetanib, and 12% of patients were discontinued from treatment due to adverse events.

Cabozantinib

Cabozantinib is an oral tyrosine multikinase inhibitor of hepatocyte growth factor receptor (MET), VEGFR-2, and RET. This drug was studied in a phase 3 clinical trial (EXAM) and designed similarly to the ZETA trial, in that patients with measurable, unresectable locally advanced or metastatic sporadic or hereditary MTC were randomly assigned in a 2:1 fashion to cabozantinib or placebo, with PFS as the primary endpoint; however, there were two important differences: (1) patients were required to have disease progression per RECIST within 14 months of study entry and (2) prior TKI therapy was allowed.[45] 330 patients were enrolled, with 21% having received a prior TKI. The estimated median PFS was 11.2 months with cabozantinib versus 4.0 months with placebo (HR, 0.28; 95% CI, 0.19 to 0.40; $p < 0.001$), and PFS benefit was maintained for patients who had received prior TKI therapy. The ORR per RECIST was 28%. Although there was no statistically significant difference in OS between the two study arms as a whole, median OS was improved with cabozantinib in the subset of patients enrolled harboring *RET* M918T mutation from 18.9 months with placebo versus 44.3 months with cabozantinib (HR, 0.28; 95% CI, 0.38 to 0.94; $p < 0.03$).[46] Grade 3 or 4 adverse events were reported in 69% of patients on cabozantinib, with the most common therapy-related adverse events including diarrhea, palmar-plantar erythrodysesthesia, weight loss, anorexia, nausea, and fatigue. Adverse events led to dose decreases in 79% and 16% treatment discontinuation in patients on cabozantinib.

Because the side effects of vandetanib and cabozantinib have the potential to affect QoL, are not curative, and no study has addressed the question of the best timing to initiate systemic therapy, a critical challenge remains regarding when a patient with MTC should start treatment. Although there is general consensus that multikinase inhibitors should be not be considered in patients who have asymptomatic, low burden, slowly progressive disease, and it is clear that patients with symptomatic and/or rapidly progressive disease need treatment started, the decision regarding the optimal timing of starting therapy for patients who are asymptomatic, but have disease progressing at a moderate pace, must be individualized for each patient.

Future Directions

RET as a driver mutation is present in essentially all hereditary MTCs, somatically mutated in a majority of sporadic MTCs, and codes for a tyrosine kinase that is constitutively activated by mutation. Thus specifically targeting RET for therapeutic effect is appealing. Recently, two new agents, BLU-667 and LOXO-292, designed to potently and specifically inhibit RET, have now entered clinical development.

BLU-667

BLU-667 is an oral, highly selective and potent RET inhibitor developed to specifically inhibit the RET kinase only and thus minimize the "off target" side effects engendered by multikinase inhibitors with their multiple targets. The drug was designed to inhibit MTC tumors driven by the spectrum of *RET* mutations as well as tumors driven by *RET* fusions, as seen in 6% of PTCs.[11] The phase 1, first-in-human study of BLU-667 (ARROW), has been reported in abstract form.[47] To date, 37 patients with MTC have been treated in the dose escalation phase and at the recommended phase 2 dose (RP2D). The drug has been well tolerated, with most adverse events grade 1 or 2. The most frequent adverse events include constipation, transaminitis, hypertension, leukopenia, diarrhea, neutropenia, increased creatinine, fatigue, and headache. In the MTC patients treated across all doses, the ORR was 49%, and thus far responses appear durable, with the longest response ongoing at 15 months. Calcitonin and CEA levels declined dramatically as well. In *RET*-fusion PTCs, BLU-667 also shows activity, with responses seen in two of five patients enrolled.[48]

LOXO-292

LOXO-292 is a second oral selective RET inhibitor similarly designed to potently and specifically inhibit the RET kinase alone. The LOXO-292 phase 1 dose escalation first-in-human trial (LIBRETTO-001) has also been reported.[49] Results from 29 *RET*-mutant MTC and 9 RET-fusion thyroid cancer patients have been reported. In keeping with the drug's specificity for RET, LOXO-292 was well tolerated, with few grade 3 or higher toxicities. Grade 1 or 2 adverse events seen in 10% of patients or more included diarrhea, fatigue, xerostomia, constipation, hypomagnesemia, cough, headache, and nausea. The ORR for the MTC group was 59%, and in *RET*-fusion thyroid cancer the ORR was 78%. In MTC, calcitonin and CEA levels declined substantially with LOXO-292. Responses were seen across all but the lowest dose levels and appear durable, with all but one MTC patient remaining in response at median follow-up period.

Taken together, the early BLU-667 and LOXO-292 experience indicates great promise for the strategy of potently and specifically targeting driver *RET* alterations in thyroid cancer. The combination of tolerability and activity are expected to usher in a whole new era of treatment for *RET*-driven cancers.

REFERENCES

For a complete list of references, go to expertconsult.com

SECTION 8

Parathyroid Surgery

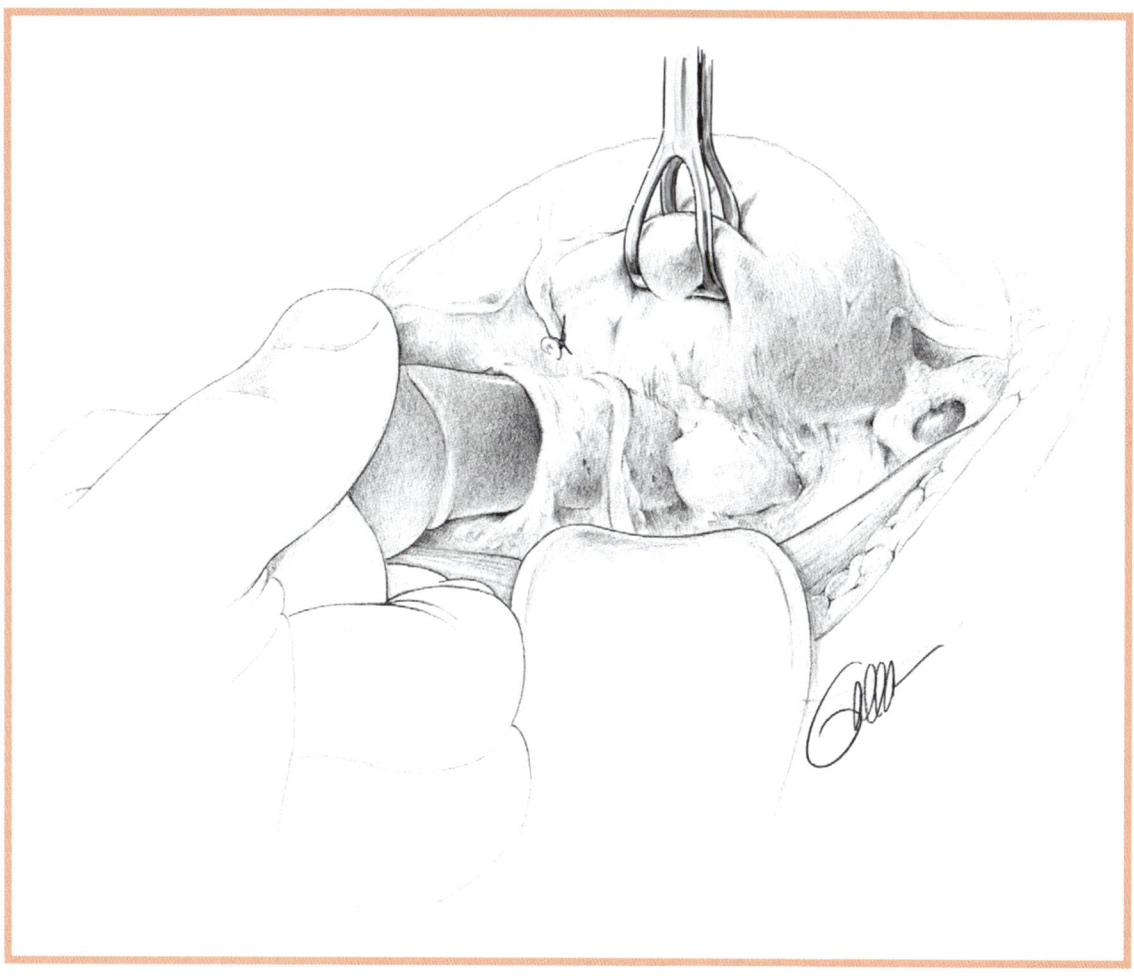

53

Primary Hyperparathyroidism: Pathophysiology, Surgical Indications, and Preoperative Workup

Shonni J. Silverberg, John P. Bilezikian

Primary hyperparathyroidism (PHPT) is characterized classically by hypercalcemia and levels of parathyroid hormone (PTH) that are frankly elevated or inappropriate in the presence of hypercalcemia. Patients with the disease today in the United States bear little resemblance to those with the severe disorder of "stones, bones, and groans" described by Fuller Albright and others in the 1930s.[1-4] Then, patients typically had skeletal manifestations described as *osteitis fibrosa cystica*, which were exemplified by brown tumors of the long bones; subperiosteal bone resorption; distal tapering of the clavicles and phalanges; and salt-and-pepper–appearing erosions of the skull on radiograph (Figure 53.1). Nephrocalcinosis was also present in approximately 80% of patients. Neuromuscular dysfunction was characterized by proximal muscle weakness. The widespread use of automated biochemical screening in the United States, starting in the 1970s, and subsequently by other countries, signaled two important changes in the recognition of this disease. It became much more common with a 4- to 5-fold increase in incidence. The second noteworthy change was the recognition that a clear majority of patients discovered in this way did not manifest the classical features of the disease. They were said to be asymptomatic. Nephrolithiasis lingered as the most common overt clinical manifestation of the disease, but its incidence fell to 15% to 20%. Radiologic manifestations became a curiosity, and neuromuscular dysfunction essentially disappeared.

Little controversy exists concerning appropriate therapy for PHPT in its classic form. In the presence of symptoms, either of hypercalcemia or overt target involvement, surgery was and still is indicated. However, with clear-cut symptoms absent in most patients whose disease was discovered by biochemical screening tests, the need for parathyroidectomy in all patients was questioned. This dilemma led to four International Workshops on the Management of Asymptomatic Primary Hyperparathyroidism, the most recent of which occurred in 2013.[5] Participants and attendees reviewed the features of the two presentations of the disease—symptomatic versus asymptomatic—with attention to technological advances that have provided over the past several decades greater insights into the extent to which asymptomatic disease could also be accompanied by subclinical manifestations of target organ involvement as well as by information about putative off-target actions of PTH in this disease. Moreover, long-term natural history studies of patients who did or did not undergo parathyroidectomy helped place revised guidelines into context.[5] Approaches to medical management with pharmacologic approaches advanced. Finally, over the past 15 years, yet another phenotype of primary hyperparathyroidism emerged, namely in those who demonstrate elevated levels of PTH in the absence of hypercalcemia. This third phenotype, normocalcemic PHPT, presented yet another challenge to the management of this disease.

In this chapter, we review the chronology of advances in the various phenotypes of primary hyperparathyroidism while providing a newer perspective, namely that technology has helped reinterpret this disease. Worldwide, all three forms of PHPT coexist today with frequencies varying by countries and their different approaches to medical care as well as to individual epidemiologic features of the population.

CLINICAL PRESENTATIONS OF PRIMARY HYPERPARATHYROIDISM

Symptomatic Primary Hyperparathyroidism

As noted earlier, this form of PHPT is historically the way this disease presented before the advent of multichannel screening technology. Symptoms were due to hypercalcemia, per se, often with levels of 13 to 16 mg/dL and with overt skeletal and/or renal manifestations. Over the years, it has become apparent that this form of PHPT can be exacerbated with regard to clinical symptomatology by vitamin D deficiency. The hypothesis of Stanbury in the early 1970s—namely that PHPT can worsen in the presence of vitamin D deficiency— has been documented clearly during the ensuing decades. The pathophysiology of this hypothesis relates to the normal physiologic relationship between vitamin D and PTH. With vitamin D deficiency, PTH levels will rise. This relationship is still evident in PHPT.[6,7] One of the best examples of this relates to a comparison of two different cohorts of patients with PHPT from New York and China.[8] The Chinese cohort was much more symptomatic; the group demonstrated average 25-hydroxyvitamin D levels of about 9 ng/mL, which was markedly low. On the other hand, the New York cohort, with much less symptomatology, had levels of 25-hydroxyvitamin D of 21 ng/mL. Giving credence to the concept that the asymptomatic variant of the disease surfaced with the use of biochemical screening, the New York cohort was identified in this way, but the Chinese cohort was identified only after patients manifested features of the disease.

EPIDEMIOLOGY OF PHPT

PHPT mainly affects people in their middle years with a peak incidence between 50 and 60 years of age. However, the disease appears from

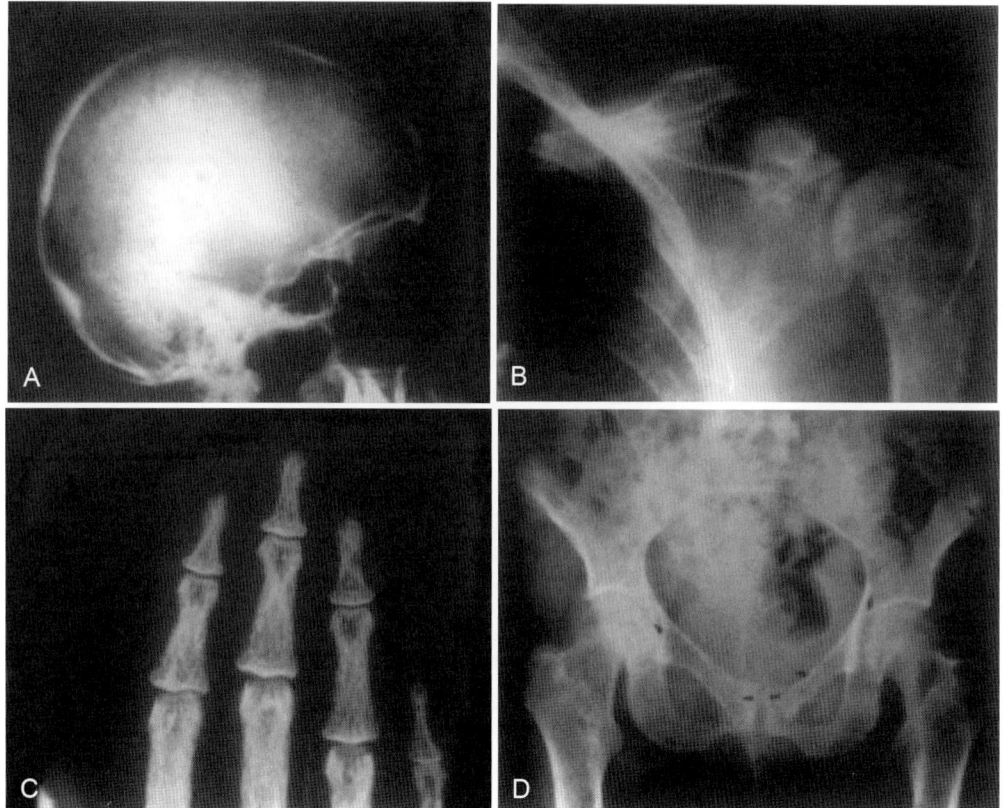

Fig. 53.1 Osteitis fibrosa cystica in classic primary hyperparathyroidism. **A,** Salt-and-pepper skull. **B,** Cystic bone disease of the clavicle. **C,** Subperiosteal bone resorption of the digits. **D,** Cortical erosions.

infancy through all stages of life. Women are affected more frequently than men, approximately 3:1 to 4:1. Typically, when biochemical screening is part of a country's healthcare system, patients are often discovered to have elevated serum calcium concentration during evaluations for an unrelated medical problem or simply though routine health screening. At the time of diagnosis, under these conditions, most patients with PHPT do not have classic symptoms or signs associated with disease. Kidney stones are uncommon, and clinical fracture events are rare. Diseases epidemiologically (although not etiologically) linked with PHPT, such as hypertension and peptic ulcer disease, are seen commonly but no more so than in unaffected individuals. Constitutional complaints, such as weakness, easy fatigability, depression, and intellectual weariness, also manifest themselves. Results of physical examination are generally unremarkable. Band keratopathy, a former hallmark of classic PHPT resulting from deposition of calcium-phosphate crystals in the cornea, is rarely seen today, even by slit-lamp examination. The neck shows no masses. The abnormal parathyroid cannot be felt. The neuromuscular system is normal on routine examination.

The differential diagnosis of PHPT includes the other major cause of hypercalcemia, malignancy, which is readily distinguished from PHPT. Patients with hypercalcemia of malignancy typically have symptoms with advanced disease that has already been diagnosed. An exception is multiple myeloma in which hypercalcemia can be the initial manifestation. Biochemically, PTH levels are suppressed in malignancy. Classic immunoassays for PTH, used widely now for more than 30 years, facilitate the distinction between primary hyperparathyroidism and hypercalcemia of malignancy. Very rarely, a patient with malignancy is shown to have elevated PTH levels resulting from the ectopic secretion of native PTH from the tumor itself. Much more commonly, the malignancy is associated with the secretion of PTH–related protein (PTHrP), a molecule that is not detected by immunoassays for PTH. It is more common for a malignancy to appear with coexisting PHPT than for hypercalcemia to be caused by ectopic PTH secretion from a malignancy.

SKELETON

Although *osteitis fibrosa cystica,* the classic radiologic depiction, is distinctly unusual in patients who have PHPT in the United States, this does not imply that the skeleton is unaffected in those with asymptomatic disease. There is now abundant evidence for skeletal involvement in the hyperparathyroid process. The availability of sensitive techniques to monitor the skeleton has given us an opportunity to address these issues in patients who have the asymptomatic variant of the disease.

BONE DENSITOMETRY

The advent of bone mineral densitometry as a major diagnostic tool for osteoporosis occurred when the clinical profile of PHPT was changing from a symptomatic disease to an asymptomatic one. Questions about skeletal involvement in PHPT could be addressed despite the absence of overt radiologic features of the disease. Dual energy x-ray absorptiometry (DXA) in PHPT has provided insight in this regard. Three-site densitometry (lumbar spine, hip, and distal 1/3 radius) has been particularly informative because of the proclivity of PTH to be catabolic at cortical sites (e.g., distal 1/3 radius) and anabolic at cancellous sites (e.g., lumbar spine). In PHPT, bone density at the distal third of the radius is diminished.[9] Bone density at the lumbar spine is only minimally reduced, typically within 5% of age-matched mean values. The

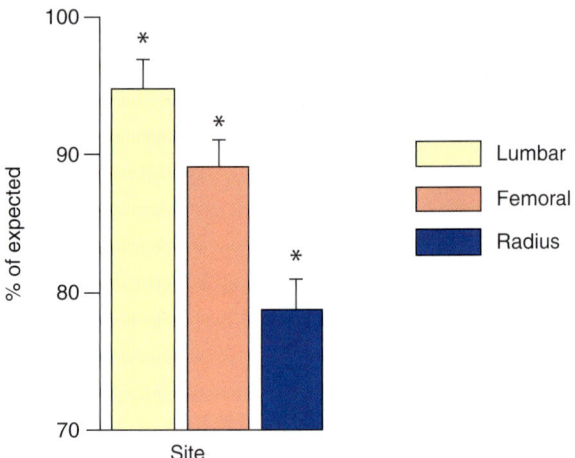

Fig. 53.2 Bone densitometry in primary hyperparathyroidism. Data are shown in comparison to age- and sex-matched normal subjects. Divergence from expected values is different at each site ($p = 0.0001$). (Redrawn from Silverberg SJ, Shane E, de la Cruz L, et al. Skeletal disease in primary hyperparathyroidism. *J Bone Miner Res.* 1989;4[3]:283–291.)

hip region, containing a relatively equal mixture of cortical and cancellous elements, shows a densitometric value that is intermediate between the cortical and cancellous sites (Figure 53.2). These observations initially supported not only the notion that PTH is catabolic in cortical bone but also the view that PTH can have anabolic properties in cancellous bone under specific circumstances.[10,11] In postmenopausal women with PHPT, the same pattern was observed.[9] Thus postmenopausal women with PHPT show a reversal of the pattern typically associated with postmenopausal estrogen deficiency—namely preferential loss of cancellous bone. These observations suggested that PHPT may help protect postmenopausal women from cancellous bone loss due to estrogen deficiency.

The bone density profile in which skeletal mass is relatively preserved at the vertebrae and diminished at the more cortical distal radius does not always appear in PHPT. A small group of hyperparathyroid patients shows evidence of vertebral osteopenia at the time of presentation. In our natural history study, approximately 15% of patients had a lumbar spine Z score (number of standard deviations away from age and sex-matched mean) of less than 1.5 at the time of diagnosis.[12] In addition, patients with PHPT can show uniform reductions in bone mineral density (BMD) at all sites, whereas others, although rare, have normal bone density at all sites.

New Insights Into the Skeleton Based Upon Imaging Technology

Although BMD is a gold standard for clinical assessment of the skeleton, it does not give direct insight into skeletal microstructure. The advent of high-resolution peripheral computed tomography (HRpQCT) permitted noninvasive assessment of skeletal microstructure in this disease. HRpQCT visualizes both the cortical and trabecular compartments of the skeleton and thus can ascertain the extent to which the trabecular skeleton can be involved in this disease. The impetus for this inquiry came from studies, noted later, that suggested from both epidemiologic and prospective data a global increase in fracture risk, not simply the nonvertebral skeleton as was suggested by DXA. By HRpQCT, we and others have shown that both the cortical and trabecular compartments of bone are adversely affected in PHPT.[13-15] Stein et al. showed even further that by individual trabecular segmentation analysis, vertically oriented rods were predominant over horizontally disposed elements. This kind of topology results in reduced bone strength, as was shown by finite element analysis in this study.

HRpQCT provides great insight into skeletal microstructure in PHPT, but it is not and will never be clinically available on a routine basis. Potentially, a method to assess skeletal microstructure clinically would provide access to this kind of information to any clinician. The trabecular bone score (TBS) is a textural analysis of the lumbar spine image obtained by DXA.[16,17] Based upon a software algorithm that can semiquantitatively determine the extent of homogeneity or heterogeneity of bone, it determines microstructural quality. As shown by Silva et al. and by Romagnoli et al., TBS scores are significantly lower in PHPT than lumbar spine bone mineral densitometry by DXA. Applied to PHPT, these new imaging technologies clearly demonstrate that both cortical and trabecular compartments of bone are affected.

BONE HISTOMORPHOMETRY

To a certain extent, analyses of percutaneous bone biopsies from patients with PHPT have confirmed the pervasive nature of skeletal involvement in PHPT. Cortical thinning and a very dynamic process associated with high turnover and accelerated bone remodeling are regularly observed. The inability to perceive trabecular involvement may speak to the possibility that the iliac crest, the site of the bone biopsy, as more direct measurements of the nonvertebral skeleton. It is of note that in HRpQCT studies, the radius and the tibia are measured.[18-20]

FRACTURES

For many years, the question of fracture incidence in PHPT was an open one. Early studies by Dauphine et al. reported an increased prevalence of vertebral fractures in patients with mild PHPT, but other studies argued otherwise.[21-23] Approximately 20 years ago, this question was addressed by a careful epidemiology survey of a well-defined cohort of PHPT patients. Kholsa et al. from Rochester, Minn., found increased incidence of vertebral, Colles' rib, and pelvic (but not hip) fractures in patients with PHPT.[23] The results of this study were initially interpreted as possibly due to selection bias, but they corresponded exactly with information from later studies in which the nonvertebral skeleton and, in particular, cortical and trabecular bone were clearly documented to be at risk in this disease, as noted earlier. Further support for the proposition that the trabecular skeleton is at risk for fracture in PHPT came from the work of Vignali et al. This group studied vertebral fractures in PHPT by x-ray and by vertebral fracture assessment.[24] Vertebral fractures were seen much more frequently in patients with PHPT (24.6%) than in the control subjects (4.0%; $p < 0.001$).

NEPHROLITHIASIS

Kidney stones remain the most common manifestation of the disease.[25] The incidence has declined over the years, but again, application of imaging technology has given us new insight into prevalence of hypercalciuria, nephrolithiasis, and nephrocalcinosis in this disease.[26]

Not surprisingly, more recent systematic evaluation of the kidneys among patients with PHPT, not known to have renal involvement, has revealed stones and/or nephrocalcinosis in 21% to 55% of patients.[27,28]

OTHER ORGAN INVOLVEMENT

Over the years, PHPT has been described as affecting many different organ systems. Perhaps, the most common complaints have been those nonspecific descriptions of weakness and easy fatigability. Classic PHPT has been associated with a distinct neuromuscular syndrome, characterized by type II muscle cell atrophy.[29] In the milder, less symptomatic form of the disease that is common today, this disorder is rarely seen.[30] The neuropsychiatric abnormalities of PHPT have long been an area of active interest.[26-28] Many patients, families, and physicians comment on features of depression, cognitive difficulties, and anxiety in those with the disease. Furthermore, many of these complaints have been described as being reversible after parathyroidectomy. The surgical literature provides further data supporting postoperative improvements.[31-34] Data on 152 patients revealed that 40% of patients reported less fatigue after surgical cure compared with thyroid surgical patients, who served as control subjects.[32] Similar findings were reported by others.[33,34] Walker et al. suggest the existence of cognitive deficiencies in postmenopausal women with PHPT, some of which normalize after parathyroidectomy.[35] However, the three randomized and controlled trials of surgery versus observation in mild PHPT have shown variable effects of surgery on psychiatric and quality-of-life measures.[36-38] Interim analysis of the largest trial (Bollerslev et al.) concluded that there was insufficient evidence of predictable improvement in these indices to recommend surgery solely for the purpose of reversing these complaints.

At the most recent international workshop on the management of PHPT, in 2013, this issue was comprehensively reviewed with the conclusion that we still do not have sufficient evident to draw conclusions about the direct relationship between PHPT and these nonspecific features.[5] As a result, most experts do not include such features as a clear guideline for operative intervention in this disease.[39]

Many other pathologic features have been described in patients with PHPT. Hypertension has been noted to be present in a higher percentage of patients than expected.[40,41] However, the hypertension does not remit with cure of the underlying hyperparathyroid process. The only randomized and controlled trial data show improvement in follow-up measurements of blood pressure in both those who had surgery and those who did not have surgery.[42] Data on cardiovascular manifestations of mild PHPT remain incomplete. Left ventricular hypertrophy, common in those with more severe disease, does not appear in those with very mild PHPT. Also, carotid intima medial thickness increases in PHPT.[43,44] The effect of surgery on these indices remains to be seen.

Associations have also been reported between PHPT and peptic ulcer disease. Today, it is felt that a significant relationship between the two conditions exists only in patients with multiple endocrine neoplasia, type 1. The association of pancreatitis with PHPT found in patients with marked hypercalcemia does not appear in those with mild elevations in serum calcium. Finally, gout and pseudogout have been described in PHPT, both in the stages of untreated disease and immediately after surgical cure.[45] Again, verifiable etiologic relationships between PHPT and uric acid or pyrophosphate arthropathy remain to be established.

NORMOCALCEMIC PRIMARY HYPERPARATHYROIDISM

After the recognition in the early 1970s that most patients with PHPT did not have classical symptoms of the disorder, 4 decades passed before the normocalcemic variant of this disease was described. This happened about 15 years ago. It was discovered in patients being evaluated for low bone mass or frank osteoporosis.[45,46] The first descriptions of normocalcemic PHPT involved patients with bone loss. Patients being evaluated for bone loss in medical centers had their PTH measured as a routine part of the evaluation for osteoporosis even with completely normal concentrations of total and ionized serum calcium. Some had elevated PTH levels in the absence of any secondary cause. We now appreciate that this normocalcemic form of PHPT can occur among unsuspecting populations as well. Thus normocalcemic PHPT can be asymptomatic or symptomatic.[47-50]

A Current View of the Variable Presentations of Primary Hyperparathyroidism

Although the three different forms of primary hyperparathyroidism have been described within a chronologic context, it is noteworthy that all three forms of this disease, namely the symptomatic, the asymptomatic, and the normocalcemic, exist concurrently in the world today. In fact, it is likely that these variants of the disease always have coexisted. The form of the disease that is most likely to be seen depends on several factors. For example, in countries like India where biochemical screening is not yet common medical practice, the symptomatic form of PHPT is most likely.[51] In North America, Western Europe, and many other parts of the world where biochemical screening is common medical practice, asymptomatic PHPT will be the most likely and recognized as a relatively common endocrine disorder. The term *asymptomatic* should probably be qualified, even if only semantically, because as we have noted, skeletal and renal imaging has detected involvement of these target organs to a much greater extent than previously thought.[52] The most recent variant of this disease, normocalcemic PHPT, will be seen most often in medical centers that specialize in metabolic bone diseases. Thus, although the history of this disease evolved into our recognition of three different phenotypes, technology has defined their coexistence, the relative incidence of which is a function of country- and practice-specific variables.

PATHOLOGY

The pathology of PHPT is discussed in detail in Chapter 65, Surgical Pathology of the Parathyroid Glands. By far the most common lesion found in patients with the disease is the single parathyroid adenoma, which occurs in 80% of patients. Risk factors identified for development of PHPT include a history of neck irradiation and prolonged use of lithium therapy for affective disorders.[53-55] However, the majority of cases of PHPT have no defined cause. Molecular abnormalities leading to clonal emergence are discussed elsewhere (see Chapter 55, Principles in Surgical Management of Primary Hyperparathyroidism; Chapter 62, Parathyroid Management in the MEN Syndromes; Chapter 64, Parathyroid Carcinoma; and Chapter 65, Surgical Pathology of the Parathyroid Glands). Although in most cases a single adenoma is found, multiple parathyroid adenomas have been reported in 2% to 4% of cases. These may be familial or sporadic. Parathyroid adenomas can be discovered in many unexpected anatomic locations. Embryonal migration patterns of parathyroid tissue account for a plethora of possible sites for ectopic parathyroid adenomas. The most common ectopic sites are within the thyroid gland, the superior mediastinum, and the thymus. Occasionally, the adenoma may ultimately be identified in the retroesophageal space, the pharynx, the lateral neck, and even the submucosa of the esophagus (see Chapter 2, Applied Embryology of the Thyroid and Parathyroid Glands; Chapter 55, Principles in Surgical Management of Primary Hyperparathyroidism; Chapter 56, Standard Bilateral Parathyroid Exploration; Chapter 57, Minimally Invasive Single Gland Parathyroid Exploration; Chapter 60, Surgical Management of Multiglandular Parathyroid Disease; Chapter 61, Surgical Management of Secondary and Tertiary

Hyperparathyroidism; and Chapter 63, Reoperation for Sporadic Primary Hyperparathyroidism).

In approximately 15% of patients with PHPT, all four parathyroid glands are involved. No clinical features differentiate single versus multiglandular disease. The etiology of four-gland parathyroid hyperplasia is multifactorial (see Chapter 60, Surgical Management of Multiglandular Parathyroid Disease). It may be associated with a familial hereditary syndrome, such as multiple endocrine neoplasia, types 1 and 2a (see Chapter 62, Parathyroid Management in the MEN Syndromes). Although the pathophysiology of the sporadic cases is unknown, the calcium set point does not seem to be altered. Instead, it seems that the increased number of parathyroid cells in the hyperplastic glands causes the excessive secretion of PTH. As in the case of parathyroid adenomas, underlying molecular mechanisms are heterogeneous.

CLINICAL COURSE WITH AND WITHOUT SURGERY

As the disease profile has changed, questions have arisen concerning the necessity of surgery in asymptomatic patients. As more data have become available, there has been a gradual evolution of the criteria used to identify which patients should routinely be sent to surgery and which might be followed safely without intervention.[5,56-58] Surgery is advised in all patients with any overt manifestation of PHPT (nephrolithiasis, *osteitis fibrosa cystica*, classic neuromuscular disease). For patients without "classical" symptoms of parathyroid disease, the 2014 International Consensus Panel Guidelines suggest surgery for those meeting the following criteria (Table 53.1):[5]

1. Calcium level: Serum calcium more than 1.0 mg/dL above the reference limit.
2. Renal Parameters: Creatinine clearance <60 cc/min; nephrocalcinosis or nephrolithiasis identified on imaging; 24-hour urine calcium >400 mg/day; or increased stone risk by biochemical stone risk analysis.
3. Bone Parameters: Osteoporosis by bone density at any site (T score ≤ −2.5); clinical fragility fracture; or vertebral compression fracture on spine imaging.
4. Age <50 years.

A reasonable list of testing to consider before surgery appears in Table 53.2.

TABLE 53.2 Evaluation Before Considering Surgery in Primary Hyperparathyroidism

Category	Test	Caveat
Serum biochemistry	Calcium, albumin, PTH, 25-hydroxyvitamin D	Ionized calcium not routine. Necessary for normocalcemic PHPT
Urinary biochemistry	24-hour urinary calcium and creatinine	Rule out FHH
Skeletal evaluation	Bone densitometry (DXA)	3 site
Genetic testing		Consider with patient/family history of other MEN disorders, age less than 40 or family history PHPT
Other imaging	Spine Kidney	Image for subclinical vertebral fracture(s) and renal stones

DXA, dual energy x-ray absorptiometry, FHH, familial hypocalciuric hypercalcemia, MEN, multiple endocrine neoplasia, PHPT, primary hyperparathyroidism, PTH, parathyroid hormone.

SURGERY

Once the decision has been made to refer for parathyroidectomy, preoperative localization is warranted (see Chapter 55, Principles in Surgical Management of Primary Hyperparathyroidism). Preoperative localization allows consideration of minimally invasive parathyroidectomy (see Chapter 57, Minimally Invasive Single Gland Parathyroid Exploration) and also permits identification of ectopic glands. Preoperative localization is also particularly helpful in the patient with previous neck surgery in whom usual anatomic landmarks may be altered. Both the localization and surgical techniques are fully discussed elsewhere (see Chapter 57, Minimally Invasive Single Gland Parathyroid Exploration and Chapter 58, Minimally Invasive Video-Assisted Parathyroidectomy).

TABLE 53.1 Current versus Prior Guidelines for Surgery in Asymptomatic Primary Hyperparathyroidism

	GUIDELINES FROM			
Criteria	1990[50]	2002[51]	2009[58]	2014[5]
Serum calcium (above normal)	1–1.6 mg/dL	1.0 mg/dL	1.0 mg/dL	1.0 mg/dL
Renal Parameters	24-hour urinary calcium >400 mg; Creatinine clearance reduced by 30%	24-hour urinary calcium >400 mg; Creatinine clearance reduced by 30%	Creatinine clearance <60 cc/min	Creatinine clearance <60 cc/min 24-hour urinary calcium >400 mg; High stone risk
Skeletal Parameters	DXA Z-score ≤ 2.0 (forearm)	DXA T-score ≤ 2.5 (any site)	DXA T-score ≤ −2.5 (any site); Fragility fracture	DXA T-score ≤ −2.5 (any site); Fragility fracture; Vertebral compression fracture on spinal imaging
Age	<50	<50	<50	<50

DXA, dual energy x-ray absorptiometry.
Modified from Bilezikian JP, Brandi ML, Eastell R, et al. Guidelines for the management of asymptomatic primary hyperparathyroidism: Summary statement from the Fourth International Workshop. *J Clin Endocrinol Metab*. 2014; 99(10):3561–3569.

After successful surgery, biochemical indices return rapidly to normal.[59] The serum calcium tends not to fall below normal, a situation characteristic of an earlier time when PHPT was a symptomatic disease with overt skeletal involvement ("hungry bone syndrome"). Transient hypocalcemia while remaining parathyroid glands recover can be prevented by giving patients several grams of calcium daily for the first weeks after surgery. Vague or constitutional symptoms may or may not improve after surgery, whereas hypertension and peptic ulcer disease, if present, are unlikely to remit. Surgery is of clear benefit in reducing the incidence of recurrent nephrolithiasis.[60,61] More than 90% of patients with stone disease and hyperparathyroidism do not form additional stones after parathyroid surgery, and those few who do are thought to have a second cause for their stone diseases. Long-term observational data confirm short-term randomized and controlled trial data demonstrating that surgery also leads to an improvement in BMD in patients with PHPT (Figure 53.3).[36-38,59,62] Parathyroidectomy leads to a 10% to 12% increase in bone density in the lumbar spine and femoral neck. The increase occurs mainly within the first years after surgery, but it may be sustained for a decade after surgery. In patients with hyperparathyroidism who have vertebral osteopenia or osteoporosis at the time of diagnosis, the postoperative increase in vertebral bone density is even greater, averaging 20% after parathyroidectomy.[12] The marked improvement seen in patients with low vertebral bone density argues for surgery in those who have cancellous as well as cortical bone loss, and it has led to the guideline supporting parathyroidectomy for patients with osteoporosis at any site (see Table 53.1).

MEDICAL MANAGEMENT

Although many patients with PHPT who do not meet any surgical guidelines experience no significant change in serum calcium, PTH, urinary calcium, or bone density, our 15-year observational study found that slightly more than one third (37%) of patients did have evidence of disease progression.[55] Lumbar spine, femoral neck, and radius BMD generally showed stability for 5 to 8 years (see Figure 53.3).[52,55] With longer follow-up, however, a significant decline in bone density has been documented at sites containing more cortical bone (hip and forearm).[62] This suggests that prolonged observation without intervention may place subjects at risk.

No clinical or biochemical features predicted which patients would have progressive disease and which would not, although those who had progressive disease tended to be younger than those who did not. Indeed, progression of disease was seen in more than 60% of patients under the age of 50 years, whereas in those over the age of 50, only 23% developed new indications for surgery while under observation.[63] These data provide evidence-based support for an age-related criterion for surgery.

Patients who do not undergo surgery must therefore be followed closely, and those who develop new indications for surgery should be offered parathyroidectomy. In patients followed without surgery, the 2014 guidelines suggest that serum calcium levels and estimated glomerular filtration rates should be obtained every 12 months, whereas bone densitometry should be repeated annually or biannually depending on availability (see Table 53.3 for all guidelines for follow-up). Current guidelines also suggest that patients with PHPT and coexisting vitamin D deficiency be treated with vitamin D to assure a 25-hydroxyvitamin D (25OHD) level above 20 ng/mL.[5] A randomized, controlled trial (RCT) of treatment with 2800 IU vitamin D daily showed a reduction of PTH levels and improved spine bone density with an increase in 25OHD from 25 to 37 ng/mL with no untoward consequences.[64]

Patients should be instructed to remain well hydrated and to avoid thiazide diuretics. Prolonged immobilization, which can worsen hypercalcemia and hypercalciuria, should also be avoided.[65] Although patients are frequently advised to limit their dietary calcium intake because of hypercalcemia, we do not advocate such a step. In patients with normal levels of 1,25-dihydroxyvitamin D_3, Locker et al. noted no

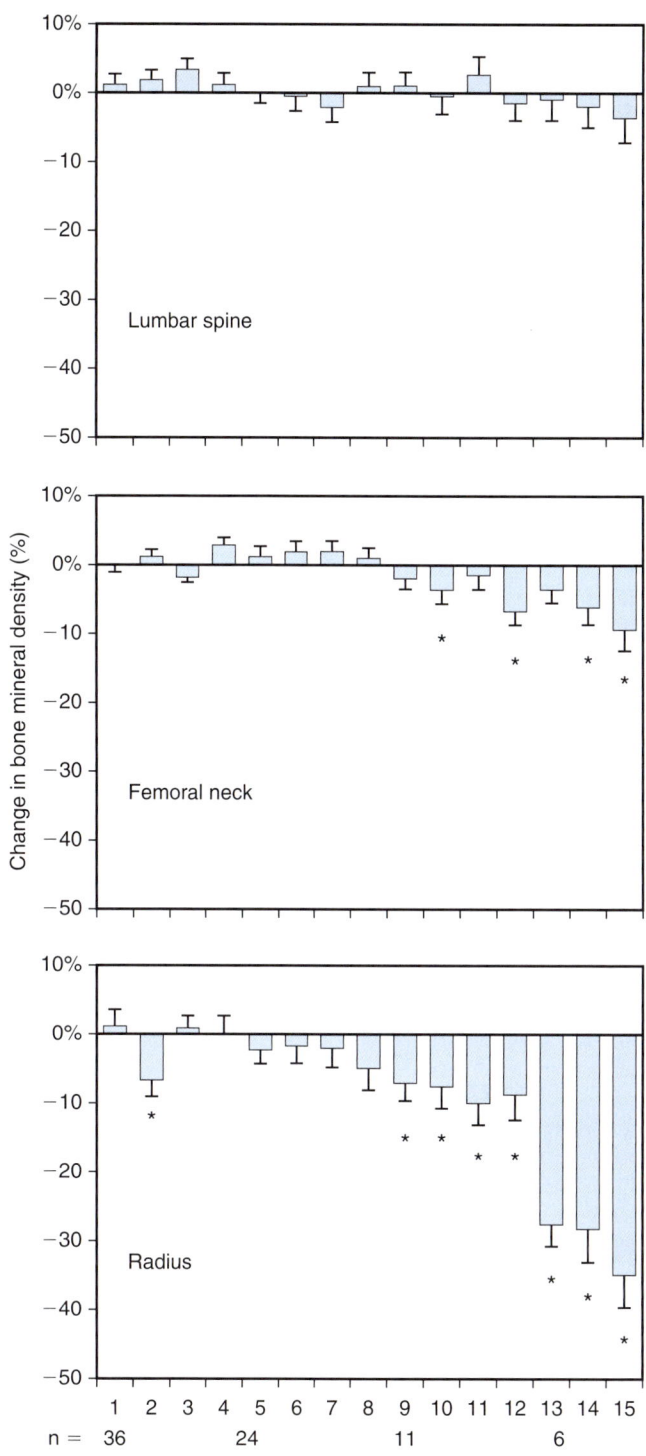

Fig. 53.3 Bone density over 15 years in primary hyperparathyroidism. Data are presented as percentage change from baseline bone density measurement by site. Significant differences from baseline at $p < 0.05$. (Modified from Rubin MR, Bilezikian JP, McMahon DJ, et al. The natural history of primary hyperparathyroidism with or without parathyroid surgery after 15 years. *J Clin Endocrinol Metab*. 2008;93(9):3462–3470.)

TABLE 53.3 Current Guidelines for Following Patients With Asymptomatic Primary Hyperparathyroidism Who Do Not Undergo Parathyroid Surgery

Measurement	Guideline
Serum calcium	Annually
Renal guidelines	Estimated glomerular filtration rate (eGFR): Annually 24-hour urinary calcium/renal imaging/biochemical stone risk profile: Only if there is clinical suspicion for stone
Skeletal guidelines	Bone density: Annually or biannually Vertebral imaging: Only if clinically indicated

Modified from Bilezikian JP, Brandi ML, Eastell R, et al. Guidelines for the management of asymptomatic primary hyperparathyroidism: summary statement from the Fourth International Workshop. *J Clin Endocrinol Metab.* 2014; 99(10):3561–3569.

difference in urinary calcium excretion between those on high (1000 mg/day) and those on low (500 mg/day) calcium-intake diets.[66] In those with elevated levels of 1,25-dihydroxyvitamin D_3, high calcium diets were associated with worsening hypercalciuria. This observation suggests that dietary calcium intake in PHPT can be liberalized to 1000 mg/day if 1,25-dihydroxyvitamin D_3 levels are not increased, but they should be more tightly controlled if those levels are elevated.

DIAGNOSIS AND COURSE OF NORMOCALCEMIC PRIMARY HYPERPARATHYROIDISM

The diagnosis of normocalcemic PHPT has been muddied in the literature by early reports that were limited by assay technology, which could falsely elevate PTH levels, and by the inclusion of many patients who actually had secondary hyperparathyroidism resulting from vitamin D deficiency, hypercalciuria, renal insufficiency, and certain forms of liver and gastrointestinal disease. In patients with PHPT, coexisting vitamin D deficiency can lower elevated serum calcium into the normal range, and it is arguably the most common explanation for elevated PTH and normal serum calcium levels. The diagnosis of normocalcemic PHPT requires that the patient have levels of 25-hydroxyvitamin D within the normal physiologic range (levels above 30 ng/mL are desirable before this diagnosis is made) and that other causes of secondary hyperparathyroidism be ruled out as well (i.e., normal urinary calcium excretion as well as renal function, liver function, and absence of malabsorption).[5] It is important that ionized calcium levels be measured (which is not necessary in hypercalcemic PHPT) and that these levels be consistently normal.[5]

Patients with normocalcemic PHPT are frequently recognized during an evaluation for low bone mass. Although some of these patients may represent the earliest manifestations of PHPT, others seem to have abnormalities that are not clearly progressive. In various series, only 0.6% to 19% of patients go on to develop hypercalcaemia.[4,47,67] These patients have higher rates of osteoporosis, fractures, and renal stones than are seen in unselected hypercalcemic PHPT cohorts, likely due to selection bias (the diagnosis is made during evaluation for one of these issues).[45,68] It should be noted that although the recommendations of the 2014 International Consensus Panel includes guidelines for surgery in patients with normocalcemic PHPT, these are not evidence based.[5] Watchful waiting is often advisable because hyperparathyroidism remits in some patients over time. Further data are necessary to allow reliable indications for and outcomes of surgery in normocalcemic disease.

DRUG TREATMENT

Oral Phosphate

Oral phosphate can lower serum calcium by up to 1 mg/dL.[69] Problems with oral phosphate include limited gastrointestinal tolerance, possible further increase in PTH levels, and the possibility of soft-tissue calcifications after long-term use. This agent is no longer an advisable treatment for PHPT.

Bisphosphonates and Denosumab

Bisphosphonates and denosumab are antiresorptive agents used in the treatment of osteoporosis. Although they do not affect PTH secretion directly, by reducing bone resorption, they may reduce serum and urinary calcium levels. Small, randomized, controlled studies of alendronate typically documented increased BMD of the lumbar spine and hip regions along with reductions in bone turnover markers with minimal effect on serum calcium levels.[70] One uncontrolled trial of risedronate found an increase in spine BMD that was less than that achieved by parathyroidectomy.[71] The a first published experienced with denosumab promise by being associated with a greater improvement in BMD than in a comparable group of euparathyroid, postmenopausal women.[72] These results suggest that these agents might be a useful treatment for low bone density in patients for whom parathyroid surgery is not to be performed.

Estrogen Therapy and Selective Estrogen Receptor Modulators

Postmenopausal women with PHPT who receive estrogen replacement therapy for symptoms of menopause can expect a beneficial effect on their bone density.[70] RCT data assessing conjugated estrogen (0.625 mg daily plus medroxyprogesterone 5 mg daily) versus placebo confirm prior reports of a salutary effect on bone density in the femoral neck and lumbar spine.[73] However, previous reports demonstrating a decline in serum calcium levels were not confirmed by RCT. The only study of the selective estrogen receptor modulator, raloxifene, was a short-term (8-week) trial in 18 postmenopausal women. Raloxifene (60 mg/day) led to a statistically significant, although small (0.5 mg/dL), reduction in the serum calcium concentration and in markers of bone turnover.[74] There are no data on bone density with raloxifene or fracture with estrogen or raloxifene in PHPT.

CALCIMIMETIC AGENTS

Calcimimetics act on the parathyroid cell calcium-sensing receptor, mimicking the effect of extracellular calcium. This leads to the activation of the receptor and subsequent inhibition of parathyroid cell function. The first-generation ligand, phenylalkylamine (R)-N-(3-methoxy-alpha-phenylethyl)-3-(2-chlorophenyl)-1-propylamine (R-568), is a calcimimetic compound that increases cytoplasmic calcium and reduces PTH secretion in vitro, and in a single-dose study, it was shown to inhibit PTH secretion and lower serum calcium concentrations in postmenopausal women with PHPT.[75] The second-generation ligand, cinacalcet, reduces the serum calcium concentration to normal in PHPT.[76-78] Although the serum calcium concentration normalizes, PTH levels decrease but do not return to normal. The urinary calcium excretion does not change nor does the average BMD, even after 3 years of administration of cinacalcet. Thus cinacalcet has not turned out to be the hoped-for alternative to parathyroidectomy. However, cinacalcet has been shown to be effective in reducing serum calcium levels in patients with intractable PHPT[79] and inoperable parathyroid carcinoma.[80] Cinacalcet was approved by the European Medicines Agency in 2008 for PHPT and by the U.S. Food and Drug Administration (FDA) in 2011 for the treatment of severe hypercalcemia in PHPT patients who cannot have surgery.

UNUSUAL PRESENTATIONS

Neonatal Disease

Neonatal PHPT is a rare form of PHPT caused by homozygous inactivation of the calcium-sensing receptor. When present in a heterozygous form, it is a benign hypercalcemic state, known as *familial hypocalciuric hypercalcemia*.[81,82] However, in the homozygous, neonatal form, hypercalcemia is severe, and the condition is fatal unless recognized early. The treatment of choice for neonatal hypercalcemia is early subtotal parathyroidectomy to remove most of the hyperplastic parathyroid tissue.

Primary Hyperparathyroidism in Pregnancy

PHPT in pregnancy is of concern primarily for its potential effect on the fetus and neonate.[83] Complications of PHPT in pregnancy include spontaneous abortion, low birth weight, supravalvular aortic stenosis, and neonatal tetany. The latter condition is a result of fetal parathyroid gland suppression by high levels of maternal calcium, which readily cross the placenta during pregnancy. Infants with this condition are used to hypercalcemia in utero; they have functional hypoparathyroidism after birth and can develop hypocalcemia and tetany in the first few days of life. Today, with most patients (pregnant or not) having a mild form of PHPT, an individualized approach to management is advised. Many patients with very mild disease can be followed safely with successful neonatal outcomes without surgery. For more severe disease, parathyroidectomy in the second trimester is recommended.

Acute Primary Hyperparathyroidism

The term *acute PHPT* (also known as *parathyroid crisis, parathyroid poisoning, parathyroid intoxication,* and *parathyroid storm*) describes an episode of life-threatening hypercalcemia of sudden onset in a patient with PHPT.[84] Clinical manifestations of acute PHPT are mainly those associated with severe hypercalcemia. Laboratory evaluation is remarkable, not only for very high serum calcium levels but also for extreme elevations in PTH approximately 20 times the normal level. Although a history of persistent mild hypercalcemia has been reported in 25% of patients, the risk of developing acute PHPT in a patient with mild asymptomatic PHPT is very low. Concurrent medical illness with immobilization may precipitate the acute event. Early diagnosis and aggressive medical management, followed by surgical cure, are essential for a successful outcome.

PARATHYROID CANCER

Parathyroid carcinoma accounts for less than 0.5% of cases of PHPT (see Chapter 64, Parathyroid Carcinoma).[85] The etiology of the disease is unknown, and no clear risk factors have been identified. No evidence supports the malignant degeneration of previously benign parathyroid adenomas. Manifestations of hypercalcemia are the primary effects of parathyroid cancer. Metastatic disease is a late finding in the course of the disease with the involvement of liver (10%); lymph node (30%); and lung (40%) most common.

The clinical profile of parathyroid cancer differs from the profile of benign PHPT in that no female predominance is seen among patients with carcinoma, and elevations of serum calcium and PTH are far greater. A palpable neck mass, distinctly unusual in benign PHPT, has been reported in 30% to 76% of patients with parathyroid cancer.

Surgery is the only effective therapy currently available for this disease. The greatest chance for cure occurs with the first operation. Once the disease recurs, cure is unlikely, although the disease may smolder for many years thereafter. The tumor is not radiosensitive, but there are isolated reports of tumor regression with localized radiation therapy. When metastasis occurs, isolated removal is an option, especially with pulmonary metastatic disease. Such isolated resections of metastatic disease are never curative, but they can lead to prolonged remissions, sometimes lasting for several years. Similarly, local debulking of tumor tissue in the neck can be palliative, although malignant tissue is often left behind. Finally, traditional chemotherapeutic agents have not been useful. Immunotherapy, which optimally raises titers of antibodies to PTH, has been reported to ameliorate previously refractory hypercalcemia, but such success is very rare and not curative.[86] If surgery is not an option, attention focuses instead on control of hypercalcemia. The intravenous bisphosphonates have been used in their capacity as agents that treat severe hypercalcemia, but they do not have a long-term effect. Cinacalcet lowers serum calcium level and decreases symptoms of nausea, vomiting, and mental lethargy, which are common concomitants of marked hypercalcemia.[80] The FDA has approved cinacalcet for the treatment of hypercalcemia in patients with parathyroid cancer. No data exist on the effect of cinacalcet on tumor growth in parathyroid cancer. Thus this agent is not an alternative to surgery. Instead, it offers an option for the control of intractable hypercalcemia when surgical removal of malignant recurrent or metastatic disease is no longer an option.

REFERENCES

For a complete list of references, go to expertconsult.com.

54

Guide to Preoperative Parathyroid Localization Testing

Carrie C. Lubitz, Quan-Yang Duh

Please go to expertconsult.com to view related video:
Video 54.1 Introduction to Chapter 54, Guide to Preoperative Parathyroid Localization Testing.
This chapter contains additional online-only content available on expertconsult.com.

INTRODUCTION

The skill of an experienced parathyroid surgeon remains the most important asset in identifying abnormal parathyroid glands. Results of initial operations for primary hyperparathyroidism (PHPT) are similar with or without preoperative imaging.[1] Historically, more than 95% of patients have been cured after bilateral cervical exploration by experienced parathyroid surgeons without the help of localization studies and was not felt to shorten operative time in experienced hands.[2-4] However, in contrast to those who undergo a first-time operation, reoperative parathyroidectomy has higher failure and complication rates. Thus localization studies are crucial for patients undergoing reoperation.

Please see the Expert Consult website for more discussion of this topic.

Over the past 15 years, trends in the approach to surgery have changed substantially from the majority of surgeons performing four-gland exploration to now, when most surgeons perform focused explorations.[8] Today, the most commonly used noninvasive imaging studies are cervical ultrasound (US), nuclear scintigraphy, computed tomography (CT), and magnetic resonance imaging (MRI).

Please see the Expert Consult website for more discussion of this topic.

It should be emphasized that imaging is not used for diagnosis. The diagnosis of PHPT is made by the concurrent elevation of serum calcium and parathyroid hormone (PTH). Positive imaging does not always confirm the diagnosis, and negative findings are not uncommon, especially with multigland disease. Invasive studies, usually reserved for reoperative cases or ectopic glands, include US or CT-guided fine-needle aspiration (FNA) with concomitant PTH assay, parathyroid angiography, and/or selective venous sampling for PTH gradient.

PHPT is most likely caused by solitary adenomas (75% to 85%); whereas multigland disease (hyperplasia: 10% to 15%; double adenomas: 2% to 12%) and carcinoma (1%) are less common.[20] Preoperative localization by imaging studies identifies candidates for minimally invasive parathyroidectomy in the majority of patients with PHPT. In this chapter, we review three types of parathyroid localization studies: radiology-based studies, nuclear medicine-based studies, and invasive procedures.

LOCALIZATION STUDIES

Please see the Expert Consult website for more discussion of this topic.

Radiology-Based Studies

Cervical Ultrasound

The sonographic appearance of a parathyroid adenoma is typically homogeneous, hypoechoic, and frequently a feeding vessel can be visualized (Figure 54.1). Parathyroid glands are most commonly oval shaped, but they can be elongated, bilobed, or multilobed.[25] Other abnormalities include parathyroid cysts, cystic components within larger solid lesions, giant adenomas, and calcifications. Parathyroid cysts are thin-walled structures that show posterior enhancement and have no internal echoes. Patients with parathyroid cysts can have fluctuating and/or normal serum PTH levels. Cystic lesions within large solid adenomas can have anechoic areas with posterior acoustic enhancement. Giant adenomas are defined as those larger than 3 cm. Calcifications, although rarely found in parathyroid adenomas, are hyperechoic and cast discrete acoustic shadows (see Figure 54.1). Finally, an inhomogeneous pattern of hyperechoic and hypoechoic images may be found corresponding to fat and hypercellular parathyroid tissue, respectively.

US has several advantages and disadvantages. Advantages include the following: (1) it is inexpensive; (2) it does not involve radiation or contrast exposure; (3) it is noninvasive; (4) it is excellent at detecting parathyroid tumors near the thyroid; (5) it identifies thyroid nodules; (6) it is a diagnostic tool that surgeons can use in their offices; and (7) it can guide needle biopsy. Disadvantages of US include the following: (1) it is operator dependent; (2) a surgeon will find it difficult to detect substernal, retrotracheal, retroesophageal, and deep-seated parathyroid tumors; and (3) it is "nonfunctional" (e.g., it can be difficult to distinguish between small lymph nodes and small abnormal parathyroid glands).

A systematic review showed that the sensitivity and positive predictive value (PPV) of US range from 51% to 96% and 50% to 100%, respectively,[26] and the accuracy of surgeon-performed US in comparison with radiologist-performed is comparable. US is less accurate for localizing multiple adenomas or parathyroid hyperplasia whether it is performed by the radiologist or by the surgeon; sensitivities range from 13% to 24%.[27,28] However, several factors decrease the sensitivity and PPV. These include concomitant thyroid nodules and multiple parathyroid adenomas or parathyroid hyperplasia.[19,23-25] If in doubt, the clinician can consider performing percutaneous FNA of the lesion(s) in question and send the specimen for PTH measurement.[19]

Please see the Expert Consult website for more discussion of this topic.

Computed Tomography

CT is another noninvasive parathyroid localization technique. The sensitivity of CT scans increases with the use of patient-positioning

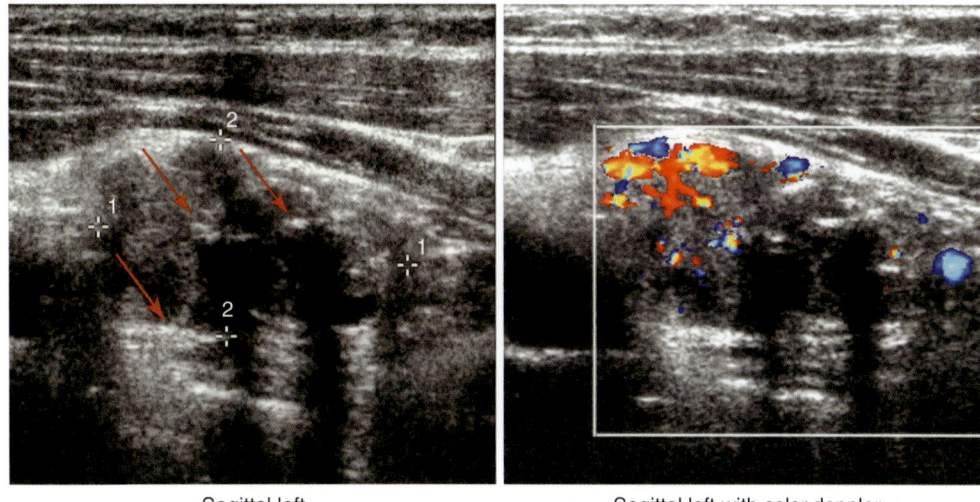

Sagittal left   Sagittal left with color doppler

Fig. 54.1 A lower left parathyroid adenoma localized by high-resolution ultrasound. A large (3.2 × 2 × 1.6 cm) lobular hypoechoic mass *(outlined by dotted white square)* with vascular flow *(seen on Doppler imagery)* and shadowing calcifications *(red arrows)* seen in the inferior aspect of the left lobe of the thyroid.

harnesses (providing improved neck extension); intravenous contrast; and high-resolution CT scanners (2.5 to 3 mm cuts). Four-dimensional CT (4D-CT) is a contrast CT protocol format that produces multiplanar images using different perfusion characteristics of parathyroid, thyroid, and lymph nodes over time.[32,33] 4D-CT can provide both anatomic and physiologic details about the abnormal parathyroid gland in a single study. The parathyroid adenomas have rapid uptake and comparatively early washout of intravenous contrast. 4D-CT scan was found in the initial report study to be more accurate at localizing the parathyroid adenoma to a particular side (sensitivity: 4D-CT 88% versus sestamibi 65% versus US 57%) and quadrant (sensitivity: 4D-CT 70% versus sestamibi 33% versus US 29%) than either US or sestamibi. The expertise of the radiologist increases the accuracy of CT scanning as well.[33,34]

CT scanning has several advantages and disadvantages in localizing abnormal parathyroid glands. At tertiary referral centers, reported sensitivity of CT scans for lateralizing parathyroid adenomas is >85% and 66% to 70% for localizing to the correct quadrant.[33-35] The sensitivity is excellent in cases where US and/or sestamibi are negative, discordant, or ectopic.[32,35,36] In cases with negative or discordant US and/or sestamibi, 4D-CT lateralized 73% of parathyroid adenomas and more than 80% in reoperations; cases of four-gland hyperplasia remain challenging.[32,37] Many clinicians are now using 4D-CT as their initial localization study.

CT is excellent for localizing ectopic glands, such as those in the anterior mediastinum or undescended parathyroid glands (Figures 54.2 and 54.3).[38] CT scanners are readily available in most hospitals, yield reproducible images, take much less time than sestamibi scanning, and can guide needle biopsy; in addition, the interpretation is less subjective than for US. The disadvantages are exposure to contrast, radiation and decreased specificity. Average effective radiation doses are comparable between 4D-CT (~10 mSv) and sestamibi scans (~7 mSv) with average annual background radiation exposure of 3 mSv/year.[39,40] Although the dose to the thyroid specifically is reportedly much higher than sestamibi, the lifetime attributable risk of cancer is extremely low for the single scan needed for diagnosis in the vast majority of cases.[39,40]

Magnetic Resonance Imaging

 Please see the Expert Consult website for discussion of this topic, including Figures 54.4 and 54.5.

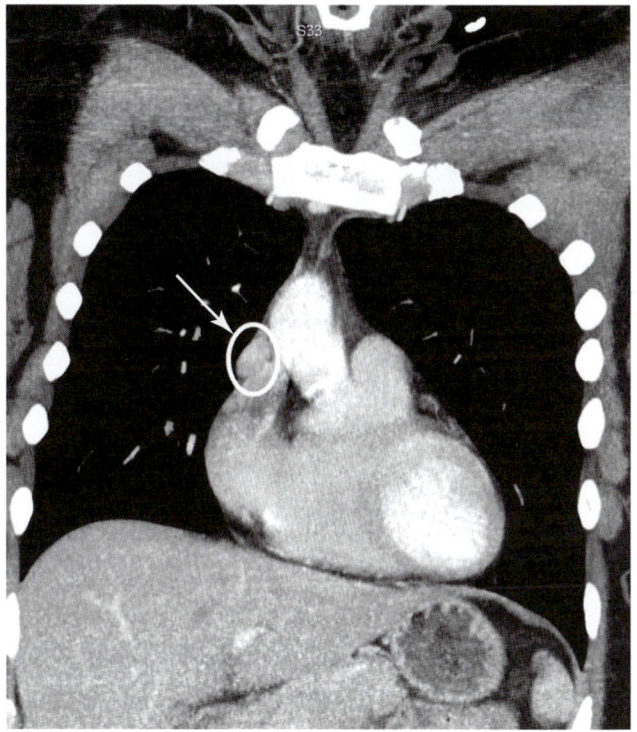

Fig. 54.2 Computed tomography (CT) scan of thorax with intravenous contrast demonstrates a 1.8 × 0.9 cm soft-tissue density adjacent to the right atrium and anterior to the superior vena cava, which corresponds to the area of increased uptake in the mediastinum on 99mTc-sestamibi (MIBI) and combined single-photon emission computed tomography (SPECT)/CT.

Nuclear Medicine-Based Studies

Nuclear medicine imaging of parathyroid glands has continued to improve since its introduction in the 1980s. Many clinicians use nuclear imaging for first-line noninvasive "functional" imaging. It is safe, and it has sensitivity and specificity similar to US in most series. Nuclear imaging techniques can find glands that cannot be seen on US, such

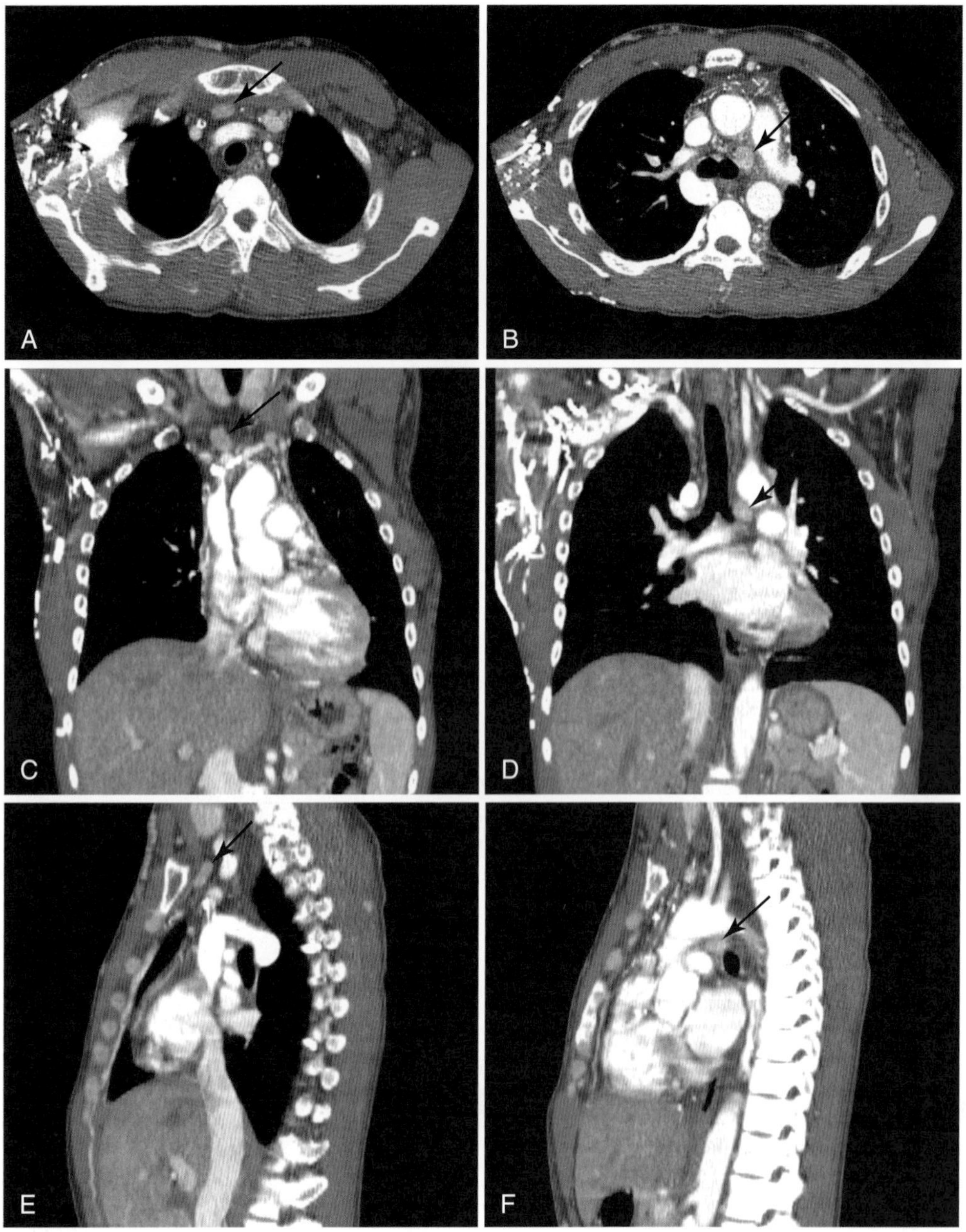

SECTION 8 Parathyroid Surgery

Fig. 54.3 Computed tomography (CT) scan with intravenous contrast in a 29-year-old man with recurrent secondary hyperparathyroidism after a prior subtotal parathyroidectomy. CT scan revealed three ectopic parathyroid glands. They are in the (1) lower left neck below the thyroid but above the clavicle (not shown); (2) upper right anterior mediastinal lesion located behind the sternum and cephalad to the brachiocephalic artery and vein with axial **(A)**; coronal **(C)**; and sagittal **(E)** views; (3) deep left mediastinal enhancing mass (1.8 × 1.3 cm) adjacent to the left mainstem bronchus with axial **(B)**; coronal **(D)**; and sagittal **(F)** views. The patient had a bilateral neck re-exploration to remove both a left neck and a right anterior mediastinal parathyroid tumor via a cervical incision. The left pulmonary hilum mass was not explored.

as those deep in the neck, posteriorly located or ectopic in the chest and mediastinum.

 Please see the Expert Consult website for more discussion of this topic, including Figure 54.6.

The use of 99mTc-sestamibi (also known as MIBI) for parathyroid imaging was first described in 1989.[48] Sestamibi is also used for cardiac perfusion studies. Unlike thallium, sestamibi accumulates in the mitochondria rather than in the intracellular potassium pool. Sestamibi washes out of parathyroid adenomas at different rates, depending on the concentration of mitochondria in the tissue. Parathyroid adenomas often have a high mitochondrial content compared with thyroid tissue, allowing for slower washout from parathyroid adenomas.

Currently, there is no parathyroid-specific radionuclide, which means all radionuclides that accumulate in the parathyroid glands also accumulate in the thyroid, thereby making it difficult to image only the parathyroid gland.[49]

Double-tracer subtraction imaging can be used to solve this problem. In this technique, the patient is given two radionuclides, one that is thyroid specific and one that accumulates in both the thyroid and parathyroid glands. The two thyroid-specific radionuclides most commonly used are radioiodine (^{123}I) and technetium pertechnetate (^{99m}Tc-pertechnetate). Images of both radionuclides are taken individually, and a computer is then used to "subtract" the "thyroid-only" image from the combined thyroid/parathyroid image, leaving only the parathyroid image (Figure 54.7). This is technically challenging because it requires the patient to maintain the same position throughout the scan. Because of difficulty with motion artifact, this technique is only useful with planar images, and it cannot be used for single-photon emission computed tomography (SPECT) images. Planar, SPECT, and subtraction imaging can be used for all radionuclide tracers.

Sestamibi can be used to image parathyroid glands by a double-phase technique (using varying washout times) or subtraction imaging (using dual isotopes ^{123}I or thallium for highlighting the thyroid tissue) with similar accuracy.[50] One study of 246 patients showed that subtraction imaging has a sensitivity of 89% for detecting single parathyroid adenomas; whereas, dual-phase imaging has a sensitivity of 73%. Specificities for both techniques were similar (90% to 95%).[50] In the double-phase technique, images are first taken at 10 minutes and then at 2 to 3 hours.

Dual-phase imaging has advantages over subtraction imaging. Dual-phase imaging is not affected by motion artifact, making it better for SPECT imaging than subtraction imaging.

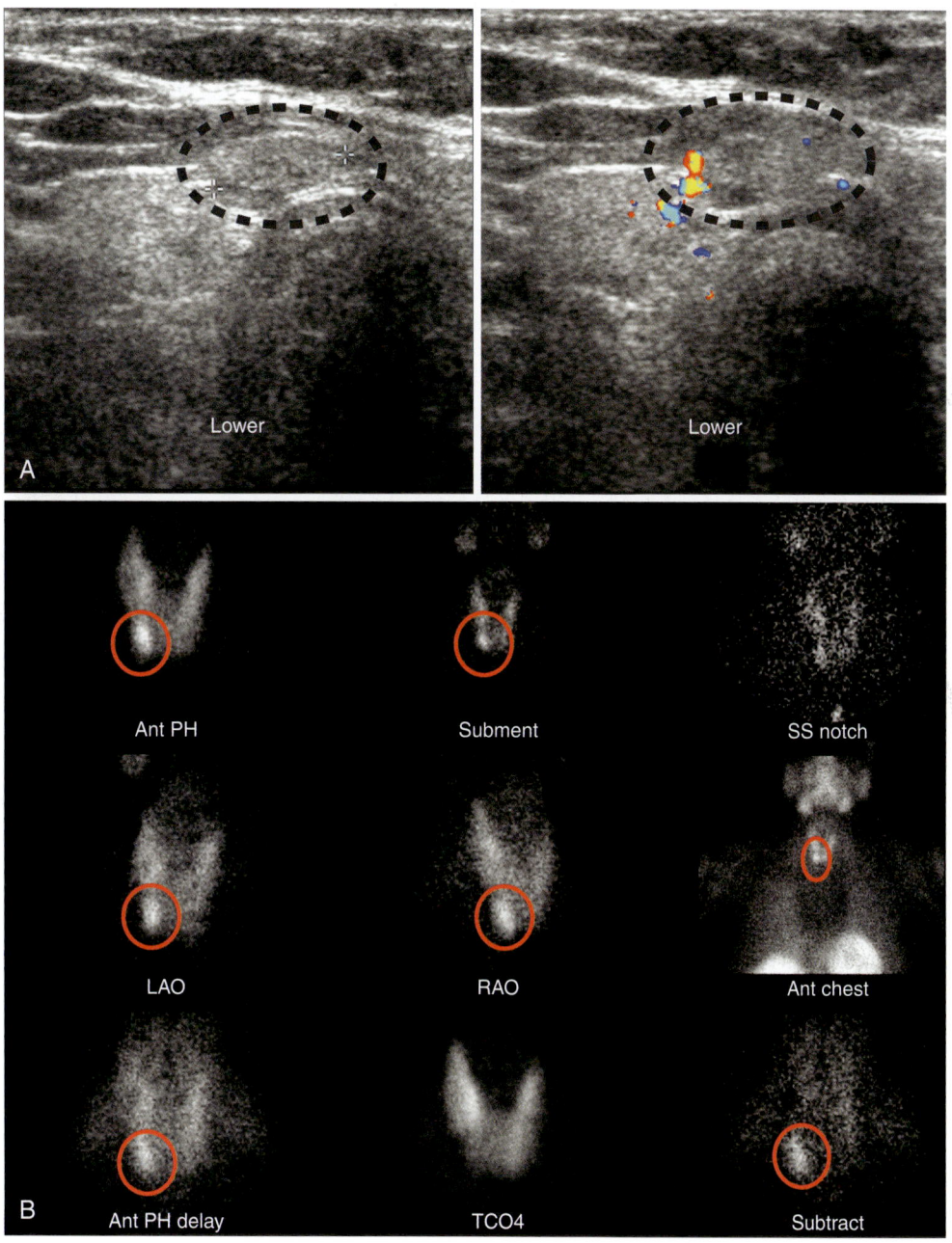

Fig. 54.7 A lower right parathyroid adenoma localized by ultrasound and sestamibi subtraction imaging. A 60-year-old woman with primary hyperparathyroidism had concordant 99mTc-sestamibi (MIBI) and ultrasound studies. She had a successful lower right parathyroidectomy via a focused anterior approach. **A,** Ultrasound showed a 2 × 1.3 × 0.8 cm hypoechoic nodule at the level of the lower right pole of the thyroid. **B,** Sestamibi subtraction imaging showed a right inferior parathyroid adenoma, consistent with ultrasound findings.

Please see the Expert Consult website for more discussion of this topic, including Figure 54.6.

Although SPECT imaging increases the sensitivity of dual-phase planar imaging, it is still less sensitive than subtraction images.[53] A planar subtraction image can be added to a dual-phase SPECT image by injecting ^{99m}Tc-pertechnetate after obtaining the dual-phase delayed images. SPECT images can also be fused with a CT image to provide better imaging and to help plan minimally invasive parathyroidectomies (Figure 54.8) and in multigland disease.[53-55] Nuclear medicine studies are operator dependent; image acquisition, patient positioning, and protocol greatly affect accuracy.[56]

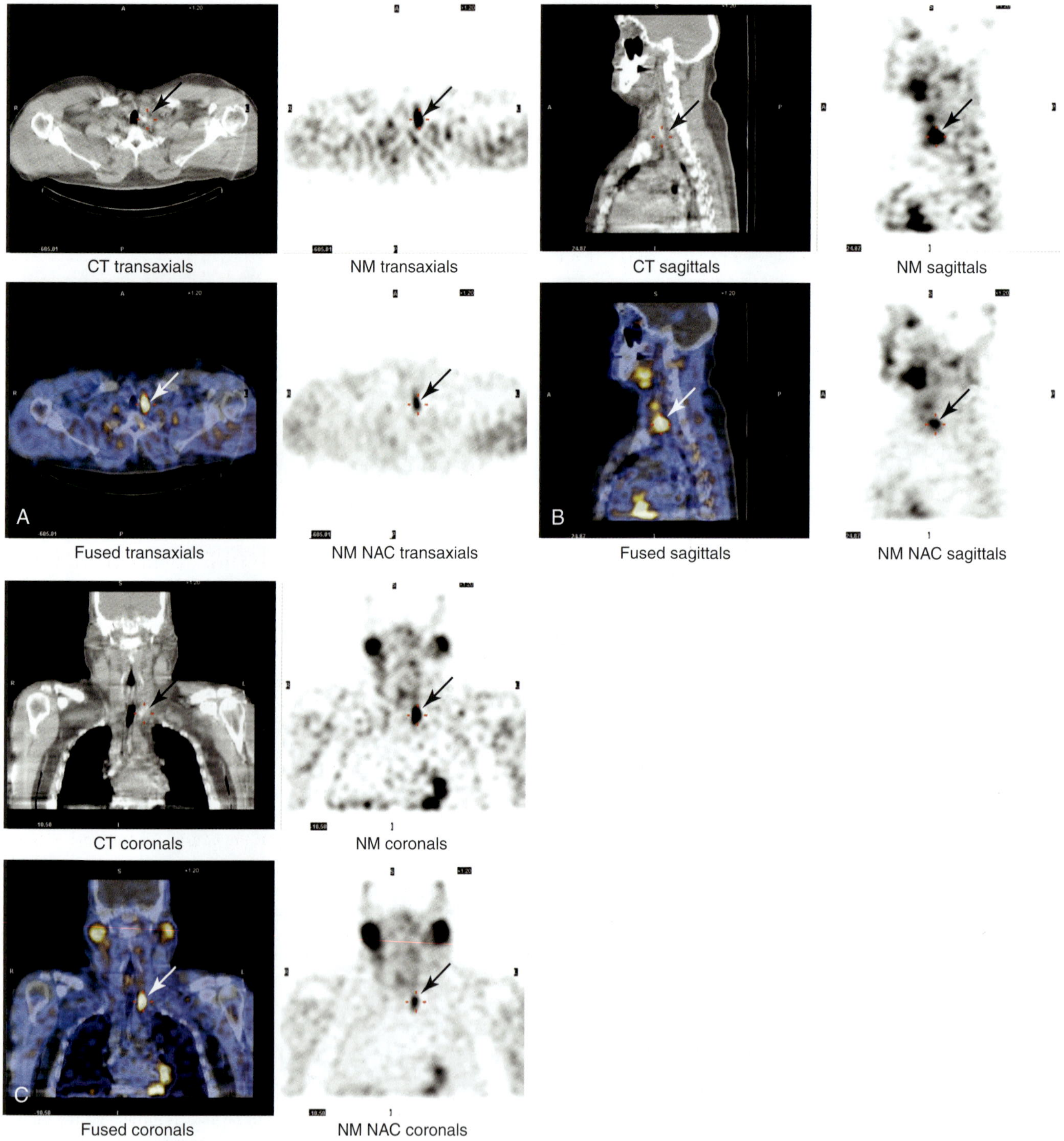

Fig. 54.8 Combined single-photon emission computed tomography/computed tomography (SPECT/CT) and sestamibi scan of a 43-year-old man with primary hyperparathyroidism. SPECT/CT views of the neck with Tc-99m sestamibi. Axial (**A**); sagittal (**B**); and coronal (**C**) views. Persistent focal uptake of sestamibi in the *lower* left thyroid bed is consistent with a parathyroid adenoma. Intraoperatively, this patient was found to have a *upper* left parathyroid adenoma.

Sestamibi has several limitations. False positives and false negatives can occur. Some solid thyroid nodules, such as Hürthle cell nodules, have a high oxyphilic content that can cause a false-positive sestamibi scan. This type of false-positive scan can be minimized by the combination of subtraction and dual-phase SPECT imaging. Sestamibi uptake by thyroid carcinomas as well as metastatic disease, lymphadenopathy, sarcoidosis, and brown fat also can cause false-positive results. False-negative sestamibi scans occur from low oxyphilic cell count in the parathyroid adenoma or increased sestamibi metabolism, causing early washout. Low oxyphilic cell count parathyroid tumors are typically associated with parathyroid hyperplasia, double adenomas, and smaller single adenomas.

Please see the Expert Consult website for more discussion of this topic.

Sestamibi: Summary

In conclusion, sestamibi is more sensitive for detecting single adenomas (sensitivity 89%) than thallium (sensitivity 72%) and is the nuclear imaging test of choice. The best method of sestamibi imaging is debatable; methods range from planar subtraction imaging, dual-phase imaging, and dual-phase SPECT imaging to SPECT/CT fusion imaging. All of these methods can be used in a single sestamibi scan to improve results. The biggest drawbacks of sestamibi are its low sensitivity for multigland disease and its inability to detect small adenomas.

Tetrofosmin

Please see the Expert Consult website for discussion of this topic.

Positron Emission Tomography

Positron emission tomography (PET) imaging using fluoro-2-deoxy-D-glucose (FDG) in the has not gained widespread use.[63]

Please see the Expert Consult website for more discussion of this topic.

^{18}F-fluorocholine-PET has also been found to be useful for localizing parathyroid adenomas that were missed by other conventional imaging studies.[68]

Invasive Procedures

Invasive localization studies should be used only for reoperative surgery when noninvasive studies have failed to identify the abnormal parathyroid gland because there is morbidity and/or potential complications from the procedures. Invasive techniques are only required in rare cases Because of improvements in accuracy of noninvasive imaging, the cost and expertise required, and the risk to the patient.

Fine-Needle Aspiration

FNA of enlarged parathyroid glands by CT or US guidance was initially described in the early 1980s.[69,70] Studies have since shown FNA to be very specific in distinguishing between parathyroid and nonparathyroid tissue. Cytology of FNA is less sensitive than measuring PTH levels of the aspirate because follicular thyroid tumors can be misinterpreted as parathyroid tissue by cytology.[71] This technique can be particularly helpful in equivocal cases and reoperative cases as well as in the rare event of a true intrathyroidal parathyroid to distinguish it from a thyroid nodule.

Selective Venous Sampling

Venous sampling for parathyroid hormone became possible after the development of the PTH radioimmunoassay. It is performed by assessing PTH levels from various cervical, vertebral, and mediastinal venous drainage locations with a "positive" noted by an increase in PTH levels of 1.5- to 2-fold compared with peripheral levels. This technique requires expert interventional radiologists and exposes a patient to a high level of radiation; it is also costly. Therefore selective venous sampling is reserved for patients needing reoperation for persistent or recurrent disease.[72,73]

Parathyroid Arteriography

In rare cases, selective angiographic injection is performed in conjunction with venous sampling by specialized interventional radiologists. Remote devastating complications have been reported; these include central nervous system embolic infarction and quadriplegia.[74] Because of the risks associated with this test and the improvements in noninvasive imaging techniques, parathyroid arteriography is rarely used today.

UNIQUE SCENARIOS

Posteriorly Located Upper Gland (PLUG) Adenomas

Please see the Expert Consult website for discussion of this topic.

Localization Studies During Pregnancy

Please see the Expert Consult website for discussion of this topic.

Localization Studies for MEN 1, Secondary Hyperparathyroidism, and Tertiary Hyperparathyroidism

Please see the Expert Consult website for discussion of this topic.

ALGORITHMS FOR FIRST-TIME OPERATIONS AND RECURRENT/PERSISTENT DISEASE

Scenarios for using localization studies in patients with hyperparathyroidism can be divided into two situations: (1) first-time operation or (2) reoperation (Figure 54.9 and Figure 54.10). Although localization studies are not necessary for first-time operations, they do allow for a limited exploration, which is desirable. On the other hand, localization studies are crucial for reoperations. Noninvasive and less expensive studies should be used before more invasive and expensive studies. The most commonly used initial parathyroid localization studies include US, sestamibi, and 4D-CT. The type, order, and/or combination of studies vary according to surgeon preference, institutional expertise, and other clinical factors. One author (CL) performs intraoffice US to assess for thyroid and parathyroid disease. If there is a clear adenoma, the patient goes to surgery without further imaging. If the US is not revealing, a 4D-CT is obtained before surgery. The other author (QD) also uses intraoffice US but routinely adds sestamibi scan before an initial operation. If the US and sestamibi yield concordant localization of a parathyroid adenoma, there is a negligible risk of multigland disease (i.e., double adenomas or hyperplasia). Depending on the results of these studies, surgical options include (1) focused exploration; (2) unilateral exploration identifying one adenoma and one normal gland on the same side; or (3) bilateral exploration identifying all four glands. Both PTH assay and US may be used as intraoperative adjuncts (see Chapter 55 Principles in Surgical Management of Primary Hyperparathyroidism; Chapter 56, Standard Bilateral Parathyroid Exploration; Chapter 57, Minimally Invasive Single Gland Parathyroid Exploration; and Chapter 58, Minimally Invasive Video-Assisted Parathyroidectomy).

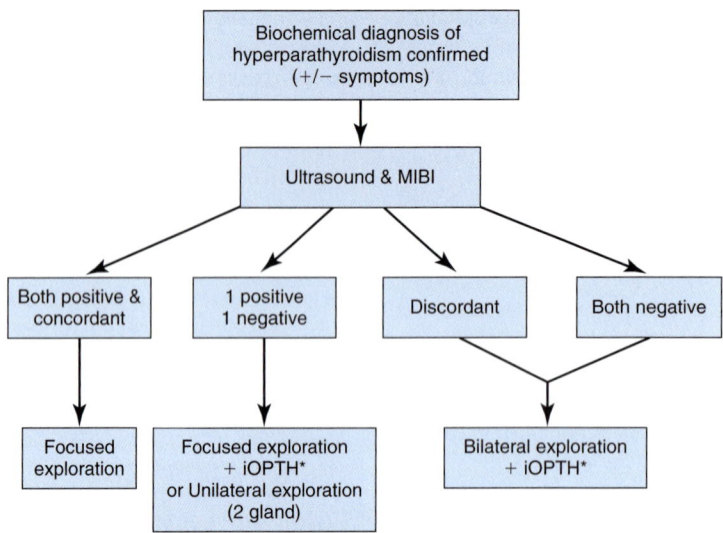

Fig. 54.9 Parathyroid localization algorithm for first-time operation used at the University of California, San Francisco.

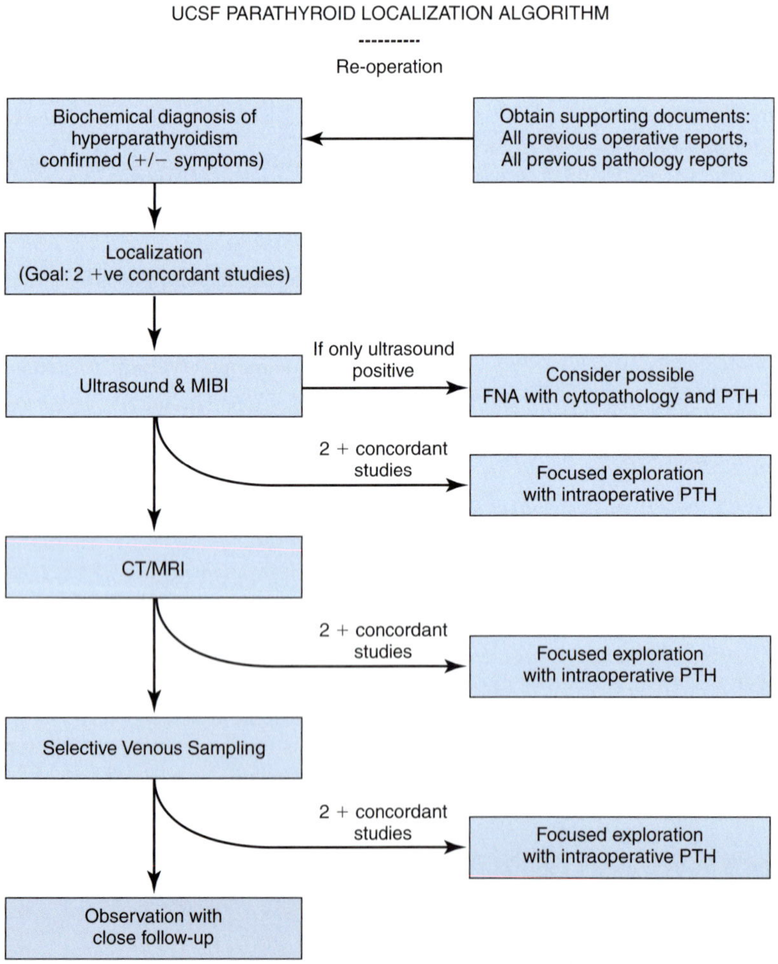

Fig. 54.10 University of California, San Francisco (UCSF) parathyroid localization algorithm for reoperation.

For reoperations, it is critical to obtain all previous operative and pathology reports to build a road map (see Chapter 63, Reoperation for Sporadic Primary Hyperparathyroidism). The localization studies required here make up a spectrum of tests from the noninvasive US, MIBI, CT, and MRI to the invasive selective venous sampling and FNA biopsy. For reoperations, we suggest that two concordant studies be obtained before proceeding with a focused exploration.

CONCLUSION

Please see the Expert Consult website for discussion of this topic.

REFERENCES

For a complete list of references, go to expertconsult.com.

55
Principles in Surgical Management of Primary Hyperparathyroidism

Nancy L. Cho, Gerard M. Doherty

"The success of parathyroid surgery must rely on the ability of the surgeon to know a parathyroid gland when he sees it, to know the distribution of the glands, where they hide and, also, to be delicate enough in technique to be able to make use of this knowledge."

Edward D. Churchill, 1931

 This chapter contains additional online-only content available on expertconsult.com.

In this chapter, we discuss the current approach to preoperative workup for primary hyperparathyroidism (primary HPT), determine appropriate surgical candidacy, review parathyroid surgical anatomy, and detail a comprehensive search algorithm for surgical exploration.

PREOPERATIVE EVALUATION

Background

Primary HPT is a common cause of hypercalcemia with approximately 100,000 new cases diagnosed in the United States each year.[1] This number may be an underestimation due to the prevalence of undiagnosed and untreated primary HPT in the general population.[2] Most cases of primary HPT are due to excess parathyroid hormone (PTH) secretion from a single adenoma (80% to 85%), followed by four-gland hyperplasia (10% to 15%), multiple adenomas (5%), and carcinoma (<1%). Primary HPT must be distinguished from other causes of hypercalcemia before surgical exploration because operating for incorrect reasons will not cure the patient and may even worsen the situation. The differential diagnosis for hypercalcemia includes malignancy, multiple myeloma, primary HPT, granulomatous disease, calcium/vitamin D supplementation, thiazide diuretics, lithium, benign familial hypocalciuric hypercalcemia, and Paget's disease.

Clinical Manifestations

Primary HPT can be associated with a wide range of symptoms as summarized by the colorful phrase "renal stones, painful bones, abdominal groans, psychic moans, and fatigue overtones." Hyperparathyroidism (HPT) complications consist of a spectrum of bony (bone/joint pain, fractures, osteitis fibrosa cystica), renal (nephrolithiasis, polyuria, renal insufficiency), gastrointestinal (nausea, vomiting, peptic ulcer disease, constipation, pancreatitis), neuropsychiatric (lethargy, "brain fog," depression, psychosis), soft tissue (calcinosis, calciphylaxis, intractable pruritus), and cardiovascular (left ventricular hypertrophy, conduction abnormalities, endothelial dysfunction, decreased QT interval) manifestations. However, in most modern series in developed regions of the world, patients generally present with asymptomatic forms of primary HPT, which are discovered in routine laboratory tests.

Preoperative History and Physical Examination

Preoperative history should include questions related to the potential etiology, symptoms, and complications of primary HPT.

History

- *Symptoms of hypercalcemia.* Weight loss, polydipsia, fatigue, memory change, depression, renal stones, hypertension, bone-joint-muscle pain, arthritis, gout, fractures, bone disease, nausea, vomiting, constipation, peptic ulcer, and pancreatitis.
- *Time course of hypercalcemia.* Gradual onset is consistent with primary HPT. More rapid onset occurs in the setting of malignancy. Hypercalcemia associated with malignancy usually occurs in relatively advanced, clinically apparent disease. Multiple myeloma is an exception where hypercalcemia might be the initial symptom. Lifelong and stable hypercalcemia is observed in benign familial hypocalciuric hypercalcemia (BFHH).
- *Age of onset.* Sporadic HPT usually occurs in older patients. Some familial HPT syndromes may present at an earlier age (see the primary HPT genetic section presented later in the chapter).
- *History related to drugs and conditions that mimic HPT.* Intake of oral calcium, vitamins D and A, thiazide diuretics, lithium, and anticonvulsants. History of vitamin D deficiency, rickets, adrenal insufficiency, hyperthyroidism, prolonged immobilization, sarcoidosis, known malignancy.
- *History of radiation exposure.* Low-dose radiation exposure can increase the risk of HPT threefold.[3]
- *Family history.* Hypertension, endocrine tumors, calcium disorders. Please see the Expert Consult website for more discussion of this topic.

Physical Examination

- Physical examination is typically unremarkable. Albright's dictum states that if a palpable nodule is present in a patient with HPT, it is an unrelated thyroid nodule. However, up to 50% of parathyroid carcinoma patients have a palpable mass.[5] A firm palpable neck mass in the setting of severe hypercalcemia and PTH elevation strongly suggests parathyroid carcinoma.
- Preoperative laryngeal examination to assess preoperative vocal cord function should be considered in patients with voice changes, preoperative evaluation suggestive of parathyroid carcinoma, or history of operation that places at risk the innervation of muscles controlling the vocal folds.[6,7]

Preoperative Laboratory Tests

- Serum calcium and intact parathyroid hormone (iPTH)
  - High calcium and high iPTH are indicative of primary HPT.
  - High calcium and normal PTH. At least 10% of surgically proven primary HPT cases have high normal serum PTH levels. This pattern of elevated calcium and inappropriately elevated PTH in the high normal range is consistent with parathyroid gland autonomy.
  - Normal calcium and elevated PTH. Normocalcemic primary HPT is considered a form of parathyroid disease, perhaps an initial form of HPT. Although normocalcemic primary HPT may be associated with symptoms or complications equivalent to those affecting patients with frankly elevated calcium, it is very important to exclude other mimicking diagnoses such as vitamin D deficiency and "renal leak" hypercalciuria as causes for PTH elevation, which in these conditions is secondary (see the discussion on vitamin D and primary HPT and normocalcemic primary HPT presented later).
  - Serum calcium of higher than 14 mg/dL raises the specter of parathyroid carcinoma and is typically accompanied by significantly elevated PTH.
- *Vitamin D-25-OH.* Vitamin D should be evaluated in patients being assessed for primary HPT. Conditions associated with vitamin D deficiency should also be considered, including Crohn's disease, cystic fibrosis, celiac disease, malabsorption after gastric bypass surgery, or renal dysfunction (with decreased ability to synthesize the active dihydroxylated form).[8]
- *24-hour urine calcium and creatinine.* Urine parameters may be measured to assess renal function and help rule out BFHH, which can mimic HPT; the diagnosis is made with low urine calcium/creatinine clearance ratio and total calcium/24-hour urine collection <100 mg.
- *Serum phosphate and chloride.* Patients with primary HPT typically have a low or low-normal phosphate. An elevated serum chloride level, with a chloride-to-phosphate ratio >33 was diagnostically helpful for HPT before accurate PTH assays.
- *Alkaline phosphatase.* Alkaline phosphatase levels may be elevated in the setting of bone disease. When elevated preoperatively, surgeons should anticipate that postoperative hypocalcemia (termed *hungry bone syndrome*), which can prolong hospitalization, may occur.
- *Bone density scan.* Patients may demonstrate osteopenia or osteoporosis as well as progressive decrease in bone density on serial imaging. Bone loss affecting the distal 1/3 radius is particularly suggestive of parathyroid disease.
- Surgeons should be knowledgeable and astute about the biochemical diagnosis of HPT. In the operating room, surgeons should be confident that the diagnosis is accurate; this implies their commitment to explore thoroughly and recognize that ≥1 abnormal glands will be amenable to curative resection through a neck incision about 98% of the time (Box 55.1).

> **BOX 55.1 Key Elements of the Biochemical Diagnosis of HPT**
>
> 1. High calcium and PTH
> 2. Normal creatinine
> 3. Low or low normal phosphate
> 4. Urinary calcium >100 mg/24 hours
> 5. Normal vitamin D-25-OH

Preoperative Genetic Assessment

Familial Syndromes and Genetic Testing

Primary HPT is predominantly sporadic but may be diagnosed in the context of an inherited syndrome. For surgeons, it is important to distinguish preoperatively if a patient with primary HPT is sporadic or syndromic in nature. The diagnosis of syndromic HPT has implications as to the number of glands involved, the extent of surgery necessary for cure, as well as important implications for family screening. Genetic testing is not recommended on a routine basis. Varying penetrance and incomplete syndromic manifestations can make the diagnosis of syndromic HPT challenging.[9] A clinician must look for clues during initial preoperative evaluation to identify when and which genetic tests should be ordered (Table 55.1).

Multiple Endocrine Neoplasia Type 1 (MEN 1)

MEN 1 is an autosomal dominant disorder of the *MEN 1* gene (encoding menin) and is also known as Wermer's syndrome.[10] It presents with tumors predominantly of the parathyroid, pancreas, and pituitary glands. HPT is the most frequent endocrine expression of MEN 1, occurring in 95% by 50 years of age. MEN 1–associated HPT presents at an earlier age, on average at 20 years, which is 30 years younger than for typical nonsyndromic primary HPT.[11] Yip found that MEN 1 is more common in young males presenting with primary HPT; he proposed a six-question panel (described on Expert Consult website).[4]

Multiple Endocrine Neoplasia Type 2A (MEN 2A)

MEN 2A is an autosomal dominant disorder resulting from mutations in the RET gene. It is also known as Sipple's syndrome and typically consists of medullary thyroid cancer, pheochromocytoma (in 50% of MEN 2A patients), and HPT (in 10% to 30% of MEN 2A patients).[12,13]

Hyperparathyroidism Jaw Tumor Syndrome (HPTJT)

This rare autosomal dominant condition is associated with the HRPT2 gene (also known as the *CDC73* gene).[9,14] HPT is the most common manifestation, which often presents with asynchronous development of multiple adenomas. Parathyroid carcinoma occurs in about 15% to 20% cases. Ossifying mandibular or maxillary fibromas, uterine polyps, and renal cysts or hamartomas also occur.

Autosomal Dominant Mild Hyperparathyroidism (ADMH)

This is a rare autosomal dominant syndrome presenting with hypercalcemia and hypercalciuria. It is associated with calcium-sensing receptor (CASR) gene mutation.[9] This syndrome usually presents in patients >40 years of age, and HPT is seen in all cases. History of failed parathyroid surgery is noted in many patients. Multi-gland excision is the treatment of choice.

Familial Hypocalciuric Hypercalcemia (FHH)

This is a rare autosomal dominant disorder presenting with asymptomatic, nonprogressive lifelong hypercalcemia with 100% penetrance.[15] It is typically diagnosed in families by the presence of hypercalcemia and relative hypocalciuria with variable PTH elevation. This represents a renal calcium set point disorder and is not managed with parathyroid surgery but needs to be preoperatively distinguished from primary HPT. It is the main reason for checking a 24-hour urine collection for total calcium and creatinine in patients preoperatively. Almost half of FHH patients have increased serum magnesium, a diagnostically-low calcium/creatinine clearance ratio (usually below 0.01), and total calcium for a 24-hour urine collection <100 mg.

FHH is the phenotype when this gene abnormality is heterozygous, whereas neonatal severe HPT is the phenotype when the gene abnormality is homozygous.

TABLE 55.1 Disorders, Characteristics, and Genetic Tests

Disorder	Age of Onset	HPT Penetrance	Associated Features	Gene Involved (Chromosomal Location)	Genetic Tests	Commercially Available Tests	Typical Appropriate Surgery
MEN 1	<30 years (usually 20–25 years)	High (90%–100%)	Pituitary adenomas; Pancreatic tumors (gastrinomas causing Zollinger-Ellison syndrome)	MEN 1 (11q13)	MEN 1	Yes	Multi-gland excision
MEN 2A	>30 years	Low (15%–30%)	MTC and pheochromocytoma	RET (10q21)	RET	Yes	Enlarged glands only
HPTJT	>30 years (Av age 32 years)	High (80%) Increased risk of parathyroid carcinoma	Fibro-osseous tumors of maxilla or mandible, increased risk of renal tumors (nephroblastomas, hamartomas, or Wilms' tumors), and uterine tumors	HRPT2 (also known as CDC73) (1q 21–32)	HRPT2	Yes	Multi-gland excision
ADMH	40–48 years	High (100%)	h/o unsuccessful parathyroid surgeries	CASR (3q21–24)	CASR	Yes	Multi-gland excision
FHH (heterozygous form)	Young (before 10 years)	High	Asymptomatic mild hypercalcemia with relative hypocalciuria, hypermagnesemia in half of the patients, low calcium/creatinine ratio with total calcium /24-hour urine collection < 100 mg	CASR (3q21–24)	CASR	Yes	Asymptomatic, no treatment
NSHPT (homozygous form)	Birth-6 months	Low (12%–14%)	Infants present with lethargy, hypotonia, failure to thrive, bony undermineralization, multiple fractures, severe skeletal deformities; if left untreated, can lead to florid rickets, devastating neurodevelopmental disorders, and often fatality	CASR (3q21–24)	CASR	Yes	Multi-gland excision

Neonatal Severe Hyperparathyroidism (NSHPT)

This is a homozygous form of FHH that manifests at birth or within the first 6 months of life.[15] There is severe symptomatic hypercalcemia with skeletal manifestations. Treatment involves prompt total parathyroidectomy.

VITAMIN D AND PRIMARY HYPERPARATHYROIDISM

Consideration of vitamin D levels is important in the preoperative evaluation of patients with presumptive HPT. First, vitamin D deficiency must be considered in the differential diagnosis. Vitamin D deficiency results in low or normal serum calcium and high PTH. In primary HPT, both calcium and PTH are high, and vitamin D levels are normal. However, normocalcemic HPT can have normal calcium and elevated PTH, which may be quite similar to vitamin D deficiency.

Second, vitamin D deficiency is common and can coexist in patients with primary HPT. Interestingly, vitamin D deficiency and insufficiency seem to be more prevalent in patients with primary HPT than in geographically matched populations.[16] Primary HPT seems to be more severe in those with concomitant vitamin D deficiency presenting with advanced disease phenotype, at least biochemically.[16-19] Coexisting vitamin D deficiency may cause the serum calcium level to fall into the normal range, which may lead to diagnostic uncertainty. The cause of vitamin D deficiency is usually multifactorial, resulting from either inadequate exposure to ultraviolet radiation, inadequate vitamin D intake (dietary), vitamin D malabsorption due to certain medical conditions such as Crohn's disease, cystic fibrosis, celiac disease, or past gastric bypass surgeries, or in the inability to synthesize the active dihydroxylated compound as in renal dysfunction.

Vitamin D–deficient patients undergoing parathyroidectomy are also at increased risk of postoperative hypocalcemia and "hungry bone syndrome," which underscores the importance of a preoperative assessment of vitamin D status in all patients with primary HPT. A postoperative rise in PTH is more likely in patients with preoperative vitamin D deficiency. Vitamin D supplementation after parathyroidectomy for primary HPT reduces the incidence of this postoperative eucalcemic PTH elevation.[20] It may be difficult to treat vitamin D deficiency in the setting of primary HPT, and close monitoring of serum and urine calcium levels is essential because limited data suggest that those levels may increase in some patients in response to vitamin D replacement therapy. If vitamin D is to be given, it should be done with care, with close follow-up, and at low doses. Data on vitamin D repletion in patients with mild primary HPT suggest that vitamin D deficiency may be corrected without worsening the underlying hypercalcemia.[17,20]

NORMOCALCEMIC PRIMARY HYPERPARATHYROIDISM

Normocalcemic primary HPT is a condition in which patients have normal serum calcium concentrations, but present with PTH levels that are consistently elevated in the absence of a secondary cause of HPT.[16,21] Some have suggested that patients with these conditions may have an early form of symptomatic primary HPT. Although total calcium levels are normal, ionized levels may be elevated in these patients. A rigorous search for the causes of secondary HPT must be done before diagnosing normocalcemic primary HPT; importantly, vitamin D deficiency must be ruled out as does renal leak hypercalciuria. A course of thiazide diuretics helps one differentiate renal leak hypercalciuria from primary HPT. In renal leak patients, the thiazide reduces renal calcium loss and PTH levels tend to normalize. In primary HPT, thiazides will tend to produce hypercalcemia and PTH levels will be stable.

Patients with true normocalcemic primary HPT are largely asymptomatic but may have more substantial skeletal involvement than is typical. These patients usually seek medical attention in the context of an evaluation for decreased bone mass. Although some patients eventually progress to overt hypercalcemic primary HPT, this transition is not inevitable, nor is there any uniform time course for the development of hypercalcemia. Many patients with normocalcemic primary HPT continue to show normal concentrations of serum calcium over time. Careful monitoring of these patients is recommended, and a proactive, surgical approach should be considered when appropriate. Data suggest that patients with normocalcemic primary HPT demonstrate improvement in bone mineral density after successful parathyroidectomy.[22]

Primary Hyperparathyroidism Surgical Guidelines

Once the diagnosis of primary HPT is made, parathyroidectomy can benefit symptomatic patients by halting or stabilizing the progression of most complications of primary HPT. Although many agree that surgery is indicated in symptomatic primary HPT, controversy exists regarding surgical indications in asymptomatic primary HPT. Surgical guidelines for patients with asymptomatic primary HPT were originally defined in 1990 by the first Consensus Development Conference on the Management of Asymptomatic Primary Hyperparathyroidism, which was sponsored by the National Institutes of Health (NIH). Subsequent conferences have revised consensus guidelines for surgical indications in asymptomatic primary HPT. The most recent (2013) guidelines are summarized and discussed in the following (see also Table 55.2):[23]

1. *Degree of hypercalcemia.* Serum calcium at more than 1 mg/dL above the upper limits of normal.
2. *Degree of hypercalciuria.* In the 1990 and 2002 guidelines, hypercalciuria above 400 mg/dL was considered an indication for surgery in asymptomatic primary HPT. In the absence of renal stones, hypercalciuria was not regarded as an indication for parathyroid surgery in 2008. The basis for this change in recommendation was that hypercalciuria had not been established as a risk factor for kidney stones in primary HPT. In 2013, the guidelines changed to recommend surgery in the presence of hypercalciuria above 400 mg/dL *and* increased stone risk by biochemical analysis. Presence of nephrolithiasis or nephrocalcinosis by x-ray, ultrasound, or computed tomography (CT) was also added as a surgical indication.
3. *Renal dysfunction.* Glomerular filtration rate (GFR) reduced to <60 mL/min. In earlier guidelines, surgery was indicated if creatinine clearance was reduced by 30% compared with age-matched normal controls.
4. *Bone density reduction.* Reduction in the bone density in women and in men over 50 years of age, with a T score of ≤−2.5 at lumbar spine, femoral neck, total hip, or distal radius. In the 2013 guidelines, vertebral fracture was added as a surgical indication.
5. *Age.* Age less than 50 years. Surgery is offered to asymptomatic young patients because multiple studies show that approximately 25% of such patients will develop complications of their disease, some of which are irreversible.
6. *Other important management factors.* Surgery is also indicated in patients for whom medical surveillance and follow-up is difficult, not desired, or not possible.

Controversy also exists regarding surgery for asymptomatic patients older than 50 years of age. Talpos, reviewing SF36 Health Survey results, reported that "asymptomatic" patients do benefit from surgery.[24] Silverberg has shown that asymptomatic patients enjoy improved and sustained lumbar spine and femoral neck (cancellous) bone density after surgery.[25] Pasieka demonstrated that surgically corrected HPT was associated with improved disease-specific symptoms,

TABLE 55.2 Comparison of New and Old Guidelines for Parathyroid Surgery in Asymptomatic primary HPT*

Measurement	1990	2002	2008	2013
Serum calcium	>1.5 mg/dL above normal	>1 mg/dL above normal	>1 mg/dL above normal	>1 mg/dL above normal
24-hour urine calcium	>400 mg/dL	>400 mg/dL	Not indicated	>400 mg/dL
Renal function	Creatinine clearance reduced by 30%	Creatinine clearance reduced by 30%	GFR <60 mL/min	GFR <60 mL/min
BMD	Z score <−2 in forearm	T score <−2.5 at any site[†]	T score <−2.5 at any site[†] or previous fracture fragility	T score <−2.5 at any site[†], previous fracture fragility, or vertebral compression fracture
Age (yr)	<50	<50	<50	<50

*Surgery is also indicated in patients for whom medical surveillance is neither desired nor possible.
[†]Lumbar spine, total hip, femoral neck, or distal third of the radius.

and patient reported health-related quality of life.[26] Zanocco demonstrated, by cost-effectiveness analysis, that parathyroid surgery was the optimal strategy for asymptomatic patients >50 years of age.[26] Currently, the trend is a much more "pro-surgery" attitude.[27]

LOCALIZATION TESTING

Please see the Expert Consult website for discussion of this topic (see also Chapter 54, Guide to Preoperative Parathyroid Localization Testing: Ultrasound, Sestamibi and 4D CT).

UNIGLANDULAR VERSUS MULTIGLANDULAR DISEASE

Primary HPT results from autonomous parathyroid glandular growth. Traditionally, clinicians have recognized two discrete forms of abnormal parathyroid growth: uniglandular and MGD. In certain circumstances, it is difficult to differentiate between these two entities. Adding further complexity to this issue is a controversial, but generally accepted, hybrid entity of "double adenoma."

Uniglandular enlargement, with three remaining uninvolved glands, represents the underlying pathology in most patients (80% to 85%) with primary HPT. The affected gland is enlarged and hypercellular, with decreased intracellular and intercellular fat. The three remaining glands are normal to small in size, not hypercellular, and have abundant fat mixed into the gland. This uniglandular enlargement represents a benign neoplasm of primarily chief cells (see Chapter 65, Surgical Pathology of the Parathyroid Glands).

In multiglandular hyperplasia, all four glands are hyperplastic and some, or all, may be enlarged. The individual glands affected by hyperplasia may vary considerably from normal size to markedly enlarged. Glands affected with hyperplasia, like single-gland adenomas, are hypercellular with decreased fat. Although histologic differences between adenomas and hyperplastic glands have been proposed (e.g., adenomas having a normal rim of parathyroid tissue around the adenoma and hyperplastic glands having a thick capsule, greater cellular atypia, a more mixed cellularity of chief cells, and oncocytes), it is generally accepted that adenomas and hyperplastic glands cannot be segregated based on histologic criteria. DeLellis has shown that only 50% of known adenomas have the "normal rim" sign.[33] Further, some hyperplastic glands affected with nodular hyperplasia may have pseudo rims. Given these histologic findings, the diagnosis of uniglandular versus multiglandular hyperplasia has generally been made with a combination of gross surgical and histologic findings (see Chapter 65, Surgical Pathology of the Parathyroid Glands).

Double Adenoma

In primary HPT, there appears to be a third, distinct, pathologic entity—double adenoma—that takes the middle ground between single-gland adenoma and four-gland hyperplasia.[33a] When explored, some patients are found to have only two enlarged glands and are durably cured upon resection of these two glands alone. Double adenoma may be considered a form of asynchronous four-gland hyperplasia, but the high, long-term cure rate associated with two-gland resection would argue toward the existence of double adenoma as a separate legitimate entity. Szabo and others have shown that the recurrence rate after initial successful surgery for double adenoma is equivalent to that after successful single-adenoma surgery (approximately 1% to 2%), with both single-gland and double adenoma recurrence rates being significantly lower than for MGD (approximately 9.2% recurrence rate).[34,35] In a series reviewing 1962 patients with primary HPT, Edis reported finding two large glands and two normal-sized glands in 1.9% of patients.[36] These patients were rendered eucalcemic through resection of only the two large glands. Most believe that double adenoma accounts for 2% to 5% of patients with primary HPT.

ASYNCHRONOUS MULTIGLANDULAR DISEASE

The occurrence of asynchronous MGD is supported by multiple studies showing that the rates of recurrent (not persistent) HPT after initial biochemical cure range from 1% to 16%. Worsey's series of 371 patients with 15-year follow-up showed that when disease recurred, it did so on average 3.8 years after an initially successful operation.[37] In such patients with asynchronous MGD, it appears that, although they have a four-gland process, the polyclonal hyperplastic tendency is weak; it is not clinically manifest, at least initially, and in some may never develop clinically. With this in mind, it is interesting to note that several milder forms of primary HPT (including single adenoma and some forms of MGD, such as double adenoma, HPT in MEN 2A, and sporadic hyperplasia) are well treated and have low recurrence rates when only grossly enlarged glands are excised. Thus, in some subset of these patients with a four-gland process, asynchronous changes may be so gradual as to never become clinically manifest; so, a conservative initial surgical plan seems optimal.

Within other forms of MGD in primary HPT (e.g., MEN 1), the tendency for all four glands to proliferate and form clones is considerably stronger.[38] This translates into a much more aggressive clinical course, as evidenced by a 50% recurrence rate in patients with MEN 1 at 12 years after successful initial subtotal parathyroidectomy.[39] A higher recurrence rate after aggressive parathyroid exploration and resection is also noted in neonatal HPT, familial HPT, and secondary HPT. Four-gland disease can be thought of as a spectrum of disease with varying degrees of penetrance and clinical aggressiveness (Figure 55.1). Changes may evolve over time, leading to recurrence through asynchronous changes in different glands. In more clinically virulent forms of MGD, even supernumerary glands develop and become clinically manifest. Excision of these supernumerary glands may require bilateral thymectomy and resection of adipose tissue surrounding the parathyroid glands.[40]

INTRAOPERATIVE PTH: FUNCTIONAL CRITERIA FOR UNIGLANDULAR VERSUS MULTIGLANDULAR DISEASE

In the past, and to some degree today, uniglandular disease was distinguished from MGD with a combination of gross surgical and histologic

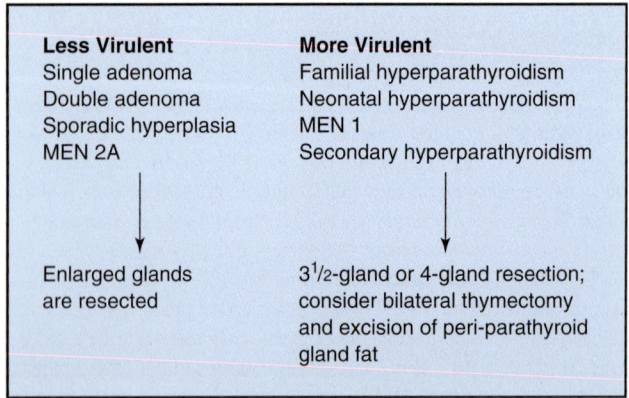

Fig. 55.1 Spectrum of clinical virulence in hyperparathyroidism.

findings. If the surgeon found that a given gland was greater than normal size and the pathologist reported there was increased cellularity and decreased stromal fat, the gland was judged to be diseased and therefore clinically significant. With these gross surgical/histologic criteria, MGD disease was found in approximately 10% to 15% of patients with primary HPT.[40a]

A new alternate test, intraoperative PTH, is available to the surgeon to facilitate the diagnosis of MGD (see Chapter 59, Intraoperative PTH Monitoring During Parathyroid Surgery). There are two options for diagnosing MGD after the first enlarged gland is removed: (1) the identification of additional grossly enlarged glands that are histologically hyperplastic, or (2) through PTH. The former is the traditional gross and histologic definition approach that requires bilateral exploration and has its advocates and claims rates of MGD of as high as 15% to 30%. The latter approach, using PTH as a biochemical test for additional hyperfunctional glands, also has its advocates and claims rates of MGD closer to 5%.[41] Those favoring PTH as the diagnostic tool believe that all enlarged or hyperplastic glands may not be clinically significant.

HISTOLOGY

Please see the Expert Consult website for discussion of this topic (see also Chapter 65, Surgical Pathology of the Parathyroid Glands).

MOLECULAR GENETICS OF PRIMARY HYPERPARATHYROIDISM

Please see the Expert Consult website for discussion of this topic (see also Chapter 65, Surgical Pathology of the Parathyroid Glands).

Clonality of Sporadic Parathyroid Tumors

Please see the Expert Consult website for discussion of this topic.

Parathyroid Oncogene Rearrangement/Overexpression

Please see the Expert Consult website for discussion of this topic.

Parathyroid Tumor Suppressor Gene Inactivation

Please see the Expert Consult website for discussion of this topic.

PARATHYROID SURGICAL ANATOMY

Normative Parathyroid Parameters

Parathyroid Number

Humans typically have four parathyroid glands. Several autopsy studies of normal individuals without HPT have reported that 3% to 6% have fewer than four parathyroid glands. Wang has suggested these data derive from inadequate dissection and that the minimum number of parathyroids should generally be regarded as four.[60-63] These same studies show that more than four glands occur in 2.5% to 6.7% of cases. Akerstrom noted that some of the supernumerary glands are very small, rudimentary glands or split glands, which typically occur within the thymus or in the fat adjacent to the normal parathyroid gland. Such small, rudimentary glands may be present in up to 13% of normal individuals. True supernumerary glands (defined as greater than 5 mg and located at some distance from the normal parathyroid gland) occur in only 5% of cases and are most often found within the thymus. In studies of patients with primary HPT, a fifth parathyroid gland is found in 0.6% to 0.7% of patients.[64,65] Supernumerary glands also occur in secondary HPT; Edis and Levitt found that 10% of persistent HPT after surgery in patients with secondary HPT resulted from supernumerary glands, a finding which persists in contemporary series.[66,67]

Parathyroid Weight

The normal weight of the parathyroid gland increases until the third to fifth decade of life and ranges from 38 to 59 mg.[68] The lower glands weigh slightly more than the upper glands.

Parathyroid Gland Characteristics

Understanding parathyroid gland embryology and intraoperative attention to detail facilitates the identification of normal and abnormal parathyroid glands. Parathyroid glands are entities distinct from the surrounding neck tissue and are recognized by a number of different characteristics. The color of the parathyroid gland is typically light brown to reddish tan. This color relates to the fat content, vascularity, and percent of oxyphil cells.[69] In obese patients, the fat content of parathyroid glands is higher. As a result, they assume a more yellowish color, which is only slightly different from surrounding fat.[33] In children, the normal parathyroid gland, which has scant fat, is darker (a pinkish brown) compared with that of adults. In adults, hypercellular glands with less fat are browner. Large glands associated with secondary HPT can be grayish. The thyroid is firm and reddish brown, whereas lymph nodes vary from gray to tan to red and are generally more firm than parathyroid glands.

Parathyroid glands also have a distinct hilar vessel (a "vascular strip"), which is visible if the surrounding fat does not obscure its hilum. The parathyroid gland has a discrete, encapsulated, and smooth surface as opposed to the more lobular surface of the thyroid; the lymph nodes have a more mottled and pitted surface. The parathyroid gland is softer to palpation than thyroid or nodal tissue. Parathyroid shape is also unique and most often leaflike or beanlike. The dissection of a small nodule on the surface of the thyroid gland, mistaken for a parathyroid gland, results in hemorrhage, whereas the dissection of a parathyroid gland closely related to the thyroid capsule demonstrates an anatomically separate organ.

The most important distinguishing feature is that the parathyroid gland, being a discrete, encapsulated organ, has a characteristic motion when the surrounding fat is gently manipulated. The discrete edge of the parathyroid gland is visible when this fat is dissected. As the surrounding fat is manipulated, the parathyroid gland glides within the fat, like a boat riding on a wave of water. This "gliding sign" is a tremendously helpful clue in parathyroid recognition during surgery.

Parathyroid Gland Symmetry

Akerstrom noted positional symmetry to the upper parathyroid glands in 80% of cases and to the inferior parathyroid glands in 70% of cases.[63] This symmetry has important implications during thyroid and parathyroid surgery. Generally, there is a similarity in shape to both upper and lower parathyroid glands. The upper parathyroid gland, however, may have a different shape than that of the ipsilateral lower parathyroid gland.

Parathyroid Glands and Plane of Recurrent Laryngeal Nerve

A very important clue in finding parathyroid glands and in differentiating upper from lower glands, which may be very close to one another on a caudal-cranial axis in some patients, is the position of the parathyroid gland relative to the recurrent laryngeal nerve (RLN). Typically, the upper parathyroid glands are dorsal (i.e., deeper in the neck), and the lower parathyroid glands are ventral (i.e., more superficial in the neck with respect to the plane of the RLN) (Figure 55.2). Migration paths of superior and inferior gland adenomas tend to respect this plane. Superior gland adenomas tend to migrate into the retropharyngeal, retrolaryngeal, and retroesophageal locations, with extension into the posterior mediastinum. Alternatively, inferior adenomas tend to be found in

Parathyroid Vascular Anatomy

The inferior thyroid artery supplies the inferior parathyroid gland. Delattre found that the inferior thyroid artery is absent, more commonly on the left, in approximately 10% of patients. In these cases, the inferior parathyroid gland may depend on a branch from the superior thyroid artery.[70] Inferior parathyroid glands that descend into the anterior mediastinum are usually vascularized by the inferior thyroid artery. If the parathyroid gland is positioned low in the mediastinum, it may rarely be vascularized by a thymic branch of the internal mammary artery or even a direct branch off the aortic arch.[71]

The superior parathyroid gland is usually vascularized by the inferior thyroid artery or by an anastomotic branch between the inferior thyroid and the superior thyroid artery. Several studies have described that in 20% to 45% of cases, the superior parathyroid gland derives significant blood supply from the superior thyroid artery. Usually, such blood supply is derived from a posterior branch of the superior thyroid artery and is given off at the level of the superior pole of the thyroid.[72] Care is required in dissecting this superior pole to preserve the posterior branch of the superior thyroid artery. The small vessels that bridge the interval between the medial surface of the parathyroid gland and the lateral surface of the thyroid are generally insufficient to vascularize the parathyroid gland.

Parathyroid Gland Position

The variability in parathyroid position arises from two discrete sources. It can be divided into (1) embryologic variability in initial descent, and (2) acquired migration. Acquired migration presumably occurs once an adenoma is formed by virtue of its mass and interaction with surrounding structures and viscera. The superior parathyroid adenomas and, to a lesser degree, inferior parathyroid gland adenomas appear to have this capability (Table 55.3).[63,65]

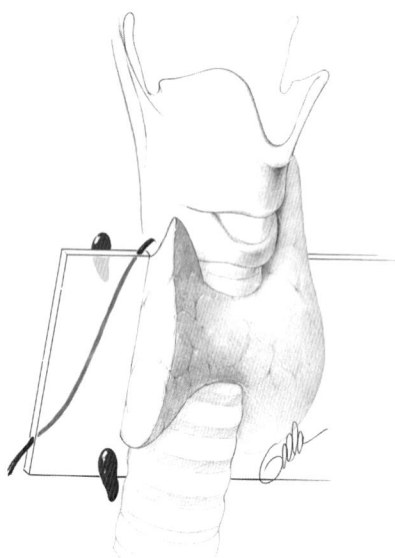

Fig. 55.2 Parathyroid gland relative to the recurrent laryngeal nerve (RLN) plane. Note that the superior parathyroid is dorsal (deep) and the inferior parathyroid is ventral (superficial) to the plane of the RLN in the neck.

the thymus and anterior mediastinum anterior/ventral to the RLN coronal plane. The relationship of the parathyroid gland to the RLN appears to be more constant than the relationship between the gland and the position of the inferior thyroid artery. When inferior parathyroid glands are ectopic because of failed embryologic descent, they are usually found within the neck more superficial than the RLN and are often associated with thymic tissue rests.

TABLE 55.3 Parathyroid Location: Normal Embryologic and Acquired Variation

	NORMAL EMBRYOLOGIC			ACQUIRED
	Normal	Expanded Normal	Ectopic	Migrated
Superior Parathyroid (PIV)	80% within 1 cm cricothyroidal cartilage junction (1 cm cranial to ITA/RLN crossing)	15% on posterolateral surface of upper half of thyroid lobe 3% retrolarynx, retroesophageal 1% above superior pole	<1% intrathyroidal <1% associated with carotid or lateral scalene fat pad	Common Para- or retropharyngeal Deep midlayer cervical fascia On prevert fascia Vascular pedicle of ITA From midpole to postmediastinum May be lower than PIII
Inferior Parathyroid (PIII)	50% within 1 cm inferior pole (inferior, lateral, posterior)	25% thyrothymic horn 12% >1 cm lateral to inferior pole 8% medial on trachea	3% anterior mediastinum, lower thymus 1% undescended Associated with carotid (bifurcation or STA takeoff) From hyoid, angle of mandible to thoracic inlet Associated with thymus remnant (parathymus) 1% subscapular/intrathyroidal	Rare Anterior mediastinum In or lateral to thymus

Percentages are for normal, nonadenomatous glands.
ITA, Inferior thyroid artery; *RLN,* recurrent laryngeal nerve; *STA,* superior thyroid artery.

EMBRYOLOGIC VARIATION

Inferior Parathyroid Gland

The inferior parathyroid gland has a longer and more variable migration path in the neck than the superior gland (see Table 55.3). The normal inferior parathyroid gland typically rests very close (within 1 cm) inferiorly, laterally, or posteriorly to the inferior pole of the thyroid in about 50% of cases (Figure 55.3). The gland typically rests in a fat lobule on or adjacent to the inferior pole. The thymic remnant (thyrothymic horn or thyrothymic ligament), when present in the adult, represents an accumulation of encapsulated fatlike tissue that appears whitish to yellowish; it arises from the thoracic inlet, and tapers toward the inferior pole of the thyroid gland. This structure represents the uppermost portion of the residual thymus, which has undergone fatty degeneration. This fat is directly beneath the strap muscles. The inferior parathyroid gland is found within the thyrothymic ligament in about 25% of cases.[63] The inferior parathyroid gland can occasionally be medial to the inferior pole on or adjacent to the trachea; alternatively, the gland may be in a discretely lateral position relative to the thyroid inferior pole.

Inferior Parathyroid Gland Ectopia

The inferior parathyroid gland may be ectopic on an embryologic basis in either a high (undescended or incompletely descended) or low (excessive migration) position. In about 3% of cases, the inferior parathyroid migration is excessive, and the gland comes to rest in the upper chest, usually in the anterior mediastinum within the lower portion of the thymus. In such circumstances, the gland typically develops a blood supply from the inferior mammary artery, a discrete thymic artery, or a direct branch from the aorta.[73] Parathyroid tissue has been found in as caudal a position as the pericardium.

High inferior parathyroid gland ectopia (i.e., failure of complete descent) occurs in approximately 1% of cases. In such cases, the inferior gland may be associated with a focus of thymic tissue emphasizing a close embryologic association with the thymus, even when ectopic.[63,74] Often, the undescended gland can be found adjacent to the carotid bifurcation, approximately 2 to 3 cm lateral to the superior pole of the thyroid gland. The undescended inferior parathyroid can extend even higher in the neck than the carotid bifurcation and can be found adjacent to the angle of the mandible near the hyoid bone. Parathyroid tissue (presumably undescended inferior parathyroid) has also been found in the submucosa of the hypopharynx.[75]

Superior Parathyroid Gland

The migration path of the superior parathyroid is shorter, and the rates of ectopia are subsequently lower than those for the inferior parathyroid (see Table 55.3). The characteristic location of the normal superior parathyroid is at the cricothyroid junction (Figure 55.4). This location is approximately 1 cm cranial to the intersection of the inferior thyroid artery and the RLN. The variability of these latter two structures makes the cricothyroid junction a more reliable landmark for the superior parathyroid. The superior parathyroid occurs at this level in 80% of cases.[60,63] At this level in the neck, the superior parathyroid is, most commonly, closely associated with the posterolateral surface of the upper half of the thyroid. The superior parathyroid is often associated with a lobule of fat and may be hidden by a layer of perithyroidal fascia, which binds it to the posterolateral aspect of the thyroid's superior pole. These fascial layers, which blend the lateral aspect of the thyroid to the adjacent inferior constrictor musculature, need to be meticulously dissected away from the thyroid capsule to reveal the superior parathyroid. In approximately 15% of cases, the superior parathyroid is actually on the posterolateral surface of the thyroid. In this location, the superior parathyroid is deep to the plane of the RLN, but it may be directly adjacent to the nerve's entry point into the larynx. As the ligament of Berry is dissected in the distalmost course of the RLN, the superior parathyroid may be revealed. In this region, the superior parathyroid may be initially obscured by a variably present nubbin of thyroid tissue, termed the *tubercle of Zuckerkandl.*

In approximately 3% of cases, the normal parathyroid gland is posteriorly located in a retrolaryngeal, retropharyngeal, or retroesophageal location. In these posterior locations, because of echo shadowing from overlying laryngeal cartilage, the diseased parathyroid may be difficult to identify by ultrasound, leading to false negative evaluations. In approximately 1% of cases, the superior parathyroid is located above the superior pole of the thyroid gland.

Superior Parathyroid Gland Ectopia

Superior parathyroid ectopia, although less common than inferior parathyroid ectopia, does occur. Some examples of superior parathyroid gland ectopia result from descent failure or laterally directed descent; this may lead to a superior parathyroid coming to rest between the thyroid gland (medially) and carotid artery (laterally), or directly adjacent to the carotid artery itself. Thompson has described finding a presumptive superior parathyroid adenoma in the scalene fat pad lateral to the carotid.[76,77] Such superior parathyroid gland ectopia occurs in less than 1% of individuals. Intrathyroidal superior parathyroid

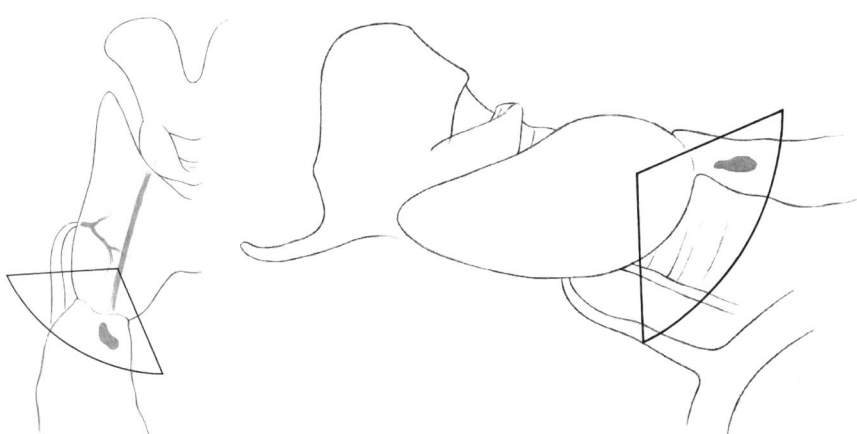

Fig. 55.3 Position of the inferior parathyroid gland. **A,** Front view distribution. **B,** Side view distribution.

SECTION 8 Parathyroid Surgery

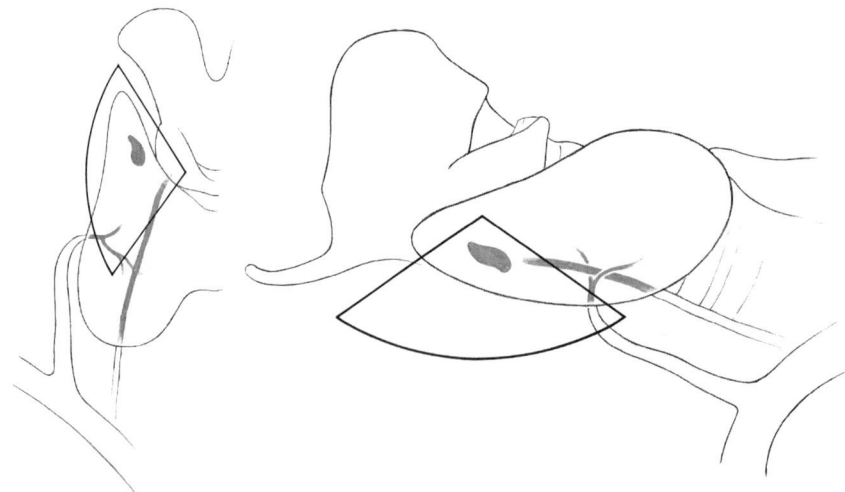

Fig. 55.4 Position of the superior parathyroid gland. **A,** Front view distribution. **B,** Side view distribution.

glands are rare and less common than intrathyroidal inferior parathyroid glands (see the section on intrathyroidal parathyroid glands presented later in the chapter).

Extreme Parathyroid Ectopia: Embryologic Rests and Supernumerary Glands

Most cases of extreme variation in parathyroid tissue position are likely related to embryologic rests of parathyroid tissue. These represent small foci of parathyroid tissue found at some distance from normal locations. Such foci of tissue may enlarge, especially in certain pathologic states characterized by an intense systemic parathyroid growth stimulus such as in MEN 1 or secondary HPT. In these circumstances, small but discrete foci of parathyroid tissue (best termed *rudimentary glands* when found near the normal parathyroid gland) can be found in the fat adjacent to the normal parathyroid gland. When these rests are identified at a greater distance from the normal parathyroid gland, they can be termed *supernumerary glands*. When present, supernumerary glands are frequently found in the mediastinal portion of the thymus. Other locations for supernumerary glands may include the pericardium, the aortopulmonary window, the neck lateral to the carotid sheath, and the laryngeal submucosa.

Acquired Migration

The variations in parathyroid gland location described previously result from variability in embryologic development. Acquired migration is another cause of ectopic location. It is the change in position of an abnormally enlarged gland secondary to the mass of the abnormal gland. Acquired migration features regional dynamics, such as repetitive muscular action of deglutition, negative intrathoracic pressure, and permissive cervicomediastinal fascial planes. Evidence for such acquired migration includes the blood supply of superior adenomas that are found in the posterior mediastinum. Although these glands are well inferior to their normal locations, they have carried their inferior thyroid arterial blood supply during their descent.

The superior parathyroid gland is felt to be especially prone to such migration. The normally located superior parathyroid, when adenomatous, migrates posteriorly and inferiorly, extending along a plane of areolar tissue on the prevertebral fascia in a para- or retroesophageal location. These abnormal glands extend behind the plane of the inferior thyroid artery and posterolateral to the RLN (Figure 55.5). Up to 40% of superior parathyroid adenomas are found in such locations. Patow has shown that the right RLN is more commonly injured than the left in patients requiring reoperative parathyroid surgery. This may in part result from this characteristic position of the migrated superior parathyroid adenoma and the more oblique orientation of the right RLN. Such adenomatous migration may occur with the inferior parathyroid, but it seems to be less frequent. When the inferior parathyroid gland migrates, it moves into the anterior mediastinum, usually into and through the thyrothymic ligament and thymus.

LOCATIONS OF MISSED ADENOMAS BASED ON REOPERATIVE SERIES

Reoperative series provide insight to the location of adenomas missed at initial surgery. Shen found that adenomas missed at the first operation occurred in the following locations (in decreasing frequency): (1) thyrothymic horn/upper thymus, (2) para- and retroesophageal (posterior mediastinum accessible through the neck), (3) intrathyroidal, and (4) associated with the carotid sheath.[78] Jaskowiak et al. found that missed adenomas occurred most often in the paraesophageal position posteriorly (27%), and that the most common ectopic sites were in the thymus (17%), intrathyroidal (10%), undescended glands above the thyroid gland (9%), in the carotid sheath (4%), and in the retroesophageal space (3%).[65]

INTRATHYROIDAL ADENOMA

In approximately 1% of all cases, the normal parathyroid gland is found within the substance of the thyroid gland and is termed *intrathyroidal*. The designation of intrathyroidal parathyroid gland requires that thyroid tissue completely encircle the parathyroid gland. Parathyroid glands that are subcapsular or partially engulfed by surface thyroid nodular change are not considered true intrathyroidal parathyroid glands. Such capsular and subcapsular glands can mimic a true intrathyroidal gland, especially in the setting of nodular goiter, where surface thyroid nodularity can envelop the adjacent parathyroid glands. The exact incidence of true intrathyroidal parathyroid gland varies from 0.5% to 4% and has been studied in autopsy, thyroid surgical specimens, and parathyroid exploration series.[62,79-81]

One would expect, according to embryology, that intrathyroidal glands would more commonly be associated with the superior parathyroid gland. However, based on pathologic data from operative specimens, the inferior parathyroid glands are more commonly intrathyroidal. Thompson found in thyroid surgical specimens that the majority of intrathyroidal glands were in the lower one-third of

CHAPTER 55 Principles in Surgical Management of Primary Hyperparathyroidism

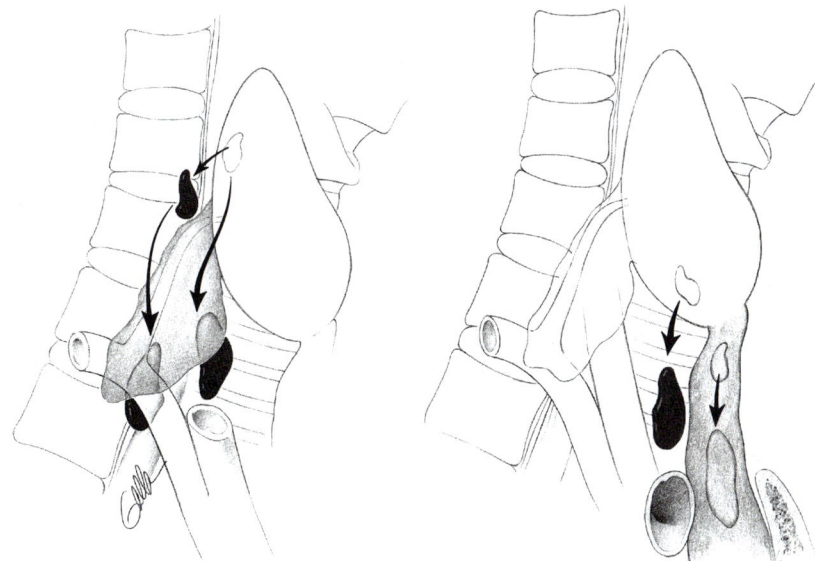

Fig. 55.5 Adenoma-acquired migration paths. **A,** Superior parathyroid adenoma migration paths, emphasizing retroesophageal locations extending to the posterior mediastinum. **B,** Inferior parathyroid gland-ectopic locations extending into the thymus and anterior mediastinum.

the thyroid lobe.[82] Wheeler and Proye, in two separate studies, judged that nearly 90% of intrathyroidal adenomas were inferior parathyroid glands.[46,79,80] True superior parathyroid intrathyroidal glands appear to be rare. Akerstrom et al., in 503 autopsy dissections, found only a 0.2% incidence.[63]

The operative strategy for an intrathyroidal adenoma should be to consider intrathyroidal adenoma during exploration if three glands are identified and normal, especially if the remaining missing gland is inferior. The near-universal use of preoperative thyroid ultrasound currently helps in the identification of intrathyroidal pathologic conditions. Thompson has shown that intrathyroidal adenoma can be excised through a small "thyroidotomy," thus avoiding the scarring and potential complications associated with a full lobectomy.[82]

THYROIDECTOMY DURING PARATHYROIDECTOMY

Given the occurrence of intrathyroidal glands, thyroidectomy is often included on the list of surgical maneuvers if the abnormal glands cannot be found during exploration. However, it is wise to avoid empiric thyroidectomy during parathyroid exploration. Thyroidectomy adds significantly to central neck scar formation, which can significantly increase complication rates at reexploration. Also, thyroidectomy increases the risk of devascularization of the remaining normal parathyroid glands; this increases the risk of permanent hypoparathyroidism at current and subsequent explorations. Indiscriminate empiric thyroidectomy often represents a final, desperate addition to a failing exploration and should be avoided.

PARATHYROID EXPLORATION: SURGICAL TECHNIQUE

This section enumerates several important principles during parathyroid exploration and is followed by a discussion of surgical technique and search algorithm (Box 55.2).

BOX 55.2 Parathyroid Exploration: General Principles

Absolutely Necessary Points
- Perform bloodless dissection.
- Consider MGD.

Helpful Points
- Low threshold to identify RLN. Depth of gland relative to RLN delineates inferior versus superior gland.
- Make use of mirror image symmetry.
- When a normal-appearing gland is found, evaluate for attached adenoma by cautious dissection.
- Follow ITA to the glands, but cautiously distally.
- Biopsy normal parathyroid only if needed.
- Replace intraoperative density tests with frozen section.
- iPTH can be helpful.

Things to Avoid
- Avoid relying completely on localization tests.
- Never remove a normal parathyroid gland.
- Avoid untargeted thyroidectomy.

General Principles

The following general principles must be kept in mind during parathyroid exploration:

1. Consider loupe-assisted bloodless dissection. A meticulous and bloodless dissection is required to discern subtle clues for parathyroid and nerve identification. Many surgeons find loupe magnification essential. The surgeon can detect and identify the pulsation of the inferior thyroid artery. Part of a normal parathyroid gland can be recognized despite the adjacent, partially encompassing adipose tissue, the subtle streak of white of the RLN can be seen underneath a band of translucent fascia.

2. Remain aware of the possible MGD, despite the result of localization tests. It is essential that the surgeon and the patient are always prepared for the potential need for bilateral exploration.
3. Palpation during parathyroid exploration has a limited but definite role. A superior parathyroid adenoma that has descended inferiorly can be palpated in the lateral thyroid region as it rests on the vertebral column and may be identified before it is visible in the field. Such adenomas are deep to the plane of the RLN and are covered by the fascia in the lateral thyroid region (middle layer of deep cervical fascia). The division of this fascia between the thyroid and the carotid artery facilitates subsequent dissection of the paraesophageal region and, more inferiorly, the retroesophageal region and posterior superior mediastinum. Palpation should be delicate enough not to result in hemorrhage, which can stain the fascial planes and make subsequent visual distinctions difficult. Palpation of discrete regions in the operative field containing the adenoma can provoke significant rise in intraoperative PTH (PTH manipulation spike) within several minutes. Rarely, the surgeon can use this spike to identify an adenoma's location before identifying the gland.
4. Have a low threshold to identify the RLN. Identifying the nerve helps to avoid injury to the nerve and aids in differentiating inferior from superior parathyroid glands. The depth of a parathyroid gland with respect to the RLN is a better indicator of its identity (inferior versus superior) than its position on a cranial-caudal axis. This relationship is especially helpful for inferiorly migrated superior parathyroid adenoma as well as undescended inferior parathyroid glands. With the former, the parathyroid gland can be very close to the lateral aspect of the RLN in this region. Surgeons can use neural monitoring of the RLN to assess the nerve just proximal to the region of dissection to evaluate whether the nerve has been injured during the exploration; this is especially helpful in revision surgery.
5. Use mirror image symmetry of the superior and inferior glands on each side. There is symmetry in location as well as in shape of the glands. Of note, the inferior gland may not look similar in shape to the ipsilateral superior gland.
6. Gently dissect a normal gland to ensure that a hidden adenoma is not attached. Dissection of any adenoma, especially one with cystic change, must be meticulous, because the spillage of such a lesion can result in multiple parathyroid gland implants (parathyromatosis) and recurrent HPT.[83,84] The dissection of the normal parathyroid gland should be performed with an understanding of the orientation of the gland's vascularity and should proceed from the distal tip toward the vascular hilum. All parathyroid glands identified during parathyroid exploration should be clearly described in the operative record. If, during dissection, a parathyroid gland is found to have a questionable vascular pedicle but has good color, it can be incised to determine whether the cut edge bleeds. Gentle technique is required to avoid undue trauma to the gland.
7. Medially following the course of the inferior thyroid artery branches can lead to identification of parathyroid glands. However, the most distal branches of these arteries can be injured easily with resultant parathyroid ischemic injury.
8. The degree to which parathyroid biopsies should be employed during parathyroid exploration is controversial. With the advent of intraoperative PTH assessment, the need for parathyroid biopsy to rule out MGD has lessened.[85] However, this occasionally still has a place in the intraoperative decision making. The distal, nonvascularized tip of the gland should be biopsied. No attempt to cauterize the gland should be made. Frozen section biopsy can sometimes distinguish between normal and abnormal (hypercellular) parathyroid glands. However, that is not reliable, and so intraoperative pathology consultation question is to distinguish parathyroid tissue from other sources (e.g., thyroid, lymph node or thymus).
9. Intraoperative tests based on differential tissue density have been used in the past, but now largely abandoned in favor of more definitive tests (pathology or intraoperative PTH measurement). These tests were based upon the observation that fat floats in saline solution, and that parathyroid tissue usually sinks.
10. Evidence of a successful parathyroid exploration with excision of an enlarged gland or glands is the sufficient drop in PTH level. When appropriately chosen PTH criteria are met, a surgeon may save time and avoid potential morbidity associated with additional dissection and normal gland biopsy. If PTH assessment is not available, frozen section of the enlarged gland and biopsy of the distal (nonhilar) tip of the ipsilateral normal parathyroid gland to rule out MGD can be performed. As noted previously, most experienced surgeons do not rely on frozen section to identify normal glands; instead, this approach should be reserved for special situations. The possibility of double adenoma is rare and even more unlikely if preoperative localization tests did not show contralateral neck findings. Cho et al. demonstrated a surgical cure rate of 97% in cases with dual localization without PTH monitoring (and 98% cure rate with intraoperative PTH); the only failures resulted from ipsilateral unidentified double adenoma, which emphasizes the importance of identifying the ipsilateral normal gland to rule out additional disease.[86]
11. Avoid excising a normal parathyroid gland during parathyroid exploration. Resection of normal parathyroid glands does not correct HPT; rather, it risks the development of hypoparathyroidism after subsequent successful resection of the adenoma. Normal glands may be identified, tagged, and even biopsied when appropriate, but never removed.

Technique of Surgery/Search Algorithm

Parathyroid exploration may be performed under general or local anesthesia. If localization studies are positive and supportive of a minimally invasive approach, local anesthesia may be offered to patients.[27,87,88] If general anesthesia is used, no paralytic agents should be used if intraoperative RLN monitoring is planned.

Exploration starts on the side suggested by localization studies (Figure 55.6). One must consider that all localization studies may be incorrect, so that the patient and the surgeon are prepared for the need for a full incision and bilateral exploration. Strap muscles are generally retracted laterally without transection. The proper plane is immediately on the posterior surface of the sternothyroid muscle, which is followed to the medial edge of the carotid sheath and then along the carotid sheath back to the prevertebral fascia. This maintains the central neck soft tissues where the parathyroid glands reside and attach to the thyroid and larynx; this simplifies the subsequent exploration. Exposure of the lateral thyroid region is sometimes facilitated through division of the middle thyroid vein. If any question exists as to the proximity of the RLN during dissection, it should be identified and protected.

The parathyroid search algorithm can be divided, after initial exposure, into step 1 (exploration of normal parathyroid locations) and step 2 (exploration for the missing gland). Exploration for the missing gland implies extending the search, beyond normal locations in a sequential and orderly way, into expanded normal locations, ectopic locations, and acquired migration sites (see Table 55.3). Successful surgery is often realized with step 1 or step 2. If four normal glands are identified during the first phase of exploration, step 3 (fifth gland

CHAPTER 55 Principles in Surgical Management of Primary Hyperparathyroidism

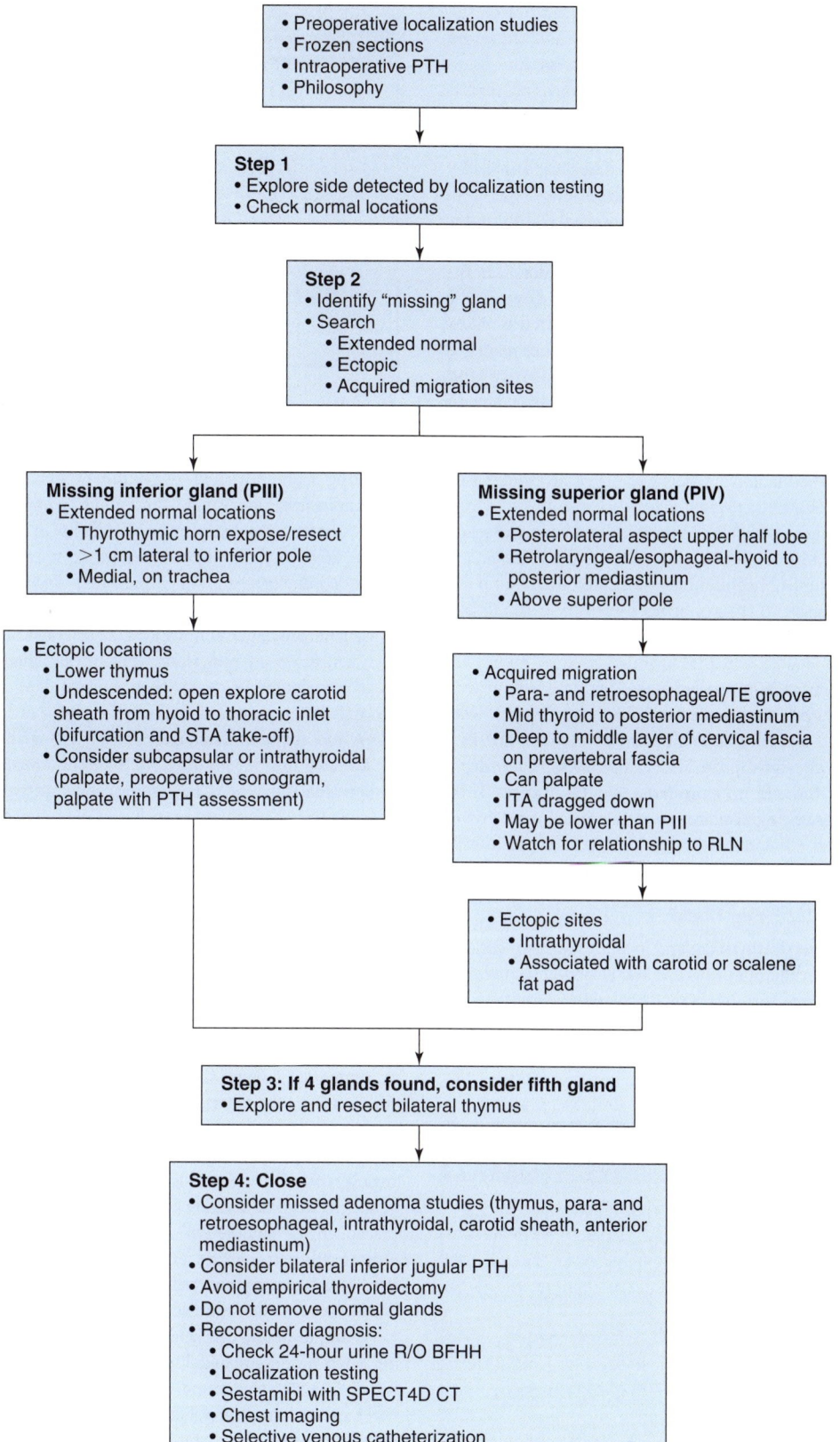

Fig. 55.6 Parathyroid search algorithm. ITA, inferior thyroid artery; PTH, parathyroid hormone; RLN, recurrent laryngeal nerve; R/O BFHH, rule out benign familial hypocalciuric hypercalcemia; SPECT, single-photon emission computed tomography; STA, superior thyroid artery; TE, tracheoesophageal groove.

dissection) is considered. Step 4 represents considerations for closure (see Figure 55.6). The specifics of this parathyroid search algorithm vary depending on surgical philosophy, use of frozen section, use of intraoperative PTH assessment, and preoperative localization studies.

Step 1: Normal Parathyroid Gland Locations

Step 1 involves a thorough exploration of the normal sites for parathyroid glands. This seems obvious, but multiple large series of revision parathyroid explorations repeatedly find most abnormal glands in normal sites. In more than 80% of cases, the superior parathyroid gland occurs within 1 cm of the cricothyroid cartilage articulation (see Box 55.3). This area can also be described as approximately 1 cm cranial to the crossing of the RLN and the inferior thyroid artery. In this region, the superior parathyroid is typically deep and often closely related to the RLN near its laryngeal entry point. The cricothyroid junction landmark is more reliable than the more variable RLN-inferior thyroid artery crossing. The superior thyroid pole vessels can be divided to mobilize the upper pole of the thyroid gland, enhancing the exposure of this region. With these maneuvers, it is best to try to preserve the posterior branch of the superior thyroid artery because this may provide for some or all of the superior parathyroid blood supply. Because the superior parathyroid can be found quite close to the RLN near its laryngeal entry point, the RLN should be specifically identified if dissection is close to the nerve. If it has not been identified, the RLN is vulnerable to injury if bleeding is encountered during adenoma resection.

The inferior parathyroid is normally located within a region 1 cm lateral, inferior, or posterior to the inferior pole of the thyroid. Here, the inferior parathyroid lies ventral to the coronal plane of the RLN and is supplied by the inferior thyroid artery (Box 55.4). The inferior parathyroid resides in this area in approximately 50% of cases. If the initial dissection is in the improper plane, a ventral inferior parathyroid may be found within fat adherent to the undersurface of the inferior aspect of the strap muscles.

Step 2: Search for the Missing Gland

Searching in these normal parathyroid gland locations leads to successful parathyroid surgery in the majority of cases. However, if complete success has not been realized through these initial maneuvers, then it is important to have an organized approach to searching for missing glands. This search should incorporate not only the embryologic

---

BOX 55.3 Superior Parathyroid/PIV Characteristics

Path	Travels with lateral anlage/C-cell complex, which forms upper portion of the lateral thyroid lobes
Location	More constant: within 1 cm of cricothyroid articulation; Less constant: 1 cm cranial to the intersection of inferior thyroid artery and RLN
Relationship to RLN	Deep
Vessel	Inferior thyroid artery or anastomotic branch formed between the inferior thyroid artery and the posterior branch of superior thyroid artery
Maneuver to identify	As the thyroid lateral lobe is dissected, thin fascial bands are taken down to maintain dissection at the level of the true thyroid capsule; superior parathyroids typically are seen in the fat lobule closely adherent to the posterior lateral aspect of lateral thyroid lobe

---

BOX 55.4 Inferior Parathyroid/PIII Characteristics

Path	Travels with thymus; position more variable than superior parathyroid
Location	Within 1 cm inferior, lateral, or posterior to inferior thyroid pole
Relationship to RLN	Superficial
Vessel	Inferior thyroid artery
Maneuver to identify	Often seen with gentle manipulation of thyrothymic fat directly underneath the strap muscles extending from the anterior mediastinum to the inferior surface of inferior thyroid pole

---

sources of variation in parathyroid location but also the variation resulting from acquired migration of enlarged parathyroid glands. To emphasize, all normal sites should be explored before one extends dissection to sites with lower probability of containing the enlarged gland. Step 2 of the algorithm represents such an organized plan of expanded exploration. When the initial exploration has revealed normal parathyroid glands but no enlarged gland, the surgeon must try to identify which gland is missing. Once a specific gland is judged missing (i.e., three normal glands have been identified and the missing gland's normal location has been thoroughly searched), then the exploration is expanded to the extended normal locations, frank ectopic locations, and acquired migration sites.

Missing inferior parathyroid gland. If an inferior gland is missing, exploration is extended to emphasize regions ventral to the RLN, with consideration for tracing branches of the inferior thyroid artery leading to the missing inferior gland (see Box 55.4). First, the extended normal sites are explored. For the inferior parathyroid gland, this means a full exploration of the thyrothymic ligament. The thymus, in the anterior mediastinum, can be slowly drawn up into the neck while watching for the brachiocephalic vein, which is deep/dorsal in the middle mediastinum. As this is done, it is important to note that small bridging veins exit the undersurface of the thymus to extend to the more dorsal brachiocephalic vein; although they are small, they require definitive control.

Expanded normal sites for the inferior parathyroid include regions greater than 1 cm lateral to the thyroid inferior pole and regions medial to the inferior thyroid pole, which are adjacent to the trachea. If these expanded normal locations are negative, exploration should extend to regions of frank embryologic ectopia known for the inferior parathyroid. These areas include the anterior mediastinum; focus should be placed on the middle and lower thymus and undescended locations. One should consider an undescended inferior parathyroid, especially if the ipsilateral thymus (which embryologically travels with the inferior parathyroid) is not present in its normal orthotopic site.

When undescended inferior parathyroid glands are identified, they are often found associated with a thymic remnant. Such undescended inferior parathyroid glands (which can be found higher than the normal superior parathyroid in a cranial-caudal axis) are usually found in association with the carotid sheath, generally medial to the sheath. A thorough search for an undescended inferior parathyroid gland involves opening the carotid sheath (i.e., dividing the investing fascia and identifying and dissecting the carotid artery, vagus nerve, and internal jugular vein) from the hyoid bone to the innominate artery on the right and an analogous caudal location on the left. The "hot spots" for such undescended inferior parathyroid glands are at the carotid bifurcation and at the takeoff of the superior thyroid artery. Parathyroid tissue has been found closely associated with the vagus nerve (even within it) and in the laryngeal pyriform sinus submucosa. These areas are difficult to palpate and explore through a standard collar incision. Finally, in considering ectopic sites, one must give attention to intrathyroidal or subcapsular inferior parathyroid glands. Review of preoperative ultrasonography or other imaging can be helpful while the surgeon considers the possibility of an intrathyroidal parathyroid adenoma at this juncture.

Thompson has shown that thyroidotomy may be more effective than thyroidectomy in the removal of an intrathyroidal adenoma.[82] Indiscriminate, untargeted empirical thyroidectomy should be avoided because it results in significant perithyroidal scarring; the scarring may lead to increased complications at subsequent exploration and potential devascularization of remaining normal parathyroid glands, which may result in hypoparathyroidism.

If exploration of extended normal locations and frank ectopic sites is unrewarding, the surgeon can consider sites of inferior parathyroid gland acquired migration. Although such migration is important for the superior gland, this source of positional variability is less important for the inferior parathyroid gland. When the enlarged inferior parathyroid migrates by force of its mass, it extends typically to the middle and lower thymus.

Missing superior parathyroid gland. If step 1 dissection suggests that a superior parathyroid gland is missing, then dissection should proceed to extended normal sites for the superior parathyroid gland; dissection should emphasize regions dorsal and lateral to the RLN, with an understanding that the vascular supply is often an anastomotic branch linking the inferior and superior thyroid artery systems (see Box 55.3). Thus the posterolateral aspect of the thyroid superior pole and just above is explored. Superior parathyroid glands are often searched for too high, too lateral, and too superficial. Adjacent retrolaryngeal and retroesophageal regions are similarly explored. These regions are deep; hence, superior pole mobilization and rotation may provide helpful exposure. If these expanded normal locations are negative, the surgeon should next consider caudal migration. Thus one should explore the retro- and paralaryngeal, and retro- and paraesophageal regions, which include tracheoesophageal groove regions from the thyroid's superior pole down to the posterior mediastinum (by opening the fascia [middle layer of the deep cervical fascia] between the carotid laterally and the airway and esophagus medially). Gentle palpation in this region can be rewarding. The inferiorly migrated superior parathyroid can come to rest at or below the ipsilateral inferior parathyroid and often takes its blood supply with it. This arterial feeding vessel can be followed downward to the inferiorly migrated gland. The gland is found deep to the overlying fascia in this region (i.e., on the underlying prevertebral fascia and vertebral column). Exploration in this region on the right must be made with an appreciation for possible nonrecurrence of the RLN. If the dissection of the superior parathyroid is still unrewarding, one may consider frank ectopic sites, which, for the superior glands, are rare. For the superior parathyroid, one may explore the carotid sheath as discussed previously and the scalene fat pad lateral to the inferior aspect of the common carotid.

Step 3: Dissection for the Fifth Gland

If all four glands have been identified through dissection and appear normal, and if the diagnosis of HPT is correct, one should consider the possibility of a fifth gland. True supernumerary parathyroid glands are defined as parathyroid tissue, located apart from the other four glands; true supernumerary thyroid glands are are greater than 5 mg in mass. These are identifiable in approximately 13% of normal individuals.[63] In the majority of such patients with HPT, the fifth gland is usually an adenoma rather than the fifth gland of MGD.[89] Such fifth gland adenomas are almost always in the mediastinal thymus; they are rarely found in other locations (such as within the mediastinum associated with the great vessels, associated with the carotid artery in the neck, or intrathyroidal). These supernumerary glands are well treated with bilateral transcervical thymic resection. In certain patients with MGD (e.g., patients with MEN 1 and secondary HPT) supernumerary glands are more common. In these disease entities, there are genetic or metabolic factors that cause parathyroid tissue (e.g., small embryologic parathyroid rests) to enlarge either due to physiologic stimulation in secondary HPT, or through neoplastic change in MEN syndromes. These may then present as apparent clinically significant supernumerary glands. In the setting of four-gland hyperplasia (both in primary and secondary HPT), a clinically significant fifth gland is more common than in uniglandular primary HPT. Bilateral thymectomy and resection of periparathyroid fat have been suggested as techniques to encompass such supernumerary glands, though the efficacy of such procedures is not entirely clear.

Step 4: Considerations for Closure

If all of the preceding dissection has not revealed parathyroid gland pathology and all four glands have been identified, halting the exploration should be considered. Ongoing and untargeted dissection puts normal parathyroid glands, their blood supply, and the RLNs (unilateral or bilateral), at risk. Normal parathyroid glands must never be removed and should be biopsied only if necessary. The surgeon should review the locations found in reoperative series to contain missed adenomas, such as thymus, para- and retroesophageal, intrathyroidal, carotid sheath, and anterior mediastinal locations. Sampling the bilateral, inferior-most jugular venous blood for intraoperative PTH can help to lateralize the abnormality if there is a differential level. Once the thorough algorithm has been completed, the exploration should be stopped; the intent should be to allow the patient to recover from the operation, to confirm the diagnosis and indications for intervention, and to determine next steps.

MEDIASTINAL ADENOMA

Mediastinal disease that cannot be safely accessed through the neck is uncommon. Wang and Clark's classic data emphasize the importance of thorough neck exploration and the high likelihood of success with a cervical incision.[90,91] Most mediastinal tumors are within or attached to the thymus; however, other locations (e.g., those associated with the ascending aorta, aortic arch, aortic arch branches, and pericardium) have been reported.[91a] The surgeon can bring the thymus up into the neck by slowly and gently retracting the thyrothymic ligament, bluntly dissecting around the thymus, and controlling any feeding blood vessels (especially those from the underlying innominate vein).

Sternotomy approaches are effective, but they are rarely necessary; they have been largely replaced by videoscopic techniques (see Chapter 7, Approach to the Mediastinum: Transcervical, Transsternal, and Video-Assisted). In cases of deep mediastinal parathyroid glands, video-assisted approaches are an effective, safe, and less invasive alternative and are the techniques of choice.[92-94] Mediastinal exploration is performed after studies (e.g., 4D-CT scan, MRI, sestamibi with single-photon emission computed tomography (SPECT), or selective venous angiography) have pinpointed the lesion; intraoperative PTH is very useful in the conduct of these procedures.

SURGICAL TECHNIQUE FOR MULTIGLANDULAR DISEASE

Please see the Expert Consult website for discussion of this topic (see also Chapter 60, Surgical Management of Multiglandular Parathyroid Disease).

PARATHYROID SURGERY FAILURE

The lower cure rates, higher complication rates, and significant cost associated with reoperation emphasize the importance of initial surgery's success.[99] Reoperative surgery is less successful than initial parathyroid exploration (see Chapter 63, Reoperation for Sporadic Primary Hyperparathyroidism). Complication rates of reoperation increase when the initial unsuccessful surgery involves extensive dissection, including thyroidectomy, due to increase in central neck scarring. Hypoparathyroidism can result following reoperation after resection of abnormal tissue due to damage to the normal parathyroid glands sustained during the initial procedure. Preoperative laryngeal examination is required to assess the mobility of both vocal cords, to accurately understand the risk of reoperation.

Reasons for Failure

Failure to cure hypercalcemia and HPT by parathyroid exploration may result from incorrect diagnosis or surgical factors. Multiple series suggest that the reasons for failure at initial parathyroid exploration include incomplete exploration with missed cervical disease, missed diagnosis of MGD or double adenoma, ectopic gland, and incorrect diagnosis.[100] The fund of knowledge and experience of the surgeon are important in avoiding incomplete exploration. Parathyroid surgery requires significant knowledge, which is not replaced by availability of localization tests or iPTH testing.

SURGICAL CONTROVERSIES

Please see the Expert Consult website for discussion of this topic.

POSTOPERATIVE ASSESSMENT

Curative parathyroidectomy is defined as normal calcium levels at 6 months after surgery. Recurrent disease is defined as the return of hypercalcemia due to HPT after at least 6 months of normocalcemia.

Measurement of Serum Calcium

Successful exploration usually results in normalization of calcium, with the nadir reached at 48 hours postoperatively. Remaining suppressed parathyroid glands, which have not been dissected or biopsied, have a prompt functional rebound.

In our practice, we discharge our patients on the day of operation, on supplemental calcium citrate (200 mg elemental calcium every 6 hours) and calcitriol (0.25 mcg daily). Most patients are asymptomatic, and these medications are discontinued once calcium and PTH levels are shown to be normal at 1 to 2 weeks after surgery. For patients with normal calcium and elevated PTH after surgery, we typically continue calcium citrate supplementation (200 to 400 mg elemental daily) while monitoring laboratory values. Some patients require additional vitamin D supplementation before PTH levels normalize. Calcium and PTH levels are checked at 3- and 6-month intervals to normality at more than 6 months postoperatively to ensure resolution.

In patients with extensive bilateral dissection and normal gland biopsy, calcium levels may drop significantly. Concomitant thyroidectomy, reoperation, and weight of the excised pathologic tissue are associated with increased rate of hypocalcemia.[105] In patients with preoperative elevated alkaline phosphatase and skeletal depletion of calcium, the postoperative course may demonstrate bone hunger and lower than expected calcium levels. Symptomatic patients may require increase in dose supplementation to alleviate symptoms. In patients with significant hypocalcemic symptoms or significantly low calcium levels, intravenous (IV) calcium should be started promptly until the oral regimen becomes effective. Hypomagnesemia can lead to less effective treatment responses; serum magnesium levels should be assessed if calcium replacement is problematic or if symptoms persist.

Postoperative Management

Normally, PTH levels decrease after successful parathyroid surgery. Mandal noticed that 71% of 78 patients had PTH levels <10 pg/mL the night of the operation, and 1 week after the operation, mean serum PTH returned to normal in 88% of patients.[106] However, even in apparently cured patients, PTH can become elevated after surgery. Multiple series have noted elevated PTH in 8% to 43% of eucalcemic patients after successful parathyroidectomy.[106-115] The elevated PTH may stabilize, increase, or decrease over time and tends to normalize or decrease by 12 to 16 months in 78% to 88% of patients. Some reports suggest that PTH levels remain increased for up to 1 to 4 years without recurrence.[116]

Postoperative elevation of PTH is more likely in cases when there is (1) higher preoperative HPT disease severity, as indicated by higher preoperative PTH, larger adenoma size, and MGD; (2) evidence of decreased peripheral sensitivity to PTH, perhaps resulting from chronic preoperative PTH elevation; (3) renal insufficiency; (4) postoperative exaggerated response to excess bone demineralization; and (5) preoperative vitamin D deficiency. Postoperative elevation of PTH is more common in older patients and in females compared with males. The surgical approach (unilateral versus bilateral) does not influence the number of patients showing elevation of postoperative PTH.

Elevated postoperative PTH does not predict failure in the majority of patients and is a poor test for postoperative disease status. Solorzano et al., in their study of 505 patients, noted that up to one third of patients developed elevated postoperative PTH, with an overwhelming majority of these patients achieving long-term eucalcemia.[116] Charlett et al. noted that elevated postoperative PTH had a sensitivity of 62.1% and a specificity of 75% for detecting operative failure.[100] Yen et al. proposed that PTH measurements after surgery for primary HPT may be misleading, costly, and not indicated in normocalcemic patients.[109]

We recommend measuring calcium and PTH at 1 to 2 weeks, 3 months, and 6 months to assess for surgical cure. For patients with normal calcium and elevated PTH after surgery, we measure vitamin D levels and replenish if needed. We advise patients to follow age and gender-specific calcium intake guidelines to support bone health. Improvement in bone density occurs at a tempo measured in years.

REFERENCES

For a complete list of references, go to expertconsult.com.

Standard Bilateral Parathyroid Exploration

Allan E. Siperstein, Antonia E. Stephen, Mira Milas

> Please go to expertconsult.com to view related video:
> **Video 56.1** Introduction to Chapter 56, Standard Bilateral Parathyroid Exploration.

Modern management of parathyroid disease has evolved with the influence of several fundamentally new and important factors. First is the reality that primary hyperparathyroidism (PHPT) is no longer a rare endocrine disorder, but the most common cause of hypercalcemia in the outpatient population; it has an estimated prevalence of 1 in 500 women and 1 in 2000 men. The incidence increases with age and is 2 to 3 times more common in women.[1] A second and related factor is a higher prevalence of asymptomatic PHPT, where a clear biochemical diagnosis of parathyroid disease exists without noticeable symptoms or clinically detectable consequences, such as bone density loss or kidney stones.[2] An additional reason that more patients are being diagnosed in an asymptomatic phase of the disease is because calcium has become a routine component of automated chemistry panels; this helps lead to incidental detection of symptomatic hypercalcemia. Conversely, more practitioners are also recognizing the need to screen patients with osteoporosis, osteopenia, and kidney stones for underlying PHPT; practitioners use not just calcium screening, but a panel that includes calcium, intact parathyroid hormone (PTH), and 25-hydroxyvitamin D levels (see Chapter 53, Primary Hyperparathyroidism: Pathophysiology, Surgical Indications, and Preoperative Workup). Finally, perhaps the most visible changes in the landscape of parathyroid disease management are the paradigm shifts in the preferred operative approach. After many years of standard bilateral explorations, there was a shift in the late 1990s to a more focused approach: the exploration of a single site of suspected parathyroid gland abnormality.[3] Many parathyroid surgeons adapted this as the favored initial approach to parathyroid surgery, guided by radiological studies and intraoperative PTH measurement (see Chapter 54, Guide to Preoperative Parathyroid Localization Testing; Chapter 57, Minimally Invasive Single Gland Parathyroid Exploration; Chapter 58, Minimally Invasive Video-Assisted Parathyroidectomy; and Chapter 59, Intraoperative PTH Monitoring during Parathyroid Surgery). More recently, however, the bilateral exploration appears to be back in favor among endocrine and head and neck surgeons. Image-directed, focused parathyroid surgery is still frequently used in appropriate patients, but the limitations of preoperative localization and intraoperative PTH levels in reliably identifying multi-gland disease is well-appreciated, and the pendulum appears to be swinging back to the middle ground of selected, focused operations and a low threshold to consider a bilateral exploration.

This technique of achieving the surgical cure of PHPT was the original operative approach preferred from the 1920s through the late 1990s[3]. At its essence, this approach can be defined as the exploration and examination of all parathyroid glands bilaterally with appropriate resection of diseased glands. It is imperative to recognize that "conventional" or "bilateral" parathyroid procedures are not obsolete; they remain essential and are at the core of successful parathyroid surgery. Bilateral parathyroidectomy will remain integral to the surgical treatment of PHPT; for appropriate patients, it is the ideal initial operation. It is also important to recognize that bilateral parathyroid examination can be performed in a minimally invasive manner. This approach requires a thorough understanding of parathyroid gland anatomy, embryology, and of specific indications based on clinical presentation, parathyroid imaging, and intraoperative findings. In this chapter, we provide the rationale for and method of bilateral parathyroid exploration, illustrated with relevant clinical examples and a strategy for addressing the problematic circumstance of finding a "missing gland" (see also Chapter 55, Principles in Surgical Management of Primary Hyperparathyroidism).

ANATOMY AND EMBRYOLOGY RELEVANT FOR BILATERAL PARATHYROID EXPLORATION

There are typically four parathyroid glands in most individuals; thus bilateral exploration ideally aims to identify all four (see Chapter 2, Applied Embryology of the Thyroid and Parathyroid Glands). A large autopsy study identified four parathyroid glands in 84% of human cadavers, ≥5 glands in 13%, and only three parathyroids in 3%.[4,5] Supranumerary parathyroids are most often located in the thymus. The possibility of having an unusual number or location of parathyroid glands has a direct effect on the success of parathyroid surgery and the potential need for bilateral parathyroidectomy, yet it remains difficult to predict such anomalies reliably. The potential for missed ectopic or supranumerary parathyroids and persistent or recurrent hyperparathyroidism (HPT) should be discussed with patients before surgery to properly inform expectations of surgery.

The key aspects of parathyroid anatomy and embryology to adapt to bilateral parathyroidectomy are illustrated in Figures 56.1 to 56.3. Normal parathyroid glands are approximately 5 to 6 mm in greatest dimension, weigh 15 to 35 mg, and can be inconspicuous with their orange-tan color embedded or flattened within a surrounding yellow fatty tissue envelope. The appearance of parathyroids can be variable even when they are biochemically functioning normally. When diseased, parathyroid glands may display variable morphological changes in size, shape, texture, and firmness. Abnormal parathyroids are generally fuller in all dimensions, have a darker brown or reddish-brown color, do not compress easily, or are significantly firm when gently probed. They may have an irregular and lobular shape, more prominent

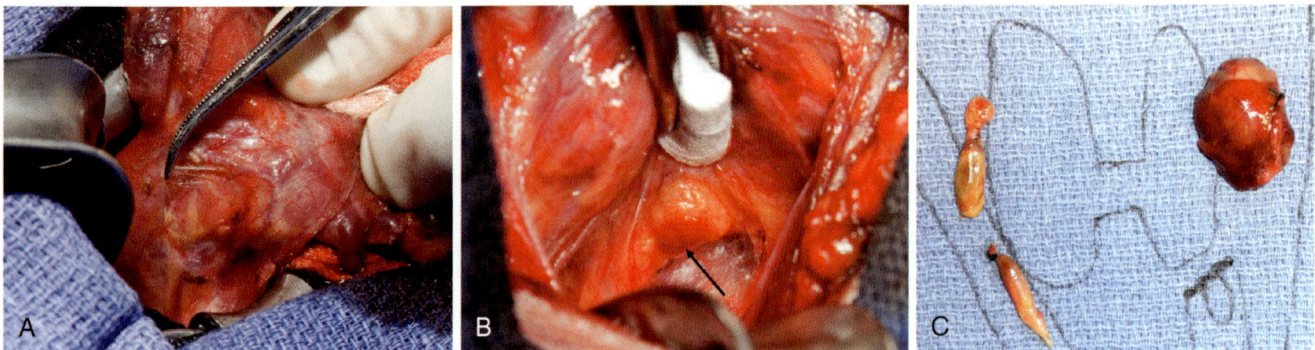

Fig. 56.1 Parathyroid anatomy can be variable. Normal parathyroids are marked with an arrow. Even normal parathyroid glands can assume irregular shapes (**A** and **B**) that should not be mistaken for adenomas or hyperplasia. Asymmetry or variable degrees of parathyroid enlargement, furthermore, exist even in multigland hyperplasia (**C**). The intraoperative photo illustrates three variably abnormal parathyroids in morphology; all were histologically hypercellular. (Reprinted with permission, Cleveland Clinic Center for Medical Art & Photography © 2008–2011. All rights reserved.)

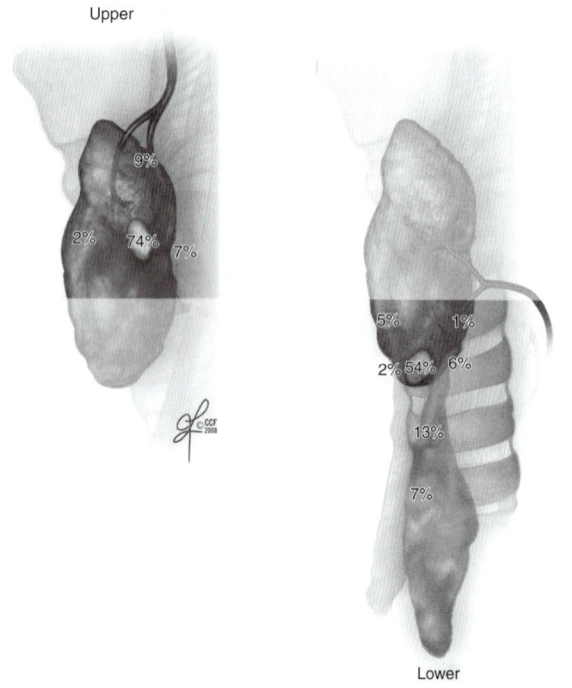

Fig. 56.2 Normally expected distribution of upper and lower parathyroid glands. (Reprinted with permission, Cleveland Clinic Center for Medical Art & Photography © 2008–2011. All rights reserved.)

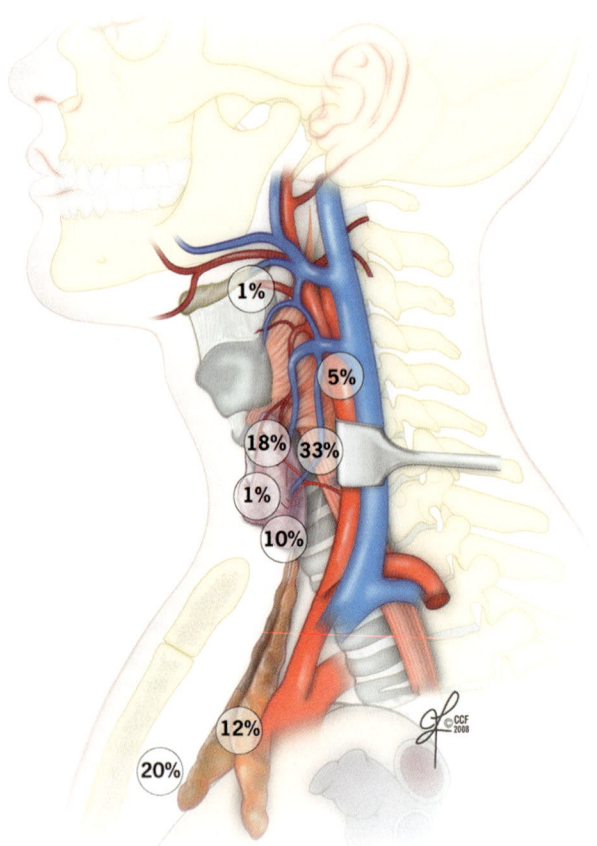

Fig. 56.3 Distribution of ectopic parathyroid glands. (Reprinted with permission, Cleveland Clinic Center for Medical Art & Photography © 2008–2011. All rights reserved.)

vascular pedicles, or a plexus of vasculature. Glands of patients with secondary and tertiary HPT may be sclerotic and light in color from fibrosis.

In cases of borderline abnormal appearance, it is helpful to determine in vivo parathyroid weight before excision of the parathyroid. This can be readily done *without* removing the gland by measuring parathyroid length (L), width (W), and height (H) using a small ruler or micrometer device. Because most glands are oval, calculating the volume of an ellipsoid using sizes in millimeters (mm) estimates parathyroid gland weight in milligrams (mg): (weight [mg] $\approx$ L $\times$ W $\times$ H mm^3 $\times$½). We have observed that the metric of the total volume of diseased glands (TVDG) is statistically the same, whether the surgical findings are single- or multigland parathyroid disease.[6] In other words, the size of a typical single adenoma will be similar to the additive size (by volume or weight) of both double adenomas or of four hyperplastic glands. This implies that there ought to be caution for the likely presence of multigland disease—and therefore the need for bilateral parathyroid exploration—when only a mildly enlarged parathyroid is encountered first. Even when imaging studies suggest a single site of parathyroid disease and intraoperative PTH falls appropriately, a parathyroid gland that is 75 to 200 mg in size will rarely be a single adenoma (see Chapter 59, Intraoperative PTH Monitoring during Parathyroid Surgery). There is ongoing interest and some controversy in defining what truly constitutes an abnormal parathyroid and whether this is a matter of purely morphological form, biochemical function, or a combination of both features (see Chapter 55, Principles in Surgical Management of Primary Hyperparathyroidism).

Embryologically, the upper parathyroids develop from the fourth branchial pouch and migrate caudally with the thyroid, whereas the lower parathyroid glands derive from the third branchial pouch and migrate with the thymus. The upper parathyroid glands have a narrower area of distribution, are fairly reliably positioned in the perithyroidal fat posterior to the superior pole of the thyroid gland, and they are near the path of the recurrent laryngeal nerve (RLN) as it enters the cricothyroid muscle (see Figure 56.2). In contrast, the lower parathyroids are more widespread around the lower pole of the thyroid gland, thyrothymic ligament, and pretracheal fat. Symmetry is usually present between parathyroid locations in the left and right sides of the neck, and this can strategically be used when trying to locate parathyroid glands. Double parathyroid adenomas, however, do not have a uniform or random distribution pattern; when only two glands are enlarged and histologically hypercellular, they tend to be on opposite sides of the neck and may tend to the upper parathyroids; this pattern is designated "fourth pouch disease."[7] (Figure 56.4).

Additional clues for parathyroid location can come from observing the patterns of vasculature in and around the expected parathyroid region. Both parathyroids typically derive some blood supply from the inferior thyroid artery. In relation to the path of the main trunk of this artery as it nears the thyroid, upper parathyroids are cranial and deeper; lower parathyroids are caudal, anterior, and medial. Unusually curved or extra branching patterns of the artery may alert to abnormal parathyroids found hanging at the ends of those branches, sometimes several centimeters away from the thyroid capsule. Within their fatty envelope, a normal parathyroid will have a leaflike branching pattern of the vascular pedicle. This is a helpful contrast to lymph nodes, fat or thymic tissues (that have no visible vascular pattern), and abnormal parathyroids whose vascular pedicle may be exaggerated. Being alert to these subtle morphological features can expedite finding parathyroids during bilateral exploration.

Migratory distribution of the parathyroids can lead to ectopic locations within the following locations: the thymus, the sheath encompassing the carotid artery, the jugular vein, the vagus nerve (even in high cervical locations), the retroesophageal region, and even within the thyroid. Some, but not all, of these areas can be accessed via the usual cervical incision during bilateral parathyroid exploration. Recently, Perrier et al. proposed novel nomenclature to further classify cervical parathyroid adenomas into regions relevant for parathyroid exploration (see Chapter 57, Minimally Invasive Single Gland Parathyroid Exploration).[8] Ectopic parathyroid locations in the anterior mediastinum, other deeper regions of the mediastinum, and even the pericardium require alternate surgical approaches, which often require collaboration with thoracic surgeons.

THE RATIONALE FOR BILATERAL PARATHYROID EXPLORATION

The cornerstones of successful parathyroid surgery are correct initial diagnosis of parathyroid disease and clear articulation of treatment goals based on an individual's clinical profile of parathyroid disease. Although, on the surface, it may appear that these processes are the same whether parathyroidectomy is approached as a focal or bilateral

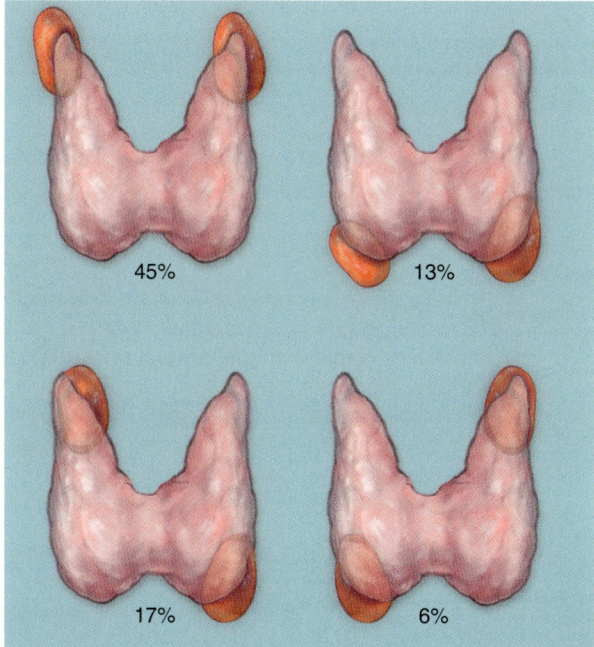
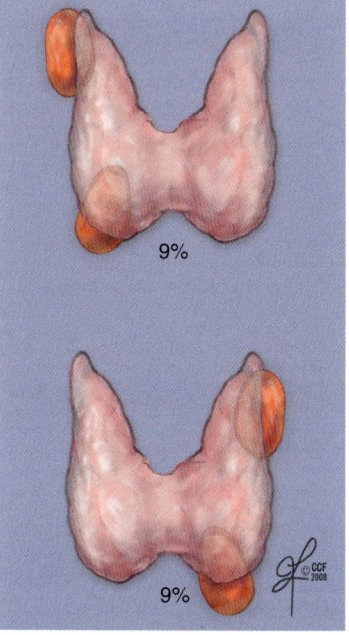

Fig. 56.4 Double parathyroid adenomas have nonuniform distribution that favors enlargement of both upper glands. Only a minority (18%) will have ipsilateral location. (Reprinted with permission, Cleveland Clinic Center for Medical Art & Photography © 2008–2011. All rights reserved.)

Diagnosis

Bilateral parathyroid exploration principally involves patients with PHPT, although it is also needed in those who have secondary or tertiary HPT from renal disease. The latter diagnoses are covered in detail in separate chapters (see Chapter 60, Surgical Management of Multiglandular Parathyroid Disease; Chapter 61, Surgical Management of Secondary and Tertiary Hyperparathyroidism; and Chapter 62, Parathyroid Management in the MEN Syndromes). Traditionally, the diagnosis of PHPT has rested on the demonstration of simultaneously elevated serum total or ionized calcium with elevated intact PTH in the setting of normal or high calcium excretion in the urine. With this combination of findings, the diagnosis of PHPT is practically definitive. In part, this is because modern measurements of PTH detect the intact molecule, reflecting the entire protein derived from the parathyroid glands and essentially eliminating confounding diagnoses from ectopic sources of PTH, such as tumors producing PTH-related peptide (PTHrp). The rare hereditary condition of benign familial hypercalcemic hypocalciuria (BFHH) is excluded by the finding of normal or high levels of calcium in a 24-hour urine collection.

Approximately 10% of patients will have unusual biochemical presentations that do not fit these classical diagnostic criteria but are nonetheless found to have PHPT. There are at least two atypical versions of the disease. Normocalcemic PHPT manifests with normal total serum calcium but high PTH and has been relatively well appreciated. Despite borderline laboratory values, patients with normocalcemic hyperparathyroidism may suffer from kidney stones, osteoporosis, and bone fractures.[9] Patients with the other form of PHPT have high calcium levels but normal PTH. Diagnosis is somewhat easier if PTH values are "inappropriately" high-normal for the degree of hypercalcemia (40 to 60 pg/mL on a scale where 60 pg/mL is maximal reference range) but can be less clear when values are as low as 5 to 15 pg/mL.

Box 56.1 provides a recommended diagnostic workup for PHPT and strategies to clarify the diagnosis in challenging scenarios. It is advisable to obtain a baseline bone density assessment with a dual energy x-ray absorptiometry (DEXA) bone scan, especially if this did not precede referral of the patient to the surgeon. Urinary calcium excretion lower than 50 mg/dL should prompt consideration of explanations that include BFHH, renal disease, and the use of thiazide diuretics, among others.

Although there can be other nonendocrine causes of hypercalcemia coexisting with PHPT, these are exceedingly rare. Separate investigations for these causes is not warranted at the outset in a patient with elevated calcium, intact PTH, and whose medical history does not have pertinent findings (e.g., hypercalcemia-associated malignancies). Such investigations may be helpful in atypical presentations. Obtaining a thorough family history is important to discern possible multiple endocrine neoplasia (MEN), and, if suspected, appropriate additional evaluation can be tailored. Routine genetic testing for MEN 1 (where 90% manifest parathyroid disease) and MEN 2 (where parathyroid disease affects <5% patients) is unwarranted as part of the initial diagnostic workup for PHPT.

A detail-oriented and meticulous determination of clinical history is essential to enhance recognition of those patients who will be better served with a bilateral exploration. Some investigators have even proposed a scoring system to aid this process, particularly for identifying MEN kindred.[10]

Treatment

Parathyroidectomy has the following operative goals: (1) achieving normocalcemic state and normal long-term PTH, (2) avoiding injury to the laryngeal nerves, (3) engendering minimal postoperative morbidity and negligible mortality, and (4) accomplishing cosmetic scar appearance acceptable to the patient. Surgery remains the most clearly demonstrated mechanism for durable cure of PHPT and symptomatic improvement, particularly related to osteoporosis, bone fractures, and

---

BOX 56.1 Diagnostic Workup for Primary Hyperparathyroidism

In a patient found to have hypercalcemia or diagnosed with conditions that can be related to PHPT (osteopenia, osteoporosis, kidney stones)
- Careful history and physical examination, including symptoms, prior head and neck radiation treatments, prior neck surgery, medications, and prior endocrine disorders in the patient and patient's family
- Initial serum biochemical profile: serum total calcium, serum ionized calcium, intact PTH, serum phosphate, 25-hydroxyvitamin D, 1,25-dihydroxyvitamin D
- If this initial profile is compatible with PHPT, complete the diagnostic workup with 24-hour urine collection for measurements of urinary volume, creatinine, and calcium
- Diagnosis is confirmed when there is elevated serum total or ionized calcium or both, in conjunction with elevated or high-normal PTH, and elevated or normal 24-hour urinary calcium
- Note that imaging studies (e.g., ultrasound, 99-Tc sestamibi scan, 4D-computed tomography) are not intended for diagnostic purposes, but as localizing studies obtained after diagnosis and the decision to proceed with surgery

In a patient with normocalcemic hyperparathyroidism (HPT)
- Repeat several serum biochemical profiles. Look for elevation in ionized calcium
- Consider underlying vitamin D deficiency or other causes of secondary HPT and treat appropriately

- Consider calculating the patient's personal upper limit of normal PTH by the formula PTH [ULN pg/mL] = 120 − (6 × serum calcium mg/dL) − (½ × 25-hydroxyvitamin D ng/mL) + (¼ × patient's age in years); the measurements of calcium, PTH, and vitamin D should be from the same blood draw; if the patient's measured serum value of PTH is higher than this calculated ULN PTH, the diagnosis of PHPT would be more likely

In a patient suspected to have other potential causes of hypercalcemia or an initial biochemical profile that shows hypercalcemia with low normal intact PTH, consider screening for
- Bony metastases, sarcoidosis, pulmonary tumors (chest radiograph)
- Multiple myeloma (serum protein electrophoresis)
- PTH-related peptide producing tumors (serum PTHrp)
- Check recent staging for cancer status if history of prior malignancy

In a patient with possible multiple endocrine neoplasia (MEN) type 1 or 2
- Screen for serum or urinary metanephrines before parathyroid surgery
- Complete investigation of endocrinopathies as appropriate for patient's history
- Genetic testing to confirm MEN 1 or 2 is not required before parathyroidectomy

BOX 56.2 Indications for Bilateral Parathyroid Exploration as the Initial Surgery for Parathyroid Disease

Absolute Indications
- Known or suspected multiple endocrine neoplasia (MEN) syndromes
- Known secondary and tertiary hyperparathyroidism (HPT) in the setting of renal failure or after kidney transplantation
- Intraoperative PTH fails to drop after resection of suspected single adenoma
- Failure to find diseased gland at location indicated by imaging studies
- Finding more than one abnormal parathyroid during intended focal or unilateral neck exploration
- Negative imaging studies
- Imaging studies suggesting multiple sites of disease
- Coexisting thyroid cancer or bilateral goiter requiring total thyroidectomy

Advisable Indications
- Discordant parathyroid imaging studies
- Unavailability of intraoperative PTH measurement
- Inability to obtain preoperative imaging
- Lithium-induced PHPT
- Non-MEN familial HPT
- Coexisting thyroid pathology that may require operative intervention
- Surgeon preference or experience

neurocognitive issues.[1] All of the newer surgical techniques that have evolved since the early 2000s share the following goals: focal and unilateral exploration with or without intraoperative PTH measurement, radioguided parathyroid surgery, and videoscopic and robotically assisted parathyroidectomy.[11] It is again important to stress that standard, bilateral parathyroid exploration meets these goals as well; however, some literature has questioned comparative performance with respect to morbidity and cosmetic outcomes.[3,12-14] Especially when performed by experienced surgeons, bilateral parathyroid exploration has an excellent long-term track record of curing PHPT and can be achieved with minimal morbidity.[15,16]

Rationale for Parathyroid Surgery and Bilateral Exploration

Recently-published guidelines for the management of PHPT suggests operative management is clearly indicated for all patients with classic symptoms or complications of PHPT.[1] More challenging has been the perspective of decision making for those patients with apparently asymptomatic PHPT. A combined panel of expert surgeons and endocrinologists issued recently modified guidelines outlining the criteria for surgical referral of patients with asymptomatic PHPT: (1), those patients <50 years of age; (2), those patients with a serum calcium level >1.0 mg/dL above the normal range; (3), those patients with T-scores < −2.5 at lumbar spine, total hip, femoral neck, or distal one-third radius or vertebral fracture on x-ray, computed tomography (CT), magnetic resonance imaging (MRI), or vertebral fracture assessment (VFA); (4), those patients with urinary calcium >400 mg/24 hour and increased stone risk; and (5), those patients with a creatinine clearance <60 cc/min.[17,18]

It is difficult to predict reliably the development, timing, and progression of disease in patients with asymptomatic HPT. Long-term nonoperative management can be costly. For these reasons, other experts have advised a more liberal approach to recommendations of parathyroidectomy beyond the criteria identified by the National Institutes of Health (NIH), provided that surgery can be performed safely and with minimal risks for a disease that, in some patients, may be minimally problematic at the time of presentation.

The indications for bilateral parathyroid exploration as the initial surgery for PHPT, once a patient has met the criteria indicated previously, are listed in Box 56.2. The guiding principle of bilateral parathyroid exploration is that some patients have significantly higher risk for multigland parathyroid disease. Therefore successfully achieving the operative goal of normocalcemia is contingent upon the evaluation of all parathyroid glands in their usual anatomical locations and upon the appropriate resection of those glands that appear abnormal.

PREOPERATIVE PLANNING: PARATHYROID LOCALIZATION STUDIES

The thoughtful, stepwise assessment of the patient to reach a diagnosis of parathyroid disease and identify the need for surgery is the most important part of preoperative planning. The remaining efforts are directed to determining that a patient is medically fit to undergo parathyroidectomy safely and to localize the site of parathyroid disease.

There is a spectrum of radiological imaging studies available for localization of abnormal parathyroid glands (see Chapter 54, Guide to Preoperative Parathyroid Localization Testing). The most frequently used modalities are neck ultrasound, 99-Tc sestamibi scans, and CT scans, or combinations of these. Normal parathyroids are not expected to be imaged, except perhaps with four-dimensional computed tomography (4D CT) scans. Scans with 99-Tc sestamibi are conducted variably among radiology departments; techniques include 2D planar scans with initial and delayed imaging, 3D single-photon emission computed tomography (SPECT) imaging, use of concomitant CT scanning with or without intravenous contrast dye, and use of ^{123}I to subtract the contribution of thyroid uptake of 99-Tc sestamibi. Surgeons may find it valuable to be familiar with the technique used by their radiologists and to review images collaboratively because reported accuracies of the various modalities range widely from 50% to 96%.[19] MRI, selective venous sampling, and occasionally positron emission tomography (PET) scans are localization techniques typically used for reoperative rather than initial preoperative evaluation. Neck ultrasound, particularly surgeon-performed ultrasound, provides the added advantage of identifying concomitant thyroid disease that may need to be addressed during parathyroid surgery. Thyroid nodular disease is seen in as many as 30% of patients, whereas 4% will have previously undiagnosed thyroid cancer detected during an evaluation for PHPT.[20]

It is valid to consider whether patients selected for bilateral parathyroid exploration require any preoperative imaging. In principle, this imaging is not essential because the risk of mediastinal or cervical ectopic parathyroid disease is rare. It is justifiable to conduct bilateral parathyroid exploration without imaging studies, and this strategy has a decades-long successful track record. Conversely, if no preoperative imaging studies are available or if they are entirely negative, bilateral rather than focal parathyroid exploration is advisable. Nevertheless, preoperative imaging with bilateral parathyroid exploration we feel is valuable because it can facilitate the conduct and speed of the operation by focusing early dissection on the region of greatest suspected abnormality. The practice of a surgeon reviewing the actual radiology images before operation is strongly encouraged. This can reveal anatomical details that may aid decision making during surgery.

SURGICAL TECHNIQUE OF BILATERAL PARATHYROID EXPLORATION

Bilateral parathyroid exploration can be accomplished with minimal invasiveness and morbidity, gentle dissection, and the use of a few delicate instruments. Most surgeons currently perform parathyroid surgery with general anesthesia, and some use local anesthetics supplemented by deep cervical nerve block and sedation. No antibiotics are needed except in reoperative cases. Deep vein thrombosis (DVT) prophylaxis is left to the judgment of the surgeon and tailored to patient need. However, in general, sequential compression stockings provide the least risk of neck hematoma while providing adequate DVT prophylaxis.

Bilateral parathyroid exploration can also be performed without the use of intraoperative adjuncts, although these may be helpful depending on the complexity of surgical findings, assessment of usefulness by the individual surgeon, or experience of the surgeon. Numerous intraoperative adjuncts have been described.[13,14] Most notably, intraoperative PTH measurement has become a fundamental part of modern parathyroid surgical practice.[13] It is used to confirm complete excision of hyperfunctioning glands (see Chapter 59, Intraoperative PTH Monitoring during Parathyroid Surgery). Intraoperative PTH, however, is least accurate in predicting multigland parathyroid hyperplasia.[15,21] Other adjuncts include frozen section histology and needle aspiration of excised tissue for measurement of PTH as a means of distinguishing parathyroid from nonparathyroid tissue. It is useful to recall that neither frozen section examination nor permanent histology can distinguish among single adenomas, hyperplasia, or various underlying parathyroid disease states (i.e., primary, secondary, or familial HPT). Intraoperative gamma probe has been applied to in vivo localization of abnormal parathyroids and ex vivo measurement of radiotracer counts as markers of normal versus abnormal parathyroids.[22,23] Intraoperative ultrasound has been suggested to facilitate incision placement. The ultimate application of these adjuncts remains surgeon-dependent, and some are more essential for focal rather than bilateral parathyroid exploration.

Once anesthetized, the patient is positioned with arms tucked at the side. Their head is gently hyperextended, which is facilitated by placement of a roll or beanbag between the scapulae. Care to have vertical alignment of the patient's chin, suprasternal notch, and center of the thyroid cartilage aids a symmetrical incision. Likewise, to optimize cosmetic results, it is helpful to mark potential incision sites while the patient is awake and sitting upright because this best reveals natural skin creases, which can move or become less visible in the supine position. The authors prefer chlorhexidine for sterile prep because it in nonflammable and avoids potential irritation and staining of the face and neck.

A transversely oriented incision is made according to the optimal site marked. In most patients, this is 1.5 to 2 fingerbreadths above the suprasternal notch. The length of the incision varies with surgeon preference and usually does not need to be longer than 4 to 6 cm. Bilateral parathyroid exploration can be performed via incisions as small as 2.5 cm positioned in the midline at the thyroid isthmus. The incision is carried down by electrocautery through the platysma muscle that is about 2 to 3 mm thick (more visible in men) and relatively free of blood vessels. Deep to the platysma is an avascular plane just above the anterior jugular veins that can be developed to aid exposure using a combination of electrocautery and blunt dissection. This subplatysmal plane is developed until the thyroid cartilage is palpable superiorly and the sternal notch inferiorly; however, it can be dissected less in thin patients. Mobilizing these flaps offers optimal exposure through small incisions by increasing the ease of retraction. Anterior jugular veins are preserved as a potential source of blood sampling for intraoperative PTH.

Once the subplatysmal flaps are created, a self-retaining retractor is placed. The avascular midline raphe of the strap muscles is opened vertically along the midline to separate the muscles and expose the thyroid. Occasionally, small vessels can cross this midline and require ligation; however, electrocautery is sufficient for dividing most of these tiny branches. The sternothyroid muscle is bluntly separated from the undersurface of the sternohyoid muscle for a short distance, again to aid mobility in lateral retraction. The loose areolar tissue between the sternothyroid muscle and thyroid is taken down with cautery at low settings or blunt dissection. It is important to separate these tissues or any pretracheal fat at the very edge of the sternothyroid muscle to avoid unintentionally displacing parathyroid tissue laterally. Traction is exerted on the thyroid lobe either by using a peanut or manually with 4 × 4 sponges (to elevate and medially rotate the lobe). This exposes the lateral and posterior thyroid surface and brings the middle thyroid vein into view. This vein is always above the plane of the carotid artery, which should now be visible or palpable. The vein courses in a medial to lateral direction, similar and often parallel to the inferior thyroid artery, which, in contrast, is always situated deep to the carotid artery. The middle thyroid vein can be isolated, ligated, and divided to facilitate exposure.

Bilateral parathyroid exploration begins by identifying the abnormal parathyroid gland in the area, suggested by preoperative imaging. Very fine instruments are used for these maneuvers and the importance of maintaining a bloodless field cannot be overemphasized. Blood staining discolors the adjacent tissue and can make parathyroids less noticeable. If parathyroid imaging is negative, the area of the lower parathyroid is exposed first because it is more accessible. Exposure of the upper parathyroid area requires an even greater degree of medial rotation of the thyroid lobe. The strategy is to identify fatty-appearing tissue along the edges of the thyroid or adjacent to the space where branches of the inferior and superior thyroid artery enter the thyroid gland. Purposeful observation of the operative field is more effective than blind dissection. Care should be taken to stay close to the thyroid to avoid injury to the RLN. The nerve does not necessarily have to be exposed or skeletonized as part of parathyroid exploration. Its presence in the vicinity and orientation relative to enlarged parathyroids should always be considered, and its path revealed just enough, if necessary, to ensure its safety during subsequent dissection. This is especially the case with large superior parathyroid glands, which can displace the RLN on the posterior or anterior capsule of the gland, requiring it to be moved away gently.

When an area of likely parathyroid abnormality is seen, careful blunt dissection is done using a fine curved hemostat to separate the overlying fatty tissue. The surgeon looks for subtle color changes (darker orange to brown) of the parathyroid. A normal parathyroid will appear flattened and have a leaflike vascular pattern absent in simple fat or thymus. It can be gently coaxed out of the areolar or fatty covering to determine its entire size and that it does not hide an enlarged segment (a "cap of normal" disguising an underlying parathyroid tumor). An abnormal or enlarged parathyroid will often appear as a mass bulging below overlying tissue or have a sliding motion back and forth beneath a film of thin areolar cover. The abnormal parathyroid should also be separated from the encasing thin areolar tissue so that its only attachment is the vascular pedicle. This can sometimes be facilitated by using a number 3 Penfield instrument, whose curvature can gently scoop out a parathyroid. Ideally, the dissection should free the enlarged parathyroid along its lateral and posterior aspects first, leaving the medially located pedicle along the thyroid last.

We have designated the search for parathyroid glands along the usual anatomical distribution of upper and lower parathyroids as the "primary parathyroid survey." It takes into consideration exploring all the regions shown in Figure 56.2 until the remaining three parathyroids have been identified. It is useful to develop a systematic order of exploration and practice it routinely. A convenient strategy is to target exposure of the most abnormal parathyroid first, the ipsilateral parathyroid second, and, finally, to explore the contralateral side. When all parathyroids have been identified, assessment about the disease process (e.g., single adenoma, double adenoma, or hyperplasia) can be made; a decision about which parathyroids to remove and in which order can be determined.

Treatment of single adenomas is simple excision of the abnormal gland. Multigland hyperplasia is ideally treated with subtotal parathyroidectomy and parathyroid cryopreservation. If only two or three of the four glands are abnormal, the abnormal parathyroids are excised while the normal parathyroids can be left in situ without resection; their location is marked with a clip. If all four glands are abnormal, the remnant should be fashioned first; the practitioner should resect all but a segment measuring approximately 6 × 4 mm or the size of a normal parathyroid (around 25 mg). This segment remains attached to the vascular pedicle and is marked with a clip across the transected surface. Parathyroids with discrete or long vascular pedicles, and those with oval rather than a globular or knobby shape, are easier to fashion into remnants. Inferior parathyroids are more suitable to use as remnants because they are easier to approach in event of future reoperation. It is wise to expose all parathyroids before embarking on excision of those encountered early because the surgeon's assessment of the disease process or preference for which parathyroid to use for remnant creation may change.

A "secondary parathyroid survey" refers to the exploration of cervical regions when parathyroid position is more unusual or ectopic and when the previously discussed primary survey has not led to conclusive findings. Important areas to examine are summarized in Figure 56.5. The most commonly missed location is a retroesophageal parathyroid that has sunken into the deep posterior space behind the tracheoesophageal groove, and often lies on the anterior surface of the spine and below the main trunk of the inferior thyroid artery. This parathyroid is embryologically derived from the upper gland; however, both intraoperatively and on imaging studies, it often appears to have a position more inferior than the actual lower gland (Figure 56.6). The secondary survey should not be performed just to locate a normal parathyroid, but a missing pathological gland. The thymus should be retracted out of the mediastinum as far as possible without avulsion, carefully examined, palpated, and removed. The middle thyroid vein should be ligated and divided, if not already done because this provides greater exposure of the trachea and esophagus. Mobilizing the upper thyroid pole, such as during thyroidectomy, can occasionally disclose ectopic parathyroids without devascularizing the thyroid gland. Thyroid lobectomy on the side of the missing abnormal parathyroid can potentially be avoided if preoperative ultrasound described a normal thyroid without nodules. Examination of the path along the carotid artery and jugular vein can be performed as widely as the incision allows. The skin incision can be enlarged to permit adequate exposure of any of these regions.

Parathyroid gland location is generally symmetrical, and knowledge of this can aid in contralateral neck exploration. A parathyroid located at the posterior midpoint of the thyroid lobe could represent either a lower gland that sits higher than usual or an upper gland that is more inferior than usual; finding the other ipsilateral gland should consider both possibilities. Double parathyroid adenomas, reported in 3% to 15% of patients, have a nonuniform distribution that favors enlargement of both upper parathyroids.

After exploration and resection are completed, the neck is irrigated with sterile water, which provides a clearer view of the surgical field than saline. Hemostasis is achieved. Each gland or remnant should be reevaluated for viability. Some mild bruising and discoloration of the parathyroids is acceptable. If parathyroid tissue has become completely black from ischemia or has questionable viability, it can be reimplanted into the ipsilateral sternocleidomastoid (SCM) muscle.

The strap muscles and platysma are reapproximated with absorbable suture, and the skin incision is closed. Drains are seldom, if ever, necessary. Our preferred technique for skin closure is 2 layers with a fine monofilament suture and either adhesive strips of surgical glue applied to the skin.

STRATEGY FOR FINDING THE "MISSING" PARATHYROID

Occasionally during bilateral parathyroid exploration, fewer than the desired number of parathyroids are identified.

Situation 1

Three parathyroid glands are identified; one is an extremely large gland with a clinical conclusion that it represents a single adenoma, and the other two glands are normal. The likelihood that the fourth parathyroid will be abnormal is small; it is comparable to the likelihood that the patient may have only three parathyroids or that the fourth is ectopic but abnormal. Thus an exhaustive search (all elements of the secondary survey) for a suspected normal parathyroid may not be indicated. Measuring intraoperative PTH may provide additional reassurance in weighing the odds of residual parathyroid abnormalities. Obviously, this is most useful if performed properly with initial preresection PTH measurements and then postresection values. Not all surgeons may routinely use intraoperative PTH during bilateral parathyroid exploration or have access to this adjunct. If it is available, however, a single measurement at the end of surgery may provide some additional "data" to aid the assessment of success before closing in this kind of ambiguous situation.

More challenging are the scenarios where a suspected enlarged or abnormal parathyroid remains undiscovered. There are practical steps to consider in the strategy of finding these "missing" glands.[24]

Situation 2

Three normal parathyroids have been identified, but either the left or the right upper parathyroid is missing. The most common location of such a missing parathyroid is deep in the tracheoesophageal groove. The space dorsal to the thyroid and anterior to the vertebral column should be opened and explored. Sometimes, digital palpation can be helpful in balloting a gland hiding in such deep spaces. The esophageal border should be inspected because (in rare cases) parathyroids may be invested with fascia and compressed to appear similar to esophageal muscle. It may be useful to ligate the superior thyroid vessels and mobilize the upper pole of the thyroid as during thyroidectomy. Parathyroids may hide in the medial deep recesses adjacent to the trachea, cricoid, and thyroid cartilages. When compared with lower parathyroids, upper parathyroid glands are less likely to be intrathyroidal; thus performing a thyroid lobectomy on the side of the missing parathyroid is rarely necessary, especially if preoperative ultrasound described a normal thyroid. However, a lobectomy on the side of this missing parathyroid remains appropriate if the other maneuvers are unrevealing. Also, exploring the other regions (e.g., carotid sheath) of the secondary survey is indicated if the prior dissection did not disclose the answer.

Situation 3

Three normal parathyroids have been identified but either a left or right lower parathyroid is missing. The most likely location of the fourth and abnormal parathyroid is in the thymus. The cervical portion of the thymus can be defined at the border of the sternothyroid muscle, and often more easily if it attaches via the thyrothymic ligament to the lower pole

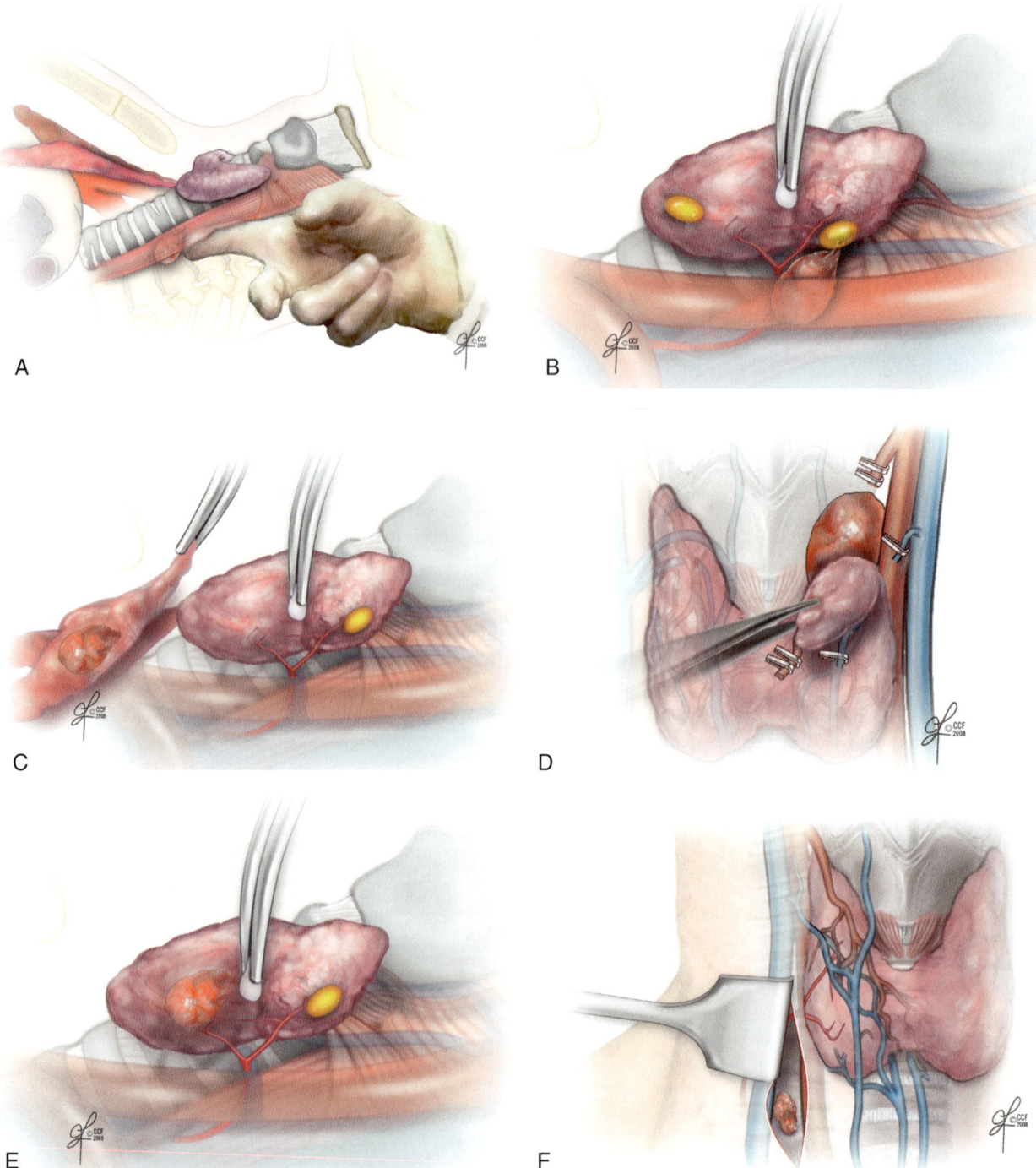

Fig. 56.5 Secondary parathyroid survey examines areas of atypical or ectopic parathyroid location when initial exploration fails to reveal all pathological glands. **A** and **B,** Examination and palpation of retroesophageal space and anterior cervical spine. A paratracheally descended upper parathyroid can be missed if a "cap of normal" gland is evident in the usual location. **C,** The cervical thymus on each side should be mobilized, retracted upward, and excised. **D,** Mobilization of the superior thyroid pole to expose parathyroid glands in high or deep parapharyngeal or paratracheal spaces. **E,** Intrathyroidal parathyroid gland location may be amenable to enucleation of parathyroid or require thyroid lobectomy. **F,** Examination of carotid sheath area. (Reprinted with permission, Cleveland Clinic Center for Medical Art & Photography © 2008–2011. All rights reserved.)

of the thyroid. The thymus has a paler yellow coloration and a smoother surface than pretracheal fat. The thymus can then be gently pulled upward; this ligates small veins and releases thin adventitial tissue as far as the tension of its mediastinal roots allows. Even parathyroids appearing significantly low in the mediastinum on imaging may be amenable to this strategy (Figure 56.7). If these maneuvers prove unrevealing, the next most likely location for a missing lower parathyroid is intrathyroidal. As has been mentioned already, a thyroid lobectomy can be avoided in the setting of a normal ultrasound. If in doubt, the thyroid parenchyma at the lower thyroid pole can be incised in

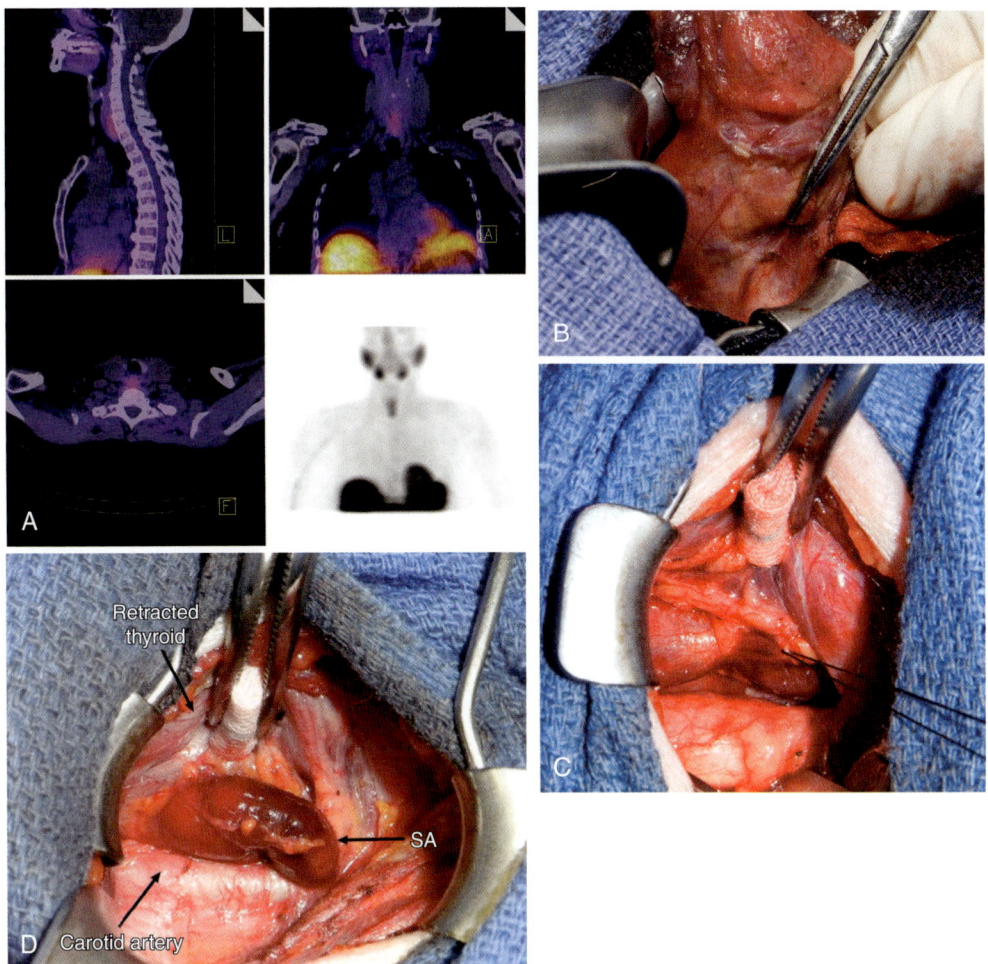

Fig. 56.6 Preoperative imaging (**A**) shows a large inferior midline signal abnormality on the grayscale 99-Tc sestamibi image. It is more precisely seen on the color SPECT views to be very posterior in the tracheoesophageal groove, thus actually representing a right upper parathyroid. A normal right lower parathyroid is at the tip of the instrument in panel **B**. The vascular pedicle of the right upper parathyroid adenoma is looped in panel **C**, and the excised specimen is oriented in vivo in panel **D**. (Reprinted with permission, Cleveland Clinic Center for Medical Art & Photography © 2008–2011. All rights reserved.)

search of the rare parathyroid that appears isoechoic on ultrasound and thus misleads localization. In the absence of preoperative ultrasound, or if palpation detects thyroid nodularity intraoperatively, ipsilateral lobectomy is a rational choice. If these top two maneuvers are unsuccessful, the surgeon should proceed to inspect other regions of the secondary survey.

Situation 4

This situation is a particular subset of the case where three normal parathyroids are identified, but either the left or right lower parathyroid is missing. The secondary survey has identified a large parathyroid; it is at the level of the superior thyroid artery, is anterior to the carotid bulb and has a fragment of thymic tissue attached. Edis and colleagues, as long ago as 1979, described this as an undescended "parathymus," which results from a fourth pouch anomaly.[25] Often, a surgeon can detect or be suspicious of this ectopic parathyroid preoperatively by careful review of imaging studies.[26]

Situation 5

Four clearly normal parathyroids have been exposed during dissection. The PTH is still elevated, confirming that there is a supranumerary parathyroid gland. Although all ectopic regions are potentially at risk for hiding the abnormality, the most likely source is the cervical thymus. Thus both the left and right tracts of the cervical thymus should be removed, and this is most readily done without significant morbidity. If that maneuver does not identify the abnormal parathyroid, the authors prefer to conclude the operation and arrange that a patient in this situation undergoes repeat imaging, which may resort to selective venous sampling among other modalities. An extensive secondary survey risks considerable dissection without prioritizing likely regions of ectopic disease, and it can be unnecessary if the abnormality is mediastinal. Care should be taken to reinspect the four parathyroids to confirm their normal appearance and to exclude the possibility that they represent a "cap of normal" tissue that hides a more distantly positioned parathyroid irregularity. In this scenario, as in the other ones, biopsy of parathyroid glands is left to a surgeon's judgment; this takes into consideration available expertise in pathology and the goal of such a biopsy. In the authors' experience, biopsy of parathyroid glands in these challenging cases is performed selectively and has the role of proving that parathyroid tissue was found where claimed. Rarely does biopsy of normal-appearing glands clarify nature of disease (e.g., potential hyperplasia) or contribute to predicting ectopic sites.

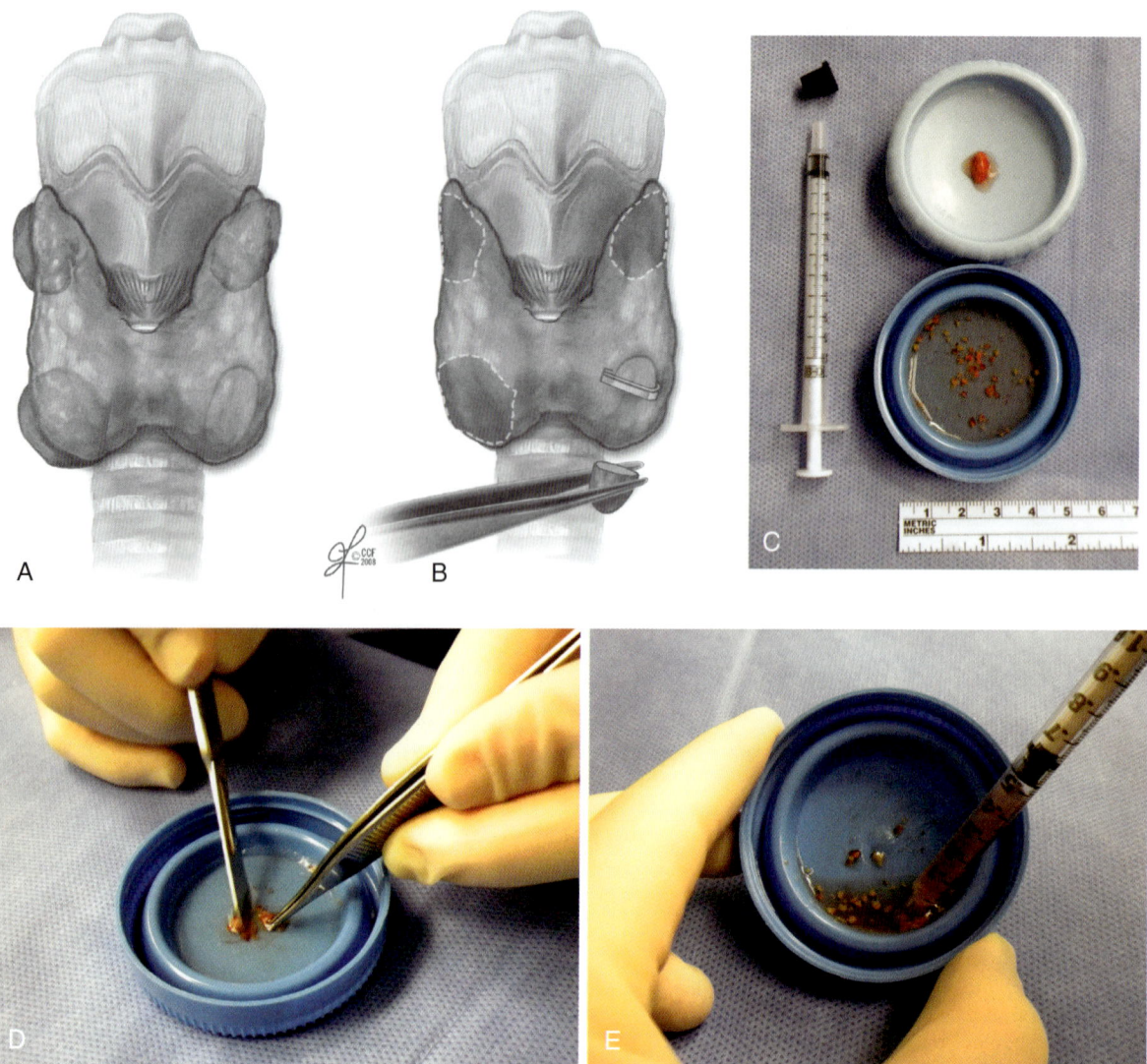

Fig. 56.7 A to E Subtotal or near-total parathyroidectomy with parathyroid cryopreservation. The small parathyroid fragments are drawn up into the syringe as a convenient way of transportation in sterile fashion to the cryopreservation facility. (Reprinted with permission, Cleveland Clinic Center for Medical Art & Photography © 2008–2011. All rights reserved.)

Situation 6

Three parathyroids are identified. Two are normal in appearance and size. The third is slightly enlarged, perhaps borderline in appearance on other morphological features. The fourth parathyroid has not been seen. This situation is challenging because of the ambiguous operative findings. In circumstances such as these, the surgeon should reflect on the correctness of the diagnosis of parathyroid disease and the specific reasons for surgery in the patient. If there is doubt in either of these, surgery should end without further potentially harmful exploration. If the patient has mild PHPT, then removing the slightly enlarged parathyroid is reasonable. Intraoperative PTH can be measured. If the postresection PTH is in the normal range, it may be reassuring to some degree. However, if it meets the criteria of >50% drop but remains above normal, or if the preresection PTH value was only mildly elevated, PTH is less accurate in predicting a cure.[21] If the patient has more severe PHPT, then the mild abnormality is unlikely to be the explanation of the disease, and a search for the missing fourth parathyroid should follow the strategies described previously.

Situation 7

This scenario could be conceived of as an "identity crisis" of the parathyroid. Two normal parathyroids are identified on one side. Contralaterally, a normal parathyroid is found at the midportion of the thyroid gland, just at the crossing of the inferior thyroid artery and the RLN. It is unclear whether this normal gland represents a "high," lower parathyroid or a lower-positioned upper parathyroid. Hence it is unclear whether a lower or upper parathyroid is missing, and both scenarios have to be considered. Some anatomical nuances can aid this process. If a coronal plane is drawn through the recurrent nerve, a lower parathyroid will be anterior to it; however, an upper parathyroid will be dorsal or posterior to it (see Figure 31.20 Chapter 31 Principles in Thyroid Surgery). This may help determine the order of a secondary survey and whether to start with the algorithm described for scenario 2 or for scenario 3.

Situation 8

These findings represent a difficult day in the operating room: only one or two parathyroid glands are identified, and their appearance is ambiguous. Strategy relies on the principles of mentally confirming that the diagnosis and indication for surgery were proper. The practitioner must pause to review any imaging available in the operating room, judge the risks of extensive secondary exploration versus the potential benefits, and must remember to do no harm while accumulating as much information as might be helpful in a subsequent operation. Consultation with a surgical partner or other experienced parathyroid surgeon intraoperatively (if possible) can be useful. A rudimentary "venous sampling" can be performed by obtaining a blood sample from the left and right internal jugular veins for intraoperative PTH measurement; the hope is for some lateralization that can guide surgery.

In all of the preceding scenarios, with anticipation of potentially unsuccessful first parathyroid surgery, marking the known parathyroid glands with large titanium clips can aid subsequent imaging and reexploration. Also, refraining from parathyroid excision until the situation is as clear as possible will minimize the risk of future hypocalcemia.

POSTOPERATIVE MANAGEMENT

Short-term postoperative management varies according to surgeon preference. After bilateral neck exploration for parathyroidectomy, most surgeons elect to observe their patients for 23 hours, but many use outpatient care.[3] Long-term management relies on diligent monitoring of calcium and PTH levels; this allows observation of durable cure of HPT. Ideally, a full biochemical panel includes calcium, PTH, and vitamin D. The full panel should be checked at 2 weeks after surgery during the first postoperative visit, then at 6 months, and then annually for the remainder of the patient's lifetime. The effect of vitamin D deficiency in causing transient secondary HPT postoperatively, in an otherwise cured patient, is well recognized. This can be seen in 20% to 30% of patients in the first year after surgery and requires reassurance (of both patient and referring physicians), treatment, and monitoring. It can be encountered after both bilateral and focal exploration.[27] It is important to ensure that the patient receives adequate calcium and vitamin D supplementation after surgery. Minimal daily calcium carbonate or citrate supplementation is 500 to 600 mg taken two to three times daily. Depending on the degree of vitamin D deficiency, some patients may require over-the-counter supplements of 800 to 2000 IU daily of vitamin D_3 cholecalciferol, whereas others need a prescription-level strength such as 50,000 IU ergocalciferol weekly (for 25-hydroxyvitamin D <20 ng/mL). Very rarely, 0.25 or 0.5 mcg daily of calcitriol (for 1,25-dihydroxyvitamin D deficiency or significant hypocalcemic symptoms) may be needed. These patients should be reevaluated with blood tests at 3 months after surgery to determine the need for ongoing vitamin D supplementation. Durable cure after bilateral parathyroid exploration means a 95% to 98% success rate, with 2% to 5% of patients at risk of developing recurrent HPT.

SPECIAL CONSIDERATIONS IN BILATERAL PARATHYROID EXPLORATION

Tissue Handling

There must be delicate tissue handling to avoid damage to normal parathyroids or disruption of abnormal glands. The actual parenchyma of these structures should never be grasped itself; rather, forceps and instruments should handle the surrounding fatty tissue, filmy adventitia, or vessels. Hypocalcemia becomes a greater risk with subtotal or near-total excision of multigland hyperplasia. A parathyroid remnant grafted on its native vascular pedicle is usually less prone to cause hypocalcemia than total parathyroidectomy with remnant implantation into the muscles of the neck or nondominant forearm.

Cryopreservation

An additional safeguard against permanent hypocalcemia can come from cryopreservation of small parathyroid fragments (see Figure 56.7). Cryopreservation is not immediately available and has to be developed as a protocol at each hospital (only about 20% of academic centers have parathyroid cryopreservation capabilities).[3] Cryopreservation allows more aggressive subtotal resection and a smaller remnant. In the absence of this capability, the surgeon should use judgment about the extent of resection in multigland hyperplasia and can consider leaving a remnant larger than 25 mg. The need to reimplant cryopreserved parathyroid tissue usually becomes evident within 6 months of surgery if the cervical remnants become nonfunctional. To be cryopreserved, a parathyroid gland is partially submitted to pathology for histological evaluation and partially submitted for cryopreservation. The portions for cryopreservation are cut into small pieces, about 1 to 2 mm in size, and brought into suspension in sterile saline. These portions are labeled (which parathyroid gland was the source) and sent to the tissue bank.

Parathyroid Reimplantation and Remnant Size

If a normal parathyroid gland has been devascularized during bilateral neck exploration (a rare event), it can be reimplanted into the ipsilateral SCM. Before doing so, a portion should be sent to pathology for frozen section for histological confirmation that it is normal parathyroid tissue. This can be done on a fragment as small as 1 to 2 mm. The remaining gland is placed on sterile ice until the end of the case, before closing the incision. The gland is then cut with a 15-blade scalpel into small pieces, approximately 1 to 2 mm in size. The SCM is exposed and small pockets are created 1 to 2 cm apart by bluntly separating the muscle fibers. Two or three pieces are placed in each pocket, and the pocket is closed with microclips to facilitate identification in case of future reoperation. This same methodology applies to auto transplantation of hyperplastic parathyroid tissue after a complete resection of all four parathyroid glands. The practice of implanting a small piece of hyperplastic parathyroid tissue into the forearm has largely fallen out of favor; instead, sites such as the SCM or anterior chest wall tissue close to the clavicle are now more frequently used.

For many surgeons, a subtotal parathyroidectomy is the procedure of choice for four-gland parathyroid hyperplasia in PHPT, secondary HPT, or tertiary HPT. Remnants are best fashioned from a lower parathyroid, as these are generally easier to approach in their more anterior positions should recurrence develop. A good vascular stalk is important to ensure viability. The remnant should be made first, before the other glands being removed. During the remainder of the gland excisions, repeated checks on the viability of the remnant should be made in case a second remnant needs to be created. The authors leave a large clip or non-absorbable stitch on the transected edge of the gland to facilitate identification of the remnant in the case of recurrent HPT.

SUMMARY

Bilateral neck exploration for four-gland parathyroid evaluation is the required surgical approach in cases of multigland hyperplasia. It applies to patients with familial HPT syndromes and those with secondary and tertiary HPT, where multigland disease is the defining clinical manifestation. In PHPT, bilateral neck exploration remains the advised treatment of choice when preoperative parathyroid imaging is equivocal, negative, discordant, and when coexisting thyroid pathology warrants a broader evaluation of the central neck. Furthermore, bilateral neck exploration is advised when a diagnosis of hyperplasia may be apparent before surgery or when findings during limited or unilateral exploration suggest additional diseased glands. Even in the modern era of focused parathyroid surgery, standard bilateral exploration is needed in at least 30% of patients.[3] Ectopic and bilateral parathyroid disease remains difficult to predict reliably before surgery. It should be emphasized that bilateral exploration can be performed using principles of parathyroid exposure and evaluation based on knowledge of anatomy and embryology: via small incisions and with minimal and gentle tissue handling. Bilateral parathyroid exploration, however, requires a more detailed and unique set of skills: familiarity with strategy to expose parathyroids in ectopic sites, knowledge of how to find "missing glands," a knowledgeable assessment of subtle parathyroid gland abnormalities (both morphological and biochemical), and experience in accomplishing subtotal parathyroid resection that balances long-term cure and the avoidance of hypoparathyroidism. Standard bilateral parathyroid exploration is a necessary technique in the armamentarium of any surgeon who seeks to specialize in the treatment of parathyroid diseases.

REFERENCES

For a complete list of references, go to expertconsult.com.

57

Minimally Invasive Single Gland Parathyroid Exploration

Sareh Parangi, T.K. Pandian, Geoffrey Thompson

> Please go to expertconsult.com to view related video:
> **Video 57.1** Minimally Invasive Parathyroidectomy.

BACKGROUND

Subsequent to the first parathyroidectomy documented in the literature (in 1925 by Felix Mandl of Vienna), four-gland exploration via a generous incision was the standard technique until the 1970s and 1980s.[1] The advent of various localization modalities since that time, coupled with the fact that approximately 85% of patients with primary hyperparathyroidism (PHPT) have a solitary adenoma, has led many surgeons to prefer minimally invasive parathyroidectomy (MIP) as their operative approach of choice.[2] The general goals of MIP are to limit operative dissection, reduce incision length, and improve postoperative recovery. Perhaps one of the greatest benefits of MIP is the potential for reduced scarring of deeper tissues, allowing for future operations, if needed, to be safer and less difficult.

There is considerable variability in the literature as to what exactly is defined as MIP;[1] in general, however, it refers to any surgical approach that preoperatively aims to identify and remove a single enlarged gland (i.e., *focused parathyroid exploration*) and may, in select circumstances, allow examination of the ipsilateral gland as well (i.e., *unilateral exploration*). Choices for incision in MIP include a standard collar incision, smaller midline incision, ectopic or lateral incision, or video-assisted approach (see Chapter 55, Principles in Surgical Management of Primary Hyperparathyroidism, Chapter 56, Standard Bilateral Parathyroid Exploration, and Chapter 58, Minimally Invasive Video-Assisted Parathyroidectomy). Intraoperative parathyroid hormone (PTH) level monitoring can be employed to confirm that excision of the gland identified preoperatively results in biochemical cure (see Chapter 59, Intraoperative PTH Monitoring During Parathyroid Surgery). Many groups recommend that intraoperative PTH monitoring be employed routinely in all cases of MIP.[2-4]

The most imperative prerequisite to MIP is adequate preoperative localization by imaging to guide the operation. This can be accomplished with a variety of modalities including ultrasound, computed tomography (CT), Tc-99m sestamibi, and positron emission tomography (PET). Imaging accuracy can be variable based on region and institution;[2,5] thus these factors should be considered in the development of preoperative localization protocols.

There are several advantages to MIP compared with traditional four-gland exploration in appropriate patients. These include the option to perform surgery under local anesthesia, reduced operative time, decreased postoperative pain, improved cosmesis, shorter time to hospital discharge, reduced complication rate, reduced deep tissue scarring, and decreased overall costs.[6-9] In addition, the majority of data would suggest long-term outcomes are comparable to the standard multigland exploration.[3,10]

This chapter addresses considerations for performing MIP, including anatomic factors, the importance of a parathyroid localization nomenclature system, the role of preoperative imaging studies, and operative preparation and techniques.

CONSIDERATIONS FOR PERFORMING MIP

Patient Selection

Many patients with PHPT may be candidates for MIP. The ideal patient should have evidence to suggest the presence of a single parathyroid adenoma. Key elements include biochemical proof of PHPT, preoperative imaging that is highly suggestive of single-gland disease with identification of parathyroid adenoma location, and access to an experienced parathyroid surgeon. Patients suspected to have multi-gland disease, such as those with multiple endocrine neoplasia type 1 (MEN 1), other familial syndromes, lithium use, chronic renal failure, or a possible diagnosis of parathyroid cancer may not be good candidates for MIP (see Chapter 60, Surgical Management of Multiglandular Parathyroid Disease; Chapter 61, Surgical Management of Secondary and Tertiary Hyperparathyroidism; Chapter 62, Parathyroid Management in the MEN Syndromes; and Chapter 64, Parathyroid Carcinoma). Pediatric patients and those younger than age Chapter 45 were originally thought to be at higher risk for multigland disease and, thus, ineligible for MIP; however, recent data suggest favorable outcomes with MIP in these populations.[10,11] Concurrent thyroid pathology that could require concomitant thyroid gland resection should be absent. A more comprehensive list of contraindications to MIP is presented in Table 57.1.

Anatomic Considerations

The focused approach of MIP requires a thorough knowledge of cervical anatomy and embryology (see Chapter 2, Applied Embryology of the Thyroid and Parathyroid Glands). Parathyroid gland location follows definite embryologically influenced patterns. Because the superior parathyroid glands share an embryologic origin with the lateral thyroid tissue in the primordium in the fourth branchial pouch, nondiseased superior parathyroid glands are invariably found close to the dorsum of the upper thyroid lobe. When a superior parathyroid gland becomes heavy, enlarged, and adenomatous, it tends to be found more posteriorly and caudally. If closely associated with the thyroid capsule, the gland will remain in contact with the posterior surface of the thyroid, in continuity with thyroid tissue. The pedicle of the superior parathyroid gland is located lateral and posterior/dorsal to the oblique course of the recurrent laryngeal nerve (RLN).

TABLE 57.1 Contraindications to Minimally Invasive Parathyroidectomy	
Absolute Contraindications	**Relative Contraindications**
Known multigland disease such as familial hyperparathyroidism or multiple endocrine neoplasia (MEN) disease	Symptomatic cervical disc disease Anticoagulation
Concurrent thyroid pathology requiring surgical intervention	Known contralateral nerve injury Previous ipsilateral cervical surgery
Discordant imaging	Lithium use or chronic renal failure

BOX 57.1 Anatomic Pearls in Minimally Invasive Parathyroidectomy

Superior glands can be inferior to the inferior gland.
Ninety percent of parathyroid glands are within 1 cm of the junction of the inferior thyroidal artery and recurrent laryngeal nerve.
Within the inferior triangle (viewed from the front, laterally defined by the RLN, with base inferior) lie most inferior glands (see Figure 57.1, A).
Within the superior triangle (viewed from the front, medially defined by the RLN with base superior) lie most superior parathyroid glands (see Figure 57.1, A).
The recurrent laryngeal nerve is more oblique on the right side.

The inferior parathyroid glands share their embryologic origin with the thymus, and both arise from the third branchial complex. An enlarged inferior parathyroid gland usually remains in close proximity to the lower pole of the thyroid, often just lateral or posterior to the lower pole. If the enlarged inferior parathyroid gland becomes heavy or caudal embryologic migration is excessive, it may descend into the thyrothymic ligament. The enlarged gland may also be present deeper within the thymus and may even reside in the mediastinum.

Experienced surgeons use the RLN as an important landmark for identifying parathyroid glands. The inferior parathyroid gland is consistently anterior or ventral to the RLN, whereas the pedicle to the superior parathyroid gland is always posterior or dorsal to the RLN.

Enlarged superior parathyroid glands are almost always found in specific sites; these are, in order of frequency of occurrence, (1) the dorsum of the upper pole of the thyroid, (2) the paraesophageal space posterior to the thyroid parenchyma (a less common location is the retropharyngeal space), and (3) descent into in the paraesophageal space caudal to the inferior pole of the thyroid.

An enlarged inferior parathyroid gland most commonly rests at the lower pole of the thyroid, within the thyrothymic ligament or in the superior-most portion of the cervical thymic tongue. Occasionally, the inferior parathyroid gland descends within the thymus into the upper mediastinum.

A common misconception is that a parathyroid gland located high in the neck is always a superior gland and that one located low in the neck is an inferior gland. In fact, a superior enlarged parathyroid gland may descend caudally and be located near the lower pole of the thyroid or even below the inferior pole of the thyroid. In this situation, the gland frequently is suspended by a long, vascular pedicle from the inferior thyroid artery. The superior gland in this case may actually be "inferior" to the inferior gland base. Surgeons must always pay attention to the location of the gland relative to the course of the RLN. Enlarged superior glands that have descended caudally still retain their normal position posterior or dorsal to the RLN, whereas enlarged inferior glands always remain anterior or ventral to the RLN. The importance of this positioning is that the superior gland will be dorsal in the neck in proximity to the deeper tracheoesophageal region.

The relationship of an enlarged parathyroid gland to the thyroid capsule is also critical to the potential position of a diseased gland. When located within the fibrous thyroid capsule, the diseased parathyroid gland expands but remains within the confines of the surgical capsule of the thyroid. When located external to the thyroid capsule, enlarged parathyroid glands may become subject to gravity and the repetitive forces of deglutition and become displaced posteriorly behind the gland in the tracheoesophageal region. A summary of anatomic "pearls" for MIP is presented in Box 57.1.

A STANDARD PARATHYROID NOMENCLATURE SYSTEM

Standardizing parathyroid nomenclature offers a universal, consistent language to communicate the precise locations of enlarged parathyroid glands among members of the multidisciplinary team, which includes radiologists, surgeons, anesthesiologists, endocrinologists, pathologists, ultrasonographers, and nuclear medicine physicians.[12] One such classification system was developed and used at the MD Anderson Cancer Center to allow a systematic approach to the most frequently encountered positions of enlarged parathyroid glands. This clinically useful classification scheme encompasses information about the parathyroid gland's pedicle and the surrounding structures, and it incorporates the relation of the RLN to the glands as discussed previously. Based on the premise that superior glands have a pedicle that originates lateral to the RLN and that inferior glands have a pedicle that originates medial to this nerve, the system considers natural descent patterns (both embryologic and acquired): superior glands descend posteriorly in the tracheoesophageal groove, and inferior glands descend anteriorly in the plane of the trachea.

The classification system is alphabetical and uses the letters A through G to describe exact parathyroid gland locations.

This system not only offers a concise, reliable means of communicating the exact location of enlarged parathyroid glands but also can facilitate surgical planning and selection of approach. The gland's letter designation has, therefore, implications for placement of the incision, patient positioning, the scope of the operation, and the selection of anesthesia. For example, precise information about the expected location of the adenoma allows for better planning by the anesthesiologist, who can determine the type of anesthesia needed based on operative complexity, depth of dissection, and projected duration of the procedure. Knowledge of the adenoma's location also helps operating room personnel anticipate technical requirements, such as the need for nerve monitoring devices, instrumentation for sternotomy or thymectomy, or intraoperative ultrasound. Common descriptors of adenoma location also facilitate communications between physicians (e.g., reviewing the report of an operation performed by another surgeon, particularly if reoperation is being planned) and in documenting an excised gland's exact location for the pathologist. In addition to describing common locations of glands, the alphabetic letters A through G are used as reminders of locations to explore when a diseased gland cannot be identified intraoperatively.

A common nomenclature also facilitates communications among institutions in situations such as registering patients for clinical trials and reporting results in the medical literature. At the MD Anderson Cancer Center, this nomenclature provides primary terminology for use in imaging reports and has been expanded and incorporated into anesthesia, nursing care, operative, and pathology reports. The authors

CHAPTER 57 Minimally Invasive Single Gland Parathyroid Exploration

BOX 57.2 Alphabetical Nomenclature System for Adenomatous Parathyroid Glands

Type A. A type **A** gland is **a**dherent to the posterior thyroid parenchyma. This gland is in the **a**ccepted, expected location of a normal gland. It is **a**lmost **a**ttached, **a**lmost intracapsular.

Type B. A type **B** gland is **b**ack **b**ehind the thyroid parenchyma. The surgeon should **b**e careful not to miss it. It is exophytic to the thyroid parenchyma and lies in the tracheoesophageal groove. An undescended gland high in the neck near the carotid bifurcation or mandible is classified as a type **B +** gland.

Type C. A type **C** gland is **c**ommonly missed; it **c**ould be mistaken for the esophagus when palpated. It is **c**audal to the thyroid parenchyma, **c**loser to the **c**lavicle, in the tracheoesophageal groove.

Type D. Dissection of a type **D** gland may be **d**ifficult because the gland is **d**angerously close to the recurrent laryngeal nerve. Preoperative images **d**on't enable **d**etermination of origin.

Type E. A type **E** gland is **e**asy to resect. It is the most **e**xternally located gland because it is not deep in the neck. **E**arly on, its **e**ase of resection gives the **e**ndocrine surgeon **e**xtra confidence.

Type F. A type **F** gland has **f**allen into the thyrothymic ligament. **F**requently it is referred to as *ectopic*. Resection can be **f**un because a type **F** gland can usually be retrieved with delivery of the superior portion of the thymus. For the inexperienced surgeon, however, resection can be **f**rightening because of the delivery of the gland from the mediastinum via the neck.

Type G. A type **G** gland **g**ot caught in thyroid tissue during descent—stuck in the starting **g**ate. A true intrathyroidal gland is rare—**g**auche **g**land!

of the system have found that it greatly improves communication, removes ambiguity, and obviates lengthy descriptions of parathyroid gland locations.

The alphabetical classification system for identifying and locating adenomatous parathyroid glands is presented here and in Box 57.2 (also see Figure 57.1):

Type A. **A**dherent to the posterior thyroid parenchyma, a type A parathyroid gland is in the expected location of a normal parathyroid gland and is in apposition to the posterior surface of the thyroid parenchyma. The gland may be compressed within the capsule of the thyroid.

Type B. **B**ehind the thyroid parenchyma, a type B gland is a superior gland that is exophytic to the thyroid parenchyma and has fallen posteriorly into the tracheoesophageal groove. There is minimal or no contact between the gland and the posterior surface of the thyroid tissue. On coronal views, the gland is posteriorly located

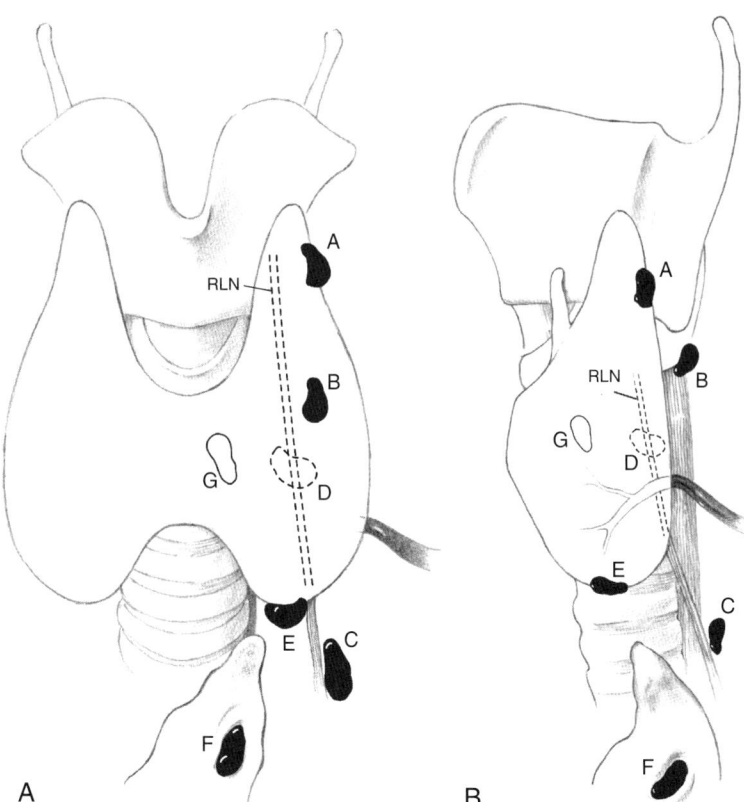

Fig. 57.1 A, The anterior-posterior view of the cervical region showing the relationship of the parathyroid glands to the recurrent laryngeal nerve (RLN). The letters depict the gland locations. *A, B,* and *C* glands are superior glands and are generally located in the superior triangle formed by the RLN medially with the triangle base superior. *E* and *F* glands are inferior glands and are generally located in the inferior triangle with the RLN laterally and the triangle base inferior. *D* glands are those closest to the RLN and cannot be easily deciphered as superior or inferior without intraoperative assessment of the pedicle in relation to the RLN. The *G* gland is intrathyroidal. **B,** Lateral view of the cervical region shows the oblique angle and anterior-posterior projections of enlarged parathyroid glands. The letters depict the gland locations.

near the esophagus. An undescended gland high in the neck near the carotid bifurcation or mandible also may be classified as a type B gland.

Type C. **C**audal to the thyroid parenchyma, a type C gland is a superior gland that has descended posteriorly and caudally into the tracheoesophageal groove. On anterior images, a type C gland is inferior to the inferior pole of the thyroid parenchyma. The type C gland is posterior to and in many cases inferior to the oblique angle of the RLN. Glands in the carotid sheath are either type B or C glands, depending on their craniocaudal relationship to the inferior pole of the thyroid gland (cranial, type B, caudal, type C).

Type D. **D**irectly over the RLN in the middle region of the posterior surface of the thyroid tissue. The dissection of the type D gland can be "difficult" or "dangerous" because of this gland's proximity to the RLN. The gland lies in the middle region of the posterior surface of the thyroid parenchyma, near the junction of the RLN and the inferior thyroid artery. The embryologic origin of a type D parathyroid adenoma may be that of either a superior or inferior gland. The distinction is made intraoperatively based on the gland's relationship to the RLN and the pedicle of the gland. Usually, the position of the pedicle cannot be determined on preoperative imaging studies.

Type E. The type E gland is an inferior gland that is proximal to the inferior pole of the thyroid parenchyma. This gland is more closely aligned with the same anterior-posterior plane of the thyroid tissue and the trachea (as opposed to more posterior glands that relate to the esophagus). The type E adenoma has a pedicle that is medial and anterior to the RLN and is the easiest to resect because of its superficial location relative to the depth of the cervical region.

Type F. The type F gland is an inferior gland that has descended into the thyrothymic ligament or superior thymus. This gland may be in the anterior mediastinum. On anterior-posterior imaging views, the type F gland is in the coronal plane of the thymus. It has "fallen" into the thyrothymic ligament, is below the inferior pole of the thyroid, and is usually superficial or immediately lateral to the trachea. A type F gland is frequently referred to as an ectopic gland, and its resection usually involves transcervical delivery of the thyrothymic ligament or superior portion of the thymus.

Type G. The type G gland is a rare, gauche gland. This gland is an intrathyroidal parathyroid gland that has thyroid tissue circumferentially around it. Resection of a type G gland may require thyroid lobectomy because the gland "got caught" within the thyroid tissue.

PREOPERATIVE IMAGING AND LOCALIZATION

Preoperative imaging is critical to successful MIP (see Chapter 54, Guide to Preoperative Parathyroid Localization Testing: Ultrasound, Sestimibi and 4D CT). It provides the surgeon with a roadmap for resection of an adenoma by providing a precise location of the gland and adjacent structures. It should be emphasized that preoperative imaging does not assist with diagnosis or in the decision to proceed with surgery. Modalities may include ultrasound, nuclear medicine studies, and CT. Many surgeons feel that two different modalities with concordant results are necessary to proceed with MIP.[4,12-15] Some groups suggest that four-dimensional CT is the most accurate imaging modality.[16,17]

As mentioned previously, the sensitivity and specificity of a particular modality can vary depending on region and institution.[2,5] This variability should be considered when deciding which modalities to pursue. We recommend that these imaging techniques be performed by dedicated imaging professionals with experience and an interest in parathyroid disease. For these purposes, securing the services of a dedicated team with a track record of performing repeated studies is desirable. The surgeon should direct the selection and sequence of the preoperative images to be obtained to tailor the most efficient and effective surgical intervention. In addition, surgeons should routinely review the images themselves before an operation; they should not rely on reading the reports only. Surgeon-performed ultrasound has a proven track record of assisting the surgeon in localizing the enlarged gland and should be emphasized in the workup where possible.[18,19] Accurate anatomic and functional data can dictate incision placement, patient positioning, and can help determine whether intraoperative nerve monitoring (IONM) may be necessary.

Preoperatively determining the accurate location of a suspected parathyroid adenoma can direct the surgical approach, minimizing dissection and maximizing efficiency during parathyroidectomy. Knowledge of the precise location of an enlarged parathyroid gland and its relationship to surrounding structures is essential for MIP and reoperation for persistent or recurrent disease. Simply put, if the imaging studies cannot localize the gland, an MIP should not be performed.

Our general approach is to use a nuclear medicine imaging study (to provide information on gland function) combined with an anatomic imaging study (to provide useful information about surrounding structures), such as ultrasound or CT. It is preferable to be able to "localize" a gland to a specific quadrant rather than just "lateralize" it.

OPERATIVE PREPARATION AND TECHNIQUES

Anesthesia Considerations

The type of anesthesia to be used in MIP should be determined by the surgeon and anesthesiologist based on the patient's surgical fitness, comorbidities, body habitus, expected procedure duration, location of the diseased parathyroid gland, and experience of the anesthesia team. Monitored anesthetic care using a combination of local anesthesia and sedation may be appropriate for thin patients who have a type E inferior gland that would be expected to require a minimal surgical procedure with a short operative time. General anesthesia may be best for a deep gland in the tracheoesophageal groove (type B or C gland) in an obese patient with minimal hyperextension and significant comorbidities. Access to a peripheral blood draw site must be identified before induction to allow easy access to peripheral blood for PTH assessment.

Operating Room Checklist

Before making an incision, the surgeon performing MIP must ensure the necessary components of a safety checklist are addressed. This includes standard verification of correct patient name, medical record number, procedure, operative laterality, presence of surgical consent, review of patient-specific studies (e.g., electrocardiogram or coagulation profile), and verbalization of anesthesia concerns. In addition to these items, review of documentation confirming biochemical proof of disease and examination of all relevant preoperative imaging should be performed in the operating room.

Operating room team members should be briefed on all necessary equipment before patient arrival. This may include an appropriate nerve monitoring equipped endotracheal tube (ET), associated supplies, and avoidance of paralysis if neural monitoring is planned. Ethylenediaminetetraacetic acid (EDTA), tubes, syringes, and the importance of rapid transport of the intraoperative PTH specimens should be discussed. At the appropriate time, operating room personnel should be clearly told which specific gland is excised to initiate appropriate specimen labels.

The anesthesiologist should be notified about the need for and anticipated timing of peripheral venous blood sampling for PTH. Some groups believe central venous sampling from the internal jugular vein is also feasible and accurate;[20,21] however, measurement of extended intraoperative PTH values may be required.[22,23] A central draw may be considered if peripheral access is difficult. If a central draw from the internal jugular vein is performed, all samples should be obtained from the same location along the vein. Our preference is to obtain peripheral venous access that can be used for blood draws as needed. There is no need for intraarterial access; a simple venipuncture at a predetermined location vetted by the anesthesia team before draping is usually adequate. Anesthesia or operating room personnel should be asked to begin a timer once the suspect gland has been excised. This may help notify the surgeon of postexcision time intervals to guide additional PTH draws.

Patient Positioning and Preparation

Natural skin creases should be marked on the patient's neck in a natural sitting position while in the preoperative holding area. Using 2 to 3 mL of blood, a baseline pre-excision PTH value can be drawn in the preoperative holding area at the time of intravenous access and sent for analysis. After ET intubation, the patient is placed in the supine position with the neck slightly extended by placing rolled surgical sheets or a thyroid bag transversely beneath the patient's shoulders. The patient's head should be supported with blankets, a sponge, or gel donut to minimize postoperative neck pain resulting from hyperextension. Anesthesia should be asked to secure the ET and direct the ET tube cephalad to keep the operative field clear. The arms are tucked at the patient's sides or secured across the patient's shoulders. Care is taken to pad pressure points on the patient's body and to avoid compression of the peripheral intravenous line or blood pressure cuff. The table is tilted 20 degrees in the reverse Trendelenburg or beach-chair position.

If preoperative ultrasound has been helpful in localization, a quick surgeon-performed ultrasound after positioning often aids in the final decision about incision placement and allows the use of the smallest incision closest to the target gland. If there is more than one option of natural skin creases, the on-table ultrasound may assist the surgeon in choosing the one best suited for the dissection. Use of this preincision ultrasound also facilitates training of residents and fellows because they receive immediate feedback on their technique for ultrasound-based localization.

The skin at the surgical site is prepared with sterile solution and draped to include the chin 3 to 4 cm below the substernal notch and the posterior margins of the sternocleidomastoid muscle. Accessories that may be used include a fiberoptic headlight unit and optical magnification. If a baseline PTH was not obtained in the preoperative holding area, 2 to 3 mL of blood is drawn just before incision in the operating room, placed in an EDTA tube, labeled, and processed as a baseline preincision PTH value. For surgeons who prefer central venous draws, this should be performed before major manipulation of the gland (see chapter 59 Intraoperative PTH Monitoring During Parathyroid Surgery). Box 57.3 presents a list of preoperative and intraoperative surgical "pearls" for MIP.

Front Door Technique

The front door technique uses a shorter version of a standard midline incision, which can then be moved cephalad or caudad as needed to best approach the localized gland. Using a midline incision allows access to virtually all localized inferior glands and many nonectopic superior glands. Advantages of this approach include familiarity for all surgeons with the anatomic planes, excellent cosmesis, and the ability to quickly convert to a bilateral neck exploration if necessary, sometimes even without extension of the skin incision (Figure 57.2).

Incision

After infiltration of a local anesthetic, a 3 to 5 cm Kocher incision is marked roughly 2 cm cephalad to the sternal notch or at the level of the thyroid isthmus. The midline of the neck and the two edges of the outlined incision are also marked with a sterile pen. The site of the incision depends on whether the adenoma is localized to the superior or the inferior parathyroid gland. For an inferior parathyroid adenoma, the medial-most portion of the outlined incision on the ipsilateral side of the neck is used as the point of entry. A 2.5- to 3-cm incision is made with a scalpel (blade number 15) (Figure 57.3). Monopolar electrocautery is used to divide the platysma. The subcutaneous tissues and platysma are elevated with two curved mosquito clamps, and the superficial (investing) layer of the deep cervical fascia is exposed. Appropriate subplatysmal flaps are then raised. The strap

---

BOX 57.3 Preoperative and Intraoperative Surgical Pearls for Minimally Invasive Parathyroidectomy

Preoperative
Peripheral venous access obtained and accessible by the anesthesia team can make intraoperative blood draws efficient.

Patient Positioning
- Tucking the patient's arms or securing the arms across the chest improves ergonomics, allowing the surgical team to avoid retracting at an angle.
- Moderate hyperextension with a gel or towel roll posterior to the shoulders allows the thyrothymic tract to ascend, delivers inferior parathyroid glands from the chest, and improves lateral access to the tracheoesophageal groove in an obese patient.
- Including the chin and sternum in the draped surgical field affords easy landmark references.

Intraoperative
Baseline PTH levels drawn just before or at the time of incision offer an easy opportunity to document the actual time of dissection.

Inferior glands can be easily accessed with a medial incision, obviating dissection across the RLN.

Superior glands can be easily accessed with a more lateral incision (i.e., "back door approach").

A timer should be started by anesthesia or operating room personnel after the diseased gland is excised, to aid in timing of intraoperative PTH draws.

Dissection
- Elevating the thyroid lobe with an up-and-over technique greatly facilitates exposure of the tracheoesophageal groove and of the posterior surface of the thyroid lobe; this helps expose an intracapsular type A gland.
- Digital palpation of the tracheoesophageal groove allows for early detection of a mobile parathyroid adenoma that has fallen posteriorly.

SECTION 8 Parathyroid Surgery

muscles are identified and separated longitudinally in the median raphe using electrocautery. A spring-loaded retractor is a simple tool that can then be used for retraction and avoids skin marks or damage.

Thyroid Mobilization

The strap muscles are carefully elevated anterior and cephalad, away from the anterior surface of the thyroid capsule with small, Teflon-coated army-navy, Green, or thyroid-Kocher retractors. The ipsilateral thyroid lobe is then exposed and grasped with two Kocher or mosquito clamps. The tips of the clamps are placed at the edges of the thyroid lobe: one at the junction of the upper and middle third of the gland and the other at the junction of the middle and lower third. The surgical assistant on the contralateral side of the table deviates the gland in an up-and-over maneuver (Figure 57.4). Alternatively, the lobe can be forcibly retracted with a peanut. Avoiding any bleeding from the thyroid or nearby structures is key when the field of dissection is so small. Blood, when mixed with fat can mislead the surgeon because parathyroid tissue can often look like orange or light brown fat. Although usually not necessary, the middle thyroid vein can be ligated to allow for adequate retraction.

Expected Location of Inferior Parathyroid Glands

The inferior parathyroid gland is usually identified at the inferior extent of the ipsilateral thyroid pole. This gland may also be found adherent to the thyroid capsule near the inferior pole. The gland is

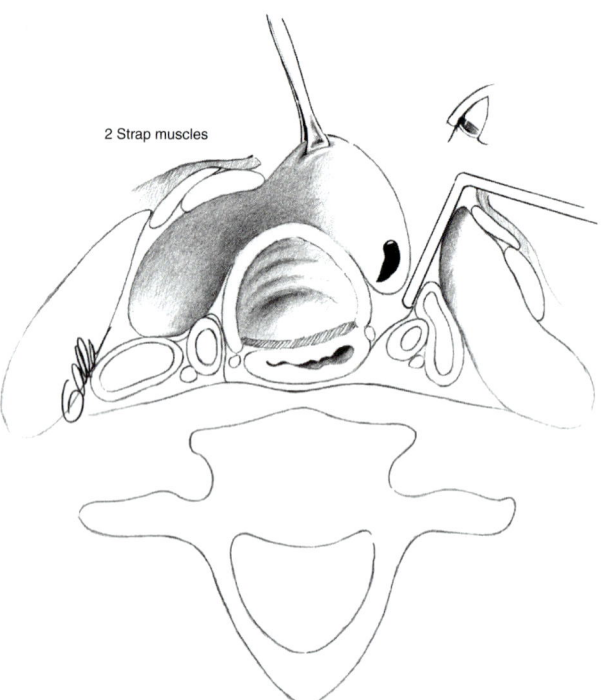

Fig. 57.2 The Front Door or midline approach. The bulge of the parathyroid gland within the confines of the thyroid capsule can be appreciated in the illustrations of this type A gland in this medial approach (strap muscle retracted left and right). The gland is touching the posterior surface of the thyroid parenchyma. Upon incision, the tissue of the soft parathyroid gland bulges and exudes from the capsule.

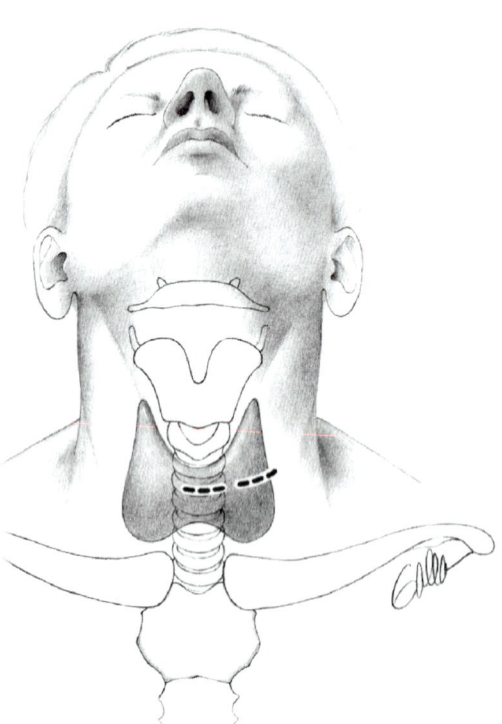

Fig. 57.3 The incision location for minimally invasive parathyroidectomy. The medial incision is used to access an inferior parathyroid gland that is anteriorly located. The lateral incision would be used to access a gland in the tracheoesophageal groove via the lateral, back door approach.

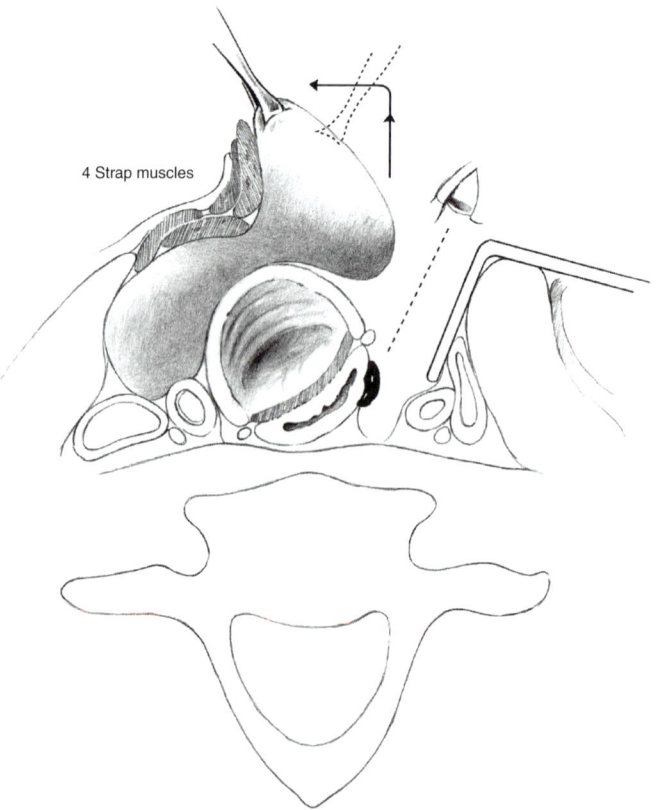

Fig. 57.4 The "back door" or "lateral" approach. The thyroid parenchyma is grasped with Kocher clamps and deviated medially in the lateral approach (all strap muscles medial). Lifting the gland "up and over" allows for inspection in the tracheoesophageal groove. It is important that the Kocher grasp be large, to avoid tearing tissue, and that the grasp be lateral to allow for maximal torque. This illustration demonstrates exposure of a superior, type B gland.

commonly in the same coronal plane as the inferior thyroid pole. An enlarged inferior parathyroid gland is usually anterior to the RLN and caudal to the inferior thyroid artery. Alternatively, enlarged inferior parathyroid glands may be located adjacent to or within the upper thyrothymic tongue.

Dissection of an Inferior Parathyroid Adenoma

Circumferential dissection is accomplished using either a fine iris or tenotomy scissors and a fine right angle clamp. Some surgeons prefer a fine-tipped forceps along with a Jacobson mosquito or fine Jake. The enlarged parathyroid gland should never be grasped and fractured. Forceps allow gentle retraction of the periphery of the gland. A fine grasp of the surrounding fatty tissue is ideal to mobilize the gland. After circumferential dissection of the gland, the venous tributary to the gland is clipped with a small hemoclip or tied. A prominent artery usually is not found, but if present, should also be divided. Care is taken at all times to assure that the RLN is not being grasped or divided. The pedicle of the superior parathyroid can be in close proximity to the RLN and, therefore, even placing a small hemoclip should be done with great caution. The adenoma is then excised (see Figure 57.2). Energy devices for ligation of the pedicle are usually not necessary but are occasionally helpful if the gland is very enlarged or has a rich blood supply.

Back Door Technique

This technique employs an incision classically used for reoperative thyroid or parathyroid surgery. Placement of the incision at the lateral border of the strap muscles avoids the scarred midline (see Figures 57.3 and 57.4). Some advocate this approach for superior parathyroid adenomas that are deep in the neck or quite lateral in their position as seen in preoperative imaging. This approach can also be used to identify inferior pole adenomas if ultrasound guidance in the preoperative position shows this to be the best placement of the incision. The back door technique does demand that the surgeon be aware of the altered anatomic approach because the thyroid is now exposed from lateral to medial view rather than the traditional medial to lateral view (see Figure 57.4).

Incision

For a superior parathyroid adenoma, the lateral-most portion of the previously outlined incision is used as the point of entry. The site is medial to the medial border of the sternocleidomastoid muscle and lateral to the lateral border of the strap muscles (see Figure 57.3). The 2.5-cm transverse incision is made with a number 15 blade scalpel through the skin and subcutaneous tissue. Monopolar electrocautery is used to divide the platysma to the superficial (investing) layer of the deep cervical fascia.

Exposure

Subplatysmal flaps are created with electrocautery. Small Richardson or army-navy retractors are placed beneath the superior and inferior flaps to expose the strap and sternocleidomastoid muscles. The fascial attachments between the lateral borders of the strap muscles and the anterior border of the sternocleidomastoid muscle are separated longitudinally using a fine right-angle clamp and electrocautery. The sternohyoid muscle is elevated off the anterior surface of the thyroid capsule. The sternocleidomastoid muscle is then retracted laterally with a small army-navy retractor. The location of the internal jugular vein is referenced. The position of the carotid artery is noted by either inspection or palpation.

Thyroid Mobilization

The ipsilateral thyroid lobe is exposed and grasped with two Kocher or mosquito clamps. To the extent possible, the tips of the clamps are placed on the lateral, dorsal-most aspect of the lobe: one tip near the upper third junction and one tip near the inferior third junction. The surgical assistant deviates the thyroid parenchyma with the so-called up-and-over technique to elevate the thyroid tissue. Alternatively, the lobe can be retracted with a peanut. The thyroid lobe is deviated medially. This maneuver expedites exposure of the superior parathyroid gland by exposing the "cotton candy" fascia posterior and lateral to the surface of the thyroid gland in the paratracheal area. Type A glands can be visualized on the posterior surface of the thyroid lobe. This technique also offers excellent exposure for type B glands that are in the tracheoesophageal groove posterior to the thyroid lobe (see Figure 57.4).

Location and Dissection of Superior Parathyroid Glands

Gentle inferior retraction toward the carotid sheath will place tension on the RLN and allow for its easier identification. The middle thyroid vein, the inferior thyroid artery, and the RLN are identified. The pedicle of the superior gland is posterior and lateral to the RLN. An enlarged parathyroid adenoma is usually seen on the undersurface of the thyroid gland near the upper half of the lobe and adherent to the parenchyma. In this case a small incision in the perithyroid fascia will often allow the delivery of the bulbous gland. Alternatively, parathyroid glands may be located separate and away from the thyroid capsule in the tracheoesophageal groove (type B gland; see Figure 57.4). Creating a dissection plane and loosening of the tissues posterior to the thyroid and parallel to the tracheoesophageal groove allows digital palpation and probing with the index finger of the dominant hand around the esophagus. This is an excellent and often underappreciated maneuver to locate these glands and, if not performed, can lead to missed glands. Once this maneuver is done, gentle finger dissection and use of a peanut allow the surgeon to distinguish between an enlarged parathyroid and the esophagus; this distinction can be challenging. The slight bulge of the gland or the inferior rim of a type B gland can be palpated with the tip of the finger and then further dissected with a peanut (Figure 57.5). If the gland has descended caudally near the mediastinum, digital palpation can identify the superior edge. Once the gland is identified and circumferentially dissected with meticulous care to avoid injury to the RLN, the pedicle is then clipped with a small

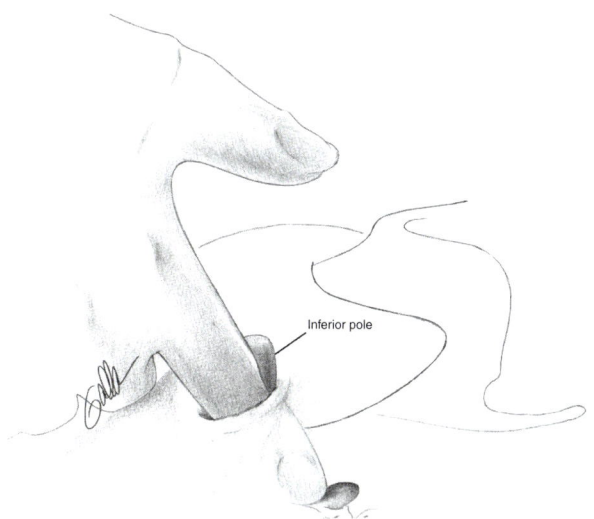

Fig. 57.5 The index finger serves as an excellent sensor to feel the parathyroid gland even before it is visualized. The soft bulge of the mobile tissue, separate from the thyroid gland, can be appreciated with gentle palpation.

hemoclip or ligated with suture and the gland is removed. Care is taken to avoid fracturing or tearing the gland by gently grasping the surrounding tissue and operating away from the gland.

Specimen Assessment and Post-Excision PTH

Specimens should be inspected in an *ex vivo* setting. Normal parathyroid glands weigh approximately 20 to 50 mg. Adenomas are larger, have a peanut butter color, and are usually soft but solid in texture. While the gland is still on the sterile field, we longitudinally divide the gland using a number 10 blade scalpel to visually inspect the parathyroid parenchyma. This blade should not be used again on the patient; this will help avoid seeding of parathyroid cells into the incision. A creamy peanut butter appearance is confirmation that the lesion is not a lymph node or a thyroid nodule. Some surgeons obtain frozen section analysis on each excised specimen, whereas others rely on surgical experience and judgment in most cases. Frozen section analysis can confirm the cellularity of the mass. Hypercellularity suggests an adenoma. The percentage of fat to cells is also an important aspect of the assessment because normal parathyroid tissue has approximately 50% fat on microscopic inspection. A 25-gauge needle and a syringe with 2 mL of saline can also be used to directly aspirate the gland. A PTH value >2500 pg/mL in the aspirate is biochemical confirmation of parathyroid tissue. If possible, the specimen is placed on a standardized template for medical photographic purposes.

Postexcision PTH values are a critical element to most surgeons who use a MIP approach (see Chapter 59, Intraoperative PTH Monitoring during Parathyroid Surgery). We prefer not to use the jugular vein for drawing intraoperative PTH blood samples because we believe spikes in the PTH level from proximity or dissection may mislead laboratory values. The intraoperative postexcision PTH level suggests to the surgeon when an adequate amount of hyperfunctioning tissue has been resected. Due to the short half-life of PTH of only 3 to 7 minutes, a precipitous PTH decline of >50% at 10 to 15 minutes (and into the normal range) suggests that the hyperfunctioning tissue has been adequately removed. More recent data would suggest that in addition to a decline of >50%, a PTH value less than 40 pg/mL reduces the likelihood of future recurrence.[24,25] Some surgeons obtain two postexcision intraoperative PTH measurements: one is drawn 5 minutes after excision of the adenoma, and the other is drawn 10 minutes afterward. Other surgeons just draw one postexcision level at 10 to 15 minutes and consider the operation a success with no need to convert to a bilateral exploration if the postexcision level is reduced by 50% and into the normal range. In single-gland disease, which is, of course, the exact patient population targeted for MIP, often the PTH drops are quite dramatic. Preincision PTH levels less than 100 pg/mL can be more challenging. Even mild renal failure can result in difficult-to-interpret intraoperative PTH results given the considerable effect on the clearance of intact PTH and PTH fragments. We prefer to see a >50% drop as well as a PTH level <40 pg/mL given more recent data on long-term recurrence when postexcision PTH is >40 pg/mL.

Wound Closure

The wound is irrigated, and a Valsalva maneuver with the patient in Trendelenburg can provide an assessment of hemostasis. Some surgeons elect to place a hemostatic agent in the resection bed routinely, although this is not necessary in the vast majority of cases and has been associated with increased rates of hematoma.[26] The strap muscles and platysma are closed with interrupted absorbable sutures. The skin is closed with running absorbable suture or with surgical glue. No drain is necessary. A sterile dressing is applied to the skin.

Nerve Monitoring and Radioguided Gamma-Probe Use

Nerve monitoring requires general anesthesia but can be useful in selected cases. If, for example, the procedure is a reoperation or the gland is suspected of being a type D gland near the nerve, the monitoring device may be helpful (see Chapter 36, Surgical Anatomy and Monitoring of the Recurrent Laryngeal Nerve). Some surgeons use nerve monitoring in every case; ultimately this decision should be left up to the discretion of the surgeon. We reserve the use of the radioguided gamma-probe technique for difficult reoperation cases such as the following: a significant amount of scar tissue is suspected, the ipsilateral nerve is at high risk for injury, and the thyroid parenchyma has been previously removed. Technical considerations pertaining to dosing and timing of the isotope injection are discussed in other chapters.

POSTOPERATIVE CARE AND FOLLOW-UP

If laboratory measurements indicate that an adequate PTH decline of >50% with a postexcision level <40 pg/mL, the patient has a high likelihood of being cured. Serum calcium levels begin to drop within hours. There is no need for serial calcium assessments if an MIP was performed without violating the remaining glands. The calcium level usually reaches nadir at 72 hours after adenoma excision. Patients should be properly educated about oral calcium supplementation should they have transient symptoms of tingling and numbness. Patients should be able to tolerate a regular diet and typically have minimal pain or nausea at the time of discharge from the hospital. We observe patients for 3 to 6 hours for signs of a hematoma. Patients who live more than 1 hour away should be counseled to stay nearby overnight, rather than travel back to their home. Patients should not be left alone the night of surgery and the companion should be able to speak English and be responsible for communication with the surgeon should any complications arise. Symptoms of dysphagia, difficulty lying supine, or anxiety should prompt a postoperative evaluation.

The dressing, if one was used, can be removed on postoperative day 1. Patients should be advised to watch for signs of rapid swelling or a firm mass in the neck, which may represent a hematoma. Erythema, fevers, discharge from the wound, or worsening tenderness may suggest an infection. However, hematoma and infection are extremely rare after this operation. Selective calcium supplementation is advised for patients whose PTH levels are expected to drop drastically, such as those with preoperative calcium levels >14 mg/dL or PTH levels >400 mg/dL. Some surgeons will routinely place all parathyroidectomy patients on a temporary course of supplemental calcium. Follow-up can be done over the phone or with a Health Insurance Portability and Accountability Act (HIPAA)-complaint virtual visit if it is more convenient for the patient. Calcium levels can be obtained 1 to 2 weeks after surgery and again at 6 months to ensure cure. Once yearly calcium thereafter to ensure there is no recurrence is probably prudent.

MIP should be considered for patients with sporadic PHPT and preoperative imaging results that suggest single gland disease. The imaging results serve as a road map for the surgeon and the intraoperative PTH level suggests the completeness of the resection. A standard parathyroid nomenclature offers a consistent means of communicating the gland location and offers a precise, reproducible system for documentation. The role of robotic surgery and other advanced technologies will continue to evolve and will open the door to even better methods of surgically curing this metabolic disease.

REFERENCES

For a complete list of references, go to expertconsult.com.

58

Minimally Invasive Video-Assisted Parathyroidectomy

Rocco Bellantone, Marco Raffaelli, Celestino Lombardi, Carmela De Crea

 This chapter contains additional online-only content, available on expertconsult.com.

Please see the Expert Consult website for more discussion of this topic.

INTRODUCTION

Bilateral neck exploration (BNE) with the identification of at least four parathyroid glands and the removal of pathologic parathyroid tissue has represented, for several decades, the standard of treatment of primary hyperparathyroidism (PHPT) (see Chapter 56, Standard Bilateral Parathyroid Exploration).[1,2] In experienced hands, this approach has a cure rate of more than 95% with minimal morbidity of usually less than 3%.[1]

In spite of the excellent results obtained with BNE, since the early 1980s, less invasive procedures (e.g., unilateral neck exploration [UNE]) have been introduced with the aim to reduce the surgical trauma and the already-low complication rate of parathyroidectomy.[3,4]

The rationale for a minimally invasive approach for parathyroidectomy derives from the fact that most patients (>85%) with PHPT have a single parathyroid adenoma, which is potentially identifiable and removable with a focused, selective cervical exploration.

The application of minimally invasive parathyroidectomy (MIP) was initially limited. Only since the early 1990s have these procedures been widely developed; this is because of the evolution of the techniques of preoperative localization (e.g., ultrasound and sestamibi scan)[5] and the introduction of quick intraoperative parathyroid hormone (PTH) assay.[6] Preoperative localization studies allow for a more targeted approach, and the intraoperative PTH assay is able to intraoperatively confirm the success of surgery.[7,8]

PREOPERATIVE LOCALIZATION STUDIES

In the case of concordant ultrasonography and scintigraphy, the overall accuracy in parathyroid localization is higher than 95%, whereas in the case of negative localization studies, the likelihood of multiglandular disease (MGD) is higher than 30%.[9,10]

Obviously, the availability of accurate preoperative localization studies allows the planning of minimally invasive surgical procedures targeting the identified affected gland(s). Imaging studies are concordant in up to 65% of patients with PHPT.[7,11] It has been well demonstrated that if more than 51% of the patients are eligible for a unilateral exploration or a focused approach, the use of preoperative localization studies is cost effective.[12] A "targeted" approach can also be proposed in cases of positivity of only one localization study.[10] In such a circumstance, the risk of an MGD is about 17%.[10]

INTRAOPERATIVE PTH ASSAY

Similar to the progress in the field of preoperative imaging techniques that allowed for targeted approaches, the development and the availability of the intraoperative PTH assay gave surgeons the opportunity to intraoperatively verify the completeness of the surgical resection as an alternative to the complete visualization of all four glands[6,8,18-21] (see Chapter 59, Intraoperative PTH Monitoring During Parathyroid Surgery). The half-life of intact PTH is 3 to 5 minutes. As a consequence, after the resection of a single adenoma, the removal of all hyperfunctioning parathyroid tissue should be confirmed by a significant reduction of PTH levels. Because rapid techniques have been developed, the intraoperative PTH assay appears to be an attractive method to intraoperatively verify the success of the surgical resection (i.e., a "biochemical" frozen section). The turnaround time has now become very short (less than 10 minutes) and can be performed by laboratory personnel in the operating room using portable machines. Several studies demonstrated a positive correlation between an adequate intraoperative PTH decrease and postoperative eucalcemia.[7]

As a consequence, intraoperative PTH assay emerged as an important adjunct to localizing studies when a focused approach has been planned. By delivering immediate feedback during surgery, intraoperative PTH monitoring allows the surgeon to decide whether unilateral exploration has been successful or if four-gland exploration is necessary.[6-8,18-20] It has been demonstrated that intraoperative PTH increases the cure rate of minimally invasive procedures from 95% to 98%, although it has also been associated with an increase of about 13% of unnecessary BNE.[9,22]

Most authors agree that intraoperative PTH monitoring is an important, essential, complementary tool in cases of minimally invasive procedures.[18-20,23,24] However, some authors have questioned its usefulness in intraoperative decision making, especially in cases with concordant localization studies that suggest one gland disease.[25-27] The position statement of the European Society of Endocrine Surgeons suggests intraoperative PTH may be best reserved for patients undergoing targeted parathyroidectomy on the basis of a single preoperative localization study (i.e., sestamibi scan[28] or ultrasonography[29]) or in cases of discordant preoperative localization studies in which the risk of MGD is higher.[17,30]

In a retrospective nonrandomized comparative study, Barczyński et al.[31] found that the routine use of intraoperative PTH significantly improves cure rates of minimally invasive, either open or video-assisted parathyroidectomy (VAP), in comparison to open image-guided UNE without intraoperative PTH. This study also suggested that intraoperative PTH can help inform the surgeon in making decisions regarding how to proceed with further neck exploration, especially in cases of only one positive imaging study.[31] Moreover, one paper demonstrated that, at least in an endemic goiter region, intraoperative PTH monitoring seems necessary even in patients with "localized" single-gland disease; abandoning it would significantly increase persistent disease (from 0.9% to 5%).[32]

Please see the Expert Consult website for more discussion of this topic.

MINIMALLY INVASIVE PARATHYROIDECTOMY

The application of endoscopic techniques to neck surgery during the late 1990s resulted in the development of minimally invasive techniques for parathyroidectomy.[53] The general trend toward less invasive procedures for parathyroidectomy is well demonstrated by the results of an international survey, which was conducted in 2000 among the members of the International Association of Endocrine Surgeons (IAES). Fifty-nine percent of the participants used a minimally invasive approach.[54] We feel this percentage may have further increased since that time.

Even if a minority of the authors still consider a standard BNE performed by an experienced endocrine surgeon to be the best treatment for patients with PHPT,[55,56] others maintain that BNE should be relegated to the past. Clearly, minimally invasive procedures for parathyroidectomy are assuming a more and more important role; in time, they may represent the new gold standard for the treatment of PHPT, at least in its sporadic form.

The consensus statement of the European Society of Endocrine Surgeons (ESES) assumed that even if BNE has excellent results and is always an option for the surgical treatment of PHPT, MIP is a safe and cost-effective procedure to treat selected patients with sporadic PHPT, especially in cases of positive preoperative localization tests.[30] Similarly, the proceedings of the third international workshop on PHPT (Orlando, Florida, 2008) reported that, "unlike previous dogma that mandated surgical identification of both pathologically enlarged and normal parathyroid glands, the current paradigm in many centers is to identify and excise the incident enlarged gland and to confirm operative cure employing a rapid intraoperative PTH assay."[52] Despite these statements, an audit from the Scandinavian quality register for parathyroid surgery showed that BNE is still performed in two thirds of parathyroid procedures.[57] Indeed, it is true that not all patients with hyperparathyroidism can be treated by a selective minimally invasive approach. Thus we feel that BNE does still maintain a relevant role in the treatment of patients with PHPT (see Chapter 56, Standard Bilateral Parathyroid Exploration).

Minimally invasive (e.g., focused, targeted, or selective) parathyroidectomy encompasses a number of different techniques, including open approaches (e.g., open minimally invasive parathyroidectomy [OMIP][58,59]), minimally invasive radio-guided parathyroidectomy (MI-RP),[60,61] VAP,[62-64] and purely endoscopic parathyroidectomy (EP).[53,65-69] As a consequence, there is no strict or unequivocal definition of what an MIP is. The term *minimally invasive* should be reserved for procedures that allow performance of a traditional operation through access and minimize trauma of the surgical exposure and dissection. BNE is associated with a very low morbidity (<3%) and high success (>95%) rates by experienced surgeons. A minimally invasive procedure should obtain at least the same results, with the main advantage of reducing the skin incision and, consequently, allowing better cosmetic results.[70,71] MIP was thus used to indicate parathyroid procedures performed through a mini-incision usually <2.5 to 3 cm.[71]

This definition is, at least, reductive, because mini-incision does not necessarily mean a minimally invasive procedure. Moreover, there are several other potential advantages of the targeted parathyroid procedures (i.e., decreased postoperative pain and complications rate), which should be mainly related to the less extensive surgical dissection.

Many studies comparing MIP/focused parathyroidectomy with standard BNE suggest that the focused techniques are safe and at least as good as BNE; these techniques have some advantages such as lower postoperative hypocalcemia, shorter operative time, earlier discharge, better cosmetic results, and reduced postoperative pain. These results were strongly confirmed by five randomized trials with short-term results[71-75] and one study with long-term results[76] that demonstrated some distinct benefits for MIP over standard BNE (see the Evidence-Based Recommendations section).

TECHNIQUES FOR MIP

Several variants of minimally invasive procedures have been described since the late 1990s, including minimally invasive procedures without endoscope (e.g., OMIP and MI-RP)[8,60,61,77-81] and with the use of the endoscope (e.g., EP and VAP).[53,62-69]

Minimally Invasive Radio-Guided Parathyroidectomy

In MI-RP, a handheld gamma probe is used to facilitate intraoperative localization, identification, and dissection of the pathologic gland(s); the probe is also used to confirm the removal of all hyperfunctioning parathyroid tissue.[60,61,81] This approach implies that technetium 99m-sestamibi is injected intravenously 2 to 4 hours before surgery. Obviously, a prerequisite for this approach is the precise coordination between the operating room, the nuclear medicine department, the surgeon, and the nuclear medicine radiologist.[27] On the operating table, the anterior portion of the patient's neck is scanned; the site with highest count is explored using the handheld probe as a guide toward the pathologic gland(s). An excised parathyroid adenoma should contain more than 20% of the postexcision background radioactivity.[82] This approach may result in reduced operative time[83] and may eliminate the need for intraoperative PTH.[61] Although this technique has been refined and validated, it has been adopted only by a minority of endocrine surgeons worldwide mainly because of the logistic requirements. Moreover, it is widely believed that MI-RP adds little information to preoperative sestamibi scan and intraoperative PTH measurement;[27,52,77] however, there is no prospective study on this topic. Some data suggest the gamma probe may be potentially misleading in certain circumstances.[79,84] At present, MI-RP is considered an alternative minimally invasive technique, which has potential advantages in reoperative cases.[30]

Open Minimally Invasive Parathyroidectomy

OMIP represents the most widespread minimally invasive technique.[52,54,85] In the IAES survey, 92% of the surgeons dealing with MIP adopted an OMIP, whereas only a minority of them (35%) relied on endoscopic (13%) or video-assisted procedures (22%).[54] A focused parathyroidectomy, performed through a small (2.5 to 5 cm) central[52] or a lateral (over the site of the adenoma and overlying the anterior border of the sternocleidomastoid muscle)[59] incision, guided by preoperative localization studies and intraoperative PTH, seems, therefore, to be the most attractive and widespread technique for the surgical treatment of PHPT.[7,8,24,52,54,58,59,77,79,80] Indeed, experienced endocrine surgeons seem to find the procedure easy to learn and reproduce in different surgical settings; it can be performed under locoregional anesthesia, with reduced operative time, and as a short stay procedure.[7,24] On the other hand, the main limitation of OMIP resides in the potential poor visualization of the neck structures because of the small size of the skin incision or, conversely, the need for a larger skin incision compared with video-assisted or endoscopic techniques. Because coexistent thyroid nodular disease is relatively common, associated thyroid resection can be performed as well, especially by this approach. Typically, resection is undertaken after conversion from regional block to general anesthesia.[24]

Video-Assisted and Endoscopic Techniques

Procedures that use the endoscope (purely endoscopic and video-assisted techniques) take advantage not only of a targeted approach but also of the endoscopic magnification with optimal visualization of the neck structures (the recurrent laryngeal nerve [RLN] and parathyroid glands, in particular); video-assisted or endoscopic techniques should be preferred mainly because of this important advantage. These procedures require dedicated surgical instrumentation, an adequate and relatively prolonged learning curve, and usually general anesthesia. Nonetheless, at least from a theoretical point of view, endoscopic or video-assisted procedures are particularly suitable for parathyroid surgery because parathyroid surgery is usually a procedure for benign disease without issues of local invasion.

Techniques that imply the use of the endoscope can be classified in endoscopic[65-69] and video-assisted procedures (see Chapter 32, Robotic and Extra Cervical Approaches to the Thyroid and Parathyroid Glands).[62-64,86,87]

Endoscopic Parathyroidectomy

Gagner first described the totally EP in 1996,[53,88] and other authors subsequently used and modified it.[65,66] It is carried out entirely under steady gas flow, using a 5-mm endoscope introduced through a central trocar, and two or three additional trocars for the instruments (Figure 58.1). The dissection is first performed beneath the platysma to obtain a good working space. The midline is then opened, and the strap muscles are retracted to expose the thyroid lobe and explore the parathyroid glands after dissecting the thyroid from the fascia.

Although this technique employs a cervical access, other procedures with an extracervical endoscopic approach have been described. These approaches gained an initial success mainly in the Asian surgical community, where avoiding any neck scar seems to be of utmost importance.[64] Several approaches have been described, including extracervical accesses from the chest wall,[67] the breast,[89] and the axilla[68] (see Figure 58.1). All the endoscopic techniques are characterized by the of continuous CO_2 insufflation[53,65-68] or mechanical external retraction[69,90-92] to maintain the operative space for dissection and for trocar positioning.

The authors who support these procedures emphasize the cosmetic result and minimize the risk of hypercarbia and subcutaneous emphysema when the gas insufflation remains below 4 mm Hg.[67,68] Surely, these procedures guarantee an optimal cosmetic result because of the small and often distant scars, but they are technically demanding and difficult to reproduce in different settings, especially by surgeons who do not have endoscopic experience. Moreover, the totally endoscopic techniques with extracervical accesses are intended to maximally improve the cosmetic outcome, but they require an extensive and difficult dissection to reach the operation site. The long operative time reported represents another major limitation for the diffusion of these approaches. Moreover, the risks related to CO_2 absorption are not

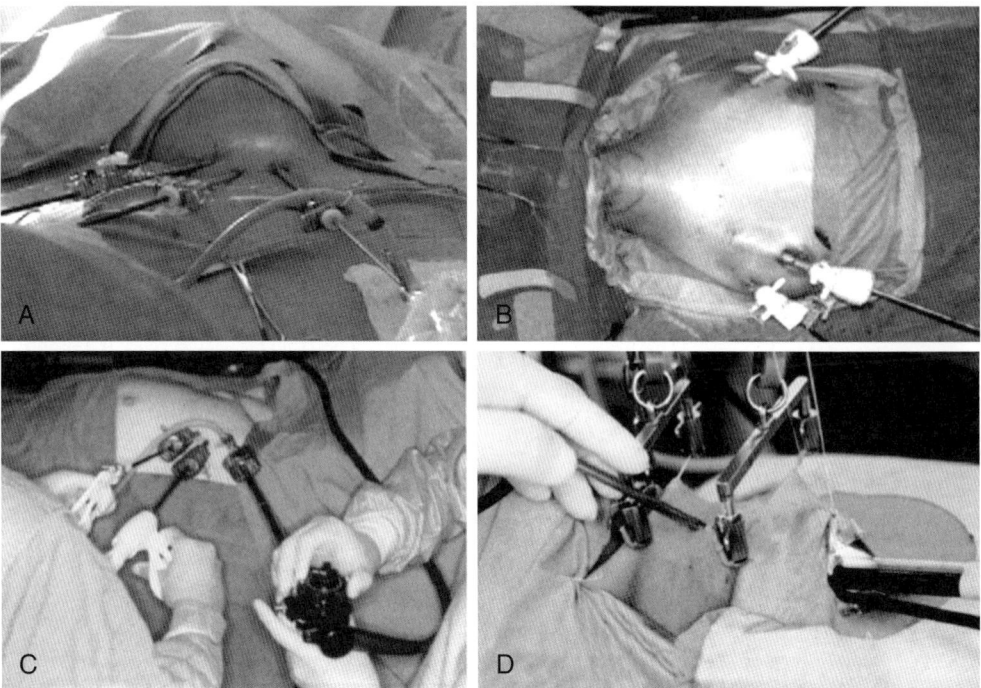

Fig. 58.1 Purely endoscopic parathyroidectomy (EP): different approaches. **A,** Cervical access. **B,** Breast access. **C,** Axillary access. **D,** Chest access–skin lifting. (**A,** From Gagner M. Endoscopic subtotal parathyroidectomy in patients with primary hyperparathyroidism. *Br J Surg.* 1996;83[6]:875. **B,** From Ohgami M, Ishii S, Arisawa Y, et al. Scarless endoscopic thyroidectomy: breast approach for best cosmesis. *Surg Laparosc Endosc Percutan Tech.* 2000;10[1]:1–4. **C,** From Ikeda Y, Takami H, Sasaki Y, et al. Endoscopic neck surgery by the axillary approach. *J Am Coll Surg.* 2000;191[3]:336–340, Fig. 1. **D,** From Shimizu K, Akira S, Tanaka S. Video-assisted neck surgery: endoscopic resection of benign thyroid tumor aiming at scarless surgery on the neck. *J Surg Oncol.* 1998;69[3]:178–180.)

completely eliminated.[88,93,94] Probably, for all these reasons, these procedures encountered only limited acceptance.

Video-Assisted Parathyroidectomy by the Lateral Approach (VAP-LA)

VAP-LA was first described by Henry et al.[63] The lateral approach is characterized by a 12-mm skin incision on the anterior border of the sternocleidomastoid muscle, which is 3 to 4 cm above the sternal notch on the side of the affected gland. Through this incision, the tissue is dissected with an open technique to reach the prevertebral fascia. Once enough space has been created, two 2.5-mm trocars are inserted on the line of the anterior border of the sternocleidomastoid muscle 3 to 4 cm above and below the first incision through which a 10-mm trocar for the endoscope (10 mm, 0 degrees) is inserted (Figure 58.2). Unilateral video-assisted parathyroid exploration and dissection are carried out with 8-mm Hg CO_2 insufflation during the whole procedure. At the beginning of the experience with this approach, the operation was with limited video-assisted techniques.[63,95,96] Indeed, after dissection of the adenoma, the trocars were removed, and the vascular pedicle was ligated and cut under direct vision, and the procedure was terminated under direct vision. After the initial learning curve, dissection was completely carried out under endoscopic vision.[97,98] After completing the dissection of the affected gland, small adenomas are directly extracted through the 10-mm trocar; large adenomas that cannot be introduced into the 10-mm trocar are extracted through the trocar site under direct vision.

In the largest retrospective series reported,[96,97] VAP-LA provided an optimal visualization of the neck structures and was particularly suitable for adenoma deeply located in the neck or in the upper and posterior mediastinum, usually affecting the superior parathyroid gland. VAP-LA seems quite easy to reproduce. It allows for an excellent 99% cure rate, is effective, safe, and has a minimal complication rate. Nonetheless, the rate of contraindications for VAP-LA appears higher than for minimally invasive video-assisted parathyroidectomy (MIVAP; 43% versus 29% respectively), which is discussed later.

Important for success with the lateral approach is the absence of nodular goiter and the demonstration of a single enlarged parathyroid gland on preoperative imaging studies.

In a series evaluating medium-term results of VAP-LA, Maweja et al.[98] reported an excellent 98.5% cure rate with one case of recurrent disease in a total of 394 endoscopic procedures, with a median follow-up of 20.5 months.

The main technical limitation of the technique is the unilateral approach that does not allow the possibility of accomplishing a bilateral exploration (when necessary) except by conversion to an open conventional procedure.

Minimally Invasive Video-Assisted Parathyroidectomy (MIVAP)

MIVAP was first described by Miccoli et al.[62] In 1998, our department adopted the procedure.[64] Early after its first description, this technique encountered large, worldwide acceptance[87,99-102] because it is easy to reproduce in different surgical settings. Actually, it reproduces in all the steps of the conventional operation, with the endoscope representing only a tool that allows one to perform the same operation through a smaller skin incision.

Indications for MIVAP

Ideal candidates for MIVAP are patients with sporadic PHPT in whom a single adenoma is suspected based on preoperative sestamibi scan and ultrasonography. Parathyroid adenomas with a maximum diameter larger than 3 cm should not be selected for MIVAP, because a difficult dissection can determine a dangerous capsular rupture and consequent parathyromatosis.[103,104] Exclusion criteria include previous conventional neck surgery, persistent or recurrent hyperparathyroidism, mediastinal adenomas, and concomitant large goiter.

With increasing experience, selection criteria for MIVAP have been refined and widened. Patients with concomitant nodular goiter requiring surgical removal can be selected for MIVAP if the inclusion criteria for the video-assisted thyroidectomy are respected.[64] We have found, based on the surgeon's experience and on a per-case basis, that patients with previous contralateral neck surgery or intrathymic/retrosternal adenomas can be selected for MIVAP. Also, in cases of suspected MGD, a video-assisted BNE can be planned. Video-assisted BNE through a central, minimal access approach is also appropriate for patients with uncertain preoperative localization.[103,104]

Previous contralateral neck surgery (i.e., contralateral thyroid lobectomy) is no longer an absolute contraindication for MIVAP. In such cases, however, a lateral approach seems preferable; it permits one to avoid the scar and fibrotic tissue consequent to the previous operation.[103,104]

The subset of patients with sporadic PHPT who are also candidates for MIVAP is largely variable in different series (37% to 71%)[64,103,104] and is mainly related to the different incidences of coexisting thyroid disease that may require a conventional approach.[64]

MIVAP has been proposed also for patients with four gland hyperplasia (i.e., familial PHPT[105] and secondary and tertiary HPT[87,106,107]). However, these findings still require validation in larger series and comparative studies.

MIVAP: Surgical Procedure

The operative technique has been previously described in detail.[108]

Patients and surgical team position. The patient, under general or locoregional anesthesia with cervical block, is positioned supine with the neck in slight extension. The surgical team is represented by the surgeon and two assistants, one of whom handles the endoscope (Figure 58.3). The need for at least three surgeons involved in the

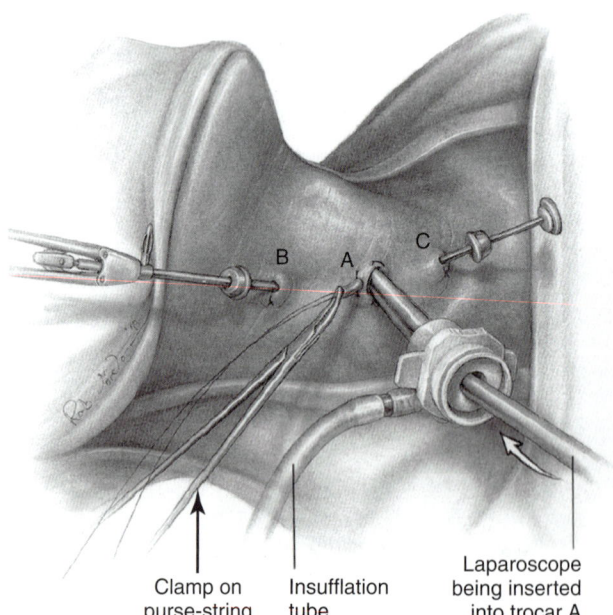

Fig. 58.2 Video-assisted parathyroidectomy by the lateral approach (VAP-LA): completed setup. (From Henry JF. Endoscopic exploration. *Op Tech Gen Surg.* 1999;1:49–61.)

CHAPTER 58   Minimally Invasive Video-Assisted Parathyroidectomy   541

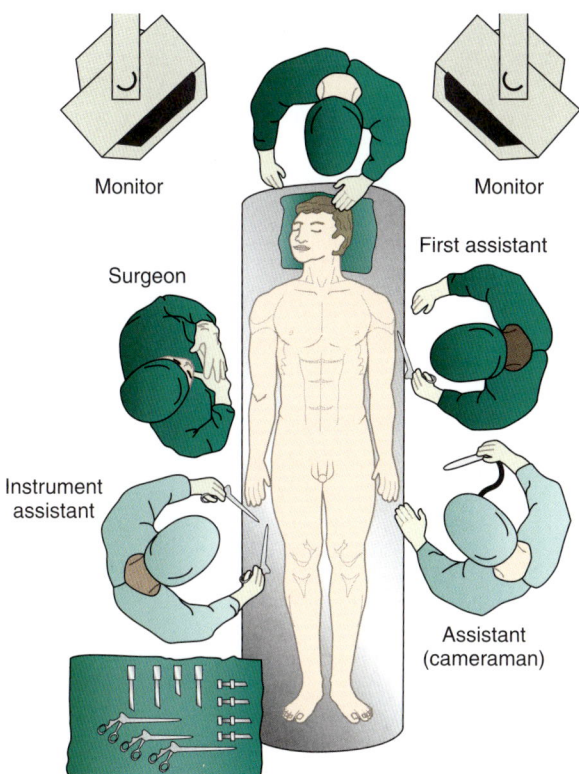

Fig. 58.3 Minimally invasive video-assisted parathyroidectomy (MIVAP): Setup of the operative room and surgical team. (From Bellantone R, Lombardi CP, Raffaelli M. Paratiroidectomia miniinvasiva video-assistita. In: *Encyclopedie Médico-Chirurgicale*, Tecniche Chirurgiche-Chirurgia Generale, 46-465-A. Paris: Elsevier SAS, 2005;1–18.)

procedure has been considered one of the main limitations to the acceptance of this approach.[7]

The monitor is positioned at the head of the patient in front of the surgeon, who is positioned on the right side of the patient. A second monitor is usually positioned in front of the assistants, who are on the left side of the patient (see Figure 58.3).

Anesthesia. In the early days, the procedure was carried out under general anesthesia with orotracheal intubation.[62,86] This could be considered a limitation of the technique compared with OMIP. With increasing experience, the feasibility of this approach under locoregional anesthesia with superficial modified[64] or deep cervical block[108,109] has been demonstrated.

Surgical technique. A small (1.5-cm) skin incision is performed between the cricoid cartilage and the sternal notch, in the midline. The skin incision is usually higher than in conventional cervicotomy and can also be modulated on the basis of the preoperative ultrasound findings (Figure 58.4).

The cervical *linea alba* is opened as far as possible. At one time, the procedure required a short CO_2 insufflation to facilitate dissection of the thyroid lobe from the strap muscles.[62] This use of insufflation now has been omitted. The thyroid lobe is separated from the strap muscles by means of small conventional retractors (Farabeuf retractors), which are also used to maintain the operative space. With this purpose, the thyroid lobe is medially retracted, and the strap muscles on the affected side are retracted laterally. The endoscope (5 mm, 30 degrees) and the dedicated small surgical instruments (2 mm in diameter) are then introduced through the single skin incision (Figure 58.5). The assistant maintains the endoscope with two hands. The absence of any external support allows for minor degrees of change of the position of the endoscope in relationship to the particular exigencies of the dissection. This represents an important advantage of the video-assisted procedure over purely endoscopic techniques. The tip of the endoscope is usually oriented toward the patient's head, but it can be changed to expose and explore the upper mediastinum, when required, in search of the mediastinal gland.

The first step of the procedure consists of completely freeing the thyroid gland from the strap muscles to expose the parathyroid sites. After identifying the inferior laryngeal nerve in the involved side, usually where it crosses the inferior thyroid artery (Figure 58.6), a targeted exploration is usually carried out to identify the abnormal gland preoperatively localized. The 2 to 3 × magnification of the endoscope permits easy identification of the nerve and the parathyroid glands, if the principles of blunt and bloodless dissection are respected. In case there is a suspicion of MGD (because of inadequate intraoperative PTH decrease, double glands enlargement at unilateral exploration, or in the case of inadequate preoperative localization studies), bilateral parathyroid exploration can be accomplished by the same video-assisted technique through the single, central skin incision. After being identified, the affected parathyroid gland is bluntly dissected under endoscopic vision by using dedicated spatulas and a spatula-shaped aspirator (KARL STORZ, Tuttlingen, Germany). The pedicle of the adenoma is usually clipped with titanium clips or ligated with conventional ligature. After the pedicle has been cut, the adenoma is extracted through the skin incision (Figure 58.7). Intraoperative PTH assay should confirm the removal of all pathologic tissue. After they have been checked for hemostasis, the strap muscles are sutured along the midline as well as the platysma. The skin is closed by means of a nonreabsorbable subcuticular running suture or by a skin sealant. No drain is employed.

Some authors proposed MIVAP variants. Lorenz illustrated a modified MIVAP[99,101] using a separate 5-mm incision caudal to the main access, which was created with a newly designed, self-cutting, blunt trocar for an additional gas insufflation port. A 5-mm, 30-degree magnifying endoscopic camera was introduced, and continuous gas insufflation during the open phase of preparation served as a coagulation smoke radiator to prevent obscured vision. Other authors have suggested performing a radio-guided video-assisted parathyroidectomy to exploit the advantages of both video- and radio-guided techniques.[110,111]

Results of MIVAP

The conversion rate is highly variable, ranging from 0.9%[64] to 43%.[112] Reasons for conversion are usually related to difficulties identifying the diseased gland(s), difficult dissection (eventually related to suspicion of malignancy), suspicion of MGD, intraoperative PTH results, and ectopic glands. Nonetheless, one should consider that proper patient selection and surgical team experience play an important role in the conversion rate. With appropriate selection criteria and adequate experience, the conversion rate to conventional BNE is usually low, even in the endemic goiter region.[64]

Operative time is largely influenced by surgical team skill; an appropriate learning curve should be considered at the beginning of the experience just as it is for other surgical procedures.[113] However, with increasing experience, operative time decreases significantly and is comparable or even shorter to that of a conventional operation.[64,104,113]

Several large retrospective series have reported on the outcome of MIVAP. In their paper reporting on 350 cases of MIVAP after 6 years of experience, Miccoli et al.[104] reported a cure rate of 98.3%. At a median follow-up of 35.1 months, persistent disease was evident in four cases, all of them resulting from false-positive results of intraoperative PTH failing to recognize MGD. In that series, complications occurred in 14 patients. The authors reported 2.7% of transient hypocalcemia,

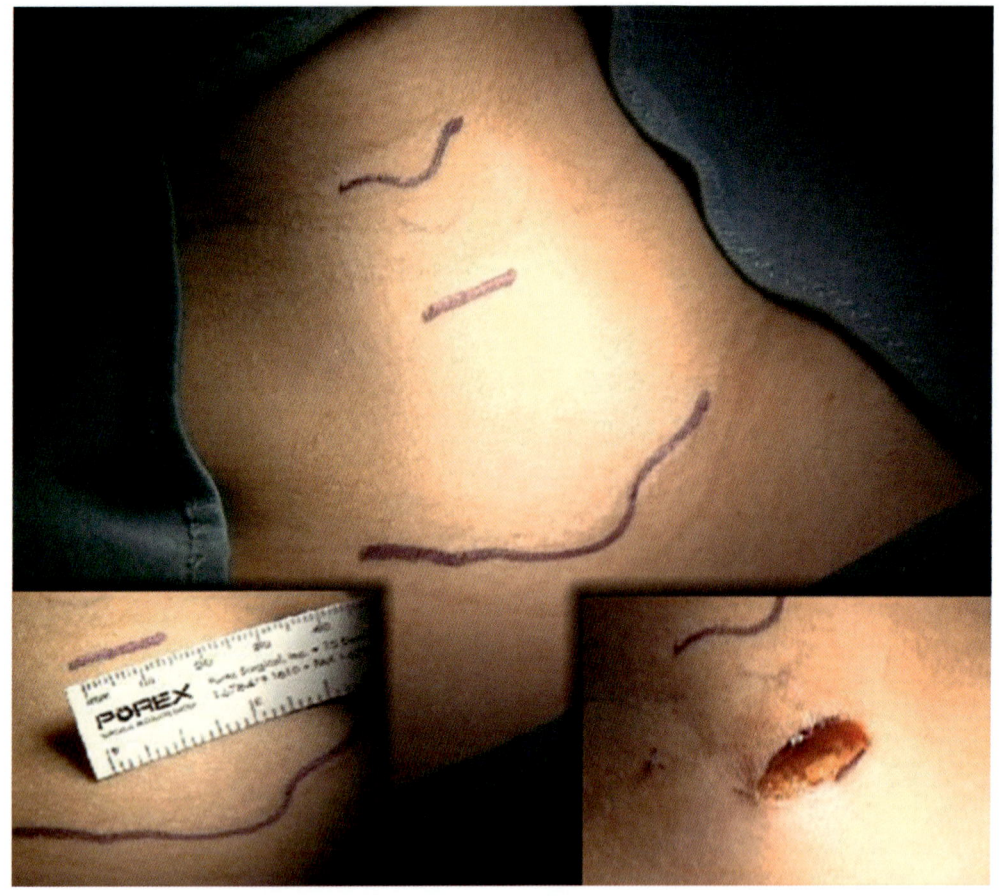

Fig. 58.4 Minimally invasive video-assisted parathyroidectomy (MIVAP): Skin incision.

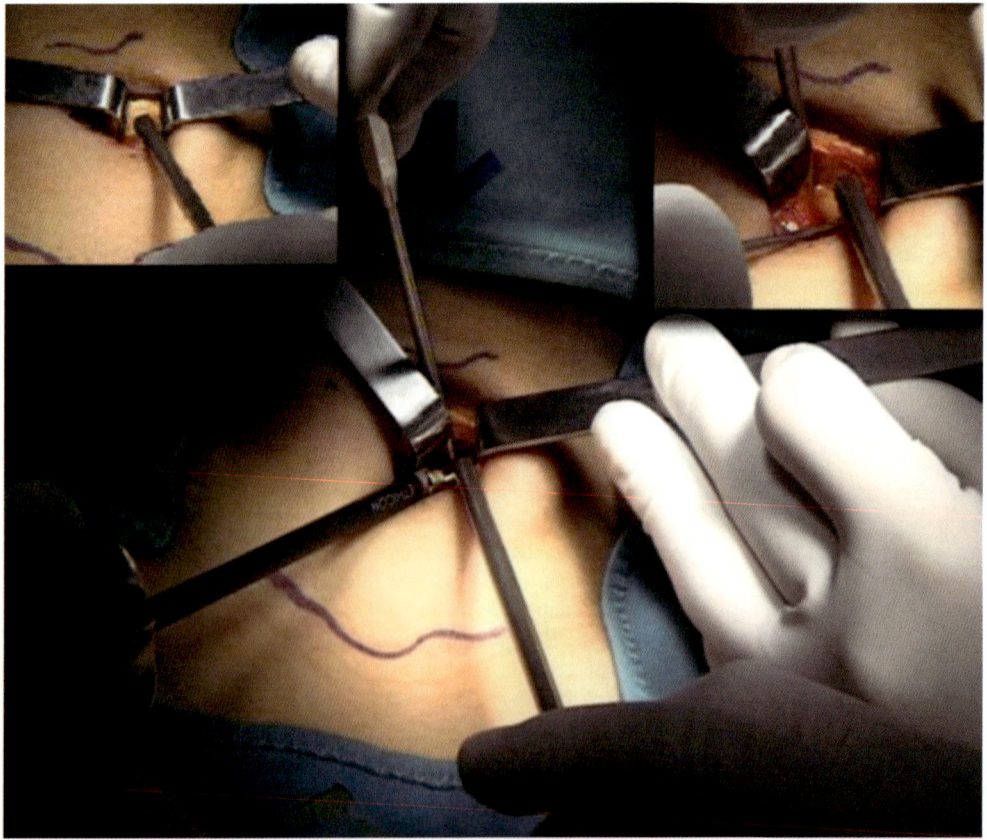

Fig. 58.5 Minimally invasive video-assisted parathyroidectomy (MIVAP): After creating the operative space, the endoscope and surgical instruments are inserted through the skin incision without any trocar use.

CHAPTER 58 Minimally Invasive Video-Assisted Parathyroidectomy

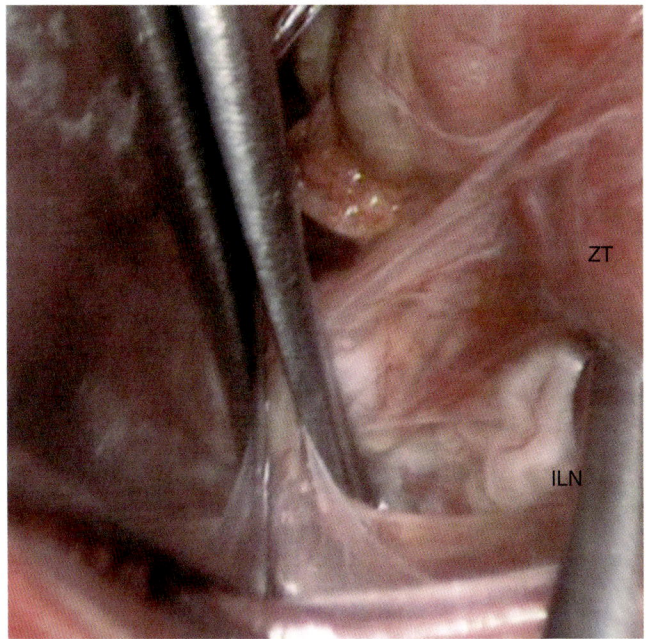

Fig. 58.6 Minimally invasive video-assisted parathyroidectomy (MIVAP): The recurrent laryngeal nerve (RLN) is well exposed and prepared thanks to the endoscopic magnification. ZT, Zuckerkandl's tubercle.

0.8 % of definitive nerve palsy (three cases), and 0.3% of postoperative bleeding. Other investigators have reported similar results even in smaller series.[87,99,101] In our previous published series of 107 cases of VAP with central access, we reported a similar success rate of 98.1% with persistent disease in two cases (1.9%).[64] We encountered a higher rate (11.1%) of temporary hypocalcemia with no cases of definitive hypoparathyroidism, whereas no other complications were observed.[64] It should be noted that long-term results evaluating recurrent disease rates are not yet available in the world literature.

Advantages and Disadvantages of MIVAP

MIVAP gained wide acceptance in several referral centers[64,73,87,99,101,104] shortly after its first description. Its success, compared with other techniques, is likely the result of several factors. First, and perhaps most important, is the advantage of endoscopic magnification. Additionally, the procedure is similar to the conventional surgery; the operative procedure reproduces the steps of the standard operation. The camera is only a tool that allows one to perform the same intervention with minimal access. From a purely technical point of view, this facilitates the operation. This method is significantly different from other endoscopic techniques, which involve access that is completely different from conventional surgery. Obviously, for obtaining the best results, surgeons should be well trained in both endocrine and endoscopic surgery. Moreover, like all other new surgical procedures, a learning period should be considered.[103,113] Excellent

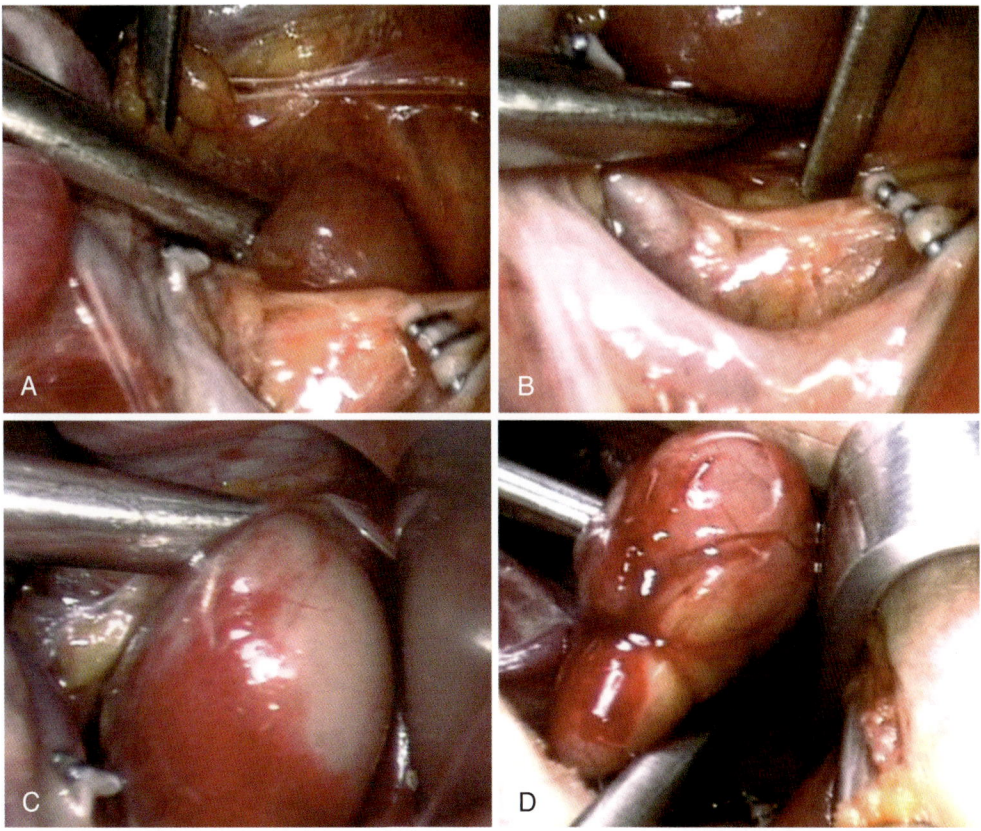

Fig. 58.7 A–D, Minimally invasive video-assisted parathyroidectomy (MIVAP): A large left superior parathyroid adenoma, migrated posterior to the inferior thyroid artery, is progressively freed.

visualization of neck structures results from the twofold to threefold endoscopic magnification, which permits an easy and prompt identification of the laryngeal nerve and parathyroid glands and reduces the risk of nerve palsy or the troublesome occurrence of capsular gland rupture. In one prospective randomized trial, the mean time for adenoma localization was significantly shorter in the group of patients who underwent MIVAP compared with patients operated on with OMIP.[73]

Another merit of the technique is the possibility of performing a BNE, when necessary, through the same central access. This characteristic, in part, explains the very low conversion rate reported in larger series (0.9% to 8%).[64,103] The possibility of performing a BNE produces two main effects on the restrictive inclusion criteria. First, at least from a theoretical point of view, MIVAP can be performed if intraoperative PTH monitoring is not available or, in the case of inadequate preoperative localization studies, given the possibility to explore all parathyroid sites through this approach.[64,86,114] One prospective randomized study[114] compared bilateral video-assisted neck exploration after the removal of enlarged glands with focused MIVAP plus intraoperative PTH to evaluate the effectiveness of the two techniques in the treatment of patients with PHPT. The bilateral video-assisted neck exploration was as safe and effective as MIVAP with intraoperative PTH, and it did not prolong the operative time of the surgical procedure.

Its minimal invasiveness and the similarity with the conventional procedure render MIVAP approach feasible also under locoregional anesthesia (cervical block),[109] at least in selected patients. Moreover, it has been demonstrated that locoregional anesthesia allows for a significant reduction of operating room time, and it is associated with significantly less postoperative pain.[109] As for other targeted approaches, MIVAP may be performed as an outpatient or same-day procedure, at least in selected cases. It should be noted that in the authors' department, we do not perform parathyroid surgery on an outpatient basis. In Italy, many patients are reluctant to be discharged early after surgery (i.e., on the same day of the operation), especially when they live a long distance from a hospital, or if they have come from another region. Moreover, the Italian National Health System does not provide facilities for a close outpatient follow-up of patients undergoing operations.

Another advantage of the central access is the possibility to also perform thyroid resection, even bilateral, when necessary. This introduces an important difference, not only if compared with other endoscopic techniques but also compared with OMIP, because conversion to a conventional approach is usually required when a bilateral thyroid resection is needed.[24] Because of the high prevalence of multinodular goiter in some countries, this minimally invasive video-assisted thyroidectomy (MIVAT)-related advantage has allowed experienced surgeons to increase the number of patients eligible for a video-assisted procedure.[64,86] In our experience, because of the high prevalence of goiter in the Italian population, this allows us (in approximately 20% of patients) to treat both parathyroid and thyroid during the same procedure.[64]

Another important advantage over other endoscopic and nonendoscopic minimally invasive techniques is the fact that MIVAP allows full exploration for deeply located inferior pathologic glands (i.e., retrosternal and intrathymic) because the endoscope is not limited in its position by any external device. Because it is handheld, it can be rotated and placed in any direction to allow exploration of all neck and upper mediastinum sites despite a very small skin incision.

The minimal access is associated with a better cosmetic result. Moreover, the absence of neck hyperextension and extensive dissections may result in less postoperative pain. Several comparative studies have demonstrated the advantages of VAP in terms of reduced postoperative pain, better cosmetic results, and higher patient satisfaction over both conventional and open nonendoscopic MIP.[73,75]

Despite these advantages and the excellent results in terms of reduced complications and better cure rates, as we discussed earlier, major concerns for the introduction and application of MIVAP in the clinical practice have been raised; these are mainly related to technical and economic issues.

First of all, the availability of specific instrumentation for VAP has been considered a source of additional costs compared with conventional surgery. However, endoscopic tools (e.g., endoscopes, videos, light sources, cameras, etc.) are now available in almost all operating rooms. Moreover, specific small instruments for MIVAP are reusable, and their cost can be amortized with use.

Operative time, which was considered one of the limitations of the technique, has been demonstrated to decrease with increasing experience and even to rival with that of conventional surgery.[103,113] Moreover, a prospective, randomized, small comparative study showed that the operative time for MIVAP was significantly shorter than that for a conventional bilateral exploration[75] and similar to that for an OMIP.[73]

Some criticism may be directed to the number of assistants needed. Indeed, two assistants are necessary to accomplish the procedure: one to hold the endoscope and the other to hold the retractors. This need can be difficult to fulfill in all surgical settings.

The possibility of performing the procedure under locoregional anesthesia, of carrying out concomitant thyroid resection, and of exploring all regions of the neck has extended the indications for MIVAP. However, they are still limited, especially in endemic goiter areas where a large thyroid gland can prevent video-assisted dissection. This is well represented in our experience in an endemic goiter area, where only 37% of patients with PHPT were eligible for MIVAP; this typically occurs because of a large multinodular goiter.[64]

Early on, another technical limitation for the application of the procedure was previous neck surgery. With increasing experience, reoperative neck surgery was also demonstrated to be feasible; patients with contralateral thyroid resection have been successfully approached by MIVAP.[64,103] Another technical limitation concerns large parathyroid adenomas (>30 mm). Indeed, the dissection and extraction of large adenomas through a small incision can result in capsule rupture with the theoretic risk of parathyromatosis. Although this presents a theoretic and significant risk, no such cases have thus far been reported.

MIP: EVIDENCE-BASED RECOMMENDATIONS

The evidence-based medical literature is frequently used to recommend specific treatments.[115,116] A well-conducted prospective randomized trial is assigned the highest level of evidence. Unfortunately, in parathyroid surgery, there are only a few prospective randomized studies (level of evidence 1b associated with a grade A level of recommendation).[117]

Four randomized trials comparing minimally invasive open parathyroidectomy with standard BNE have been published.[71,72,74,76] These studies strongly demonstrated that UNE, under both general[71,74,76] and locoregional anesthesia,[72] is associated with shorter operative time,[71,72] with the same cure rate at short-[74] and long-term follow-up.[76]

One prospective randomized trial (level of evidence 1b, grade of recommendation A) compared MIVAP with BNE in terms of operative time, postoperative pain, complications, cosmetic result, and costs.[75] MIVAP is associated with a significant decrease in operative time, postoperative pain, and postoperative inactivity period. The personal satisfaction relating to the cosmetic outcome was significantly superior in the group of patients who underwent MIVAP. No significant differences between the two procedures were found in terms of overall costs.[75]

A larger nonrandomized case control study with historical controls matched for age and sex has been designed by Henry et al.[95] (level III evidence, grade of recommendation B) to compare the results of VAP-LA versus BNE. Statistically significant advantages were registered in favor of the VAP-LA group with regard to the analgesic requirement and patient satisfaction with cosmetic outcome.

On the basis of these five studies, MIP should be considered as the initial, safe, and cost-effective surgical approach for the treatment of at least a portion of patients with sporadic PHPT. Single-gland excision through a limited, selective exploration does not imply an increased risk of persistent/recurrent PHPT compared with BNE. Importantly, the prevalence and severity of postoperative hypocalcemia seem to be lowered by MIP (grade A recommendation).[30]

Please see the Expert Consult website for more discussion of this topic.

It is important to understand that MIVAP allows for BNE without converting the procedure to open conventional surgery. This allows for the option of avoiding intraoperative PTH. A randomized trial (level of evidence 1b, grade of recommendation A)[114] compared bilateral neck MIVAT exploration versus focused parathyroidectomy plus intraoperative PTH reviewing outcomes, operative time, and costs. The results of the study prove that endoscopic bilateral exploration can be performed while avoiding the time and the costs of intraoperative PTH with the same effectiveness of endoscopic-focused parathyroidectomy with intraoperative PTH monitoring. The major drawback of such an approach consists of the potential risk of unjustified removal of enlarged but not pathologic parathyroid glands.[114]

Finally, only two prospective randomized trials compared the two most widely accepted approaches for MIP: OMIP and MIVAP. In the first paper, published by Barczyński et al.,[73] the two minimally invasive techniques showed similar results with regard to cure and morbidity rates, operative time, postoperative hospital stay, and long-term satisfaction with the cosmetic outcome. In the MIVAP group, there was an easier recognition of the RLN, a significantly lower pain intensity within the 24 hours after surgery, a lower analgesic request rate and analgesic consumption, and shorter scar length. Moreover, the MIVAP group was characterized by significantly better physical functioning and a higher early cosmetic satisfaction rate at 1 month after surgery. On the other hand, costs were significantly higher for MIVAP because of the use of endoscopic tools. The second multiinstitutional trial included 143 patients who were randomized to the open (OMIP = 75 patients) or the video-assisted approach (n = 68 patients), by either a central (MIVAP = 26 patients) or a lateral approach (VAP-LA = 42 patients).[112] OMIP was found to be a quicker operation than the video-assisted technique. No significant difference was found in terms of postoperative outcome measures. However, the main limitations of this study reside in its multiinstitutional design and in the fact that at least some of the surgeons involved had not yet reached an adequate level of experience in video-assisted procedures at the time of the study. This could explain the high conversion rate in the video-assisted group (43% overall for the video-assisted group, 25% to BNE, 18% to OMIP) and also the effect of the significant difference in operative time between the two groups.[112]

In conclusion, in the heterogeneous field of MIP, there is evidence suggesting that MIVAP is preferable to OMIP due to better cosmetic outcome, better visualization of the neck structures, and improved pain control.[117] There is also low-level evidence that MIVAP has some advantages over other purely endoscopic procedures for parathyroidectomy and VAP-LA in terms of technical difficulties, the ability to perform a bilateral exploration, and associated procedures on the thyroid gland.[117] Although these data concerning initial results are encouraging, longer follow-up studies to confirm the safety of this procedure in terms of cure with respect to conventional surgery are needed.

It has been demonstrated that MIVAP is also feasible in cases of secondary and familial hyperparathyroidism.[87,105-107] However, additional well-designed studies are necessary to demonstrate its real advantages over conventional BNE in MGD.

REFERENCES

For a complete list of references, go to expertconsult.com.

59

Intraoperative PTH Monitoring During Parathyroid Surgery

Denise Carneiro-Pla, Phillip K. Pellitteri

INTRODUCTION

Intraoperative parathyroid hormone monitoring (IPM) has been used since the 1990s to guide the excision of abnormal parathyroid glands in patients with sporadic primary hyperparathyroidism (SPHPT). Currently, many high-volume parathyroid surgeons use IPM, selectively or routinely, to guide parathyroidectomy in patients with primary hyperparathyroidism (PHPT).[1]

This surgical adjunct has helped change the operative approach to parathyroidectomy from the traditional bilateral neck exploration (BNE) (which had visualization of all parathyroids and excision of enlarged glands based on the surgeon's subjective judgment of gland size) to a minimally invasive parathyroidectomy with removal of only the hypersecreting gland(s); this helps preserve all normally functioning tissue. This less invasive approach to parathyroidectomy, safely achieved with the help of IPM, is not only as successful as BNE but also allows for surgery in an ambulatory setting with less neck dissection, often with fewer glands excised, shorter operative time, and fewer postoperative complications (see Chapter 56, Standard Bilateral Parathyroid Exploration).

The goals of this chapter are the following: (1) to discuss the practical issues regarding the use of intraoperative PTH monitoring during parathyroidectomy, (2) to suggest guidelines for interpreting intraoperative PTH levels based on the available published data and the authors' personal experiences, and (3) to give an overview of the current controversies associated with the use of this surgical adjunct.

HISTORY OF INTRAOPERATIVE PTH MONITORING

Since the 1990s, a significant volume of information has been gleaned regarding the application of this methodology as well as its influence on the conduct of parathyroidectomy in various parathyroid disorders. The basic premise justifying the use of such a test resides in the ability to rapidly measure the hyperfunction of abnormal parathyroid tissue in the operating room.

The discovery of parathyroid hormone (PTH) and the subsequent development of assays to accurately measure levels in both the physiologic and pathologic state has been earmarked by a number of major events, which together have led to the current application of the intraoperative measurement of PTH in managing surgical parathyroid disease. In 1923, a general surgeon, A.M. Hanson, was the first to demonstrate presence of the hormone. The extract of the hormone, which he developed from bovine parathyroid glands, was used successfully in treating experimental tetany.[2,3] Nearly 3½ decades after its initial discovery, two groups working independently were able to further characterize this extract as PTH. Rasmussen and Craig from the Rockefeller Institute in New York, as well as G.D. Aurbach in Boston, extracted a stable parathyroid polypeptide and demonstrated that the hypercalcemic properties previously described resided in a single hormonal substance.[3-5] Berson and Yalow, working at the Bronx VA Hospital in 1963, in collaboration with Aurbach and John Potts from the National Institutes of Health (NIH), described a radioimmunoassay for PTH.[6] In an effort to raise an antibody that recognized human PTH specifically, Eric Reiss and Janet Canterbury, working at the Michael Reese Hospital in Chicago in 1965, harvested bovine parathyroid glands and injected the extract into various experimental animals. These early efforts were unsuccessful. However, after many trials, an antibody to bovine parathyroid was obtained that had a high affinity for human PTH in experimental chickens.[7] Using this antibody, these investigators developed an assay with satisfactory identification of PTH concentrations in humans.[7]

In 1988, Nussbaum et al. modified the original immunoradiometric assay (IRMA) by increasing the temperature of incubation and employing a kinetic enhancer; these changes decreased the turnover time to approximately 15 minutes.[8] In this initial report, these investigators described the first use of PTH monitoring during parathyroidectomy, although the patients in their series underwent BNE, and PTH was measured postoperatively. Although the reporting of this clinical experience appeared to be of interest clinically, it was not readily accepted as an alternative to the existing practice of conventional BNE, especially given that operative success rates in the treatment of PHPT were approximately 95%. Flentje et al. modified the PTH assay by decreasing the laboratory turnaround time to 1 hour and attempted to use it perioperatively in 1990.[9] They described PTH level changes during parathyroidectomy and, although measured after the operation, it was clear that PTH levels dropped after excision of the abnormal parathyroid gland. In 1990, Chapuis et al. reported on their series of 13 patients in whom the PTH dropped >70% in 20 minutes after parathyroidectomy by using the IRMA for intraoperative PTH measurement.[10]

An early advocate of the use of IPM in the United States was Dr. George Irvin from the University of Miami. Irvin's initial venture into adding the intraoperative assessment of PTH levels to his surgical practice, by his own admission, came from an operative failure in the early 1990s. After the initial failed parathyroidectomy in this patient, a reexploration was performed at which time a contralateral thyroid lobectomy for an occult second intrathyroidal parathyroid adenoma was carried out. Using a modification of the technique described by Nussbaum, Irvin was able to demonstrate a rapid decline in PTH levels measured intraoperatively after removal of the second parathyroid adenoma.[11] In 1991, Irvin et al. described for the first time a series of 21 patients who had their parathyroidectomies guided exclusively by IPM using an immunoradioisotopic method.[12]

With George Irvin's help in 1996, this rapid assay was converted to an immunochemiluminescence method, and the "quick" PTH assay became commercially available for intraoperative use, which is still the methodology used today. After Irvin's initial publication, which provided impressive clinical justification for the implementation of this methodology, the literature has been replete with increasing reports describing numerous investigations on the use of intraoperative PTH measurement for parathyroid exploration. These pioneers, and especially Dr. Irvin, have changed the surgical management of PHPT as IPM-guided parathyroidectomy has become the approach of choice of many specialized surgeons in the treatment of parathyroid disease.

WHICH PATIENTS BENEFIT FROM IPM-GUIDED PARATHYROIDECTOMY?

IPM has been extensively described and studied in patients with SPHPT, whereas its use in patients with secondary and tertiary hyperparathyroidism as well as in multiple endocrine neoplasia (MEN) requires further investigation as the studies are limited. Postoperative long-term follow-up of these patients to determine which is the optimal intraoperative criteria and protocol to predict cure in these distinct forms of HPT is necessary to establish the use of IPM in these patients.[13-17] IPM can be used to guide parathyroidectomy in isolated familial hyperparathyroidism (HPT) with an acceptable accuracy.[18] However, the results of this surgical adjunct in predicting operative success in patients with parathyroid cancer are not as encouraging.[19] The data and suggested guidelines for the use of IPM methodology discussed in this chapter are best applied for treatment of only SPHPT.

INTRAOPERATIVE PTH MONITORING AS AN ADJUNCT DURING PARATHYROIDECTOMY

The authors use the information of IPM to do the following:
1. Confirm complete excision of all hyperfunctioning parathyroid tissue before the operative procedure is finished, without visualization of normally functioning parathyroid glands.
2. Point out the presence of additional hypersecreting tissue by an insufficient PTH drop, indicating that further neck exploration is required in an attempt to prevent operative failure.
3. Differentiate parathyroid from nonparathyroid tissues by using biochemical fine-needle aspiration (FNA), to be described in detail later in this chapter.
4. Lateralize the side of the neck harboring the most hypersecreting parathyroid gland by performing differential jugular venous sampling in patients with negative or equivocal preoperative localization studies.

The accuracy of this adjunct in correctly guiding the surgeon to the desired outcome (complete excision of all hyperfunctioning glands and achievement of postoperative eucalcemia) is strongly related to the criteria used to predict such an outcome. Intraoperative PTH assays only measure PTH levels at specific time points during the procedure as determined by the surgeon. It is therefore essential to understand hormone dynamics during parathyroidectomy to properly request blood sampling during the procedure.

IPM PROTOCOL FOR INTRAOPERATIVE BLOOD SAMPLING

A peripheral access with a 16-gauge catheter or arterial line for blood sampling during the procedure is obtained either in the holding area or in the operating room. It is important to ensure that blood can be drawn after access is obtained, especially after the patient's arms are tucked in; positioning may affect satisfactory sampling from an adequately placed line. This access is kept open with saline infusion throughout the procedure, and an intravenous (IV) extension is used to give the anesthesiologist access to the tubing for blood collection at times requested by the surgeon. It is important to instruct the anesthesia team about discarding 10 cc of blood with saline to avoid sample dilution potentially leading to falsely lower PTH levels. Three to 5 cc of whole blood are collected for PTH measurement and are placed in an ethylenediaminetetraacetic acid (EDTA) tube at specific times, including the following:

1. in the operating room before the skin incision is made (preincision),
2. when all blood supply to the suspicious gland is ligated (preexcision or time zero),
3. 5 minutes,
4. 10 minutes, and
5. occasionally, 20 minutes after excision of the suspected abnormal gland.

When peripheral PTH values drop >50% from the highest, either preincision or preexcision levels (10 minutes after removal of all abnormal parathyroid glands), postoperative normal or low calcium levels are predicted with excellent accuracy.[20] While waiting for PTH results to be reported by the laboratory (which can range between 8 and 15 minutes depending on the assay used), the surgeon may proceed with closure of the cervical incision, avoiding manipulation of the remaining parathyroid glands in an effort to minimize the chance of falsely elevating PTH levels, which could result in a delay in hormone drop. Although the 10-minute PTH level fall of >50% is the definitive measurement of postoperative success, the PTH fall of >50% at the 5-minute interval also will be seen in the majority of surgically cured patients. Given this, some surgeons prefer to check a 5-minute level, which if reduced >50% allows the termination of the procedure without further neck exploration or visualization of the remaining, normally-secreting parathyroid glands; this allows the patient to be extubated and sent to the recovery room earlier. By this time, the 10-minute PTH level is reported, confirming operative success. Conversely, if the criterion is not met in the 10-minute sample, the neck is reexplored and the protocol for blood sampling is repeated for each additional excised gland until all hypersecreting tissue is removed as indicated by meeting the criteria.

In cases where the PTH percent drop is not quite sufficient in 10 minutes, but it is significant (~40%), a 20-minute sample can be collected for PTH measurement before the neck is reexplored. However, if there is no significant PTH drop in 5 or 10 minutes, the cervical incision should be reopened promptly to identify and excise additional hypersecreting tissue.

INTRAOPERATIVE SCENARIOS AND TROUBLESHOOTING

1. *Adequate PTH drop after excision of a suspicious gland.* Figure 59.1 shows the hormone dynamic after excision of a single hypersecreting parathyroid gland resulting in adequate PTH drop and operative success. When such a PTH fall is seen, the surgeon can proceed with closure of the cervical incision without visualization or biopsy of the remaining normally secreting parathyroid glands. Frozen section of the excised parathyroid gland is also not necessary because parathyroid tissue excision is confirmed by the adequate PTH drop.
2. *Insufficient PTH drop after excision of a suspicious gland pointing out the presence of multiglandular disease.* Figure 59.2 shows the hormone dynamics in a patient with multiglandular disease. After excision of the first parathyroid gland, the PTH level did not drop adequately, guiding the surgeon to further explore the cervical area for additional hyperfunctioning tissue. Note that the same

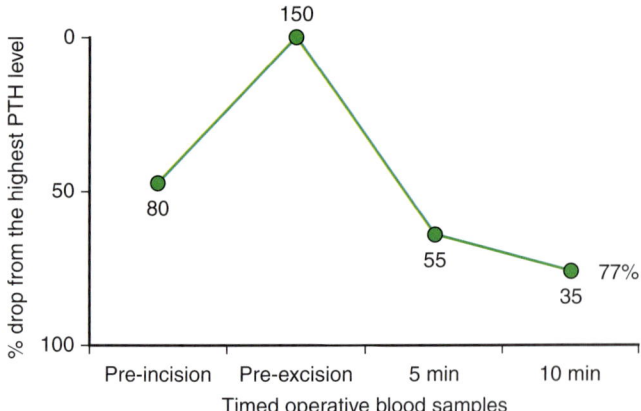

Fig. 59.1 PTH dynamic during excision of a single parathyroid gland resulting in adequate PTH drop correctly predicting operative success for at least 6 months. min, minutes; PTH, parathyroid hormone.

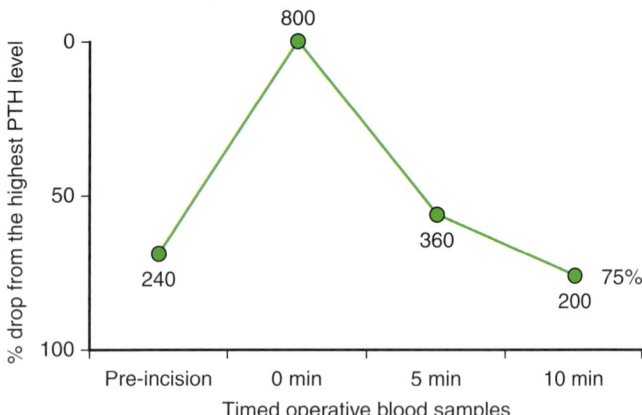

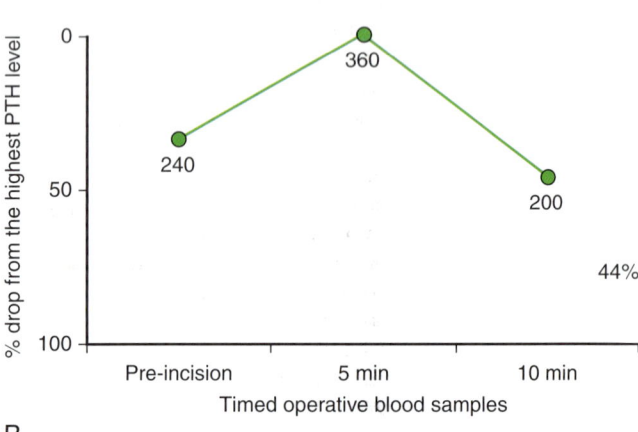

Fig. 59.3 A, The increase in parathyroid hormone (PTH) level at the 0-minute sample as a result of manipulation during parathyroid gland dissection. **B,** An *apparent* insufficient PTH drop if the 0-minute sample was not collected during the parathyroidectomy of this same patient.

protocol for blood sampling is repeated for each excised suspicious tissue until the IPM criterion is met. The PTH level selected to calculate a sufficient PTH drop after an extensive neck dissection should be the last preexcision level or the preincision level, whichever is greater.

3. *Elevation of PTH level at the preexcision/0-minute sample.* Figure 59.3, A, shows the intraoperative hormone dynamic of a patient in whom the manipulation of an abnormal gland during dissection increased the PTH level significantly in the preexcision/0-minute sample. In patients like this, which are seen in about 16% of cases, the importance of collecting both samples (preincision and preexcision/0 minute) to calculate the PTH decline accurately is evident.[20] Figure 59.3, B, shows the same patient's PTH levels and the consequence of not collecting the 0-minute sample leading to a falsely inadequate PTH drop. In such patients, by not registering the peak of the PTH level during manipulation of the parathyroid gland, this *apparent* insufficient PTH drop can lead to unnecessary BNE. The same issue is possible if the preexcision/0-minute sample is obtained too early in the dissection, which will also result in missing the peak of PTH level.

4. *Sufficient PTH drop on the preexcision/0-minute level.* Figure 59.4, A, shows the intraoperative PTH dynamics of a patient in whom the PTH level already met the criterion at the 0-minute sample. This finding indicates that the parathyroid gland's main blood

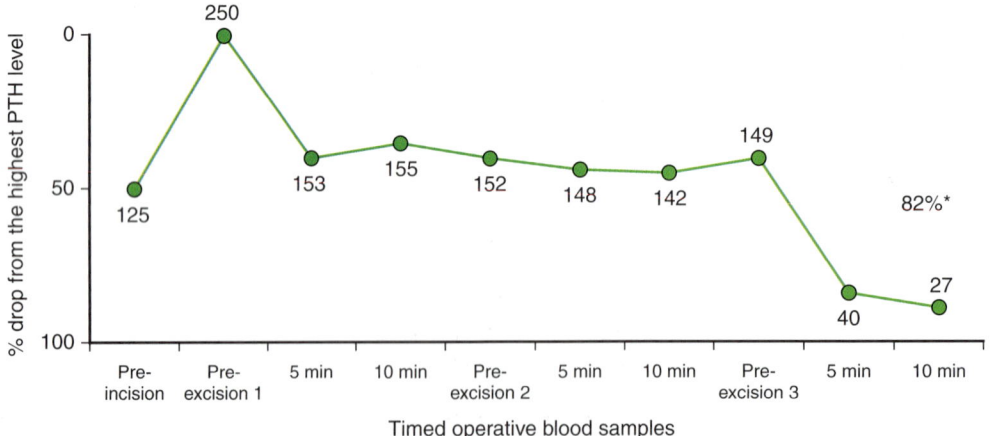

Fig. 59.2 Intraoperative parathyroid hormone (PTH) dynamic of patient with multiglandular disease and insufficient PTH drop after excision of two parathyroid glands. After excision of a third and final hypersecreting gland, PTH drops significantly, assuring complete excision and operative success. min, minutes; PTH, parathyroid hormone. *Note that the percentage PTH drop in this prolonged and extensive neck exploration is calculated from the last preexcision or initial preincision sample.

CHAPTER 59 Intraoperative PTH Monitoring During Parathyroid Surgery

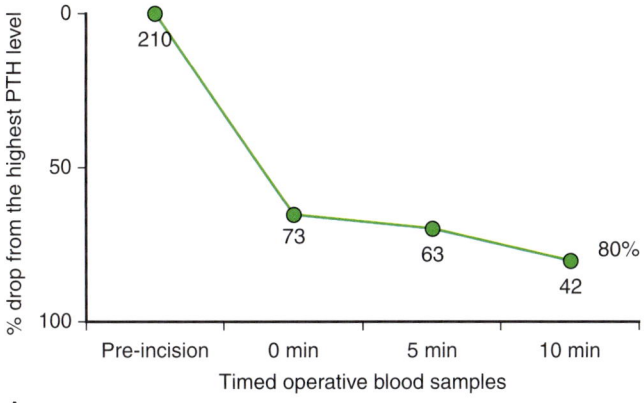

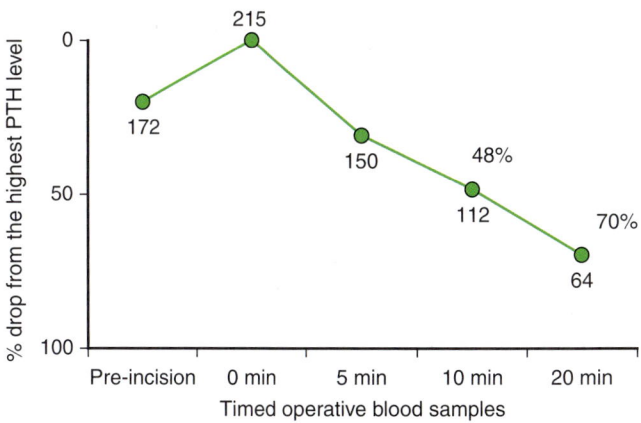

Fig. 59.5 The intraoperative parathyroid hormone (PTH) dynamic of a patient in whom the PTH level does not drop sufficiently in 10 minutes after excision of a suspicious gland; however, sample collection in 20 minutes meets the criteria correctly predicting operative success.

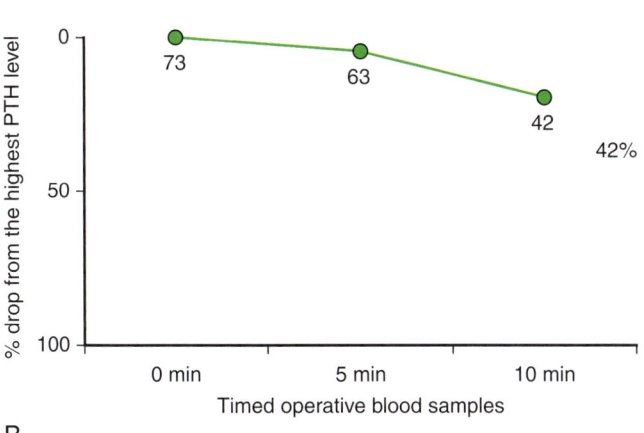

Fig. 59.4 A, The hormone dynamic of a patient in whom the parathyroid hormone (PTH) dropped significantly at the 0-minute sample. **B,** An *apparent* insufficient PTH drop if preincision level would not have been measured.

> **BOX 59.1 Intraoperative PTH Monitoring Recommended Criteria**
>
> **Baseline Values**
> 1. Baseline preincision sample.
> 2. Baseline preexcision sample, taken just before the fully dissected adenoma's vessel is ligated and adenoma is resected.
>
> **Excision Values**
> 1. Five-minute postexcision—majority of patients cured will be >50% of either #1 or #2 (whichever is higher).
> 2. Ten-minute postexcision—most accurate predictor of patients cured if >50% of either #1 or #2 (whichever is higher).
> 3. Twenty-minute postexcision—may be necessary if the 10-minute fall is significant but doesn't fully meet the >50% criteria.

supply was ligated early in the dissection and the PTH has already dropped. In this case, it is clear by the preexcision/0-minute sample that this is the only hypersecreting parathyroid gland, thereby allowing the surgeon to finish the procedure safely. Figure 59.4, B, demonstrates that in cases where the PTH level has already declined significantly in the 0-minute sample (15% of the cases), not measuring the preincision sample might result in an *apparent* insufficient PTH drop, potentially leading to unnecessary further neck exploration.[20]

5. *Delay of intraoperative PTH drop after successful excision of a single hypersecreting parathyroid gland.* Figure 59.5 shows the intraoperative hormone dynamics in a patient with a delayed PTH drop after excision of a single hypersecreting parathyroid gland. In these situations, the PTH declines significantly but does not meet the criteria in the 10-minute sample; a 20-minute value might be helpful in preventing further neck exploration. The 20-minute sample might also be useful to surgeons who require a drop in PTH level >50% and a return to normal range to predict operative success. When the PTH level is very high in the 0-minute sample, it is biochemically impossible for the PTH to return to normal limits in a period of 10 minutes; however, it often occurs 20 minutes after excision of all hypersecreting parathyroid glands (Box 59.1 and Figure 59.6). This scenario may be encountered as well in a patient with preexisting renal insufficiency, whereby metabolic changes can result in a delayed decline in PTH levels

INTRAOPERATIVE CRITERIA IN PREDICTING OPERATIVE SUCCESS

IPM is only as good as the surgeon's interpretation of the intraoperative hormone dynamics and the criteria used to predict a certain outcome. Some have evaluated IPM to predict the size of the remaining glands, postoperative PTH levels associated with eucalcemia, and recurrence of HPT. In the authors' opinion, the goal of parathyroidectomy guided by IPM should be the same as without IPM (i.e., operative success measured by achievement of eucalcemia for at least 6 months after the procedure). Conversely, operative failure is defined by hypercalcemia associated with elevated PTH levels occurring within 6 months of the operation caused by insufficient excision of hypersecreting parathyroid glands. Patients who develop recurrent HPT have hypercalcemia and elevated PTH levels 6 months after a period of eucalcemia; therefore this condition is not a result of insufficient parathyroid tissue excision and operative failure. These definitions are important, not only for surgical outcomes but also in determining the accuracy of IPM in guiding parathyroidectomy in patients with SPHPT. Using these definitions, the accuracy of IPM and the ">50% PTH drop" in predicting postoperative calcium levels are shown in Table 59.1. True positive (TP) is defined as correct prediction of postoperative normal calcium levels for at least 6 months (>50% PTH drop 10 minutes after gland excision); true negative (TN) is the correct prediction of incomplete excision (<50% PTH

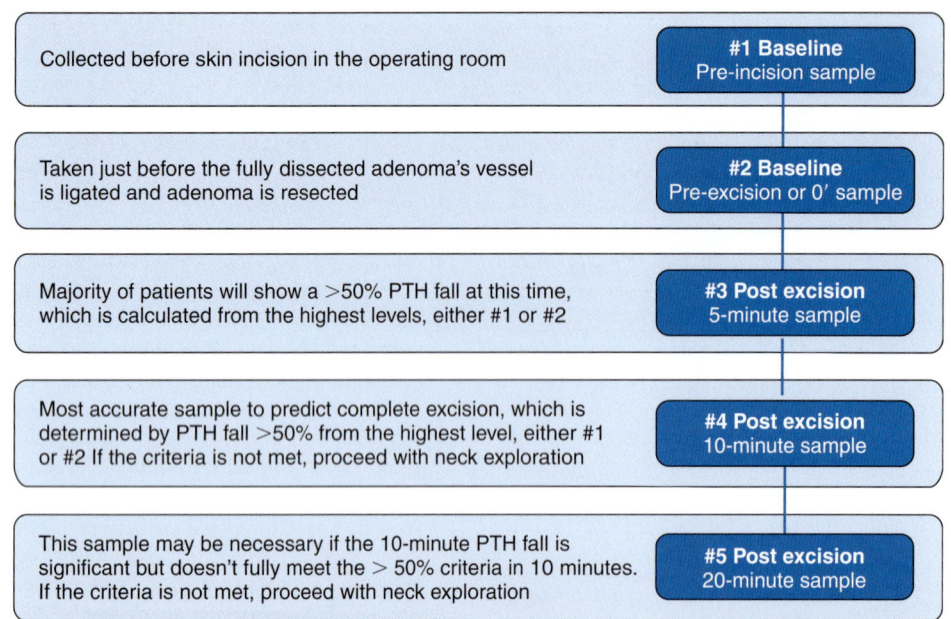

Fig. 59.6 Intraoperative parathyroid hormone (PTH) monitoring recommended criteria.

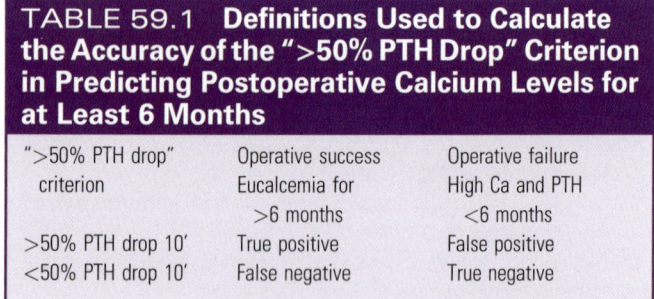

TABLE 59.1 Definitions Used to Calculate the Accuracy of the ">50% PTH Drop" Criterion in Predicting Postoperative Calcium Levels for at Least 6 Months

">50% PTH drop" criterion	Operative success Eucalcemia for >6 months	Operative failure High Ca and PTH <6 months
>50% PTH drop 10′	True positive	False positive
<50% PTH drop 10′	False negative	True negative

10′, 10-minute sample that is collected 10 minutes after gland excision; Ca, total serum calcium level; PTH, parathyroid hormone level.

drop) either by resection of an additional gland(s) or postoperative failure; false positive (FP) is incorrect prediction of eucalcemia (>50% PTH drop) with subsequent postoperative persistent hypercalcemia and high PTH levels within 6 months of the operation; and false negative (FN) is the incorrect prediction of incomplete excision (<50% PTH drop) followed by postoperative eucalcemia without excision of additional hypersecreting glands. Because the intraoperative IPM criteria used is based on the 10-minute sample, any delayed PTH fall in 20 minutes after gland excision with subsequent postoperative eucalcemia should be considered an FN result.

LIMITATIONS OF INTRAOPERATIVE PTH MONITORING WITH THE ">50% PTH DROP" CRITERION

Prediction of Size of the Remaining Normally Secreting Parathyroid Glands

It has been shown that parathyroidectomy guided by the previously described criterion or any more conservative criteria does not predict the macroscopic size of the remaining normally secreting parathyroid glands. Some have used IPM during BNE and have demonstrated that 9% to 19% of the patients will have another enlarged gland found after a sufficient PTH drop after the first gland excision.[21-25] This finding is not surprising because enlarged, albeit normally functioning, parathyroid glands are left in situ after a minimally invasive parathyroidectomy. These enlarged glands in normal patients are often found incidentally during thyroidectomy. The rate of multiglandular disease (MGD) is much lower when parathyroidectomy is guided by function instead of parathyroid gland size (3% to 9% versus 14% to 30%).[13,26-39] However, from the excellent cure rates reported using this modality in guiding the extent of resection, it would appear that those studies advocating conventional BNE and resection of enlarged glands do not necessarily prove that morphologically enlarged glands contribute to operative failure if not excised. Furthermore, it is known that abnormal secretion is not necessarily associated with parathyroid gland size.[40] Despite these reports, no studies using the intraoperative assessment of PTH levels to guide the extent of parathyroidectomy have described a higher operative failure or recurrence rate owing to missed multiglandular disease. In a prospective study by Genc et al., patients with a single positive focus on Tc-99m sestamibi scan or ultrasound scanning underwent either conventional BNE or minimally invasive parathyroid exploration guided exclusively by IPM. With similar operative success rates in both groups, those patients who underwent minimally invasive parathyroidectomy demonstrated a significantly lower incidence of MGD compared with the BNE group, thereby suggesting that not all enlarged glands are physiologically hypersecretory and do not contribute to hypercalcemia.[41] A possible explanation is that one parathyroid tumor may be functionally dominant in some patients, and other enlarged parathyroid glands are relatively quiescent. This concept was illustrated in a prospective randomized study of 40 patients by Miccoli et al.; they evaluated morphologic criteria versus functional criteria in guiding the extent of parathyroidectomy. These investigators found that patients who had parathyroidectomy guided by gland size during BNE demonstrated a higher incidence of MGD (10%) than patients who had parathyroidectomy guided by functional criteria with intraoperative PTH monitoring (0%).[42] Although fewer parathyroid glands were excised in the latter group, the operative success rate was equitable, which suggests that abnormal glands determined by morphologic criteria may not be sufficient to characterize hyperfunction.

The same findings are seen when stricter criteria are used. For example, if the surgeon requires a >50% PTH drop as well as a return to normal range in 10 minutes after excision of a single parathyroid gland, 24% of the patients will be unnecessarily reexplored and only 0.5% will in fact have additional hypersecreting glands that need to be excised to achieve cure.[20] As the criteria become more strict, BNEs are performed more frequently and a greater number of enlarged but normally secreting parathyroid glands are found and excised.[43-45] The disadvantages of BNE are potentially higher complication rates and the development of fibrotic tissue in the central neck, increasing the complexity of a second neck exploration either for thyroid or parathyroid disease. Furthermore, the presence of fewer parathyroid glands and uncertainty of the function of these previously explored glands are critical factors when a second cervical procedure is needed.

Prediction of PTH Levels in Postoperative Normocalcemic Patients

There has been an attempt to predict postoperative PTH levels in eucalcemic patients with IPM.[46] It is known that despite the specific operative approach used (BNE or focused parathyroidectomy guided by IPM), PTH levels are found to be elevated in 8% to 30% of eucalcemic patients after successful parathyroidectomy.[47-50] The majority of these patients will return to normal PTH levels months later, demonstrating that their remaining glands are not autonomously functioning. Bergenfelz and others have suggested that these high PTH levels are compensatory: parathyroid glands are responding to a deficit in total body calcium as well as in some cases vitamin D deficiency.[47,51] Interestingly, there is no difference in intraoperative hormone dynamics found in eucalcemic patients presenting with normal or high postoperative PTH levels.

Late Recurrence

There is no significant difference in intraoperative PTH dynamics between patients with long-term postoperative eucalcemia and those who developed recurrent hypercalcemia.

Secretion of the First Gland Excised in Patients With Multiglandular Disease

The function of the first excised parathyroid gland cannot be determined whether the PTH levels remained elevated after its excision. Intraoperative PTH levels can only determine the function of the glands left in situ and not the secretion status of the initially excised gland(s), which could potentially be an enlarged, normally functioning parathyroid gland(s).

Prevent Operative Failure in All Patients

Unfortunately, operative failure will eventually occur in about 2% to 3% of the patients even when IPM is used. This operative adjunct predicts, but does not prevent, operative failure in patients whose hypersecreting gland(s) could not be found despite careful BNE performed by an experienced surgeon. Furthermore, it cannot prevent operative failure caused by misdiagnosis. It should be noted that operative failure caused by false positive IPM results occurs in only 0.9% of patients using the ">50% PTH drop" criteria.[20]

Protocol and Criteria Dependence

The accuracy of IPM in guiding parathyroidectomy is not only based on the surgeon's interpretation of the intraoperative PTH levels and protocol used, but also on the ever-changing definition of MGD. As we have described previously, some workers determine gland abnormality by size, whereas others use function to determine which glands are abnormal. There are several protocols and criteria used with IPM. Some studies use criteria that require a drop in the PTH level of 60% or 70%, 10 or 15 minutes after gland resection to predict operative success.[8,52,53] Others require a drop in the PTH level and its return to the assays' normal range to predict cure.[31,43,44,54] The different criteria used for evaluating hormone dynamics have different sensitivities and specificities in predicting operative outcome; some are more sensitive and others are more specific. It is up to the surgeon to choose the criteria that best fit his or her practice.

Currently, the authors use a dual set of criteria slightly more stringent to decrease FP and FN results. These include: (1) >50% PTH drop from the highest preoperative level and a return to normal range, or a >65% PTH drop 10 minutes after gland(s) removal predicts complete excision and operative success. If part 1 of the criteria is not met, a 20-minute level is collected and part 2 is applied: (2) >50% PTH drop from the highest baseline levels and a return to normal range 20 minutes after all hyperfunctioning tissue is removed; this predicts operative success.[55,56]

IPM Cost

This surgical adjunct is still costly. However, the use of IPM compensates for its cost by shortening operative time, obviating the need for frozen sections (in most situations), and allowing these procedures to be done in an ambulatory setting. To decrease the cost of IPM, some hospitals place the assay cart at the central laboratory where the system can be used for other purposes, and the technician does not need to be dislocated to the operative room. This surgical adjunct is most helpful in reducing operative times when used as a point-of-care system inside or in close proximity to the operating room, where PTH levels can be reported as soon as possible, allowing real-time operative decisions based on PTH dynamics.

RESULTS OF PARATHYROIDECTOMY GUIDED BY IPM

The implementation of intraoperative PTH monitoring in determining the extent of parathyroidectomy in patients with SPHPT has been demonstrated to be a successful adjunct modality delivering excellent short- and long-term results.[26,31,32,36,57-60] Such intraoperative monitoring of PTH has been accurate in predicting the complete excision of all hyperfunctioning parathyroid glands, with little variation among investigators that use this modality exclusively to guide the extent of resection. The success rate after parathyroidectomy performed by an experienced surgeon exceeds 95% in studies describing traditional BNE.[61,62] Minimally invasive parathyroidectomy guided by IPM results in cure rates similar to conventional bilateral exploration; in some centers, even higher operative success rates are described when IPM is used.[26,31,36,39,57-60] Operative success of minimally invasive parathyroid exploration guided by an IPM range from 97% to 99%, with a lower reported incidence of MGD (3% to 9%) compared with conventional BNE(14% to 30%) (see Chapter 55, Principles in Surgical Management of Primary Hyperparathyroidism).[13,26-39]

Successful parathyroidectomy is achieved with unilateral neck exploration in >80% of patients, usually performed with smaller incisions, less neck dissection, and as ambulatory procedures.

The presence of MGD may be suspected in a subset of patients for whom the preoperative baseline index level of serum intact PTH is low. Patients with low levels (<100 pg/mL) were found to demonstrate a 20% incidence of MGD compared with an 8% incidence in those patients exhibiting higher baseline index PTH levels above 100 pg/mL in this investigation. Further, the kinetic profile of patients with a low baseline level demonstrated a significantly lower percentage decline after removal of the last identified abnormal parathyroid gland, which suggests that correlation between intraoperative PTH findings and complete resection may be inconsistent in predicting operative success in this population. Careful evaluation of preoperative biochemical profiles represents an important consideration in surgically managing patients with HPT. It is clear from the current body of information gleaned from the experience, with IPM as a guide to determine the extent of parathyroid gland resection, that this modality is highly accurate in predicting a successful outcome after neck exploration for the majority of patients with PHPT.

OTHER APPLICATIONS FOR INTRAOPERATIVE RAPID PTH ASSAYS

Biochemical Fine-Needle Aspiration

This useful technique differentiates parathyroid gland from other tissues during parathyroidectomy.[63,64] PTH levels are measured in the tissue sample obtained from FNA and differentiate parathyroid glands from other structures such as thyroid nodules and lymph nodes with a specificity of 100%. A 25-gauge needle attached to a syringe is used to collect the tissue sample. The aspirated content in the needle is diluted with 1 cc of saline solution, centrifuged for 10 seconds, and the supernatant is used for PTH measurement. This technique is faster than frozen section if the rapid assay is used as a point-of-care system, which can be very helpful when gland identification is difficult—for example, in the case of an intrathyroidal parathyroid or a lesion that could be a thyroid nodule versus a subcapsular parathyroid gland.

Differential Internal Jugular Venous Sampling

This technique, which is positive in 70% to 81% of cases, can guide the surgeon to the side of the neck harboring the most hypersecreting parathyroid gland in patients with negative or equivocal preoperative localization studies.[65-69] Before skin incision, and in a vein location as caudal as possible, 3 mL of whole blood is collected from both internal jugular veins under ultrasound guidance. PTH levels are then measured in both jugular vein samples as well as on the initially collected sample from the peripheral access. Figure 59.7 demonstrates a positive differential jugular venous sampling in a patient with a right-sided hypersecreting parathyroid gland. This intraoperative method of lateralization allows unilateral neck exploration in most patients with preoperative negative localization studies when associated with IPM. Recently, this lateralization method was brought to the office setting; this allows the surgeon to identify the side of the neck containing the most hypersecreting parathyroid gland with an overall accuracy of 84% in patients with negative or equivocal preoperative localization studies.[70]

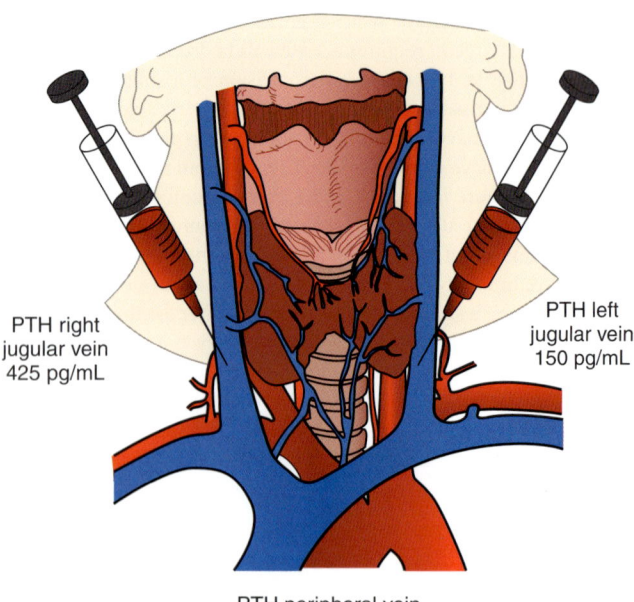

Fig. 59.7 The results of intraoperative parathyroid hormone (PTH) differential jugular venous sampling in a patient with a preoperative negative localization study and a hypersecreting parathyroid gland on the right side.

SUMMARY

IPM is a useful surgical adjunct during parathyroidectomy for the treatment of PHPT and is becoming the standard of care in many centers specializing in parathyroid surgery. There are many advantages of parathyroidectomy guided by IPM, namely, focused dissection with similar or even higher operative success rates compared with traditional BNE. This less extensive operative approach is usually performed with shorter operative times as well as with fewer risks and complications. However, to achieve such excellent results, the surgeon needs to be aware of hormone dynamics during parathyroidectomy and carefully choose the protocol and IPM criteria that best fit his or her practice. Understanding the nuances of IPM will provide intraoperative confidence in predicting operative success and preventing failure in cases of unsuspected MGD while safely limiting neck exploration in most patients with SPHPT. Parathyroidectomy guided by IPM for the treatment of SPHPT is safe, highly successful, less invasive, and associated with lower risks than BNE; therefore IPM represents an ideal option for the treatment of primary hyperparathyroidism.

REFERENCES

For a complete list of references, go to expertconsult.com.

Surgical Management of Multiglandular Parathyroid Disease

Michael Stechman, Anders Bergenfeltz, David Scott-Coombes

Albright's 1934 description of primary water clear cell hyperplasia, that involving all four parathyroids represents the first recognition of the concept of primary hyperparathyroidism (PHPT) due to multiple gland disease (MGD) rather than single-gland disease.[1] Although the incidence of this now-unusual condition was to decline, the "New Entity in the Surgery of Hyperparathyroidism," known as primary chief cell hyperplasia, was described in Cope's landmark 1958 paper.[2] Even then, both authors postulated that the phenomenon of hyperparathyroidism (HPT) due to MGD might be the result of an extrinsic stimulus acting on the parathyroids. Cope also commented on the histologic similarities of adenomas and chief cell hyperplasia and the diagnostic uncertainty that this occasioned. In his later description of the surgical management of 104 cases of PHPT due to hyperplasia, he demonstrated that subtotal resection of 3.5 glands (which left a remnant of 30 to 50 mg of viable tissue) was the treatment of choice for this condition.[3]

Since then, the advent of preoperative parathyroid localization has resulted in a paradigm shift in the approach to single-gland disease: from bilateral cervical exploration (BCE) to a focused approach. The shift has resulted in fewer four-gland explorations. Conversely, patients with negative localization are more likely to have smaller parathyroid tumors and more often have MGD. The diagnosis of PHPT with mild aberration or even normal serum calcium levels means that patients with negative imaging now account for one-fifth of patients referred with PHPT. One national study that investigated the outcomes for parathyroidectomy in unlocalized disease reported a 13% negative exploration rate and persistent HPT (surgical failure) in 18%.[4]

Therefore parathyroidectomy for MGD is complex and associated with a higher operative failure compared with single-gland disease. Surgery in this setting poses several challenges; the diagnosis is often not clear until well into the neck exploration because preoperative localization is rarely helpful. Furthermore, hyperplastic glands are typically much smaller than solitary parathyroid adenomas; therefore they are more difficult to identify. At times, it can be difficult to distinguish a small hyperplastic gland from a normal parathyroid. Lastly, subtotal resection with or without thymectomy requires more surgical experience and judgment compared with excision of a solitary adenoma. For these reasons, consideration should be given toward centralizing the management of patients predicted to have MGD, including those with negative preoperative localization, to high-volume centers.

In this chapter, we discuss the pathology and etiology of sporadic multiglandular parathyroid disease and the rationale for the different surgical approaches used in the management of this specific condition.

DEFINITION AND INCIDENCE

Although 80% to 90% of patients presenting with PHPT have disease that is due to a single adenoma, the remainder of patients will have more than one diseased gland encountered at surgery, termed MGD. A systematic review of more than 22,000 patients determined the incidence of MGD PHPT to be 9.84% with 5.74% patients affected by multiple gland hyperplasia and 4.14% affected by double adenomas.[5] However, despite the large number of patients included in this study, its results highlight the wide variation in the reported incidence of MGD (9% to 26%, Table 60.1)[6-11] and the varying definitions of MGD. This disparity is due, in part, to whether parathyroid glands are designated abnormal based upon their macroscopic appearance, pathologic criteria, genetic differences, or endocrine functionality. Data are further confounded by the extent to which abnormal glands are sought in the era of more limited parathyroid exploration.

MACROSCOPIC AND MICROSCOPIC PATHOLOGY OF ABNORMAL GLANDS

Visual appearance has long been the standard for identifying abnormal parathyroid glands via BCE. Although it is reliable, the technique necessitates extensive surgical experience, a sound knowledge of parathyroid embryology, and knowledge of the likely location of eutopic and ectopic glands.

The normal parathyroid measures 6mm in length, is pale-tan in color, oval-shaped, and possesses a well-defined capsule, allowing it to "float" independently in the perithyroidal fat. The average weight is 40 to 60 mg. In contrast, pathologic, glands are enlarged (weighing ≥80 to 100 mg) and assume a more rounded, bilobed, or even multi-lobulated appearance (Figures 60.1 and 60.2). The softer consistency and yellow-brown or brown-reddish color on sectioning of parathyroid tissue sets it apart from the grayish cut surface of a lymph node and the firmer consistency of the dark brick red thyroid gland (Figure 60.3). The finding of one enlarged gland in the presence of three other normal glands is indicative of single adenoma or uniglandular disease. Conversely, it can usually be presumed that the presence of two, three, or four enlarged glands signifies MGD.

Double Adenoma

Encountered in between 3 and 12% of explorations for PHPT,[7,9,12,13] there is debate as to whether this entity represents the synchronous or asynchronous occurrence of two distinct adenomas or asymmetric four-gland hyperplasia.[14] It is argued that, because the hypercalcemia rates after double adenoma excision are similar, albeit slightly higher

TABLE 60.1 Variation in Reported Incidence of Multiple Gland Disease

Year	Center	Operative Approach	Intraoperative PTH used?	No. of Patients Studied	Double Adenoma (%)	Hyperplasia (%)	Overall MGD	Ref.
1956–1990	Uppsala, Sweden	BCE	No	659	77 (11.7)	54 (8.2)	19.9%	12
1982–1992	San Francisco, USA	BCE	No	416	49 (11.8)	58 (13.9)	25.7%	9
2001–2013	Wisconsin, USA	Focused and BCE	Yes	1402	124 (8.8)	181 (12.9)	21.7%	6
1999–2009	Ann Arbor, USA	Focused	Yes	1855	Not stated		13%	8
1990–2013	Sydney and Melbourne, Australia	Focused and BCE	No	4569	519 (11.3)	181 (3.9)	15.2%	10
1993–2010	Leuven, Belgium	BCE	No	698	46 (6.6)	17 (2.4)	9%	7
2004–2014	Cardiff, United Kingdom	BCE and Focused	Yes	552	Not stated		10.8%	11

BCE, bilateral cervical exploration; PTH, parathyroid hormone; MGD, multiple gland disease.

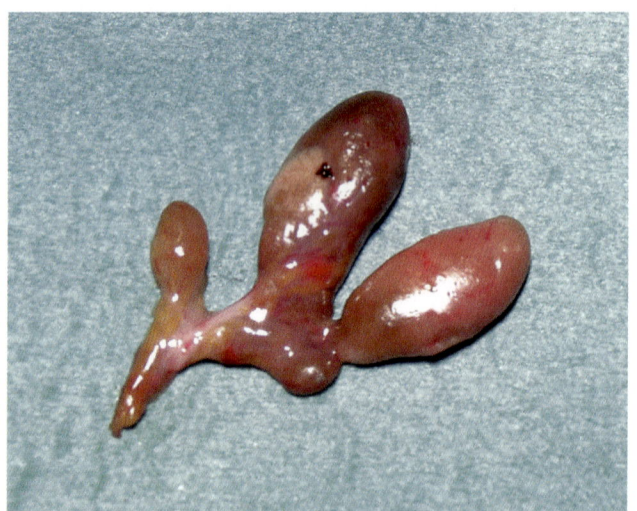

Fig. 60.1 Multilobulated diseased parathyroid gland. Part of this gland may easily be missed during parathyroid surgery.

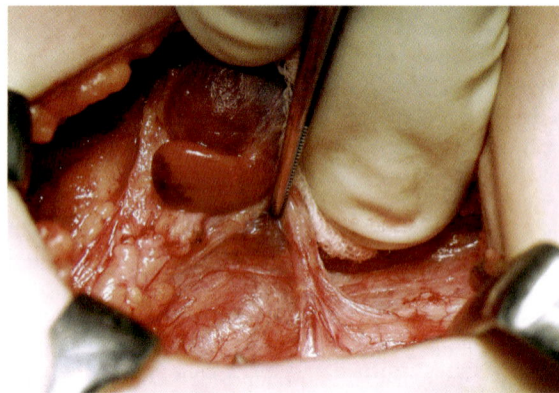

Fig. 60.3 Pathologic glands in a 13-year-old patient with secondary HPT. Initially, the inferior gland is inferiorly descended and hidden by the pretracheal fascia from where it can be pulled up.

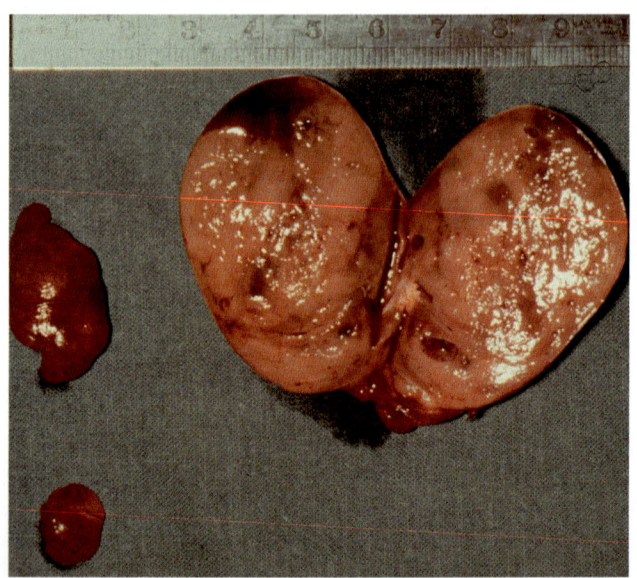

Fig. 60.2 Asymmetric glandular enlargement in a patient with MEN 1-associated HPT (ruler in centimeters).

than those observed in patients with uniglandular disease (2% to 4% for double adenoma versus 1% to 2% for single adenoma), it is most likely that patients with double adenoma comprise a heterogenous group of patients with true adenomas and asymmetric four-gland hyperplasia.[6]

Four-Gland Hyperplasia

The most frequent manifestation of MGD in primary HPT, chief cell hyperplasia affecting all 4 glands, is sporadic in approximately 75% of the patients; however, it may develop from a background of long-term lithium therapy for bipolar illness, or it may be inherited as part of a multiple endocrine neoplasia (MEN) syndrome (see Chapter 62, Parathyroid Management in the MEN Syndromes). Secondary four-gland parathyroid hyperplasia also develops as an inevitable result of chronic renal failure (see Chapter 61, Surgical Management of Secondary and Tertiary Hyperparathyroidism). In chief-cell hyperplasia, size-discrepancy between individual glands is usually marked; enlarged, obviously abnormal glands will commonly be found to coexist with smaller, apparently normal ones (Figures 60.2 and 60.4). Nodularity and variable growth patterns are generally more obvious in the enlarged hyperplastic glands; frequently, one or several nodules appear to have

CHAPTER 60 Surgical Management of Multiglandular Parathyroid Disease

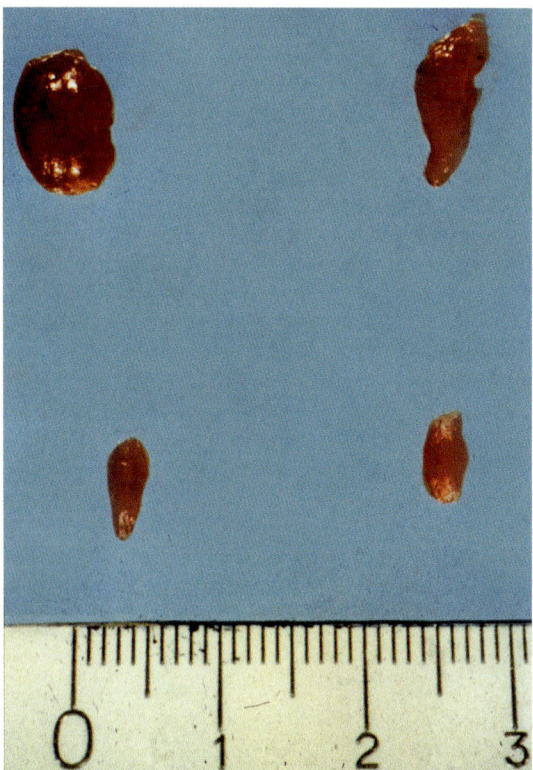

Fig. 60.4 Parathyroid glands in patient with borderline hypercalcemia and hyperplasia with minimal glandular enlargement (autopsy case) (ruler in centimeters).

EXTENT OF PARATHYROID EXPLORATION AND DIAGNOSIS OF MGD

The presence of MGD can be reliably diagnosed as BCE if more than one enlarged gland is present. However, it is less clear whether all enlarged glands are hyperfunctioning. The modern-day preeminence of scan-directed parathyroidectomy has raised questions about whether functionality can be assumed based upon appearance and whether it is clinically relevant.[20] Historically, centers that undertake BCE have tended to quote higher rates of MGD (>20%)[12,21,22] compared with centers undertaking focused surgery based on preoperative localization scans (i.e., minimally invasive parathyroidectomy [MIP] or unilateral exploration), where the rate of MGD is reported to be around 5% to 10%.[11,23] The accepted explanation for this discrepancy is that enlarged-yet-nonfunctioning glands are left in situ during scan-directed surgery. This is borne-out by the observations that normocalcemia rates after BCE and focused surgery are approximately equivalent[24] (2.3% and 3.7% respectively) and that the recurrence rate after focused surgery with intraoperative PTH is less than 3% during long-term follow-up of 10 years, rather than the 10% to 15% predicted by experience with BCE.[13,20] These data suggest that although it is highly likely that enlarged glands remain in situ after targeted surgery, they are not the cause of recurrent disease in any clinically significant way.

Therefore the definition of MGD may implicitly depend on the extent of surgical exploration (e.g., minimally invasive, unilateral or bilateral), whether intraoperative PTH levels decline after parathyroidectomy, and the failure to obtain postoperative normocalcemia, despite removal of a pathologic gland.

acquired more pronounced growth advantage or may even occupy the entire gland.[15] Cases with modest hypercalcemia commonly exhibit less pronounced glandular enlargement and less variability between glands (see Figure 60.4) but typically still show signs of micronodular hyperplasia in the smaller glands.[16]

HISTOPATHOLOGICAL CRITERIA FOR ADENOMA AND HYPERPLASIA

Pathologic examination of excised parathyroid tissue can determine whether or not it is abnormal. Normal parathyroids are composed of chief cells rich in cytoplasmic fat droplets, which are notable for their positive Oil-red O staining; these droplets are interspersed with stromal fat, which increases with age and patient obesity.[15] Conversely, parathyroid adenomas excised from patients with PHPT demonstrate encapsulated nodules composed of chief cells, a prominent absence of cytoplasmic lipid droplets, and may exhibit a rim of compressed and lipid-rich parathyroid tissue, which is best seen at the vascular pole of the gland.[17] The presence of these changes is pathognomonic of parathyroid adenoma, although the absence of a rim does not exclude adenoma.[18]

Parathyroid hyperplasia affects multiple glands, usually all four. Typically, the glands are enlarged with diffuse, nodular or mixed, predominantly chief cell hyperplasia. They may also frequently contain foci of oxyphil cells and very occasionally clear cells. Larger nodules may exhibit reduced fat content and mimic adenomas by flattening a rim of suppressed tissue at their boundary. For this reason, distinguishing histologically between adenoma and hyperplasia may be difficult or impossible. The distinction may be particularly difficult if only one gland is sent for evaluation, and the status of the remaining glands is unknown to both surgeon and pathologist,[19] which is often the case in focused exploration (Figure 60.5).

TUMOR CLONALITY IN UNIGLANDULAR AND MULTIPLE GLAND DISEASE

The somatic mutation theory of tumorigenesis predicts that parathyroid adenomas in sporadic PHPT are monoclonal expansions derived from one transformed parathyroid cell, whereas parathyroid hyperplasia describes a reactive polyclonal expansion due to an exogenous stimulus.[19,25] Therefore clonality would be expected to distinguish adenoma and hyperplasia. However, genetic studies have yielded conflicting results, with some authors determining that parathyroid adenomas are polyclonal,[26] monoclonal and polyclonal,[27] purely monoclonal,[28] and predominantly polyclonal with only a minority found to be truly monoclonal.[29] Although it is possible that the differences in results derived in these studies may in part be due to the research methodologies employed, they also involved small numbers of patients. A more recent prospective study examining the clonal status of more than 100 patients with apparent adenomas determined that up to 46% were polyclonal.[25] The study also examined clinical, operative, and pathologic data on those with mono- and polyclonal tumors; no statistically significant differences were found in terms of age, race, body mass index (BMI), bone mineral density, preoperative biochemistry, and localization results between patients with monoclonal and polyclonal tumors. However, as might be expected, the incidence of MGD was significantly greater in the polyclonal group (23% versus 7%, $p = 0.039$), and patients with polyclonal tumors undergoing unilateral exploration were less likely to have MGD identified at surgery than those undergoing BCE (1 of 16 patients versus 8 of 14 patients, $p = 0.025$). The authors concluded that focused surgery in patients with polyclonal tumors was likely to result in abnormal glands being left in situ, but patients with polyclonal tumors were not discernably different in terms of their preoperative parameters.

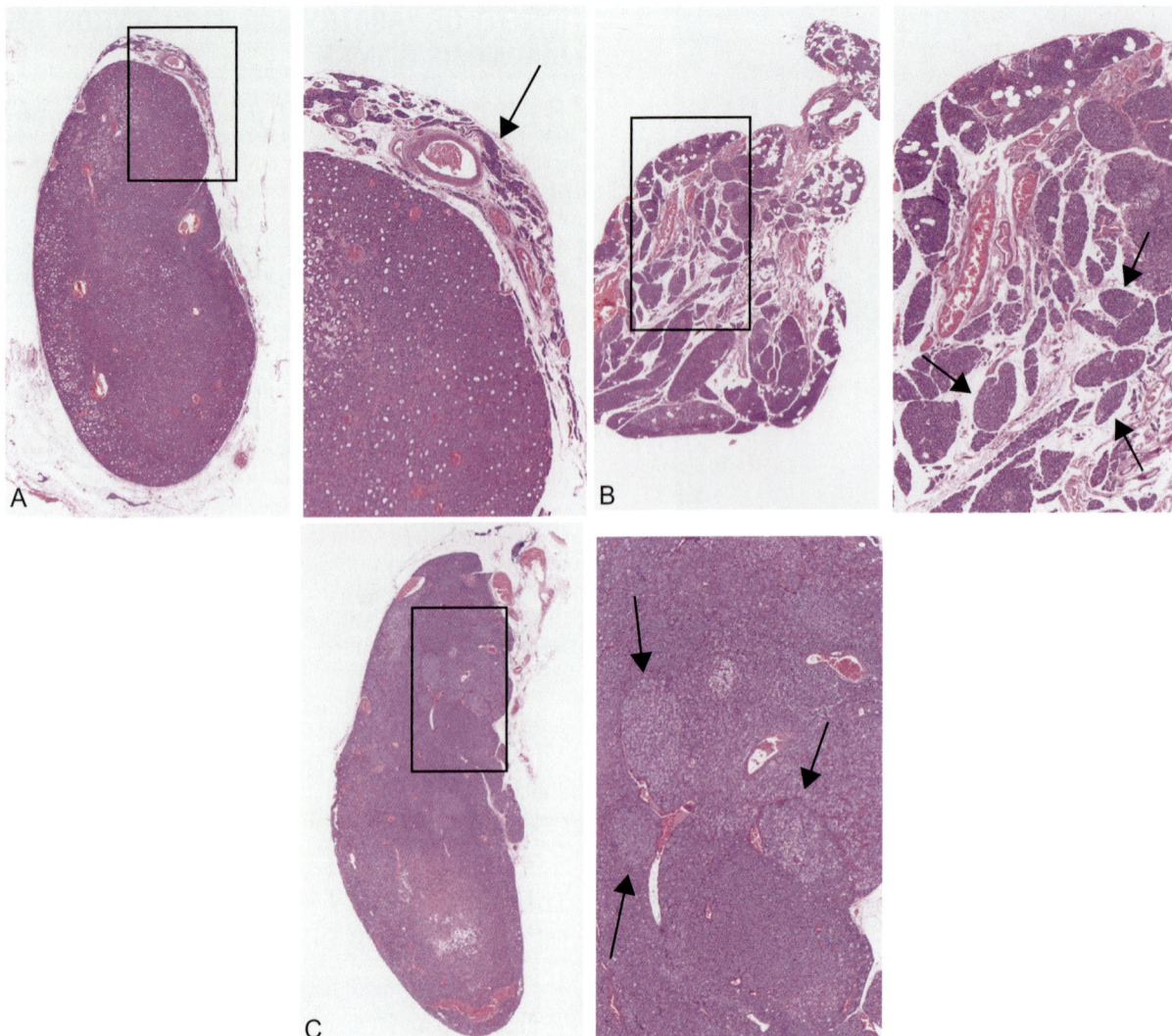

Fig. 60.5 Distinguishing a chief cell parathyroid adenoma (**A**), with a clear rim of compressed normal parathyroid (**A**, right panel, *arrow*), from a nodular hyperplastic gland (**B**), with multiple separate hyperplastic nodules (**B**, right panel, *arrows*), is usually straightforward. Tumor (**A**) weighed 2110 mg and was excised from a 66-year-old male patient with PHPT. A single enlarged parathyroid was seen on MIBI and USS. Tumor (**B**) was one of four enlarged parathyroids seen at surgery in a 63-year-old female patient with PHPT. She was successfully treated with a subtotal parathyroidectomy. Panel (**C**) shows a 780 mg tumor removed from a 30-year old female patient with renal stones and a single enlarged gland on MIBI and USS. Although it is composed predominantly of chief cells, there is some nodularity (**C**, right panel, *arrows*) with scattered oxyphil cells, and no compressed rim of normal parathyroid tissue. Such appearances may be compatible with an adenoma if the other three glands are normal. However, those glands were not seen at surgery because a focused parathyroidectomy was performed. This exemplifies the difficulty with which pathologists are often faced, particularly if operative information is limited. All three patients were normocalcemic on review ≥6 months after surgery. (Images courtesy Dr. A.M. Boyde, Consultant Histopathologist, University Hospital of Wales, Cardiff.)

ETIOLOGY AND RISK FACTORS FOR MGD

Age and Gender

Because of the preponderance for MGD in inherited PHPT, one might suppose that four-gland hyperplasia would be more common in younger patients. Indeed, in one series 465 patients, MGD was found to be twice as common in patients aged less than 40 years compared with those older than 40 years of age (22.9% versus 11% respectively).[30] However, this difference disappeared once patients with inherited disease were removed from the analysis (12.5% versus 10%), and no gender difference was noted either. Double adenomas have been observed to occur in older patients and cited as a factor in recurrent PHPT in two large studies.[6,9] The evidence on increasing age as a factor in hyperplastic MGD is mixed; in both of the latter studies on double adenoma, hyperplasia occurred in slightly younger patients (median age less than 60 years). In contrast, a more recent study reported that the rate of MGD in patients older than 65 years was double that of those patients under 65 years of age (24% versus 12%, $p = 0.001$).[31] During follow-up, older patients also had a lower normocalcemia rate (93% versus 95%, $p = 0.27$). Again, there were no gender differences. The authors suggested that planned BCE should be considered in older patients, especially if a small gland was localized on preoperative scans. Therefore when considered as a whole, the evidence suggests that increasing age is a risk factor for MGD, particularly double adenoma.

Diet and Digestive Disorders and Diabetes

It is well recognized that vitamin D deficiency, chronically low calcium intake,[32] and raised BMI[33] result in compensatory secondary HPT usually in the presence of eucalcemia. For nearly 60000 women in a prospective cohort study of nearly that lasted 22 years, the risk of PHPT was found to be inversely related to calcium intake; a high calcium intake was protective against the onset of PHPT (RR 0.56, 95% CI 0.37 to 0.86). A retrospective review of more than 1300 consecutive patients with PHPT treated surgically, of whom 15% had MGD, found raised BMI to be associated with MGD (BMI 30 to 39.9: OR 1.5, 95% CI 1.2 to 2.5 and BMI $\geq$40: OR 1.8, 95% CI 1.3 to 3.1).[34] Furthermore, gastrointestinal malabsorption secondary to celiac disease,[35] bariatric surgery, chronic pancreatitis, and diabetes are also risk factors for PHPT.[36] Recently, a Scandinavian study demonstrated an independent association between diabetes and MGD (OR 2.97, 95% CI 1.4 to 6.3).[37] However, although population-based studies suggest a causal link between these disorders and HPT, the underlying mechanisms by which a normal physiologic response to an exogenous stimulus results in dysregulated PTH secretion and hypercalcemia remains elusive. Furthermore, although one would expect MGD hyperplasia to be more prevalent in patients who develop PHPT on the background of such metabolic alterations, apart from the findings in obese patients and those with diabetes, the data are inconsistent. Similarly, there are no clear mechanistic insights into to how these disorders lead to MGD PHPT at present.

Exposure to Radiation

A causal link between radiation exposure to the neck and PHPT was first postulated when patients treated with radiotherapy for tuberculous adenitis in the 1930s and 1940s were followed-up with in the 1970s; up to 15% of the patients had evidence of HPT;[38] which appeared to be dose-related and may explain why other investigators have failed to demonstrate a link.[39] The subsequent report that 25% of the so-called "liquidators" (i.e., clean-up workers) for the Chernobyl accident developed PHPT 10 to 20 years later seems to substantiate this link.[40] More detailed clinical studies that examined the presentation, biochemistry, and demographic characteristics of patients treated for PHPT between 1982 and 1993, found the factors to be similar regardless of prior history of radiation exposure; the incidence of MGD was similar (26% versus 28%).[41] However, the incidence of concomitant thyroid pathology was much greater in the irradiated group (multinodular goiter 27% versus 7% and papillary thyroid cancer (PTC) 14% versus 0.3%). It seems highly likely, therefore, that radiation does induce PHPT, but the incidence of MGD does not appear to be increased and it remains to be elucidated why any putative field change brought about by radiation exposure does not appear to increase the risk of four-gland disease compared with single-gland disease.

Lithium

Lithium compounds have been used to modulate and stabilize mood for several decades, in particular, for the treatment of hypomania and bipolar disorder.[42] Long-term therapy requires therapeutic monitoring because of its narrow therapeutic window. Despite this, lithium may be associated with endocrine and metabolic side effects, even at therapeutic concentrations. These include weight gain, hypothyroidism, nephrogenic diabetes, and HPT.[43] Hypercalcemia typically develops after years of treatment, is generally mild, and has an accompanying, slight elevation of PTH. The condition is often reversible if lithium is withdrawn, but this is not always possible. Lithium-associated HPT arises through the interaction of lithium with the calcium sensing receptor (CaSR). It is proposed that this process alters the set-point of the CaSR and raises the threshold at which calcium-mediated negative feedback occurs.[44,45] If treatment continues for several years, PHPT results. Although the exact pathway is poorly understood, treatment with cinacalcet (a calcimimetic) has shown the process to be reversible, with normalization of serum calcium and PTH levels, in selected patients.[46,47] The reported prevalence of lithium-associated HPT is between 2.7% and 23.2%.[48] If the hypercalcemia is marked or persists after lithium withdrawal, or if the patient needs to continue lithium therapy, parathyroidectomy is generally recommended. Series of patients treated surgically have demonstrated that there is an increased incidence of MGD in patients with lithium-associated HPT that ranges from 25% to 50%.[49-52] The most recent systematic review analyzed more than 200 patients treated surgically and determined that 51% had MGD, OR 3.44 (95% CI 2.59 to 4.56, $p < 0.0001$).[52]

Thiazide Drugs

Treatment of hypertension with thiazide diuretics commonly induces hypercalcemia; the likely mechanism is increased renal tubular reabsorption of calcium, which results in reduced urine calcium excretion. Therefore it is advised that thiazides are discontinued for 2 to 3 months before definitive diagnosis of PHPT.[53] In a recent epidemiologic study, hypercalcemia was noted a median of 5 years after thiazide initiation, and it was reversible after cessation in just under 30% of patients.[54] Twenty-four percent of the cohort was subsequently diagnosed with PHPT; of these patients, 43% had at least one pathologic gland excised. Intermittent postoperative hypercalcemia was noted in 30% of the group, raising the possibility that MGD was present at a much higher rate than expected for sporadic disease. Despite this putative link with MGD, the authors concluded that thiazides are more likely to unmask PHPT rather than cause it.[54]

PREOPERATIVE DIAGNOSIS OF MGD

Clinical Presentation and Biochemistry in MGD

The preoperative identification of patients with MGD is desirable for several reasons: it will confer a strategy of BCE; it allows better planning because the procedure will take longer; the patient may be counseled for an increased risk of recurrent disease and risk of further surgery; and due to the complex nature of the problem, it allows referral to a high-volume parathyroid surgery center. For these reasons, a good deal of effort has been directed at determining diagnostic criteria that might guide decision making before the patient undergoes surgery. To date, numerous studies have aimed predict MGD pre-operatively with varying degrees of success.[55-59]

The dichotomous, so-called CaPTHUS scoring system was based on data from 238 patients treated in San Francisco and validated in a further 492 patients.[56] The system assigns one point each: for serum Calcium >12 mg/dL, serum PTH > twice the upper limit of normal, single localized gland on cervical ultrasound, single localized gland on sestamibi (MIBI) scan and concordant localization scans (maximum score, 5). A resulting score of $\geq$3 yields a positive predictive value of 97% to 100% for single-gland disease; this allows targeted parathyroidectomy without intraoperative PTH.[60] Conversely, scores of $\leq$2 selected a group of patients in which the incidence of MGD was more than 30%; within these patients, BCE was more likely to be required.

Preoperative clinical information is another aspect that has been examined with mixed findings. Although small-scale studies have not discerned any difference in presentation between those patients with single adenoma and those with MGD in terms of their presenting calcium and PTH concentrations,[57] detailed analyses of larger cohorts of patients have determined some significant differences between the two groups. By use of machine learning to interrogate a database of some 2010 patients treated surgically for PHPT (single adenoma 76% and MGD 24%), a clinical decision-support tool has been developed that can predict MGD with 94% overall accuracy (sensitivity 94%, specificity 83.8%, PPV 94%).[58] Although, age, sex, and BMI were not found to be significantly different in single-gland disease and MGD groups, a statistically significant set of characteristics of patients with MGD was determined; the set included the following: lower preoperative calcium levels (10.4 ± 0.86 versus 10.9 ± 0.83 mg/dL, $p < 0.001$), lower urinary calcium excretion (243 ± 157 versus 300 ± 209 mg/day, $p < 0.001$), higher vitamin D levels (33 ± 14.7 versus 30 ± 12.9 ng/mL, $p < 0.001$), and a significantly greater incidence of renal stones (21% versus 16.5%, $p < 0.016$). The principal advantage of such an algorithm is that it allows clinicians to determine the risk of MGD and does so well before surgery; the algorithm can even help omit unnecessary imaging, which may add little to the preoperative planning.

The theme of low preoperative serum PTH concentrations has been addressed in two other studies involving a total of 1692 patients.[61,62] Analysis of subgroups with hypercalcemia and normal preoperative PTH (≤69 pg/mL), demonstrated that the incidence of MGD was between 36 and 58.8%; this signifies that low serum PTH (alone) is a valuable portent of MGD. Therefore it may be that individual risk-stratification of patients into high- and low-risk for MGD will permit more tailored preoperative consent, appropriate choice of imaging, choice of surgical procedure, and direction of high risk cases to higher-volume centers.[63]

Preoperative Localization With Ultrasound and ^{99m}Tc-Sestamibi in MGD

A number of preoperative imaging modalities are now in common use for patients who are surgical candidates for parathyroidectomy. It is accepted that, although these tests may aid in choice of operative strategy, they play no part in the diagnosis of PHPT (see Chapter 54, Guide to Preoperative Parathyroid Localization Testing: Ultrasound, Sestimibi and 4D CT).[64] To date, the focus has been determining whether preoperative imaging can select patients for less invasive, targeted parathyroidectomy with or without intraoperative PTH measurement, with an acceptable degree of success. The utility and accuracy of these techniques has been systematically reviewed[5,65-68] in the setting of single-gland and MGD; the results are summarized in Table 60.2.

Perhaps the most widely used method is high resolution cervical ultrasound scanning (USS); it is quick, noninvasive, allows concurrent assessment of pathology in the thyroid and cervical lymph nodes, and involves no ionizing radiation. Meta-analysis has shown that its overall sensitivity for detecting single pathologic parathyroid glands is 76% to 79% (95% CI: 70 to 81%)[5,66] with a specificity of 91% to 96%;[69,70] however, it is less sensitive in people with obesity and is of limited use in detecting ectopic glands in the thorax. However, in the setting of MGD, the sensitivity decreases significantly to 35% (95% CI: 30% to 40%); in double adenoma, it is even lower: 16% (95% CI: 4% to 25%).

Scintigraphy with ^{99m}technetium (^{99m}Tc)-labeled MIBI is also commonly used. MIBI localizes abnormal glands by virtue of its positive charge and lipophilic properties that result in its rapid accumulation and prolonged washout from the mitochondria of parathyroid cells.[71] Whereas one of its advantages over USS includes its ability to detect ectopic glands, it does involve a dosage of ionizing radiation, it does

TABLE 60.2 Sensitivity (%) for Neck Ultrasound, ^{99m}Technetium-Labeled Sestamibi (MIBI) and MIBI SPECT/CT in Detecting Single and Multiple Gland Disease (MGD)

Modality	Single-Gland Disease	MGD	Overall
High resolution USS	76–79	35	70
^{99m}Tc-sestamibi	88–97	44–61	83
Sestamibi SPECT/CT	79–98	66	88

Data from Ruda JM, Hollenbeak CS, Stack BC. A systematic review of the diagnosis and treatment of primary hyperparathyroidism from 1995 to 2003. *Otolaryngol Head Neck Surg*. 2005;132(3):359–372; Cheung K, Wang TS, Farrokhyar F, Roman SA, Sosa JA. A meta-analysis of preoperative localization techniques for patients with primary hyperparathyroidism. *Ann Surg Oncol*. 2012;19(2):577–583; Nichols KJ, Tomas MB, Tronco GG, Palestro CJ. Sestamibi parathyroid scintigraphy in multigland disease. *Nucl Med Commun*. 2012;33(1):43–50; Nichols KJ, Tronco GG, Palestro CJ. Influence of Multigland Parathyroid Disease on 99mTc-Sestamibi SPECT/CT. *Clin Nucl Med*. 2016;41(4):282–288.

not allow concomitant assessment for thyroid pathology, and some benign and malignant thyroid nodules exhibit MIBI-uptake. The overall sensitivity for single-gland disease from systematic review is 88% (95% CI: 87% to 89%). Similar to USS, this is much lower for MGD and lower still for double adenoma (44%, 95% CI: 41% to 48% and 30%, 95% CI: 2% to 62%, respectively).[5]

More recently, MIBI scintigraphy has been combined with three-dimensional single-photon emission computed tomography (SPECT) and computed tomography (CT) overlay to provide better visualization of posterior tumors. The addition of SPECT/CT yields sensitivity for single-gland disease of nearly 80% and a greater sensitivity for MGD of 66%.[68]

The reasons for the reduced ability of these modalities to detect MGD probably relates to the reduced gland volume of individual hyperplastic glands compared with single adenomas in the case of USS, and reduced avidity for MIBI in hyperplastic glands compared with adenomas.[67,68] Indeed, it has been observed that MIBI SPECT sensitivity is inversely related to the number of lesions present.[68]

Given the relatively poor positive predictive value of USS and MIBI at detecting MGD, what can be inferred when the results of these investigations are negative? Studies examining this outcome have consistently come to the same conclusion: negative localization studies are themselves associated with a rate of MGD that may be over 35%.[4,11,2-75] Furthermore, almost without exception, these series have reported that patients with negative scans have smaller tumors, a higher rate of negative exploration, and much poorer rates of postoperative normocalcemia, ranging from 82% to 91% compared with 96% to 97.5% for patients with at least one positive scan. In the largest study, based upon the Scandinavian Quality Register for Thyroid and Parathyroid Surgery, the rate of persistent PHPT was 18%, and the negative exploration rate was 13.3%. However, this outcome was 2.5-fold less likely if intraoperative PTH was employed.[4]

In summary, the predictive value of USS and MIBI in MGD is much lower than in uniglandular disease, and negative scans are associated with much higher rates of MGD and with poorer outcomes, particularly if both modalities are negative. Conversely, concordant scans for a single enlarged gland are highly predictive of single-gland disease, although there is debate about the utility of intraoperative PTH in this scenario. Preoperative indices that predict MGD are summarized in Table 60.3.

TABLE 60.3 Summary of Preoperative Factors That May Predict an Increased Risk of MGD at Surgery

Predictive factor	% Incidence of MGD (if known)	DA or HA	References
Radiation	20–25%	HA	38
Lithium therapy	50%	HA	50
Mild hypercalcemia at diagnosis	Risk not stated but increased	HA	58
PTH in normal range at diagnosis	36–59%	HA	58,61,62
Mild hypercalciuria	Risk not stated but increased	HA	37,58
Negative MIBI and USS	24–37%	HA and DA	4,11,63,74
BMI >40	OR 1.8 (95%CI 1.3–3.1)	HA	34
Diabetes	OR 2.97 (95% CI 1.4–6.3)	HA and DA	37
High calcium diet	OR 0.5 (95%CI 0.37–0.86)	Protective	32

DA, double adenoma; HA, hyperplasia; PTH, parathyroid hormone; MIBI, 99mTc-Sestamibi; USS, ultrasound scan; BMI, body mass index; OR, odds ratio; CI, confidence interval.

Other Imaging Modalities

Although imaging modalities such as CT, magnetic resonance imaging (MRI), and ^{18}Fluorodeoxyglucose (FDG) and ^{18}Fluorocholine (FCH) positron emission tomography (PET) have been described in the localization of parathyroid glands.[76-79] Their use is most commonly reserved for those patients undergoing evaluation for reoperative surgery after failed exploration or for those in whom ectopic glands are suspected. Furthermore, they are of most utility in patients with single-gland disease where sensitivities range from 40% to 70% for CT and MRI and are in excess of 80% for PET. Additionally, ^{11}C-Methionine-PET/CT has been described; although its sensitivity is 83% for single-gland disease, it is also of use in MGD, where its sensitivity is close to 70%.[80] Despite these results, it is likely that cost and resource limitations will continue to restrict the more widespread use of PET for parathyroid localization at the current time.

More recently, there is emerging data on the use of four-dimensional CT (4DCT), both in preoperative planning after failed exploration for PHPT and also in the diagnosis of MGD. A scoring system composed of a points for the Wisconsin index (WIN) (product of preoperative serum calcium and PTH values: >1600 = 0; 800 to 1600 = 1; <800 = 2), the number of lesions seen on 4DCT (single lesion = 0; multiple = 2 and none = 2), and the size of the largest lesion (>13 mm = 0; 7-13 mm = 1, <7 mm = 2) was found to have sensitivities of 81%, 93% and 98% for detection of MGD for scores of ≥4, ≥5, and ≥6 respectively.[81] In the setting of patients with a low baseline PTH, 4DCT has also shown promise, with a sensitivity of >80% for detecting MGD in this high-risk group,[82] which has prompted the authors to suggest that 4DCT may be advised in such patients and/or those with inconclusive USS and MIBI results. Although radiation exposure to the neck from 4DCT is still relatively high and, therefore, limits its use as a first-line investigation in the evaluation of PHPT, a combination of restricting the number of CT phases required and improvements in scan resolution may allow a change in practice in the future.[83]

INTRAOPERATIVE ADJUNCTS IN MGD

Intraoperative PTH

The assaying of serum PTH levels intraoperatively before and after the excision of hyperfunctioning parathyroid tissue is an established technique, yet its use is controversial (see Chapter 59, Guide to Preoperative Parathyroid Localization Testing: Ultrasound, Sestimibi and 4D CT). This is especially true in patients with concordant USS and MIBI who would be strongly predicted to have single-gland disease (incidence of MGD, 1% to 3.5%);[84] the value added is subsequently low.[85] However, its use in the challenging subgroup of patients with MGD has been examined extensively.[86-88] In patients with discordant imaging, the rate of MGD approaches 20%; therefore intraoperative PTH is invaluable for excluding other functioning glands for those patients in whom a minimally invasive route is planned.[89] In terms of detection of MGD intraoperatively, the sensitivity of intraoperative PTH depends on the specific criteria applied. The most widely used is the Miami criterion of >50% decline in intraoperative PTH at 10 minutes from whichever is the greater of the baseline or preexcision intraoperative PTH values.[90] This has been demonstrated to possess the optimal balance between positive predictive value at detecting MGD (99.6%) and negative predictive value (70%). Application of other criteria, such those described in Halle and Rome, although highly sensitive, result in a higher rate of false positive conversion to BCE in the absence of MGD.[84]

The converse to this is what to deduce about the utility of intraoperative PTH when there is a failure of PTH levels to decline after excision of a diseased gland. "Operative failure" as it has been termed, has been examined in more 2000 patients and found to be associated with rates of MGD of >30%, smaller glands, and, if there is persistent disease, an association with significantly smaller decreases in intraoperative PTH.[91] Interestingly, about half of 'operative failure' patients described in this study were still normocalcemic at 6 months. Lastly, the predictive value of intraoperative PTH levels at 5 minutes has also been studied. In a series of >1000 patients with a MGD rate of 17.8%, it was found that those with MGD had decline in intraoperative PTH at 5 minutes; the decline was much smaller in magnitude compared with those patients with single-gland disease (24.9% versus 85.3%, $p < 0.01$). Consequently, it was concluded that when the intraoperative PTH level does not drop by at least 35% at 5 minutes after excision, the surgeon should consider further exploration rather than waiting for additional PTH levels.[88]

The Wisconsin Index (WIN)

The WIN and WIN nomogram are additional tools that can be used to guide intraoperative decision making during focused surgery by providing a prediction of the risk of MGD.[92] Derived from a series of more than 1200 consecutive patients, WIN is based upon the product of preoperative serum calcium and PTH values; patients are subdivided into three WIN categories (<800, 801 to 1600 and >1600). The weight of the first gland is used to determine the risk of MGD. Thus for a gland of 500 mg is excised from a patient with a WIN value of <800, the risk of MGD is 9%, whereas if a 500 mg gland is excised from patient with a WIN of >1600, the risk is 61%. This allows the surgeon to decide whether to proceed with BCE or await the outcome of intraoperative PTH values.

SURGICAL TREATMENT

Sporadic MGD

Operative Strategy in Nonlocalized Disease

The standard approach for nonlocalized disease is BCE.[64] This is recommended because not only is the site of the tumor unknown preoperatively, but the rate of MGD (when localization is negative) is in the order of 20% to 35%.[4,72,74] An alternative strategy is to perform a unilateral exploration and use an intraoperative PTH assay when a tumor is identified during the first side of a BCE and intraoperative PTH falls by at least 50% postexcision. Using a "left-side first" approach, it has been shown that this can be achieved in 27% of cases, but BCE remains the prevailing approach for the majority (73%).[11]

Intraoperatively, the diagnosis of MGD is either simply determined by visual identification of more than one enlarged parathyroid gland, or from the failure of intraoperative PTH to adequately fall after removal of the (first) parathyroid tumor. In both scenarios a BCE is undertaken (as detailed in Chapter 56, Standard Bilateral Parathyroid Exploration). Smaller tumors identified at operation should raise suspicion for MGD and surgeons should have a lower threshold to perform a BCE.

The principles of BCE are to first identify all four glands and search sites of ectopic cervical locations when necessary. Resection or removal of any enlarged gland or glands is postponed until at least four glands have been visualized. At this point, the surgeon will be able to determine whether the patient has four-gland hyperplasia or a double adenoma.

Double Adenoma

Cure is achieved when both glands are excised. In the majority of patients, the tumors are bilateral. A recent series of double adenomas reported that in about half of patients the adenomas are of a similar size and in half, the enlargement is asymmetric.[93] Reliance should not be placed on intraoperative PTH especially when the tumors are asymmetric and the larger tumor is resected first.[93,94] Although long-term follow-up has demonstrated a high cure rate after excision of both tumors;[94] others have shown that the rate of persistent HPT is higher than that of single adenoma and hyperplasia (4% versus 1.3% and 2.2%); the presence of a double adenoma should alert the surgeon to the possibility of four-gland hyperplasia.[95]

Four-Gland Hyperplasia

The recommended operation is a subtotal parathyroidectomy.[64] After all four glands have been identified the surgeon is best able to compare the sizes and gross features of all glands and can then select the smallest and most normal appearing gland as remnant. If the smallest gland is normal in size, it may be left in situ. If the gland is enlarged, it should be partially resected to leave a well vascularized remnant of approximately 50 mg (Figure 60.6). Resection is performed with a knife with careful preservation of the vascular supply. Spillage of parathyroid tissue during glandular transection is avoided by cutting against a gauze sponge. Bleeding from the remnant will quickly stop with gentle compression. If the viability of the remnant or unresected gland is unequivocal, the other glands are removed. If, however, the remnant tissue has questionable viability, it has to be removed and the next, least enlarged parathyroid is selected to serve as a remnant. In cases of recurrent HPT, the surgeon should be prepared for reexploration. Therefore the site of the remnant is marked with both a clip and a nonabsorbable (polypropylene) suture (to the thyroid). Where the surgeon is faced with a choice about which gland to select as a remnant, many surgeons advocate the selection of an inferior parathyroid gland because it is more often further from the recurrent laryngeal nerve (RLN), and its discovery in reoperation avoids a deeper dissection. An accurate record of the operation must be kept in the medical records, and an intraoperative photograph may be useful.

Subtotal parathyroidectomy has been reported to provide long-term cure in 85% to 90% of patients with sporadic MGD HPT.[96,97] Failure

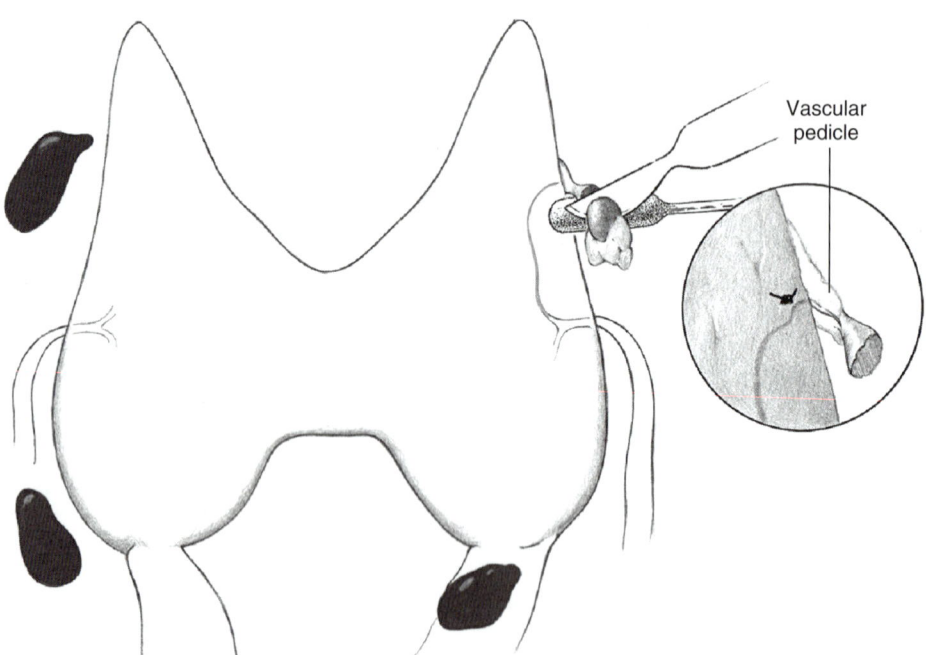

Fig. 60.6 Technique of subtotal parathyroidectomy. After all four parathyroid glands have been visualized, the smallest anodular gland is selected as a remnant and resected to a size of approximately 50 mg. When the viability of the remnant is ensured, the other glands are removed. The region of the remnant should be marked with a suture or a clip.

resulting in persistent disease has been related mainly to the presence of overlooked supernumerary glands, whereas remnant recurrence generally has been rarer or developed later during follow-up.[96] The risk of hypoparathyroidism generally should be less than 1%.[98]

The Role of Routine Thymectomy

Up to 13% of people have more than four parathyroid glands[99] and the thymus is a common site for supernumerary glands. As the only cure for hyperplastic HPT is parathyroidectomy, it is important that all diseased glands are removed. Leaving behind parathyroid tissue may contribute to persistent or recurrent HPT. For that reason, routine thymectomy has been a standard component of a BCE and subtotal parathyroidectomy. The evidence to support this strategy is weak because most studies include mixed populations of sporadic and familial PHPT as well as secondary HPT; often, the numbers are small. A recent retrospective study of 328 patients with PHPT showed a trend to a better cure rate with thymectomy (99%) versus without thymectomy (95%); however, this did not reach statistical significance.[100] For those who underwent thymectomy, supernumerary glands were present in 9% of specimens. Currently, there is no consensus about the role of routine thymectomy with subtotal PTX, but if thymic tissue can be identified, there is no evidence to suggest that its excision is harmful.

The surgeon performs the thymectomy by dissecting close to the thymic capsule and exploring first the cervical portion of the gland (Figure 60.7, A and B). Traction is then applied with the aid of two surgical forceps grasping the tissue further and further down. Then, there is mainly blunt dissection under the sternum and careful ligation of veins, which drain into the innominate vein; as much as possible of the thymus is delivered, until it tends to rupture with a featherlike ending. Clearance of fat in the central part of the neck should be done cautiously to avoid jeopardizing the circulation of normal parathyroids.

The Role of Total Parathyroidectomy Alone

Historically, a total parathyroidectomy alone was considered in secondary HPT because of high recurrence rates. However, this strategy was soon abandoned, because the aparathyroid condition was claimed to result in adynamic bone, low turnover bone disease with occasionally increased bone pain, and increased risk of hypercalcemia. It was later

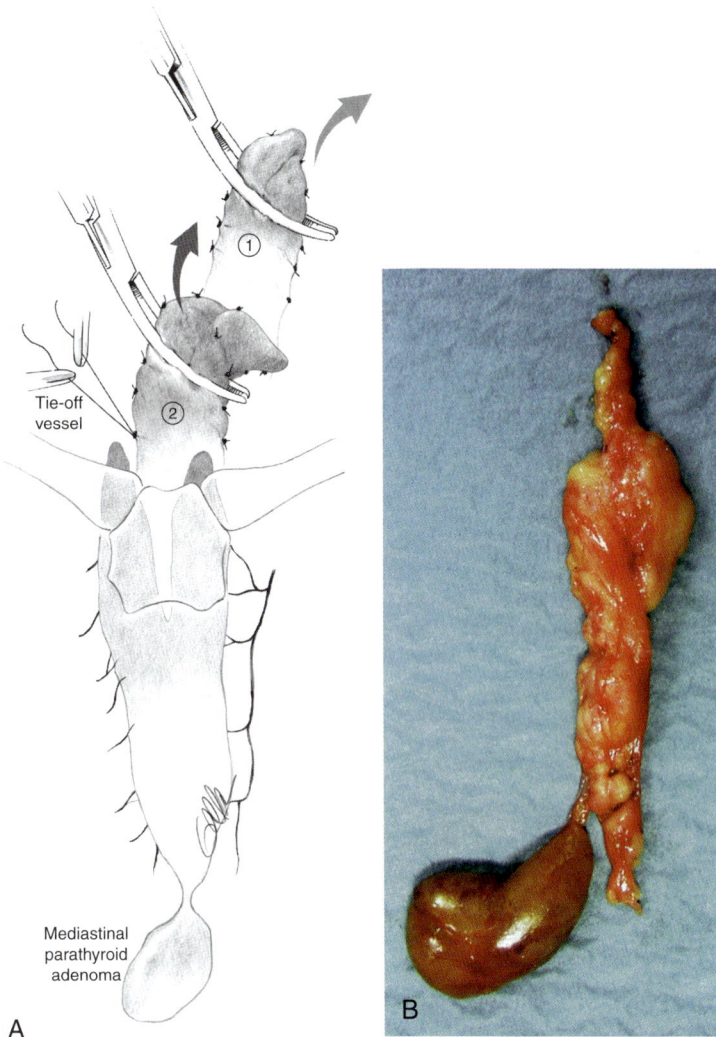

Fig. 60.7 A, Part of the mediastinal thymus is delivered by continuous traction applied by two surgical forceps, grasping farther and farther down on the delivered thymus, concomitant with finger dissection close to thymic capsule and continuous clipping of veins, which drains into the innominate vein. **B,** Figure illustrates a large pathologic gland delivered from the mediastinum; up to 14 cm of the thymus can be delivered in this way.

demonstrated that parathyroid glands, after resection, retained their function when autotransplanted to the sternocleidomastoid muscle in the treatment of patients with thyroid carcinoma; total parathyroidectomy with autotransplantation was recommended in patients with primary parathyroid hyperplasia.[101] Therefore there is no role for total parathyroidectomy alone in treating MGD.

The Role of Total Parathyroidectomy and Autotransplantation

With this procedure, all four parathyroid glands are visualized and removed. Historically, the identity of each gland is confirmed histologically by frozen section examination, but confirmation by FNA and intraoperative PTH assessment of the gland aspirate are more recent methods.[102] Concomitantly, the cervical thymus is removed (see previous). Tissue slices with an estimated weight of 60 to 80 mg (i.e., somewhat larger than initially recommended) are cut from the smallest and most normal-appearing (i.e., least nodular) gland.[103,104] The tissue slices are cooled in iced physiologic saline solution and cut with a knife into 0.5- to 1-mm pieces, which are autotransplanted into 20 separate pockets in the brachioradialis muscle (Figure 60.8). Each pocket is closed with 5-0 nonabsorbable suture, and the transplant area is marked with hemostatic clips.

With this method, a period of postoperative hypocalcemia will be experienced, because graft function depends on vascularization from the surrounding muscle. Appropriate graft function is generally delayed 2 to 3 months postoperatively or longer; until then, the patients need to be maintained on vitamin D and calcium supplementation. A patient who remains normocalcemic is likely to have undergone incomplete parathyroidectomy, which may result from presence of supernumerary parathyroid tissue in the neck or mediastinum.[105] Intraoperative PTH is unreliable in predicting the early PTH status in this population.[106] Failure and permanent hypoparathyroidism may occur somewhat more often than after subtotal parathyroidectomy, but the incidence should be low with appropriate handling of the tissue used for transplantation. Late failure of parathyroid autografts has been reported.

The Role of Total Parathyroidectomy, Cryopreservation and Delayed Autotransplantation

Since the development of cryopreservation in the 1970s, this was a popular technique in units that possessed the necessary technology. The goal of cryopreservation is to provide a curative option for patients experiencing hypocalcaemia after parathyroidectomy. Although rates of preservation in USA are high, both the actual usage of the cryopreserved tissue (1%) and the success of delayed autotransplantation (10%) are low.[107] Its continuing practice is therefore questionable.[64]

OPERATIVE STRATEGY IN LOCALIZED DISEASE (UNILATERAL EXPLORATION/LATERAL APPROACH)

Any surgeon undertaking parathyroidectomy must be adaptive to the spectrum of pathology that is encountered in HPT.[108] There will be occasions when the surgeon has selected a targeted approach on the basis of positive preoperative localization. A decision to convert to BCE may arise when no tumor is found (false positive scan), when there is a failure of the intraoperative PTH to fall adequately after excision of an enlarged gland, or even when a second enlarged gland is identified on the ipsilateral side.

Lithium-Associated HPT

The proportion of patients with a solitary adenoma versus micronodular parathyroid hyperplasia is as high as 50:50.[49,109] For this reason, some surgeons advocate BCE, whereas others favor a selective approach (based on whether or not there is positive preoperative localization)

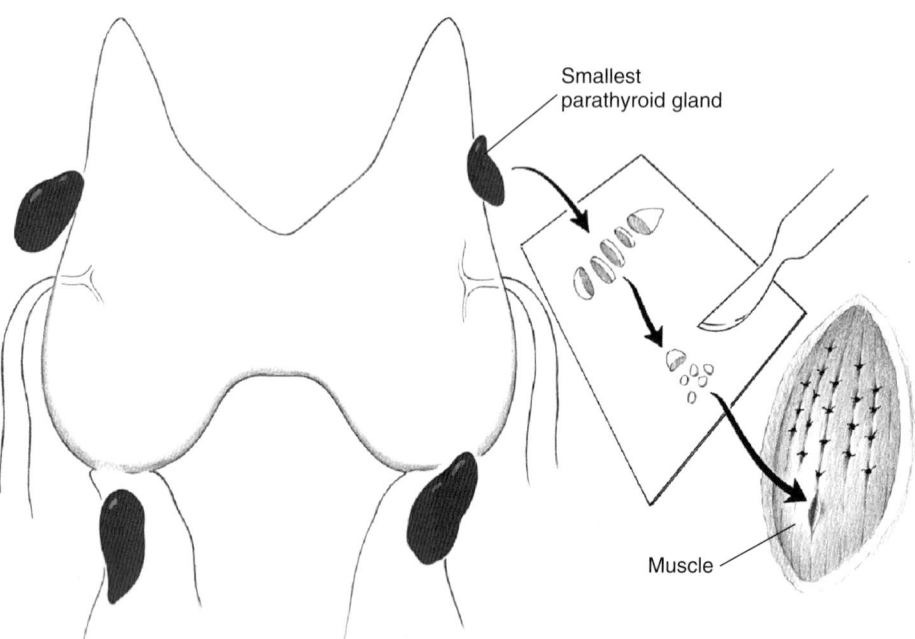

Fig. 60.8 Technique of total parathyroidectomy and autotransplantation. Complete neck exploration is undertaken with visualization of all parathyroid glands. All glands are removed, and cervical thymectomy is performed. Part of the smallest gland (approximately 60 to 80 mg) is used for autotransplantation after biopsy and frozen section confirmation that it is a parathyroid. This tissue is sliced with a knife and cooled in iced physiologic saline before being cut into 0.5- to 1-mm pieces, which are implanted into separate pockets in brachioradialis muscle. Each pocket is closed with 5-0 nonabsorbable sutures, and the transplant area is marked with hemostatic clips.

using intraoperative PTH. The evidence to support either strategy is weak because of the small numbers reported in studies. The European Society of Endocrine Surgeons Consensus Statement[110] and AAES Guidelines[64] support either surgical strategy.

Bilateral Cervical Exploration

Glandular involvement is typically asymmetric and may appear as single-gland disease. As with sporadic HPT, tumors are typically smaller.[111] One reason to consider BCE in all patients with lithium-associated HPT is due to frequent misleading or discordant localization studies associated with this disorder.[112] During exploration, if the first abnormal gland is <200 mg in weight, there should be heightened suspicion of MGD, which also presages a tenfold higher failure rate.[113] Patients with MGD are at a higher risk of persistent/recurrent disease.[110]

Targeted Parathyroidectomy

Other studies have reported excellent outcomes (100% cure) for a selective surgical approach directed by intraoperative PTH measurement.[49,111,114] An alternative approach would be to remove both parathyroid tumors on the side of the adenoma, thus clearing one side of the neck in case of recurrence (akin to the approach adopted by some units when treating patients with MEN-1 HPT).

Some patients develop hypercalcemia shortly after the initiation of lithium treatment and may have primary HPT unmasked by the therapy. These patients generally harbor a parathyroid adenoma and three normal glands.

Expected Outcomes

The general trend is that large series report cure rates similar for MGD compared with single adenomas.[115] In a study comparing the outcomes of parathyroidectomy with a whole gland remnant or a partial gland remnant, there was no difference in either the cure rate or recurrence rate.[116] Although there is no evidence base, a policy of following-up patients with MGD for a longer period of time (compared with single adenoma) seems justified.

REFERENCES

For a complete list of references, go to expertconsult.com.

61

Surgical Management of Secondary and Tertiary Hyperparathyroidism

Yoshihiro Tominaga

> Please go to expertconsult.com to view related video:
> **Video 61.1** Total Parathyroidectomy with Forearm Autograft for Patients with Advanced Secondary Hyperparathyroidism.
> **Video 61.2** Total Parathyroidectomy with Forearm Autograft for Patients with Advanced Secondary Hyperparathyroidism: Usefulness of IONM.

SECONDARY HYPERPARATHYROIDISM

Definition

Secondary hyperparathyroidism (SHPT) refers to the situation in which a derangement in calcium homeostasis leads to a compensatory increase in parathyroid hormone (PTH) secretion.[1] SHPT requiring parathyroidectomy (PTx) occurs more commonly in progressive chronic kidney disease (CKD)[2] but also may occur in long-term lithium therapy[3] and certain disorders of gastrointestinal absorption, deficiency of vitamin D, liver disease, and pseudohypoparathyroidism. The term *tertiary hyperparathyroidism* (THPT) is associated with clinically persistent hypercalcemia in SHPT after successful renal transplantation (RTx).[4-6]

Epidemiology and Rate of PTx for SHPT

Multivariate analysis showed that younger age, female gender, white race, absence of diabetes, long duration of hemodialysis, use of intravenous vitamin D, previous RTx, and several other comorbid conditions represent risk factors for requirement of PTx in patients with SHPT. Mook et al. found an abrupt decline in the rate of PTx for SHPT over the past decade after introduction of cinacalcet, with stabilization of rates from 2006 to 2011. In hospitals, the mortality rate declined steadily over that timeframe, which suggests either improved surgical and perioperative medical care or an improvement in patient selection (Figure 61.1).[7,8] The Parathyroid Surgeon's Society of Japan (PSSJ) has studied the annual number of PTx for SHPT. The annual number of PTx for SHPT increased until 2007, but the rate remarkably decreased when cinacalcet became available in Japan in 2008 (Figure 61.2).[9] The same clinical results have been reported in European countries through The Dialysis Outcome and Practice Pattern Study (DOPS). The overall cost and the cost utility of medical therapy (including cinacalcet) may, to some extent, limit the use of this new therapy; it may, in turn, influence the future rates of PTx in different countries.[9,10] The Japanese Society for Dialysis Therapy (JSDT) reported that in Japan, the frequency of PTx was about 10% in patients who had had hemodialysis for more than 10 years, and about 30% among those being treated with hemodialysis for more than 20 years.[11]

Pathogenesis, Histopathology, and Pathophysiology

A summary of pathogenesis of SHPT due to CKD is presented in Figure 61.3.[12,13] The dominant etiologic factors are hypocalcemia, reduced renal production of 1,25-dehydroxy vitamin D, and hyperphosphatemia (through phosphate retention), which directly acts on parathyroid cells to stimulate PTH secretion, synthesis, and proliferation of parathyroid cells. Recently, a novel phosphaturic hormone fibroblast growth factor (FGF) 23 has been identified. FGF23 is secreted by osteocytes, and the serum level of FGF23 becomes progressively elevated in CKD. Furthermore, it has recently been shown that FGF23 directly acts on parathyroid cells and mediates secretion of PTH in the presence of Klotho as cofactor.[14]

There are numerous derangements in calcium pathways in CKD, which are complex and not completely understood. It has been confirmed that there is diminished expression of calcium sensing receptor (CaSR) in parathyroid cells in patients with CKD.[15,16] These patients also have skeletal resistance to PTH due to diminished expression of PTH/PTHRP receptor in osteoblasts.[17]

The characteristic histopathological findings of parathyroid glands in patients with CKD include varying degrees of asymmetric enlargement, nodularity, and increase in oxyphilic and transitional oxyphilic cells. Patterns of parathyroid hyperplasia in SHPT are classified into four categories (Tominaga's classification). They include: (1) diffuse hyperplasia, (2) early nodularity in diffuse hyperplasia, (3) nodular hyperplasia, and (4) single nodular gland (Figure 61.4). Almost all glands exceeding 500 mg display nodular hyperplasia.[18-21] It has been hypothesized that in CKD patients have polyclonal diffuse hyperplasia which transforms into nodular hyperplasia. In these nodules, parathyroid cells proliferate monoclonally with high growth potential. It has been speculated that the different genetic events known to occur in sporadic primary adenoma may occur in nodular SHPT. The exact nature of these genetic changes and their role in this morphologic progression of SHPT is still unclear.[22-24]

It has been confirmed that expression of vitamin D receptor (VDR) and CaSR is diminished in these clonal nodules; cells within these clonal nodules have resistance to calcitriol and hypercalcemia. It has therefore been hypothesized when at least one parathyroid gland progresses to nodular hyperplasia, SHPT may be refractory to medical treatments (Figure 61.5).

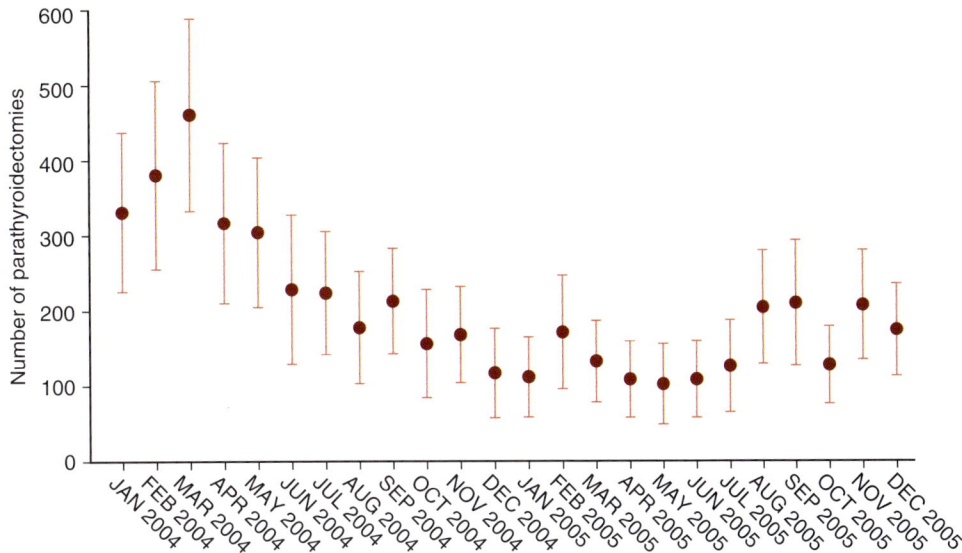

Fig. 61.1 Rate of parathyroidectomy (PTx) for secondary hyperparathyroidism (SHPT) in the U.S. (Redrawn from Kim SM, Long J, Montez-Rath ME, Leonard MB, Norton JA, Chertow GM. Rates and outcomes of parathyroidectomy for secondary hyperparathyroidism in the United States. Clin *J Am Soc Nephrol.* 2016;11[7]:1260-1267.)

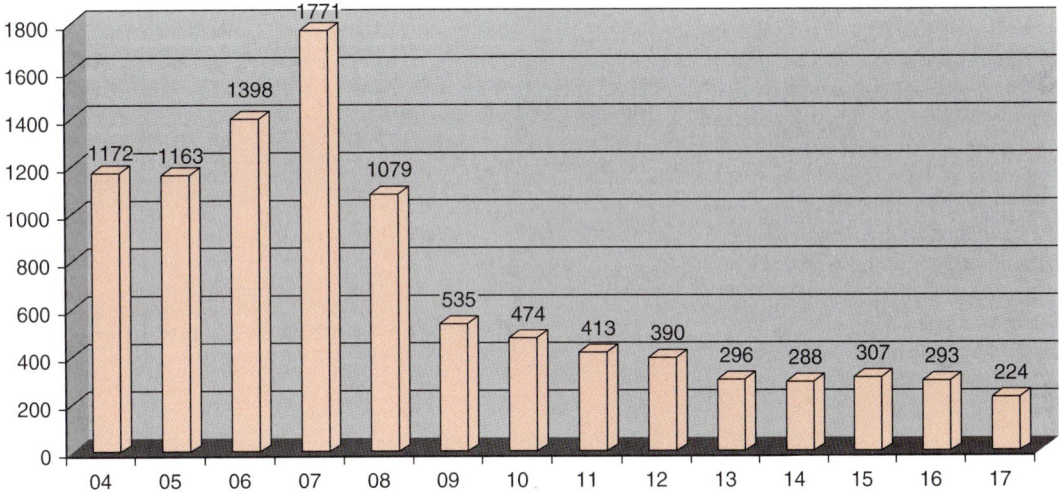

Fig. 61.2 Annual number of parathyroidectomies for secondary hyperparathyroidism (SHPT) and Tertiary hyperparathyroidism (THP). (Data from Parathyroid Surgeon's Society of Japan.)

Medical Treatment

A number of various medical treatment options exist to control SHPT (Box 61.1).

First, calcium concentration in dialysate should be optimized. High (3.0 mEq/L), middle (2.75 mEq/L), and low (2.5 mEq/L) calcium dialysates are available (see Box 61.1). Calcium carbonate, calcium acetate, and calcium lactate have been prescribed for calcium replacement. This administered calcium acts on the parathyroid cell CaSR to increase inositol phosphate levels in parathyroid cells and increase intracellular calcium level; it serves to suppress PTH secretion as well as parathyroid cell proliferation. Calcium carbonate and calcium acetate are also phosphate binders and can induce ectopic calcifications.

Hyperphosphatemia is one of the causes of ectopic calcification, cardiovascular complication, and mortality. Therefore control of hyperphosphatemia is an essential element of treatment in CKD. Limitation of phosphate in diet and adequate hemodialysis and phosphate binders are fundamental for the treatment. Recently, new phosphate binders (without calcium content) have become available as high molecular polymer (Sevelamar hydrochloride), lantana carbonate, or ferric containing phosphate binders. GI symptoms are sometimes problematic side effects of these drugs.[25,26]

Deficiency of active vitamin D is one of the main pathogenetic factors for SHPT. Calcitriol and alpha calcidol are common active vitamin D products; however, they induce hypercalcemia and hyperphosphatemia. It was hoped that maxacalcitol (OCT) and paricalcitol, new derivatives of active vitamin D, may allow suppression of PTH without hypercalcemia and hyperphosphatemia. It seems, however, that some degree of elevation of serum calcium and phosphate levels cannot be avoided.[26]

Calcimimetics (Cinacalcet hydrochloride)

Calcimimetics have been divided into two types: Type I, which mimic extracellular ionized calcium and directly stimulates the CaSR; and Type II, which are positive allosteric modulators.

SECTION 8 Parathyroid Surgery

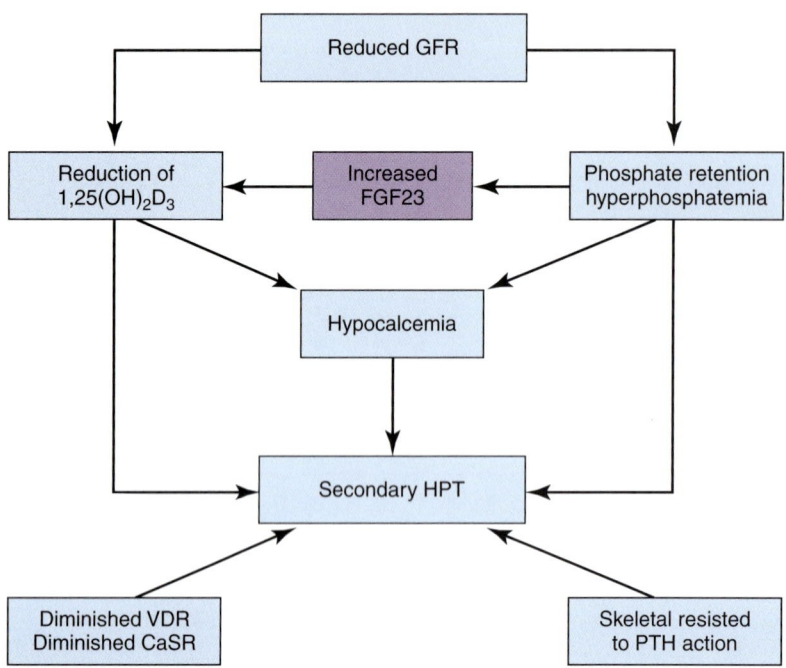

Fig. 61.3 Pathogenesis of secondary hyperparathyroidism (SHPT). GFR, glomerular filtration rate, FGF, fibroblast growth factor, HPT, hyperparathyroidism, VDR, vitamin D receptor, CaSR, calcium sensing receptor, PTH, parathyroid hormone.

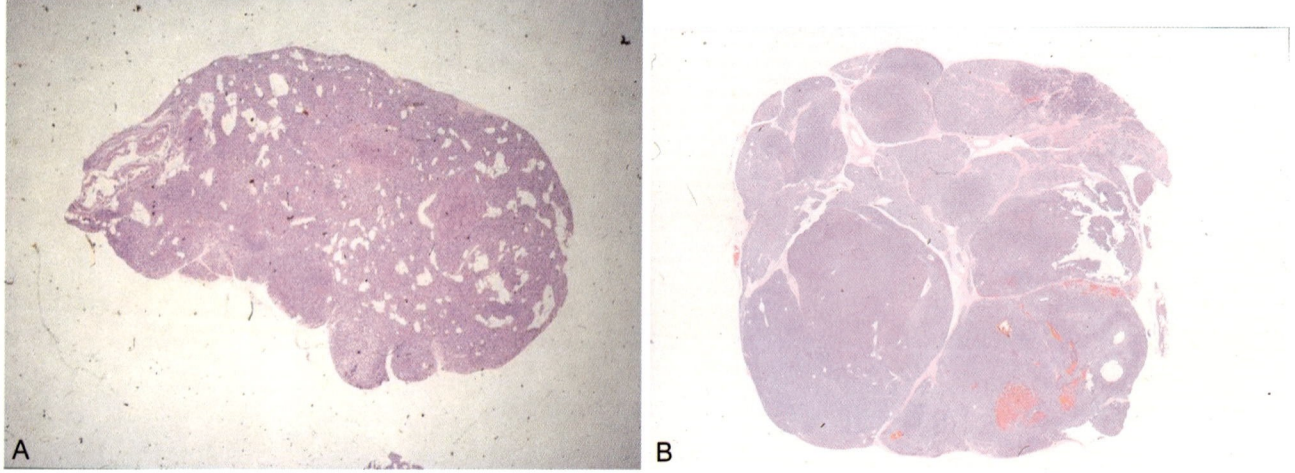

Fig. 61.4 A, Diffuse hyperplasia. Parathyroid parenchymal cells, mainly chief cells proliferate diffusely with lobular structure. **B,** Nodular hyperplasia. In nodular hyperplasic gland that contains well circumscribed encapsulated nodules, each nodule usually consisting of a single cell type.

Common calcimimetics include cinacalcet hydrobromide (a second generation Type II calcimimetic available since 2004), etercalcetide (a positive allosteric 3rd generation calcimimetic), and evocalcet (the most recently available calcimimetic), which has gastrointestinal (GI) symptoms comparable to cinacalcet. Cinacalcet hydrochloride acts on CaSR by allosteric action and enhances sensitivity to extracellular calcium and intracellular calcium signaling. This, in turn, serves to suppresses PTH section and parathyroid cell proliferation. Some patients complain of nausea and vomiting, which can limit cinacalcet compliance.[27-30]

The majority of patients with SHPT can be managed by the medical treatments that are outlined in Box 61.1. Kidney Disease Improving Global Outcome (KDIGO), an international workshop, recently proposed clinical practice guideline for CKD-related mineral and bone disease (CKD-MBD).[31] The guideline recommends normalizing serum phosphorus levels. It also recommends that in patients undergoing hemodialysis intact PTH levels should be no higher than two to nine times the upper limits of normal levels for the given assay.[32-35]

To control hypocalcemia, dialysate containing high calcium concentration usually is used and oral calcium containing phosphate binders (i.e., calcium carbonate or calcium acetate) are taken. Hyperphosphatemia is controlled by removal of phosphorous by adequate hemodialysis, limitation of dietary phosphate intake, and administration of phosphate binders. Treatment for lowering PTH include calcitriol, vitamin D analogues, and calcimimetics. VDR activators easily induce hypercalcemia and hyperphosphatemia and sometimes SHPT may be resistant to these medicines.

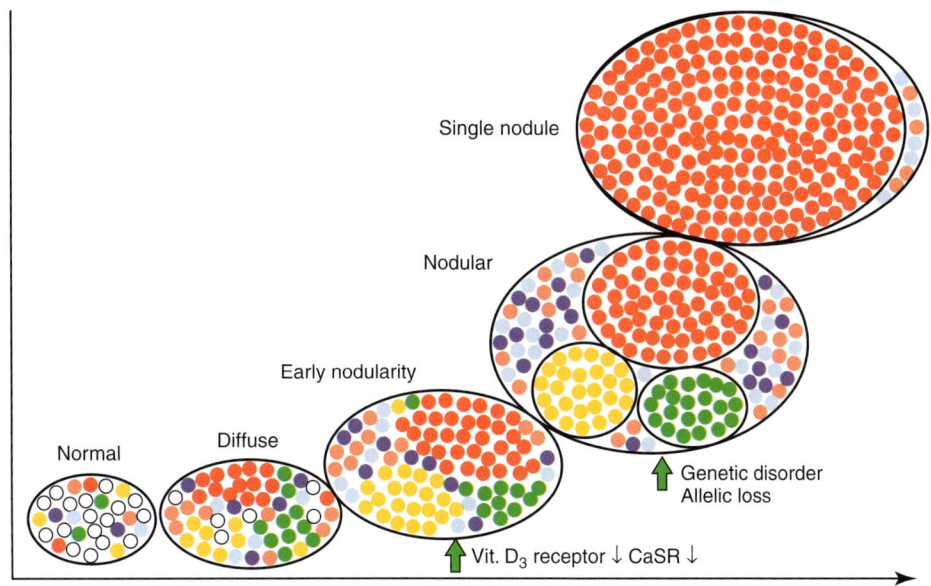

Fig. 61.5 Progression of parathyroid hyperplasia in secondary hyperparathyroidism (SHPT) resulting from chronic kidney disease.

BOX 61.1 Available Therapeutic Modalities for Secondary Hyperparathyroidism

1. Phosphate binders
   Calcium carbonate, calcium acetate
   Sevelamer hydrochloride
   Lanthanum carbonate
   Ferric contained binder
   (Ferric citrate hydrare, sucroferric oxyhydroxide)
2. Active vitamin D sterols, vitamin D receptor activators
   Calcitriol
   22-Oxacalcitriol
   Falecalcitriol
   Alphacalcidol
   Paricalcitol
   Doxercalciferol
3. Calcimimetics
   Cinacalcet HCl
   Etelcalcetide
   Evocalcet

BOX 61.2 Clinical Symptoms of Secondary Hyperparathyroidism

1. High turnover bone, osteitis fibrosa
   Bone pain, arthralgia, bone loss, skeletal deformity, fracture
2. Ectopic calcification
   Vascular and valvular calcification, tumoral calcinosis, calciphylaxis, calcification in lung, intestine, and stomach
3. Neuromuscular psychiatric symptoms
   Muscular weakness, gait disturbance, irritability, sleeplessness, loss of concentration, depression, etc.
4. Anemia resistant to ESA, malnutrition, itching, cough
5. Heart failure (DCM like heart)

ESA, erythropoietin stimulating agent, DCM, dilated cardiomyopathy.

Based on existing clinical evidence, Kidney Foundation of the USA proposed the Kidney Disease Outcomes Quality Initiative (K/DOQI) clinical practice guideline for bone metabolism and disease.[32] The guideline recommends in hemodialysis patients for whom serum calcium level is 8.4 to 9.5 mg/dL, serum phosphorus level is 3.5 to 5.5 mg/dL, calcium phosphorous product is less than 55, and intact PTH level is between 150 and 300 pg/mL. This is done to avoid ectopic calcification and cardiovascular complications.

Clinical Symptoms and Findings of Secondary Hyperparathyroidism

Box 61.2 shows the clinical symptoms and findings of SHPT.[36] Laboratory examination typically reveals remarkably high serum PTH level, hyperphosphatemia, and high bone metabolic markers (total alkaline phosphatase [Al-P], bone specific Al-P, and osteocalcin). Serum calcium level is usually low; however, it is easily influenced by medical treatment.

Neuromuscular psychiatric symptoms usually are more severe in SHPT than in primary hyperparathyroidism (PHPT). Patients frequently complain on muscular weakness, irritability, sleeplessness, itching, cough, and other symptoms. Ectopic calcification of vessels and heart valves induce cardiovascular complications and high mortality. Calciphylaxis, cutaneous necrosis induced by calcific uremic arteriolopathy, involves progressive skin necrosis and constitutes a condition of considerable mortality.[27-29,35]

Skeletal abnormalities, most often caused by PTH-induced bone resorption, occur relatively early in patients with CKD. These bone disorders come in multiple forms, including classic osteitis fibrosa cystica. Patients often experience skeletal deformation and frequent fracture. Clinically, these patients may demonstrate subperiosteal resorption in digital pharynxes clavicular head, (salt and pepper skull), lumbar osteosclerosis, (rugger jersey spine), and skeletal cystic formation with brown tumor.

Parathyroid Gland Intervention

Percutaneous Ethanol Injection Therapy (PEIT) was established in Japan and is widely used. Selective PEIT has been used especially for patients with CKD.[37-40] In the JSDT guideline, PEIT is recommended for patients who have only one enlarged nodular gland. After the enlarged gland is ablated by PEIT, aggressive medical treatment should be continued. After introduction of cinacalcet, the number of PEIT procedures remarkably decreased. If the patient suffers from advanced SHPT and concomitant cardiovascular disease, PEIT should be considered. Recurrent nerve paralysis and hemorrhage after the procedure should be kept in mind as complications of PEIT.

Surgical Indications

Surgical indications for SHPT are controversial especially after introduction of calcimimetics. Unfortunately, it is unclear as to which particular groups of patients might benefit best from cinacalcet-based medical therapy, and which patients are better treated by expeditious PTx (see Box 61.3). Some feel PTx is most optimal as an initial treatment, and cinacalcet therapy becomes an alternate therapy for patients where SHPT is difficult to manage after surgical treatment.[41-45]

The surgical indications have been influenced by practical guidelines which vary geographically. All guidelines propose that surgery should be considered when severe SHPT is resistant to medical therapy. PTx for SHPT is a very beneficial treatment; it can stop the progression of cardiovascular complications and improve quality of life and survival.

Previously, surgical indications in SHPT have mainly been based on clear cut severe symptoms or evidence of bone disease. KDIGO guidelines define bone disease (MBD) as a pathologic entity, which includes certain laboratory findings, ectopic calcification, bone fracture. They term this constellation of findings *CKD-MBD*.

Currently, surgical treatment is seen in the context of the many new forms of medical treatment. VDR agonists, calcimimetics, and phosphate binders without calcium have been documented to suppress PTH secretion and bone turnover. One must, however, keep in mind that medical treatment may induce persistent hypercalcemia and/or hyperphosphatemia; the treatment may be associated with cardiovascular complications which can affect survival.

Although surgical guidelines vary geographically, they all tend to propose that surgery should be considered when SHPT is severe and resistant to medical therapy. PTx has been shown to demonstrate a beneficial effect on survival by reducing cardiovascular complications. PTx performed by expert surgeons generally results in marked sustained reduction in levels of serum calcium, and phosphate.

K/DOQI guidelines from the U.S. Kidney Foundation have proposed that PTx should be recommended in patients with severe SHPT (i.e., patients with persistent serum levels of intact PTH >800 pg/mL), which is associated with hypercalcemia or hyperphosphatemia and refractory to medical therapy.

A European guideline of clinical algorithms for renal osteodystrophy recommends PTx when a high PTH level (>50 pmol/L) has not decreased by more than 50% after 2 months of medical therapy, or when there are persistent clinical symptoms and the parathyroid gland diameters estimated by parathyroid imaging are over 1 cm.

JSDT guidelines for medical and surgical treatment for SHPT in 2006 and 2012 (Box 61.4) recommend PTx for severe SHPT refractory to medical treatment and PEIT, if only one parathyroid gland is enlarged, and it is located at a site suitable. The guidelines propose that severe SHPT is present when intact PTH levels >500 pg/mil is also levels if hyperphosphatemia and/or hypercalcemia are difficult to manage with medical treatment. These guidelines define severe SHPT when high serum PTH vales are present, but it is important to mention that PTH is modified by serum calcium level and influenced by VDR antagonists and calcimimetics.

The size of enlarged parathyroid gland is an important factor to predict the efficacy of the medical treatment. Therefore our clinic recommends determination of the size of parathyroid gland by ultrasound (US) before aggressive medical treatment. A gland with volume exceeding 500 mm^3 or 1 cm, is likely to have developed nodular hyperplasia. SHPT might, as a result, be resistant to medical treatment in such patients. and PTx may be preferred to medical management (see Box 61.3).

BOX 61.3 Surgical Indications for Secondary Hyperparathyroidism in the Era of Cinacalcet

1. When SHPT is refractory to vitamin D or vitamin D analogues and long-term survival can be expected
2. When quality of life is highly impaired due to severe SHPT
3. When cinacalcet treatment cannot be continued due to adverse effects, poor compliance, or other reasons
4. When sufficient reduction in PTH cannot be achieved with cinacalcet administration
5. Thyroidectomy for thyroid disease, especially papillary thyroid carcinoma is required concomitantly

SHPT, secondary hyperparathyroidism, PTH, parathyroid hormone.

BOX 61.4 Surgical Indications for Secondary Hyperparathyroidism Modified by JSDT Guideline

Essential Components

1. Persistent high serum level of intact PTH level >500 pg/mL
2. Hyperphosphatemia (serum P >6.0 mg/dL) and/or hypercalcemia (serum Ca >10.0 mg/dL) which is refractory to medical therapy.
3. To detect estimated volume of the largest gland >300-500 mm^3 or long axis >1 cm

Clinical Findings

If patients have one of these factors, parathyroidectomy should be absolutely recommended:

1. Deformity, fracture or progressive reduction in bone mineral content
2. Ectopic calcification
   vessels and valvar calcification, tumoral calcinosis, calciphylaxis, calcification in lung, intestine and stomach
3. Neuro-muscular psychiatric symptoms
   muscular weakness, gait disturbance, irritability, sleeplessness, loss of concentration, depression, etc.
4. Anemia resistant to ESA, malnutrition, itching, cough
5. Heart failure (DCM like heart)
6. Severe osteitis fibrosa, high bone turnover bone pain, arthralgia, bone loss, skeletal symptoms (bone and joint pain, arthralgia, muscle weakness, irritability, itching, depression, etc.)

JSDT, Japanese Society for Dialysis Therapy, PTH, parathyroid hormone, ESA, erythropoietin stimulating agent, DCM, dilated cardiomyopathy.

Preoperative Image Diagnosis

Historically, preoperative localization studies for PHPT were usually considered to be less important than the skill of the experienced parathyroid surgeon. Approximately 95% of patients were cured after bilateral cervical exploration by experienced parathyroid surgeons without help of localization studies. Recently, focused exploration has been popularized for patients with PHPT, which is, in turn, facilitated by preoperative localization. For patients with multiglandular disease (MGD) including SHPT, some expert parathyroid surgeons do not require preoperative imaging; however, in our department, we have routinely performed preoperative image diagnosis for the localization and detection of nodular hyperplastic parathyroid glands.

There are several modalities for detecting enlarged parathyroid glands including US, computed tomography (CT), scintigram, magnetic resonance imaging (MRI), and positron emission tomography (PET). (See Chapter 54, Guide to Preoperative Parathyroid Localization Testing). Three dimensions of the affected parathyroid glands can be measured by US, and the volume of glands can be estimated using the formula height: a × width b × depth c × π/6. US has its advantages and disadvantages. Advantages include it is inexpensive, involves no radiation or contrast exposure, is noninvasive, can identify thyroid pathology, and allows for needle biopsy as needed. Disadvantages include it is operator-dependent, and it may miss substernal parathyroid glands or glands that are located in retrotracheal or retroesophageal locations. US allows for fine-needle aspiration biopsy (FNA) and measurement of PTH values.

Four-dimensional computed tomography (4DCT), single-photon emission computed tomography (SPECT), and CT have recently been available and may be beneficial in identification of feeding arteries of parathyroid glands and, perhaps, in detecting smaller glands.

Surgical Procedures for SHPT

As noted earlier, treatment varies based on geographic area and regional philosophies. For SHPT, subtotal PTx, total PTx with autograft and total PTx without autograft have all been widely accepted. In addition, some institutes routine thymectomy at the initial operation.[40-43]

Rhothmund et al. performed a randomized study comparing subtotal PTx and total PTx with autograft; they found no significant difference with respect to efficacy and recurrence rate between the two operative procedures. Others have found similar results.[46-54]

Thus the method used for the surgical treatment of SHPT may depend on surgeon's preference. In the opinion of this author, total PTx with autograft is suitable operative procedure for patients in whom long survival is expected and in whom hemodialysis treatment will be ongoing without the expectation of RTx. In these patients, the risk of recurrent HPT is the main issue, and that risk is negligible after total PTX and autotransplantation.[5,55] However, in patients expecting kidney transplantation, subtotal PTX is optimal in that it preserves some parathyroid glandular function for the posttransplant, normalized metabolic milieu.[56,57]

After identification of all parathyroid glands, remnant size should be tailored to the underlying diagnosis. For subtotal PTx, a volume equivalent to one normal parathyroid gland should be left in patients undergoing dialysis; a volume equivalent to four normal parathyroid glands should be left in patients with successful kidney grafts.

SHPT is a typical MGD due to stimulation to the parathyroid cells, and it will persist to some extent after PTx. Therefore, to avoid reoperation, all parathyroid glands (including supernumerary glands) should be identified. After PTx, adequate medical treatment is required to avoid recurrent SHPT.[56,57]

Advantages and disadvantages in each operative procedure are shown in Box 61.5. There are many options relating to autografting,

> **BOX 61.5 Subtotal Parathyroidectomy**
>
> **Advantages of subtotal PTx:**
> 1. To keep normal parathyroid function after the initial operation
> 2. The procedure is simple
>
> **Disadvantages of subtotal PTx:**
> 1. Retaining adequate parathyroid tissue might be difficult
> 2. Risk of dissemination of parathyroid cells (parathyromatosis)
>
> **Advantages of total PTx with autograft**
> 1. Adequate amount of parathyroid tissue can be retained (transplanted)
> 2. At recurrence, it is easy to resect parathyroid tissue noninvasively
>
> **Disadvantages of total PTx with autograft**
> 1. Hypoparathyroidism immediately after PTx requires significant postop Ca replacement
> 2. Possible risk of dissemination of parathyroid cells into muscular tissue
>
> PTx, parathyroidectomy, Ca, calcium.

such as timing, location, amount of tissue grafted, and type of hyperplastic tissue grafted. Delayed transplant means that after confirmation of hypoparathyroidism, cryopreserved parathyroid tissue is autografted. Because autograft of cryopreserved, parathyroid tissue is logistically challenging, expensive, and may result in failure. Delayed autografting has not been widely accepted.

Several sites for autograft have been proposed. The original autograft site described by Wells was the brachioradialis muscle.[47] It is possible to evaluate function of autografted parathyroid tissue by measuring PTH levels after sampling from both antecubital veins. Some surgeons prefer to autograft into the sternocleidomastoid muscle, abdominal muscle, or into the subcutaneous fat of the forearm, abdomen, or presternal area. Recently, autograft into the tibialis anterior muscle has been reported.[57] At graft-dependent recurrence it has been suggested that it may be easier to remove autografted tissue from fat tissue than from muscle. No prospective randomized control studies have presented evidence demonstrating strong preference for autografting site.

Selection of parathyroid tissue for autograft has been an important issue. Our group previously reported that when transplanting nodular hyperplastic tissue, the frequency of graft-dependent recurrence was significantly higher than when diffuse hyperplastic tissue was autografted.

The amount of autografted parathyroid tissue is another issue. It has been proposed by that 10 to 15 pieces of 1 × 1 × 3 mm of parathyroid tissue should be autografted in patients with MEN Type 1. Because optimal PTH levels might be higher in patients with CKD, our group has been transplanting 30 pieces corresponding to about 90 mg of parathyroid tissue.

Another question is whether there is a role for total PTx without autograft. An advantage of this procedure is that the treatment is simple, and that risk of recurrence is very low. The disadvantage is the risk of hypoparathyroidism, in which a large amount of calcium replacement is required and, in turn, ectopic calcification and cardiovascular complication may be induced; hypoparathyroidism resulting from the procedure may increase mortality. Because of the risks of hypoparathyroidism and uncontrollable hypocalcemia after kidney transplant, KDQI and JSDT guidelines recommend that total PTx without autograft should be avoided for patients anticipating kidney transplant.[21,51,58-65]

At present, we cannot determine which procedure is the most suitable operative procedure for patients with advanced SHPT.

The decision may depend on the surgeon's preference and clinical status of the patients (i.e., whether the patient is a candidate for kidney transplantation, the patient's age, and the patient's expected survival after PTx), as well as the patient's compliance with medicines.[66]

In our experience, subtotal PTx is frequently followed by recurrent HPT due to residual parathyroid tissue in the neck. When reexploration of the neck is required, there is higher risk to injure the recurrent laryngeal nerves (RLNs) than at the initial operation. Such revision surgery also carries some risk of parathyromatosis. For patients who require long-term hemodialysis after PTx, the risk for recurrence is not negligible. Because it is easier and safer to remove residual parathyroid tissue from the forearm at recurrence compared with a neck reexploration, total PTx with forearm autograft is, according to our opinion, recommended in a patient who has to continue hemodialysis for long periods after the operation without RTx.

Preoperative Examination and Management

Generally, PTx for SHPT is performed under general anesthesia. Because patients on hemodialysis frequently have comorbid cardiovascular disease, careful preoperative evaluation is mandatory. Adequate preoperative hemodialysis, especially to prevent hyperpotassemia and overhydration, is required before the operation. The operation can be performed under local anesthesia in these patients because of high risk of general anesthesia.[67]

Surgical Approach

In SHPT, the underlying metabolic stimuli act on all parathyroid glands and tissue and fundamentally all glands including supernumerary glands are hyperplastic. Thus, to avoid persistent/recurrent HPT, all parathyroid glands including supernumerary glands should be detected. It has been reported that the frequency of supernumerary glands detected at surgery for SHPT is as high as 15% to 20%. To remove supernumerary glands, resection of surrounding fat tissue of original parathyroid glands is essential. In our series, the frequency of rudimentary or split type glands was 24.8%. It is not so difficult to detect these type glands at the operation because the glands are usually located surrounding original glands. True supernumerary glands most commonly occur in the thymus and can be detected histopathologically after the operation. Also, up to 40% of inferior glands can be located in thymic tongue. Thus removal of thymic tissue from neck incision is important to avoid missing glands. The second and frequent location of supernumerary glands is the left paratracheal, paraoesophageal area. Careful searching of these areas is necessary.

To detect parathyroid glands, junction between RLN and inferior thyroid artery is a very useful landmark (Figure 61.6) (see Chapters 36, Surgical Anatomy and Monitoring of the Recurrent Laryngeal Nerve, and 55, Principles in Surgical Management of Primary Hyperparathyroidism). The superior glands are most frequently located superior to the artery nerve crossing point and dorsal to the RLN (see Figure 61.6, *area A*). If the gland cannot be identified in the area, the area ventral to the RLN (see Figure 61.6, *area C*) should be searched. Superior glands may sometimes drop into the paraesophageal area and may extend caudally to toward the posterior mediastinal direction (Figure 61.7). The gland may be identified dissecting along the inferior thyroid artery. This course may lead to the descent of the superior gland. If the superior gland is missed, the ipsilateral upper pole of thyroid lobe is mobilized, and the posterior surface of thyroid lobe, the area of superior thyroid artery, the space anteromedial RLN (surrounding Berry's ligament) as well as lateral and posterior to esophagus, and the carotid sheath are searched. If the gland cannot be identified, an ipsilateral thyroid partial lobectomy can be performed.

The inferior parathyroid gland most frequently is located inferior to the artery-nerve crossing point landmark and lies ventral relative to the RLN. If the inferior gland cannot be discovered, dissection of paratracheal fat tissue is performed (as one does in a central lymph node dissection). If the gland cannot be found, an exploration of the thyro-thymic ligament can be performed. If undescended thymus can be detected, the thymic tissue should be resected carefully because the inferior gland can sometimes be located in undescended thymus (Figure 61.8). The surrounding carotid artery should be dissected.

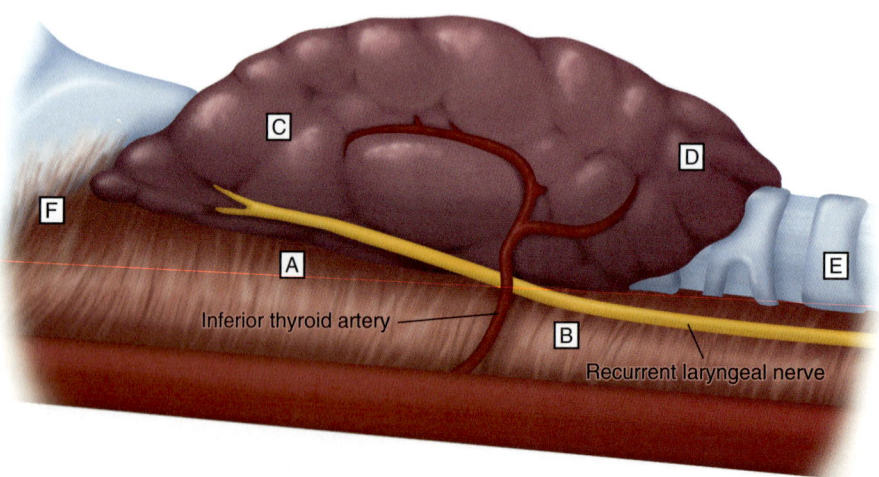

Fig. 61.6 Location of parathyroid glands. **A,** superior from the junction between recurrent laryngeal nerve and inferior thyroid artery (landmark) and dorsal from recurrent laryngeal nerve. **B,** Inferior from the junction and dorsal from the nerve. **C,** Superior from the junction and ventral from the nerve. **D,** Inferior from the junction and ventral from the nerve. **E,** Paratracheal area including the thyrothymic ligament and thymic tongue. **F,** Superior from upper pole of thyroid lobe

CHAPTER 61 Surgical Management of Secondary and Tertiary Hyperparathyroidism 571

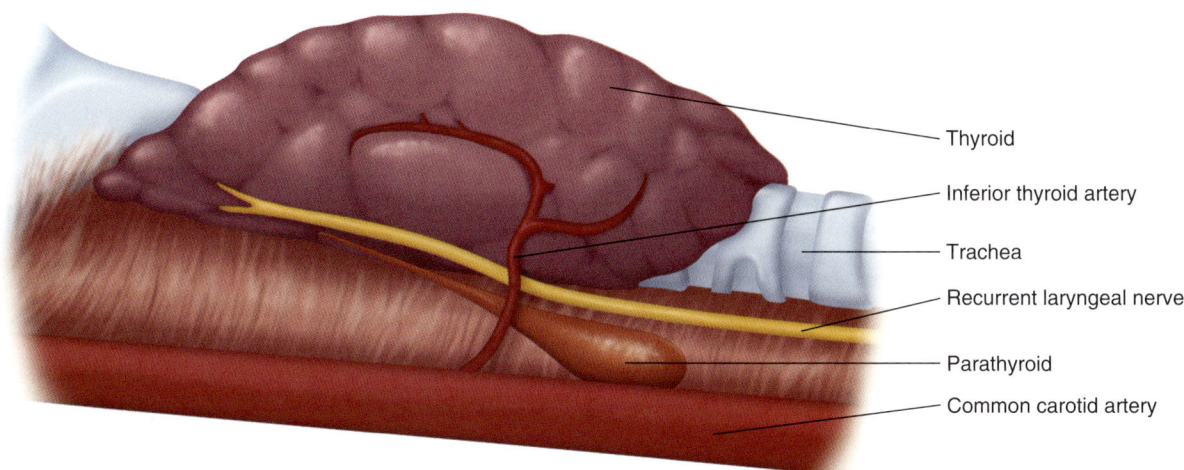

Fig. 61.7 Superior parathyroid gland uncommonly descends to mediastinum.

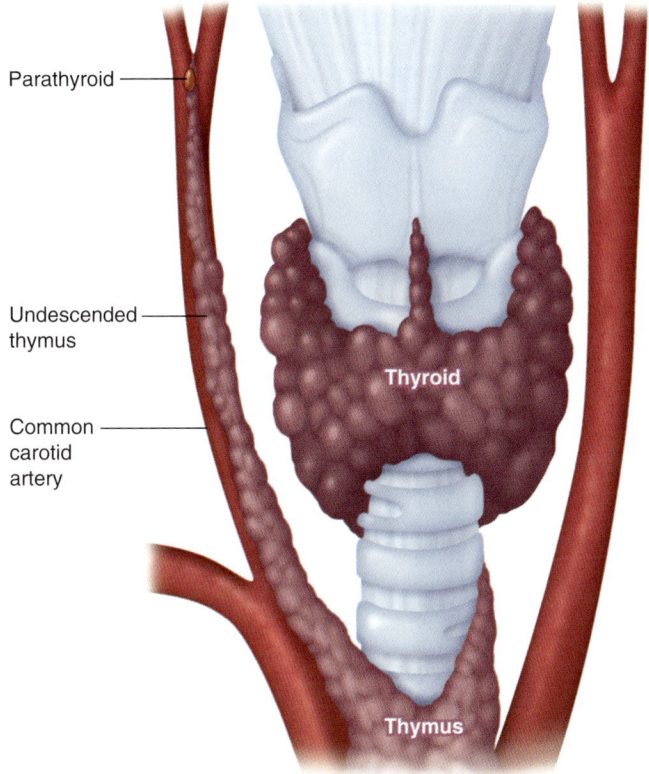

Fig. 61.8 Undescended thymus with parathyroid gland located on top of undescended thymic tongue.

If the gland cannot be discovered by these procedures, the ipsilateral thyroid lobe can be resected. It is very important to avoid injury and rupture of parathyroid capsule to prevent dissemination of parathyroid cells surrounding tissue.[68,69]

In treating patients who will continue long-term hemodialysis treatment after parathyroid surgery and who are expected to have extended survival, we prefer total PTx with forearm autograft and resection of thymic tissue from neck incision.

Intraoperative PTH monitoring is useful to recognize adequacy of removal of pathologic parathyroid tissue gland in SHPT. However, we should keep in mind that PTH is metabolized partially in kidney and the half-life of 1-84 PTH is therefore affected by uremia. In our experience, if the intact PTH level drops under 30% of the level at the beginning of the operation, resection should be judged as complete.[70]

After identification of all parathyroid glands, the remnant size should be tailored to the underlying diagnosis. For subtotal PTx, a volume equivalent to one normal parathyroid gland should be left in patients undergoing dialysis; and a volume equivalent to four normal parathyroids should be left in patients with successful kidney graft.

It is very important to select hyperplastic parathyroid tissue for autograft to prevent graft-dependent recurrent HPT. We have reported that when transplanting nodular hyperplastic tissue, the frequency of graft-dependent recurrence was significantly higher than when diffuse hyperplastic tissue was autografted. The site and method for performing autografts is another issue. In the most widely accepted method small parathyroid parenchymal pieces are autografted to the muscle of the forearm. Some surgeons prefer to autograft into the sternocleidomastoid muscle, the subcutaneous forearm tissue, to a subcutaneous, presternal position, or to the abdomen or tibial muscle. As noted earlier, there have been no prospective randomized control studies presenting evidence for a preferable site for autografting.

Resected parathyroid glands are preserved in cold saline after the removal (Figure 61.9). After pathologic confirmation, 1 × 1 × 3 mm slices are made from diffuse hyperplastic tissue for autograft[21,51,65] (Figure 61.10). We make a pocket in the brachioradial muscle of forearm without A-V fistula and put a piece in each muscle pocket using nonabsorbable suture. We perform that same procedure at 30 times. In total, about 90 mg of parathyroid tissue is autografted (Figure 61.11).

Postoperative Management

Several issues may need to be addressed after PTx for SHPT, such as monitoring for postoperative hemorrhage, assessment of vocal cord function, and monitoring for overhydration, hyperkalemia, and hypocalcemia.

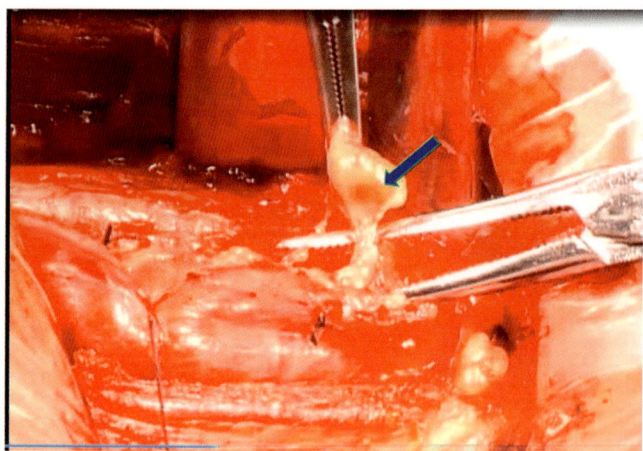

Fig. 61.9 Small parathyroid gland located in fatty tissue surrounding lower pole of thyroid lobe was resected en bloc with fatty tissue.

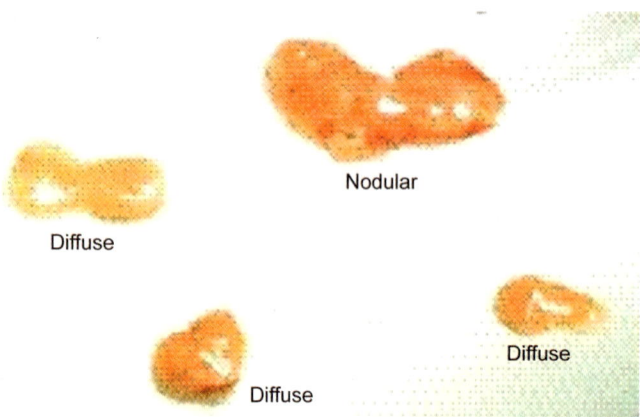

Fig. 61.10 From diffuse hyperplastic parathyroid gland, 1 × 1 × 3 mm slices were made.

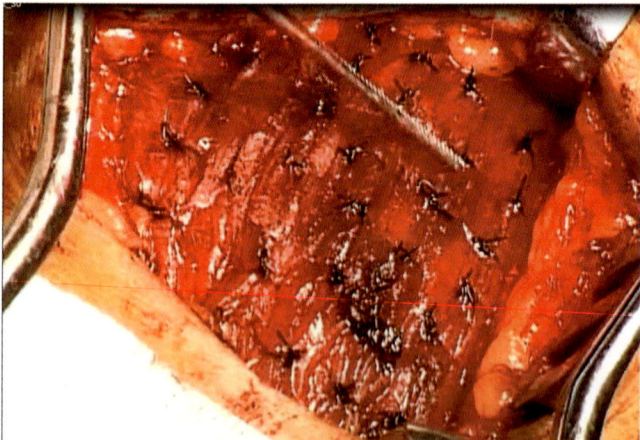

Fig. 61.11 30 parathyroid slices were autografted into brachioradial muscle.

Dialysis patients have an increased risk of bleeding. To prevent postoperative hemorrhage, careful hemostasis should be performed during operation. Drains and hemostatic materials can be considered. Despite these efforts, hemorrhage cannot always be avoided; hemorrhage occurs in 1 out of 500 cases in our experience. Careful follow-up is required after the operation.

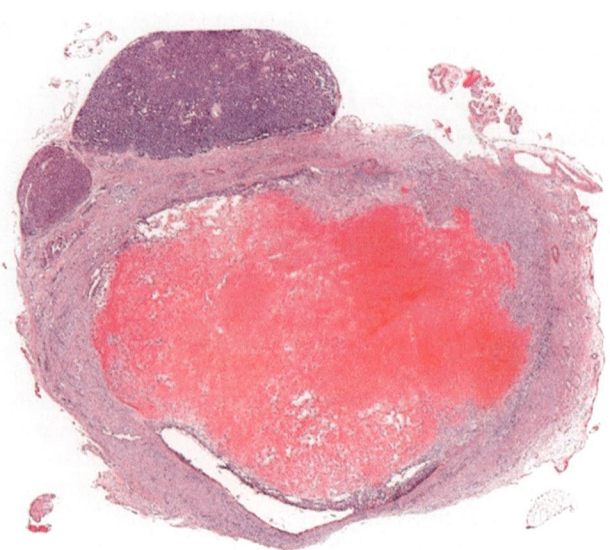

Fig. 61.12 Hemorrhagic infarction and fibroses are encountered frequently after exposure of cinacalcet.

Injury to the RLN is a significant issue. After administration of cinacalcet, fibrosis and hemorrhage with infarction in the parathyroid gland may frequently occur. The later may induce adhesions around the parathyroid glands that lead to difficult dissection and paralysis of the RLN (Figure 61.12). We have found that intraoperative neural RLN monitoring is useful to prevent injury to the RLN, especially in patients who already have a unilateral paralysis of the RLN before PTx (see Chapter 36, Surgical Anatomy and Monitoring of the Recurrent Laryngeal Nerve).

After PTx, serum calcium level drops rapidly because patients usually have severe hungry bone syndrome; calcium and phosphorus move to bone from blood as bone formation becomes prominent. It is of note that autografted parathyroid tissue begins functioning only 2 to 3 weeks after PTx. Each institute has individualized protocols to supplement calcium. We initiate calcium replacement therapy when the serum calcium level decreases under 9.0 mg/dL. If the Al-P level before PTx is more than 500 IU/L, which implies the patient will have severe hungry bone syndrome postoperatively, we initiate 1200 mg/day intravenous (IV) calcium replacement via central venous line, as well as oral supplementation (i.e., alphacalcidol 3 mcg/day, and calcium carbonate 12 g/day). If Al-P level is less than 500 IU/L, IV calcium supplementation can generally be omitted with the initiation of only oral calcium and vitamin D replacement. We adjust the dose of calcium agent and vitamin D to obtain a serum calcium level of between 8 to 9 mg/dL. Recently, it has been shown that in patients with administration of VDR antagonists and/or cinacalcet, the incidence of severe hungry bone has decreased. Sometimes, emergent hemodialysis is required because of hyperpotassemia and/or overhydration.

Careful follow-up is needed. After PTx serum calcium (Ca), P, and PTH level should be kept in target ranges by adequate medical treatment to prevent recurrent HPT, adynamic bone disease, and ectopic calcification.[71-74] Medical treatment after PTx is important to prevent recurrent HPT and adynamic bone disease. When intact-PTH level less than 100 pg/mL, serum calcium level should be controlled within 8 to 9 mg/dL. When intact-PTH level exceeds 100 pg/mL, serum calcium level should be controlled between 9 and 10 mg/dL to prevent recurrent HPT. Physicians must be aware of the development of adynamic bone disease both due to low PTH levels (especially after aggressive PTX) and also due to bone resistance to PTH inherent in CKD, which may be associated with ectopic calcification.

Function of Autografted Parathyroid Tissue

Function of grafted parathyroid tissue can be recognized by measuring PTH levels sampled from both antecubital veins. PTH gradient is defined as PTH level of grafted arm per PTH level from nongrafted arm. If the gradient exceeds to 1.5, the autograft is judged as "functioning." In our series, almost all grafted parathyroid tissue was functioning.[75]

The effect of PTx is dramatic and remarkable. After PTx, serum calcium and phosphorus have generally achieved recommended target values in the treatment of SHPT for at least 3 years. Symptoms of SHPT (i.e., bone pain, depression, itching, easy fatigue, etc.) are generally relieved by PTx. Bone metabolism has been clearly improved by PTx. The bone mineral content in cortical bone measured by x-ray absorptiometry increases after PTx. Bone biopsy has shown that bone resorption is immediately suppressed, and bone formation is accelerated after PTx. Fracture risk has been lower among hemodialysis patients who underwent PTx when compared with matched control subjects.[10,76-78]

It is well known that calciphylaxis and tumoral calcinosis are generally remarkably improved by PTx. Unfortunately, vascular and valvular calcifications are usually not affected, even by successful PTx.[75,79-85] It is therefore important that PTx should be performed at an early stage before the calcification can become progressive. Beneficial effects by PTx on anemia,[86,87] muscle strength, nutritional state,[78,88] cognition,[89] 22-immune system,[90,91] and blood pressure[92] have been reported.

Mortality and Complications

PTx is expected to improve survival in hemodialysis patients with advanced SHPT.[93-97] In a retrospective, observational study, Kestenbaum et al. evaluated a large series of patients. Using an American database, they showed that at about 560 days, survival of the PTx group surpassed that of the non-PTx group.[98] Costa-Hong studied cardiovascular events and mortality in hemodialysis patients with advanced SHPT and reported that PTx was associated with reduced incidence of major cardiovascular events and overall mortality. Recently, Komaba et al. have evaluated mortality of Japanese hemodialysis patients who underwent PTx; the clinicians compared these patients with patients who had advanced SHPT without PTx. The clinicians reported that patients in the PTx group had better overall 10-year survival than patients in the non-PTx group. It has been proposed that PTx has beneficial influence on reducing mortality; this is mainly because of prevention of cardiovascular complications. Healthier and relatively younger patients can reach long-term survival with hemodialysis treatment after PTx.[99-102]

In our series, mortality is defined as death within 1 month after PTx, occurred in 3/3500 (0.09%) patients. Three patients in our hospital suffered from chronic heart failure before PTx. Paralysis of the RLN is usually <1%. Wound bleeding and reoperation is less than 0.3%. Incidentally, 5.8% of patients undergoing PTx also were found to have thyroid carcinoma. When thyroid carcinoma is speculated by US before the operation, thyroidectomy should be performed concomitantly.[103,104]

Persistent and Recurrent HPT

It is difficult to define SHPT as recurrent or persistent because serum calcium level is easily changed by medical treatment after PTx. We routinely measure intact PTH level day 1 after PTx. When the lowest PTH levels is more than the upper normal range (60 pg/mL), we define it as persistent HPT, whereas when the PTH becomes elevated over time, we define the condition as recurrent HPT.[105]

The number of parathyroid glands removed at initial PTx in our series is presented as the following: in 3.9% of patients, fewer than four glands were removed, and supernumerary glands were detected in 17.3% cases that underwent initial PTx at our institute.[106-108] Based on the previously stated definition, the incidence of persistent HPT was 4.0%. Mediastinal parathyroid glands were the most common cause of persistent HPT. The most common location of mediastinal parathyroid glands was the aortic-pulmonary window.

As for recurrent HPT, we should consider several factors as possible origins of oversecretion of PTH after total PTx with forearm autograft. The factors are the following: autograft hyperfunction, residual gland in neck or mediastinum, distant metastasis of parathyroid carcinoma, and local regional implantation surrounding thyroid gland (parathyromatosis) (Box 61.6).

For reoperation, detection of a targetable surgical lesion preoperatively, through imaging, is essential (see Chapter 63, Reoperation for Sporadic Primary Hyperparathyroidism). First, one must determine whether the recurrence is graft-dependent by PTH gradient and/or Casanova's test. When PTH levels do not drop significantly by grafted arm tourniquet, it is recognized that the origin is not autograft but residual gland in neck or mediastinum. If the recurrence is graft-dependent, the enlarged graft should be evaluated by MRI or US. Autografted parathyroid tissue should be removed en bloc with surrounding muscle to prevent re-removal of autograft (Figures 61.13 and 61.14). With this muscle/parathyroid tissue debulking, typically, parathyroid tissue can be identified microscopically within the remaining graft bed and hypoparathyroidism can be avoided. The frequency of

---

BOX 61.6 Possible Origins of Oversecretion of PTH after initial PTx for SHPT

1. Autograph excess function
2. Residual gland in neck or mediastinum (mediastinal, intrathyroidal, undescended gland, etc.)
3. Parathyromatosis
4. Parathyroid carcinoma (distant metastasis)

PTH, parathyroid hormone, PTx, parathyroidectomy, SHPT, secondary hyperparathyroidism.

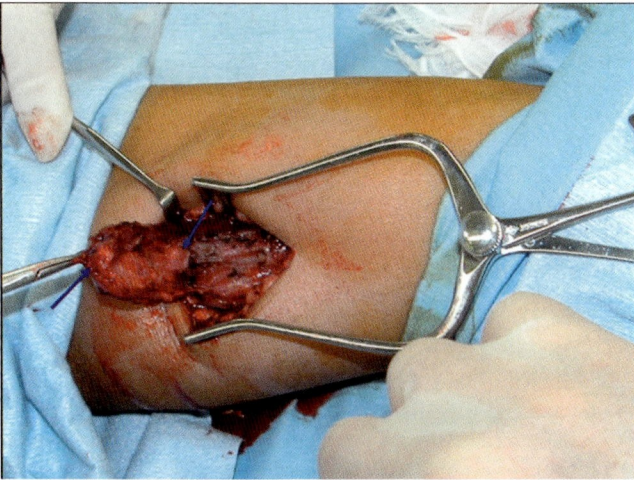

Fig. 61.13 Graft-dependent recurrent secondary hyperparathyroidism (SHPT). Enlarged autografts are resected en bloc with surrounding muscle to avoid reoperation.

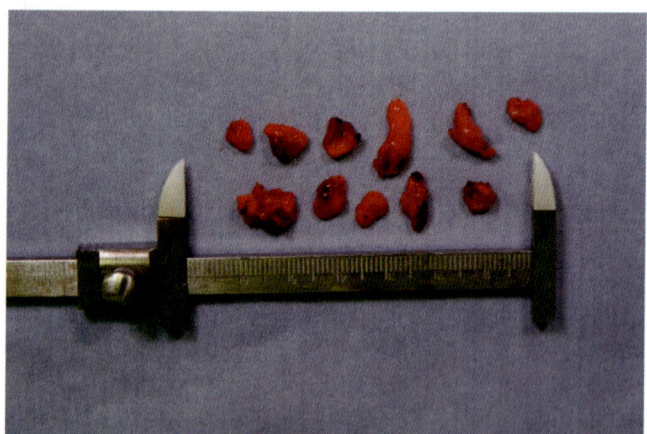

Fig. 61.14 Removed autografted nodules.

TABLE 61.1 Incidence of Ectopic Parathyroid Gland(s) Detected Both at Initial Operation and Reoperation in Our Series

Undescended gland	0.97%
Intrathyroidal	2.2%
Surrounding Berry's ligament	1.3%
Mediastinal*	1.38%
Parathyromatosis	0.3%
Parathyroid carcinoma**	0.14%

*Gland located in mediastinum removed with sternotomy or endoscopic procedure
**With distant metastasis

graft-dependent recurrence has increased gradually (about 17.5% at 10 years after initial PTx in our series).

If the recurrence is not graft-dependent, residual glands should be evaluated by at first US and then scintigram. The incidence of recurrent HPT due to residual glands in neck or mediastinum was only 1.4% in our series. The common locations of residual glands in patients with recurrent HPT were left paratracheal, intrathymus, intrathyroidal, and undescended glands. The incidence of glands removed at the initial PTx and reoperation in each ectopic site in our series is shown in Table 61.1.[109]

Neck reexploration in patients, who had their initial operation performed at other hospitals, can be problematic because it can be difficult to detect RLNs. We feel it is very important to review all records available from the initial operation and to use nerve monitoring to identify RLNs in these difficult revision cases. The remaining glands are frequently located at usual sites, such as the thymic tongue. Undescended glands and glands located surrounding Berry's ligament are also sometimes found in these revision circumstances.[110]

Parathyromatosis is defined as multiple foci of benign hyperfunctioning parathyroid tissue in the neck or mediastinum. Parathyromatosis is usually induced by rupture of capsule of parathyroid glands during surgical exploration or PEIT. It is usually very difficult to diagnose parathyromatosis by image diagnosis; in spite of reoperative en-bloc resection with thyroid, high PTH levels persisted sometimes.

We recommended chest CT examination for patients whose origin of PTH oversecretion cannot be found by common radiographic diagnostic procedures. In some patients with parathyromatosis, distant metastasis of parathyroid carcinoma, HPT cannot be controlled by surgical treatment. In these cases, cinacalcet is useful to control hypercalcemia.[111-114]

TERTIARY HYPERPARATHYROIDISM

Hyperparathyroidism after Successful Kidney Transplantation

Clinical Manifestation

Hyperparathyroidism (HPT) after successful kidney transplantation is termed THPT. Disturbance in bone metabolism with bone loss, high risk of fracture, and cardiovascular events are common complications that affect patients after successful RTx and represent important causes of morbidity and mortality. Three major components contribute to bone metabolism disturbances in patients after RTx include preexisting renal osteodystrophy at time of RTx, effects from immunosuppressive agents, and reduced renal function after transplantation.[115-119] Advanced SHPT can therefore persist after successful kidney transplantation, and PTx sometimes is required in these patients.[120]

Requiring surgical intervention occurs in 1% to 5% of patients with SHPT after successful kidney transplantation. Long-term dialysis before RTx and detection of enlarged nodular parathyroid glands are predictive factors for requirement of PTx for THPT. Laboratory investigation reveals hypercalcemia, hypophosphatemia, moderately elevated PTH level, and a usually increased Al-P level. In majority of patients with HPT after kidney transplantation, hypercalcemia and hypophosphatemia usually resolve within the first year.[121,122]

Patients with THPT may suffer from bone pain, joint pain, fractures, bone loss, nephrolithiasis, and soft tissue or vascular calcification (including nephrocalcinosis which can in turn sometimes influence kidney graft function). Usually, through imaging (e.g., US or MIBI scintigram), an enlarged parathyroid gland can be detected.[123]

Medical Treatment and Surgical Indication

Recently, cinacalcet has been used for patients with THPT. It has been found that cinacalcet can control HPT and hypercalcemia among patients with THPT with a low incidence of side effect. However, at present, the use of cinacalcet in patients with CKD stage 3 or 4 and THPT has yet to be approved, and its treatment in this particular clinical setting remains controversial.[123-125]

As for dialysis patients with advanced SHPT, PTx is most successful treatment for resolving advanced HPT in patients with THPT. However, the surgical indications for THPT and the timing of the operation are problematic because hypercalcemia can spontaneously resolve within 1 year after RTx. When parathyroid hyperplasia progresses to nodular hyperplasia, SHPT cannot be relieved by successful RTx. Evaluation of gland size by ultrasound informs the surgeon as to the likelihood of response to RTx surgery. The factors listed in Box 61.7 have been accepted as indications for PTx in patients with THPT.[126,127]

BOX 61.7 Indications for Parathyroidectomy (PTx) in Patients With THPT

1. Persistent hypercalcemia more than 6 months after kidney transplant
2. Low bone mineral density
3. Renal stone or nephrocalcinosis
4. Deterioration of kidney graft due to THPT
5. Symptomatic HPT (bone and joint pain, bone fracture, purities, fatigue, depression, irritability, sleeplessness, peptic ulcer, etc.)
6. Enlarged parathyroid gland detected by US

PTx, parathyroidectomy, THPT, tertiary hyperparathyroidism, HPT, hyperparathyroidism, US, ultrasound.

Surgical Procedures

Subtotal PTx and total PTx with autograft are widely accepted for THPT. Total PTx without autograft cannot be accepted for patients with THPT because of persistent uncontrollable hypocalcemia. A majority of surgeons prefer subtotal PTx for patients with THPT; surgeons recommend a volume equivalent to four normal parathyroid glands, which should be maintained (assuming successful kidney graft function) to prevent hypoparathyroidism and hypocalcemia.[128-131]

Deterioration of kidney graft function after PTx for THPT has been described. It has been hypothesized that transient hypoparathyroidism may be a possible explanation for impairment of kidney graft function. PTH has vasodilatory effect on preglomerular vessels. Renal graft deterioration occurs during the first week after the PTx, but usually renal function shows slow-but-steady improvement over a number of years toward their former baseline. For the treatment of THPT, subtotal PTx, rather than total PTx with autograft, has been recommended to prevent kidney function deterioration.

REFERENCES

For a complete list of references, go to expertconsult.com.

Parathyroid Management in the MEN Syndromes

Tracy S. Wang, Douglas B. Evans

Primary hyperparathyroidism (PHPT) is the presence of elevated serum calcium levels combined with inappropriate suppression of parathyroid hormone (PTH). It is most commonly a sporadic disease; however, in a small subset of patients, it can be part of a familial syndrome. These inherited disorders include multiple endocrine neoplasia (MEN) type 1, MEN type 2A, hyperparathyroid-jaw tumor syndrome, familial isolated hyperparathyroidism, and benign familial hypocalciuric hypercalcemia. This chapter focuses on the surgical management of HPT in patients with MEN 1 and MEN 2A.

MULTIPLE ENDOCRINE NEOPLASIA (MEN) TYPE 1

MEN 1 is an autosomal dominant disease with a prevalence of 2 to 3 persons per 100,000 population; it is equally common among men and women.[1,2] MEN 1 is clinically defined as the presence of any two of the three most common tumors in a single patient: parathyroid tumors (manifested as PHPT); pituitary tumors; and pancreatic neuroendocrine tumors (pNETs), most commonly gastrinoma, insulinoma, and nonfunctioning pNETs (Figure 62.1). Other MEN 1-associated tumors include facial angiofibromas, lipomas, carcinoid tumors, thyroid neoplasms, nonfunctional adrenocortical adenomas, and rarely, pheochromocytomas.[3,4] Familial MEN 1 is defined clinically as an index case of MEN 1 and at least one first-degree relative with tumors in one or more of these sites.

GENETIC TESTING IN MEN 1

MEN 1 is caused by a germline mutation in the *MEN 1* gene, which is located at chromosome 11q13; it encodes the 610-amino acid protein referred to as *menin*. The menin protein has a role in DNA replication and repair, and it is involved in transcriptional regulation. *MEN 1* gene mutations generally result in a truncated menin protein, and the mechanism of tumor formation appears to occur according to the *two-hit* hypotheses; the first genetic hit is inherited and is present in all cells. When the second copy of *MEN 1* is mutated in any one cell, a neoplastic clonal expansion is initiated, which leads to the development and manifestation of MEN 1–related tumors.

More than 1300 mutations of the *MEN 1* gene were identified within the first decade after the gene was identified, including 1133 germline and 201 somatic mutations; these mutations have been found in 70% to 90% of families with MEN 1.[1,5] Despite this diversity in mutations of the menin gene, studies of patients with MEN 1 have supported the theory that the MEN 1 trait arises from the same chromosomal locus because >90% of tumors exhibit loss of heterozygosity (LOH) on 11q13; therefore the tumors result from mutations in the menin gene.[3] The heterogeneity of mutations has made mutational analysis in MEN 1 challenging. In addition, at least 10% of *MEN 1* germline mutations arise *de novo*.[3] From a clinical perspective, this heterogeneity has resulted in the lack of a population-level genotype-phenotype correlation (as opposed to MEN 2A). A specific *MEN 1* mutation does not appear to be associated with the development and biologic behavior of tumors or the clinical features of disease, such as patient age or sites of tumor development.[1,4,6] A review of the literature has demonstrated that, in general, different families with the same clinical manifestations have had diversity in mutations and, likewise, different families with different clinical manifestations have been found to have the same *MEN 1* mutation.[4,7-9] However, the specific mutation type and location may be associated with the expression of a relatively constant phenotype within an individual family kindred of MEN 1 patients.[4]

Genetic testing allows affected patients with a known germline mutation to be followed prospectively, which facilitates earlier surgical intervention and potentially decreases morbidity and mortality. Furthermore, patients with a negative genetic test can be spared annual clinical testing and are assured that there is no risk of passing a mutation on to their children.[1,4] The most recent guidelines for the management of patients with MEN 1 include the following recommendations for genetic counseling and *MEN 1* germline mutational analysis: (1) an index case with ≥2 MEN 1-associated endocrinopathies (parathyroid, pancreas, or pituitary); (2) all first-degree relatives of a known *MEN 1* mutation carrier; or (3) in patients with suspicious or atypical features which may be consistent with MEN 1. This latter category would include all patients <30 years of age already diagnosed with PHPT, multigland PHPT, gastrinoma syndrome, multiple pNETs (at any age), or patients with ≥2 MEN 1-associated tumors that are not part of the classical triad of MEN 1-associated tumors (e.g., PHPT and adrenal tumor).[3,10] The age threshold that should prompt genetic testing for patients with PHPT is not absolute; some experts have suggested genetic testing for patients with PHPT at <40 years of age.[11]

Periodic screening for MEN 1-associated endocrine tumors in *MEN 1* carriers (known germline mutation) is likely to be beneficial because earlier diagnosis and appropriate timing of any necessary treatment may help reduce morbidity and mortality. Age-related penetrance for all features is near zero in patients younger than 5 years of age, greater than 50% by age 20, and above 95% by age 40.[3] In the majority of patients with MEN 1, PHPT will be the first manifestation of the disorder; in approximately 15% of patients, hyperprolactinemia (sometimes asymptomatic) will present first. MEN 1 consensus guidelines currently recommend biochemical screening at least annually to

CHAPTER 62 Parathyroid Management in the MEN Syndromes

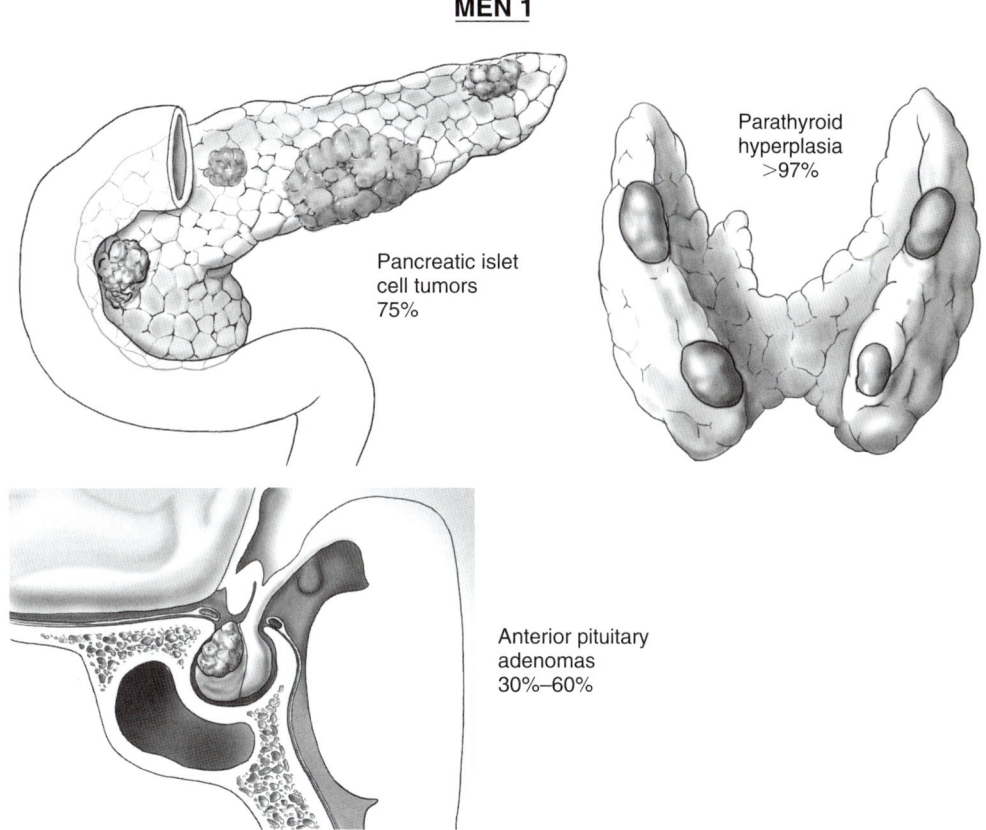

Fig. 62.1 The most common clinical features of multiple endocrine neoplasia type 1 (MEN 1). (Printed with permission from © brysonbiomed.com.)

include serum calcium and intact PTH levels beginning by age 8. Other biochemical evaluation would include prolactin, chromogranin A, IGF-1, and gastrointestinal hormones (e.g., gastrin, insulin with a fasting glucose, glucagon, VIP, and pancreatic polypeptide). In addition, imaging studies (i.e., magnetic resonance imaging (MRI) or computed tomography (CT) of the pancreas, adrenal glands, and pituitary) every 1 to 3 years are recommended.[3]

MEN 1–ASSOCIATED HYPERPARATHYROIDISM

MEN 1-associated HPT accounts for 2% to 4% of all cases of PHPT. It is characterized by multigland disease (MGD) with the clonal, asymmetric enlargement of all parathyroid glands.[2,3,12,13] The typical age of onset of MEN 1-associated PHPT is in the third or fourth decade and is often the first manifestation of MEN 1. Importantly, there is near complete penetrance (>90%) of PHPT by age 50.[3,14,15] MEN 1-associated HPT occurs approximately 30 years earlier than in patients with sporadic PHPT.

Symptoms in patients with MEN 1-associated PHPT are similar to those in patients with sporadic PHPT; they include the following: nephrolithiasis, decrease in bone mineral density, muscle weakness, aches and pains, and neurocognitive symptoms of fatigue, depression, mood changes, sleep impairment, and difficulty with memory and concentration. Patients with MEN 1-associated PHPT may have a long asymptomatic phase but often have more aggressive disease due to recurrent HPT. Even if asymptomatic, gene carriers have a detectable decrease in bone mass density by age 35.[2,14,16] MEN 1 can cause simultaneous PHPT and Zollinger-Ellison syndrome (gastrinoma), and hypercalcemia increases the secretion of gastrin from gastrin-secreting tumors of the pancreas and duodenum.

Given the two-hit etiology of MEN 1-associated PHPT, parathyroid gland involvement is often asynchronous and asymmetric. Macroscopically-normal parathyroid glands have been reported in 12% to 55% of patients at the time of initial surgery, particularly in younger patients.[2,5,14] It has been postulated that the prospect of having simultaneous *second hits* in each of the parathyroid glands is extremely low, but that the probability that the second hit would occur in a parathyroid gland increases with time. Therefore the likelihood of having a phenotypically normal-appearing parathyroid gland decreases with age.[17] Supernumerary (more than four) and ectopic parathyroid glands have also been reported in up to 20% of affected patients; these glands may be found intrathymic, intrathyroidal, or in the anterior mediastinum. This may be related to the presence of parathyroid rests (embryonic parathyroid remnants) that are stimulated.[5,14] Malignant progression of MEN 1-associated PHPT (parathyroid carcinoma) has not been reported.

INDICATIONS FOR SURGERY

Indications for parathyroidectomy are no different in patients with MEN 1 than for those with sporadic PHPT.[3,5,11-13,18] Parathyroidectomy is recommended for patients with symptomatic PHPT (nephrolithiasis, peptic ulcer disease, fragility fractures), particularly those with hypergastrinemia due to Zollinger-Ellison syndrome (even if asymptomatic) because successful surgery may markedly reduce gastrin secretion.[19-21] Recent guidelines for the management of patients with asymptomatic PHPT recommend surgery for patients with (1) serum calcium levels 1 mg/dL (0.25 mmol/L) above reference range; (2) age <50 years; (3) renal effects, including creatinine clearance <60 mL/min, 24-hour urine calcium >400 mg/day, increased stone risk by biochemical stone risk analysis, presence of nephrolithiasis or nephrocalcinosis on imaging studies; or, (4) skeletal effects, including bone mineral density by dual energy x-ray absorptiometry (DXA) consistent with a T score of >2.5 at any site or a vertebral fracture on imaging studies.[11,18] The American Association of Endocrine Surgeons (AAES) guidelines for the management of PHPT also recommend (strong recommendation, low-quality evidence) parathyroidectomy for patients with neurocognitive and/or neuropsychiatric symptoms thought to be attributable to PHPT.[11]

For patients with MEN 1-associated PHPT, it is unclear if earlier surgical treatment reduces morbidity or mortality, particularly in those patients who are asymptomatic or minimally symptomatic. Early parathyroidectomy, especially in younger patients, would decrease the long-term effects of PHPT, particularly with reference to skeletal effects. Bone mineral density evaluation should therefore play an important role in the planning and timing of surgery.[12,14,16,22] Earlier intervention may also improve the symptoms of other concomitant endocrinopathies, such as hypergastrinemia.[14] However, postponing surgery may facilitate the initial procedure by increasing the likelihood of finding all parathyroid glands as they may be larger and easier to locate, including the presence of supernumerary/ectopic glands. Delayed intervention may also decrease the likelihood of persistent/recurrent disease and the need for a future reoperative parathyroidectomy.[14]

The use of preoperative localization studies (e.g., technetium-99m sestamibi with single photon emission computed tomography cervical ultrasonography, or CT [Tc99m MIBI-SPECT/CT]) before initial parathyroidectomy solely for localization of abnormal parathyroid gland(s) in patients with MEN 1-associated PHPT remains debated when considering the high likelihood of multigland hyperplasia and the need for bilateral exploration and intraoperative identification of all parathyroid glands. However, imaging studies may be helpful in the identification/localization of ectopic or supernumerary glands. Therefore some investigators (including the authors) prefer to use localization studies to prevent a missed ectopic gland from being the cause of a failed operation. In addition, recent studies have advocated for unilateral clearance in select patients with preoperative imaging suggestive of single gland disease. There may also be a role for cervical ultrasonography in all patients; recent guidelines recommend evaluation for any concurrent thyroid pathology that may necessitate thyroidectomy.[11,23]

SURGICAL TREATMENT OF MEN 1–ASSOCIATED HPT

The early and late outcomes of surgical treatment of MEN 1-associated PHPT are inferior to those for sporadic PHPT, because of the development of hyperplasia in parathyroid glands that appeared macroscopically normal at initial surgery (and were left in situ) or in hyperplastic remnants, which over time hypertrophy.[14] The goals of initial surgery are to (1) successfully correct hypercalcemia while minimizing the risk of persistent or recurrent PHPT, (2) avoid permanent hypoparathyroidism, and (3) facilitate the anticipated future surgical treatment of recurrent PHPT. Reasonable options for the initial operation in patients with MEN 1-associated PHPT are subtotal parathyroidectomy (with consideration of transcervical thymectomy) or total parathyroidectomy with heterotopic autotransplantation of resected parathyroid tissue (Table 62.1). More recently, unilateral clearance of both ipsilateral parathyroid glands and thymectomy has been described for young patients with localized disease on preoperative imaging. Resection of only macroscopically enlarged glands has been shown to be associated with significantly higher rates of persistent/recurrent disease.[21,24-34]

Less Than Subtotal Parathyroidectomy

Subtotal parathyroidectomy is defined as the removal of 3-3.5 parathyroid glands. Therefore less than subtotal parathyroidectomy is the removal of ≤2.5 parathyroid glands, leaving at least 1.5 presumably normal-appearing glands in situ and marked with titanium clips or nonabsorbable stitches to facilitate identification in a subsequent operation. Less than subtotal resection has been associated with an unacceptably high frequency of persistent or recurrent PHPT in patients with MEN 1-associated PHPT, with reported rates of 35% and 61%, respectively.[24,25,27,31,33-35] In a review of 79 patients by Arnalsteen and colleagues, the rate of reoperation in patients who underwent resection of only grossly enlarged glands at initial parathyroidectomy was 30%, compared with 7% in patients who underwent initial subtotal parathyroidectomy ($p = 0.02$).[27]

A single-institution review of 73 patients who underwent parathyroidectomy for MEN 1-associated PHPT in the Netherlands found rates of persistent/recurrent disease of 53% in patients who underwent less than subtotal parathyroidectomy, 17% after subtotal parathyroidectomy, and 19% after total parathyroidectomy with autotransplantation.[28,31] In a 12-study meta-analysis of patients who underwent less than subtotal parathyroidectomy, compared with those who underwent subtotal or total parathyroidectomy, patients who underwent less than subtotal parathyroidectomy had an odds ratio for recurrent PHPT of 3.11 (95% confidence interval [CI] = 2.00 to 4.84).[34] In a review of 92 patients with MEN 1 who underwent initial parathyroidectomy, the 13 (14%) who had less than subtotal parathyroidectomy had a shorter median recurrence-free survival rate compared with the patients who underwent either subtotal or total parathyroidectomy (7 versus 16.5 years; $p = 0.03$). The actuarial 1-, 5-, and 10-year recurrence-free survival was 92%, 69%, and 37%, respectively, for patients after less than subtotal parathyroidectomy and 100%, 80%, and 61%, respectively, after subtotal or total parathyroidectomy.[25]

Given the improved accuracy of preoperative imaging and the routine use of intraoperative PTH monitoring during parathyroidectomy, the possibility of a less extensive initial parathyroidectomy has been studied in patients who have concordant preoperative imaging studies suggesting unilateral disease.[32] In an initial report, 8 patients had "unilateral clearance," defined as removal of both parathyroid glands on the same side of the neck and cervical thymectomy; 16 patients had subtotal parathyroidectomy. After a mean follow-up of 47 months in the unilateral clearance group and 68 months in the subtotal parathyroidectomy group, the rates of persistent disease were 13% (n = 1) and 6.3% (n = 1); the rate of recurrent disease was 13% (n = 1) and 31% (n = 5; $p = 0.62$). Although unilateral clearance has the potential advantage of leaving one side "untouched" and thereby facilitating a future reoperation by avoiding having to reopen a scarred anatomic field, it should be noted that the one patient with persistent disease in the unilateral group had persistence on the ipsilateral side, which was likely due to a supernumerary gland.[32] The current data remains too limited to routinely endorse this approach.

Subtotal Parathyroidectomy

Subtotal parathyroidectomy involves the removal of 3 to 3.5 parathyroid glands, it remains the preferred operative approach at the time of initial surgery in patients with MEN 1–associated PHPT, with a "strong recommendation with moderate quality evidence" in recent management guidelines.[11-13,25,27,36,37] The goal of subtotal parathyroidectomy is to achieve long-term eucalcemia while minimizing the risks of permanent hypoparathyroidism. In one of the largest studies

TABLE 62.1 Guide to the Operative Management of HPT in Patients With MEN 1 and MEN 2A

Clinical Scenario	Operation Performed	Preoperative Localization	Parathyroid Autograft	Autograft Location
MEN 1 first operation	Subtotal parathyroidectomy, transcervical thymectomy	Encouraged; to look for ectopic glands	Not performed in the absence of total parathyroidectomy or intraoperative PTH <10 pg/mL	Forearm
MEN 1 reoperation for recurrent HPT	Resect localized gland(s), extent of operation guided by intraoperative PTH (see text)	Yes	Yes (unless intraoperative PTH fails to drop to ≤10 pg/mL, which suggests additional parathyroid remains in the neck)	Forearm
MEN 2A, calcium normal	Prophylactic thyroidectomy	No	No	NA
MEN 2A, calcium normal	Therapeutic thyroidectomy for invasive MTC	No	Yes, strongly encouraged	Depends on *RET* mutation; if mutation associated with HPT, then use forearm
MEN 2A and HPT	Prophylactic or therapeutic thyroidectomy planned, and HPT is noted—remove abnormal parathyroid glands and leave the normal appearing ones assuming intraoperative PTH normalizes; consider transcervical thymectomy	Encouraged; to look for ectopic glands	Yes, in all patients with invasive MTC and in patients who undergo a prophylactic thyroidectomy and have an intraoperative PTH <10 pg/mL	Forearm
MEN 2A, S/P total thyroidectomy and HPT noted	Resect localized gland(s)	Yes	Yes, if intraoperative PTH <10 pg/mL	Forearm
MEN 2A, S/P total thyroidectomy and parathyroidectomy and recurrent HPT	Resect localized gland(s)	Yes	Yes, if intraoperative PTH <10 pg/mL	Forearm

HPT, hyperparathyroidism; *MEN 1*, multiple endocrine neoplasia type 1; *MEN 2A*; multiple endocrine neoplasia type 2A; *MTC*, medullary thyroid cancer; *PTH*, parathyroid hormone.

comparing different surgical approaches in 174 patients with MEN 1–associated PHPT over three time periods, the rate of postoperative hypercalcemia decreased (47%, 15%, 19%; $p < 0.0001$) as the use of subtotal parathyroidectomy increased (25%, 59%, 51%; $p = 0.0004$). The increased rate of hypocalcemia (5%, 15%, 15%) was not statistically significant.[38]

In a cohort of 79 patients who had at least three parathyroid glands resected at initial surgery, the rate of recurrent PHPT was 33% after subtotal parathyroidectomy and 23% after total parathyroidectomy. The authors advocated subtotal parathyroidectomy as the initial procedure of choice rather than total parathyroidectomy. Total parathyroidectomy was associated with significantly higher rates of severe hypoparathyroidism; it required long-term treatment with calcium and vitamin D or delayed parathyroid autotransplantation in comparison with subtotal parathyroidectomy (46% versus 26%).[25] A randomized, prospective single-center trial of subtotal parathyroidectomy versus total parathyroidectomy and autotransplantation was performed in 32 patients, with mean follow-up of 7.5 ± 5.7 years.[30] Recurrent PHPT occurred in 6 (19%) patients, 4 (24%) of 17 patients who underwent subtotal parathyroidectomy, and 2 (13%) of 15 patients who underwent total parathyroidectomy ($p = 0.66$). There was no difference in the rates of transient hypoparathyroidism (47%, total parathyroidectomy versus 35%, subtotal parathyroidectomy). Permanent hypoparathyroidism occurred in 2 (12%) patients treated with subtotal parathyroidectomy and 1 (7%) treated with total parathyroidectomy. The authors advocated subtotal parathyroidectomy overall as the procedure of choice.[30]

A retrospective cohort study of 37 patients with MEN 1-associated PHPT found recurrent PHPT in 20 patients (65%) at a median of 4 years after initial surgery; 16 patients (75%) <3 parathyroid glands resected at the time of initial surgery and the remaining 4 patients had a subtotal parathyroidectomy. Of these 20 patients, 16 underwent an additional 24 parathyroid-related operations; recurrent HPT was found in 7 patients (35%) at the time of last follow-up. Of 25 parathyroid autografts performed in 22 patients, four patients remained permanently hypoparathyroid, which highlights the importance of finding a balance between the risks of recurrent PHPT and permanent hypoparathyroidism, particularly in patients with MEN 1–associated PHPT, which usually develops early in life.[12]

In a study that examined the causes, timing, and treatment of 69 patients with recurrent MEN 1–associated PHPT, all 69 patients had initial subtotal parathyroidectomy and 60 patients also underwent cervical thymectomy. After initial surgery, 15 patients had a single, normal-appearing gland remaining in the neck, and 54 patients had an estimated 50- to 70-mg remnant of an abnormal gland. Recurrent PHPT was found in 9 (13%) of the 69 patients within a mean of 85 months (range, 12 to 144 months); five occurred in a parathyroid remnant, three patients in a previously "normal" gland, and one recurrence was in a remnant of a supernumerary gland. Two patients had a second recurrence also resulting from a supernumerary gland. Recurrence was associated with a longer follow-up time (115 months versus 66 months, $p = 0.005$), which demonstrates that MEN-1 associated PHPT recurs in the neck (especially if a thymectomy was not performed) or at the site of an autograft, at some point in time, because all parathyroids are genetically abnormal.[37]

Our recommended initial surgical procedure is subtotal parathyroidectomy and transcervical thymectomy (see Table 62.1). Subtotal parathyroidectomy is performed by identification of all four parathyroid glands and any supernumerary or ectopic glands (facilitated by the use of MIBI and/or CT imaging before surgery). The most normal-(smallest) appearing parathyroid gland should be left undisturbed, in situ, and should not be greater than two times normal size (approximately 40 mg). Partial resection should be undertaken for glands larger than this size, taking care not to seed the local region and place the patient at risk for parathyromatosis within the thyroid bed, sternocleidomastoid muscle, sternothyroid muscle, or the wall of the esophagus. If a gland is to be partially resected, a large metallic clip should be gently placed across the parathyroid gland and the gland sharply divided at that level; the clip also will allow for easy identification of the gland if a future reoperation is necessary. If a gland is partially resected, it should be done before resection of the remaining parathyroid glands in case the gland is devascularized. Before proceeding with resection of the other remaining glands, the in situ gland should be carefully inspected for viability—if nonviable, another of the parathyroid glands can be chosen for partial resection.

A transcervical thymectomy is performed because of the potential for the patient to have an ectopic or supernumerary gland. A parathyroid autograft, in the nondominant forearm, is not routinely performed at the initial operation if the intraoperative PTH level remains detectable (above 10 pg/mL). This avoids the risk for the future development of autograft hyperfunction and the need to determine whether recurrent PHPT is secondary to the autograft or to residual cervical parathyroid tissue (as parathyroid tissue is in both the neck and the arm). When PHPT recurs in the future, after a previous subtotal parathyroidectomy, total parathyroidectomy with forearm autografting should be completed. Because delayed autograft function is a well-known problem with MEN 1–associated PHPT, some investigators prefer to perform a forearm autograft at the time of initial subtotal parathyroidectomy; this is an unresolved controversy.

Total Parathyroidectomy With Forearm Autograft

Total parathyroidectomy includes the removal of all four parathyroid glands, including any ectopic/supernumerary glands. This aggressive approach, designed to avoid cervical recurrence of HPT, must be accompanied by autologous parathyroid autotransplantation to avoid permanent hypoparathyroidism. Advocates of total parathyroidectomy for MEN 1–associated PHPT cite the low rates of recurrent disease; when recurrence does develop in a forearm autograft, it can be "debulked" under local anesthesia—much simpler than a reoperative procedure on the neck. Tonelli et al. studied 51 patients, including 45 patients who underwent initial total parathyroidectomy. At the time of last follow-up, no patient had developed cervical recurrence and five recurrences (10%) in the forearm were observed after a mean of 7 years. However, permanent hypoparathyroidism occurred in 10% of patients after initial surgery.[22] Similarly, Lambert et al. found no cervical recurrences in five patients who underwent total parathyroidectomy.[12]

Parathyroid autotransplantation can be performed immediately upon completion of total parathyroidectomy from fresh autologous tissue; it can be performed days later, if PTH levels are not detectable, using cryopreserved tissue.[14,39,40] However, few centers currently permit cryopreservation of parathyroid tissue due to the institutional complexities associated with the short-term preservation of human tissues. Parathyroid tissue that is to be autografted should be obtained from the most normal-appearing parathyroid gland based on volume, color, and texture of the gland. The parathyroid tissue should be minced into small pieces. The optimal site of autotransplantation is within the brachioradialis muscle of the nondominant forearm to prevent a potential cervical reoperation if the graft becomes hyperfunctional. During follow-up, serum PTH levels obtained from right and left basilic veins (antecubital level) can be used to confirm/monitor the function of the autotransplantation. The autograft is performed by incision of the fascia of the brachioradialis muscle; the muscle fibers are gently divided to create a small pocket into which fragments of parathyroid tissue are placed. The pocket is then sutured with a nonabsorbable suture (we use a blue 5-0 Prolene) and marked with a metallic clip. The reported optimal number of fragments to autograft has ranged from 5 to 25.[39,41,42] If autografting is performed in a delayed setting, the vials containing the cryopreserved parathyroid fragments should be placed in a 37° C water bath until the medium is thawed and subsequently washed to eliminate toxicity of the preservation fluid. Before autotransplantation, a piece of tissue should be submitted for frozen section to confirm parathyroid tissue.

Outcomes from parathyroid forearm autotransplantation have varied, perhaps because of the experience of the surgeons and the varied techniques employed for autografting. Autografts may take years to develop function. Up to 40% of autografts may fail and result in permanent hypoparathyroidism[12,25,42]—hence the concern with total parathyroidectomy as the initial treatment for MEN 1–associated PHPT. Lambert and colleagues described their experience with 25 parathyroid autografts in 22 patients; 11 autografts were performed in 10 patients who underwent subtotal parathyroidectomy, and 14 autografts were performed in 12 patients who underwent resection of four or more parathyroid glands. At the time of last follow-up, 15 (60%) autografts were functional, 1 was nonfunctional, and 6 (24%) were unable to be assessed. Despite autografting, four patients (18%) were permanently hypoparathyroid. Two patients required emergency treatment of hypocalcemia and frequent outpatient visits for assessment of serum calcium levels. After autograft revision with cryopreserved parathyroid tissue, one patient remained hypoparathyroid at the time of last follow-up.[12]

Patients are also at risk for recurrent HPT within the forearm autograft. When this occurs, forearm debulking should be performed. It has been our experience that intraoperative ultrasound guidance aids in the debulking of the parathyroid autograft to an optimal size. Ultrasound guidance combined with the use of intraoperative PTH can facilitate the management of a hypertrophied forearm autograft. In a study of 234 patients who underwent subtotal parathyroidectomy or total parathyroidectomy with autotransplantation for MEN 1-associated PHPT or end-stage renal disease, 8 MEN 1 patients had total parathyroidectomy with autotransplantation. This included 6 patients who underwent total parathyroidectomy with autotransplantation at the time of initial surgery; the patients also underwent initial subtotal parathyroidectomy and required salvage total parathyroidectomy with autotransplantation for recurrent HPT. Of these eight patients, five developed recurrent HPT at the site of autotransplantation (all in the initial total parathyroidectomy group), which required six procedures for either parathyroid hyperplasia (n = 3) or parathyromatosis (n = 3).[43]

The Role of Transcervical Thymectomy

We routinely perform transcervical thymectomy because of the potential for an ectopic parathyroid gland within the thyrothymic ligament, the presence of which would increase the likelihood of recurrent HPT. Up to 30% of patients with familial PHPT will harbor enlarged supernumerary/ectopic glands; in addition, for patients with MEN 1, thymectomy may prevent the development of a thymic carcinoid.[3,13] Powell et al. retrospectively identified 66 patients who underwent initial subtotal parathyroidectomy and transcervical thymectomy for MEN 1-associated PHPT. In 17 (53%) of 32 patients, in whom fewer than four parathyroid glands were found in orthotopic positions, parathyroid tissue was identified within the thymic tissue.[44] Thymectomy at the time of initial parathyroidectomy has been associated with a decreased likelihood of recurrent HPT.[37] A bilateral thymectomy can be safely performed through a cervical incision. After mobilization of the cervical portion of the thymic tongue, gentle traction can be applied to the thymic tissue to remove as much of the thymus as possible through a cervical incision. Median sternotomy is not performed for prophylactic thymectomy.

TREATMENT OF PERSISTENT OR RECURRENT MEN 1–ASSOCIATED PHPT

Up to 50% of patients with MEN 1–associated PHPT will develop persistent PHPT (hypercalcemia within 6 months of surgery) or recurrent PHPT (hypercalcemia that develops >6 months after the initial surgery and after a period of normocalcemia).[24-26,36,38] After biochemical confirmation of recurrent disease, the site of recurrence must be determined. Recurrent disease can occur from the growth of remnant tissue after subtotal parathyroidectomy, from supernumerary or ectopic tissue in the neck or mediastinum not removed at the first operation, or from autograft hyperfunction.

Indications for reoperation are similar to the indications for initial neck exploration. However, the risks of potential patient morbidity must be balanced with the likelihood of postoperative normocalcemia. In contrast to the approach to the first operation, localization of hyperfunctioning parathyroid tissue is critically important before reoperative parathyroidectomy. We routinely perform technetium Tc99m MIBI-SPECT/CT, cervical ultrasonography, and four-dimensional computed tomography (4D-CT) imaging. If localization is still not successful, angiography with selective venous sampling can be considered.[12,45,46] All patients with persistent or recurrent MEN 1–associated PHPT, who have parathyroid tissue in the neck, should undergo completion total parathyroidectomy with parathyroid autografting in the nondominant forearm. In general, parathyroid tissue should not be intentionally left in the neck at the time of reoperation. In addition, intraoperative PTH monitoring should be routinely used.[11,47] In a study of 30 patients with MEN 1–associated persistent/recurrent PHPT, 5 (17%) patients were found at reoperation to have additional enlarged glands not visualized on preoperative imaging; intraoperative PTH levels did not decrease until after resection of these glands.[47] At the time of reoperation, if the intraoperative PTH does not decline into the normal range after removal of the gland(s) seen on preoperative imaging, the extent of further neck exploration/dissection becomes a dilemma (the solution of which should be individualized based on a thorough knowledge of the individual patient). The correct approach is derived from a detailed knowledge of all prior operations, an appreciation for the difficulty of further dissection in a reoperative field, and the risk for nerve injury. If the thymus was not removed at the first operation, a transcervical thymectomy would be an obvious next step. If the intraoperative PTH remains elevated, then assessment of bilateral internal jugular vein PTH levels would be appropriate. If there is an obvious step-up in PTH level on one side (>10% at a minimum), then removing the thyroid gland and associated soft tissue (assuming patient consent) would be reasonable. However, simply trying to reopen both central compartments without a defined strategy is usually ill-advised. Figure 62.2 demonstrates the CT scan of a 28-year-old patient with recurrent MEN 1–associated HPT and ureterolithiasis after two previous cervical operations and resection of a total of two enlarged parathyroid glands. Although ultrasonography and technetium Tc99m MIBI scans did not localize parathyroid tissue, a 1.4-cm hyperplastic

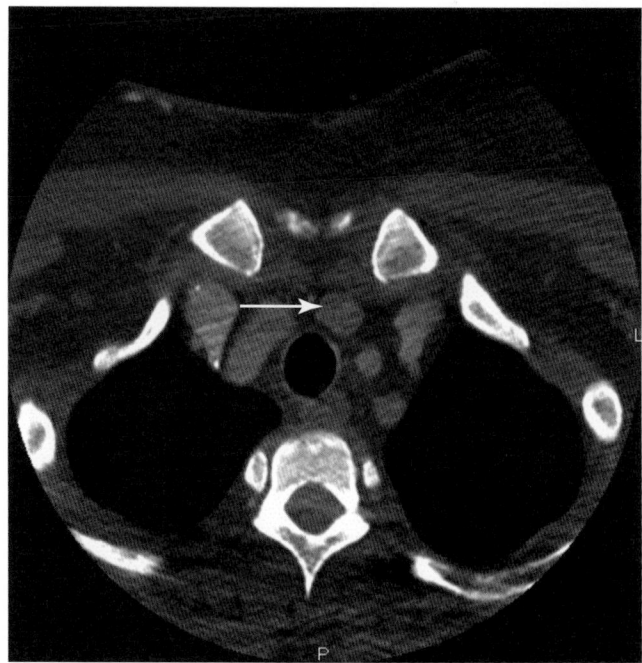

Fig. 62.2 Computed tomography (CT) scan of recurrent hyperparathyroidism in a patient with multiple endocrine neoplasia type 1 (MEN 1). A 1.4-cm hyperplastic parathyroid was identified within the left thyrothymic ligament *(arrow)*.

parathyroid was identified within the left thyrothymic ligament on CT. The patient underwent successful surgery with removal of two additional intrathymic parathyroid glands and forearm autotransplantation; the patient remains on low-dose calcium supplementation postoperatively.

The reported incidence of recurrent disease resulting from the autonomous function of parathyroid autografts ranges from 3% to 30%.[39,42,48-50] To detect recurrence in the forearm autograft when parathyroid tissue remains in the neck, one can simply obtain bilateral antecubital PTH levels. The Casanova test can also be performed but is rarely necessary in our experience.[51] Patients with hyperfunction of a forearm autograft should undergo debulking under local anesthesia using intraoperative ultrasonography and the intraoperative PTH assay to guide the extent of debulking.

MULTIPLE ENDOCRINE NEOPLASIA TYPE 2A

MEN 2A is an autosomal dominant disorder that has been recognized in approximately 500 to 1000 kindreds (see Chapter 27, Syndromic Medullary Thyroid Carcinoma: MEN 2A and MEN 2B).[13,52] It is characterized by medullary thyroid cancer (MTC), pheochromocytoma, and PHPT; uncommon variants include cutaneous lichen amyloidosis and Hirschsprung disease (Figure 62.3).[2,52] There is a high penetrance of MTC in all variants of MEN 2A (>90% penetrance); pheochromocytomas are observed in ~50% and HPT in 15% to 30% of gene carriers.[2,14,52]

GENETIC TESTING IN MEN 2A

MEN 2A is caused by a germline mutation in the rearranged during transfection *(RET)* proto-oncogene on chromosome 10q11.2; this condition affects 1 per 30,000 individuals.[2] The *RET* gene contains 21 exons and encodes a single-pass transmembrane tyrosine kinase receptor. Missense mutations result in the transformation of a single amino

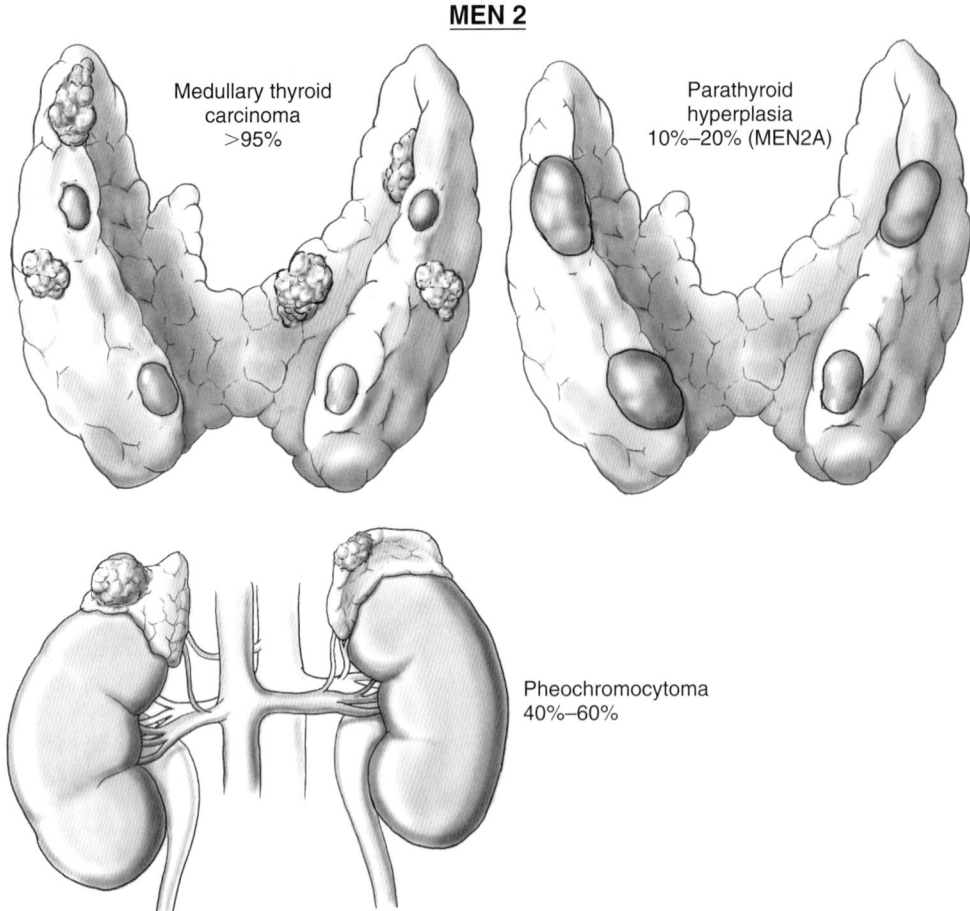

Fig. 62.3 The most common clinical features of multiple endocrine neoplasia type 2 (MEN 2). (Printed with permission from © brysonbiomed.com.)

acid and production of a dominant, transformed protein *(RET)* with oncogenic activity. Depending on the specific codon mutation, different areas of the receptor are activated with differing levels of transforming activity. For example, alteration in the intracellular catalytic core (i.e., mutation of codon 918) has the highest transforming activity, whereas interference with ATP binding (i.e., mutations in codons 768, 790, 791, 804, and 891) has lower transforming activity.[2,52,53] Progression of disease and the development of MTC, pheochromocytoma, and PHPT correlates with the transforming activity of the *RET* mutation but also requires additional second hits.

DNA sequencing for the *RET* mutation is very accurate and widely available; 98% of MEN 2 index cases have an identified mutation, and a limited number of MEN 2–associated mutations have been identified. Therefore the current American Thyroid Association (ATA) guidelines recommended testing of exon 10 (codons 609, 611, 618, and 620), 11 (codons 620 and 634), 8, 13, 14, 15, and 16 at the time of initial genetic testing. The remaining 15 exons are sequenced only if the initial sequencing is negative or if there is a discrepancy between the MEN 2 phenotype and expected genotype.[52] Genetic testing for *RET* germline mutation carriers is currently recommended for the following people: all patients diagnosed with MTC, first-degree relatives of patients with proven hereditary MTC, parents whose infants or children have the classic phenotype of MEN 2B, patients with cutaneous lichen amyloidosis, and infants or children with Hirschsprung's disease.[52]

In contrast to MEN 1, there is a strong relationship between a specific *RET* codon mutation and the phenotypic expression of disease.

PHPT occurs in 15% to 30% of patients with MEN 2A. It is most common in patients with the codon 634 mutation (cysteine-to-arginine amino acid substitution) and less common with mutations in codons 609, 611, 618, 620, 790, and 791.[53-55] This genotype-phenotype correlation is important in the clinical management of MEN 2A patients because identification of a mutation associated with the development of PHPT may alter the initial approach to the management of the parathyroid glands at the time of prophylactic/therapeutic thyroidectomy.

MEN 2A–ASSOCIATED PHPT

PHPT is the most variable component of the MEN 2A syndrome. MEN 2A–associated PHPT is generally milder than in patients with MEN 1, with often only a slight elevation of serum calcium.[2,56,57] The majority of patients (up to 85%) have asymptomatic disease at the time of diagnosis and few patients have nephrolithiasis or neurocognitive symptoms.[2,57,58] Previous studies have shown that the median age of diagnosis for MEN 2A–associated PHPT is 38 years.[57-59] ATA guidelines currently recommend that the surveillance for PHPT begin at the time of screening for the presence of a pheochromocytoma, which is usually 11 years of age in carriers of *RET* mutations 634 and 883 and by 16 years of age in carriers of other MEN 2A–associated *RET* mutations. Surveillance is easy; it consists of annual albumin-corrected calcium or ionized serum calcium measurements with serum intact PTH.[52]

As with other forms of familial HPT, including MEN 1, it is generally thought that MEN 2A–associated PHPT involves multiple glands;

however, single adenomas and asymmetric gland enlargement have been more often reported in MEN 2A than MEN 1.[2,54,56,58,60] In a multicenter study of 56 patients with MEN 2A and PHPT, the final pathology consisted of 24 single adenomas, 4 double adenomas, and 25 patients with multigland hyperplasia.[58] The incidence of supernumerary and ectopically located parathyroid glands is much lower than that associated with MEN 1, but supernumerary and ectopic glands have been reported.[60]

INDICATIONS FOR SURGERY

Indications for parathyroidectomy are no different in patients with MEN 2A than for those with sporadic PHPT or MEN 1–associated PHPT.[3,5,13,52] However, in contrast to MEN 1, the majority of patients diagnosed with MEN 2–associated PHPT will have undergone previous thyroidectomy and often central compartment neck dissection as either prophylactic or therapeutic surgery for MTC. Preoperative evaluation must include a thorough review of previous operative notes and pathology reports (to determine how many parathyroid glands were identified at the initial procedure), intraoperative assessment of size and morphology, and which (if any) glands were biopsied, removed, or autotransplanted. As with other reoperative cervical procedures, preoperative laryngoscopy to document normal vocal cord mobility should be performed in all patients.[11,61] Also, all patients with MEN 2A should undergo biochemical evaluation for pheochromocytoma with assessment of plasma-free metanephrines and normetanephrines. If a pheochromocytoma is present, adrenalectomy should occur before parathyroidectomy. However, it has been our experience that the two procedures can be performed under the same anesthesia induction, with resection of the pheochromocytoma (cortical sparing) occurring first, followed by parathyroidectomy.[52]

SURGICAL TREATMENT OF MEN 2A–ASSOCIATED PHPT

The goal of surgical management of MEN 2A–associated PHPT is to avoid hypoparathyroidism, particularly in patients who have undergone previous thyroidectomy. However, surgical therapy, rather than medical management, is still preferred because of the high rate of biochemical cure in MEN 2A patients; the exception to this preference is in cases of excessive surgical risk or limited life expectancy. In patients who have *not* had previous neck surgery and who are diagnosed with PHPT at the time of planned prophylactic or therapeutic thyroidectomy for MTC, initial surgery should always include a strategy for intraoperative management of the parathyroid glands.[52] Surgical options include (1) resection of only visibly enlarged glands, (2) subtotal parathyroidectomy leaving one or part of one parathyroid gland in situ, or (3) total parathyroidectomy with forearm autograft (see Table 62.1).[2,11,14,52,57,60,62] Patients who undergo prophylactic or therapeutic thyroidectomy with no preoperative biochemical evidence of PHPT, but in whom grossly enlarged parathyroid glands are discovered at the time of surgery, should undergo resection of only visibly enlarged parathyroid glands.[11,52] If all glands are abnormal, subtotal parathyroidectomy is preferred. Parathyroid forearm autotransplantation should be considered, particularly in patients with invasive MTC because they are at risk for recurrence, which may require a reoperation on the central neck compartment.[11] In contrast, for patients who undergo prophylactic thyroidectomy at a time when invasive MTC is unlikely (based on age, mutation status, and serum level of calcitonin), a forearm autograft is not necessary.

During thyroidectomy for MTC, normal parathyroid glands may be accidentally resected or devascularized. Normal parathyroid tissue should be left in the patient, whenever possible, either in situ on an adequate vascular pedicle.[52,63] If a normal appearing parathyroid gland is devascularized at the time of thyroidectomy for invasive MTC, an autograft should be performed because such patients are at risk for recurrent MTC in the central neck compartment. Reoperation on the central neck may result in devascularization/resection of all remaining parathyroid tissue, which will render the patient permanently hypoparathyroid. The location of the autograft depends on the *RET* mutation; for patients with MEN 2A in whom there is a strong family history of PHPT or an *RET* mutation known to carry a significant risk of PHPT (i.e., codon 634 mutation), parathyroid tissue should be placed in the forearm. Patients with an *RET* mutation harboring a low risk of PHPT, or those patients with *RET* mutations consistent with MEN 2B or familial MTC, may undergo autograft of a normal appearing parathyroid gland in either the forearm or the sternocleidomastoid muscle.

There is no apparent benefit to prophylactic parathyroidectomy (removal of normal appearing glands) at the time of prophylactic or therapeutic thyroidectomy because only 20% to 30% of MEN 2A patients will develop PHPT; those patients at risk are identified by their *RET* mutation status. Rates of permanent hypoparathyroidism after thyroidectomy by experienced surgeons are low (i.e., 1% to 2%), although the incidence is slightly higher in patients who undergo central neck lymphadenectomy.[64-66] These low rates do not justify the risk of prophylactic total parathyroidectomy and autotransplantation because prophylactic thyroidectomy is performed in young patients who would potentially be subject to lifelong hypoparathyroidism.[67] Decker et al. performed prophylactic thyroidectomy in 11 children (2 to 12 years of age) with MEN 2A mutations and no preoperative biochemical evidence of PHPT; intraoperatively, normal parathyroid glands were identified and left in situ. Postoperatively, 10 (91%) children were normocalcemic.[67]

Patients who develop PHPT after previous thyroidectomy should not undergo a neck exploration without preoperative localization studies.[11,46,68-70] In general, reoperation should be directed at only localized, hypertrophied parathyroid glands.[52] Surgical principles are identical to those discussed for patients with recurrent HPT.

TREATMENT OF PERSISTENT OR RECURRENT MEN 2A–ASSOCIATED PHPT

Persistent or recurrent HPT has been reported in up to 40% of patients with MEN 2A–associated PHPT.[35,57,58,60] Management of patients with recurrent HPT is similar to patients with recurrent MEN 1–associated HPT; confirmation of disease and subsequent localization is crucial (see Table 62.1). Figure 62.4 shows the CT scan of a 40-year-old patient with a codon 634 mutation and recurrent MEN 2A–associated HPT after initial resection of a single hyperplastic parathyroid gland and autograft of a devascularized normal appearing gland into the sternocleidomastoid muscle of the neck. Preoperative localization confirmed recurrence within the autograft (arrow) as well as an enlarged, left inferior parathyroid (arrowhead). The patient underwent resection of both the enlarged parathyroid and the hypertrophied autograft; the patient was eucalcemic postoperatively.

USE OF INTRAOPERATIVE ADJUNCTS DURING PARATHYROIDECTOMY FOR MEN–ASSOCIATED PHPT

The role of intraoperative PTH monitoring in the initial surgical management of MEN 1–associated PHPT remains debatable, given the need

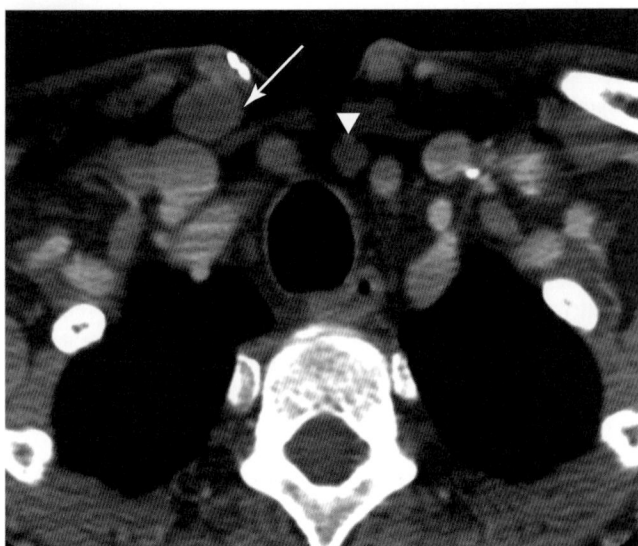

Fig. 62.4 Computed tomography (CT) scan of recurrent hyperparathyroidism in a patient with multiple endocrine neoplasia type 2A (MEN 2A). Hyperplastic parathyroid tissue is located within the previously autografted remnant *(arrow)* and an enlarged left inferior parathyroid *(arrowhead)*.

for bilateral exploration in these patients. However, although intraoperative PTH monitoring may not alter the surgical approach (when subtotal parathyroidectomy is planned), it may help guide the extent of subtotal resection of the parathyroid gland chosen to remain in situ.[5,12,14] The optimal intraoperative PTH criteria that reliably predict long-term eucalcemia in this subset of patients remains to be defined. However, there is consensus that more stringent criteria than is used for sporadic PHPT may be required to reduce the risk of persistent HPT in MEN 1 patients.[12,71-73] Intraoperative PTH monitoring should be used in all patients who undergo reoperative surgery for persistent or recurrent MEN–associated HPT.

Studies on the use of radioguided parathyroidectomy for inherited syndromes are limited. The use of radioguided parathyroidectomy has not been widely adopted in the management of patients with sporadic or familial HPT because studies have shown that its use does not provide significant additional information that is not obtained by preoperative imaging studies and intraoperative PTH monitoring.[45,74-76]

NONSURGICAL MANAGEMENT OF PERSISTENT OR RECURRENT MEN–ASSOCIATED PHPT

There are no approved medical treatments for PHPT, although nonsurgical alternatives are desirable for patients with persistent or recurrent disease who are high-risk for surgery because of medical comorbidities or multiple previous cervical explorations. Cinacalcet, the oral calcimimetic, has been approved for use in the treatment of patients with secondary HPT that results from end-stage renal disease; the drug is approved for the treatment of patients with severe hypercalcemia who are unable to undergo parathyroidectomy. Cinacalcet has been shown to be effective in reducing serum calcium levels, but it has not been associated with a lasting effect or any improvement in bone mineral density.[77-80]

Percutaneous sonographically guided ethanol ablation has been reported as an alternative treatment for PHPT in patients at prohibitive surgical risk that results from medical comorbidities or multiple reoperations and in whom there is a single remaining enlarged parathyroid gland, which has been accurately localized.[81,82] In an initial study of 36 patients with PHPT, Harman et al. attempted complete ablation in 29 patients and partial ablation in 7 patients. Eucalcemia was achieved in 10 (34%) and 2 (29%) patients, respectively.[82] In a follow-up study from the same institution, 22 patients with MEN 1 who had undergone previous subtotal parathyroidectomy and had clinical evidence of recurrent HPT resulting from a single enlarged parathyroid gland underwent attempted ethanol ablation. A total of 41 treatments were performed, including ablation of a forearm autograft. Overall, 34 treatments (83%) resulted in normal or below-normal serum calcium levels; 11 patients required additional treatments. One patient developed long-term hypocalcemia; no patients had permanent recurrent laryngeal nerve (RLN) injury. Thus ethanol ablation may offer a reasonable alternative to reoperation in a certain subset of patients who have successful localization of the hyperplastic gland.[81]

CONCLUSIONS

PHPT resulting from MEN 1 or MEN 2A is a relatively uncommon cause of PHPT. However, it is important that the physicians treating patients with inherited PHPT be well versed in the management of this condition. The diagnosis of MEN 1 should be considered in patients with ≥2 MEN 1–related tumors or a clinical history otherwise suggestive of MEN 1. PHPT is often the first clinical manifestation of disease in the proband of an MEN 1 family or in at-risk members of a known MEN 1 kindred. The diagnosis of MEN 2A is typically made before the onset of PHPT because of the near 100% penetrance of MTC. Genetic testing (before surgery on the neck) is particularly important in patients with MEN 2A because of the strong genotype-phenotype correlation of the specific *RET* mutation identified. We prefer to know the *RET* status of the patient before thyroid/parathyroid surgery because it will indicate the location of a parathyroid autograft if one is performed. Indications for surgery in MEN–associated PHPT are no different than indications for sporadic PHPT. The goals of initial parathyroidectomy in patients with MEN–associated PHPT are to achieve eucalcemia and minimize the risk of immediate hypoparathyroidism. Forearm autografting of remnant parathyroid tissue should be considered for all patients with MEN 2A–associated PHPT, invasive MTC, and all patients with inherited PHPT who undergo reoperative neck surgery.

REFERENCES

For a complete list of references, go to expertconsult.com.

Revision Parathyroid Surgery

Michael C. Singer, Ayaka Iwata, Brendan C. Stack, Jr.

INTRODUCTION

As many as 10% of patients who had previous operations for primary hyperparathyroidism (PHPT) will experience persistent or recurrent disease after surgery (Box 63.1).[1] Due to the sequelae of PHPT, some of these patients will require reoperative parathyroid surgery. Unfortunately, in contrast to primary parathyroid surgery, which is extremely safe and has a high success rate, reoperative parathyroid surgery is associated with significant risks. Reoperative parathyroid surgery is a complex exercise that requires specialized skills and understanding to optimize outcomes. These reoperative procedures should be image driven, when possible, and the form of imaging available will vary by region and individual center. Surgeons performing reoperative parathyroid surgery need to be facile with a range of operative techniques to address the challenges that can present in these patients.

WHY?

One cause of unsuccessful primary parathyroid surgery is failure to diagnose the patient correctly. Although laboratory assessment in many patients with PHPT is clear and conclusive, in others the diagnosis can be challenging.

Several factors may influence biochemical results and lead to confusion in patient assessment. Vitamin D deficiency and calcium deficiency, particularly if severe, may mask PHPT because these patients may have a normal calcium level. In addition, 24-hour urine calcium excretion may be low in severely calcium-deficient individuals, and the PHPT biochemical picture can even mimic secondary hyperparathyroidism. Correction of any documented deficiencies and repeat testing after replacement therapy may reveal the true diagnosis of PHPT.

The use of thiazide diuretics and lithium, which may raise parathyroid hormone (PTH) and cause mild hypercalcemia, may mimic the diagnosis of PHPT. These medications should be discontinued when possible and the biochemical evaluation repeated 6 weeks after medication washout. Nonparathyroid-mediated hypercalcemia (i.e., lymphoma, granulomatous diseases, hyperthyroidism, metastatic bone disease, multiple myeloma, vitamin D toxicity, and milk-alkali syndrome) is distinguished from PHPT by an appropriately suppressed PTH paired with elevated calcium. PTH-related peptide (PTHrP) can be assayed when PTH is suppressed in the presence of hypercalcemia and there is a suspicion of malignancy.

Familial hypocalciuric hypercalcemia (FHH) must also be excluded with a 24-hour urine collection and estimation of the calcium-creatinine clearance ratio. This can be done based on a low urinary calcium-creatinine excretion ratio of <0.01. If below 0.01, a genetic mutational analysis of the calcium-sensing receptor (CaSR), and possibly G alpha 11 and AP2S1 may be pursued. Conversely, a renal leak of calcium (hypercalciuria) can result in a compensatory raise in PTH, and it would cause persistent hyperparathormonemia, even after successful surgery for hyperparathyroidism.[2]

In patients correctly diagnosed with PHPT, primary parathyroidectomy can fail for several reasons. Persistent hyperparathyroidism (HPT) is typically due to unsuccessful or inadequate surgery. Most commonly this occurs with a missed single adenoma, most frequently in a normal embryologic location rather than an ectopic location. Ectopic adenomas are found in common places (tracheoesophageal grove and thyrothymic ligament) that often are not dissected well by an occasional parathyroid surgeon. Intrathyroidal adenomas are infrequent causes for failed parathyroid surgery (<1%). In the case of four-gland hyperplasia, a less than complete excision (<3 glands) can result in a failure to cure. This often happens when all four parathyroid glands are never located during the initial surgery.

Recurrent HPT is usually due to a lack of appreciation for the underlying disease process, most commonly an asynchronous second adenoma or an unappreciated four-gland hyperplasia.[3,4] Recurrent HPT in MEN-1 can be an expected outcome after adequate primary surgery that was initially successful. Recurrent HPT patients are more likely to have a family history of hyperparathyroidism and/or have had their initial parathyroid surgery performed at a young age.

WHO?

Any patient with persistent elevated calcium or elevated PTH levels in the face of inappropriately normal calcium levels after a parathyroidectomy procedure is a potential candidate for reoperative parathyroidectomy. The biochemical diagnosis of persistent and recurrent PHPT is the same as for the initial diagnosis of PHPT.[1,5-7] Persistent HPT is defined as hypercalcemia within 6 months of the initial parathyroidectomy; whereas, recurrent HPT is defined as hypercalcemia recurring 6 months or more after a successful parathyroidectomy.

National data sets reveal lower cure rates with reoperative parathyroid surgery—84% compared with 95% for first-time surgery. Not only are cure rates lower, but also, complication rates are higher with a sixfold increase in vocal cord paralysis and a doubling of the amount of bleeding compared with primary surgery.[8] Permanent hypoparathyroidism rates of between 10% to 20% are also reported.[9]

Institutional experience has been shown to influence operative success with higher volume institutions having more favorable outcomes.[10,11] Regarding PHPT, surgeons having an annual volume in excess of 50 cases have better outcomes compared with lower volume surgeons, but there are no studies examining this question for reoperative surgery.[12]

Due to the increased surgical risk of operating in a challenging, scarred surgical field, the threshold for reoperative surgery should be

> **BOX 63.1 Summary of AHNS Guidelines on Revision Surgery**
>
> A set of guidelines published in 2018 was the first international multisociety and multidisciplinary effort to aggregate best practices and evidence to guide surgeons and patients on revision of surgery in cases of previously failed parathyroid surgery.
>
> 1. a) The first step in the evaluation of the reoperative parathyroid patient must include complete biochemical confirmation of primary hyperparathyroidism with hypercalcemia, relative or absolute hyperparathormonemia, and preferably hypercalciuria before reoperation.
>   b) The diagnosis of hyperparathyroidism must be secured through exclusion of nonparathyroid causes of hypercalcemia and/or hyperparathormonemia.
> 2. Detailed review of past surgical and pathologic data is essential to optimize surgical success.
> 3. Assessment of patient's current health status and previous surgical complications, if any, must be made before planning for reoperative surgery.
> 4. Preoperative laryngeal assessment is required in all patients before reoperative parathyroid surgery.
> 5. a) Preoperative imaging of reoperative parathyroid surgical patients is mandatory.
>   b) Using the imaging modality that is readily available, most reliable, and cost effective in a given health system is recommended. This will vary depending on location.
> 6. Reoperative parathyroid surgery should be performed in the setting of an identified target gland(s) on preoperative imaging studies.
> 7. Parathyroid reoperations are challenging and should be undertaken by experienced surgeons.
> 8. Parathyroids should be approached through nondissected planes; when possible, most heavily scarred regions should be avoided.
> 9. Intraoperative adjuncts, such as neural monitoring and PTH assay, should be used during reoperative parathyroid surgery. Radioguidance, visible tracers, or ultrasound can be used, based on surgeon experience and availability.
> 10. During reoperative parathyroid surgery when postoperative hypoparathyroidism is a concern, primary auto transplantation should be considered after frozen section confirmation. Parathyroid cryopreservation can also be considered if available.
> 11. Nutritional and pharmacologic optimization should be performed in patients refusing or in patients who are not candidates for reoperative parathyroid surgery. Treatable metabolic abnormalities should also be addressed in operative patients.

AHNS, American Head and Neck Society; PTH, parathyroid hormone.
Data from Stack BC Jr, Tolley NS, Bartel TB, et al. AHNS Series: Do you know your guidelines? Optimizing outcomes in reoperative parathyroid surgery: definitive multidisciplinary joint consensus guidelines of the American Head and Neck Society and the British Association of Endocrine and Thyroid Surgeons. *Head Neck.* 2018;40[8]:1617–1629.

higher than for first-time surgery. Patients who have had parathyroid surgery typically meet one or more of the generally accepted guidelines for surgery. In these patients, the indications for surgery have not changed, except now that they have had unsuccessful parathyroid surgery, the increased risks associated with the reoperative procedure must be considered. In patients who underwent parathyroid surgery but didn't meet any specific guidelines, the decision to consider another parathyroid operation should be even more carefully contemplated. Asymptomatic patients with PHPT have been followed for up to a decade without overt evidence of clinically significant disease progression.[1]

As described earlier, an improper diagnosis of PHPT can lead to unsuccessful primary parathyroidectomy. Therefore critically, the first step for considering someone a candidate for reoperative surgery is to reaffirm conclusively the diagnosis of PHPT. Once confirmed, a determination of disease severity and possible clinical effects of the continued or recurrent HPT is required. An assessment of the degree of hypercalcemia [such as a serum calcium greater than 3.0 mmol/l (12.0 mg/dL)] may be complemented by an evaluation of kidney function (especially the glomerular filtration rate); renal imaging (abdominal ultrasound or computed tomography for nephrolithiasis or nephrocalcinosis); somatic symptoms (musculoskeletal aches and pains); assessment of bone health (with dual energy x-ray absorptiometry, [DEXA]); and an assessment of cardiovascular risk (computed tomography [CT] calcium cardiac scoring).

The decision to move forward with reoperative parathyroid surgery is nuanced, and it demands extensive counseling of the patient and close coordination between the patient's physicians.

WHEN?

Typically, reoperative parathyroid surgery is elective, like the first parathyroid surgery. This is often true for both the need and the timing of the surgery. Extreme hypercalcemia, advanced osteoporosis (especially with a high risk of fractures or after a recent fracture), and unrelenting renal lithiasis with severe renal colic may make revision parathyroid surgery more acutely required.

HOW?

The need for precision is imperative in reoperative parathyroid surgery, so having a specific imaged target(s) is essential.[13] Often, thorough and more comprehensive parathyroid (cervical and upper thoracic) imaging than that which was used for the initial operation is the basis for successful parathyroid reoperation.[14,15] Focused exploration and excision based on a preoperative image in conjunction with intraoperative PTH is the most effective way to manage the reoperative parathyroid patient. Unguided bilateral exploration of what can be a significantly scarred central neck is not recommended because it is challenging, often results in a second failure to treat hyperparathyroidism, and risks complications, such as hypoparathyroidism and bilateral vocal cord paralysis as well as tracheal and cervical esophageal injury.

If the first parathyroid operation was done by an inexperienced parathyroid surgeon who missed a well-localized adenoma, reoperation can be rather straightforward, because the first surgeon failed to go deep enough in to the neck for a superior adenoma or inferior enough within the thymus for an inferior parathyroid adenoma.[16-18] A number of approaches are available to the reoperative parathyroid surgeon through less-dissected planes, which can make reoperation more likely to be successful and, at the same time, minimize the risks of complications.

Original Midline Approach

If a patient has undergone a previous minimally invasive or targeted parathyroidectomy on one side and additional glands are localized on the contralateral side, it is perfectly reasonable to go through an original midline approach, especially if the strap muscles on the side in question have not been badly scarred to the underlying thyroid.[19,20] If after dealing with an abnormal gland(s) on the previously unoperated side, the intraoperative PTH level does not fall appropriately, then it may be best to approach the original side by a lateral dissection (between straps and sternocleidomastoid [SCM] muscle) to avoid bleeding from peeling the scarred strap muscles off the thyroid.[21]

Lateral Approach

The lateral approach is ideal for missed superior parathyroid glands in patients who have previously undergone a standard midline approach (Figure 63.1).[22] One of the most commonly missed parathyroid adenomas is the superior adenoma posterior to the recurrent laryngeal nerve (RLN) deep within the tracheoesophageal groove or retroesophageal/prevertebral region. With this approach, a plane is developed between the sternocleidomastoid and the lateral strap muscle on the side in question. The contents of the carotid sheath are then retracted laterally, thus exposing the prevertebral fascia and the tracheoesophageal groove. Typically, the previously undisturbed RLN can be easily identified via this approach in a previously undissected plane and can be retracted medially. The lateral approach may be more difficult after prior low anterior cervical spine surgery because its plane of dissection is similar; however, this alone should not contraindicate the lateral approach.

Superior Approach

If preoperative localization identifies an undescended inferior parathyroid gland at the level of the carotid bifurcation, ultrasound can

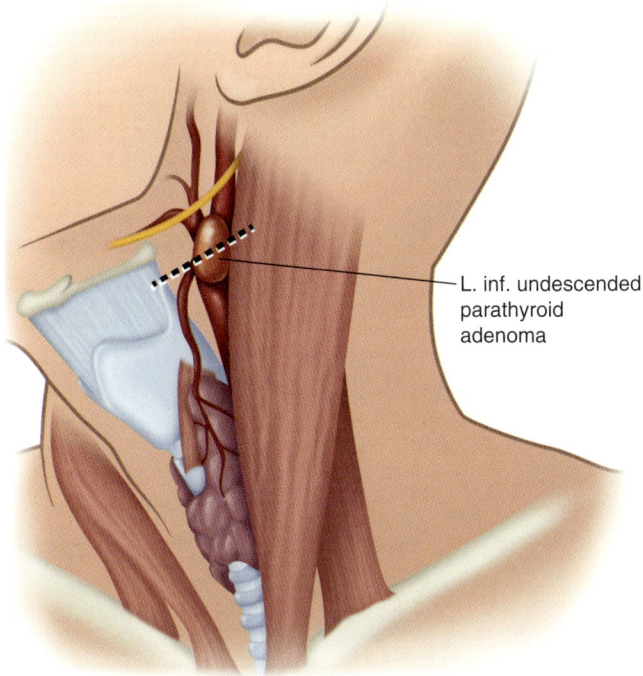

Fig. 63.2 The superior approach. (Redrawn and modified from Thompson GB. "No frills" image-guided exploration. *Oper Tech Gen Surg.* 1999;1 [1]:34–48.)

determine the most direct route to this missing gland.[22] One can make a small incision in a skin crease directly overlying the gland, and using a focused approach through previously nondissected planes, one easily can identify the adenoma and remove it (Figure 63.2). Care must be taken to avoid injury to the nearby vagus, superior laryngeal, and hypoglossal nerves. Intraoperative nerve monitoring is an effective tool to identify these structures and to protect them from dissection trauma.

Inferior Approach

An inferior adenoma within the upper portion of the thymus and/or superior mediastinum can be approached through a previously nondissected plane once the original incision is reopened (Figure 63.3).[22] There is no need to mobilize the thyroid gland on either side. The lower thyroid pole can be exposed along with the thyrothymic ligament. The thyrothymic ligament can then be separated from the inferior pole and gently retracted upward, often exposing the missed inferior parathyroid adenoma. A map of typical locations for parathyroid discovered at reoperation is presented (Figure 63.4).[15]

COMMON REOPERATIVE OR CHALLENGING PRIMARY OPERATIVE SCENARIOS

The challenging nature of reoperative parathyroidectomy has been discussed throughout this chapter. Even those reoperative cases that appear likely to be relatively straightforward preoperatively can at the time of surgery confound even the most skilled and experienced surgeons. However, even among these demanding cases, certain clinical scenarios present particular difficulties that need to be addressed. In these cases, the likelihood of success and risk of complications are often elevated.

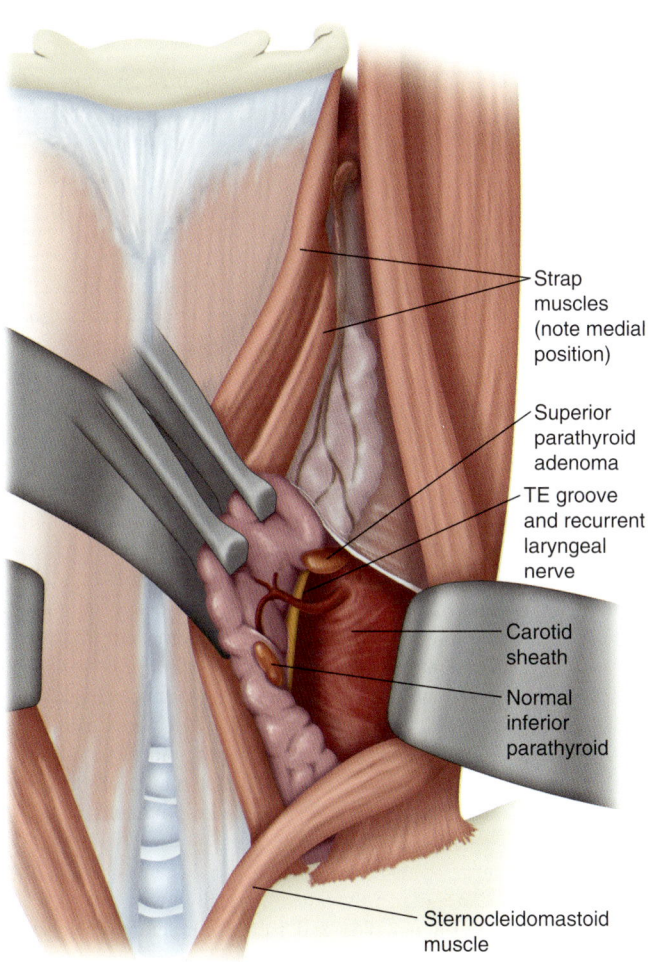

Fig. 63.1 The lateral approach. (Redrawn from Thompson GB. "No frills" image-guided exploration. *Oper Tech Gen Surg.* 1999;1[1]:34–48.)

588 SECTION 8 Parathyroid Surgery

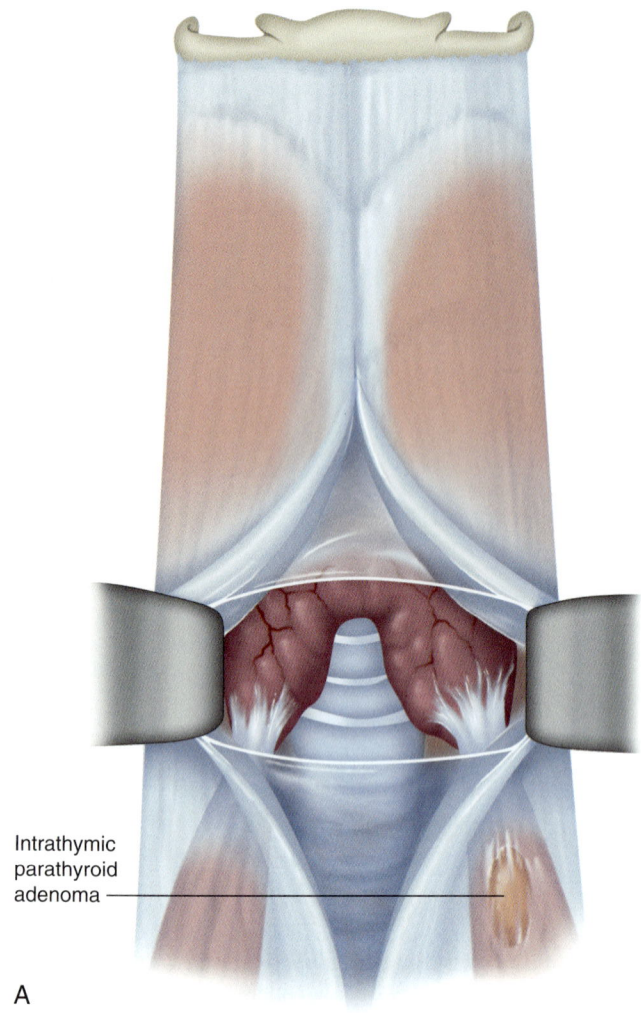

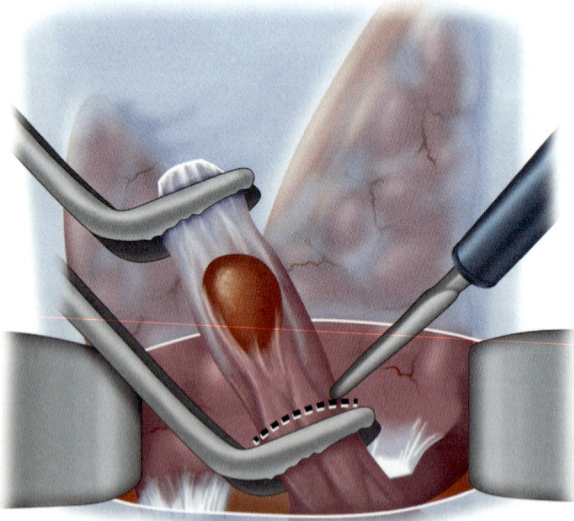

Fig. 63.3 A, Inferior approach, initial view of inferior thyroid lobes. **B,** The thyrothymic ligament is retracted superiorly to deliver the parathyroid adenoma. (Redrawn from Thompson GB. "No frills" image-guided exploration. *Oper Tech Gen Surg.* 1999;1[1]:34–48.)

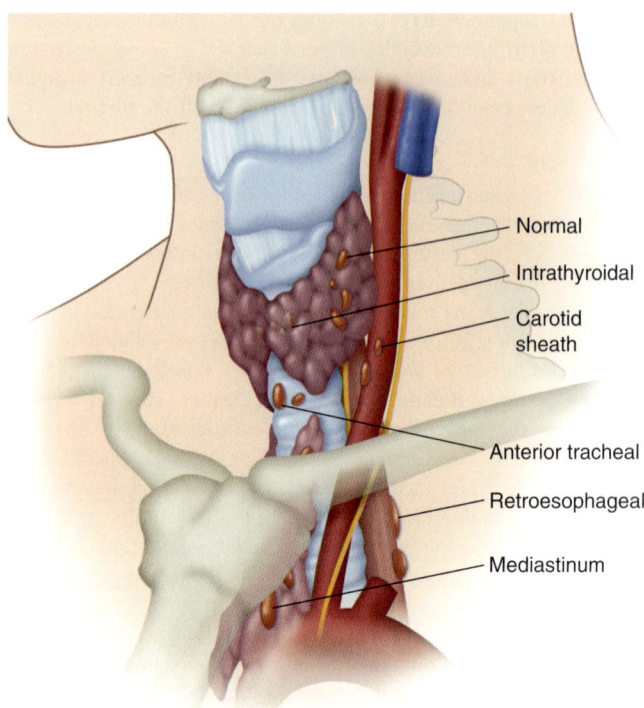

Fig. 63.4 Location of ectopic parathyroid glands found on reoperation.

Case #1

A patient has persistent PHPT after unsuccessful bilateral neck exploration for presumed four-gland hyperplasia. Pathologic assessment of the glands that were removed describes them as "hypercellular."

Challenges

These patients can have undergone excision of one, two, or even three glands. Despite their removal, a patient's laboratory results do not improve after surgery. Often at the time of the first surgery, an extensive search will have been conducted to identify the remaining glands, thereby creating extensive scar tissue throughout the neck. Additionally, as the unidentified gland(s) is often in a eutopic position, it often rests in an area disturbed during primary surgery. The difficulty of this case is magnified by the nonlocalizing nature of many hyperplastic parathyroid glands. As mentioned earlier, the rate of successful localization in cases of hyperplasia is markedly lower than in adenomatous disease.

Tips for Success

Uncured four-gland hyperplasia represents one of the most problematic scenarios for reoperative parathyroidectomy, especially when more than one gland remains *in situ*. As with all reoperative cases, a detailed review of all available data, particularly the operative and pathology reports, is crucial (Figure 63.5).

Although localizing studies are frequently unsuccessful in patients with parathyroid hyperplasia, they should still be obtained. All modalities of imaging, including computed tomography and magnetic resonance imaging scans, should be considered. Unfortunately, other forms of localization, such as selective venous sampling and intraoperative radioguidance, are also rarely beneficial with four-gland hyperplasia.

Given the extreme difficulty of this type of case, reoperative surgery should be reserved only for those who have severe disease sequelae. If no localizing information is available and surgery is required, proximal ligation of the thyroid arteries, particularly the inferior vessel, can be attempted to "blindly" devascularize the gland(s). Importantly, this maneuver puts the patient at risk of permanent hypoparathyroidism.

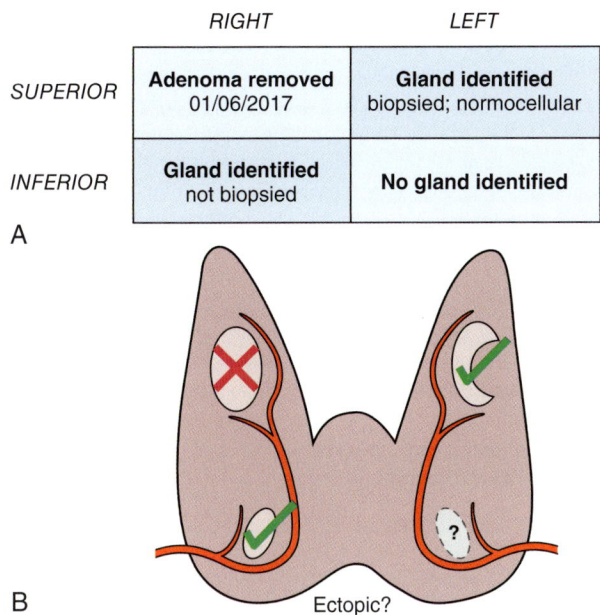

Fig. 63.5 A and **B,** Technique for "forensic" localization of likely adenoma based on previous pathology and operative reports. Information can be recorded as shown in figure B to focus the surgeon's interest on a particular quadrant of interest in the reoperative neck. Thyroid biopsy should be judiciously employed. (Redrawn from an illustration by Andrew M. Hinson, MD.)

is a challenging endeavor because it is often difficult to excise the precise amount of tissue to allow for a desired reduction in PTH levels without crossing over into hypoparathyroidism. Also, although perhaps lowering PTH levels sufficiently (at least for some period of time), if a subtotal resection is planned, it is crucial for the patient to understand that the remaining tissue is pathologic and may regrow and cause recurrent hyperparathyroidism in the future. In this situation, an arduous second reoperation might become necessary to remove additional tissue from a scarred location.

An alternative approach is to remove the remaining pathologic gland in its entirety. A part of this gland can then be reimplanted into the sternocleidomastoid muscle or a subcutaneous pocket just adjacent to the incision. This implanted tissue should be clearly marked with a suture or surgical clips to facilitate identification if the need arises for further excision. This approach ensures that the patient will be cured of hyperparathyroidism. However, the success rate of transplanting parathyroid tissue is unclear; the patient may be left permanently hypoparathyroid. An additional precaution that may be taken is to cryopreserve some of the excised gland. If the transplanted tissue does not function, future attempts can be made to reimplant the cryopreserved tissue. Secondary auto transplantation of cryopreserved parathyroid tissue is not uniformly successful.

Case #2

A patient presents with persistent PHPT after unsuccessful bilateral neck exploration. At surgery, three glands were identified and removed despite having a relatively normal appearance. A fourth gland was never discovered. Pathology suggests normocellular parathyroid glands. On subsequent imaging studies, what appears to be the likely adenomatous remaining gland is well localized.

Challenges

In some instances when not all glands have been found during an initial exploration, a well-intentioned surgeon will remove those glands that have been identified in an effort to achieve a cure. If the pathologic gland is not included, this provides no benefit for the patient and only sacrifices normal parathyroid tissue. Unfortunately, if all the normal glands have been excised (or simply devascularized during dissection), removal of the pathologic gland during reoperation likely will lead to permanent hypoparathyroidism and hypocalcemia.

Tips for Success

Regarding the patient described in this scenario, in light of clear localizing information, reoperation likely will be successful, but it also will result in hypoparathyroidism. The effect of hypoparathyroidism on a patient's quality of life is significant and should not be minimized. This outcome needs to be discussed extensively with the patient and weighed against the risks of continued hyperparathyroidism.

Several approaches can be considered to try to avoid permanent hypoparathyroidism. A subtotal resection of the remaining gland can be attempted. This

Case #3

A patient has PHPT and requires treatment. The patient has never had attempted parathyroid surgery but did undergo an anterior cervical discectomy and fusion (ACDF) one year earlier.

Challenges

Any surgery involving the central neck will result in the development of significant scar tissue. Patients who have undergone an ACDF will often have a robust inflammatory reaction to the dissection and the hardware placed during the surgery. This scar tissue can lead to the loss of normal tissue planes and can cause alterations in normal anatomy.

Tips for Success

Even if excellent preoperative localizing information is available, any parathyroidectomy performed in a patient who has previously undergone a cervical surgery is likely to have a higher failure and complication rate. Extra care is required in these cases to prevent injury to the RLN, esophagus, and trachea.

Several methods can be employed in these patients to reduce the risk of complications and facilitate dissection. First, many surgeons do not routinely use intraoperative neuromonitoring during parathyroidectomy. However, in any reoperative case, nerve monitoring can be extremely beneficial because identifying the RLN can be quite challenging. Second, blunt, rather than sharp, dissection should be used in these cases. Blunt dissection is less likely to lead to an inadvertent tear or perforation of the aerodigestive tract. Finally, as discussed earlier in this chapter, a lateral (or "back door") approach used to avoid the scarred central aspect of the neck, is often the safest route to the targeted area in these patients.

Case #4

A patient has PHPT requiring treatment but never had attempted parathyroid surgery. However, 10 years earlier, the patient was diagnosed with Graves' disease and treated with radioactive iodine (RAI) ablation of the thyroid. Imaging studies all suggest the presence of a right superior parathyroid adenoma.

Challenges

Although this patient has not undergone any central neck surgery, the RAI ablation potentially increases the risks of this parathyroidectomy. In some patients after treatment with RAI, the thyroid tissue becomes fibrotic but remains an identifiable landmark. However, in others the ablation results in the apparent loss of any identifiable thyroid tissue.

This "absence" of the thyroid gland is important for several reasons. The thyroid gland serves as a clear landmark during parathyroid surgery and orients the surgeon to the general position of the parathyroid glands. Loss of this anatomic guide can be disorienting during the procedure. Additionally, when the thyroid is absent, the carotid sheath structures tend to move medially toward the trachea. This positioning is critical to recognize to avoid inadvertent injury to the carotid artery or jugular vein. Perhaps most hazardous is the lack of any thyroid tissue to protect the RLN. Without the thyroid overlying it, the nerve is fully exposed almost immediately after the strap muscles are retracted. Often during parathyroidectomy, surgeons will place a retractor on the thyroid lobe and retract it medially. If a similar maneuver is performed on a patient such as this, the retractor can be easily placed directly onto the nerve, leading to injury.

Tips for Success

Parathyroid surgery after RAI ablation can be readily performed in a safe manner. The key to success is to be familiar with the possible changes in anatomy that can occur after ablation. The unprotected RLN is most at risk because a retractor can be placed before the area is well exposed. In these patients, surgeons need to consider the location of the nerve as soon as the midline raphe is divided and the strap muscles are retracted laterally.

Case #5

A patient has PHPT after an unsuccessful bilateral neck exploration performed one year earlier. At surgery three glands were identified that were normal in appearance. A fourth gland was never discovered. During the course of the dissection, the right RLN was injured. Recent imaging studies all suggest the presence of a left overly descended superior parathyroid adenoma. Importantly, fiberoptic laryngoscopy reveals a paralyzed right vocal cord.

Challenges

In this scenario, reoperative surgery is likely to be successful given the precise localizing information available. However, the apparent adenoma is located on the side of the only functioning RLN. Critically, a nerve injury on the contralateral side (the side of the suspected adenoma), even if temporary, would be devastating because the patient could develop airway obstruction and might require a tracheostomy. Although recurrent nerve injuries are uncommon during parathyroidectomy, they do occur. This risk is increased with dissection of superior glands, as the nerve is superficial to them and sometimes needs to be significantly manipulated.

Tips for Success

Several elements of the care of this patient are crucial. Most importantly, the vocal cord paralysis must be recognized before any surgery on the contralateral side. Although these injuries can sometimes be recognizable by symptoms (hoarseness, difficulty swallowing, etc.), vocal cord paralysis can also be relatively asymptomatic. In these patients, only laryngoscopy will reveal the issue. Thus before a second operation, for any patient who has previously undergone any type of neck surgery, preoperative laryngoscopy is mandatory.

Once recognized, the implications of this injury need to be discussed at length with the patient. Given the potential for a disastrous outcome, if the second nerve were to be injured, the strength of the indication for surgery must be carefully weighed. If the decision to proceed with surgery is made, avoiding a nerve injury is imperative. Certainly, as in many cases of reoperative parathyroidectomy, intraoperative neuromonitoring can be helpful. In this specific scenario, further consideration should be made to use continuous intraoperative neuromonitoring (discussed elsewhere in this textbook). This method of neuromonitoring may be particularly advantageous as it may help further minimize the risk of even temporary nerve dysfunction.

SUMMARY

Reoperative parathyroidectomy can often be performed successfully, particularly if imaging directs the surgeon to a specific target. However, surgeons need to approach these cases with caution and carefully weigh the risk-benefit ratio of proceeding with the patient and physicians. Although a range of techniques can be employed to address the challenges encountered in reoperative surgery, select cases can be particularly precarious, even for the most experienced surgeon.

REFERENCES

For a full list of references, go to expertconsult.com.

64

Parathyroid Carcinoma

Rita Y.K. Chang, Brian H.H. Lang

Please go to expertconsult.com to view related video:
Video 64.1 Parathyroid Carcinoma: Management Principles with an Illustrative Case

BACKGROUND

Parathyroid carcinoma (PC) is a rare but ominous cause of primary hyperparathyroidism (HPT).[1,2] It accounts for less than 1% of the cases of primary HPT. In a retrospective study of two European cohorts of primary HPT from 2005 to 2014, the incidence of PC in patients with HPT was 0.3% and 2.1%, respectively. This difference was perhaps related to selection and referral biases.[3] In a systematic review of 22,225 cases of primary HPT reported from 1995 to 2003, PC accounted for 0.74%.[4] Interestingly, the reported incidence appears to be higher in some countries, like Japan and Italy (around 5%).[5] In Europe, the incidence was reported to be 1.25 to 2.0 cases per 10,000,000 persons.[6,7] In the Surveillance, Epidemiology, and End Results (SEER) cancer registry data from 2000 to 2012, the incidence rate was 0.41.[8] Due to its rarity and the paucity of large-scale published patient series, there is still a lack of understanding of the natural course and prognostic implications of this disease. In addition, there is still no clear consensus on its management and follow-up (see Chapter 65 Surgical Pathology of the Parathyroid Glands).

Although primary HPT is more commonly associated with females (4:1),[9] there is no gender difference in PCs. Males may have a slightly worse prognosis.[10,11] It is usually diagnosed after age 30, and the mean age of diagnosis is 50 years old, which is 10 years earlier than benign parathyroid adenomas.[11-14]

RISK FACTORS AND ETIOLOGY

The etiology of PC remains largely unknown. A few risk factors have been identified based on epidemiology studies; however, mechanisms and causal relationships still remain poorly understood. Recently, some advances in molecular biology have shed light on the plausible pathogenesis of PC. Clinical risk factors are reviewed here.

Prior Neck Irradiation

Like many other cancers, ionizing radiation exposure has been implicated as a cause or risk factor for PC.[15-17] However, it should be noted that the majority of patients with PC do not appear to have any prior history of radiation exposure to the head and neck region.

Chronic Renal Failure

Some reports have suggested chronic renal failure to be a possible risk factor of PC.[18,19] Mechanisms are largely unknown. Clonal analysis showed that in chronic renal failure, parathyroid glands could initially grow diffusely and polyclonally, after which the foci of nodular hyperplasia become monoclonal neoplasia,[19] although the exact mechanism remains to be elicited. Currently, there is no evidence that PC arises from malignant transformation of preexisting parathyroid lesions. A few case reports regarding PC associated with renal HPT have been published.[20-22] It has been shown that PC arising in the setting of renal parathyroid hyperplasia does not have HRPT2/CDC73 alterations and no parafibromin loss.[23]

Genetic Mutations

The disease may occur as part of a syndrome. The potential genes are listed here (see also Table 64.1):

HRPT2/CDC73: The observation of *HRPT2/CDC73* gene mutations in sporadic PC and hereditary hyperparathyroid jaw tumor syndrome (HPT-JT) leads to the understanding of plausible molecular pathogenesis of PC. HPT-JT is a rare autosomal-dominant disorder, causing one or more parathyroid gland neoplasms. Patients are predisposed to ossifying fibromas of the jaw, cystic and neoplastic renal lesions, uterine tumors, and parathyroid neoplasia with an increased risk of parathyroid cancer. Approximately 15% of patients who have HPT-JT develop PC.[24] It is associated with inactivating germline mutations in the *HRPT2* gene,[25] which encodes parafibromin. Some sporadic PCs also have defects in this gene, mostly with somatic or clonal mutations.[26-28] Unsuspected germline mutations can be discovered in patients who presented clinically with sporadic PC, suggesting that these patients have HPT-JT or a phenotypic variant.[26]

PRUNE2: Inactivating mutations have been found in 18% of PCs. It is located in chromosome 9q21.2 and encodes a protein that suppresses oncogenic cellular transformation.[29]

MEN1: Mutations of the *MEN1* gene can occasionally be seen, although rarely, in PCs. Only one case has been reported in a series of 348 cases of MEN 1 (0.28%) from the Mayo Clinic from 1977 to 2013. The clinical features are similar to PC in patients without MEN 1.[30] Somatic mutations in the *MEN1* gene in chromosome 11q13 have been found in up to 30% of sporadic PC.[31-34]

Epigenetics

Aberrant DNA methylation signatures and a microRNA expression profile have recently been identified for PCs.[35]

CLINICAL PRESENTATION

Most PCs are functional and hypersecrete parathyroid hormone (PTH). Patients with a PC typically present with severe hypercalcemia

TABLE 64.1 Aberrant Gene Expression and Related Molecular Mechanisms in Parathyroid Carcinoma

Gene ID	Chr. Map	Gene function	Variation in PCs	Frequency in PCs	Reference
HRPT2/ CDC73	1q31.2	Transcribe parafibromin, which is involved in regulating gene transcription in nucleus. Parafibromin is a tumor suppressor gene	Loss of function	70%	Sharretts and Simonds[24]
MEN1	11q12	Provides instructions for making a protein called MENIN, which is a tumor suppressor; associated with MEN 1 syndrome	Loss of function	13%	Haven et al.[31]
PRUNE2	9q21.2	Tumor suppressor gene involved in suppressing RAS homolog family member A activity	Loss of function	18%	Yu et al.[29]

CDC73, cell division cycle 73; HRPT2, hyperparathyroidism 2 with jaw tumors; MEN 1, multiple endocrine neoplasia type 1; PC, parathyroid carcinoma; PRUNE2, prune drosophila homolog of 2.

TABLE 64.2 Clinical Features of Parathyroid Carcinoma Compared With Benign Primary Hyperparathyroidism

	Parathyroid Adenoma	Parathyroid Carcinoma
Age of diagnosis	50–60	40–50
Sex (female:male)	3–4:1	1:1
Palpable neck mass	Seldom	50%
Concomitant renal and bone diseases	Seldom	Common
Serum calcium level	Elevated	>14 mg/dL (3.5 mmol/L)
Parathyroid hormone level	1.5–2 times of normal	5–10 times of normal
Size of tumor (cm)	<3	>3
Invasion to surrounding tissues	Seldom	Common

with overt dehydration. Renal (32% to 70%) and bone disease (34% to 73%), gastrointestinal complications including ulcers and pancreatitis (15%), and even parathyroid crisis (12%) are relatively common.[5,13,14,36-39] Concomitant renal and bone complications can be found in 50% of patients with PC at diagnosis.[38] The serum calcium level is usually above 14 mg/dL (3.5 mmol/L), and serum PTH concentration can be 5- to 10-fold higher than the upper normal limit (Table 64.2).[40,41]

A palpable neck mass is present in approximately 50% of PCs, which is not found in benign parathyroid adenomas or hyperplasia unless there is a concomitant thyroid nodule.[5,13] Invasion to surrounding structures is not uncommon (34% to 75%). Strap muscles and the surrounding soft tissues are most often involved by the tumor bulk. Invasion to the recurrent laryngeal nerve (RLN) is seen in approximately 7% to 13% of patients with a PC. Tracheal involvement occurs in 11% of the patients and esophageal or carotid sheath involvement occurs in 2% of patients.[42] Distant metastases at presentation are uncommon. Ultimately, lymph node (LN) metastasis (<5%) and distant metastasis (<2%), usually involving liver, lung, and bone, may occur.[13] Inferiorly located parathyroid glands are much more commonly affected than superiorly located glands.[5,13,43] Multiglandular carcinoma is extremely rare with only a few case reports.[44,45]

Occasionally, PC can be nonfunctional (2% to 7%). To date, only 32 cases of nonfunctional PC have been reported in the literature.[46,47] An older age for presentation in 60 to 70 year olds is observed, and half of these patients are presented with a neck mass between 5 and 11 cm in size.[47,48] Understandably, they are diagnosed at a more advanced stage, with more locally aggressive tumor and more distant metastasis to lungs, cervical LN, liver, and bone. Diagnosis of these patients is based entirely on histologic findings, as they are normocalcemic with normal levels of PTH. In contrast to the more typical functional PC, these patients usually die of mass effect and tumor burden rather than hypercalcemia.[12,48,49]

Diagnosis and Workup

The biochemical workup is similar to that of primary HPT. PC is generally not confirmed before surgery but should be suspected in patients suffering from parathyroid crisis, marked hypercalcemia, very high PTH concentrations, or a neck mass. The diagnosis of PC is typically made at the time of surgery or after surgery through histology.

Biochemical Tests

The serum calcium concentration is usually more than 14 mg/dL (3.5 mmol/L), and serum PTH concentration can be 5- to 10-fold, higher than the upper limit of normal. Alkaline phosphatase (ALP) levels have also been shown to be significantly higher than in benign disease—with levels under 300 IU/L making carcinoma unlikely.[50] Interestingly, raised baseline serum and urinary human chorionic gonadotrophin (hCG) levels are also observed in some reports,[51,52] although the measurement is not routinely performed for diagnosing PC.

Imaging Studies

Unlike adenomas, localization studies have less of a role in PC. However, traditional imaging studies can provide some information regarding the stage of the PC. Although imaging can rarely distinguish benign adenoma from PC, tumors which are large in size, invasive to surrounding structures, or have metastasized to distant sites are more likely to be malignant.

Ultrasound (US) of the neck is considered the first imaging study. It is readily available, safe, and noninvasive and can provide the most essential information regarding tumor size, location, and extent. Typical features suggestive of malignancy include inhomogeneity, hypoechogenicity, and irregularity of borders.[53]

Technetium (99mTc) sestamibi (or MIBI) scanning can identify parathyroid tissue in ectopic areas.[54] Other useful imaging includes a higher resolution computed tomography (CT) scan with contrast and magnetic resonance imaging (MRI) as they can assess the relationship of the tumor with the surrounding structures.[55] MRI with gadolinium and fat suppression allows for accurate soft tissue imaging of the neck.[54]

In a retrospective analysis with 20 patients who diagnosed with PC, the sensitivity of single preoperative imaging, whether by US, CT, or

MIBI, was approximately 80%. Combining CT with MIBI and US could increase the sensitivity to 95% or better, and therefore multiple imaging modalities are important in the preoperative evaluation of PC.[56]

In the setting for recurrent PC with hypercalcemia, preoperative imaging is mandatory to assess location of recurrence and the relationship to surrounding structures. In the case of suspected metastatic disease, systemic workup, including MIBI, CT, or MRI scan, can detect the location of a metastasis and locoregional recurrence.[54]

Fluorodeoxyglucose-positron emission tomography (FDG-PET) has been described in the management of PC.[57-60] Increased FDG uptake on the basis of suspicious anatomic features may suggest PC.[54] Some studies have assessed dual isotopes (^{11}C-choline and Fluorine-18-fluorodeoxyglucose [FDG]) as substrates for PET/CT studies, and they found them to be more accurate than standard FDG-PET/CT in detecting abnormal parathyroid tissue.[61,62]

Other Investigations

If axial imaging cannot localize the parathyroid lesion, selective venous catheterization together with PTH measurement can be used but is rarely needed in PC.[63] If PC is suspected, preoperative cytology with fine-needle aspiration is not necessary and should be avoided due to risk of dissemination of tumor and tumor seeding.[64,65] Similarly, excisional biopsy is not recommended. Frozen sections are of no value in distinguishing benign from malignant disease.

HISTOPATHOLOGY

Given that imaging studies cannot reliably distinguish PC from adenoma, the diagnosis of PC often relies on clues or hints observed during the operation. Findings of a large, grayish white and hard tumor, which is adhesive to surrounding structures, raise the possibility of PC. If there are any doubts, a more radical approach (e.g., en bloc resection with a hemithyroidectomy) is often advised.

To date, there has been no gold standard test to confirm PC (see Chapter 65, Surgical Pathology of the Parathyroid Glands). Histologic features of PC, although present, may be variable, making the malignant diagnosis challenging. Table 64.3 summarizes the diagnostic and molecular features of PC to aid diagnosis. Features that correlate best with cancer diagnosis are gross invasion beyond capsule or extracapsular vascular or lymphatic invasion.[10,36] Classic pathologic features for PC also include trabecular pattern, mitotic figure, and thick fibrous bands. In 1973, Shantz and Castleman, based upon an analysis of 70 cases of PC, established a set of criteria for the histologic diagnosis of this malignancy (Table 64.4).[66] However none of the features are pathognomonic for PC, and some are present in benign adenomas.[67,68]

Other diagnostic techniques are available to increase diagnostic accuracy. Electron microscopy of PC tissue reveals nuclear and mitochondrial alterations, with nuclear diameter greater than adenomas.[66] Flow cytometry can be used to measure nuclear DNA content to predict the invasive potential of tumors.[37] Mean nuclear DNA content is greater, and an aneuploid DNA pattern is more common in PC than in adenomas; when present, aneuploidy appears to be associated with a poorer prognosis.[69]

Because PC is difficult to diagnose even on histology, the 2004 World Heath Organization (WHO) classification defined a category of "atypical parathyroid adenomas," which represents parathyroid neoplasms without concrete signs of vascular or capsular invasion, but with some morphologic features suspicious for PCs, including broad fibrous bands with or without hemosiderin deposits, mitoses, and neoplastic cell groups in a thickened fibrous capsule.[70]

In this subgroup of atypical parathyroid adenomas, the use of immunohistochemical biomarkers may be helpful, but these tests are not widely available. For example, in one study, patients with PC were found to have abnormal expression of retinoblastoma (RB) protein (a complete or predominant absence of nuclear staining for the protein), whereas none of the adenomas had abnormal staining for RB protein.[71] Ki-67, a marker of cell proliferation, has been found to be useful in distinguishing PC from adenoma; more intense staining in the malignant cases has been observed. However, there is significant overlap between groups of tumors so Ki-67 is not suitable for definitive differentiation between benign and malignant tumors.[72,73] The HRPT2 gene product, parafibromin, is often absent in PC;[74,75] HRPT2 gene mutations are also frequently found in PC. In a study of HRPT2 mutation analysis in 60 parathyroid tumors, HRPT2 somatic mutations were detected in four of four sporadic PC samples, and germline mutations were found in five of five HPT-JT parathyroid tumors.[28] The use of an immunohistochemical panel that includes loss-of-expression of parafibromin, galactin-3, PGP9.5, and Ki-67 has been suggested from a small series to aid in diagnosis of PC, with a sensitivity of 80% and specificity of 100%.[76]

Stratification and Staging

Before the latest (8th) edition of the Tumor, Node, Metastases (TNM) cancer manual from the combined American Joint Committee on Cancer (AJCC) and the Union for International Cancer Control (UICC), there was no staging system for PC. Talat and Schulte proposed a classification system in 2010 based on a retrospective literature review of 330 patients,[10] which divided patients according to an anatomy-based system resembling the TNM system. Separation of patients into low- and high-risk groups identifies a 3.5- to 7.0-fold higher risk of

TABLE 64.3 Histopathological Features of Parathyroid Carcinoma

Diagnostic features	Gross vascular, capsular or perineural invasion
	Gross invasion to surrounding structures
	Distant metastasis
Suspicious features (atypical adenoma)	Solid growth pattern
	Broad fibrous band with or without hemosiderin deposits
	Increased mitotic activity
	Macronucleoli
	Nuclear atypia
	Necrosis
Biomarkers	Loss of parafibromin
	Loss of retinoblastoma protein
	Ki 67 >5%
	Galactin-3, PGP9.5

TABLE 64.4 Pathologic Features of Parathyroid Carcinoma

Macroscopic Features	Microscopic Features
Large >3 cm, 2-10 g	Uniform sheets of cells arranged in lobular pattern, separated by dense fibrous trabeculae
Grayish white	
Adherent to adjacent tissue	
Irregular and firm	Mitotic figures within the parenchymal cell
More common in inferior gland and occasionally in ectopic site	
	Vascular and capsular invasion
	Chief cell-predominant cell type
	Cellular atypia

TABLE 64.5 Parathyroid Carcinoma: Proposed TNM Definitions

Tumor

Tx	Primary tumor cannot be assessed
Tis	Atypical parathyroid neoplasm (neoplasm of uncertain malignant potential)
T1	Localized to the parathyroid gland with extension limited to the soft tissue
T2	Invade the thyroid gland
T3	Surrounding structures such as recurrent laryngeal nerve, esophagus, or trachea
T4	Major blood vessels/spine

Node

Nx	Regional LN cannot be assessed
N0	Absence presence of disease in the central (N1a) or lateral (N1b) neck LN
N1	Presence of disease in the central (N1a) or lateral (N1b) neck lymph nodes
N1a	Metastasis to level VI (pretracheal, paratracheal, and prelaryngeal/Delphian lymph nodes) or superior mediastinal lymph nodes (level VII)
N1b	Metastasis to unilateral, bilateral, or contralateral cervical (levels I, II, III, IV, or V) or retropharyngeal nodes

Metastasis

M0	Absence of disease outside of the neck
M1	Evidence of disease not confined to the neck

Prognostic Staging

There are not enough data to propose anatomic stage and prognostic groups for parathyroid carcinoma (see text below).

TNM, Tumor, Node, Metastases, Tis, in situ cancer; LN, lymph node. Used with the permission of the American College of Surgeons. Amin, M.B., Edge, S.B., Greene, F.L., et al. (Eds.) *AJCC Cancer Staging Manual.* 8th Ed. New York: Springer; 2017.

recurrence and death for the high-risk group.[10] Later, Schulte et al. validated the results of the prognostic classification systems and further classified high-risk cancer into vascular invasion alone (class II), nodal metastasis or organ invasion (class III), and distant metastasis (class IV).[77]

Recently, PC has been included in the 8th AJCC and UICC TNM cancer manual (Table 64.5). The proposed staging system includes with variables like age at diagnosis, gender, race, size of primary tumor, location of tumor, presence of invasion into the surrounding structures, distant metastatic disease, number of nodes removed, number of positive nodes, highest preoperative calcium, highest preoperative PTH, presence of lymphovascular invasion, histologic grade (high grade or low grade), weight of primary tumor, mitotic rate, and time to recurrence.[78] The aim is to facilitate the development of a more suitable staging system in the future.

PREOPERATIVE MANAGEMENT

To date, the only curative treatment for parathyroid carcinoma is complete surgical excision of the tumor and any possible metastatic deposits. Before operation, control of the hypercalcemia is necessary because uncontrolled hypercalcemia may cause severe dehydration. This usually entails aggressive fluid replacement with volume expansion and diuresis with diuretics. If these are not adequate, bisphosphonate may be used to achieve a reduction in serum calcium level. Occasionally hemodialysis is required. In addition to hypercalcemia, other complications of primary HPT, such as bone disease, acute renal failure, and renal stones, may require early detection and treatment.

Surgical Management

Surgery offers the only realistic chance of curing PC. A summary of clinical management for PC is shown in Table 64.6. The aim of the initial operation is to remove the tumor en bloc with clear excision margins.[79] This almost always involves ipsilateral hemithyroidectomy.[27,80] If there is an obvious tumor invasion of the RLN, the nerve should be excised together with the tumor (i.e., en bloc resection).[81] Overlying strap muscles, paratracheal lymphatics, and adjacent soft tissue should also be excised en bloc when they are involved.

From the SEER database from 1988 to 2010, only one-tenth of patients had concomitant nodal positivity at the time of diagnosis. Tumors ≥ 3 cm were associated with a greater chance of nodal metastasis, but interestingly, nodal metastasis is not associated with disease-specific survival.[82] Thus regional nodal metastasis is rare and prophylactic central or lateral neck dissection is not advocated and has not been shown to improve outcomes.[83] However, if any regional nodes are enlarged and suspicious, an ipsilateral selective neck dissection should be performed.

During resection, great care should be taken to avoid rupture of the parathyroid gland capsule to prevent tumor seeding.[84] The use of intraoperative PTH measurement is advocated, if available, to confirm biochemical cure. However, it should be noted that PC generally would have a higher intraoperative PTH baseline value and a greater percentage intraoperative PTH drop after excision than adenomas.[85] If intraoperative PTH remains elevated after resection of the tumor, this may mean residual surrounding soft tissue involvement (incomplete resection) and/or occult metastases. Rarely, there may be PC in a background of parathyroid hyperplasia, concomitant parathyroid adenoma, or multiglandular carcinoma, especially in patients with familial HPT of *HRPT2* gene mutation. There is no consensus on whether four-gland exploration should be performed in the setting of suspected PC. Concerns exist for tumor seeding to the contralateral normal neck for bilateral neck exploration. It is of note that PC involving two or more glands has been reported.[45] In patients with known *HRPT2* gene mutations or HPT-JT, because they are potentially at a higher risk of multiglandular disease, bilateral exploration may be advised. Guidelines and recommendations on the precise extent of dissection and operative approach are not available due to the rarity of the disease. In principle, an en bloc resection with clear surgical margins and removal of involved nodes are considered adequate.[86]

About 20% of the PCs are not expected either during preoperative workup or at the time of operation.[87,88] If PC is only diagnosed after initial parathyroidectomy, the patient's biochemical profile and tumor histology should be carefully reassessed. If there are persistent hypercalcemia or HPT, presence of gross vascular or capsular invasion, and incomplete resection margins, reoperation is indicated.[89,90] If a patient remains normocalcemic and histology only shows microscopic evidence of PC, close follow-up with serum calcium, PTH, and US to detect local recurrence should follow.[87]

Postoperative Care and Surveillance

In the early postoperative period, hypocalcemia from hungry bone syndrome can be quite profound, so careful oral and/or intravenous calcium replacement is required.

All patients with proven PC should undergo lifelong follow-up with serum calcium and PTH levels. Recurrence is common in some studies

TABLE 64.6 Summary of Clinical Management for Patients With Parathyroid Carcinoma

Clinical Condition	Consideration
Initial Surgery	
En bloc resection with ipsilateral hemithyroidectomy +/− central neck dissection +/− lateral neck dissection	• Neck dissection is required only when nodal metastasis is present • RLN should be resected if involved by tumor • Intraoperative PTH might be useful to confirm oncological completeness
Unanticipated Parathyroid Carcinoma Diagnosed After Parathyroidectomy	
Low risk: Microscopic evidence of parathyroid carcinoma Serum PTH and calcium normal	Close surveillance with serum calcium, PTH, and US neck
High risk: Presence of gross vascular or capsular invasion Incomplete resection margins Serum PTH and calcium high	Revision surgery for complete resection
Surveillance After Complete Resection	
PTH excess or hypercalcemia	Repeat imaging to localize recurrent disease
Recurrence/Incomplete Resection	
Resectable neck recurrence	Revision surgery for complete resection
Nonresectable neck recurrence	Radiotherapy
Resectable distant metastasis	Resection or ablative treatment
Nonresectable distant metastasis	Ablative treatment if possible Medical therapy to control hypercalcemia
Genetic Counseling and Testing Offered to Patients With Diagnosed Parathyroid Carcinoma	
HRPT2/CDC73 germline mutations	Offer genetic test to family Additional investigations (jaw radiograph, abdominal US) to look for manifestation of HPT-JT
MEN1 mutations	Offer genetic test to family Additional investigations to look for MEN 1 associated tumor
Mutations negative	Continue surveillance

HPT-JT, hyperparathyroidism-jaw tumor syndrome; MEN 1, multiple endocrine neoplasia type 1; PTH, parathyroid hormone; RLN, recurrent laryngeal nerve; US, ultrasound.

up to 50%, mostly within the first 2 to 3 years of operation,[2,13] although recurrence many years later has been reported. Early recurrence usually manifests as elevated serum calcium and PTH levels. Patients may become symptomatic when tumor load is high. Local recurrence in the thyroid bed and paratracheal areas is most common. Other forms of recurrences include more diffuse tumor seeding (parathyromatosis), nodal metastasis, and distant metastases.[91] If recurrence is suspected, restaging by neck US, CT, and/or MRI is necessary.

Follow-up recommendations for atypical parathyroid adenomas are more difficult. The long-term behavior of these tumors is less well-defined. Close surveillance with regular serum calcium and PTH is generally recommended to eliminate the chance of missing malignant and recurrent diseases.

RESECTION OF RECURRENCE

Although reoperative neck surgery is associated with higher morbidity (most notably RLN injury) and rarely leads to complete cure, it is the most effective way to control hypercalcemia via reducing tumor load.[2] There is no consensus on neck reoperation; however, the best chance of cure is in the first two explorations[92] as an increasing number of neck operations may provide only limited benefits. In the case of distant metastasis, resection or ablation of pulmonary or hepatic metastases may also provide palliation.[2,92]

Adjuvant Treatment

Results of adjuvant treatment for PC are limited. Trials of chemotherapeutic agents, either alone or in combination, such as nitrogen mustard; vincristine, cyclophosphamide and actinomycin D; adriamycin, cyclophosphamide, and 5-fluorouracil; and adriamycin alone, have generally been disappointing.[38] Sorafenib has been stated to be useful in reduction of tumor load in PC with lung metastasis in an isolated case report.[93]

Locoregional external radiation (RT) after operation is generally well tolerated and has minimal long-term side effects.[94] Patients treated with postoperative RT may have a lower risk of locoregional disease progression, and thus it may be used to manage local recurrence and improve disease-specific survival.[94,95] However, no benefit for overall survival has been clearly demonstrated. RT is also used as a way of palliation in locally advanced disease or in the presence of distant disease.[11,13,96,97]

Other ablative/embolization treatments such as radiofrequency embolization or transarterial catheter embolization, of distant metastatic disease have been reported, but the number of cases is limited.[98,99] Likewise, isolated reports of ethanol ablation temporarily decreasing serum calcium and PTH levels for palliation of PC exists. However, caution should be taken with ethanol injection in the central neck as it may cause permanent damage to the RLN.[100]

Medical Therapy for Hypercalcemia

Uncontrolled hypercalcemia is one of the most important causes of death in patients with recurrence and metastatic disease. Aggressive tumor resection can mitigate hypercalcemia, but this must be balanced against the operative morbidity.[2] Medical therapy remains the first-line treatment. In the acute phase, this involves volume loading and diuresis with a calcium-wasting loop diuretic. In the longer term, bisphosphonates, calcitonin, and calcimimetics might be added. Denosumab remains an option in refractory hypercalcemia after bisphosphonates and calcimimetics; however, its efficacy in PC is evidenced by isolated case reports only.

Bisphosphonate: This is the analog of pyrophosphate and can bind to hydroxyapatite in bone matrix. It prevents osteoclast attachment to the bone matrix and osteoclast recruitment and viability. Among currently available bisphosphonates, intravenous zoledronic acid or pamidronate are the preferred agents.[101] Pamidronate inhibits both normal and abnormal bone resorption without interfering with bone formation and mineralization and has been reported to improve hypercalcemia in individual cases of PC.[101] Zoledronic acid is more potent than pamidronate in treating hypercalcemia in malignancy,[102] although this effect has not yet been documented specifically in PC.

Calcitonin: This is a human calcitonin analog that promotes renal excretion of calcium and decreases bone resorption via interference with osteoclast function,[103] thus making it effective in hypercalcemia caused by multiple myeloma, carcinoma, or primary HPT. The onset of action is approximately 2 hours and the effects may last 2 to 5 days, but tachyphylaxis can be a problem. It is usually administered in cases of severe hypercalcemia to rapidly bring down the calcium level while coadministering bisphosphonate.

Calcimimetics: These agents bind to and modulate the parathyroid calcium-sensing receptor, increase sensitivity to extracellular calcium, and reduce PTH secretion.[104] Cinacalcet is one of the calcimimetics, which was approved by the U.S. Food and Drug Administration (FDA) for the treatment of hypercalcemia in PC, secondary HPT associated with renal failure, and severe hypercalcemia in patients with primary HPT unable to undergo parathyroidectomy.[105] In an open-label study for inoperable PC, cinacalcet can effectively reduce serum calcium concentration by at least 1 mg/dL in two-thirds of patients.[104] Common side effects include nausea, vomiting, headache, and dehydration.

Denosumab: It is a monoclonal antibody against receptor activator of NF-κB (RANKL) and subsequently inhibits the development of osteoclasts and prevents breakdown of bone. In case reports, monotherapy with denosumab is effective in hypercalcemia refractory to surgery, bisphosphonates, and calcimimetics.[106-108] High-dose monthly denosumab is required to reduce severely elevated serum calcium levels.[109,110] Stabilization of serum calcium may last for a few weeks or as long as 2 years.[110] The most common side effects are joint and muscle pain in the arms or legs.

Anti-PTH immunotherapy: It is postulated that the inhibition of PTH hormone activities could be achieved by potent PTH antibodies. The theory has been tested in a patient with metastatic PC with severe bone disease and extreme hypercalcemia who is resistant to conventional therapy. It is shown that successful induction of anti-PTH antibodies, using PTH peptide fragments for immunization, could normalize serum levels of calcium as well as improve clinical symptoms over 6 months.[111] Besides controlling hypercalcemia, immunotherapy has caused tumor shrinkage in isolated cases of advanced PC.[112] Similar results have been replicated in a Japanese patient.[113]

GENETIC TESTING

Patients diagnosed with PC, either sporadic or associated with familial HPT or HPT-JT, should be considered for mutational analysis including *MEN1* and *HRPT2*. The presence of mutations carries important implications for diagnosing/excluding HPT-JT and familial endocrine neoplasia syndromes and for the management of patients and family members at risk.[26] If the *HRPT2* mutation test is detected in sporadic PC, such patients may have classic HPT-JT, or its phenotypic variant. Thus they should be assessed and screened for the relevant tumors in HPT-JT. The management for the index patient, regarding whether to perform total parathyroidectomy or four-gland exploration, is controversial. Family members who have the mutation screened positive should be advised to have surveillance for the particular disease such as MEN and HPT-JT and have surveillance targeted to PC with serum PTH and calcium.[74] However, the efficacy of such surveillance is unknown due to the scarcity of the condition.

OUTCOME AND PROGNOSIS

PC is generally an indolent tumor.[12] Survival can be long even when the disease has recurred or metastasized. Hypercalcemia remains an important cause of disease-related morbidity and mortality.

The recurrence rate after initial operation is high, approximately 50%, even after seemingly curative surgery. Most of the recurrence occurs 2 to 3 years after the first operation, but still a significant number of patients die of recurrence years later. In one study, among 22 patients who had normal serum calcium concentrations after surgery, the recurrence rate at 1, 5, and 10 years was 27%, 82%, and 91%, respectively.[14]

Survival has varied widely in the literature, with 5-year survival ranging from 20% to 85% and 10-year survival from approximately 15% to 80%. The National Cancer Database survey (1985 to 1995) with their series of 286 patients reported 5- and 10-year survival rates of 55.5% and 49%, respectively.[9] An updated report from 1985 to 2006 with a total of 733 patients revealed 5- and 10-year overall survival rates of 82.3% and 66%, respectively.[96] SEER cancer registry (1988 to 2003 and 2000 to 2012) reported 10-year survival rates of 64.8% (1988 to 2003) and 65.4% (2000 to 2012).[8,11] Young age, female gender, recent year of diagnosis, smaller tumor size, and absence of distant metastases were associated with improved survival.[9,96,114]

SUMMARY

PC is an extremely rare endocrine malignancy that typically presents with the clinical sequelae of extremely elevated serum calcium levels. To stage the tumor more accurately, at least one imaging study is recommended. Needle or excisional biopsy is generally not recommended for fear of causing tumor seeding. A better understanding of molecular biology, specifically the association of *HPRT2* gene mutations and other mutations in PC, has improved the overall management of this rare tumor. However, despite these advances, a high index of clinical suspicion is required to appropriately tailor the correct management of patients. Complete en bloc resection of the tumor in the very first operation remains the best chance of a cure. Radiotherapy could be a useful adjuvant or palliative treatment. Disease recurrence after operation is common; a combination of palliative resection and medication to control hypercalcemia can limit, improve quality of life and prolong survival.

REFERENCES

For a full list of references, go to expertconsult.com.

65

Surgical Pathology of the Parathyroid Glands

Mahsa S. Ahadi, Anthony J. Gill

This chapter contains additional online-only content available on expertconsult.com.

DEVELOPMENT AND ANATOMY

Please see the Expert Consult website for more discussion of this topic.

The parathyroid glands have parenchymal and fat-rich stromal components and are enveloped by a thin capsule which extends into the parenchyma, dividing it into multiple lobules.[6] The parenchymal cells are arranged in nests or cords and are separated by richly vascular stromal elements (Figure 65.1). There are four main types of parenchymal cells: chief cells, oxyphil cells, transitional cells, and clear cells. The chief cells (also known as principal cells) are 8 to 10 μm, polyhedral with centrally placed round nuclei, and have dense chromatin and inconspicuous nucleoli. The cytoplasm of the chief cells is faintly eosinophilic and may appear clear due to intracytoplasmic accumulation of glycogen or lipid, particularly in inactive cells. More lipid is found in the cytoplasm of chief cells in adults than children.[10]

Oxyphil cells (also known as oncocytes) are larger than chief cells, measuring 12 to 20 μm, and have abundant granular eosinophilic cytoplasm with abundant mitochondria and nuclei that are larger and more vesicular than those of chief cells. These cells are not found in childhood, but their numbers increase with age.[10] Oxyphil cells may coalesce into nodules or masses in later adulthood and morphologically they may be difficult to distinguish from the Hürthle cells of the thyroid with which they share the finding of prominent cytoplasmic mitochondria (Figure 65.2). Transitional cells, also known as transitional oncocytes, can be considered intermediate between chief cells and oxyphils in both size and morphology. Clear (water clear) cells are 10 to 15 μm in diameter and demonstrate clear cytoplasm often with relatively pyknotic or eccentric nuclei.[11]

The distribution of fat and parenchymal cells in the parathyroid gland is not uniform, so biopsy specimens from normal glands may predominantly consist of fat, parenchymal cells, or an equal mixture of both. Stromal fat cells tend to be concentrated toward the polar regions of the glands.[12,13]

The amount of stromal fat is also variable and related to age and nutritional status. Although parathyroid glands in children contain only very small amounts of stromal fat; by early adulthood, stromal fat cells make up approximately 20% of the volume of the glands.[14]

In some circumstances, parathyroid tissue can histologically resemble thyroid tissue, particularly if it is arranged in a follicular-like architecture surrounding secreted parathyroid hormone (PTH), which can resemble thyroid colloid. The observation that parathyroid parenchymal cells have well-defined cytoplasmic membranes compared with the indistinct membranes of thyroid epithelium as well as the absence of oxalate crystals in the parathyroid (which are common in the thyroid) may be useful in this distinction.

HYPERPARATHYROIDISM

Please see the Expert Consult website for further discussion of this topic.

In most patients with PHPT, the disease is sporadic, without a personal or family history of PHPT or other endocrinopathies. These patients are predominantly female and present typically in the sixth decade with uniglandular involvement. The heritable forms account for 10% to 15% of cases of PHPT and represent a clinically and genetically heterogenous group of disorders (see Chapter 60, Surgical Management of Multiglandular Parathyroid Disease; and Chapter 62, Parathyroid Management in the MEN Syndromes). Common hereditary forms of disease include familial cancer predisposition syndromes (multiple endocrine neoplasia type 1 [MEN 1], MEN 2A, MEN 4, and hyperparathyroidism-jaw tumor [HPT-JT] syndrome) and hereditary "hypercalcemic" syndromes (familial hypocalciuric hypercalcemia [FHH-1, FHH-2, FHH-3], and neonatal severe HPT [NSHPT]). Familial isolated hyperparathyroidism (FIHPT) is a rare and nonsyndromic cause of heritable PHPT.

PRIMARY HYPERPARATHYROIDISM

Parathyroid Adenoma

A single parathyroid adenoma (PA) accounts for the overwhelming majority of cases of primary hyperparathyroidism (PHPT); 80% to 85% of cases. Adenomas can occur at any age, although most become evident clinically in the fourth decade. They occur more commonly in females, with a female-to-male ratio of 3:1 to 4:1.[15,17,26,27]

Please see the Expert Consult website for more discussion of this topic.

Most adenomas are ovoid or reniform and have a smooth surface, but occasional tumors may be multilobate and therefore at higher risk for recurrence because they may be removed incompletely during initial surgery. On cross-section, adenomas are encapsulated and soft in consistency, with a tan to orange-brown color. Foci of cystic change are common, particularly in large adenomas. Cystic parathyroid tumors may be associated with prominent pericapsular fibrosis attributable to previous episodes of rupture and repair. Adherence of fibrotic tissue from a previously ruptured cystic adenoma to the adjacent thyroid or soft tissues may lead to a clinical suspicion of carcinoma at surgical exploration.

Fibrosis is also seen in some patients with multiple endocrine neoplasia (MEN) syndromes and also after procedures on parathyroid glands, such as fine-needle aspiration (FNA; for PTH measurement and/or cytologic examination) and ethanol injection.

597

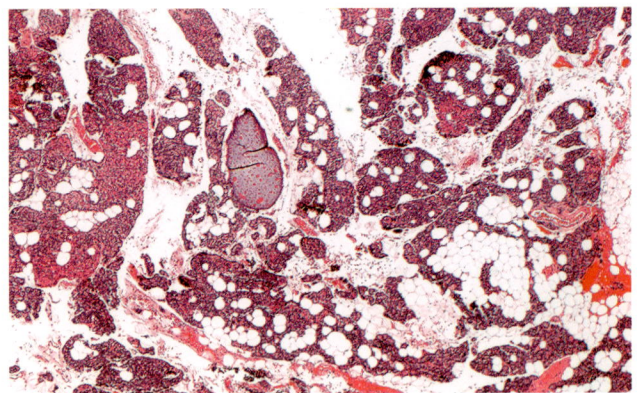

Fig. 65.1 Normal parathyroid gland from a middle-aged adult consisting of a mixture of chief cells and stromal fat cells.

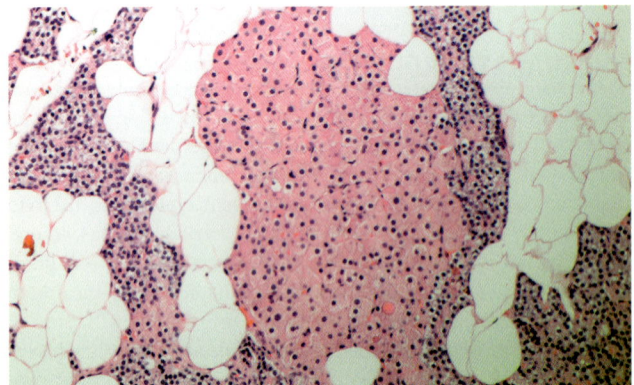

Fig. 65.2 Normal parathyroid gland from a middle-aged adult containing small oncocytic nodules. The oncocytes have abundant eosinophilic cytoplasm.

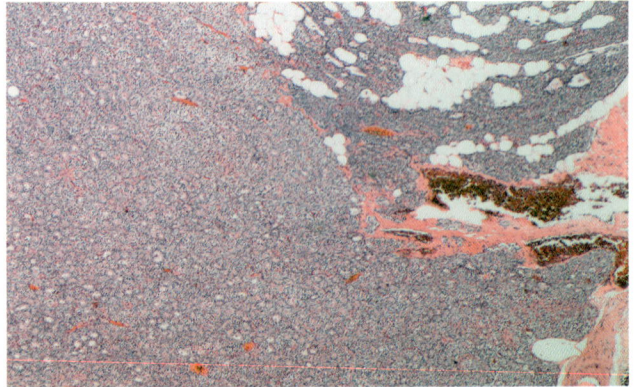

Fig. 65.3 Parathyroid chief cell adenoma *(left)* is sharply demarcated from the adjacent normocellular parathyroid gland *(right)*.

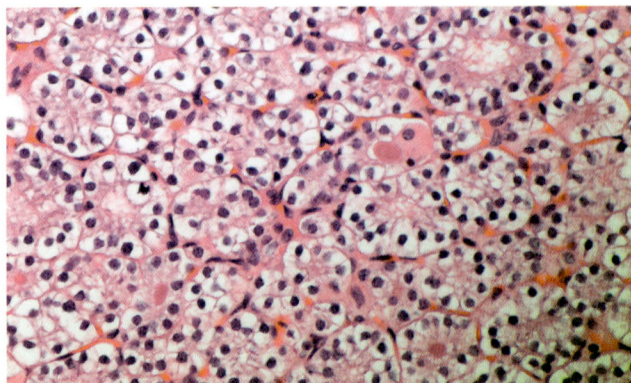

Fig. 65.4 Parathyroid adenoma contains an area where chief cells are arranged in nests and follicle formations with focal colloid-like material.

PAs are composed of variable proportions of chief cells, clear cells, oxyphilic cells, or transitional cells; however, chief cell adenomas are the most common type (Figures 65.3 and 65.4).[16,26,27] The tumor cells can be arranged in cords, nests, sheets, papillary, pseudopapillary, and follicles with palisaded appearances around blood vessels.[26] The follicle-like structures often contain a densely eosinophilic colloid-like material morphologically similar to colloid found in the thyroid, and the distinction between parathyroid and thyroid tissue in such instances may be particularly difficult, if not impossible, at frozen section. However, colloid in thyroid tissue frequently contains birefringent oxalate crystals, which are absent from the colloid-like material in parathyroid tumors.[34] The colloid-like material in parathyroid often stains with Congo red with green birefringence under polarized light.[35] Focal calcification of the luminal parathyroid colloid may also occur, which is similar to that seen in oncocytic thyroid neoplasms.

The nuclei of neoplastic cells often appear round and central and are generally larger than those in the adjacent normal gland. These contain dense chromatin and occasionally small nucleoli.[26,27] The cytoplasm of neoplastic chief cells is faintly eosinophilic but may appear clear because of the accumulation of glycogen deposits. Scattered pleomorphic and hyperchromatic nuclei as well as multinucleate cells are relatively common and occasionally may form nodular aggregates.[16,27]

Although scattered mitotic figures may be present in most cases, the proliferative index of most adenomas as assessed by Ki-67 (MIB-1) is generally <5%.[16,26,36,37]

Adenomas also may contain other cell types, including groups of oncocytes and transitional oncocytes and can even display a multinodular appearance, with individual nodules of chief cells or oncocytes. The nodules often have a higher proliferative index than the non-nodular portions of the adenoma.[38]

A rim of residual normal or even atrophic gland is present in approximately 50% of adenomas (see Figure 65.3). The rim is often separated from the adenomas by a capsule, but in some cases, the cells of the rim appear to merge imperceptibly into the adenoma. The probability of finding a rim of normal gland is greater in smaller adenomas than in larger tumors. Typically, the cells within the rim are smaller than the adenoma cells and often contain a single large lipid droplet. If lipid is present within the adenoma cells, it tends to be more finely distributed within the tumor cells. The parathyroid chief cells within the rim generally contain more abundant immunoreactive PTH and messenger RNA than do the adenoma cells.[39]

The absence of a rim of normal gland does not exclude the diagnosis of adenoma because the preexisting normal gland may have been overgrown or the rim may have been lost during sectioning.[13] Although adenomas have traditionally been described as having no stromal fat, some tumors may contain stromal fat cells distributed diffusely throughout the tumor.[27] In some instances, a small biopsy of an adenoma may be misinterpreted as a normal gland because of the abundant fat. Knowledge of the size of the gland would circumvent this potential pitfall. Occasional adenomas may contain abundant fibrous tissue, chronic inflammation, and hemosiderin deposits.

Several adenoma variants have been described.

Oxyphilic adenomas (also known as *oncocytic adenomas*) make up approximately 5% of all PAs.[40] A cutoff of 75% of neoplastic cells demonstrating oxyphil differentiation has been proposed to define this entity (Figure 65.5). Experience is limited, but oxyphilic adenomas have been reported to be more frequently associated with symptomatic patients, and with higher preoperative serum calcium and PTH levels.

These adenomas are also more difficult to localize on preoperative ultrasound examination.[41]

Water-clear cell adenomas are rare and characterized by the presence of cells with multiple cytoplasmic vacuoles, similar to those seen in clear cell hyperplasia.[42] Their primary significance is that they may mimic metastatic clear cell renal carcinoma on histologic examination (Figure 65.6).

Lipoadenomas (hamartomas) are rare tumors and are characterized by the proliferation of both parenchymal and stromal elements.[43] The stromal elements include abundant fibroadipose tissue with varying degrees of myxoid change and variable numbers of lymphocytes (Figure 65.7). The parenchymal components are usually present in the form of compressed cell cords. Lipoadenomas should be distinguished from so-called *large normal* or *fat rich* parathyroid glands by the presence of increased acinar tissue as well as adipose tissue.

Microadenomas can be defined as tumors measuring less than 0.6 cm in diameter and/or weighing less than 200 mg.[44-46] They may be overlooked on surgical exploration and frozen section. In several reported cases, microadenomas became apparent only after serial sectioning of paraffin-embedded samples. Some studies have shown that when the first resected abnormal parathyroid gland is small (<200 mg), the likelihood of multiglandular disease and operative failure is higher.[46]

Double adenomas are rare and have been reported in less than 2% of patients with PHPT.[32,33] Patients who have been diagnosed with double adenomas are more likely to relapse after surgery either with a third or fourth adenoma or multiglandular hyperplasia. Differentiation between adenomas and asymmetric nodular hyperplasia, based on morphology alone, may be somewhat arbitrary at times. In addition, emerging molecular data suggest that the nodules in parathyroid nodular hyperplasia commonly represent clonal proliferation and as such, are more closely related to adenomas. Therefore, distinction between multiple adenomas and nodular hyperplasia has become more controversial.[26]

Atypical adenomas represent a controversial pathologic entity. These tumors show some histopathological features of parathyroid carcinoma, such as band forming fibrosis, increased mitotic activity, cytologic atypia, and the presence of tumor cells within a thickened capsule, but they lack the definite diagnostic features of malignancy[26,47,48] (Figure 65.8).

It should be noted that fibrosis can occur in many situations, including previous manipulation (post-FNA biopsy), MEN syndromes, lithium intake, long-standing chronic renal failure-related parathyroid hyperplasia, in the setting of parathyroiditis, or in large adenomas undergoing episodes of rupture/infarction and repair. Fibrotic bands at the periphery of a parathyroid that does not have a true anatomic capsule may be a pitfall and mimic a tumor cell within a thickened capsule.[26]

Given the significant interobserver variability and lack of clinicopathological correlations in most cases, these borderline tumors cannot be classified with certainty. However there is good evidence that the majority of atypical adenomas do not recur.[49] Advances in molecular pathology and the use of new ancillary tests may help better refine these tumors and identify those with an increased risk of recurrence. Features reported to be associated with an increased risk of recurrence include an elevated Ki-67 proliferative index, loss of parafibromin expression by IHC, galectin-3 positivity, PGP9.5 positivity, retinoblastoma protein (Rb) loss, bcl2 loss, decrease in p27, hTERT expression, decrease in mdm2, and Adenomatous polyposis coli (APC) loss of function.[20,50-57]

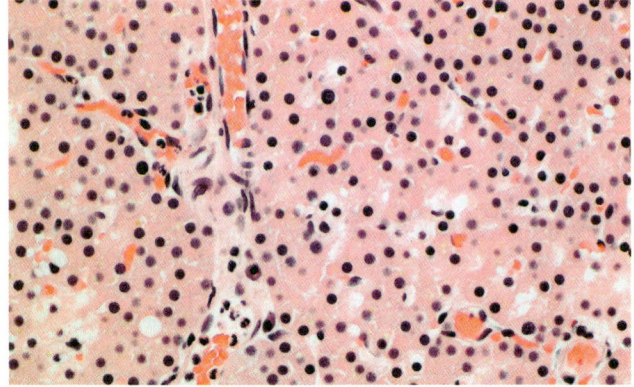

Fig. 65.5 Parathyroid oncocytic adenoma composed of large cells with abundant eosinophilic cytoplasm.

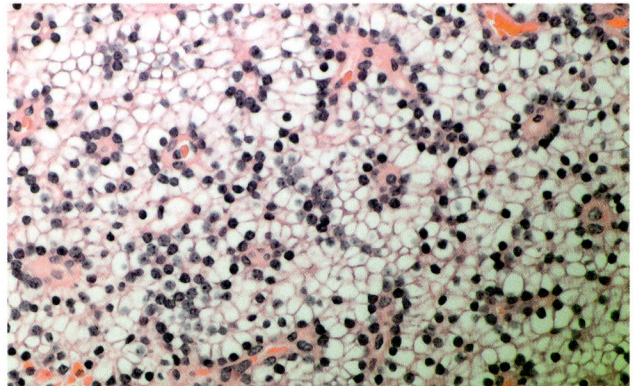

Fig. 65.6 Parathyroid water-clear cell adenoma composed of cells with multiple cytoplasmic vacuoles.

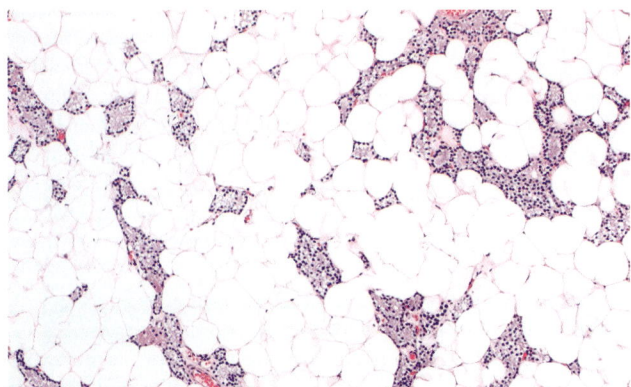

Fig. 65.7 Parathyroid lipoadenoma characterized by proliferation of both parenchymal and stromal elements.

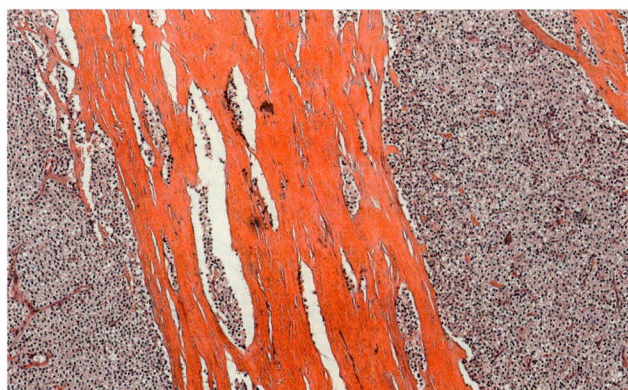

Fig. 65.8 Atypical parathyroid adenoma showing extensive areas of fibrosis. There was no evidence of invasion of adjacent structures or blood vessels.

CDC73 Mutations and Parafibromin-Deficient Parathyroid Tumors

Hyperparathyroidism-jaw tumor (HPT-JT) syndrome is a rare complex autosomal-dominant disorder characterized by the presence of parathyroid tumors, including PAs, parathyroid carcinomas, and fibro-osseous lesions of the maxilla or mandible. These patients harbor pathogenic germline mutations of the cell division cycle protein 73 (*CDC73* gene, previously known as *HRPT2*) that maps to 1q31.2 and encodes the protein parafibromin. *CDC73* functions as a genuine tumor suppressor gene that is involved in the regulation of p53 and also as a component of the human PAF1 complex, which controls RNA polymersase II-mediated transcription.[20,24,58,59]

In HPT-JT syndrome, hyperparathyroidism (HPT) commonly occurs at a young age with median first onset between the third and fourth decade. These patients also have an increased risk of developing parathyroid carcinoma, ranging from 15% to 37.5% in different case series.[24,60,61]

Somatic-only biallelic *CDC73* mutation/inactivation is also strongly associated with parathyroid carcinoma occurring outside the setting of HPT-JT syndrome.[20]

The combined result of multiple studies in parathyroid carcinomas with unequivocal histologic features of malignancy and biological evidence of malignant behavior (i.e., recurrence or metastasis) show a *CDC73* mutation frequency of up to 77%. However, the relationship between *CDC73* mutation and malignancy is much less strong when malignancy is defined by histologic criteria alone, perhaps reflecting the difficulty in making a correct histologic diagnosis of malignancy prospectively. In any case, the incidence of *CDC73* mutation in unselected parathyroid tumors is much less than 1%.[20,62]

Loss of immunohistochemical expression of parafibromin has been used as a marker of biallelic *CDC73* mutation inactivation in parathyroid tumors. However, the use of parafibromin IHC has been associated with difficulties and controversies. Although some groups have found parafibromin IHC to be useful both in differential diagnosis of atypical parathyroid tumors and as a marker of underlying *CDC73* mutation, others have found it technically difficult to perform and interpret.[20,24,53,59,60,63-65]

The parafibromin-deficient parathyroid neoplasms have been recently suggested to represent a distinct subgroup of parathyroid tumors that display a distinct morphology. These tumors are characterized by a sheet-like growth of neoplastic cells, frequently interrupted by an arborizing vasculature. These cells, at least focally, have eosinophilic cytoplasm with a quality distinct from typical granular cytoplasm of the oxyphil cells. There is nuclear enlargement and distinctive perinuclear cytoplasmic clearing, speckled chromatin, and sometimes prominent nucleoli (Figure 65.9, *A* and *B*). Clinically, these patients are usually younger, have larger tumors, and have more marked hypercalcemia. These neoplasms show complete loss of nuclear immunostaining with parafibromin. The reported incidence of large-scale germline deletions of *CDC73* in these tumors is up to 35%, and often both sequencing and multiplex ligation-dependent probe amplification assay (MLPA) studies may be required to identify these mutations.

Although there is extensive literature linking *CDC73* mutations with parathyroid carcinoma, the role of *CDC73* mutation as a marker of malignancy in atypical parathyroid tumors remains controversial. In one study, 40% of parafibromin IHC-negative parathyroid tumors also fulfilled histologic criteria for parathyroid carcinoma, and it was recommended that a lower threshold for malignancy may be appropriate in parafibromin-deficient tumors.[62] Although isolated case reports of morphologically benign tumors with parafibromin loss and *CDC73* mutation that have metastasized have been presented, metastasis in the absence of invasive disease is rare.[20,62] The primary significance of identifying parafibromin-deficient parathyroid tumors is therefore the association with malignancy, to identify potential hereditary disease, and to initiate surveillance in view of the risk of metachronous disease.[49,62]

Differential Diagnosis

Please see the Expert Consult website for more discussion of this topic.

Accurate diagnosis of parathyroid proliferations at the time of the intraoperative assessment can be difficult or even impossible. The primary role of the intraoperative pathologic examination is to confirm the presence of parathyroid tissue in the resected specimen and also to confirm the glandular abnormality (enlarged cellular gland) in patients with HPT. The evaluation of a second parathyroid gland or performing fat stains on frozen tissue was a common approach in the past, but the recent development and adoption of rapid intraoperative PTH assay appears to be a more precise tool to distinguish adenoma from hyperplasia.[26,27] (see Chapter 59 Intraoperative PTH Monitoring During Parathyroid Surgery).

With the exception of rare double adenomas, PAs and carcinomas are almost always solitary lesions, whereas hyperplasia represents multiglandular proliferation that can be asymmetric and asynchronous. The presence of an atrophic rim of hypocellular nontumorous parathyroid tissue adjacent to a cellular proliferation often helps in accurate diagnosis of PA in the appropriate clinical and biochemical context, but an enlarged parathyroid gland, lacking a normal/atrophic rim, should be classified as an "enlarged cellular parathyroid gland," as hyperplasia cannot be excluded. A diagnosis of PA can be rendered after surgery if biochemical cure is achieved and carcinoma is excluded.

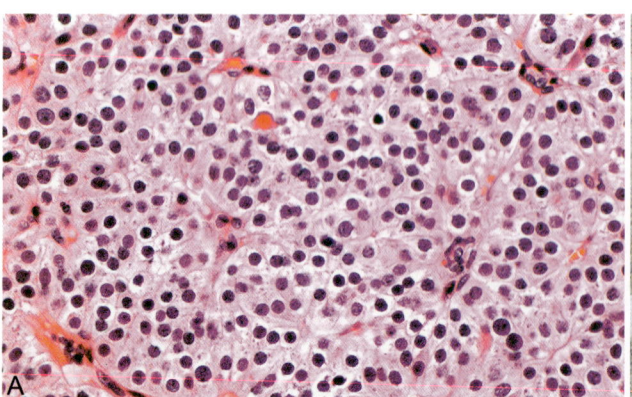
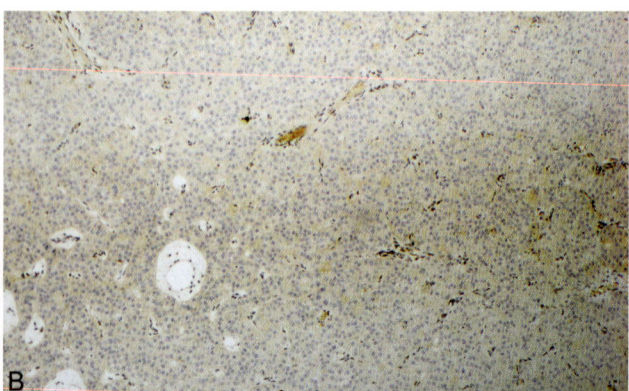

Fig. 65.9 Parafibromin-deficient parathyroid neoplasm **(A)** composed of cells with eosinophilic cytoplasm, enlarged nuclei, and perinuclear cytoplasmic clearing. **B,** Loss of nuclear expression of parafibromin by immunohistochemistry.

It should be noted that hyperplastic glands can also present small areas of normocellular tissue, which is indistinguishable from those surrounding PAs.[26]

In one study of more than 600 cases,[71] a small subgroup of patients with enlarged glands (double adenoma or hyperplasia) who were not diagnosed using ^{99m}Tc-sestamibi scintigraphy, ultrasound, or intraoperative PTH could only have been discovered with the traditional four-gland exploration approach.

This raises the question as to whether enlarged glands that are not hypersecreting at initial surgery will cause recurrent HPT in the future. Follow-up studies have demonstrated a cure rate of 98% with the focused approach; however, some studies have questioned the validity of this approach (see Chapter 59, Intraoperative PTH Monitoring During Parathyroid Surgery).[72]

Please see the Expert Consult website for more discussion of this topic.

PARATHYROID CARCINOMA

Parathyroid carcinomas are rare neoplasms, accounting for less than 1% of all cases of PHPT in most large series (see Chapter 64, Parathyroid Carcinoma).[75,76] The incidence of this tumor is variable in different parts of the world, probably representing a combination of true geographic differences and variations in the pathologic criteria for the diagnosis of parathyroid carcinoma. The diagnosis of parathyroid carcinoma rests on demonstrating an unequivocally invasive growth pattern manifested by invasion into adjacent organs, perineural growth, or vascular space invasion. Most cases occur in the fourth to sixth decades of life, and in contrast to the female predominance observed for adenomas, there are no sex differences in the incidence of carcinomas. Very rarely, these tumors have been reported in the pediatric age group, usually in association with germline *CDC73* mutation (HPT-JT syndrome).[20,62,77]

Parathyroid carcinoma is associated with significant morbidity and mortality related to PTH-mediated-hypercalcemia. Nonfunctioning carcinomas are exceedingly rare and usually present with signs and symptoms of local growth and invasion.

As mentioned before, patients with HPT-JT syndrome have an increased risk of developing parathyroid carcinoma. The lifetime risk of parathyroid carcinoma in patients with HPT-JT syndrome has been estimated to be as high as 15%.[20,62]

Somatic inactivation of *CDC73* is also a major driver in sporadic parathyroid carcinomas and reported in >70% of cases in some series.[20,26,54,62,73,78,79] It is noteworthy that approximately 30% of patients with apparently sporadic parathyroid carcinomas have been found to have germline mutations of *CDC73* even in the absence of features suggesting hereditary disease. Therefore it has been suggested that genetic counseling/testing should be considered in all patients with parathyroid carcinoma.[20,24]

It is suggested that β-catenin represents a "hub" in parathyroid tumor development. In the setting of parathyroid carcinoma, activation of the Wnt/β-catenin signaling pathway is possibly mediated by *APC* inactivation through promoter methylation. Promoter methylation of several other genes and repressive histone H3 lysine 27 trimethylation by EZH2 of the *HIC1* gene may also contribute to parathyroid tumorigenesis, and it is possible that a common pathway exists for parathyroid tumor development (i.e., in PAs, parathyroid carcinomas, and secondary HPT tumors).[23]

An increased risk of parathyroid carcinoma has also been reported in patients with isolated familial HPT, some of whom may be better classified as having HPT-JT syndrome.[80] Carcinoma occurs extremely rarely, if at all, in a setting of MEN 1 and MEN 2, particularly when strict pathologic criteria are applied and the difficulty in distinguishing benign recurrent disease from carcinoma both clinically and pathologically are considered.[20,81-83] Similarly, parathyroid carcinoma has been reported in the setting of tertiary HPT due to renal failure[78]; however, many of these reported cases may simply represent locally recurrent benign disease. It is therefore not our practice to make a diagnosis of parathyroid carcinoma in the setting of MEN 1, MEN 2, or tertiary HPT when the disease is confined to the neck and lacks vascular invasion.

Parathyroid carcinomas are typically large (mean diameter of 3 cm and mean weight of 6.7 g), irregular, grayish-white, hard (see Chapter 64, Parathyroid Carcinoma), and often densely adherent to the adjacent soft tissues or thyroid gland. The latter feature is a valuable clue for the surgeon. However, in some series, only approximately 50% of cases are recognized as being adherent to or invading adjacent structures.[78,84]

Microscopically, parathyroid carcinomas are usually composed of chief cells arranged in solid sheets or trabecular patterns (Figure 65.10). Tumors containing a predominance of clear (vacuolated) chief cells or oncocytes also occur, and carcinomas containing an admixture of the various cell types are not uncommon.

Although the diagnosis of carcinoma is restricted to cases that demonstrate unequivocal invasive growth, some features classically reported to be associated with malignancy include the presence of thick fibrous bands, mitotic activity, capsular invasion, and vascular invasion.[85] However, these findings are not as frequently present as initially reported, and fibrosis, mitotic activity, or trabecular growth on their own do not connote malignancy.[48] Areas of fibrosis, for example, may be prominent in large adenomas, particularly those with cystic change and in cases of secondary hyperparathyroidism (S-HPT).[27] Moreover, mitotic activity occurs in a substantial portion of adenomas and hyperplasias. The presence of collections of neoplastic chief cells in the capsules of parathyroid neoplasms (entrapment) cannot be used as a criterion of malignancy because this feature occurs commonly in adenomas.

Histopathological diagnosis of parathyroid carcinoma is challenging, and unequivocal invasion of the surrounding soft tissue and/or metastasis is required for a diagnosis of carcinoma, which was also emphasized in the latest World Health Organization (WHO) 2017 criteria for the diagnosis of endocrine tumors (Figures 65.11 and 65.12).[76,86]

Because of these difficulties, considerable efforts have been directed toward developing other ancillary methods, such as immunohistochemistry and DNA analysis.[87]

Please see the Expert Consult website for more discussion of this topic.

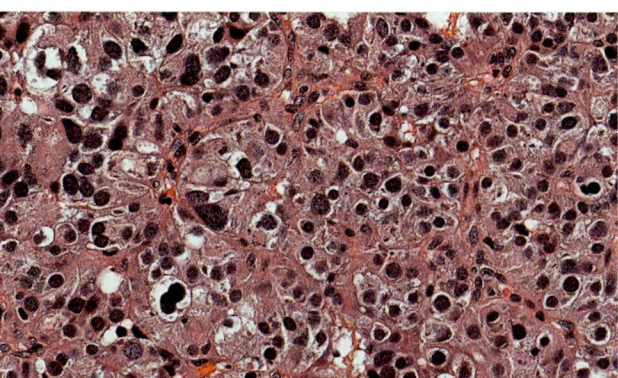

Fig. 65.10 Parathyroid carcinoma composed of cells with pleomorphic nuclei containing prominent nucleoli.

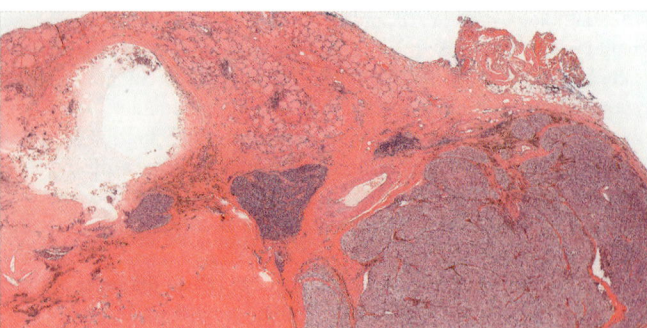

Fig. 65.11 Parathyroid carcinoma with invasion into adjacent soft tissue.

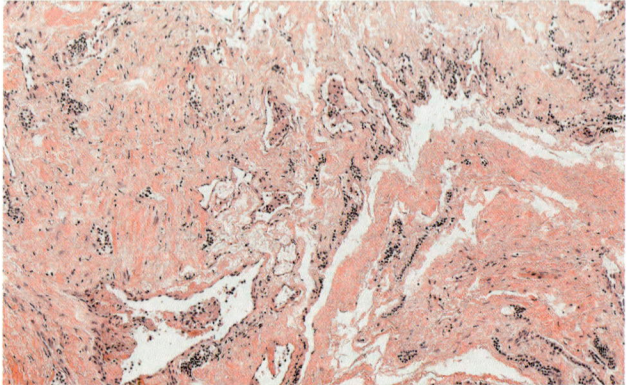

Fig. 65.12 Vascular invasion at the periphery of a parathyroid carcinoma.

The diagnosis of carcinoma is most often suggested by the presence of an enlarged gland that adheres to the adjacent thyroid or soft tissue. In these instances, an en bloc resection with removal of the adjacent thyroid is the treatment of choice. The distinction between retrogressive changes in an adenoma and parathyroid carcinoma may be impossible at the time of frozen section.

PRIMARY CHIEF CELL HYPERPLASIA

Primary chief cell hyperplasia (P-CCH) is responsible for approximately 15% of all cases of PHPT and is more common in women than in men. This disorder is characterized by an absolute increase in parenchymal cell mass, resulting from a proliferation of chief cells, oncocytes, and transitional oncocytes in multiple parathyroid glands in the absence of a known stimulus for PTH hypersecretion.[92] This disease may occur sporadically (75% of cases) or may occur as a manifestation of one of the heritable HPT syndromes (Table 65.1). With the development of increasingly more sensitive diagnostic molecular tests, the proportion of recognized familial cases is likely to increase.[16] Virtually all patients with MEN 1 will have evidence of PHPT, whereas only approximately 20% to 30% of patients with MEN 2A will have this disorder.[93,94] Primary parathyroid hyperplasia does not occur in patients with MEN 2B or in those patients with familial (isolated) medullary thyroid carcinoma (FMTC) (see Chapter 60, Surgical Management of Multiglandular Parathyroid Disease; and Chapter 62, Parathyroid Management in the MEN Syndromes).

Relatively recently, a subset of patients with multiglandular disease and overlapping features of MEN 1 and MEN 2 were identified. These patients were subsequently given the diagnosis of MEN 4 syndrome (also known as "MEN X syndrome") and found to have germline mutations in *CDKN1B* (12p13.1; encoding the CDKI, p27kip1, implicated in cyclin D1 signaling).[24]

Please see the Expert Consult website for more discussion of this topic.

Symmetric enlargement of all parathyroid glands occurs in approximately 50% of all patients with P-CCH, whereas the remaining patients have asymmetric enlargement.[101,102] The former pattern has been referred to as *classic hyperplasia*; the latter has been termed *pseudoadenomatous hyperplasia*. The distinction between asymmetric hyperplasia and adenoma may at times be extremely difficult if not arbitrary. The term *occult hyperplasia* refers to those cases in which there is minimal enlargement of all glands.

The predominant cell type in P-CCH is the chief cell, although varying proportions of oncocytes, transitional oncocytes, and vacuolated chief cells may be present (Figure 65.13).[27] The numbers of stromal fat cells are markedly reduced overall, but there may be considerable variation in the numbers of fat cells in different areas of the glands. Accordingly, a small biopsy of an enlarged gland may give a low ratio of chief cells to stromal fat cells. Occasional cases of P-CCH may have increased numbers of stromal fat cells throughout; this entity has been referred to as *lipohyperplasia*.[43,103]

In cases of P-CCH, the proliferation of chief cells can occur in diffuse, nodular, or mixed diffuse/nodular patterns.[26] The nodular pattern is more common and may be more evident in the early phases of the disease. Hyperplastic chief cells are usually arranged in solid sheets, cords, or follicles. Aggregates of chief cells may also be present in the soft tissues of the neck or mediastinum and may also undergo hyperplastic changes in patients with P-CCH. These lesions have been referred to as parathyromatosis and may be responsible for persistent or recurrent HPT in patients treated by parathyroidectomy for P-CCH.[104] Both chronic inflammation and cyst formation can occur in cases of P-CCH, and a rare cystic variant of P-CCH has been described.[105-107]

The distinction between P-CCH and adenoma is usually not difficult if multiple parathyroid glands are examined. An important clue when only a single gland is present is the presence of a prominent multinodular growth pattern. Some hyperplastic nodular glands may have a "pseudorim", mimicking adenoma.

Please see the Expert Consult website for more discussion of this topic.

OTHER FAMILIAL HYPERPARATHYROIDISM SYNDROMES

Please see the Expert Consult website for discussion of this topic.

Primary Clear Cell Hyperplasia

Primary water-clear cell hyperplasia is a rare variant of parathyroid hyperplasia characterized by the proliferation of water-clear cells in multiple glands.[27,31,116] There is no association with familial syndromes. Generally, there is more florid HPT, and the degree of hypercalcemia is greater than in those patients with P-CCH. Typically, all four glands are involved, although the upper glands tend to be somewhat larger than the lower glands. The often grossly enlarged glands are red-brown and may contain foci of cystic change and hemorrhage. The proliferating cells have multiple small cytoplasmic vacuoles derived from Golgi vesicles that are responsible for the clear appearance of the cytoplasm. The nuclei are round to ovoid and hyperchromatic; multinucleate cells are relatively common in this disorder. Of note, similar water-clear cell adenomas have also been reported, with the possibility of asymmetric hyperplasia being the actual diagnosis in some cases. The molecular basis underlying this morphologic variant remains unclear.[26,117]

TABLE 65.1 Heritable Hyperparathyroidism Disorders and Syndromes

Disorder/Syndrome	Gene (Locus) and Molecular Pathology	Parathyroid Pathology	Other Features
Multiple endocrine neoplasia (MEN) 1	*MEN1* (11q13) Loss of function	Hyperplasia (90%)	Pituitary adenomas, pancreatic endocrine tumors, carcinoid tumors, adrenocortical tumors, facial angiofibromas, collagenomas, lipomas
Multiple endocrine neoplasia (MEN) 2A	*RET* (10q11.2) Gain of function	Hyperplasia (30%)	Medullary thyroid carcinoma, pheochromocytoma
Multiple endocrine neoplasia (MEN) 2B	*RET* (10q11.2) Gain of function	Normal	Medullary thyroid carcinoma, pheochromocytoma
Multiple endocrine neoplasia (MEN) 4	*CDKN1B* (12p13.1) Expression of cyclin-D1	Multiglandular hyperplasia	
Familial medullary thyroid carcinoma (FMTC)	*RET* (10q11.2) Gain of function	Normal	Medullary thyroid carcinoma
Hyperparathyroidism-jaw tumor (HPT-JT) syndrome	*CDC73 (HRPT2)* (1q25–q32) Loss of function	? Cystic adenoma, carcinoma (15%)	Ossifying jaw fibromas, renal cysts, carcinomas, Wilms' tumor, parathyroid carcinoma
Familial hypocalciuric hypercalcemia (FHH)	*CaSR*/heterozygous (3q13.3q21) Loss of function	Mild hyperplasia	
Neonatal severe primary hyperparathyroidism	*CaSR*/homozygous (3q13.3–q21) Loss of function	Severe hyperplasia	
Familial isolated hyperparathyroidism (FIHPT)	*GCM2* (suggested) (6p24.2) Gain of function (*CDC73, MEN1, CaSR* mutation testing negative)	Hyperplasia, carcinoma (occasional)	
Familial hypercalcemic hypercalciuric (autosomal-dominant mild HPT)	*CaSR* Loss of function	Hyperplasia, adenoma	

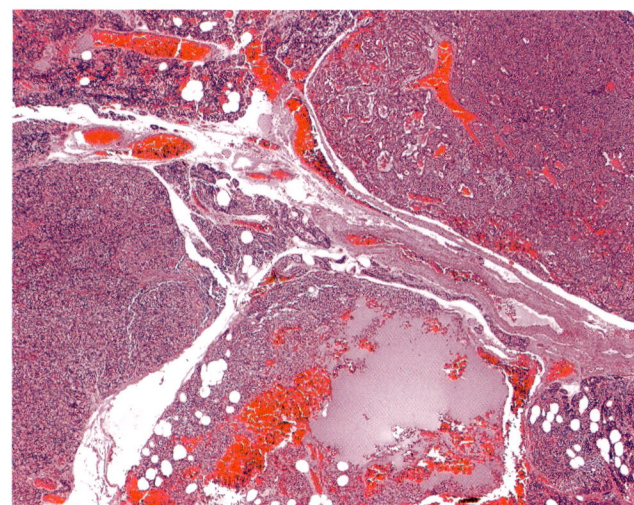

Fig. 65.13 Primary parathyroid hyperplasia associated with multiple endocrine neoplasia type 1 (MEN 1). This gland shows diffuse and nodular hyperplasia. There is focal cystic change.

Secondary and Tertiary Hyperparathyroidism

Secondary hyperparathyroidism (S-HPT) generally represents diffuse parathyroid hyperplasia as an adaptive increase in the synthesis and secretion of PTH and results from hypocalcemia of diverse etiologies, including chronic renal failure, vitamin D deficiency, and intestinal malabsorption (see Chapter 61, Surgical Management of Secondary and Tertiary Hyperparathyroidism).[17] Tertiary (T)-HPT refers to the development of autonomous parathyroid hyperfunction, characterized by hypercalcemic HPT in patients with preexisting S-HPT. The clinical manifestations of these disorders include bone pain and skeletal deformities (renal osteodystrophy), muscle weakness, growth retardation, and extraskeletal calcifications.

Generally, parathyroid glands in patients with S-HPT have greater uniformity in glandular size than those in patients with P-CCH, particularly in early stages of the disease.[118,119] With progression of the disease, gland size tends to become more variable. In a large series of cases of S-HPT reported by Roth and Marshall, the weight of the glands varied from 120 mg to 6 g.[119] The earliest microscopic changes are an increased number of chief cells with a concomitant decrease in stromal fat cells. The proliferating chief cells are arranged in diffuse sheets, but foci of cordlike, acinar, and trabecular growth may be prominent. Some cases may feature prominent mitotic activity. With further progression, there is usually a proliferation of oncocytes and transitional oncocytes. Both the chief cells and oncocytes may have a strikingly nodular growth pattern (Figure 65.14). Fibrous capsules may surround foci of nodular proliferation, simulating multiple adenomas. Areas of hemorrhage, calcification, chronic inflammation, and cyst formation typically occur in large, hyperplastic glands. Clinically, this histopathological progression from diffuse to nodular hyperplasia is associated with the development of refractory HPT and new hypercalcemia in patients with previously controlled S-HPT.[26] Although the parathyroid changes in patients with S-HPT have been classified as hyperplasias, molecular studies indicate a

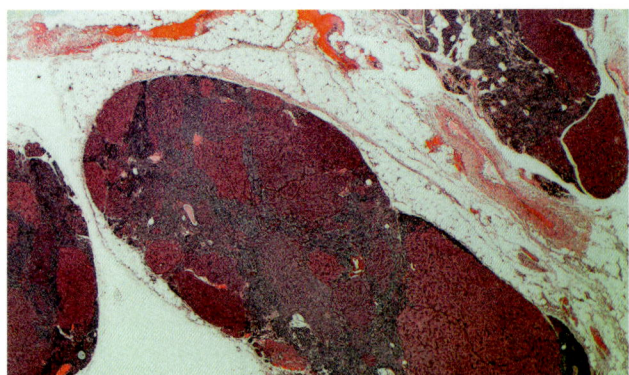

Fig. 65.14 Secondary parathyroid hyperplasia associated with chronic renal failure. The gland shows evidence of diffuse and nodular hyperplasia.

clonal transformation from diffuse polyclonal hyperplasia due to decreased *CaSR* signaling from hypercalcemia.[26,120] Generally, primary and secondary hyperplasia cannot be distinguished based on a morphologic assessment alone. The clinical history is essential in making this distinction. On occasion, parathyroid glands from patients with longstanding S-HPT may be impossible to distinguish from carcinoma based on pathologic examination alone because both conditions may exhibit fibrosis and mitotic activity. Pragmatically, despite the frequent finding of a growth pattern that appears invasive, it is not our practice to make a diagnosis of parathyroid carcinoma in the setting of tertiary renal failure unless there is unequivocal vascular invasion or distant metastasis outside the neck.

Parathyromatosis

Developmental rests of parathyroid tissue are relatively common in the soft tissue of the neck and mediastinum, often in proximity to normally situated parathyroid glands. In patients with primary or secondary hyperplasia, the rests may also become hyperplastic, a phenomenon that has been referred to as *parathyromatosis*.[104] Parathyromatosis is a rare cause of persistent or recurrent HPT after parathyroidectomy or incomplete excision of a hyperplastic or adenomatous gland,[121] and although some authors believe that this entity results from spillage of parathyroid tissue during surgery, others believe that it reflects local recurrence, hyperplasia of ectopic rests of parathyroid tissue, and/or parathyroid malignancy.[26] The distinction of parathyromatosis from parathyroid carcinoma is challenging and in some cases arbitrary. In patients with previously untreated primary or secondary hyperplasia, foci of parathyromatosis are unassociated with desmoplasia. However, in patients who have had prior surgery, parathyromatosis may be associated with considerable fibrosis, "invasion" of skeletal muscle and soft tissues, and mitotic activity, features that are similar to parathyroid autotransplants.[122] Clinical information, presence or absence of invasive growth (particularly angioinvasion) and ancillary tools such as parafibromin, Ki-67, Rb, and galectin-3 may be helpful in making this distinction.[26,53] Vascular invasion is absent in cases of parathyromatosis, and its presence excludes the diagnosis in favor of parathyroid carcinoma. Recent studies indicate that the molecular profiles of parathyromatosis are similar to those of benign parathyroid tumors with respect to the expression of parafibromin, Ki-67, Rb, and galectin-3.[53]

CYSTS

Please see the Expert Consult website for discussion of this topic.

SECONDARY TUMORS

Please see the Expert Consult website for discussion of this topic.

HYPOPARATHYROIDISM

Please see the Expert Consult website for discussion of this topic.

REFERENCES

For a complete list of references, go to expertconsult.com.

INDEX

Note: Page numbers followed by *f* indicate figures, *t* indicate tables, and *b* indicate boxes.

A

Abis, Abdul Kasan Kelebis, 2
Ablative procedure, ultrasound guidance and, 164. *See also* Ethanol ablation
Abnormal/continued descent, thyroid anomalies and, 17, 23–24
Absorption, 167
Accessory thyroid gland, 110
Accreditation Council for Graduate Medical Education (ACGME), 427
Acoustic radiation force impulse (ARFI) imaging, 165
Acquired migration, 510
ACR. *See* American College of Radiology (ACR)
Acropachy, 80
Active surveillance
  papillary microcarcinoma (PMC)
    management strategy, clinical framework for, 201–202, 201*f*
    practical application, 203
    to surgical intervention, indications, 202–203, 202*b*
  reoperative thyroid surgery, 464
Acute primary hyperparathyroidism, 493
Acute suppurative thyroiditis. *See also* Infectious thyroiditis
  clinical manifestations of, 46
  introduction to, 41*b*, 46–47
  management of, 47
  pathogenesis of, 46
Adenolipoma, 392
Adenomas, 609
  as benign neoplasm, 391
  double, 506
  toxic and pretoxic
    percutaneous ethanol injection (PEI) for, 475–476
Adenomatous nodule, as benign neoplasm, 391
Adenomatous parathyroid gland
  classification system for, 531–532, 531*b*
Adjunctive techniques, in revision surgery
  preoperative and intraoperative investigations, 470
  radioguided revision thyroid surgery, 470–471
  ultrasound-guided revision thyroid surgery, 470
Adjuvant therapy/treatment
  parathyroid carcinoma (PC), 595
  radioactive iodine (RAI), 448
Advanced laryngeal invasion, 369, 370*f*
Advertising, ethics in, 434–435
Aerodigestive tract injury, 422–423
Afirma®, 127
  Gene Expression Classifier (GEC), 121
  Gene Sequencing Classifier (GSC)
    clinical validation, 125
    Hürthle cell cell neoplasm index classifier, 125
    Hürthle cell index classifier, 125
    NGS technology, 121–125
    RNA-Seq, 121–125
    sample report, 125, 126*f*
  for indeterminate cytopathology, 119–120*t*, 121
Age
  Hurthle cell carcinoma and, 226
  primary hyperparathyroidism and, 505
  PTC patient variables and, 189
  sporadic medullary thyroid carcinoma and, 230
  thyroid nodule risk and, 100–101
Airway assessment, in thyroid disease, 57, 57*b*

Airway complications
  difficult intubation as, 423, 423*f*
  tracheomalacia as, 423–424
Airway management, anaplastic thyroid cancer and, 250
AIT. *See* Amiodarone-induced thyrotoxicosis (AIT)
Alcohol ablation
  of malignant metastatic lymphadenopathy in thyroid cancer, 476–477
Alcohol injection, 472, 475
  risks and side effects of, 477
  into solid nodules, 475–476
Alkaline phosphatase (ALP), 503, 592
Allelic loss of heterozygosity (LOH), 521
Amelita Galla-Curci nerve, 281–283, 316
American Academy of Otolaryngology Head and Neck Surgery (AAO/HNS), 160–161
American Board of Surgery (ABS), 431–432
American College of Radiology (ACR), 102
American College of Radiology Thyroid Imaging Reporting and Data System (ACR TI-RADS) Committee, 103
American College of Surgeons (ACS), 426–427
American College of Surgeons National Surgical Quality Improvement Program (ACS NSQIP), 431–432
American Head and Neck Society (AHNS), 161
American Joint Committee on Cancer (AJCC)
  anaplastic thyroid cancer staging system and, 247
  differentiated thyroid cancer and, 218
  medullary thyroid cancer, 231, 231*t*
  risk stratification, 220*f*
American Medical Association (AMA), 434
American Thyroid Association (ATA), 35, 37, 113, 194, 428
  active surveillance, 199
  central neck dissection
    recommendations and, 149
  differentiated thyroid cancer and, 118, 218, 448, 449*f*
  external beam radiation, 454
  intermediate-risk patients, 450–451
  intermediate to high- and high-risk patients, 450
  laryngeal exam guidelines and, 161
  low-risk papillary thyroid cancer, disease progression during active surveillance of, 199–200, 200*t*
  low-risk thyroid cancer, 450
  MTC guidelines, 482
  papillary thyroid microcarcinoma and, 195–196
  risk of tumor recurrence, 440, 441*t*
  risk stratification, 220*f*, 223–224
  standard of care guidelines and, 436–437
  thyroid nodule management guidelines, 118
Amiodarone-induced thyrotoxicosis (AIT), 45
Anaplastic carcinoma
  surgical pathology of thyroid gland and, 397–398
Anaplastic lymphoma kinase (ALK) translocations, 481
Anaplastic thyroid cancer (ATC), 119, 127–131
  airway management and, 250
  clinical course and prognosis, 247–251
    surgery, initial assessment for, 248–251
    treatment planning, 248
  enlarging neck mass, patient evaluation, 246
  enteral access maintenance and, 250
  epidemiology, 247

605

Anaplastic thyroid cancer (ATC) *(Continued)*
  external beam radiotherapy and, 456–457, 456f, 457t
  growing neck mass, pathological evaluation, 246
  negative predictive value, 121
  neoadjuvant approach for unresectable primary disease and, 248
  pathology, 247
  positive predictive value, 121
  primary thyroid lymphoma
    clinical diagnosis and imaging, 253–254
    epidemiology, 252
    histopathology, 252–253
    treatment, 254
  radiotherapy
    concurrent chemoradiotherapy, 251–252
    failure patterns and follow-up, 252
    palliative systemic therapies, 252
  staging, 247
  surgical checklist for, 249b
Anaplastic thyroid carcinoma (ATC)
  chemoradiotherapy, 251–252
  external beam radiotherapy and, 248, 254
  failure patterns and follow-up, 254
  fine-needle aspiration and, 115–116, 115f
  initial assessment for surgery and, 248–251
    airway management, 250
    enteral access, maintenance of, 250
    surgical approach, 250–251
    surgical complications, management of, 251
  molecular pathogenesis of, 182
  palliative systemic therapies, 252
  pathology of, 247
  staging for, 247
  surgery, initial assessment, 248–251
  treatment planning, 248
  ultrasound characteristics of, 140, 162f
Anatomy
  bilateral parathyroid exploration and, 517–519, 518–519f
  considerations for MIP and, 529–530, 530b, 530t, 531f
  parathyroid glands and, 507–508, 597
  superior laryngeal nerve, 316–320, 317–318f
Anechoic cysts, 474
Anesthesia
  history of, 3
  for minimally invasive parathyroidectomy, 532
  for minimally invasive video-assisted parathyroidectomy, 541
Aneuploidy, 611
Ann Arbor modification of Rye classification system, 254t
Anterior mediastinal goiter (substernal goiter type I), 53
Antimicrosomal antibodies, 31
Anti-PTH immunotherapy, 596
Antisepsis, history of, 3–4
Antithyroid drugs (ATDs), 81–83
Apathetic hyperthyroidism, 79
Artifact, principles of ultrasound and, 133–134, 133f
Aspirate, thyroid nondiagnostic, 109–110, 111f
Aspiration parathyroid hormone (PTH) rinsing, 147–148
Asynchronous multiglandular disease, 506, 506f
ATDs. *See* Antithyroid drugs (ATDs)
Attenuation coefficient, 167
Atypia of undetermined significance (AUS), 112, 112–113f, 118
Atypical adenoma, 599, 599f
Autografted parathyroid tissue
  function of, 573
  hyperplastic parathyroid tissue, 571
Autoimmune thyroiditis. *See* Hashimoto's thyroiditis

Autonomous functioning thyroid nodules (AFTNs), 170–171
  complications, 170–171
  radiofrequency ablation (RFA), 167
  thermal ablation, 170
Autosomal dominant mild hyperparathyroidism (ADMH), 503, 504t
Autotransplantation, 12
Awake injection, 411–413, 412f, 413t
Axial CT scanning, 57b, 58, 59b
Axial resolution, 132–133

B

Back-door approach, 95, 96f
Back-door technique, for minimally invasive parathyroidectomy, 534f, 535–536
  exposure, 535
  incision, 535
  post-excision PTH, 536
  specimen assessment for, 536
  superior parathyroid gland and, 535–536
  thyroid mobilization, 535
Barium swallow study, 58, 58.e2
Bayesian network meta-analysis, 181–166
Benign call rate (BCR), 121, 125
Benign cold thyroid nodule, 168–170
Benign familial hypocalciuric hypercalcemia (BFHH), 502, 520
Benign multinodular goiter (BMNG), 92–93, 106
Benign neoplasm, 391
Benign thyroid disease reoperation
  after thyroidectomy, 94–95, 96f
  aggressive benign nodular recurrence after total thyroidectomy, 92–93
  bilateral subtotal procedure for multinodular goiter, 90–91, 91f
  epidemiology of, 89
  inadequate partial resection or enucleation for, 90
  introduction to, 89
  operative strategy for, 94–95
  postoperative complications for, 95
  postoperative management and prevention for, 95–97
  preoperative evaluation for, 93–94
  recurrent disease in embryologic remnant and, 91–92, 92f, 107f
  recurrent Graves' disease management and, 97–98
  recurrent nodular goiter clinical presentation and, 89–90, 90f
  thyroid lobectomy with recurrent contralateral disease, 90
Berry picking, 372–373
Beta-blockade, 420
Bilateral cervical exploration (BCE), 553, 563
Bilateral neck exploration (BNE), 537–538, 544. *See also* Bilateral parathyroid exploration
  intraoperative parathyroid monitoring and, 550–551
Bilateral parathyroid exploration
  anatomy and embryology for, 517–519
  diagnosis of, 520, 520b
  introduction to, 517
  localization studies for, 521
  postoperative management of, 527
  rationale for, 519–521
  special considerations in, 527
  strategies for missing glands of, 523–527
  summary for, 527–528
  surgical techniques for, 521–523
  treatment of, 520–521
Bilateral subtotal thyroidectomy, 90–91
  Graves' disease and, 83
  thyroidectomy nomenclature and, 280–281
Bilateral vocal fold immobility, 417, 418f
Billroth, Albert Theodor, 4–5, 4f, 7–8
  modern thyroid surgery and, 4–5
Bilobar multinodular disease, 93
Biochemical cure, 232–233

Bisphosphonate, 492, 595
Blood sampling, IPM protocol for, 551
BLU-667, 484
BMNG. *See* Benign multinodular goiter (BMNG)
Body mass index (BMI), 158
Bone densitometry, 487–488, 488f
Bone density, primary hyperparathyroidism and, 505
Bone disease, 12
Bone histomorphometry, 488
Bone mineral density (BMD), 488
BRAF
   Afirma BRAF, 121
   follicular variant of papillary thyroid cancer, 118–119
   genetic alterations in PTC and, 183, 183t
   V600E mutations, 197, 200
Branchial complex stage, 16f
Branchial pouch, 606
B-rapidly accelerated fibrosarcoma (BRAF) point mutations, 258
Breathiness, 157
British Association of Endocrine and Thyroid Surgeons (BAETS), 156, 158, 160
British Thyroid Association (BTA), 161

C
Cabozantinib, 127–131
   and differentiated thyroid cancer (DTC), 480–481
   and medullary thyroid carcinoma (MTC), 483
Calcimimetic agent
   primary hyperparathyroidism and, 492–493
Calcimimetics, 492–493, 565–567, 596
Calcitonin, 101, 455, 483, 596
Calcitonin testing, 232
Calcitriol, 527
Calcium acetate, 565
Calcium carbonate, 565
Calcium deficiency, 11–12
Calcium lactate, 565
Calcium replacement therapy, 572
Calcium sensing receptor (CaSR), 557, 564, 614
   chronic kidney disease and, 564
   familial hypocalciuric hypercalcemia and, 614
Cancer
   incidence of, 102
Cancer Care Ontario (CCO), 428–429, 429t
Capsular invasion
   parathyroid carcinoma and, 593–594
Carboplatin, 456–457
Carboxymethylcellulose injection, 413
Carcinoembryonic antigen (CEA), 455, 483
Carcinogenic embryonic antigen (CEA), 232
Carcinoma
   mucoepidermoid, 399
   poorly differentiated, 397
   showing thymus-like differentiation (CASTLE), 399
Carney complex, 182, 256, 266–267
Carotid artery
   exposure of, 468–469, 468f
Carotid sheath dissection, 61, 62–63f
Casanova's test, 573–574
Caudal pharyngeal complex, 23
C-cell, 229
C-cell hyperplasia (CCH)
   medullary thyroid cancer and, 229, 231
CCND1/PRAD1 gene, 608
CDC73 gene mutations, 591, 600
Centers for Medicare & Medicaid Services (CMS), 431
Central neck compartment
   anatomic and surgical boundaries of, 467
   anatomy of, 372, 373f

Central neck compartment *(Continued)*
   bilateral paratracheal dissection, 378
   elective/prophylactic, 373–375
   indications for, 375, 375b
   introduction to, 372
   operative techniques for, 468–470
   preoperative evaluation, 375–376, 376–377f
   surgical technique, 376–378
   terminology, 372–373
   therapeutic central lymph node dissection, 373
Cernea EBSLN Classification Scheme, 317–318, 318f
Cervical goiter
   history of, 56
   physical examination for, 56–57
Cervical lymph nodes, 103, 454, 457
Chemotherapy. *See also* Cytotoxic chemotherapy
   Hurthle cell carcinoma and, 228
Chernobyl nuclear power station, 100. *See also* Thyroid cancer
Chest radiography, 58, 58.e2
Chief cell
   differentiation of, 23
   neoplastic, 598
   parathyroid adenoma composition and, 598, 598f
   primary chief cell hyperplasia and, 602
Chloride, 503
Cholecalciferol, 527
Chronic infectious thyroiditis, 48–49
Chronic kidney disease (CKD)
   and calcium sensing receptor (CaSR), 564
   secondary hyperparathyroidism and, 564
   and vitamin D receptor, 564
Chronic lymphocytic thyroiditis (CLT), 40–41, 111, 112f
Chronic renal failure, 591
Chyle leak, 424
Cinacalcet, 492–493, 564–568, 567–568b, 574
Cisplatin, 456–457
Clinical decision-making modules (CDMM), 464
Code of ethics, 434
Collaborative Endocrine Surgery Quality Improvement Program (CESQIP), 431
Colles' fracture, 488
Columnar cell variant, 394
Combined modality therapy (CMT), 458
Comet tail artifact, 133–134, 134f
Common carotid artery (CCA), 473
Complete remission rates (CRRs), 480
Completion thyroidectomy, 118
   Hurthle cell carcinoma and, 227
   papillary thyroid microcarcinoma and, 196
   for PTC detected on lobar specimen, 276
      hypoparathyroidism and, 277
      RLN paralysis and, 277
      surgical complications and, 276–278
   reoperative surgery and, 467
   timing of, 467
Comprehensive parathyroidectomy, 517
Computed tomography (CT), 72f, 102, 152, 176, 255, 256f
   axial imaging, 463
   with contrast, 151
   preoperative parathyroid localization testing and, 494–495, 495–496f
   preoperative radiographic evaluation and, 150
   ultrasound and, 151–153, 152–155f, 155t
Continuous neural vagal monitoring (C-IONM), 352–353
Contralateral lobe palpation, 467
Cope, Oliver, 12–14
Core-needle biopsy (CNB), 109, 163–164
Corneal nerves, thickened, 242
Cowden syndrome, 182
   familial papillary thyroid cancer and, 266

C-reactive protein (CRP), 43
Cricoid invasion, 368–369, 369f
Cricothyroid muscle (CTM). *See also* Vocal fold
    external branch of superior laryngeal nerve and, 316–317, 317f
Crile, George, 7, 7f
Crile's pneumatic antishock suit, 7, 7f
CRP. *See* C-reactive protein (CRP)
Cryopreservation, 526f, 527, 562
CT. *See* Computed tomography (CT)
Cutaneous lichen amyloidosis (CLA), 237, 241
Cyclin D1, 521
Cystic thyroid nodules
    percutaneous ethanol injection (PEI), 473–474
Cysts, 473–474, 473f
    anechoic, 474
    aspiration using intravenous (IV) cannula and extension tube, 475, 475f
    injection, 474
    of parathyroid gland, 133–134, 133f, 174, 604, 615
    of thyroid gland, 138, 155, 155f
        nondiagnostic aspirates and, 110
Cytotoxic chemotherapy, 446

D

Dabrafenib, 127–131, 457
    and differentiated thyroid cancer (DTC), 480
da Vinci, Leonardo, 2
Deep vein thrombosis (DVT), 521–522
Definitive form stage, 36
Delayed autotransplantation, 562
Delivered energy, 167
Delphian node, 13
Denosumab, 596
    primary hyperparathyroidism and, 492
De Quervain's thyroiditis. *See* Subacute thyroiditis
de Quervain's thyroiditis, 41–44
Dialysis Outcome and Practice Pattern Study (DOPS), 564
DICER syndrome, 182
DICER1 syndrome, 256
Dictation, thyroidectomy surgical steps and, 293
Differentiated thyroid cancer (DTC), 100
    anaplastic lymphoma kinase (ALK) translocations, 481
    BRAF-MEK targeted therapies, 480
    cabozantinib and, 480–481
    case examples for
        follow-up scenario 1, 222
        follow-up scenario 2, 222–223
    dabrafenib and, 480
    dynamic risk assessment and, 221–222
    external beam radiotherapy
        resected disease, 452–455, 453t, 453f
        unresectable disease, 452, 453f
    follicular thyroid cancer as, 204
    immunotherapy
        pembrolizumab and lenvatinib combination, 481
        pembrolizumab monotherapy, 481
    inherited tumor syndromes associated with, 256, 256t
    initial risk stratification for, 218–219
    introduction to, 218
    lenvatinib and, 479–480
    neurotropic tyrosine receptor kinase (NTRK), 481
    ongoing clinical trials for, 481t
    postoperative management of
        follow-up, 443–444
        goals, 440
        prognosis, 444–445
        treatment according to risk of cancer recurrence, 440–442
        treatment of distant metastases, 445–446
    predicting clinical outcomes for, 223–224

Differentiated thyroid cancer (DTC) *(Continued)*
    RAI-refractory, 479
        genotyping in, 482
    rearranged during transfection (RET), 482
    response to therapy assessment and, 219–221, 221t
    risk stratification for, 262, 262t
    sorafenib and, 480
    standard of care, 479–480
    subtypes, 479–482
    summary for, 224
    thyroid tumorigenesis and progression, 258
    vemurafenib and, 480
Differentiated thyroid carcinoma (DTC), 127–131
    follicular thyroid carcinomas, 118–119
    follicular variant of papillary thyroid cancer, 118–119
    Hürthle cell carcinoma, 118–119
    incidence
        current rates, 174
        international trends, 176
        mortality trends, papillary thyroid cancer, 176–177
        papillary thyroid carcinoma (PTC), 174
        United States, 174–176
    mortality trends of
        autoimmune thyroid disease, 178
        diagnostic cascade, 177
        dietary nitrates, 178
        estrogen, 178
        iodine deficiency and excess, 177
        ionizing radiation, exposure to, 177
        new/increased risk factors hypothesis, 177–178
        obesity and diabetes, 177–178
        papillary thyroid cancer, 176–177
        threshold for evaluation, 177
        thyroid specimens, management of, 177
    overdiagnosis and overtreatment of, 158, 179t
    papillary thyroid carcinomas, 118–119
    thyroid cancer, increased incidence of
        associated cost burden, 178–179
        guideline changes, 179
        noninvasive follicular thyroid neoplasm with papillary-like nuclear features (NIFTP), 180
        treatment side effects, 179
Diffuse follicular variant of papillary cancer, 393
Diffuse hyperplasia, 564, 566f
Diffuse large B-cell lymphoma (DLBCL), 458–459, 459f
Diffuse sclerosing variant, 402
Diffuse sclerosing variant papillary thyroid cancer (DSVPTC), 256–257, 256–257f
DiGeorge syndrome, 15, 617
Dissection
    bilateral paratracheal, 378
    paratracheal, 377–378
    prelaryngeal, 377
    pretracheal, 377
Distant metastases (DM)
    localized treatments, 445
    radioactive iodine, 445, 445b
    systemic treatments, 445–446
Distant mets, systemic therapy and, 233–234
Diverticulum, 15
Dominant nodule, 103
Donabedian model, 428, 428t
Doppler ultrasonography, 87–88, 134, 135f, 141
    neck nodes sonography and, 141
Double adenoma, 506, 553–554, 599, 609
    surgical treatment, 560
Double parathyroid adenomas, 519, 519f
Double-tracer subtraction imaging, 496–497

Doxorubicin, 456–457
Drug-induced thyroiditis
  introduction to, 45–46, 45t
  management of, 46
DTC. See Differentiated thyroid cancer (DTC)
Dual energy x-ray absorptiometry (DEXA), 487–488, 520, 577–578
Dunhill procedure, 90–91
Dunhill, Thomas Peel, 8
Dynamic risk assessment, 221–222, 442–443, 443t
Dysarthria, 50
Dyshormonogenetic goiter, 92–93
Dysphagia, 50, 246, 250
Dysphonia, 102

E
Echogenicity, 133
Ectopia, thyroid, 17, 17–19f
Ectopic localization, acquired, 25, 38
Ectopic thyroid tissue (ETT), 51–52, 51t, 400
Edema, laryngeal, 60
Elasticity imaging. See Elastography, thyroid
Elastogram, 141, 165f
Elastography
  lymph node metastases and, 145
  thyroid and, 135, 137, 141, 156, 164–165, 165f, 167–174, 174f
Elderly patient
  hyperthyroidism and, 79
Electromyography, 317
Electronic noise, 152
Embryologic rests, 510
Embryology
  applied
    parathyroid glands and, 22
    recurrent laryngeal nerve and, 21
    superior laryngeal nerve, 21–22
    thyroid gland and, 15–21, 16t, 16f
  bilateral parathyroid exploration and, 517–519
Encapsulated angioinvasive carcinoma, 396
Encapsulated follicular variant of papillary thyroid cancer (EFVPTC), 159
Encapsulated variant, 393
Endemic goiter regions, 53
Endocrine neck surgery, 419
Endocrine surgery, 8
Endoscopic parathyroidectomy (EP), 539–540, 539f
Endoscopic procedure, 539
Ergocalciferol, 527
Erythrocyte sedimentation rate (ESR), 43
Esophageal invasion, 369–370
Estrogen receptor modulators, 492
Estrogen therapy, 492
Ethanol, 472
Ethanol ablation (EA), 163, 165–166, 584
Ethanol extravasation, 477
Ethanol injection
  solitary toxic nodule and, 88
Ethical issues
  advertising and, 434–435
  optimizing informed consent and, 433
  surgical innovation and new technology as, 433–434
ETT. See Ectopic thyroid tissue (ETT)
European Society of Endocrine Surgeons (ESES), 538
Euthyroid sick syndrome, 28, 29f
Excision
  scar, 468
Exposure time, 167
External beam radiation therapy (EBRT), 233
External beam radiotherapy (EBRT), 442
  anaplastic thyroid carcinoma, 248, 254
  thyroid hormone suppression and, 228
  for thyroid malignancy
    aggressive histology lymphomas and, 459, 459f
    anaplastic thyroid cancer (ATC) and, 456–457, 456f, 457t
    differentiated thyroid cancer (DTC) and, 452–455, 453f, 453t
    indolent lymphoma and, 459
    introduction to, 452
    lymphoma and, 457–458
    medullary thyroid cancer (MTC) and, 455–456, 455f, 456t
    metastatic disease and, 457, 458f
    technique for, 459–460
    toxicity from, 460
External branch of superior laryngeal nerve (EBSLN), 156–158.
    See also Superior laryngeal nerve (SLN)
  classification of, 317
  diagnosis of paralysis for, 324
  incidence of injury to, 324
  treatment of injury to, 324
Extrathyroidal extension (ETE), 174, 188

F
Fabricus, Wilhelm, 2
False thyroid capsule, 284–285
Familial adenomatous polyposis (FAP), 182, 256
  causes of papillary thyroid cancer and, 187
  familial papillary thyroid cancer and, 266
Familial hypocalciuric hypercalcemia (FHH), 493, 503, 504t, 585, 597, 603t, 614
Familial isolated hyperparathyroidism (FIHPT), 597, 603t
Familial medullary thyroid cancer (FMTC)
  gene carrier evaluation for surgery and, 240–242
  genotype presentation for, 235–240
  MEN 2A and, 240–241
  neuroendocrine components in, 236
  nonendocrine components in, 236–237
Familial medullary thyroid carcinoma (FMTC), 234, 603t
Familial nonmedullary thyroid cancer (FNMTC), 204
  causes of papillary thyroid cancer and, 187
  classification of, 264–265, 265t
  clinical features of, 265
  epidemiology of, 264
  genetics and, 266–268
  pediatric thyroid cancer and, 255–256
  prognosis/outcome for, 268, 269t
  screening and surveillance, 268
  syndromic, 266–267
  treatment of, 268
  tumor histology of, 266
Fatty lobules, 23
FDG-PET. See F-fluorodeoxyglucose-positron emission tomography
F-fluorodeoxyglucose-positron emission tomography (FDG-PET), 246, 253f, 444
  fine-needle aspiration and, 108
Fiber tip shape, 167
Fibroblast growth factor (FGF), 564
Fibroblast growth factor receptors (FGFR), 479–480
Fibrosis, 597
Fifth gland dissection, 515
Fine-needle aspiration (FNA), 87–88, 100, 104–105, 105f.
    See also Fine-needle aspiration biopsy (FNAB)
  atypia/follicular lesion of undetermined significance and, 118
  Bethesda system, 118
  biochemical, 552
  biopsy
    anaplastic thyroid cancer and, 246
  follicular neoplasm/suspicious for follicular neoplasm (FN/SFN), 118
  goiter assessment and, 59

Fine-needle aspiration (FNA) *(Continued)*
  Hurthle cell tumors and, 227
  and molecular testing, for indeterminate cytopathology
    Afirma®, 119–120t, 121–125
    case examples for, 127
    clinical utility of, 119–120
    future applications, 127–131
    molecular techniques, 119
    principles of, 118–120
    selection of, 127
    ThyGeNEXT®-ThyraMIR®, 119–120t, 125–127
    thyroid cancer, molecular alterations in, 118–119
    ThyroSeq®, 119–120t, 120–121
  pediatric thyroid cancer and, 259
  preoperative parathyroid localization testing and, 499
  reoperative thyroid surgery and, 464
  thyroid gland and
    accuracy of, 109
    atypia/follicular lesion of undetermined significance and, 112, 112–113f
    benign conditions and, 110–112
    Bethesda System and, 109, 110t, 110b
    complications of, 117
    Hürthle cell neoplasms and, 113–114, 114f
    indications for, 108–109
    introduction to, 108
    malignant tumors and, 114–117, 116f
    nondiagnostic thyroid aspirates and, 109–110, 111f
    suspicious follicular neoplasm and, 112–113, 113f
    techniques for, 109
  thyroid surgery and
    atypia of undetermined significance, 273
    benign biopsy and, 273
    diagnostic for medullary carcinoma, anaplastic carcinoma,lymphoma and, 273–274
    diagnostic for papillary carcinoma and, 274
    follicular/Hurthle cell neoplasm and, 273
    follicular lesion of undetermined significance, 273
    nondiagnostic biopsy and, 273
    suspicious for malignancy and, 273
  ultrasound-guided, 135, 153
Fine-needle aspiration biopsy (FNAB), 157, 435
  follicular thyroid cancer and, 206
  as ultrasound guided, 118, 141, 163
Flat tip technique, 168, 184f
Flow volume loop analysis, 58, 58.e1, 57.e3
  chest radiography and barium swallow study, 58.e2
  MRI scanning, 58.e3
  scintigraphy, 58.e4
  sonography, 58.e4
Fluorodeoxyglucose-positron emission tomography (FDG-PET), 593
FNA. *See* Fine-needle aspiration (FNA)
Follicle formation, 27
Follicular adenoma, 87
  genetic alterations associated with, 184
  variants of
    atypical follicular adenoma as, 391
    hyalinizing trabecular adenoma as, 391–392
Follicular-derived familial tumors, 398
Follicular lesion of undetermined significance (FLUS), 112, 112–113f, 118
  negative predictive value, 121
  positive predictive value, 121
Follicular neoplasm (FN), 105–106, 112–113, 118, 164
  negative predictive value, 121
  positive predictive value, 121
Follicular thyroid cancer (FTC), 257
  diagnosis of, 206–207
    clinical presentation of, 206
    cytopathology for, 206–207

Follicular thyroid cancer (FTC) *(Continued)*
    histopathology of, 205–207, 205f
    molecular diagnostics for, 206–207
  epidemiology of, 204
  etiology of, 204–206
  introduction to, 204
  molecular pathogenesis of, 181
  prognosis for, 209–211, 209–212t
  specific genetic alterations in, 183t
  summary of, 212
  surgical management of, 260
  treatment of, 207–209
    medical therapy and, 208–209
    surgery and, 207–208
Follicular thyroid carcinoma, 118–119, 174. *See also* Minimally invasive follicular carcinoma
  ultrasound characteristics of, 140, 159f
Follicular tumor, well-differentiated of undetermined/uncertain malignant potential, 396
Follicular variant of papillary thyroid carcinoma (FVPTC), 115, 115f, 118–119, 127, 256, 258, 393
Foramen cecum, 15
Forearm autograft, 580–581, 583
Foss, Harold, 8
Four-dimensional computed tomography (4D CT), 511, 521
  multiple gland disease (MGD), 559
Four-gland hyperplasia, 554–555, 554–555f
  subtotal parathyroidectomy, 560–561, 560f
  surgical treatment, 560–561
Fourth pouch disease, 519
Fractures, primary hyperparathyroidism and, 488
"Free-hand" technique, 477
Friedman EBSLN Classification Scheme, 318–319, 320f
Front door technique, for minimally invasive parathyroidectomy, 533–535, 534f
  incision, 533–534
  inferior parathyroid adenoma dissection, 535
  location of inferior parathyroid gland and, 534–535
  thyroid mobilization, 534, 534f
Frozen section (FS)
  intraoperative, 227
  thyroid nodule assessment and, 400
Full sternotomy, 73–75

G

Galen, 8–9, 9f
Galen's anastomosis, 331
Ganglioneuroma, 241–242
Gardner's syndrome, 266
  causes of papillary thyroid cancer and, 187
Gelfoam injection, 413
Gene expression analysis, 106
Gene Expression Classifier (GEC), 121
Gene Sequencing Classifier (GSC)
  clinical validation, 125
  Hürthle cell cell neoplasm index classifier, 125
  Hürthle cell index classifier, 125
  NGS technology, 121–125
  RNA-Seq, 121–125
  sample report, 125, 126f
Genetic assessment
  familial syndromes and, 503
  MEN 1 and, 504t
Genetic control, 15
  and evolutionary model, 23, 34–35
Genomic classifier (GC) score, 120
Genomic sequencing classifier (GSC), 106
German Association of Endocrine Surgeons, 161
Giant cell, 41–42

INDEX

Glial cell missing 2 (GCM2) transcription factor, 610
Glide sign, 288–289, 507
Glottic exam, 158
Glucocorticoid therapy, 45, 48
Goiter. *See also* Cervical goiter; Multinodular goiter; Posterior mediastinal goiter; Substernal goiter
   acute airway compromise of, 79–57.e1f, 57.e1, 57.e2
   clinical presentation of, 56–57
   definition of, 53
   early history of, 2
   Hashimoto's thyroiditis and, 40
   intubation and, 60
   isolated mediastinal, 53.e3
   natural history of, 56
   nodular, 90
   nontoxic nodular, 89
   pathogenesis of, 56, 56.e2, 56.e3
   prevalence of, 56
   recurrent goiter, 69, 68.e1
   retrotracheal cervical, 63–65, 64–65f
   risk of malignancy, 60, 59.e2
   surgery for
      complications of, 68
      extent of, 60–61, 61*b*
      Hashimoto's thyroiditis, 61
   surgical technique for, 61–68, 69.e6
      carotid sheath and, 61, 62–63f
      incision as, 61
      parathyroid preservation during, 65
      recurrent laryngeal nerve and, 61–63, 63f
      strap muscles and, 61
      substernal goiter and, 65–67, 66f
      superior goiter extent and, 65
      vagal monitoring during, 67–68, 67f
      ventral recurrent laryngeal nerve and, 63–65, 64–65f
   thyroid fine-needle aspiration and, 110–111, 111f
   toxic, 111–112
   toxic nodular goiter (TNG), 83
   ultrasound and, 140, 152
   workup for
      acute airway compromise and, 57
      airway assessment in thyroid disease and, 57
      introduction to, 57, 57*b*
      upper airway compromise evaluation and, 57–59
Graves' disease, 2
   clinical presentation of, 79–80, 82*b*
   diagnosis and evaluation for, 80
   epidemiology of, 79
   pathogenesis of, 79
   recurrent
      management of, 97–98, 114
   treatment of, 80–83
   ultrasound and, 140
Grayscale sonography, 141
GSC. *See* Gene Sequencing Classifier (GSC)

H

Halsted, William S, 5, 6–7f, 7, 11
Harmonic imaging, 152
Hashimoto's thyroiditis (HT), 61, 116–117, 158, 61.e1
   clinical manifestations of, 40–41
   introduction to, 40–41, 41*b*
   management of, 41
   pathogenesis of, 40
   ultrasound and, 140–141, 163f
Hashitoxicosis, 40–41
Healthcare Research and Quality (AHRQ), 426
Hematoma, 420–421, 421f

Hemithyroidectomy, 217*b*, 280–281
Hemorrhage
   thyroid surgery complications and, 420–421, 421f
Hemorrhagic infarction, 572, 572f
Hemostasis
   history of, 4
   reoperative surgery and, 470
Hereditary medullary thyroid carcinoma
   complications and outcomes after surgery for, 245
   introduction to, 235
   prophylactic surgery for asymptomatic carriers of, 244
   reoperation for, 243f
   surgery for carriers of, 240–242
   synchronous with hyperparathyroidism, 242
   synchronous with pheochromocytoma, 242
Heredity syndromes, 187
Heritable hyperparathyroidism disorders and syndromes, 603*t*
High-intensity focused ultrasound (HIFU), 163, 171
High-resolution peripheral computed tomography (HRpQCT), 488
Hirschsprung's (HSCR) disease, 236–237, 241
Hoarseness, 157
Horner's syndrome, 71–72, 424, 424f
HoxA3, 29
HPT. *See* Hyperparathyroidism
HRPT2 mutation
   parafibromin and, 593, 600
   parathyroid cancer and, 591
HT. *See* Hashimoto's thyroiditis (HT)
Human chorionic gonadotrophin (hCG), 592
Hungry bone syndrome, 491
Hürthle adjuvant therapy
   radioactive iodine, 227
   targeted therapy, 228
   thyroid hormone suppression, 228
Hürthle cell carcinoma (HCC), 118–119, 140, 160f
   Afirma®
      GEC validation, 121
      GSC classifier, 125
      ThyroSeq v3, validity of, 121
Hürthle cell index classifier, 125
Hürthle cell neoplasm index classifier, 125
Hürthle cell neoplasms (HCN), 105–106, 113–114, 114f
Hurthle cell tumors (HCTs)
   adjuvant therapy and, 227–228
   fine-needle aspiration and, 227
   follow-up for, 228
   genetics of, 226
   intraoperative frozen section and, 227
   introduction to, 225
   pathology of, 225
   preoperative evaluation for, 227
   presentation and natural history of, 225–226
   RET/PTC rearrangements and, 226
   staging and prognostic factors for
      age and, 226
      distant metastases for, 226
      extent of surgery and, 227
      invasiveness, 226–227
      lymph node and distant metastases for, 226
      size and, 226
   summary for, 228
   surgery for, 227
   ultrasound and other imaging modalities for, 227
Hyalinizing trabecular neoplasm, 391–392
Hydrocortisone, 420
Hydro-dissection technique, 163, 165, 166f, 171
25-hydroxyvitamin D (25OHD), 491–492

INDEX

Hypercalcemia
　familial hypocalciuric, 503
　medical therapy for, 595–596
　parathyroid carcinoma and, 595–596
　pHPT surgical guidelines and, 505, 505t
Hypercalcemia of malignancy, 487
Hypercalciuria, pHPT surgical guidelines and, 505
Hyperparathyroidism (HPT), 171
　autosomal dominant mild, 503
　biochemical diagnosis of, 503b
　complications, 502
　FMTC/MEN 2A and, 241
　FMTC/MEN 2B and, 236
　history of, 12–13
　localization studies
　　first-time operations and, 499–501, 500f
　　recurrent/persistent disease and, 499–501
　neonatal severe, 504
　persistent, 573–574
　recurrent, 573–574, 573b
　surgical pathology of, 597, 598f
　ultrasound and, 147–148, 147f, 174, 174f
Hyperparathyroidism-jaw tumor (HPT-JT) syndrome, 503, 504t, 591, 596, 600, 603t
Hyperphosphatemia, 565
Hyperplasia
　chief cell, 554–555, 556f, 566f
　classic, 602
　diffuse, 564, 566f
　occult, 602
　percutaneous ethanol injection (PEI), 477
　pseudoadenomatous, 602
　water clear cell, 553
Hyperplastic parathyroid tissue, 571
Hypertension, 489
Hyperthyroidism, 59, 102
　etiologies of, 35, 35b
　pregnancy and, 37
　serum thyroid antibodies in, 36
　signs and symptoms of, 35, 35b
　subclinical, 36
　surgical management of
　　Graves' disease and, 79–83
　　introduction to, 79, 80–82f
　　solitary toxic nodule and, 87–88
　　toxic multinodular goiter and, 84–87
　　toxic nodular goiter and, 83
　thyroid function testing in, 35–36
　thyroid imaging in, 36–37, 36t
　treatment of, 37
Hypertrophic scar, 422
Hypocalcemia
　treatment for, 420
Hypoparathyroidism, 47, 94–95, 106
　complications of thyroidectomy and, 278
　permanent, 562
　reoperative surgery and, 233
　surgical pathology of parathyroid glands and, 604, 617
　thyroid surgery complications and, 419–420, 420t
Hypothyroidism, 29–30
　etiologies of, 33–34, 34b
　pregnancy and, 37
　risk factors for, 34b
　serum thyroid antibodies in, 34
　signs and symptoms of, 33, 33b
　subclinical, 34
　thyroid function testing in, 34
　thyroid imaging in, 35

Hypothyroidism (Continued)
　thyroid surgery complications and, 420
　treatment of, 35

I

Imaging
　axial CT scanning and, 58, 59b
　chest radiography/barium swallow study and, 58
　modalities, 103
　MRI scanning and, 58
　radiographic evaluation/regional symptomatology and, 58
　recurrent disease and, 94
　sonography/scintigraphy and, 58
Immunoradiometric assay (IRMA), 546
Immunotherapy
　differentiated thyroid cancer (DTC), 481
IMRT (intensity-modulated radiation therapy), 454–455, 459–460
Incision for thyroid and parathyroid surgery
　best practices, 390
　drain placement for, 387, 399, 399f
　general principles of, 386–388
　　individualizing incisions and, 386, 395–396f
　　location of, 386–387, 387f
　　skin closure and, 387–388, 388f
　　skin management and, 387, 387f
　historical perspectives of, 386
　introduction to, 386
　specific procedure considerations for, 388–390
Incision line, reoperation and, 468
Indocyanine green (ICG) angiography, 279, 280–281f
Indolent lymphoma
　external beam radiotherapy and, 459
Infection
　thyroid surgery complications and, 422, 422f
Infectious thyroiditis
　clinical manifestations of, 46
　introduction to, 41b, 46–47
　management of, 47
　pathogenesis of, 46
Inferior approach
　reoperative surgery and, 94–95, 96f
Inferior parathyroid gland
　ectopia of, 509
　embryology of, 16f, 22–25
　identification of, 570–571
　if missing, 514–515
　thyroidectomy nomenclature and, 285, 288t, 289b
Inferior thyroid artery
　parathyroid identification and, 570
Informed consent, 433
Infranumerary gland, 25, 37
Innominate vein, 73
Institutional review board oversight, 433–434
Intact parathyroid hormone (iPTH), 503
Intensity-modulated radiation therapy (IMRT), 251, 454–455, 459–460
Internal jugular vein (IJV), 464
Internal jugular venous sampling, 552, 552f
Intestinal ganglioneuromatosis, 241–242
Intraoperative adjuncts
　in multiple gland disease (MGD), 559
Intraoperative blood sampling, IPM protocol for, 547
Intraoperative parathyroid hormone (IOPTH)
　biochemical fine-needle aspiration as, 552
　differential internal jugular venous sampling as, 552, 552f
　monitoring
　　as adjunct during parathyroidectomy, 547
　　blood sampling protocol for, 547
　　criteria for predicting operative success for, 550t

INDEX

Intraoperative parathyroid hormone (IOPTH) *(Continued)*
    history of, 546–547
    intraoperative rapid PTH assays and, 552
    introduction to, 546
    limitations of, 550–551
    MEN-associated HPT and, 583–584
    parathyroidectomy guided results for, 551–552
    parathyroidectomy patient benefit, 547
    scenarios and troubleshooting for, 547–549, 548–550*f*, 549*b*
    summary for, 552
  parathyroid surgery malpractice and, 437–438
  surgery and, 537–538
  testing for, 506–507
Intraoperative parathyroid monitoring (IPM)
  as adjunct during parathyroidectomy, 547
  blood sampling protocol for, 547
  criteria for predicting operative success for, 550*t*
  history of, 546–547
  intraoperative rapid PTH assays and, 552
  introduction to, 546
  limitations of, 550–551
  MEN-associated HPT and, 583–584
  parathyroidectomy guided results for, 551–552
  parathyroidectomy patient benefit, 547
  scenarios and troubleshooting for, 547–549, 548–550*f*, 549*b*
  summary for, 552
Intrathyroidal adenoma, 510–511
Intrathyroidal parathyroid gland, 24–25
Intrathyroidal thymoma, 399
Intubation
  of the goiter patient, 60
  thyroid surgery complications and, 423
Invasive fibrous thyroiditis
  clinical management of, 47–48
  introduction to, 47–48
  management of, 48
  pathogenesis of, 47
Invasive surgical approaches, 50
Iodine
  deficiency, 89
  follicular thyroid cancer and, 204
  history of use of, 2–3
  supplementation for, 97
Iodine-131 therapy (^{131}I)
  Graves' disease and, 82
  solitary toxic nodule and, 88
  toxic multinodular goiter and, 85
Ionizing radiation, 100
IONM, 100, 466
  algorithms, 349, 351*f*
  anesthesia, 341–345, 342*b*, 343*f*
  basic system setup for, 341, 341–342*f*
  informed consent and patient counseling, 352
  intraoperative stimulation errors, 345–346
  introduction to, 340–341
  loss of signal, 349, 350*f*
  mechanism of injury, 349–351
  monitoring safety, 351
  neural monitoring indications, 352
  nonrecurrent laryngeal nerve, intraoperative identification of, 352
  normative human monitoring data, 346–349
  timing of completion surgery, 349
  validity of noninvasive monitoring, 351
IPM. *See* Intraoperative parathyroid monitoring
Ipsilateral thyroid lobe, 535
Isolation stage, 36
Isthmusectomy, 280–281

J
Japanese Society for Dialysis Therapy (JSDT), 564, 568, 568*b*

K
Keloid, thyroid surgery complications and, 422
Ki 67 antigen, 593, 604
Kidney Disease Improving Global Outcome (KDIGO), 566, 568
Kidney Disease Outcomes Quality Initiative (K/DOQI), 567–568
Kidney graft function, 574–575
Kidney stones, 486–488
Kierner EBSLN Classification Scheme, 317–318, 319*f*
Kissing pairs, 24
Kocher, Emil Theodor, 5–8, 5–6*f*
  laryngeal nerve and, 10
Korean Society of Thyroid Radiology (KSThR), 163, 167

L
Lahey, Frank, 10, 12
Lahey incision, 393, 394*f*
Laryngeal electromyography, 410–411
Laryngeal exam
  guidelines for, 160–161
  rationale for postoperative exam and, 161
  rationale for preoperative exam and, 160
  summary for, 162
  in thyroid and parathyroid surgery, 156–162
    introduction to, 156
Laryngeal invasion
  anterior, 368
  lateral, 367–368, 367–368*f*
Laryngoscopy
  flexible, 161–162, 161*b*, 162*f*
  preoperative fiberoptic
    recurrent disease and, 94
Larynx
  goiter intubation and, 60
  invasive thyroid cancer and
    imaging for, 361–362
    introduction to, 360, 361*f*
    mechanisms of involvement in, 362–363, 375–380*f*
    recurrent laryngeal nerve management, 365–366
    signs and symptoms of, 360–361
    surgical management of, 363–365
LASER. *See* Light amplified stimulated emission of radiation (LASER)
Laser ablation (LA). *See also* Percutaneous laser thermal ablation (PLA)
  thyroid gland and, 185–170
    benign cold nodules, 168–170
    complications
      marginal regrowth, 187
      mechanism of action, 167–168, 168*f*, 183*f*
      procedure and techniques, 167–168, 169*f*, 184*f*
Laser fiber, 167, 169*f*, 183*f*
Lateral aberrant thyroid, 8
Lateral/backdoor approach, 468, 468*f*
  reoperative surgery and, 95, 96*f*
Lateral neck dissection
  anatomy of, 379, 380*f*
  closure and postoperative care, 384
  complications, 384–385
  differentiated thyroid cancer, 381
  lymph node metastases
    effect on disease outcome, 380–381
    risk factors for, 380
  medullary thyroid cancer, 381
  N + lateral neck management, 381
  radioactive iodine, 381
  reoperative surgery and, 467–468
  technique

Lateral neck dissection *(Continued)*
    flap elevation, 382
    incision, 382, 382f
    level I, 382
    levels II, III and IV, 383, 383–384f
    levels V, 383–384
    thyroid gland lymphatics, 379–380
    types of, 381–382
Lateral resolution, 132–133
Lateral thyroid anlage, 15
    anomalies of, 16t, 17
Lateral thyroid region, thyroidectomy exposure and, 285, 286f
Lebsche knife, 73
Lenvatinib, 127–131
    and differentiated thyroid cancer (DTC), 479–481
    distant metastases (DM), 446
Levothyroxine, 443–444
    hypothyroidism, 420
Lidocaine infiltration, 472
Light amplified stimulated emission of radiation (LASER), 167
Linea alba, 541
Lingual thyroid, 19, 19f
Liothyronine (LT3), 440
Lipoadenoma, 392, 599, 599f
Lipohyperplasia, 602
Liquid-based cytology (LBC), 109
Lister, Joseph, 3–4
Lithium, 45, 557
Lithium-associated hyperparathyroidism, 562–563
Lobectomy, 118
    Hurthle cell carcinoma and, 227
    partial, 280–281
    pediatric thyroid cancer and, 260
    subtotal, 90
    thyroidectomy nomenclature and, 280–281
    total, 278, 278f, 280–281, 285f, 292
    unilateral thyroid, 88
Localization study
    for minimally invasive surgical procedures, 537
    for preoperative parathyroid planning
        bilateral parathyroid exploration and, 521
        invasive procedures for, 499
        nuclear medicine-based studies for, 495–499
        during pregnancy, 515
        radiology-based studies for, 494
Loss of heterozygosity (LOH), 226
Loupe-assisted bloodless dissection, 511
Low-risk papillary thyroid cancer, 199–200, 200t
LOXO-292, 484
Lymphadenopathy, metastatic cervical, 250–251
Lymph node
    dissection of
        clinically apparent-MTC surgery and, 245
        familial nonmedullary thyroid cancer and, 268
        prophylactic or therapeutic debate, 190
        radioactive iodine therapy, indications for, 190
    macrometastases and micrometastases, 149
    metastasis
        CT scanning with contrast for, 151
        effect on disease outcome, 380–381
        introduction to, 149
        papillary thyroid cancer and, 189, 189f
        physical examination for, 150
        preoperative radiographic evaluation for, 150
        risk factors for, 380
        ultrasound for, 150–151, 150–151f
    surgery of, 188
Lymphoma
    aggressive histology of, 459, 459f
    diffuse large B-cell (DLBCL), 116–117, 116f
    external beam radiotherapy and, 457–458
    indolent (low-grade), 459
    malignant, 116–117, 116–117f
    MALT type, 116–117, 117f
    ultrasound characteristics of, 134f, 140

M

MacFee incision, 393, 394f
Macrofollicular variant, 394
Macroscopically positive nodes
    vs. microscopically positive metastasis, 149
    preoperative radiographic detection of, 149
Magnetic resonance imaging (MRI), 58, 102, 151, 176, 200, 58.e3
    preoperative parathyroid localization testing and, 495, 507–508f
    reoperative thyroid surgery and, 463–464
Maintenance of Certification (MOC), 431–432
Malignancy, risk factors for thyroid nodules and, 100–101
Malignant thyroid neoplasm, 392
Malignant thyroid nodules, management of, 107
Malpractice
    litigation
        lawsuits and, 436
        legal basis of, 436
    in thyroid and parathyroid surgery
        legal basis of, 436
        malpractice claims and parathyroid glands as, 437–438
        standard of care and, 436–437
Mandl, Felix, 12, 12f
Massachusetts General Hospital (MGH)
    history of anesthesia and, 3
    history of endocrine surgery at, 12–14, 13f
May-Grunwald Giemsa, 111
Mayo, Charles, 7–8
Mayo Clinic, 196
    micropapillary cancer series and, 195
MD Anderson Cancer Center, 530–531
Medial superior pole approach, 95, 96f
Median thyroid anlage, anomalies of, 15, 16t
Mediastinal adenoma, 515
Mediastinal exposure
    indications of, 70–73
    surgical options for, 73–77
Mediastinal lymph node metastasis, 72, 72f
Mediastinal parathyroid glands, 72–73, 72f
Mediastinoscopy, 76–77
Mediastinum, indications of exposure, 70–73
Medical therapies
    reoperative thyroid surgery, 464–465
Medullary carcinoma
    surgical pathology of, 398–399
Medullary thyroid cancer
    MEN type 2A and, 236
Medullary thyroid cancer (MTC), 28
    external beam radiotherapy and, 455–456, 455f, 456t
    pediatric thyroid cancer and, 257
        postoperative management and complications, 261
Medullary thyroid carcinoma (MTC), 119, 127–131, 482–484. *See also* Hereditary medullary thyroid carcinoma; Sporadic medullary thyroid carcinoma
    Afirma MTC, 121
    cabozantinib and, 483
    carcinoembryonic antigen doubling times, 482–483
    CT, 482–483
    fine-needle aspiration and, 116, 116f
    hereditary, 482

Medullary thyroid carcinoma (MTC) *(Continued)*
    microcalcifications, 136–137
    molecular pathogenesis of, 182
    natural history, 482–483
    RET and, 182, 184
    sporadic, 482
    standards of care, 483
    systemic therapy, 483
    ultrasound and, 140, 161*f*
    vandetanib and, 483
Medullary thyroid microcarcinoma (microMTC). *See* Sporadic medullary thyroid carcinoma
Memorial Sloan Kettering Cancer Center (MSKCC), 199–202
MEN 1 (multiple endocrine neoplasia type 1), 477, 603*t*
    conclusion for, 584
    genetic testing in, 576–577
    hyperparathyroidism
        intraoperative adjuncts during parathyroidectomy for, 583–584
        nonsurgical management of, 584
        parathyroid management in, 577
        surgical treatment for, 578–581
        treatment of persistent or recurrent, 581, 581*f*
    hypoparathyroidism
        asymmetric glandular enlargement, 554*f*
    indications for surgery and, 577–578
    localization studies for, 499, 516
    operative management of HPT, 579*t*
    parathyroid management in, 576, 577*f*
    preoperative genetic assessment and, 503, 504*t*
    primary hyperparathyroidism and, 520*b*
MEN 2 (multiple endocrine neoplasia type 2), 256, 258
MEN 2A (multiple endocrine neoplasia type 2A), 258, 603*t*
    familial medullary thyroid cancer and, 235
    genetic testing in, 581–582
    hyperparathyroidism
        parathyroid management in, 582
        surgical treatment for, 583
        treatment of persistent or recurrent, 583
    indications for surgery for, 583
    medullary thyroid cancer and, 235–236
    nonendocrine components of, 236–237
    operative management of HPT, 579*t*
    parathyroid management in, 581, 582*f*
    preoperative genetic assessment and, 503, 504*t*
    presentation by genotype and, 235–240
    treatment for persistent or recurrent, 583, 584*f*
MEN 2B (multiple endocrine neoplasia type 2B), 603*t*
    gene carrier evaluation for surgery and, 240–242
    genotype-phenotype correlations, 240, 240*t*
    germline mutations, 258
    introduction to, 235
    nonendocrine components of, 237–240, 238*t*
MEN1 gene mutations, 576, 591
MEN 1 germline mutation analysis, 576
MENIN, 608, 612
Merit-based Incentive Payment System (MIPS), 431
Messenger RNA (mRNA), 119
Meta-analysis, 97
Metastasis, age, completeness of resection, invasion, and size (MACIS) scoring, 227
Metastatic disease
    external beam radiotherapy and, 457, 458*f*
Metastatic lymph node ratio (MLNR), 429
Methimazole (MMI), 81–82, 420, 475–476
Methylene blue, 424
MGH. *See* Massachusetts General Hospital (MGH)
Microadenoma, 599
Microcalcification, 133–134, 133*f*

Microcarcinoma, 392
Microscopically positive nodes, 149
Microwave ablation (MWA), 163, 171
Middle thyroid vein, thyroidectomy exposure of, 282*f*, 285, 286*f*
Midline airway, thyroidectomy surgical steps and, 278*f*, 284–285
Mikulicz, Jan, 8
Minimally invasive, 396, 538
Minimally invasive endoscopic thyroidectomy (MIVAT), 294
Minimally invasive follicular carcinoma, 204, 207–208
Minimally invasive parathyroidectomy (MIP)
    advantages, 529
    anatomic considerations in, 529–530, 530*b*, 531*f*
    considerations for, 529–530
    contraindications, 530*t*
    introduction to, 529
    operative preparation and techniques for, 532–536, 533*b*
    parathyroid surgery and, 538
    patient selection, 529, 530*t*
    postoperative care and follow-up for, 536
    preoperative imaging & localization, 532
    techniques for, 538–544
Minimally invasive radio-guided parathyroidectomy, 538
Minimally invasive thyroidectomy, 387*f*, 388
Minimally invasive video-assisted neck dissection, 315
Minimally invasive video-assisted parathyroidectomy (MIVAP), 311. *See also* Minimally invasive parathyroidectomy (MIP)
    advantages and disadvantages of, 543–544
    evidence-based recommendations for, 544–545
    indications for, 540
    intraoperative PTH assay and, 537–538
    introduction to, 537
    as MIP technique, 540–541
    preoperative localization studies for, 537
    results of, 541–544
    surgical procedures for, 540–541
    surgical techniques for, 541, 542–543*f*
Minimally invasive video-assisted thyroidectomy (MIVAT), 311
    evidence-based recommendations, 315
    indications for, 311
    instruments for, 311, 312*f*
    operative technique for
        anesthesia, 312, 312*f*
        equipment, 313
        patient position, 312–313, 312*f*
        surgical steps, 313–314, 313–315*f*
    personal experience, 315
Mirror image symmetry, 512
Missing parathyroid, bilateral exploration and
    situation 1 of, 523
    situation 2 of, 523
    situation 3 of, 523–525
    situation 4 of, 525
    situation 5 of, 525
    situation 6 of, 526
    situation 7 of, 526
    situation 8 of, 526–527
Mitogen-activated protein kinase (MAPK) pathway, 118–119, 188
MIVAT. *See* Minimally invasive video-assisted thyroidectomy (MIVAT)
MNG. *See* Multinodular goiter (MNG)
Molecular testing, 106
    for indeterminate cytopathology
        Afirma®, 119–120*t*, 121–125
        clinical utility of, 119–120
        future applications, 127–131
        molecular techniques, 119
        principles of, 118–120
        selection of, 127
        ThyGeNEXT®-ThyraMIR®, 119–120*t*, 125–127

Molecular testing *(Continued)*
    thyroid cancer, molecular alterations in, 118–119
    ThyroSeq®, 119–120*t*, 120–121
Morselization, 65–66
Moving shot technique, 164–165, 165–166*f*
MRI. *See* Magnetic resonance imaging (MRI)
Mucosa-associated lymphoid tissue (MALT), 459
Mucosal wave, 156
Multidisciplinary Cancer Conferences (MCCs)/Tumor Boards, 427
Multiglandular disease (MGD)
   asynchronous, 506
   bilateral exploration and, 512
   surgical technique for, 516, 522
   uniglandular *vs.*, 506
Multinodular goiter (MNG), 103, 475–476
   bilateral subtotal procedure for, 90–91, 91*f*
   ultrasound and, 140
Multinodularity, size, growth pattern, and, 103
Multiple endocrine neoplasia (MEN) 4, 603*t*
Multiple endocrine neoplasia (MEN) 2B. *See* MEN 2B (multiple endocrine neoplasia type 2B)
Multiple endocrine neoplasia (MEN) syndrome, 140, 145, 554–555, 597, 612
Multiple endocrine neoplasia type 1. *See* MEN 1
Multiple endocrine neoplasia type 2A. *See* MEN 2A
Multiple gland disease (MGD)
   abnormal glands, macroscopic and microscopic pathology of, 553–555, 554*f*
   bilateral cervical exploration, 563
   biochemistry in, 557–558
   clinical presentation, 557–558
   definition, 553
   diagnosis of, 555
   double adenoma, 553–554
   etiology and risk factors for, 556–557
     diabetes, 557
     diet and digestive disorders, 557
     exposure to radiation, 557
     lithium, 557
     thiazide drugs, 557
   four-gland hyperplasia, 554–555, 554–555*f*
   histopathological criteria for adenoma and hyperplasia, 555
   imaging modalities, 559
   incidence, 553, 554*t*
   intraoperative adjuncts in, 559
   introduction to, 553
   lithium-associated HPT, 562–563
   operative strategy in localized disease, 562–563
   parathyroid exploration, 555
   preoperative diagnosis of, 557–559
   preoperative localization
     with ultrasound and 99mTc-Sestamibi, 558, 558–559*t*
   surgical treatment, 560–562
   targeted parathyroidectomy, 563
   tumor clonality in, 555
   unilateral exploration/lateral approach, 562–563
Multiplex ligation-dependent probe amplification assay (MLPA), 600

N

National Academy of Medicine (NAM), 426
National Cancer Data Base, 196
National Comprehensive Cancer Network (NCCN), 161, 429
National Inpatient Sample (NIS), 430
National Priorities Partnership (NPP), 426
National Thyroid Cancer Treatment Cooperative Study Group (NTCTCSG), 196
Natural orifice transluminal endoscopic surgery (NOTES), 301
Neck
   cross section of, 473, 473*f*
   pain, 42–43
   reexploration, 574

Neck dissection
   compartment-oriented, 232
     sporadic medullary thyroid carcinoma and, 231
Neck ultrasonography, 222–223
Negative predictive value (NPV), 106, 120–121
   atypia/follicular lesion of undetermined significance, 121
   follicular neoplasm/suspicious for follicular neoplasm, 121
Neonatal primary hyperparathyroidism, 493
Neonatal severe hyperparathyroidism (NSHPT), 504, 504*t*, 597, 603*t*
Neonatal severe primary hyperparathyroidism, 603*t*
Nephrolithiasis, 488
Nerve monitoring, minimally invasive parathyroidectomy, 535
Nerve of Amelita Galli-Curci, 158
Neuber, Gustav, 3–4
Neural crest, 33
Neuromuscular dysfunction, 486
Neuromuscular psychiatric symptoms, 567, 567*b*
Neurotropic tyrosine receptor kinase (NTRK), 481
Next-generation sequencing (NGS), 118–119, 482
N+ lateral neck management, 381
N-nitroso compounds (NOCs), 158
Nodal assessment
   sonography of, 141–145, 142*f*
Nodal border, 145, 145*f*, 167*f*
Nodal disease, 149
Nodal distribution
   contrast enhancement and, 145, 168
   echogenicity of, 144*f*, 145
   intranodal calcification and, 145, 145*f*
   intranodal echogenic hilus and, 144–145, 144*f*
   intranodal necrosis and, 145, 145*f*
   shape of, 144, 144*f*
   size of, 144
   ultrasound and, 142, 167, 167*f*
   vascularity of, 145, 146*f*
Node
   central neck, 149
   dissection of, 196–197
   lateral neck, 150
   malignant, 142–145, 142–144*t*
   papillary thyroid carcinoma and, 149–150
Nodular disease, aggressive benign
   bilobar multinodular disease, 93
   extent of initial surgery, 93
   family history and, 93
   level of experience of surgeon, 93
   patient age, 93
   recurrence and, 93
Nodule. *See also* Solitary toxic nodule
   hyperfunctioning, 87
Noninvasive follicular thyroid neoplasm with papillary-like nuclear features (NIFTP), 105–106, 120, 127, 159, 182
   definition, 213
   diagnosis
     clinical presentation, 214
     cytology, 214
     histopathology, 214–216, 214*b*
     molecular diagnostics, 216
   epidemiology, 213
   etiology, 213
   hemithyroidectomy, 217*b*
   prognosis, 217
   ThyroSeq v3, 120–121
   treatment
     follow-up, 216–217
     surgery, 216
Nonlocalized disease, operative strategy in, 560
Nonrecurrent inferior laryngeal nerve (NRILN), 21, 32
Nonsteroidal antiinflammatory drugs (NSAIDs), 44

Nonsyndromic familial nonmedullary thyroid cancer, 267–268, 267t
Nonthyroidal illness
　thyroid physiology in, 28, 29f
Nontoxic nodular goiter, 101
Normal parathyroid gland
　anatomy of, 517–518, 518f
　dissection of, 512
　locations of, 514b, 519
Normative parathyroid parameter
　number and, 507
　weight and, 507, 518–519
Normocalcemic primary hyperparathyroidism, 489, 505–506, 520, 520b
　diagnosis & course of, 492
NPV. See Negative predictive value (NPV)
NRILN. See Nonrecurrent inferior laryngeal nerve (NRILN)
NSAIDs. See Nonsteroidal antiinflammatory drugs (NSAIDs)
NTRK1, 183
Nuclear grooves, 114, 115f
Nuclear medicine imaging
　double-tracer subtraction imaging, 496–497
　dual-phase imaging, 497
　introduction to, 506f
　positron emission tomography (PET), 499, 513
　sestamibi and, 496–497, 497f, 499, 511
　single-photon emission computed tomography (SPECT), 496–498, 498f, 510
　tetrofosmin and, 499, 512

O

Obesity
　papillary thyroid cancer and, 186
Occult papillary cancers, 194
Oncocyte
　as Hurthle cells, 225
　parathyroid gland anatomy and, 597–598, 598f
Oncocytic adenoma, 598–599, 599f
Oncocytic tumor. See Hurthle cell tumors (HCTs)
Oncocytic tumors, 396
Oncogene, papillary thyroid cancer and, 188
Open minimally invasive parathyroidectomy (OMIP), 538–539, 545
Ophthalmopathy
　Graves' disease and, 80, 80f
Optic fiber, 168
Oral phosphate, 492
Oral stigmata, 242
Organification, 26
Organs at risk (OARs), 460
Osteitis fibrosa cystica, 486–487, 487f
Output power, 167–168, 184f
Oxidative phosphorylation (OXPHOS), 226
Oxyphil cells, 597
Oxyphilic adenomas, 598

P

Paclitaxel, 456–457
Palpation
　nodal disease detection and, 149
　during parathyroid exploration, 512
Palpation thyroiditis, 49
Papanicolaou staining, 111, 111f
Papillary cancer, variants of, 393–395
Papillary microcarcinoma (PMC)
　active surveillance
　　management strategy, clinical framework for, 201–202, 201f
　　practical application, 203
　　to surgical intervention, indications, 202–203, 202b
　　histopathological study of, 200
　　observational clinical trial of, 199
　　observational management approach, 199
　　research needs, 203

Papillary thyroid cancer (PTC). See also Follicular variant of papillary thyroid carcinoma (FVPTC)
　biochemical incomplete response, 190–191
　classic, 186–187
　DTC, mortality trends of
　　imaging techniques, increased use of, 177
　　overdiagnosis hypothesis, 176–177
　epidemiology of, 186
　excellent response, 190
　factors influencing prognosis for
　　age at diagnosis, 189
　　BRAF, 188–189
　　distant metastases, 188
　　extrathyroidal extension, 188
　　lymph node metastases, 188
　　multifocality, 187–188
　　oncogenes, 188
　　telomerase reverse transcriptase (TERT), 189
　　tumor histology, 187
　　tumor size, 187
　family history, 186
　indeterminate response, 191
　initial treatment for
　　completion thyroidectomy, 190
　　initial thyroid surgery, 190
　　lymph node dissection, 190
　　lymph node surgery and, 188
　　preoperative imaging, 189–190
　　radioactive remnant ablation, 190
　　radioiodine therapy, 190
　　therapeutic/prophylactic lymphnode dissection as, 190
　　thyroid hormone suppression therapy and, 191–192
　introduction to, 186
　long-term management and surveillance
　　imaging, 193
　　serum thyroglobulin, 192
　　stimulation testing, 192
　　thyroid-stimulating hormone suppression therapy, 191–192
　pediatric thyroid cancer and, 256–257
　percutaneous ethanol injection (PEI), 476
　risk factors
　　exposure to radiation, 186
　　hereditary syndromes, 187
　　obesity, 186
　　polybrominated diphenyl ethers (PBDEs), 186
　structural incomplete response, 191
　tumor staging systems for, 188
　tumor variables for
　　columnar cell variant and, 187
　　distant metastases and, 188
　　follicular variant of PTC, 187
　　tall cell variant and, 187
　　thyroglossal duct and, 50–51
　　tumor size and, 187
Papillary thyroid carcinoma (PTC), 50–51, 118–119, 127, 149, 174
　fine-needle aspiration and, 114–115, 114–115f
　genetic alterations associated with, 183–184, 183t
　microcalcifications, 136–137, 138f
　surgical pathology of, 392–393
　ultrasound characteristics of, 139, 139f
　unique features of
　　cervical lymph node micrometastasis vs. macrometastasis/clinically apparent disease, 274
　　prognostic risk grouping segregation as, 274–275, 274t
　　small lesions and, 274
Papillary thyroid microcarcinomas (PTMC), 103
　BRAF, 197
　clinical incidence, 194–195
　clinical series of patients with, 195, 195t

Papillary thyroid microcarcinomas (PTMC) *(Continued)*
  completion thyroidectomy and, 196
  initial surgery for, 196
  node dissection and, 196–197
  observational data and active surveillance, 195–196
  postoperative surveillance of, 197
  prevalence of, 194–195
  radioiodine and, 197
  summary and recommendations for, 197–198
Parafibromin, 591, 593, 599–600, 600*f*
Parafibromin-deficient parathyroid neoplasm, 600, 600*f*
Paraganglioma-like adenoma, 391–392
Paralyzed vocal fold, 404–406
Parathymus complex, 22–24, 172
  undescended, 289
Parathyroid adenoma (PA)
  differential diagnosis for, 600–601
  laser and radiofrequency treatment of, 163–171
  percutaneous ethanol injection (PEI), 477
  primary hyperparathyroidism and, 597–601, 598–599*f*
Parathyroid anatomy, and physiology, 11–12
Parathyroid arteriography, 499
Parathyroid autotransplantation, 580
Parathyroid biopsy, 512
Parathyroid cancer, 493
Parathyroid carcinoma (PC)
  aberrant gene expression, 592*t*
  biochemical tests, 592
  chronic renal failure, 591
  clinical presentation of, 591–593, 592*t*
  diagnosis and workup, 592
  epigenetics, 591
  etiology, 591
  genetic mutations, 591
  genetic testing, 596
  histopathology, 593–594, 593*t*
    staging, 593–594
    stratification, 593–594
  imaging studies, 592–593
  incidence of, 591
  introduction to, 591
  molecular mechanisms, 592*t*
  neck irradiation, 591
  postoperative care and surveillance, 594–595
  preoperative management, 594–595
  prognosis, 596
  resection of recurrence
    adjuvant treatment, 595
    medical therapy for hypercalcemia, 595–596
  risk factors, 591
  surgical management, 594
  surgical pathology of, 601–602, 601–602*f*
Parathyroid crisis. *See* Acute primary hyperparathyroidism
Parathyroid cysts (PCs), 171, 494
Parathyroidectomy, 491. *See also* Minimally invasive video-assisted parathyroidectomy (MIVAP); Subtotal parathyroidectomy; Total parathyroidectomy; Video-assisted parathyroidectomy by lateral approach
  definition of, 564
  IPM accuracy and, 551
  IPM cost and, 551
  IPM-guided patient benefits and, 550
  MEN 2A-associated HPT and, 583
  operative goals of, 520–521
  procedure considerations for, 389
  prophylactic, 583
  secondary hyperparathyroidism and, 569
  targeted, 563

Parathyroid ectopia, extreme, 510
Parathyroid embryology, 24–25
Parathyroid exploration
  closure for, 515
  general principles of, 511–512, 511*b*
  multiple gland disease (MGD), 555
  preoperative imaging and, 532
  surgical technique/search algorithm and, 512–515, 513*f*
Parathyroid glands, 419, 494
  acquired ectopic localization of, 25, 38
  advances and autotransplantation of, 12
  anatomy of, 11–12, 597, 598*f*
  anomalies in number of, 25
  anomalous development of, 32–33
  autofluorescence of, 278
  with borderline hypercalcemia and hyperplasia with minimal glandular enlargement, 554–555, 555*f*
  characteristics of, 507
  cysts and, 604, 615
  development process of, 23, 36
  ectopic position of, 146, 518*f*
  embryology of, 22, 146
  generalities for, 22
  genetic control and evolutionary model of, 23, 34–35
  goiter surgery and, 65, 68
  history of, 12
  hyperparathyroidism and, 597–601
  hypoparathyroidism and, 604, 617
  intraoperative, 506–507
  intrathyroidal parathyroid glands and, 24–25
  location of, 514, 570, 570*f*
  multilobulated diseased, 554*f*
  normal anatomy of, 146, 171, 171*f*
  other familial hyperparathyroidism syndromes an, 602, 614
  parathyroid carcinoma and, 601–602, 601–602*f*
  parathyroid surgery, 12
  physiology of, 11–12
  position, migration, ectopias of, 24*f*
  position of normal parathyroid glands, anomalies of embryologic migration, and congenital ectopias, 23–25, 23–24*f*
  preservation of, 466
  primary chief cell hyperplasia, 602, 603*f*
  resected, 571, 572*f*
  with secondary hypoparathyroidism, 554*f*
  secondary tumors and, 604, 616
  size prediction of normally secreting, 550–551
  symmetry of, 24, 507
  technical considerations, 146–147
  ultrasound for, 145–148
  undescended thymus with, 570–571, 571*f*
  vascular pattern, 146
Parathyroid gland surgery
  controversy in, 516
  failure of, 516
  malpractice claims and, 437–438
  missing gland search and, 514–515
  plane of recurrent laryngeal nerve and, 507–508, 508*f*
  position of, 508, 508*t*
  postoperative complications and, 68–69
  rationale for, 521, 521*b*
  reoperation of, 95, 516
  search algorithm for, 512–515, 513*f*
  surgical indications for, 505, 505*t*
Parathyroid hormone (PTH), 419, 486–488, 517, 546
Parathyroid hormone drop criterion
  IPM cost and, 551
  late recurrence and, 551
  postoperative normocalcemic PTH levels and, 551

Parathyroid hormone drop criterion (Continued)
  prevention of operative failure and, 551
  protocol and criteria dependence and, 551
  secretion of first gland excised in MGD and, 551
  size of normally secreting parathyroid glands and, 550–551
Parathyroid hormone level
  in multiglandular disease and, 551
  in postoperative normocalcemic patient, 551
Parathyroid hyperplasia, in secondary hyperparathyroidism (SHPT), 567f
Parathyroid III (PIII), 22–24, 24f. See also Thymic parathyroid
  symmetry of, 22–24
Parathyroid intoxication. See Acute primary hyperparathyroidism
Parathyroid IV (PIV), 23, 23f. See also Superior parathyroid gland
  symmetry of, 23–24
Parathyroid lesion, 610, 612
Parathyroid localization testing, 506
Parathyroid nomenclature system, 530–532, 531f, 531b
Parathyroid number, anomalies in, 37
Parathyroid poisoning. See Acute primary hyperparathyroidism
Parathyroid reimplantation, 527
Parathyroid remnant size, 527
Parathyroid storm. See Acute primary hyperparathyroidism
Parathyroid surgery, 12
Parathyroid surgical anatomy, 507–508
Parathyroid tissue, 37
  autografted, 569, 572–573
  autotransplantation of, 466–467
  reimplantation, 470
Parathyroid tumor
  oncogene rearrangement/overexpression and, 521
  sporadic, 521
  suppressor gene inactivation of, 507, 521
Parathyroid vascular anatomy, 508
Parathyroid vascularization, by parathyroid angiography, 278–280
Parathyromatosis, 37, 570, 573–574, 573b, 574t, 604
Paratracheal dissection, 377–378, 469–470. See also Central neck compartment
Parry, Caleb Hillier, 2
Pars obliqua, 320
Pars recta, 320
Partial sternotomy (sternal split), 73, 73–74f
Partial thyroidectomy, 105
Path of descent, 50
Patient positioning
  for minimally invasive parathyroidectomy, 533, 533b
  for minimally invasive video-assisted parathyroidectomy, 540–541, 541f
  for thyroidectomy, 283, 283f
Patient preparation
  and positioning, for central neck dissection, 468–470
Patient-reported outcome measures (PROMs), 428
Patient-Reported Outcomes Measurement Information System (PROMIS), 428
Paucicellular variant of ATC, 247
Pax-8, 29
Pediatric thyroid cancer
  etiology of, 255–256
  genetics of, 257–258
  introduction to, 255
  medullary thyroid cancer and, 257
  molecular genetics of, 258, 258t
  pathology of, 256–257
  presentation and preoperative evaluation
    clinical presentation, 258
    fine-needle aspiration and, 259
    flexible fiberoptic laryngoscopy (FFL), 258–259
    genetic testing, 259–260
    preoperative imaging, 259
    ultrasound vocal cord visualization, 259

Pediatric thyroid cancer (Continued)
  radioactive iodine, 259
    for children, 261–263
      diffuse sclerosing variant PTC, 262–263
      follow-up, 262
      summary for, 263
      surgical management of, 260
      thyroidectomy for, 260
    treatment of
      risk stratification for, 262, 262t
PEI. See Percutaneous ethanol injection (PEI)
Pemberton's sign, 56.e4
Pembrolizumab monotherapy
  and differentiated thyroid cancer (DTC), 481
Pendred syndrome
  familial nonmedullary thyroid cancer and, 267
Peptic ulcer disease (PUD), 486–487, 489, 491
Percutaneous ethanol injection (PEI), 164
  complication recognition, 477–478
  cyst injection, 474, 474–475f
  for functional and nonfunctional solid and solid thyroid tumors, 475
  in head and neck endocrine tumors, 473–474, 473f
  malignant metastatic lymphadenopathy
    alcohol ablation of, 476–477
    cost effectiveness, 477
  materials used, 477
  mitigation, 477–478
  of parathyroid adenoma and hyperplasia, 477
  practical considerations, 477
  reducing risk of ethanol extravasation and tissue damage, 477
  risks and side effects of, 477
  safety policies, 477–478
  into solid nodules, 475–476
  techniques, 477
  for toxic and pretoxic adenomas, 475–476
  and tumors, 472
  ultrasonography-guided, 472
  ultrasonography imaging anatomy of head and neck, 473, 473f
Percutaneous ethanol injection therapy (PEIT), 568
Percutaneous laser thermal ablation (PLA), 164
Perithyroidal lidocaine injection, 164, 165f
Perithyroidal sheath, 284–285
Persistent hyperparathyroidism, 578, 583–584
Persistent thyroid cancer, RAI therapy of, 448
PET. See Positron emission tomography (PET)
Pheochromocytoma (PCC), 236, 241
Phonotherapy, 324
Phosphate, pHPT lab work and, 503
Physical examination
  lymph node metastasis and, 150
  primary hyperparathyroidism and, 502–503
Piezoelectric crystals, 151
Piriform fossa, 37
Pirogov, Nikolaiy Ivanovich, 3
Plan, do, study, act (PDSA) cycles, 432
Platelet-derived growth factor receptor alpha (PDGFR-α), 479–480
Plexus thyroideus impar, 284
Ploidy analysis, 611
Plummer's disease, 83. See also Toxic nodular goiter (TNG)
Pneumothorax, mediastinal exposure and, 73
Poiseuille's law, 57.e3
Polymerase chain reaction (PCR), 119
Poorly differentiated thyroid carcinomas (PDTCs), 182
Positive predictive value (PPV), 120
  atypia/follicular lesion of undetermined significance, 121
  follicular neoplasm/suspicious for follicular neoplasm, 121
Positron emission tomography (PET), 102, 156, 499, 513
  with 18-fluoro-2-deoxy-D-glucose/CT scanning, 463–464

INDEX

Posterior enhancement, 133–134, 133f
Posteriorly located upper gland (PLUG) adenomas, 499, 514
Posterior mediastinal goiter, 63–65, 64–65f
   substernal goiter type II, 53–54, 54t, 54–56f
Posterior mediastinal thyroid, 71–72
Posterior shadowing, 133–134, 133f
Postoperative thyroxine, 113
Postpartum thyroiditis (PPT), 33–34
   clinical manifestations of, 44
   introduction to, 44–45
   management of, 45
   pathogenesis of, 44
Potassium iodine, 97
Power Doppler, 134, 135f, 137, 146–147, 147f, 166, 173
PPT. *See* Postpartum thyroiditis (PPT)
Prealbumin, 26
Precision medicine, 127–131
Pregnancy
   and hyperthyroidism, 37
   and hypothyroidism, 37
   localization study during, 515
   primary hyperparathyroidism in, 493
Prelaryngeal dissection, 377
Prelaryngeal node, 13
Preprimordial stage, 36
Pretibial myxedema, 80
   Graves' disease and, 80
Pretoxic solitary adenoma (PTA), 475–476
Pretracheal dissection, 377
Primary chief cell hyperplasia (P-CCH), 602, 603f
Primary hyperparathyroidism (PHPT). *See also* Hyperparathyroidism; Minimally invasive parathyroidectomy (MIP)
   bone densitometry, 487–488, 488f
   bone histomorphometry, 488
   characteristics and, 507
   clinical course with and without surgery for, 490, 490t
   clinical presentation of, 486
   clonality of sporadic parathyroid tumors and, 507, 521
   drug treatment for, 492
   embryologic variation and, 509–510
   epidemiology of, 486–487
   fractures and, 488
   histology of, 520
   intraoperative PTH and, 506–507
   intrathyroidal adenoma and, 510–511
   introduction to, 502
   localization testing, 506, 519
   mediastinal adenoma and, 515
   medical management of, 491–492, 491f, 492t
   MEN 1-associated hyperparathyroidism and, 577
   missed adenomas and, 510
   molecular genetics of, 507, 521
   multiglandular disease and, 522
   nephrolithiasis and, 488
   no previous neck surgery and, 583
   normocalcemic, 489, 505–506
   oncogene rearrangement/overexpression and, 507, 521
   other organ involvement and, 488–489
   parathyroid adenoma as, 597–600
   parathyroid exploration and, 511–515
   pathology of, 489–490
   patient selection for MIP and, 529, 530t
   percutaneous ethanol injection (PEI), 477
   plane of recurrent laryngeal nerve and, 507–508
   position and, 508
   postoperative assessment for, 516
   in pregnancy, 493
   preoperative evaluation for, 502–504

Primary hyperparathyroidism (PHPT) *(Continued)*
   preoperative localization testing for
     algorithms for, 499–501
     conclusion for, 501
     introduction to, 494
     localization studies for, 494–499, 516
     unique scenarios, 514
   skeleton and, 487
   suppressor gene inactivation and, 521
   surgery for, 490–491
   surgical anatomy, 507–508
   surgical controversies and, 516, 523
   surgical failure and, 516
   surgical guidelines, 505–506, 505t
   surgical management of asynchronous multiglandular disease, 506
   symmetry and, 507
   symptomatic, 486
   thyroidectomy during parathyroidectomy and, 511
   uniglandular *vs.* multiglandular disease and, 506
   unusual presentations of, 493
   vascular anatomy and, 508
   vitamin D and pHPT, 504–505
Primary thyroid lymphoma, ATC
   clinical diagnosis and imaging, 253–254
   epidemiology, 252
   histopathology, 252–253
   treatment, 254
     airway protection, 254
     chemotherapy, 254
     failure patterns and follow-up, 254
     radiotherapy, 254
     surgery, 254
Primitive pharynx, 15, 16f
Primordial stage, early, 16f, 36
Program death inhibitor 1 (PD-1), 481
Progression-free survival (PFS), 479–480
Prophylactic central neck dissection (pCND), 149
PRUNE2 gene mutations, 591
Psammoma body, 114
Pseudocyst, 473–474, 473f
Pseudo-Hirschsprung's disease, 239f, 240–241
Pseudohypoparathyroidism, 617
Pseudonodule, 41
PTC. *See* Papillary thyroid carcinoma (PTC)
PTEN hamartoma tumor syndrome (PHTS), 256
PTH–related protein (PTHrP), 487
PTMC. *See* Papillary thyroid microcarcinomas (PTMC)
Pyramidal lobe, 20, 108

Q

QUADAS-2, 121
Quality assurance (QA), 426, 427f
Quality indicators (QIs), 427–429

R

Radiation
   ionizing, 100
   pediatric thyroid cancer and, 255
   therapy, MTC, 233
Radiation-associated thyroiditis, 49
Radiation exposure, 502
   family history and, 100
Radiation therapy (RT), 255
Radioactive iodine (RAI), 429
   ablation, 447
   adjuvant therapy, 448
   administered activity, choice of, 451
   aims of, 448t

Radioactive iodine (RAI) *(Continued)*
  clinical indications for, 450*t*
  Hurthle cell carcinoma and, 227
  for nodal metastases, 381
  pediatric thyroid cancer and, 259
    for children, 261–263
      diffuse sclerosing variant PTC, 262–263
      follow-up, 262
  of persistent thyroid cancer, 448
  postoperative disease assessment, 449
  role of, 447–448
  selective use approach, 448–451
  for thyroid cancer management, 447–448
  thyroid hormone withdrawal *vs.* recombinant thyroid-stimulating hormone, 451
Radioactive iodine (^{131}I) therapy, 440–442, 442*t*
Radiofrequency ablation (RFA), 163–164
  thyroid gland and
    autonomous functioning thyroid nodules, 167
    benign nonfunctioning thyroid nodules, 165, 180
    complications, 167, 182*f*
    cystic and predominantly cystic thyroid nodules, 165–166
    equipment, 164, 164*f*
    inclusion criteria, 163–164
    mechanism of action, 163, 174*f*
    patient preparation, 164, 164*f*
    postprocedure care, 165, 179
    preprocedural workup, 164, 176, 176*t*, 176*b*
    recurrent thyroid cancers, 167, 175, 187
    technique and procedure for, 164–165, 165*f*, 177*f*
Radiofrequency (RF) generator system, 164, 164*f*
Radiographic evaluation, 57*b*, 58
Radioguided gamma-probe, minimally invasive parathyroidectomy, 535
Radioguided parathyroidectomy
  syndromes, 584
Radioguided revision thyroid surgery, 470–471
Radioiodine, 59, 106–107, 59.e1
  ablation
    familial nonmedullary thyroid cancer and, 268
    as therapy, 82
  Graves' disease and, 82
  nuclear imaging
    reoperative thyroid surgery and, 463
  papillary thyroid microcarcinoma and, 197
  solitary toxic nodule and, 88
  toxic multinodular goiter and, 85
Radionucleotide scan, 101
Radiotherapy
  parathyroid carcinoma and, 596
RAI-refractory differentiated thyroid cancer (DTC), 479
  genotyping in, 482
Raloxifene
  and primary hyperparathyroidism (PHPT), 492
Ramus anastomoticus. See Galen's anastomosis
RAS gene, 258
  follicular thyroid cancer and, 205–206
  follicular thyroid carcinoma and, 182
  follicular variant of papillary thyroid cancer, 118–119
  papillary thyroid carcinoma and, 182
Rearranged during transfection (RET), 157, 258, 482
  medullary thyroid carcinoma and, 182, 184
  mutation
    MEN 2A and, 581–582
    sporadic medullary thyroid carcinoma and, 230
Recombinant human thyrotropin-stimulating hormone (rhTSH), 440
  vs. thyroid hormone withdrawal, 451

Recurrent disease
  embryologic remnants and, 91
  medullary thyroid carcinoma and, 232–233
  preoperative evaluation for, 93–94
Recurrent laryngeal nerve (RLN), 102, 112, 201–202, 519
  abductor and adductor fibers, 331
  anatomy of, 328–329, 328*f*
  anomalous development of, 21, 22*f*
  displacement of, 330
  embryology for, 21, 21*f*
  extralaryngeal branching, 330–331
  goiter and, 61–63, 63*f*
  history of, 8–11, 9–10*f*
  inferior thyroid cartilage cornu, 333
  injury of, 357–358, 358*f* (*see also* Recurrent laryngeal nerve (RLN), injury pathophysiology of)
  injury pathophysiology of
    configuration of paralyzed vocal fold and, 404–406, 405–406*f*
    introduction to, 404
    muscle compartments and laryngeal motion for, 408, 408*f*
    preferential reinnervation, 408
    reinnervation and, 407–408
    transected nerve, 409
    variations in symptoms for, 404
  invasive disease and, 466–467
  ligament of berry, 332–333, 333*f*
  microanatomy, 329
  microdissection of, 466, 469
  monitoring of
    categories of benefits for, 338–339
    evidence based discussion on effect of, 338
    guidelines and current standards for, 338
    management of infiltrated nerve, 353–357
    past techniques as, 339
    surface recording, new expanded options for, 340, 340*f*
  nonrecurrent, 329–330
  paralysis and, 158, 277, 326
  parathyroid gland exploration and, 511–512
  surgery and, 68, 95, 282*f*, 286–288, 287*f*, 466, 469
    (*see also* Recurrent laryngeal nerve (RLN), surgical anatomy and monitoring of)
  surgical anatomy and monitoring of
    introduction to, 326–327
    management of infiltrated nerve and, 327*f*, 353–357, 356*f*
    monitoring of, 337–340
    neural injury and, 357–358
    SLN monitoring and, 359
    surgical anatomy of, 327–329
    surgical approaches to, 333–336
    surgical tips and pitfalls for, 334*f*, 336–337
    visual appearance of, 329–333
    vocal cord recovery and, 358–359
  tubercle of zuckerkandl, 330
  visualization of, 327
  voice and, 156–157
Recurrent nerves, 8
Recurrent nodular goiter
  clinical presentation of, 89–90, 90*f*
Reflection, laser light and, 167
Regional symptomatic assessment, 57–58
Regional symptomatology, 58
Remnant, embryological, 91–92, 92*f*, 107*f*
Remote-access approaches, 294
Remote-access thyroid surgery, 302–303
Renal cell carcinoma, 117, 117*f*
Renal dysfunction, 505

INDEX

Reoperation
  of benign disease, 89
  of the neck, 232–233
  of residual or recurrent medullary thyroid carcinoma, 233
Reoperative surgery, 94–95, 98
  adequate treatment of disease at primary surgery and, 467
  central neck dissection-paratracheal/superior mediastinal dissection and, 467–471
  completion thyroidectomy, 467
  parathyroid surgery
    AHNS guidelines on, 586b
    challenging nature of, 587–589, 588–590b
    inferior approach, 587, 588f
    lateral approach, 587, 587f
    midline approach, 586–587
    superior approach, 587, 587f
  RLN invasion and, 466–467
  surgery techniques for, 467
  timing of, 467
Resected disease, external beam radiotherapy, 452–455, 453t, 453f
Res ipsa loquitur, 436
Rests. *See* Thyroid rests
Retrotracheal cervical mediastinal goiter, 63–65, 64–65f
Reverse transcription polymerase chain reaction (RT-PCR), 119
Revision surgery
  adjunctive techniques for, 470–471
  definitions, 461–462
  indications for, 461–462
  radioguided, 470–471
  recurrence rates and patterns, 462
  for recurrent disease, 471
  ultrasound-guided, 470
Riedel's thyroiditis (RT), 47–48
  clinical management of, 47–48
  introduction to, 47–48
  management of, 48
  pathogenesis of, 47
Riedel thyroiditis (RT)
Rituximab, 48
RLN. *See* Recurrent laryngeal nerve (RLN)
RNA sequencing (RNA-Seq), 119, 121–125
Robot-assisted thoracoscopy, 77–78
Robotic endoscopic retroauricular (facelift) thyroidectomy, 295–296, 296f
Robotic endoscopic thyroidectomy
  complications, 300, 300t
  contraindications for, 295, 295t
  patient selection, 294–295
Robotic endoscopic transaxillary thyroidectomy, 296–299, 297–299f
RT. *See* Riedel's thyroiditis (RT)
Rultract retractor, 75

S

SAT. *See* Subacute thyroiditis (SAT)
Scandinavian Quality Register for Thyroid and Parathyroid Surgery (SQR), 158
Scapula retractor, 75–76
Scattering, backward and forward, 167
Scintigraphy, 58, 81–82f, 509, 58.e4
Sclerosing mucoepidermoid carcinoma with eosinophilia, 399
Secondary hyperparathyroidism (SHPT)
  localization studies for, 499, 516
  surgical management of, 477
    autografted parathyroid tissue function and, 573
    calcium replacement therapy, 572
    clinical symptoms and findings of, 567, 567b
    definition of, 564
    epidemiology of, 564
    graft-dependent recurrent, 573f
    medical treatment of, 565–567, 567b

Secondary hyperparathyroidism (SHPT) *(Continued)*
    mortality and complications of, 573
    parathyroid gland intervention, 568
    parathyroid hyperplasia in, 567f
    pathogenesis, histopathology, pathophysiology of, 564, 566–567f
    persistent and recurrent HPT and, 573–574
    postoperative management, 571–573
    preoperative examination for, 570
    preoperative image diagnosis, 569
    rate of parathyroidectomy (PTx) for, 564, 565f
    surgical approach for, 570–571, 570–572f
    surgical indications for, 568, 568b
    surgical procedures for, 569–570
    surgical pathology of, 603–604
Secondary parathyroid survey, 523, 524f
Secondary tumors
  surgical pathology of parathyroid glands and, 604, 616
Second hits, 577
Selumetinib
  and differentiated thyroid cancer (DTC), 480
Selvan EBSLN Classification Scheme, 319
Seroma, 422
Serotonin reuptake inhibitors (SRIs), 424
Serum calcium
  measurement of, 516
  parathyroidectomy postoperative assessment of, 516
  primary hyperparathyroidism and, 503
Serum free T4, 31, 32t
Serum thyroglobulin (Tg), 32–33, 443–444
  level of, 462–463
Serum thyroid antibodies, 31–32
  in hyperthyroidism, 36
  in hypothyroidism, 34
Serum thyroid hormones, 30–31
Sestamibi
  nuclear medicine imaging and, 496–497, 497f, 499, 511, 519
  and ultrasound assessment, 519
Severed nerve, 357
Sex, thyroid nodule risk and, 100–101
Shear wave elastography (SWE), 141
Shear wave imaging, 165
Signet-ring cell follicular adenoma, 392
Significant goiter, 53
Single-photon emission computed tomography (SPECT), 174, 496–498, 498f, 510, 515
Sistrunk operation, 31
Sistrunk procedure, 50
Skeleton
  primary hyperparathyroidism (PHPT) and, 487
  PTH-induced abnormalities of, 567
Skin flap elevation, 468
SLN. *See* Superior laryngeal nerve (SLN)
Solid thyroid tumors
  percutaneous ethanol injection (PEI), 475
Solid variant, 394
Solitary toxic nodule
  clinical presentation and evaluation of, 87–88, 87f
  pathogenesis of, 87
  treatment of, 88
Somatostatin
  chyle leak, 424
Sonography, 58, 58.e4
  neck nodes and, 141–145, 142f
Sorafenib, 127–131
  and differentiated thyroid cancer (DTC), 480
Sound waves, 132–133, 151
Spindle-cell follicular adenoma, 392
Spindle epithelial tumor with thymus-like differentiation, 399

INDEX

Spongiform nodules, definition of, 103
Sporadic medullary thyroid carcinoma
  clinical course for, 230
  conclusion for, 234
  diagnostic considerations, workup and staging, 230–231
  distant metastatic disease and systemic therapy, MTC
    diarrhea and other secretory complications, management of, 234
    isolated distant metastases, management of, 233–234
    systemic cytotoxic chemotherapy, 234
    tyrosine kinase inhibitor targeted therapy, 234
  follow-up and surveillance, 232
    calcitonin, carcinoembryonic antigen and ultrasound, 232
    calcitonin doubling time, 232
  genetics and, 230
    clinical presentation and usual clinical course, 230
    sporadic *vs.* hereditary, 230
  introduction to, 229
  pathophysiology
    calcitonin and carcinoembryonic antigen, 229–230
    histology and C-cells, 229
  primary surgical treatment
    extent of surgery, 231–232
  radiation therapy and, 233
  reoperation for, 233
  surgical management of recurrent disease, 232–233
  surgical treatment of, 231–232
  unilateral surgery for, 232
Sporadic parathyroid tumor, 521
Sporadic primary hyperparathyroidism (SPHPT)
  intraoperative parathyroid hormone monitoring an, 546
  MIVAP and, 540
Sporadic silent thyroiditis (ST)
  clinical manifestations of, 44
  introduction to, 44–45
  management of, 45
  pathogenesis of, 44
Spreader, sternal, 73
Standard of care, 436–437
Staphylococcus aureus, 46
Stereotactic body radiotherapy (SBRT), 457
Sternocleidomastoid (SCM) muscle, 465
Sternothyroid muscle, 522
Sternotomy
  full, 73–75
  partial, 73
  for substernal goiter, 66–67
Sternum, 73
Strain elastography, 141
Strap muscle
  goiter surgery and, 61
  management of, 468
  thyroidectomy steps and, 284–285, 285f
Streptococcus pyogenes, 46
Stromal fat cell, 597–598, 602
Strongyloides stercoralis, 48–49
Struma fibrosa, 47
Struma lymphomatosa, 40
Struma ovarii, 44, 52
Subacute thyroiditis (SAT)
  clinical manifestations of, 3f, 42–44
  introduction to, 41–44, 42b, 42f
  management of, 44
  pathogenesis of, 42
  ultrasound and, 141
Subclinical hyperthyroidism, 36
Subclinical hypothyroidism, 34
Subplatysmal flaps, 535

Substernal goiter, 57, 95, 56.e4
  anterior mediastinal goiter (substernal goiter type I), 53
  cervical goiter and, 54t, 56–57
  clinical presentation of, 54t
  definition of, 53, 53.e2
  incidence of, 56.e1
  isolated mediastinal goiter (substernal goiter type III), 54–56
  mediastinal exposure and, 70, 71f
  posterior mediastinal goiter (substernal goiter typeII), 53–54, 54t, 54–56f
  rate of occurrence for, 56
  sternotomy for, 66–67, 66f
  surgery for, 60, 60.e1, 60.e2
  techniques for delivery of, 65–67, 66f
  treatment options for, 59–60, 59–60b
Substernal goiter type II. *See* Posterior mediastinal goiter
Substernal goiter type III. *See* Goiter, isolated mediastinal
Substernal nodular goiter, 84f
Subtotal parathyroidectomy
  four-gland hyperplasia, 560–561, 560f
  less than, 578
  MEN 1-associated HPT surgery and, 578–580
  parathyroid hyperplasia and, 613
  secondary hyperparathyroidism, 569–570, 569b
  tertiary hyperparathyroidism and, 575
Subtotal thyroidectomy, 89, 97, 60.e2
Sulcus terminalis, 15
Superior goiter extent, 97–63.e5f, 63.e5
  goiter surgery and, 65
Superior laryngeal nerve (SLN), 11, 21–22, 329
  anatomy for, 316–320, 317–318f
  Cernea EBSLN Classification Scheme, 317–318, 318f
  conclusion for, 325
  Friedman EBSLN Classification Scheme, 318–319, 320f
  history of, 316
  incidence of EBSLN injury and, 324
  Kierner EBSLN Classification Scheme, 317–318, 319f
  monitoring of, 322–325, 323–325f
  physiology and pathophysiology of, 320
  Selvan EBSLN Classification Scheme, 319
  surgical technique for, 320–324, 321–322f
  thyroidectomy surgery and, 282f, 285f, 290–291
  treatment of EBSLN injury and, 324
Superior mediastinal dissection, 467–471. *See also* Central neck compartment
Superior parathyroid gland, 570, 571f
  acquired migration and, 510
  ectopia of, 509–510, 514b
  if missing, 515
  position of, 16f, 23
  thyroid surgery and, 289–290, 289b
Superior pole
  superior laryngeal nerve and, 282f, 285f, 290–291, 291f
  surgical approach to, 320
Supernumerary gland, 25, 37, 507, 510, 515
Suppressive therapy, 59, 58.e5
Surgeon responsibility, 435
Surgery
  bilateral parathyroid exploration and, 521–523
  clinically apparent hereditary MTC and, 242–243, 243f
    lymph node dissection, extent of, 242–243
    synchronous MTC and HPT, 242
    synchronous MTC and PCC, 242
    thyroidectomy, extent of, 242
  contralateral, 292
  FMTC/MEN 2A-MTC gene carrier evaluation for, 235–236
  goiter and, 60
  Graves' disease and, 82–83, 83b, 83f
  parathyroid carcinoma and, 594

Surgery (Continued)
  primary hyperparathyroidism (PHPT) and, 490–491
  prophylactic, 245
  rationale and indications of, 59–60, 59–60b
  solitary toxic nodule and, 88, 88f
  for substernal goiter, 60
  thyroid/parathyroid incisions for, 386
  toxic multinodular goiter and, 85–87, 86f
Surgical bed preparation, 470
Surveillance, Epidemiology, and End Results (SEER)
  Hurthle cell tumors and, 225–226
  papillary thyroid microcarcinoma and, 194
  parathyroid carcinoma and, 591, 594
Suspicious for follicular neoplasm (SFN), 112–113, 113f, 118
  negative predictive value, 121
  positive predictive value, 121
Suspicious for malignancy (SFM), 118
Swallowing, 160
Swallow therapy, 411
Syndromic familial nonmedullary thyroid cancer, 265t, 266–268
Syndromic medullary thyroid carcinoma
  MEN 2A
    clinical presentation by genotype and, 235–240
    evaluation of gene carriers for surgery and, 240–242
    introduction to, 235
  MEN 2B, 237
    surgery and, 241–242
Synoptic reporting, thyroidectomy surgical steps and, 293
Systemic therapy, medullary thyroid carcinoma (MTC), 483

T
Tall cell variant, 394
Tamoxifen, 48
TBG. See Thyroxine binding globulin (TBG)
Tearless crying, 242
Technetium pertechnetate (^{99m}Tc-pertechnetate), 496–497
Technetium sestamibi, 174
Tertiary hyperparathyroidism
  clinical manifestation of, 574
  localization studies for, 499, 516
  medical treatment and surgical indications for, 574, 574b
  surgical pathology of, 603–604
  surgical procedures for, 575
TERT promoter mutations, 200
Tetany, post thyroidectomy, 8
Tetrofosmin, 499, 512
TGDCs. See Thyroglossal duct cysts (TGDCs)
THBR. See Thyroid hormone binding ratio (THBR)
The Bethesda System for Reporting Thyroid Cytopathology (TBSRTC), 105–106, 105t, 108–109, 110t, 110b, 118, 214
The Cancer Genome Atlas (TCGA), 183
Thermal ablation, 175
  autonomously functioning thyroid nodules and, 170
Thioamides, 420
Third pharyngeal pouch cyst, 615
Thoracotomy, 75–76
ThyGeNEXT®-ThyraMIR®, 127
  background, 125
  clinical validation, 125–126
  for indeterminate cytopathology, 119–120t, 125–127
  practical considerations, 127
  sample report, 127, 128–130f
Thymectomy
  routine, 561
  transcervical, 578, 580–581
Thymic parathyroid, 22–23
Thymic remnant, 509
Thymus, dissection of, 469

Thyroglobulin (Tg), 101, 150, 447
Thyroglossal duct, 15, 50
Thyroglossal duct cysts (TGDCs), 20, 20f, 50–51, 51f, 400, 474
  embryology of, 50
Thyroglossal tract, 15, 108
Thyroid
  physiology of
    introduction to, 26–28
    nonthyroidal illness and, 28, 29f
    pregnancy and, 27–28
  as site of cancer metastases, 140
  tests for
    serum thyroglobulin, 32–33
    serum thyroid autoantibodies, 31–32
    serum thyroid hormones, 30–31
    serum TSH, 29–30, 29–31f
    thyroid imaging, 33
  ultrasound for, 134–138, 135b
  ultrasound-guided procedures for, 141
Thyroid and parathyroid surgery
  ethics and malpractice in
    ethical issues in, 433–435
    malpractice issues in, 435–438
    surgeon's responsibility and, 435
  non-neural complications of
    aerodigestive tract injury and, 422–423, 423f
    airway complications for, 423–424
    chyle leak and, 424
    hematoma as, 420–421, 421f
    hemorrhage as, 420–421, 421f
    Horner's syndrome and, 424, 424f
    hypertrophic scar as, 422
    hypoparathyroidism and, 419–420, 420t
    hypothyroidism and, 420
    infection and, 422, 422f
    keloid as, 422
    methylene blue and, 424
    mortality, 424–425
    rare complications of, 424
    seroma and, 422
    thyrotoxic storm and, 420
  quality in, 429–430
    defined, 427–430
    evidence-based methods, 432
    improvement, 426–427, 431–432
    indicators, 427–429
    measurement, 430–431
    surgical quality assurance, tools for, 431–432
Thyroid antibody, 34
  Hashimoto's thyroiditis and, 41
Thyroid cancer, 89, 194. See also Differentiated thyroid cancer (DTC); Pediatric thyroid cancer
  alcohol ablation of malignant metastatic lymphadenopathy in, 476–477
  molecular alterations in, 118–119
  risk of, 101
  thyroid metastases and, 140
Thyroid carcinoma
  epidemiology of, 181
  germline genetics of, 182
  pathology, 181–182
  prognosis for, 182
  somatic genomics of
    FTC, 184
    Hürthle cell thyroid carcinoma, 184
    molecular diagnostics, 184
    MTC, 184
    PDTC and ATC, 184
    predictive biomarkers, 184–185

Thyroid carcinoma *(Continued)*
    PTC, 183–184
        treatment-related biomarkers, 185
Thyroid cartilage, 108f
Thyroid cysts
    percutaneous ethanol injection (PEI), 473–474
Thyroid descent, embryology of, 107f
Thyroid dissection, 307–309, 307–310f
Thyroidectomy, 419. *See also* Bilateral subtotal thyroidectomy; Total thyroidectomy
    with central neck dissection, 400
    extent of, 272–280
    hereditary MTC surgery and, 242, 243f
    history of, 2
    with lateral neck dissection, 388–389
    near-total, 280–281
    nomenclature for, 280–281
    during parathyroidectomy, 511
    pediatric thyroid cancer and, 260
    postoperative voice change and, 156
    in pregnancy, 279–280
    standard pen, 388
    subtotal, 280–281
    surgical steps for, 282f, 285f, 288–290, 288t, 289f
        closure and final steps for, 292–293
        dictation and synoptic reporting for, 293
        incision and flap for, 283–284, 283–284f
        inferior parathyroid and, 285
        initial surgical considerations for, 283
        introduction to, 278f, 281–293, 282f
        isthmus and, 291–292
        lateral thyroid region exposure-middle thyroid vein and, 285, 286f
        parathyroid glands and, 288–290
        patient positioning for, 283, 283f
        recurrent laryngeal nerve and, 286–288
        strap muscles and midline airway for, 284–285, 285f
        superior pole and EBSLN for, 290–291
        thyroid bed uptake after total lobectomy and, 292
Thyroid Eye Disease, 80f
Thyroid follicle, 26, 27f
Thyroid function
    recurrent disease and, 93–94
    testing for, 59
        in hyperthyroidism, 35–36
        in hypothyroidism, 34
        in pregnancy, 37
Thyroid gland, 2
    accessory, 110
    applied embryology of
        anomalous development of, 15–21, 16t
        normal development of, 15, 16f
    gross examination of specimens and, 401–402
    histopathologic reporting of tumors and, 402
    immunohistochemistry of papillary carcinoma and, 395
    intraoperative assessment of nodules and, 400–401
    introduction to, 391
    laser ablation in, 167–170
    malignant neoplasms and, 392
    medullary carcinoma and, 398–399
    molecular pathology of follicular carcinoma and, 396
    oncocytic tumors and, 396
    papillary carcinoma and, 392–393
    poorly differentiated carcinoma and, 397
    primary nonepithelial tumors and, 399–400
    surgical pathology of
        anaplastic carcinoma and, 397–398
        benign neoplasms and, 391
        carcinoma in thyroglossal duct cyst and ectopic thyroid tissue, 400

Thyroid gland *(Continued)*
        follicular carcinoma and, 395–396
        follicular-derived familial tumors and, 398
    tumors with thymic or related branchial pouch differentiation and, 399
    variants of follicular adenoma and, 391–392
    variants of papillary cancer and, 393–395
    well-differentiated follicular "tumors of undetermined/uncertain malignant potential" and, 396
Thyroid hormone
    suppression of, 228
    synthesis and regulation, 26–27, 27–28f
Thyroid hormone binding ratio (THBR), 31
Thyroid hormone nuclear receptor (THR), 26–27
Thyroid hormone replacement therapy, 52, 442–443
Thyroid hormone withdrawal (THW)
    vs. recombinant thyroid-stimulating hormone, 451
Thyroid imaging, 33
    in hyperthyroidism, 36–37, 36t
    in hypothyroidism, 35
Thyroid Imaging, Reporting and Data System (TI-RADS), 104
Thyroid isthmus, 291–292
Thyroiditis. *See also* Infectious thyroiditis; Invasive fibrous thyroiditis; Postpartum thyroiditis; Sporadic silent thyroiditis; Subacute thyroiditis
    acute suppurative/infectious, 46–47
    chronic infectious thyroiditis, 48–49
    drug-induced, 45–46
    Hashimoto's thyroiditis (chronic lymphocytic thyroiditis), 40–41
    introduction to, 40, 41t, 41b
    invasive fibrous/Riedel thyroiditis and, 47–48
    palpation, 49
    radiation-associated thyroiditis, 49
    sporadic silent/postpartum thyroiditis and, 44–45
    subacute thyroiditis (de Quervain's thyroiditis), 41–44
    thyroid fine-needle aspiration and, 111, 112f
    ultrasound and, 140–141, 163f
Thyroid lobe, 317f, 320
Thyroid lobectomy (TL), 207–208
    with recurrent contralateral disease, 90
Thyroid malignancy, 70–71
Thyroid Microcarcinoma. *See* Papillary microcarcinoma
Thyroid mobilization
    back-door technique, for minimally invasive parathyroidectomy, 535
    front door technique, for minimally invasive parathyroidectomy, 534, 534f
Thyroid needle biopsy, 13–14
Thyroid neoplasia
    anaplastic thyroid carcinoma and, 182
    conclusions for, 185
    follicular thyroid carcinoma and, 184
    genetic alterations in papillary thyroid carcinoma and, 183–184
    genetic alterations with thyroid tumors and, 182
    introduction to, 181
    medullary thyroid carcinoma and, 184
Thyroid nodule
    in children, 262
    evaluation and management of, 106–107
        American College of Radiology (ACR), 102
        cervical lymph nodes, 103
        cytology and bethesda classification, 105–106, 105t
        fine needle aspiration, 104–105, 105f
        imaging modalities, 103
        introduction to, 100
        laboratory testing, 101, 102f
        malignant thyroid nodules, 107
        molecular testing, 106
        observation strategies, 106
        risk factors for malignancy and, 100–101
        risk stratification of, 104
        screening for, 101–102

Thyroid nodule *(Continued)*
    signs, symptoms, and physical examination, 101
    size, growth pattern, and multinodularity, 103
    treatment for benign thyroid nodules and role of diagnostic lobectomy, 106–107
    ultrasound evaluation for, 103
    US Preventative Services Task Force (USPSTF), 102
  incidental, 108–109
  indications for fine-needle aspiration for, 108–109
  intraoperative assessment of, 400–401
  laser and radiofrequency treatment of, 163–171
  ultrasound characteristics of
    calcifications and, 133–134, 133*f*, 136–137, 138*f*
    capsular contact and, 137, 139*f*
    echogenicity of, 136, 138*f*
    echo structure and, 136, 138*f*
    margins and halo/rim of, 136, 136*f*
    shape of, 136, 137*f*
    size of, 136
    vascular pattern and, 137, 139*f*
Thyroid pain, diagnosis of, 42*b*
Thyroid parathyroids, 23
Thyroid physiology
  in nonthyroidal illness, 28
Thyroid rests, 91, 109
  classification of, 17–19
  description of, 17–19, 17–19*f*
  embryologic remnants and, 91, 92*f*
Thyroid scintigraphy, 79
Thyroid-stimulating hormone (TSH), 97, 101, 195, 200, 420, 447, 475
  receptors, 111
Thyroid-stimulating immunoglobulin (TSI), 44
Thyroid storm, 83
  solitary toxic nodule and, 88
Thyroid surgery
  autopsy series and incidental finding, 194
  history of
    early years of, 2–3, 3–4*f*
    laryngeal nerves and, 8–11, 9–10*f*
    modern development of, 4–8, 4*f*
    parathyroid glands and, 11–12
    revolution of, 3–4
    surgery at Massachusetts General Hospital and, 12–14, 13*f*
  pre- and postoperative laryngeal exam for
    introduction to, 156
    recurrent laryngeal nerve paralysis and, 158
  principles in
    extent of thyroidectomy and, 272–280
    fine-needle aspiration results and, 272–280
    introduction to, 272
    nomenclature for thyroidectomy and, 280–281
    thyroidectomy surgical steps and, 281–293
  reoperative
    active surveillance, 464
    anatomic changes after thyroidectomy, 465–466
    central neck dissection, 467–471
    completion thyroidectomy and, 467
    complications, 470
    CT axial imaging with contrast and, 463
    fine-needle aspiration, 464
    indications for revision surgery, 461–462
    introduction to, 461
    lateral neck dissection and, 467–468
    management options, 464–465
    medical therapies, 464–465
    other imaging modalities and, 463–464
    parathyroid gland preservation and, 466
    parathyroid tissue autotransplantation and, 466–467

Thyroid surgery *(Continued)*
    paratracheal and superior mediastinal dissection, 467–471
    postoperative management of, 470
    postoperative surveillance, 462–464
    preoperative documentation, 465
    principles, 466
    recurrence rates and patterns, 462
    revision surgery adjunctive techniques and, 470–471
    RLN invasion, 466–467
    serum thyroglobulin levels and, 462–463
    surgical management, 465–467
    thyroglobulin washout, 464
    ultrasonography and, 463
Thyroid testing, diagnosis of, 29–33
Thyroid tissue
  ectopic, 17–19*f*
  lateral aberrant, 52
Thyroid transcription factor (TTF)-1, 610
Thyroid tumor
  primary nonepithelial, 399–400
  secondary, 117, 117*f*
  with thymic or related branchial pouch differentiation, 399
Thyroplasty, 158
ThyroSeq®, 127
  background of, 120
  CBLPath, 121
  clinical validation, 120–121
  for indeterminate cytopathology, 119–120*t*, 120–121
  sample report, 121, 122–124*f*
  ThyroSeq *Preserve*, 121
Thyrotoxicosis
  hyperthyroidism and, 79
  low radioactive iodine uptake, 44
Thyrotoxic storm, 420
Thyrotropin-stimulating hormone (TSH), 26, 28
Thyroxine (T4), 97, 158
Thyroxine binding globulin (TBG), 26–27
TI-RADS. *See* Thyroid Imaging, Reporting and Data System (TI-RADS)
Tissue handling, 527
Tissue structure, 167
TKIs. *See* Tyrosine kinase inhibitors (TKIs)
TNG. *See* Toxic nodular goiter (TNG)
TNM (tumor-node-metastases) staging system, 593–594, 594*t*
Total parathyroidectomy
  and autotransplantation, 562, 562*f*
  with forearm autograft, 580
  multiple gland disease (MGD), 561–562
  parathyroid hyperplasia and, 613
  tertiary hyperparathyroidism and, 575
Total thyroidectomy (TT), 30, 103, 118, 127
  additional considerations for, 276
  aggressive benign nodular recurrence after, 92–93
  familial nonmedullary thyroid cancer and, 268
  follicular thyroid cancer and, 207–208
  for goiter, 92–93
  Graves' disease and, 82–83
  papillary thyroid carcinoma and, 51
  in patients with indeterminate nodules, 273
  postoperative management and, 95–97
  recurrent disease in embryologic remnant and, 91–92, 92*f*, 107*f*
  recurrent disease operative strategy and, 94
  sporadic medullary thyroid carcinoma and, 231–232
Total thyroxine (T4), 26, 43
Total triiodothyronine (T3), 26, 43
Total volume of diseased gland (TVDG), 518–519
Toxic adenomas (TAs)
  percutaneous ethanol injection (PEI), 475
Toxicity, external beam radiotherapy and, 460

INDEX

Toxic multinodular goiter
　clinical presentation of, 84, 84–85f
　diagnosis and evaluation of, 85, 85–86f
　pathogenesis of, 84
　treatment of, 85–87
Toxic nodular goiter (TNG), 83
Trabecular bone score (TBS), 488
Tracheal injury, 423, 423f
Tracheal invasion, 366–367, 366–367f
Tracheoesophageal groove, 360, 361f
Tracheomalacia, 68–69, 423–424
Tracheotomy/Tracheostomy, 421, 65.e1
　anaplastic thyroid cancer and, 250
Trametinib, 127–131
　and differentiated thyroid cancer (DTC), 480
Transducer, 132–133, 151
Transisthmic approach method, 164–165, 165f
Transoral endoscopic parathyroidectomy vestibular approach (TOEPVA), 294
Transoral endoscopic thyroidectomy vestibular approach (TOETVA), 294
　contraindications for, 295, 295t
　indications for, 295, 295t
　steps in, 299
Transoral robotic parathyroidectomy vestibular approach (TORPVA), 294
Transoral robotic thyroidectomy (TORT), 301–302
Transoral robotic thyroidectomy vestibular approach (TORTVA), 294
Transoral thyroidectomy
　contraindications, 304–305
　future directions, 310
　history of, 301–302
　informed consent, 305
　notable preclinical developments in, 301, 302t
　outcomes, 310
　patient positioning, 305, 305f
　patient selection, 304–305
　preoperative workup, 305
　process improvement, 302
　remote-access thyroid surgery, 302–303
　robotic vs. endoscopic approaches, 303, 304b
　thyroid dissection, 307–309, 307–310f
　trocar placement, 305–306, 305–307f
　working space creation, 307, 307f
Trapdoor incision, 75, 75–77f
T3 resin uptake (T3RU), 31
Triiodothyronine (T3), 158
TSH. See Thyroid-stimulating hormone (TSH)
TSI. See Thyroid stimulating immunoglobulin (TSI)
Tubercle of Zuckerkandl, 107
　classification of, 20–21
　description of, 17–19f, 20–21
　recurrent disease and, 91–92, 92f, 109f
Tumor clonality
　in uniglandular and multiple gland disease, 555
Tumor, node, metastases (TNM)
　classification, 441b
　stage grouping, 441b
T3 uptake (T3U), 31
Two-hit hypotheses, 576
Type II muscle cell atrophy, 488–489
Tyrosine kinase inhibitors (TKIs), 46, 440, 445–446

U

Ultrasonography
　percutaneous ethanol injection (PEI)
　　head and neck, 473, 473f
　　preoperative parathyroid localization testing and, 494, 495f, 505–506
　　reoperative thyroid surgery and, 463
Ultrasound (US), 85, 150
　ablative procedure guidance and, 164

Ultrasound (US) (Continued)
　benign thyroid nodule characteristics and, 133–138, 134f, 136f, 157f
　CT scanning and, 151–153, 152–155f, 155t
　ectopic position and, 146
　embryology and, 146
　evaluation, for thyroid nodules, 103
　Hurthle cell tumors and, 227
　imaging, 46
　limitations of, 132
　malignant lesions characteristics and, 139–141
　neck, 444
　nodal distribution and, 142–145
　normal anatomy and, 146, 171, 171f
　office-based ultrasound, 151
　other issues of, 148, 174f
　parathyroid gland and, 145–148
　preoperative evaluation for nodal disease and, 150–151, 150–151f
　sonography of neck nodes and, 141–145, 142f
　summary for, 148
　thyroid and parathyroid glands, 134–138, 135b, 153
　　guided procedures for, 141
　　introduction to, 132
　　other diseases of, 140–141
　　physics and principles of, 132–134
　　technique and measurements for, 135, 155–156, 155f, 164–165, 165f, 167–174, 171f, 174f
　thyroid imaging, 150
　thyroid nodule and
　　characteristics of, 135–137, 135t, 154
　　elastography of, 135, 137, 141, 156, 164–165, 165f, 167–174, 174f
　　evaluation of, 135
　　radiofrequency ablation (RFA), 177, 177f
Ultrasound elastography, 103
Ultrasound-guided biopsy, 157
Ultrasound-guided revision thyroid surgery, 470
Undifferentiated carcinoma. See Anaplastic thyroid carcinoma
Uniglandular disease, 506–507
Unilateral laryngeal paralysis, 404
Unilateral neck exploration (UNE), 537
Unilateral vocal fold paralysis
　evaluation of, 410
　laryngeal electromyography, 410–411
　laryngeal reinnervation, 416
　　ansa cervicalis-to-recurrent laryngeal nerve anastomosis, 416–417
　　indications and timing of, 416
　management of
　　awake injection, 411–413, 412f, 413t
　　laryngeal framework surgery, 413–416, 414–415f
　　voice and swallow therapy, 411
　videolaryngoscopy, 410
University of Sydney Endocrine Surgical Unit, 104
Unresectable disease, external beam radiotherapy, 452, 453f
Upper airway evaluation
　flow volume loop analysis and, 58
　imaging and, 58
　regional symptomatic assessment and, 57–58
　thyroid function tests/fine-needle aspiration and, 59
Upper neck papillary thyroid carcinoma (UPTC), 50–51
Urine calcium/creatinine, pHPT lab work and, 503
US-guided percutaneous ethanol injection
　of cysts and tumors, 472
US Preventative Services Task Force (USPSTF), 101

V

Valsalva maneuver, 421
Vandetanib, 127–131
　and medullary thyroid carcinoma (MTC), 483
Vascular ablation techniques, 177

Vascular endothelial growth factor (VEGF), 158
Vascular endothelial growth factor receptors (VEGFR), 479–481
Vascular invasion, 593–594
VATS. *See* Video-assisted thoracoscopic surgery (VATS)
Vemurafenib
   and differentiated thyroid cancer (DTC), 480
Venous sampling, 499
Ventral diverticulum, 23
Ventral recurrent laryngeal nerve (ventral RLN), 63–65, 64–65*f*
Vesalius, 9
Video-assisted parathyroidectomy (VAP), 537–538
Video-assisted parathyroidectomy by lateral approach (VAP-LA), 540, 540*f*
Video-assisted thoracoscopic surgery (VATS), 77–78
Videolaryngoscopy, 410
Videolaryngostroboscopy, 324
Vitamin D
   deficiency, 486
      lab work and, 503
      primary hyperparathyroidism and, 492, 503–505
   receptor
      chronic kidney disease and, 564
      secondary hyperparathyroidism and, 565
Vocal cord paralysis (VCP), 156
   without voice symptoms, 160
Vocal fold
   mobility of, 159–160
   paralysis of
      preoperative laryngeal exam and, 160
      without voice symptoms, 160
   unilateral paralysis of, 410–411
Voice
   anatomy and, 156–158, 157*t*, 157*f*
   glottal exam and, 158
   symptoms with normal vocal fold mobility and, 159–160, 159*t*
Voice Handicap Index (VHI), 159
Voice production, 320
Voice therapy, 411
Volumetric-modulated arc therapy (VMAT), 454–455
von Eiselsberg, Anton, 5, 8, 12
von Recklinghausen, Frederick, 12

W

Wang, Chiu-an, 13–14
Warthin-like papillary carcinoma, 394
Water-clear cell adenoma, 599
Wavelength, 167
Wells, Spencer, 4
Werner syndrome (adult progeria), 182. *See also* MEN 1
   familial papillary thyroid cancer and, 266
Wisconsin index (WIN), 559
World Health Organization (WHO), 53.e1
   papillary thyroid cancers, definition of, 194
Wound closure, 470, 536

Y

"Y sign", 32

Z

Zollinger-Ellison syndrome, 577–578
Z-track technique, 474, 474*f*